W9-CPC-143

The APhA Complete Review
for Pharmacy

502 416 5922

Notices

The authors, editors, and publisher have made every effort to ensure the accuracy and completeness of the information presented in this book. However, the authors, editors, and publisher cannot be held responsible for the continued currency of the information, any inadvertent errors or omissions, or the application of this information. Therefore, the authors, editors, and publisher shall have no liability to any person or entity with regard to claims, loss, or damage caused or alleged to be caused, directly or indirectly, by the use of information contained herein.

The inclusion in this book of any product in respect to which patent or trademark rights may exist shall not be deemed, and is not intended as, a grant of or authority to exercise any right or privilege protected by such patent or trademark. All such rights or trademarks are vested in the patent or trademark owner, and no other person may exercise the same without express permission, authority, or license secured from such patent or trademark owner.

The inclusion of a brand name does not mean the authors, the editors, or the publisher has any particular knowledge that the brand listed has properties different from other brands of the same product, nor should its inclusion be interpreted as an endorsement by the authors, the editors, or the publisher. Similarly, the fact that a particular brand has not been included does not indicate the product has been judged to be in any way unsatisfactory or unacceptable. Further, no official support or endorsement of this book by any federal or state agency or pharmaceutical company is intended or inferred.

NAPLEX® is a trademark of the National Association of Boards of Pharmacy® (NABP®), and NABP® in no way endorses, authorizes, or sponsors this guide.

The APhA Complete Review for Pharmacy

Eighth Edition

Dick R. Gourley, PharmD, FAPhA
Editor-in-Chief
Dean and Professor
University of Tennessee College of Pharmacy
Memphis, Tennessee

James C. Eoff III, PharmD
Associate Editor-in-Chief
Executive Associate Dean and Professor, Clinical Pharmacy
University of Tennessee College of Pharmacy
Memphis, Tennessee

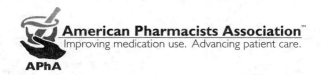

American Pharmacists Association™
Improving medication use. Advancing patient care.
APhA

Washington, D.C.

Acquiring Editor: Sandra J. Cannon
Managing Editors: Linda Stringer, Ashley Young, and Mary-Ann Moalli, Publications Professionals LLC
Copyeditors: Laura Glassman, Jennie Golden, and Mary-Ann Moalli, Publications Professionals LLC
Proofreaders: Liz Horowitz and Ben Justesen, Publications Professionals LLC
Composition: Circle Graphics
Cover Design: Richard Muringer, APhA Creative Services

©2011 by the American Pharmacists Association
Published by the American Pharmacists Association
2215 Constitution Avenue, NW
Washington, DC 20037-2985
www.pharmacist.com www.pharmacylibrary.com

APhA was founded in 1852 as the American Pharmaceutical Association.

To comment on this book via e-mail, send your message to the publisher at aphabooks@aphanet.org

Library of Congress Cataloging-in-Publication Data

The APhA complete review for pharmacy / Dick R. Gourley, PharmD, FAPhA, Editor-in-Chief, Dean and Professor, University of Tennessee College of Pharmacy, Memphis, Tennessee ; James C. Eoff III, PharmD, Associate Editor-in-Chief, Executive Associate Dean and Professor, Clinical Pharmacy, University of Tennessee College of Pharmacy, Memphis, Tennessee. — Eighth edition.
       p. ; cm.
  Complete review for pharmacy
  Includes bibliographical references and index.
  ISBN 978-1-58212-159-8 (alk. paper)
  1. Pharmacy—Outlines, syllabi, etc. 2. Pharmacy—Examinations, questions, etc. I. Gourley, Dick R., 1944- editor.
II. Eoff, James C., III, 1946- editor. III. American Pharmacists Association, issuing body. IV. Title: Complete review for pharmacy.
  [DNLM: 1. Pharmacy—Examination Questions. 2. Pharmaceutical Preparations—Examination Questions. QV 18.2]
  RS98.A64 2011
  615'.1076—dc22
                                        2010048956

How to Order This Book
Online: www.pharmacist.com/shop_apha
By phone: 800-878-0729 (770-280-0085 from outside the United States)
VISA®, MasterCard®, and American Express® cards accepted

Contents

Preface

It is indeed an honor to have again been asked to serve as editor-in-chief of *The APhA Complete Review for Pharmacy*. We are now publishing the eighth edition and sincerely appreciate the continued support of the American Pharmacists Association (APhA). The faculty of the University of Tennessee College of Pharmacy and I appreciate the confidence that APhA has demonstrated by allowing us this opportunity to assist pharmacy students in preparing for the NAPLEX examination. This project is very important to pharmacy students across the United States, and we know they appreciate the support of APhA.

As pharmacy students prepare to take the NAPLEX examination, it is imperative that they have available to them the most up-to-date and relevant information concerning the practice of pharmacy. The information explosion is such that facts change daily, and approximately 30 new drugs are marketed each year. The amount of information that any student in pharmacy must master is significant and doubles every two to three years.

The board examination is the culmination of at least six years of university work. It is impossible to go back to the beginning and review all aspects of pharmacy education to prepare for it. Therefore, we have developed a comprehensive review of pharmacy for students preparing to take the NAPLEX examination.

The format for this book was designed and adapted by Dr. Greta Gourley to meet the student's (or practitioner's) need for easy use and for focused details on pharmacy practice.

In this new eighth edition, new information related to medications has been added in a new chapter (chapter 38).

This study guide has attempted to summarize the information in a user-friendly manner. Our faculty and a panel of 10 pharmacy residents believe the information included to be the most important information needed for the NAPLEX exam. The review includes educational material, which synthesizes the most salient points; key points, which further delineate the most important factors; references; and, finally, self-study questions.

This book is also an excellent review for practicing pharmacists as they continue to expand their therapeutic knowledge and for foreign graduates interested in obtaining licensure in the United States. The case studies and more than 900 questions and annotated answers contained in the book will give students valuable practice exam experience.

It is highly recommended that any student preparing for the NAPLEX examination review the instructions on the NABP Web site (www.nabp.net). Students should also read the current literature in journals and review areas where they feel they have a weakness.

My thanks and appreciation go to my associate editor, James C. Eoff III, PharmD, executive associate dean of the University of Tennessee College of Pharmacy.

DICK R. GOURLEY, PHARMD, FAPHA
DEAN AND PROFESSOR
UNIVERSITY OF TENNESSEE COLLEGE OF PHARMACY
MEMPHIS, TENNESSEE

November 2010

Acknowledgments

We would like to thank the faculty of the University of Tennessee College of Pharmacy, who participated in preparing this comprehensive review, and Karin Ingram, executive assistant to the dean, for coordinating the preparation of the review book. We also wish to thank APhA for recognizing the need of pharmacy students for this review book. Working with Sandy Cannon and Julian Graubart at APhA has been an absolute pleasure. APhA's willingness to provide this book to all senior members of the Academy of Student Pharmacists who are pharmacy graduates in the United States is a true service to the profession of pharmacy.

We also appreciate the efforts of the following contributors for the case studies and questions and answers they prepared: Mollie Cannon, PharmD; L. Paige Clement, PharmD; Amy B. Gamlin, PharmD; Tameka W. Lucas, PharmD; Kristi Nesler, PharmD; Laura Pounders, PharmD; Kristie Ramser, PharmD; and Katie Wassil, PharmD.

Contributors

Hassan Almoazen, PhD
Assistant Professor, Department of Pharmaceutical
    Sciences
University of Tennessee College of Pharmacy

W. Andrew Bell, PharmD
Assistant Professor, Department of Clinical
    Pharmacy
University of Tennessee College of Pharmacy

Ronald L. Braden, PharmD
Associate Professor, Department of Clinical
    Pharmacy
University of Tennessee College of Pharmacy

Lawrence M. Brown, PharmD, PhD
Associate Professor, Department of Pharmaceutical
    Sciences
University of Tennessee College of Pharmacy

Rex O. Brown, PharmD, BCNSP
Professor and Executive Vice Chair, Department of
    Clinical Pharmacy
Director of Experiential Education
University of Tennessee College of Pharmacy

Joyce E. Broyles, PharmD, BCNSP
Associate Professor, Department of Clinical
    Pharmacy
University of Tennessee College of Pharmacy

Jason Carter, PharmD
Associate Professor, Department of Clinical
    Pharmacy
University of Tennessee College of Pharmacy

Peter A. Chyka, PharmD, FAACT, DABAT
Professor, Department of Clinical Pharmacy
Executive Associate Dean, Knoxville Campus
University of Tennessee College of Pharmacy

Catherine M. Crill, PharmD, BCPS, BCNSP
Associate Professor, Departments of Clinical
    Pharmacy and Pediatrics
University of Tennessee College of Pharmacy and
    College of Medicine

L. Brian Cross, PharmD, CDE
Associate Professor, Department of Clinical
    Pharmacy
University of Tennessee College of Pharmacy

Benjamin Duhart, Jr, MS, PharmD
Assistant Professor, Department of Clinical
    Pharmacy
Director, Transplant Pharmacy Services
University of Tennessee College of Pharmacy

Shannon Finks, PharmD, BCPS (AQ Cardiology)
Associate Professor, Department of Clinical
    Pharmacy
University of Tennessee College of Pharmacy

Walter L. Fitzgerald, Jr, BPharm, MS, JD
Dean, Pharmacy Education Program Development
South College, Knoxville, Tennessee
University of Tennessee College of Pharmacy

Stephanie A. Flowers, PharmD
Infectious Diseases Pharmacotherapy Fellow
University of Tennessee College of Pharmacy

Joni Foard, PharmD, CDE
Assistant Professor, Department of Clinical
    Pharmacy
University of Tennessee College of Pharmacy

Stephan L. Foster, PharmD
Professor, Department of Clinical Pharmacy
University of Tennessee College of Pharmacy

Andrea S. Franks, PharmD, BCPS
Associate Professor, Department of Clinical
    Pharmacy
University of Tennessee College of Pharmacy

Kevin L. Freeman, PharmD, BCNSP
Assistant Professor, Department of Clinical
    Pharmacy
University of Tennessee College of Pharmacy

Christa M. George, PharmD, BCPS, CDE
Assistant Professor, Department of Clinical
    Pharmacy
University of Tennessee College of Pharmacy

Benjamin Gross, PharmD, BCPS
Assistant Professor, Department of Clinical
    Pharmacy
University of Tennessee College of Pharmacy

Gale Hamann, PharmD, BCPS, CDE
Associate Professor, Departments of Clinical
    Pharmacy and Medicine
University of Tennessee College of Pharmacy and
    College of Medicine

Amanda Howard-Thompson, PharmD, BCPS
Assistant Professor, Department of Clinical
    Pharmacy
University of Tennessee College of Pharmacy

Joanna Q. Hudson, PharmD, BCPS, FASN
Associate Professor, Departments of Clinical
    Pharmacy and Medicine (Nephrology)
University of Tennessee College of Pharmacy and
    College of Medicine

Anne M. Hurley, PharmD
Assistant Professor, Department of Clinical
    Pharmacy
University of Tennessee College of Pharmacy

Jaclyn S. King, PharmD
Hematology/Oncology Pharmacy Resident
Walter Reed Army Medical Center, Washington, D.C.

Ram I. Mahato, PhD
Professor, Department of Pharmaceutical Sciences
University of Tennessee College of Pharmacy

Charles N. May, BSPh, MSHP
Assistant Professor, Department of Pharmaceutical
    Sciences
University of Tennessee College of Pharmacy

Trevor McKibbin, PharmD, MS, BCPS
Assistant Professor, Department of Clinical
    Pharmacy
University of Tennessee College of Pharmacy

Bernd Meibohm, PhD
Professor, Department of Pharmaceutical Sciences
Associate Dean for Graduate Programs and Basic
    Research
University of Tennessee College of Pharmacy

Elizabeth S. Miller, PharmD
Assistant Professor, Department of Clinical
    Pharmacy
University of Tennessee College of Pharmacy

Carrie S. Oliphant, PharmD, BCPS
Assistant Professor, Department of Clinical
    Pharmacy
University of Tennessee College of Pharmacy

Robert B. Parker, PharmD, FCCP
Professor, Department of Clinical Pharmacy
University of Tennessee College of Pharmacy

Stephanie J. Phelps, PharmD, BCPS
Associate Dean for Academic Affairs
Professor, Departments of Clinical Pharmacy and
    Pediatrics
University of Tennessee College of Pharmacy and
    College of Medicine

William Nathan Rawls, PharmD
Professor, Department of Clinical Pharmacy
University of Tennessee College of Pharmacy

Shaunta' M. Ray, PharmD, BCPS
Assistant Professor, Departments of Clinical
    Pharmacy and Family Medicine
University of Tennessee College of Pharmacy and
    College of Medicine

Kelly C. Rogers, PharmD
Associate Professor, Department of Clinical
    Pharmacy
University of Tennessee College of Pharmacy

P. David Rogers, PharmD, PhD, FCCP
First Tennessee Chair of Excellence in Clinical
    Pharmacy
Associate Dean for Translational Research
University of Tennessee College of Pharmacy

Timothy H. Self, PharmD
Professor, Department of Clinical Pharmacy
University of Tennessee College of Pharmacy

Katie J. Suda, PharmD, MS
Associate Professor and Director, Drug
    Information Center
Department of Clinical Pharmacy
University of Tennessee College of Pharmacy

Mina Tadrous, PharmD, MS
PhD Student, Department of Pharmaceutical
    Sciences
Leslie Dan Faculty of Pharmacy
University of Toronto

Laura A. Thoma, PharmD
Professor, Department of Pharmaceutical
    Sciences
Director, Parenteral Medications Laboratories
University of Tennessee College of Pharmacy

Jeremy Thomas, PharmD, CDE
Assistant Professor, Department of Clinical
    Pharmacy
University of Tennessee College of Pharmacy

Camille W. Thornton, PharmD
Associate Professor, Department of Clinical
    Pharmacy
University of Tennessee College of Pharmacy

J. Aubrey Waddell, PharmD, FAPhA, BCOP
Associate Professor
University of Tennessee College of Pharmacy
Oncology Pharmacist
Blount Memorial Hospital, Maryville, Tennessee

G. Christopher Wood, PharmD, FCCP, BCPS
with added qualifications in infectious diseases
Associate Professor, Department of Clinical
    Pharmacy
University of Tennessee College of Pharmacy

Charles R. Yates, PharmD, PhD
Associate Professor, Department of Pharmaceutical
    Sciences
University of Tennessee College of Pharmacy

Eoff's NAPLEX Study Guide

Welcome to *The APhA Complete Review for Pharmacy*. With so many different academic backgrounds, such a variety of learning experiences, and the increasing volume of information taught at U.S. colleges of pharmacy, it is impossible to cover all materials from each course you have taken while in pharmacy school. Therefore, the primary purpose of *The APhA Complete Review for Pharmacy* is to provide a summary of therapeutics as well as other basic pharmaceutical principles (dosage forms, math, biopharmaceutics, kinetics, basic and parenteral compounding, among others) that will be valuable in your preparation for the NAPLEX and also be a resource as you enter practice.

This review book is not an exhaustive discussion of the topics presented; it uses an abbreviated outline format to enable you to review and organize the material in an efficient manner for easy recall and recognition. The NAPLEX is a difficult exam, and it covers a tremendous amount of material. In recent years, the NAPLEX has become even more relevant to professional practice, with less emphasis on the basic sciences and more emphasis on drug therapy and pharmaceutical care.

Your success in pharmacy school has been due to diligence and hard work. You should have confidence that your pharmacy education has prepared you for the NAPLEX, and you should not have anxieties about the exam. However, your self-confidence should not prevent you from being meticulous about preparation for the NAPLEX. Realizing that approximately 10% of students fail to achieve a passing score on their first attempt at the NAPLEX, do not take this exam lightly.

The following are helpful hints that will improve your success on this examination:

1. *Positive attitude:* You are encouraged to approach preparation for the NAPLEX with a positive attitude. Study to learn and understand concepts, not just memorize enough facts to pass the exam. Remember that in addition to being a minimum standard required for entry into pharmacy practice, the NAPLEX is the comprehensive review, and an important benefit of taking the NAPLEX is that it will make you a better pharmacy practitioner. Without the NAPLEX, few pharmacy graduates would spend the time and effort to review the entire discipline immediately prior to completing their studies. You should be confident that you have the knowledge to pass the exam if you have prepared diligently.

2. *Planning ahead:* Do not delay your review and preparation for the NAPLEX until the last week before your scheduled exam date. Although the total amount of time varies greatly from student to student, it is recommended that you start a serious review no less than 4–6 weeks before you plan to take the exam. However, if you have limited pharmacy work experience, you should start much earlier, especially learning generic and trade names. Be conscientious about scheduling specific times to prepare for the NAPLEX over this time period. Cramming the last few days before the NAPLEX will potentially increase your anxiety and could also confuse you with such a large volume of material. Read one or two chapters per day for 4 or 5 days per week, and review the generic and trade names daily.

3. *Generic and trade names:* The first place to begin your preparation is to learn the generic and trade names for the top 200 drugs. The

importance of this basic recommendation cannot be overemphasized. Without this base, you will experience tremendous difficulty on the NAPLEX, which is traditionally over half trade names. In addition, you will also need to learn the generic and trade names for unique drugs that may not be among the top 200 drugs (e.g., Cogentin and Artane, which are used to manage the extrapyramidal side effects of psychotherapeutic agents; Tofranil, which is used to treat enuresis; Tapazole, which is used to treat hyperthyroidism). Most of the patient medication profiles contain numerous drugs that may be listed by either the generic or the trade name. Therefore, knowledge of generic and trade names is essential to identify therapeutic duplication (e.g., the patient who is prescribed Corgard who is already taking the β-blocker propranolol). You will also be expected to determine potential causes for adverse effects, as well as screen for drug interactions and drug–disease interactions, from either drugs on the profile or the new prescriptions. In some cases, drugs will be listed by their generic names, and in other cases, by their trade names.

4. *Math:* Other than generic and trade names, pharmacy math is the most important single area to review. You should practice working several examples of each type of math problem to be sure you are comfortable and confident in your ability. Although some therapeutic topics may not be covered extensively, the large number of math questions on the NAPLEX makes studying pharmacy math a high priority. Many students struggle with math on the NAPLEX. Therefore, it is recommended that you schedule several math study sessions. The metric system is emphasized, but you must know the other systems and be able to make conversions. Although the apothecary system is used infrequently, the avoirdupois system (sometimes called the household system) is still used (e.g., prepare 1 pound of ointment). When apothecary or avoirdupois measures are used, you should usually convert them to metric.

5. *Competencies:* You should review the areas of emphasis defined in the NAPLEX competency statements that are available on the NABP Web site, www.nabp.net. As you review the top 200 drugs, you should ask yourself the following questions:

- What is the therapeutic category of this drug?
- What is the mechanism of action?

- What type of patient counseling information should be provided?
- What are the major adverse effects (side effects and toxic effects)?
- What is the dosage schedule (frequency)?
- What are the major drug interactions and disease contraindications?

These topics should also be the priority areas as you review each therapeutic class of agents.

6. *Dosage schedules:* Summary charts of the major categories of drugs are provided in each of the therapeutic chapters of this book. You will find the generic as well as trade names, along with commonly available dosage forms, dosage, and frequency of use. The frequency of use is emphasized more on the NAPLEX than are the specific dosages. The following therapeutic lists with multiple agents should also be emphasized in your studying: β-blockers, calcium channel blockers, angiotensin-converting enzyme inhibitors, benzodiazepines, cephalosporins, quinolones, aminoglycosides, nonsteroidal anti-inflammatory drugs, H_2 blockers, protease inhibitors, oral antidiabetics, and statins. Be able to recognize the agents within these categories, and know how to compare the differences within the category (e.g., duration of action, dosage schedules, side effects, and distinct advantages in patients with certain diseases).

7. *Appendixes:* Many tables that can help you recall or recognize answers for NAPLEX questions are included in the appendixes, such as the major drug–drug interactions, the drugs that should not be crushed, and the top 200 over-the-counter agents. Other important tables are included throughout the book, such as the table of common antidotes for poisons and overdosages in Chapter 35, the toxicology chapter. By reviewing these therapeutic agents by categories and in tables, you will increase your recall of them on the exam.

8. *Chronic and common diseases:* The NAPLEX emphasizes the more common and chronic diseases and their therapy. Although it is a good idea to have a general knowledge of the disease process, remember that the NAPLEX is heavily weighted toward drug therapy. Therefore, you should not devote the majority of your study time to the disease process (e.g., etiology, pathophysiology, diagnosis, and signs and symptoms) at the expense of the therapy (including nondrug therapy). Although it is helpful to review your areas of strength, you should concentrate more on your areas of weakness. The less familiar you

are with a topic, the more time you should give to reviewing the topic.

9. *Priorities:* Several areas should *not* be emphasized in your review: (1) the manufacturer of the specific drug (e.g., Zithromax manufactured by Pfizer); (2) chemical structures; and (3) identification or physical descriptions (e.g., color, shape). These areas are covered only minimally on the NAPLEX.

10. *Review questions:* Reviewing sample exam questions is very helpful. However, to make your learning experience more effective, study the explanations along with their answers. Do not look only at the correct answer, but also at distractors and learn why they are incorrect. Therapeutics reference texts may also be helpful in your NAPLEX review; they provide more detailed information and may assist you with difficult or complex material. Studying such texts will also reinforce learning points about material covered in your review.

11. *Exam format:* The NAPLEX consists of 185 multiple-choice questions in a computer adaptive format that is individualized to each candidate's level of ability. The computer-adapted test system selects your next questions depending on your response to previous questions; thus, each question must be answered before you can proceed. The 150 questions that have been pretested for validity are the basis for your evaluation. In addition, 35 questions that are being evaluated for use in future exams are distributed throughout the exam.

12. *Question format:* You should log on to the NABP Web site (www.napb.net) to review the format for exam questions and the patient profiles. NABP also offers a "pre-NAPLEX" test for a fee. This pretest will allow you to practice with the computerized format. It will help allay your anxiety and be especially beneficial if you are not comfortable with exams given in a computer format.

All questions on the NAPLEX have five choices with only *one* "best" answer. You may not continue the exam until you have answered the question. You may not skip the question and come back. Therefore, you will be unable to leave any question blank. The question is superimposed at the bottom of the screen below the patient medication record. After deciding on the best answer, you will:

1. Highlight the answer.
2. Request the next question.

3. Confirm that you want the next question, which will finalize your answer.

You cannot go back to change an answer after step 3.

There are two types of multiple-choice questions:

1. The traditional single-answer type, as in the example below:

The agent of choice for the initial treatment of contact dermatitis, whether irritant or allergic, is a

A. topical antihistamine
B. oral antihistamine
C. topical corticosteroid
D. local anesthetic
E. coal tar product

2. The combined-response ("K" type) question with one, two, or three components listed, as in the example below:

The most common side effects of isotretinoin include which of the following?

I. Cheilitis
II. Acute depression
III. Decreased night vision

A. I only
B. II only
C. III only
D. I and II
E. I, II, and III

13. *Patient medication record:* The patient medication record is usually followed by 10–15 questions. You must refer to the patient profile for many of the questions. However, some questions may be answered as presented or "stand alone." You will not be able to see the entire profile on the top of the screen without scrolling down to review the whole profile. You may want to write down the significant points from the profile, such as allergies, age of the patient, and preexisting diseases, on scrap paper. Note carefully if the patient has multiple diseases, and for females, look for pregnancy or nursing, or for the likelihood of becoming pregnant. Some test takers prefer to read the questions prior to reviewing the profile, but you could miss an important fact like a drug allergy, a drug–disease contraindication, or an adverse effect being treated currently that resulted from a previously prescribed drug. In such a case,

you could answer the question without all of the necessary information. Therefore, always conduct a quick review of the profile prior to answering the questions.

14. *Testing center location:* If you are not familiar with the exact location of the testing center, locate it no later than the day before the exam. Arrive at the testing site at least 30 minutes prior to the scheduled time so that you are as calm as you can be. You do not want to be caught in traffic or to get lost trying to find the testing center and panic immediately prior to taking the exam.

15. *The night before the exam:* Do not study the night before the exam; last-minute cramming will only add to your anxiety and will not improve your test score. I recommend that you take a night off from study the evening before the exam. Go out for a relaxing dinner or a movie. Be sure to get to bed early, especially if you are scheduled for a morning exam, so your ability to reason, recognize, and recall information is sharp.

16. *Afternoon exam:* If your exam is scheduled in the afternoon, fatigue can dull your test-taking abilities. Be on guard against fatigue by having a light lunch, preferably with coffee, tea, or some caffeine-containing beverage, to be sure that you stay sharp for the afternoon session.

While you are taking the exam, keep these factors in mind:

1. Read all directions carefully. Read each question a minimum of two times to determine the nature of the question and the point of asking the question. Note any modifying terms like *always, all, never, most,* or *usually;* any double negatives; and anything else about the way the question is worded that may change the meaning of the question. Modifiers like *always* and *never* mean what they say.

2. Read all the choices thoroughly before you answer the question. Attempt to eliminate the distractor choices or incorrect answers. Two or three answers can usually be eliminated for one reason or another, and the final choice is between two answers. The more distractors you identify and eliminate, the more you increase your probability of obtaining the best answer. Then select the *single best answer.* Your first instinct is generally the best choice. Be cautious about reading multiple possibilities into

questions; the questions are straightforward and are not designed to trick you.

3. If you are positive that you do not know the answer, eliminate any distractors and guess intelligently, making the best choice of the remaining answers. If you can limit your guess to two possible correct answers, your score will be much better than if you try to guess the correct answer from five possible choices. By proceeding in this fashion over the course of the exam, you can increase your success if you guess consistently. Although blind guessing is not recommended, intelligent guessing is definitely recommended once you have narrowed the possibilities.

4. Pace yourself, but do not rush through the exam. The 4 hours and 15 minutes scheduled for the NAPLEX are more than adequate, and the majority of students have plenty of time to complete the exam. You need to proceed at a reasonable pace and need to answer approximately 45–50 questions per hour to finish comfortably in the time available. A timer is visible at the corner of the screen with your remaining exam time. If you notice that you have completed only 40 questions in the first hour, you should increase your speed.

5. Some of the math questions may be weighted more heavily, and some will take several minutes to answer. Take the time to answer the math questions correctly. Incorrect answers may lead to additional math questions (e.g., missing the first milliequivalent question could lead to more milliequivalent questions on your exam). Use the scrap paper provided for your calculations. Be sure to include units as you complete the math questions on your scrap paper.

6. It is important to remember that you cannot return to a previous question after you have confirmed an answer. There is no need to get upset over a previous question that you realize you have missed as you proceed through the exam. Do not get nervous during the exam or panic, or you may lose your ability to recall or recognize common information. Remain calm and do the best you can. Best of luck with the test!

JAMES C. EOFF III, PHARMD
EXECUTIVE ASSOCIATE DEAN AND PROFESSOR
UNIVERSITY OF TENNESSEE COLLEGE OF PHARMACY
MEMPHIS, TENNESSEE

November 2010

+62,000 Strong
Join the American Pharmacists Association and Help Build a Stronger Tomorrow

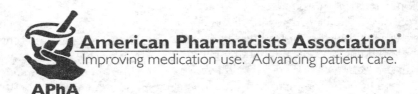

American Pharmacists Association®
Improving medication use. Advancing patient care.
APhA

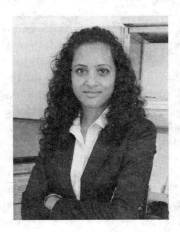

"Being active in APhA helps me put things in perspective: I can see the immediate benefits from the networking opportunities and up-to-date information on practice issues provided by APhA, and I am empowered to help shape the future of pharmacy. I look at APhA membership as an important investment, in understanding what has been, realizing what is, and influencing what will be."

—Vibhuti Arya, PharmD, *2010–11 Chair,*
APhA New Practitioner Advisory Committee,
New York, New York

At the American Pharmacists Association (APhA), we're excited about the future of pharmacy and the arrival of our new practitioner members! We see a profession rich with innovation and future-focused perspectives on patient care that oftentimes come from our new practitioner members—**the rising stars of pharmacy!**

Most likely, you currently are or have been a member of APhA's Academy of Student Pharmacists and are acquainted with the many valuable benefits of membership in APhA: special discounts on books and products, timely news and information from our periodicals, and a variety of other programs designed to supplement your education. As you begin to practice in your chosen community and practice setting, you'll find that you need to rely on these assets more than ever.

Now that you're about to make the transition to professional practice, this is the perfect time to discover how APhA can support your career! New practitioners are welcomed into APhA through a special category of membership called the APhA New Practitioners Network (APhA-NPN). Becoming a member of APhA-NPN means you'll receive the same benefits regular members receive *plus* benefits specifically tailored to new practitioners with modified pricing based on your graduation date! Even those in postgraduate and residency programs qualify for a discounted rate to help with the transition.

APhA-NPN resources cover three main areas that have proven over the years to help new pharmacists jump-start and attain the momentum early in their careers. You'll benefit from

- *Quality news and information resources* to help you stay on point with trends in the profession as well as work–life balance issues.
- *Networks of like-minded professionals* to help you navigate the daily challenges of a practicing pharmacist.
- *Additional educational resources* useful for gaining new perspectives or simply fulfilling licensure requirements when the time comes.

Sound interesting? Let's take a closer look . . .

APhA provides quality news and information you can trust.

When you need reliable information at your fingertips to help you respond to the new demands of your career, who better to trust than the organization that has been helping tens of thousands of pharmacists meet their professional challenges for more than 150 years? APhA has a solid history of leading the profession, in part by providing periodicals containing information you can use right away or keep as a reference.

Transitions: Exclusively for pharmacist members of APhA-NPN, *Transitions* is the quarterly newsletter that provides insight on your personal and professional life such as career advice, financial planning, maintaining work–life balance, and more. At a time when moving from one life stage to another can involve focusing on multiple priorities at once, *Transitions* can help you find ways to become acclimated to life's new events.

Pharmacy Today: Reading this monthly publication from APhA provides you with comprehensive news on new drug products and drug regimens, developments in innovative practice and medication therapy management, trends in health care that affect pharmacists, and legal and regulatory updates. *Pharmacy Today* will help prepare you to meet the day-to-day challenges of your career.

Pharmacy Today Health-System Edition (HSE): This special edition of *Pharmacy Today* provides unique and specialized medication therapy management (MTM) information to pharmacists practicing in hospitals and health systems, ambulatory care clinics, federal facilities, and long-term care facilities, including nursing homes and hospices. The magazine profiles effective MTM practices and techniques that serve patients in these areas. Readers can use these profiles as models to develop and improve their own MTM practice in these business settings, increase patient adherence, and build patient loyalty.

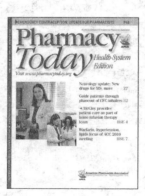

Journal of the American Pharmacists Association (JAPhA): The official peer-reviewed journal of APhA

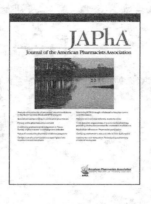

publishes research on pharmacy practice, in-depth feature articles, columns, and informed opinions. Keeping *JAPhA* on your short list of professional resources will help you stay in touch with your profession and gain new perspectives from others making great strides in improving medication use and advancing patient care. Current and past issues of *JAPhA* are available online at www.japha.org.

Journal of Pharmaceutical Sciences: This journal focuses on two major questions of importance to pharmaceutical scientists: (1) What are the physical and biological barriers that limit the access of drugs to their therapeutic targets? (2) How can drugs, dosage forms, and delivery systems be designed to maximize therapeutic efficacy? A subscription to the *Journal of Pharmaceutical Sciences* is a benefit of APhA membership. However, members may select a subscription to either the *Journal of Pharmaceutical Sciences* or the *Journal of the American Pharmacists Association.*

PharmInfoNow: This tool provides free access* to the most comprehensive literature update service available to help busy pharmacists stay current with both pharmacy practice and medication therapy management. *PharmInfoNow* is an online information management tool that provides immediate and customized access to the most current book and journal literature from the most comprehensive and trusted sources.

APhA DrugInfoLine: When you need the latest information on drug therapy developments and major therapeutic research, time is of the essence! As an APhA member, you won't have to worry because you'll have the *APhA DrugInfoLine*, which allows you to quickly and easily access "what you need to know" and "what your patients need to know" *when you need to know it.* Published monthly, *APhA DrugInfo Line* sets the standard for offering timely clinical and drug information useful in daily practice. See the

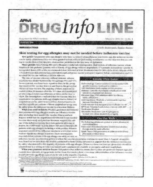

*Note: This service is available to 4th- and 5th-year new practitioners only.

Publications link at www.pharmacist.com for current and past issues of *APhA DrugInfoLine.*

Get involved! Stay connected! And get the support you deserve!

As you focus on becoming the best pharmacist you can be while balancing your personal life, you can easily get lost in the daily grind. But you don't want to miss out on relationships with peers! APhA makes it easy to stay connected to colleagues, old and new, as well as keep up with the latest trends in pharmacy through APhA Academies, e-Communities, and social networking sites.

APhA Academies are free to members and offer an opportunity to more closely align your APhA membership with the areas of practice or research that you're most interested in pursuing. By indicating your Academy preference, you will receive information tailored to your interests and be able to connect with others on issues specifically related to your practice setting. If you haven't already, consider joining one of APhA's Academies:

- APhA Academy of Pharmacy Practice and Management (APhA-APPM)
- APhA Academy of Pharmaceutical Research and Science (APhA-APRS)

APhA e-Communities offer a quick, easy way to engage with like-minded professionals and solicit feedback on APhA and pharmacy-related issues while learning about some of the hottest areas of pharmacy. In addition, APhA has established Facebook pages and LinkedIn sites to foster networking, which is vital for healthy career growth. If you want to keep up with the movers and shakers in pharmacy, then you'll want to participate in one of the following members-only virtual communities:

- Medication Therapy Management e-Community
- Nuclear Pharmacy e-Community
- APhA House of Delegates e-Community
- Health Care Reform e-Community
- APhA-APPM Hospital/Institutional Practice e-Community
- Immunizing Pharmacists e-Community

Your education is just beginning!

As your career progresses, you'll eventually need ongoing professional development and continuing education to stay on top of the latest trends and maintain licensure. Furthermore, many new practitioners take advantage of APhA's free educational opportunities as a way to *become more marketable to potential employers* by becoming more knowledgeable in their profession. APhA is the best resource for a wide variety of *quality education.* Whether you're interested in continuing education monographs, comprehensive certificate training programs, or live educational programming, you can rest assured that APhA's programs are designed to keep you on the fast track to success!

Continuing education: Convenient, accessible, and free to members, the APhA Online CPE Center at www.pharmacist.com offers more than 80 valuable and relevant continuing education activities. You'll also find information on state licensure requirements, instant Statements of Credit, and online personal transcript storage that automatically maintains a record of your CPE.

APhA's Annual Meeting & Exposition: The nation's only education-based conference for pharmacists in all practice settings is held annually in the spring. Participants can select from numerous programs geared toward the latest drug therapies and innovations in patient-centered pharmacy practice, make or enhance professional relationships, take advantage of networking opportunities, and explore various career opportunities. In addition, there are "new practitioner only" events, including financial planning strategies workshops and several social events. APhA members benefit from discounted registration rates, and all attendees are sure to have a memorable experience. Visit www.aphameeting.org for the latest information.

Certificate Training Programs: These innovative and interactive practice-based educational programs are designed to help pharmacists develop the skills needed to become confident, successful disease-state managers. Thousands of pharmacists have benefited from APhA's Certificate Training Programs. When you're ready to develop the advanced skills needed for disease management, advocate disease prevention, or assist patients with improving medication use, APhA's Certificate Training Programs are ready for you. For more information regarding programs on becoming an immunizing pharmacist, providing pharmaceutical care for patients with diabetes, or providing medication therapy management, go to www.pharmacist.com/education.

Whether you're looking to interact with other like-minded professionals, explore additional topics in pharmacy, or keep up with the latest pharmacy news, information, and trends, be sure to visit us online at www.pharmacist.com/membership to *renew* your membership. Or if you've never had a membership with APhA, *join today* so that you, too, can have the quality resources necessary to stay competitive with those who already enjoy being a part of APhA.

Join APhA! You'll be right at home where the rising stars of pharmacy are improving medication use and advancing patient care!

American Pharmacists Association
2215 Constitution Avenue, NW
Washington, DC 20037-2985
800-237-2742

For additional information about APhA and the latest pharmacy news, drug information, career information, and continuing education, or to shop the APhA store, go to www.pharmacist.com, the nation's premier Web site for practicing pharmacists.

Pharmacy Math

Hassan Almoazen, PhD

1-1. Units of Measure

Calculations in pharmacy may involve four different systems of measure: the metric system, the apothecaries' system, the avoirdupois system, and the household system.

Metric System

The fundamental units of the metric system are the gram, the liter, and the meter. Prefixes are used extensively to express quantities much greater and much less than the fundamental units. Some of the most commonly used prefixes are provided in Table 1-1.

Apothecaries' System

Although the metric system is the official system of measure for pharmacy today, the apothecaries' system is the traditional system, and some elements might sometimes be found in prescriptions. Units of the apothecaries' system are presented in Table 1-2.

Avoirdupois System

The avoirdupois system of measure for weight is used in ordinary commerce. Here, the ounce corresponds to 437.5 grains. The avoirdupois grain unit is equal to the apothecaries' grain unit. Sixteen ounces (7,000 grains) correspond to 1 pound. Note that the avoirdupois ounce (473.5 grains) and pound (7,000 grains) measures are not equal to the apothecaries' ounce (480 grains) and pound (5,760 grains) measures.

Household Measures

A tablespoon is equivalent to 15 mL, and a teaspoon is equivalent to 5 mL.

Conversion Factors

A short list of convenient conversion factors follows:

1 inch = 2.54 cm
1 fl oz = 29.57 mL
1 g = 15.4 grains
1 kg = 2.20 lb (avoirdupois)
1 lb (avoirdupois) = 454 g
1 gal (U.S.) = 3,785 mL

1-2. Significant Figures

All measured quantities are approximations. The accuracy of a given measurement is conveyed by the number of figures that are recorded. The number of significant figures in a measurement includes the first approximate figure. The last recorded digit to the right of a measured quantity is taken to be an approximation. For example, the weight 13.24 g has four significant figures, and the final digit, 4, is approximate. Calculations should be conducted so as to carry the correct numbers of significant figures.

Frequently, the different quantities in a given calculation have different numbers of significant figures. When that occurs, the following rules apply.

Addition and Subtraction

When adding or subtracting decimal numbers, round all measurements so that they have the same number of decimal places as the least in the set. For example, 13.78 mL and 53.5 mL would be added as 13.8 mL + 53.5 mL = 67.3 mL, using and retaining only one decimal place.

Table 1-1. Metric System Prefixes

Prefix	Meaning
mega-	one million times the base unit (10^6)
kilo-	one thousand times the base unit (10^3)
deci-	one-tenth the base unit (10^{-1})
centi-	one-hundredth the base unit (10^{-2})
milli-	one-thousandth the base unit (10^{-3})
micro-	one-millionth the base unit (10^{-6})
nano-	one-billionth the base unit (10^{-9})
pico-	one-trillionth the base unit (10^{-12})

Multiplication and Division

When multiplying or dividing decimal numbers, round the measurements to include the number of significant figures contained in the least accurate number. For example, 25.678 mL × 1.24 g/mL would be multiplied as 25.7 mL × 1.24 g/mL = 31.9 g, using and retaining three significant figures in each number.

Handling Zero

The digit zero may or may not be counted as a significant figure, depending on where it appears in the measured number. If zero occurs at an interior position in the number (e.g., 3,052 or 2.031), it is significant. If zero occurs as the last digit to the right of the decimal (e.g., 44.50), it is significant. If zero occurs as the first digit to the right of the decimal in a number that is less than 1, it is not significant. For example, in 0.078 there are only two significant figures. If zero occurs as the last digit, or digits, in a whole number (i.e., no decimal is expressed), its significance is unknown without further information. For example, 3,500 might have two, three, or four significant figures.

Table 1-2. Apothecaries' System of Measure

Weight	Volume
20 grains = 1 scruple	60 minims = 1 fluidram
3 scruples = 1 dram	8 fluidrams = 1 fluid ounce
8 drams = 1 ounce	16 fluid ounces = 1 pint
12 ounces = 1 pound	2 pints = 1 quart
	4 quarts = 1 gallon

1-3. Ratios and Proportions

The most frequently encountered calculations in pharmacy use ratios and proportions. In mathematics, a ratio is the quotient of one quantity divided by another quantity of the same kind, and a proportion is an equality between ratios. Thus, a proportion involves a relationship among four quantities. You can always solve for one of those quantities when the other three are known. If the ratio x/y is equal to the ratio a/b, then the proportion $x/y = a/b$ exists, and x can be obtained by algebraic manipulation ($x = ay/b$, etc.). Such problems frequently are encountered when adjusting dosages.

One common source of error in proportion problems involves writing one of the ratios upside down (e.g., writing $x/y = b/a$, when it should be written $x/y = a/b$). A disciplined approach to setting up such problems can help. For example, you might establish a rule in which you express each ratio as the quotient of like quantities. Then, when you equate the two ratios, if the numerator of one ratio is smaller (or larger) than its denominator, the same should be true of the other ratio as well.

Another source of error involves using mixed units (e.g., using one number expressed in grams and the other in milligrams). To guard against that kind of error, always write the units into the equation along with the numbers. All unit expressions should cancel except those required for the quantity being solved for (dimensional analysis).

Example: If 300 mL of a preparation contains 250 mg of drug, what weight of drug (x) is contained in 1,800 mL of the preparation?

Equate the ratios x:250 mg and 1,800 mL:300 mL to solve for x:

$$\frac{x}{250 \text{ mg}} = \frac{1,800 \text{ mL}}{300 \text{ mL}}$$

$$x = \frac{250 \text{ mg} \times 1,800 \text{ mL}}{300 \text{ mL}} = 1,500 \text{ mg}$$

Note that because the new volume is six times greater, the new weight should be six times greater as well.

1-4. Specific Gravity and Density

At times, you will be required to convert a volume measure to a weight measure, or vice versa. To do so, you will need to use either the specific gravity or the density of the material. The specific gravity (SpGr) is a ratio of the weight of the material to the weight of the same volume of a standard material. For liquids, the standard material is water, which has a density of 1 g/mL. Specific gravity is unitless. Density is the quotient of any measure of the weight of a sample of the material divided by any measure of the volume of the sample. The units must be explicitly expressed (e.g., g/mL, lb/gal, etc.). When density is expressed in grams per milliliter, it is numerically equal to specific gravity. Algebraically, density (weight/volume) is easier to work with than the corresponding expression for specific gravity.

Example: What is the weight of 750 mL of concentrated hydrochloric acid (SpGr = 1.20)? From the specific gravity definition, and using the volume of 750 mL,

$$\text{SpGr}(\text{HCl}) = \frac{(\text{weight of 750 mL HCl})}{(\text{weight of 750 mL } H_2O)}$$

Rearranging and noting that the density of H_2O is 1 g/mL,

$$\text{weight of 750 mL HCl} = (\text{SpGr})$$
$$\times (\text{weight of 750 mL } H_2O)$$
$$= 1.20 \times 750 \text{ g} = 900 \text{ g}$$

Alternatively, specific gravity is numerically equal to density expressed in grams per milliliter. Thus,

$$\text{density} = 1.20 = \frac{\text{weight HCl}}{\text{volume HCl}}, \text{ or}$$
$$\text{weight HCl} = \text{density} \times \text{volume HCl}$$
$$= 1.20 \text{ g/mL} \times 750 \text{ mL} = 900 \text{ g}$$

1-5. Percentage Error

Because all measurements are approximations, one must characterize the extent of error involved, or *percentage of error,* which is defined as

$$\% \text{ error} = \frac{(\text{error} \times 100\%)}{(\text{quantity desired})}$$

The term *error* in the numerator indicates the maximum potential error in the measurement (error = larger quantity – smaller quantity), while the term *quantity desired* in the denominator represents the total amount

measured. Percentage of error may be calculated for either a weight or a volume measurement.

Example: A quantity of material weighs 5.810 g on a prescription balance. Using a much more accurate analytical balance, the quantity weighs 5.893 g. What is the percentage of error for the original weighing?

$$\text{error} = 5.893 \text{ g} - 5.810 \text{ g} = 0.083 \text{ g}$$

The quantity desired is 5.810 g. Thus,

$$\% \text{ error} = 0.083 \text{ g} \times \frac{100\%}{5.810} = 1.4\%$$

Example: Suppose you wish to weigh out 75.0 mg of an ingredient but mistakenly weigh 65.0 mg instead. Based on the quantity desired, what is the percentage of error?

$$\% \text{ error} = \frac{(\text{error} \times 100\%)}{(\text{quantity desired})}$$
$$= \frac{(10.0 \text{ mg} \times 100\%)}{75.0 \text{ mg}} = 13\%$$

1-6. Minimum Measurable

By regulation, weighings by a pharmacist cannot exceed a percentage of error greater than 5%, which requires that the sensitivity of the balance be known and limits the smallest quantity that can be weighed. *Balance sensitivity* is defined in terms of the *sensitivity requirement* (SR), which is the weight of material that will move the indicator one marked unit on the index plate of the balance. For a class A prescription balance, SR = 6 mg. The minimum weighable quantity for a given balance can be calculated using the percentage of error formula: replace the "error" term with the SR (e.g., 6 mg), replace the percentage of error term with 5%, and replace the "quantity desired" term with "minimum weighable quantity" as follows:

$$5\% = \frac{(\text{SR} \times 100\%)}{\text{minimum weighable quantity}}, \text{ or}$$
$$\text{minimum weighable quantity} = \frac{(\text{SR} \times 100\%)}{5\%}$$

Example: For a balance that has an SR of 4 mg, what is the minimum weighable quantity to ensure a percentage of error no greater than 2%?

$$\% \text{ error} = \frac{(\text{error} \times 100\%)}{\text{quantity desired}}$$

$$= \frac{SR \times 100\%}{\text{minimum weighable quantity}}$$

$$\text{minimum weighable quantity} = \frac{(SR \times 100\%)}{\% \text{ error}}$$

$$= 4 \text{ mg} \times \frac{100\%}{2\%}$$

$$= 200 \text{ mg}$$

Example: What is the SR for a balance with a percentage of error of 5% when weighing 120 mg?

$$\% \text{ error} = \frac{(SR \times 100\%)}{\text{quantity desired}}$$

$$SR = \frac{(\% \text{ error} \times \text{quantity desired})}{100\%}$$

$$= \frac{(5\% \times 120 \text{ mg})}{100\%} = 6 \text{ mg}$$

1-7. Patient-Specific Dosage Calculations

Drugs with a narrow therapeutic range often are dosed on the basis of patient weight or body surface area. For patients with renal impairment, some drugs are dosed on the basis of creatinine clearance.

Dosing Based on Body Weight

Weight-based dosing might involve using the patient's actual body weight (ABW), ideal body weight (IBW), or perhaps an adjusted ideal body weight that is a function of IBW and ABW. Those weights are invariably expressed in kilograms.

Example: A patient weighing 180 lb is to receive 0.25 mg/kg per day amphotericin B (reconstituted and diluted to 0.100 mg/mL) by intravenous (IV) infusion. What volume of solution is required to deliver the daily dose?

$$\text{patient weight} = \frac{180 \text{ lb}}{2.20} = 82 \text{ kg}$$

$$\text{daily dose} = 82 \text{ kg} \times 0.25 \text{ mg/kg}$$

$$= \frac{20.5 \text{ mg} \times \text{mL}}{1 \text{ mL}}$$

$$= \frac{20.5 \text{ mg}}{0.100 \text{ mg}} \times = 1 \text{ mL}$$

$$\times \frac{20.5 \text{ mL}}{0.100 \text{ mg}} = 205 \text{ mL}$$

A commonly used equation for calculating IBW is

$$\text{IBW (kg)} = (\text{sex factor})$$

$$+ (2.3 \times \text{height in inches over 5 feet}),$$

where the sex factor for males is 50.0 and the sex factor for females is 45.5.

Example: The recommended adult daily dosage for patients with normal renal function for tobramycin is 3 mg/kg IBW given in three evenly divided doses. What would each injection be for a male patient who weighs 185 lb and is 5 feet, 9 inches tall?

$$\text{IBW (kg)} = 50 + (2.3 \times 9) = 50 + 21$$

$$= 71 \text{ kg (ignore ABW of 84 kg)}$$

$$\text{daily dose (tid)} = 71 \text{ kg} \times 3 \text{ mg/kg} = 213 \text{ mg (per day)}$$

Thus, each injection = 213 mg/3 = 71 mg

In the absence of other information, the usual drug doses are considered generally suitable for 70-kg individuals. Thus, in the absence of more specific information, an adjusted dosage for a notably larger or smaller individual may be obtained by multiplying the usual dose by the ratio of patient weight to 70 kg (Clark's rule).

Example: If the adult dose of a drug is 100 mg and no child-specific dosing information is available, what would the weight-adjusted dose be for a child who weighs 40 kg?

$$\text{child dose} = 100 \text{ mg} \times \frac{40 \text{ kg}}{70 \text{ kg}} = 57 \text{ mg}$$

Dosing Based on Body Surface Area

Dosing based on body surface area requires an estimation of the patient's body surface area (BSA) expressed in square meters (m²). That parameter might be estimated from a nomogram using height and weight or, for adults, by using one of several equations such as:

$$\text{BSA} = \left[\frac{(\text{height in centimeters})}{(\text{weight in kilograms})}{3,600} \right]^{\frac{1}{2}} \text{m}^2$$

Example: What is the computed BSA for an adult who weighs 88 kg and is 5 feet, 10 inches tall?

$$\text{height} = 70 \text{ inches} \times 2.54 \text{ cm/inch} = 178 \text{ cm}$$

$$\text{BSA} = \left[178 \text{ cm} \times \frac{88 \text{ kg}}{3,600} \right]^{1/2} \text{m}^2 = 2.09 \text{ m}^2$$

The average adult BSA is taken to be 1.73 m². That value can be used to obtain an approximate child's dose, given the usual dose for an adult and the child's estimated BSA.

Example: If the adult dose of a drug is 50 mg, what would the BSA-adjusted dose be for a child having an estimated BSA of 0.55 m²?

$$\text{child dose} = 50 \text{ mg} \times \frac{0.55 \text{ m}^2}{1.73 \text{ m}^2} = 16 \text{ mg}$$

Dosing Based on Creatinine Clearance

For many drugs, the rate of elimination depends on kidney function. Creatinine clearance (CrCl) is a measure of the volume of blood plasma that is cleared of creatinine by kidney filtration per minute, and it is expressed in milliliters per minute. Creatinine clearance can be calculated using the Cockcroft-Gault equation as a function of patient sex, age, body weight, and serum creatinine.

For males:

$$\text{CrCl} \, (\text{mL/min}) = (140 - \text{age in years})$$

$$\times \frac{(\text{body weight in kg})}{\left(\begin{array}{c} 72 \times \text{serum creatinine} \\ \text{in mg/dL} \end{array} \right)}$$

For females:

$$\text{CrCl} = 0.85 \times \text{CrCl for males}$$

Example: Using the Cockcroft-Gault equation, calculate the creatinine clearance rate for a 76-year-old female weighing 65 kg and having a serum creatinine of 0.52 mg/dL.

$$\text{CrCl} = 0.85 \times (140 - 76 \text{ years}) \times \frac{65 \text{ kg}}{(72 \times 0.52 \text{ mg/dL})}$$

$$= 94 \text{ mL/min}$$

Alternatively, creatinine clearance may be estimated using the Jelliffe equations.

For males:

$$\text{CrCl} = \left[98 - 0.8 \times \frac{(\text{patient age in years} - 20)}{\text{serum creatinine in mg/dL}} \right]$$

For females:

$$\text{CrCl} = 0.9 \times \text{CrCl for males}$$

The normal value for creatinine clearance is taken to be 100 mL/min. Sometimes one must adjust CrCl to the patient's BSA, which is calculated as:

$$\text{adjusted CrCl} = \text{CrCl} \times \frac{\text{BSA}}{1.73}$$

The maintenance dose for some drugs is based on IBW and CrCl. See Chapter 6 for more detailed information.

1-8. Using Batch Preparation Formulas

The relative amounts of ingredients in a pharmaceutical product are specified in a formula. A pharmacist may be required to reduce or enlarge the formula to prepare a lesser or greater amount of product. A given formula might specify either the actual amount (weight or volume) of each ingredient for a specified total amount of product or just the relative amount (part) of each ingredient. In the latter case, the ingredients must all be of the same measure (e.g., weight in grams).

Example: From the following lotion formula, calculate the quantity of triethanolamine required to make 200 mL of lotion.

Triethanolamine	10 mL
Oleic acid	25 mL
Benzyl benzoate	250 mL
Water to make	1,000 mL

$$\frac{x}{10 \text{ mL}} = \frac{200 \text{ mL}}{1,000 \text{ mL}}$$

$$x = 10 \text{ mL} \times \frac{200 \text{ mL}}{1,000 \text{ mL}} = 2.0 \text{ mL}$$

Example: From the following formula, calculate the quantity of chlorpheniramine maleate required to make 500 g of product.

Chlorpheniramine maleate	6 parts
Phenindamine	20 parts
Phenylpropanolamine HCl	55 parts

Note that the formula will give a total of 81 parts, which will correspond to the desired quantity of 500 g. Then,

$$\frac{x}{500 \text{ g}} = \frac{6 \text{ parts}}{81 \text{ parts}}$$

$$x = 500 \text{ g} \times \frac{6 \text{ parts}}{81 \text{ parts}} = 37 \text{ g}$$

1-9. Conventions in Expression of Concentration

In pharmacy, one will encounter a diversity of conventions for expressing drug concentrations. One must be prepared to calculate drug concentration units directly from their definitions and to interconvert among them.

Percentage Strength

Percentage, strictly speaking, specifies the number of parts per 100 parts. In pharmacy, percentage comes in three varieties:

- Percent weight-in-weight = %(w/w) = grams of ingredient in 100 grams of product (assumed for mixtures of solids and semisolids)
- Percent volume-in-volume = %(v/v) = milliliters of ingredient in 100 milliliters of product (assumed for solutions or mixtures of liquids)
- Percent weight-in-volume = %(w/v) = grams of ingredient in 100 milliliters of product (assumed for solutions of solids in liquids)

Example: What is the concentration in %(w/v) for a preparation containing 250 mg of drug in 50 mL of solution? Note that %(w/v) is defined as g/100 mL. Thus,

$$\text{concentration} = 0.250 \text{ g} \times \frac{100}{50 \text{ mL}} = 0.50\% \text{ (w/v)}$$

Parts (Ratio Strength)

Concentrations may be expressed in "parts" or ratio strength when the active ingredient is highly diluted. Assumptions concerning (w/w), (v/v), and (w/v) ratios are identical to those for percentages.

Example: What is the concentration in %(v/v) of a solution that has a ratio strength of 1:2,500 (v/v)?

$$x \text{ mL} : 1 \text{ mL} = 100 \text{ mL} : 2,500 \text{ mL}$$

$$x = 100 \text{ mL} \times \frac{1 \text{ mL}}{2,500 \text{ mL}} = 0.04\% \text{ (v/v)}$$

Millimoles

By definition, a 1 molar solution contains 1 gram molecular weight (1 GMW = 1 mole = weight in grams of Avogadro's number of particles) per liter of solution. The molarity expresses the number of moles per liter. The millimolarity (millimoles/liter) is 1,000 times the molarity of a solution.

Example: What is the millimolar concentration of a solution consisting of 0.90 g of sodium chloride (GMW = 58.5) in 100 mL of water? The quantity of 0.9 g in 100 mL corresponds to 9.0 g in 1,000 mL.

$$\text{molarity} = \frac{1 \text{ mole}}{1,000 \text{ mL}} = \left(9.0 \text{ g}/58.5 \text{ g/mole}\right)$$

$$= 0.154$$

$$\text{millimolarity} = 1,000 \times \text{molarity} = 154$$

Milliequivalents

By definition, the equivalent weight of an ion is the atomic or formula weight of the ion divided by the absolute value of its valence. Thus, the equivalent weight of ferric ion, Fe^{3+} (atomic weight 55.9, valence 3), is 18.6. A milliequivalent is 1,000th of an equivalent weight (i.e., 1,000 milliequivalent weights equal 1 equivalent weight). For a molecule, the equivalent weight is obtained as the GMW (formula weight) divided by the total cation *or* the total anion charge. For example, the equivalent weight of $MgCl_2$ (atomic weight of Mg^{2+} = 24.3, with a valence of +2; atomic weight of Cl^{1-} = 35.5, with a valence of −1) is (24.3 + 2 × 35.5)/2 = 47.7 g. Its milliequivalent weight is 0.0477 g, or 47.7 mg. In the case of a nondissociating (nonionizing) molecule (e.g., dextrose or tobramycin), the equivalent weight is equal to the formula weight.

Example: What is the concentration, in milliequivalents per liter, of a solution containing 14.9 g of KCl (GMW = 74.5 g) in 1 liter? Note that the valence of potassium is 1+, so the equivalent weight equals the molecular weight. Accordingly,

$$\text{mEq/L of KCl} = \text{mEq/L of K}^+ = \text{mEq/L of Cl}^-$$

$$= 1,000 \times \frac{(14.9 \text{ g/L})}{(74.5 \text{ g/mEq})} = 200 \text{ mEq/L}$$

Example: What weight of $MgSO_4$ (GMW = 120) is required to prepare 1 liter of a solution that is 25.0 mEq/L in Mg^{2+}? One must have 25.0 mEq of

MgSO$_4$ to obtain 25.0 mEq of Mg. The valence of Mg (and total positive charge) is 2+; therefore, the equivalent weight of MgSO$_4$ is 120/2 = 60 g. Accordingly, 60 mg corresponds to 1 mEq of MgSO$_4$. Then,

$$x : 60 \text{ mg} = 25 \text{ mEq} : 1 \text{ mEq}$$

$$x = 60 \text{ mg} \times \frac{25 \text{ mEq}}{1 \text{ mEq}} = 1,500 \text{ mg} = 1.50 \text{ g}$$

Example: How many milliequivalents of Ca^{2+} are contained in 100 mL of a solution that is 5.0%(w/v) in CaCl$_2$ (GMW = 111, atomic weight of Ca^{2+} = 40, atomic weight of Cl$^-$ = 35.5)? Note that the valence of calcium is 2+. The solution contains 5.0 g CaCl$_2$ per 100 mL, which corresponds to (5.0 g/111) × 2 = 0.090 equivalents of CaCl$_2$, as well as Ca^{2+}. Accordingly, 100 mL of the solution contains 90 mEq of Ca^{2+}.

Milliosmoles

Osmotic concentration is a measure of the total number of particles in solution and is expressed in milliosmoles (mOsm). Thus, the number of milliosmoles is based on the total number of cations *and* the total number of anions. The milliosmolarity of a solution is the number of milliosmoles per liter of solution (mOsm/L), where:

$$\text{mOsm/L} = (\text{moles/L}) \times \text{number of species}$$

$$\times 1,000 \text{ moles}$$

number of species = number of ionic species upon

complete dissociation

(e.g., dextrose = 1 specie,

NaCl = 2 species, MgCl$_2$)

The total osmolarity of a solution is the sum of the osmolarities of the solute components of the solution. When calculating osmolarities, in the absence of other information, assume that salts (e.g., NaCl, etc.) dissociate completely (referred to as the *ideal osmolarity*). You should be aware of the distinction between the terms *milliosmolarity* (milliosmoles per liter of solution) and *milliosmolality* (milliosmoles per kilogram of solution).

Example: What is the concentration, in milliosmoles per liter, of a solution that contains 224 mg of KCl (GMW = 74.6 g) and 234 mg of NaCl (GMW = 58.5) in 500 mL? What is the number of milliosmoles per liter of K$^+$ alone?

$$\frac{\text{mOsm KCl}}{500 \text{ mL}} = \left(\frac{0.224 \text{ g}}{74.6}\right) \times 2 \times 1,000$$

$$= 6.0 \text{ for } 500 \text{ mL}$$

$$\frac{\text{mOsm NaCl}}{500 \text{ mL}} = \left(\frac{0.234 \text{ g}}{58.5}\right) \times 2 \times 1,000$$

$$= 8.0 \text{ for } 500 \text{ mL}$$

$$\text{total mOsm/L} = 2 \times (6.0 \text{ mOsm KCl} + \text{mOsm NaCl})$$

$$= 28.0 \text{ mOsm/L}$$

$$\text{mOsm/L of K}^+ = \text{mOsm/L of } \frac{\text{KCl}}{2} = \frac{12.0}{2} = 6.0$$

Milligrams per 100 Milliliters and Milligrams per Deciliter

Traditionally, some lab test values are reported as the number of milligrams per 100 milliliters (mg%) or, equivalently, milligrams per deciliter (mg/dL).

Example: What is the %(w/v) concentration of glucose in a patient with a blood glucose reading of 230 mg/dL? Note that 1 dL = 100 mL and that 230 mg = 0.230 g. Then,

$$\text{glucose concentration} = \frac{0.230 \text{ g}}{100 \text{ mL}} = 0.230\% \text{ (w/v)}$$

"Units" and Micrograms per Milligram

The concentrations for some drugs whose production involves incomplete isolation from natural sources might be expressed in terms of "units" of activity or micrograms per milligram (mcg/mg) as determined by a standardized bioassay.

Example: A preparation of penicillin G sodium contains 2.2 mEq of sodium (atomic weight = 23, valence = 1+) per 1 million units of penicillin. How many milligrams of sodium are contained in an IV infusion of 5 million units? The 5 million unit dose will contain 5 × 2.2 mEq = 11.0 mEq.

$$\text{mEq weight of sodium} = 23 \text{ mg}$$

$$\text{weight of sodium} = (23 \text{ mg/mEq}) \times 11.0 \text{ mEq}$$

$$= 253 \text{ mg}$$

Parts per Million and Parts per Billion

Very low concentrations often are expressed in terms of parts per million (ppm) (the number of parts of ingredient per million parts of mixture or solution) or parts per billion (ppb) (the number of parts of ingredient per billion parts of mixture or solution). Thus, ppm and ppb are special cases of ratio strength concentrations.

Example: Re-express 1:25,000 in terms of parts per million.

$$x \text{ parts} : 1 \text{ part} = 1,000,000 \text{ parts} : 25,000 \text{ parts}$$

$$x = 1,000,000 \times \frac{1}{25,000} = 40 \text{ parts}$$

$$\left(\text{i.e., the concentration is 40 ppm}\right)$$

1-10. Dilutions and Concentrations

Simple Dilutions

In simple dilutions, a desired drug concentration is obtained by adding more solvent (or diluent) to an existing solution or mixture. Mathematically, the key feature of this process is that the initial and final amount of drug present remain unchanged. The amount of drug in any solution is proportional to the concentration times the quantity of the solution. Thus, taking the initial concentration as C_1, the initial quantity of solution as Q_1, the final concentration as C_2, and the final quantity of solution as Q_2, one has the relationship: $C_1 \times Q_1 = C_2 \times Q_2$. When provided with values for any three of those variables, the fourth variable can be calculated. (Because the equation can be rearranged to $C_1/C_2 = Q_2/Q_1$, it sometimes is referred to as an *inverse proportionality*.)

Example: How much water should be added to 250 mL of a solution of 0.20%(w/v) benzalkonium chloride to make a 0.050 %(w/v) solution?

$$C_1 = 0.20\% \left(w/v\right)$$
$$Q_1 = 250 \text{ mL}$$
$$C_2 = 0.05\% \left(w/v\right)$$
$$Q_2 = x$$
$$x = Q_2 - 250 \text{ mL}$$
$$C_1 \times Q_1 = C_2 \times Q_2$$
$$Q_2 = \frac{C_1 \times Q_1}{C_2} = 0.20\% \times \frac{250 \text{ mL}}{0.05\%} = 1,000 \text{ mL}$$
$$x = Q_2 = 250 \text{ mL} = 1,000 \text{ mL} - 250 \text{ mL}$$
$$= 750 \text{ mL of water to be added}$$

Alcohol Solutions

The preceding treatment of dilutions assumes that solution and solvent volumes are reasonably additive. For dilutions of concentrated ethyl alcohol in water, that is not the case, because a contraction in volume occurs on mixing. Consequently, you cannot extend the calculation to determine the exact volume of water to add to the initial alcohol solution. That is, the volume of water to be added cannot be obtained simply as $Q_2 - Q_1$. Rather, you can specify only that sufficient water be added to the initial concentrated alcohol solution (Q_1) to reach the specified or calculated final volume (Q_2) of the diluted alcohol solution.

Example: How much water should be added to 100 mL of 95%(v/v) ethanol to make 50%(v/v) ethanol?

$$C_1 = 95\% \left(v/v\right)$$
$$Q_1 = 100 \text{ mL}$$
$$C_2 = 50\% \left(v/v\right)$$
$$Q_2 = x$$
$$C_1 \times Q_1 = C_2 \times Q_2$$
$$Q_2 = \frac{C_1 \times Q_1}{C_2} = 95\% \times \frac{100 \text{ mL}}{50\%} = 1,000 \text{ mL}$$
$$= 190 \text{ mL} \left(\text{the final total volume}\right)$$

Thus, to the 100 mL of 95%(v/v) ethanol add sufficient water to make 190 mL. The sufficient quantity of water will be more than 90 mL because of the contraction that occurs when concentrated alcohol is mixed with water.

Concentrated Acids

Concentrated mineral acids (hydrochloric, sulfuric, nitric, and phosphoric) are manufactured by bubbling the pure acid gas into water to produce a saturated solution. The manufacturer specifies the concentration as a %(w/w). However, when preparing diluted acids for compounding, the pharmacist must express the concentration as a %(w/v), which requires use of the specific gravity of the concentrated acid.

Example: What volume of 35%(w/w) concentrated HCl (SpGr 1.20) is required to make 500 mL of 5%(w/v) solution?

First, determine the weight of HCl required for the dilute solution. Because the dilute solution is 5%(w/v), it will contain 5 g in each 100 mL, or 25 g in 500 mL.

Next, one must determine what weight, x, of the 35%(w/w) solution contains 25 g of HCl. By proportion,

$$x : 100 \text{ g} = 25 \text{ g} : 35 \text{ g}$$

$$x = 100 \text{ g} \times \frac{25 \text{ g}}{35 \text{ g}}$$

$$x = 71.4 \text{ g of the concentrated solution}$$

Finally, use the specific gravity of the concentrated solution to convert the weight to volume. Here, recall that specific gravity is numerically equal to density when the latter is expressed in grams per milliliter. Thus,

$$\text{density} = 1.20 \text{ g/mL} = \text{weight/volume}$$

Rearranging,

$$\text{volume} = \text{weight}\Big/\text{density} = \frac{71.4 \text{ g}}{1.20 \text{ g/mL}} = 59.5 \text{ mL}$$

Triturations

Triturations are simply 10%(w/w) finely powdered (triturated) mixtures of a drug in an inert substance.

Example: What weight of colchicine trituration is required to prepare 30 doses of 0.25 mg each of colchicine?

For the trituration, 10 mg of the mixture contains 1 mg of drug. Thus,

$$x \text{ mg of trituration} : 10 \text{ mg of trituration}$$

$$= \left(30 \times 0.25 \text{ mg drug}\right) : 1 \text{ mg drug}$$

$$x = 10 \text{ mg trituration} \times \frac{\left(30 \times 0.25 \text{ mg drug}\right)}{1 \text{ mg drug}}$$

$$= 75 \text{ mg trituration}$$

Alligation Alternate Method

Sometimes a drug concentration is required that is in between the concentrations of two (or more) stock solutions (or available drug products). In that case, the alligation alternate method may be used to quickly obtain the relative parts of each of the stock solutions needed to yield the desired concentration. If stock solutions of concentrations A% and B% (A% > B%) are to be used to make a solution of concentration C%, one sets up the following diagram to obtain the relative parts of solutions A and B.

A%		(C% − B%) parts of A
	C%	
B%		(A% − C%) parts of B

Example: In what proportion should 20%(w/v) dextrose be mixed with 5%(w/v) dextrose to obtain 15%(w/v) dextrose? How much of each is required to make 75 mL of 15%(w/v) solution?

20%		10 parts of 20%
	15%	
5%		5 parts of 5%

Thus, combine the stock solutions in the ratio of 10 parts of 20%(w/v) dextrose:5 parts of 5%(w/v) dextrose (i.e., 2:1). Accordingly, to make 75 mL of 15% solution, mix 50 mL of 20% solution with 25 mL of 5% solution.

Alligation Medial Method

Sometimes one may need to know the final concentration of a solution obtained by mixing specified volumes of two or more stock solutions. In that case, the alligation medial method may be used.

Example: What is the concentration of a solution prepared by combining 100 mL of a 10% solution, 200 mL of a 20% solution, and 300 mL of a 30% solution? Proceed as follows:

$$10\% \times 100 \text{ mL} = 1,000 \text{ \%mL}$$
$$20\% \times 200 \text{ mL} = 4,000 \text{ \%mL}$$
$$30\% \times 300 \text{ mL} = 9,000 \text{ \%mL}$$
$$\quad 600 \text{ mL} \quad 14,000 \text{ \%mL}$$

$$\text{Mixture concentration} = \frac{14,000 \text{ \%mL}}{600 \text{ mL}} = 23.3\%$$

1-11. Isotonic Solutions

In pharmacy, the preparation of many solutions requires attention to osmotic pressure, a colligative property that is especially relevant for membrane transport. Other colligative properties include freezing point depression and boiling point elevation. Those properties are a function of the total number of particles dissolved in the solution, regardless of the identity of the particles. Here, the term *particles* corresponds to cations, anions, and neutral undissociated molecules. A solution that has the same osmotic pressure as bodily fluids (blood or tears) is said to be *isotonic* (and *isosmotic*). As points of reference, 5.0%(w/v) dextrose, a nondissociating molecule, and 0.9%(w/v) sodium chloride, a dissociating molecule, are isotonic.

Dissociating Solutes

Preparing solutions of specific tonicities requires knowledge of the dissociation properties of the solutes involved. One must know if the solute in question dissociates and, if so, to what extent and into how many particles. For example, in weak solutions, sodium chloride dissociates about 80% into two particles, yielding a solution containing Na^+ ions, Cl^- ions, and undissociated NaCl molecules. A measure of the extent of dissociation is provided by the dissociation factor, *i*, which is defined as the ratio of the total number of particles following dissociation to the number of molecules prior to dissociation. For example, 100 molecules of sodium chloride (prior to dissociation) will dissociate 80% to produce 80 particles of Na^+, 80 particles of Cl^-, and 20 particles of NaCl, or 180 particles in all. The dissociation factor, *i*, for NaCl, then, is 180/100 = 1.8. A nondissociating molecule (such as dextrose or tobramycin) is assigned a dissociation constant of 1.0. If measured dissociation information is not available, one can assume approximately 80% dissociation for weak solutions of salts. In that case, salts (including drugs) that dissociate into two ions (such as sodium chloride and ephedrine hydrochloride) will have a dissociation factor of 1.8; salts that dissociate into three ions (such as ephedrine sulfate) will have a dissociation factor of 2.6; salts that dissociate into four ions (such as sodium citrate) will have a dissociation factor of 3.4.

Example: What is the dissociation factor (*i*) for a compound that dissociates 60% into three ions?

   For each 100 undissolved molecules, one will obtain the following on dissolution:

$60 \times 3 = 180$ particles of ions + 40 particles of undissociated molecules = a total of 220 particles

Thus, the dissociation factor = $i = 220/100 = 2.2$.

Example: What is the dissociation factor for dextrose, a nondissociating compound?

   For each 100 undissolved molecules, one will obtain the following on dissolution:

0 particles of ions + 100 particles of undissociated molecules = a total of 100 particles

Thus, the dissociation factor = $i = 100/100 = 1.0$.

Sodium Chloride Equivalents or E value

When preparing isotonic drug solutions, one must take the tonicity contribution of the drug into consideration. That can be accomplished by using the *sodium chloride equivalent* (E value) for the drug, which is defined as the number of grams of sodium chloride that would produce the same tonicity effect as 1 gram of the drug. If the value of the sodium chloride equivalent is not provided, it can be calculated using the molecular weights (MWs) and dissociation factors of sodium chloride and the drug in question:

$$\text{sodium chloride equivalent} = (\text{MW of NaCL})$$
$$\times \frac{(\text{drug dissociation factor})}{(\text{MW of drug}) \times (\text{sodium chloride dissociation factor})}$$
$$= \frac{(58.5)(i)}{(\text{MW of drug})(1.8)}$$

Example: What is the sodium chloride equivalent of demecarium bromide (GMW = 717, *i* = 2.6)?

$$\text{sodium chloride equivalent} = \frac{(58.5 \times 2.6)}{(717 \times 1.8)} = 0.12$$

Thus, each gram of demecarium bromide is equivalent to 0.12 g sodium chloride. So how does one proceed to prepare a drug solution that must be made isotonic? Using the total volume of isotonic solution to be prepared, first calculate the hypothetical weight, *x*, of sodium chloride (alone) that would be required to make that volume of water isotonic (0.9%). Next, using the weight of drug to be incorporated in the solution and its sodium chloride equivalent, calculate the weight of sodium chloride, *y*, that would correspond to the weight of the drug. Then, calculate the true weight of sodium chloride, *z*, to be added to the preparation as $z = x - y$.

Example: What weight of sodium chloride would be required to prepare 50 mL of an isotonic solution containing 500 mg of pilocarpine nitrate (sodium chloride equivalent = 0.23)?

   Because isotonic saline requires 0.9 g/100 mL, 50 mL of isotonic saline will require 0.45 g (i.e., $x = 0.45$ g). The 500 mg of pilocarpine nitrate will correspond to 500 mg × 0.23 = 115 mg sodium chloride (i.e., $y = 0.12$ g). Thus, the weight of sodium chloride needed to make an isotonic solution = $z = x - y = 0.45$ g $- 0.12$ g $= 0.33$ g.

Example: A (fictitious) new drug, Utopical (MW = 175, dissociation factor i = 3.4), is to be provided as 325 mg in 60 mL of solution made isotonic with sodium chloride. What is the required weight of sodium chloride?

Here, the sodium chloride equivalent of the drug is not given and must be calculated from the information provided.

$$\text{sodium chloride equivalent of Utopical} = \frac{(58.5 \times 3.4)}{(175 \times 1.8)}$$

$$= 0.63$$

Because isotonic saline requires 0.9 g/100 mL, 60 mL of isotonic saline will require 0.54 g (i.e., x = 0.54 g). The 325 mg of Utopical will correspond to 0.325 g × 0.63 = 0.20 g of sodium chloride (i.e., y = 0.20 g). Thus, the weight of sodium chloride needed to make an isotonic solution = z = $(x - y)$ = (0.54 g − 0.20 g) = 0.34 g.

1-12. Intravenous Infusion Flow Rates

A physician may specify the rate of flow of IV fluids in drops per minute, amount of drug per hour, or the duration of time of administration of the total volume of the infusion. Therefore, to program an infusion pump to give the medication at the correct rate, one may need to calculate the infusion rate in per minute or per hour increments.

Example: If 250 mg of a drug is added to a 500-mL D_5W bag, what should the flow rate be, in milliliters per hour, to deliver 50 mg of drug per hour?

$$x \text{ mL/h} : 500 \text{ mL/h} = 50 \text{ mg/h} : 250 \text{ mg/h}$$

$$x = (500 \text{ mL/h}) \times \frac{(50 \text{ mg/h})}{(250 \text{ mg/h})} = 100 \text{ mL/h}$$

Example: If an infusion flow rate is 100 mL/h and the infusion set delivers 15 drops/mL, what is the rate of flow in drops per minute?

$$15 \text{ drops/mL} = \times 100 \text{ mL/h} = 1,500 \text{ drops/h}$$

$$= 25 \text{ drops/min}$$

Example: If 500 mL of an infusion is to be delivered using an IV administration set that delivers 10 drops/mL and the flow rate is set at 1.25 mL/min, how long will it take to deliver the 500 mL?

$$\text{Total time of delivery} = \frac{500 \text{ mL}}{1.25 \text{ mL/min}} = 400 \text{ min}$$

$$= 6.7 \text{ h}$$

(The 10 drops/mL is superfluous information.)

1-13. Buffers

Buffer solutions are used to reduce pH fluctuations associated with introduction of small amounts of strong acids or bases. Typical buffer solutions are composed of a weak acid or weak base plus a salt of the acid or base. Solution pH in the presence of a buffer can be calculated using the Henderson–Hasselbalch equations.

For weak acids, $\text{pH} = \text{pK}_a + \log(\text{salt/acid})$

For weak bases, $\text{pH} = \text{pK}_w - \text{pK}_b + \log(\text{base/salt})$

where $\text{pK}_w = 14$

Example: What is the pH of a buffer solution prepared to be 0.50 moles (M) in sodium acetate and 0.05 M in acetic acid (pK$_a$ of acetic acid = 4.76)?

For weak acids, $\text{pH} = \text{pK}_a + \log(\text{salt/acid})$.

$$\text{Thus, pH} = 4.76 + \log\left(\frac{0.50}{0.05}\right) = 4.76 + \log(10)$$

$$= 4.76 + 1 = 5.76$$

Example: What is the pH of a buffer solution prepared to be 0.5 M in ammonia (pK$_b$ = 4.74) and 0.05 M in ammonium chloride?

Ammonia forms a base in aqueous solution.

$$\text{pH} = \text{pK}_w - \text{pK}_b + \log(\text{base/salt}) = 14.00 - 4.74$$

$$+ \log(0.50/0.05) = 14.00 - 4.74 + 1.00 = 10.26$$

1-14. Temperature

Frequently, one must convert temperature from Fahrenheit (F) to Centigrade (C), and vice versa. The following formula can be used: $9°C = 5°F - 160$.

Example: A patient has an oral temperature of 100°F. What is that temperature in °C?

$$9°C = 5°F - 160$$

$$C = \frac{(5°F - 160)}{9} = \frac{(5 \times 100 - 160)}{9} = 37.8°C$$

1-15. Questions

1. If 100 capsules contain 340 mg of active ingredient, what is the weight of active ingredient in 75 capsules?

   A. 453 mg
   B. 340 mg
   C. 255 mg
   D. 128 mg
   E. 75 mg

2. What is the weight of 500 mL of a liquid whose specific gravity is 1.13?

   A. 442 mg
   B. 565 g
   C. 442 g
   D. 885 mg
   E. 221 g

3. A pharmacist weighs out 325 mg of a substance on her class A prescription balance. When she subsequently checks the weight on a more sensitive analytical balance, she finds it to be only 312 mg. What is the percentage of error in the original weighing?

   A. 4%
   B. 5%
   C. 6%
   D. 10%
   E. 12%

4. What is the minimum weighable quantity for a maximum of 5% error using a balance with a sensitivity requirement of 6 mg?

   A. 80 mcg
   B. 100 mg
   C. 120 mg
   D. 150 mg
   E. 240 mg

5. A patient weighing 175 lb is to receive an initial daily intramuscular (IM) dosage of procainamide HCl (500 mg/mL vial) of 50 mg/kg

(ABW) to be given in divided doses every 3 hours. How many milliliters should each injection contain?

   A. 3.98 mL
   B. 0.49 mL
   C. 8.23 mL
   D. 1.87 mL
   E. 0.99 mL

6. What is the ideal body weight of a female patient whose height is 5 feet 8 inches?

   A. 68 kg
   B. 64 kg
   C. 150 lb
   D. 121 lb
   E. 53 kg

7. What is the approximate BSA of an adult patient who weighs 154 lb and is 6 feet tall?

   A. 1.73 m²
   B. 3.15 m²
   C. 1.89 m²
   D. 0.70 m²
   E. 2.67 m²

8. If the adult dose of a drug is 125 mg, what is the dose for a child whose BSA is estimated to be 0.68 m²?

   A. 485 mcg
   B. 318 mg
   C. 85 mg
   D. 49 mg
   E. 33 mg

9. What is the creatinine clearance for a 65-year-old female who weighs 50 kg and has a serum creatinine level of 1.3 mg/dL?

   A. 34 mL/min
   B. 40 mL/min
   C. 26 mL/min
   D. 82 mL/min
   E. 100 mL/min

10. Using the formula that follows, determine how much zinc oxide is required to make 750 g of mixture:

Zinc oxide	150 g
Starch	250 g
Petrolatum	550 g
Coal tar	50 g

A. 200 g
B. 188 g
C. 413 g
D. 113 g
E. 38 g

11. Using the formula that follows, determine the weight of kaolin that would be required to produce 500 g of mixture:

Kaolin   12 parts
Magnesium oxide   3 parts
Bismuth subcarbonate   5 parts

A. 83 g
B. 300 g
C. 208 g
D. 333 g
E. 250 g

12. How much dextrose is required to prepare 500 mL of an aqueous 10% solution?

A. 250 mg
B. 500 mg
C. 10 g
D. 25 g
E. 50 g

13. What weight of hexachlorophene should be used in compounding 20 g of an ointment containing hexachlorophene at a concentration of 1:400?

A. 25 mcg
B. 50 mcg
C. 50 mg
D. 80 mg
E. 5 g

14. What weight of magnesium chloride ($MgCl_2$, formula weight = 95.3) is required to prepare 200 mL of a solution that is 5.0 millimolar?

A. 191 mg
B. 95.3 mg
C. 19.1 mg
D. 477 mcg
E. 95 g

15. What weight of magnesium chloride ($MgCl_2$, formula weight = 95.3; Mg^{2+}, atomic weight = 24.3; Cl^{1-}, atomic weight = 35.5) is required to prepare 1,000 mL of a solution that contains 5.0 mEq of magnesium?

A. 238 mg
B. 4.76 g
C. 1.19 g
D. 60.7 mg
E. 476 mcg

16. What is the milliosmolarity (ideal) of normal saline (NaCl, formula weight = 58.5)?

A. 100 mOsm/L
B. 154 mOsm/L
C. 254 mOsm/L
D. 287 mOsm/L
E. 308 mOsm/L

17. How much water for injection should be added to 250 mL of 20% dextrose to obtain 15% dextrose?

A. 333 mL
B. 83 mL
C. 250 mL
D. 166 mL
E. 58 mL

18. What volume of a 5% dextrose solution should be mixed with 200 mL of a 20% dextrose solution to prepare 300 mL of a 15% dextrose solution?

A. 150 mL
B. 200 mL
C. 100 mL
D. 50 mL
E. 250 mL

19. What is the final concentration obtained by mixing 200 mL of 20% dextrose with 100 mL of 5% dextrose?

A. 10%
B. 15%
C. 7.5%
D. 12.5%
E. 17.5%

20. Magnesium chloride ($MgCl_2$) is a 3-ion electrolyte that dissociates 80% at the relevant concentration. Calculate its dissociation factor (i).

A. 1.8
B. 2.2
C. 2.4
D. 2.6
E. 3.2

21. Tobramycin (formula weight = 468) has a dissociation factor of 1.0. What is its sodium chloride equivalent?

    A. 0.069
    B. 0.0092
    C. 0.117
    D. 0.286
    E. 0.782

22. What weight of sodium chloride should be used in compounding the following prescription for ephedrine sulfate (formula weight = 429, dissociation factor = 2.6, sodium chloride equivalent = 0.23)?

    Ephedrine sulfate   0.25 g
    Sodium chloride   qs
    Purified water ad   30 mL
    Make isoton. sol.

    A. 1.22 g
    B. 784 mcg
    C. 212 mg
    D. 527 mcg
    E. 429 mg

23. A patient is to receive an infusion of 2 g of lidocaine in 500 mL D_5W at a rate of 2 mg/min. What is the flow rate in milliliters per hour?

    A. 2.0 mL/h
    B. 6.5 mL/h
    C. 15 mL/h
    D. 30 mL/h
    E. 150 mL/h

24. What is the pH of a buffer solution prepared with 0.05 M disodium phosphate and 0.05 M sodium acid phosphate (pK_a = 7.21)?

    A. 4.55
    B. 5.23
    C. 6.18
    D. 7.05
    E. 7.21

25. Convert 104°F to Centigrade.

    A. 22°C
    B. 34°C
    C. 40°C
    D. 46°C
    E. 54°C

26. Calculate the amount of water (in grams) in 100 mL of 65% (w/w) syrup that has a density of 1.313.

    A. 30 g
    B. 75 g
    C. 45.95 g
    D. 65.25 g
    E. 35 g

27. How much boric acid will be needed to prepare an isotonic solution of the following prescription?

Phenacaine HCl	1%	E value for phenacaine HCl is 0.20
Chlorobutanol	0.5%	E value for chlorobutanol is 0.24
Boric acid	qs	E value for boric acid is 0.52
Purified water ad	60mL	

    A. 0.55 g
    B. 0.67 g
    C. 0.75 g
    D. 1.2 g
    E. 2.2 g

28. How many milligrams of sodium chloride are required to make 30 mL of a solution of 1% dibucaine HCl isotonic with tears?

    Note: The freezing point depression of 1% dibucaine HCl solution is −0.08°C, and the freezing point depression of an isotonic solution is −0.52°C.

    A. 1.2 g
    B. 0.950 g
    C. 0.450 g
    D. 0.228 g
    E. 0.850 g

29. How many milliequivalents of Na^+ are contained in a 30 mL dose of the following solution?

Disodium hydrogen phosphate	18 g	$Na_2HPO_4\ 7H_2O$ (MW 268)

Sodium   48 g NaH_2PO_4 $4H_2O$
  biphosphate   (MW 138)
Purified   100 mL
  water ad

A. 144.63 mEq
B. 104.34 mEq
C. 40.29 mEq
D. 100 mEq
E. 52 mEq

30. How many grams per liter are needed to prepare 2N (normality) of H_2SO_4?

A. 25 g
B. 35 g
C. 78 g
D. 49 g
E. 98 g

31. How many milliequivalents of magnesium sulfate are represented in 1 gram of anhydrous magnesium sulfate ($MgSO_4$) (MW 120)?

A. 122 mEq
B. 16.67 mEq
C. 12 mEq
D. 10 mEq
E. 19 mEq

32. What is the concentration (g/mL) of a solution containing 4 milliequivalents of $CaCl_2$ $2H_2O$ per milliliter (MW 147)?

A. 0.345 g/mL
B. 0.986 g/mL
C. 0.389 g/mL
D. 0.294 g/mL
E. 0.545 g/mL

Questions 33–37 are related to the following problem:
An IV infusion for a patient weighing 132 lb calls for 7.5 mg of drug/kg of body weight to be added to 250 mL of 5% dextrose injection solution.

33. What is the patient's weight in kilograms?

A. 75 kg
B. 25 kg
C. 120 kg
D. 55 kg
E. 60 kg

34. How much drug is needed?

A. 250 mg
B. 350 mg
C. 150 mg
D. 450 mg
E. 900 mg

35. What is the total number of milliliters the patient receives per day if the IV solution runs at 52 mL/h?

A. 1,350 mL
B. 1,248 mL
C. 256 mL
D. 1,000 mL
E. 1,500 mL

36. What is the infusion rate in drops per minute (1 mL = 20 drops)?

A. 25 drops/min
B. 22 drops/min
C. 17 drops/min
D. 30 drops/min
E. 15 drops/min

37. How many IV bags does the patient receive per day?

A. 10 bags
B. 12 bags
C. 2 bags
D. 5 bags
E. 8 bags

38. If 50 mg of drug X is mixed with enough ointment base to obtain 20 grams of mixture, what is the concentration of drug X in ointment (expressed as a ratio)?

A. 1:300
B. 1:400
C. 1:200
D. 1:600
E. 1:100

39. When 23 mL of water for injection are added to drug-lyophilized powder, the resulting concentration is 200,000 units/mL. What is the volume of the dry powder if the amount of drug in the vial was 5,000,000 units?

A. 2 mL
B. 4 mL

C. 1 mL
D. 5 mL
E. 9 mL

40. If 20 grams of salicylic acid are mixed with enough hydrophilic petrolatum to obtain a concentration of 5%, how much ointment was used to prepare the prescription?

   A. 400 g
   B. 380 g
   C. 250 g
   D. 480 g
   E. 280 g

1-16. Answers

1. **C.**

$$x \text{ mg} : 340 \text{ mg} = 75 \text{ cap} : 100 \text{ cap}$$

$$x = 340 \text{ mg} \times 75 \text{ cap} / 100 \text{ cap} = 255 \text{ mg}$$

2. **B.** A specific gravity of 1.13 corresponds to a density of 1.13 g/mL.

   density = weight/volume; thus, weight

   $$= \text{density} \times \text{volume} = 1.13 \text{ g/mL}$$

   $$\times 500 \text{ mL} = 565 \text{ g}$$

3. **A.**

$$\% \text{ error} = \frac{(\text{error} \times 100\%)}{\text{quantity desired}}$$

$$= (325 - 312) \times \frac{100}{325} = 4\%$$

4. **C.**

$$\text{minimum weighable quantity} = \frac{SR \times 100\%}{5\%}$$

$$= 6 \text{ mg} \times \frac{100\%}{5\%}$$

$$= 120 \text{ mg}$$

5. **E.**

$$\text{daily dosage} = 50 \text{ mg} \Big/ \text{kg} \times \frac{175 \text{ lb}}{2.2 \text{ lb/kg}} = 3,977 \text{ mg}$$

$$\text{single IM injection} = (3,977/8) \text{ mg} \times \frac{1}{500 \text{ mg/mL}}$$

$$= 0.99 \text{ mL}$$

6. **B.**

$$\text{IBW} = 45.5 + (2.3 \times 8) = 64 \text{ kg}$$

7. **C.**

$$\text{weight} = \frac{154 \text{ lb}}{2.2 \text{ lb/kg}} = 70 \text{ kg}$$

$$\text{height} = 6 \text{ ft} \times 12 \text{ in/ft} \times 2.54 \text{ cm/in} = 183 \text{ cm}$$

$$\text{BSA} = \text{square root} \left[70 \times \frac{183}{3,600} \right]$$

$$= \text{square root} [3.56] = 1.89 \text{ m}^2$$

8. **D.**

$$\text{child dose} = \text{adult dose} \times \frac{\text{child BSA}}{1.73} = 125 \text{ mg}$$

$$\times \frac{0.68 \text{ m}^2}{1.73 \text{ m}^2} = 49 \text{ mg}$$

9. **A.**

$$\text{CrCl} = 0.85 \times (140 - 65) \times \frac{50}{(72 \times 1.3)}$$

$$= 34 \text{ mL/min}$$

10. **D.** Note that the formula is designed to produce a total of 1,000 g of the mixture. Then, by proportions:

$$x \text{ g ZnO} : 150 \text{ g ZnO} = 750 \text{ g mix} : 1,000 \text{ g}$$

$$x = 150 \text{ g} \times \frac{750 \text{ g}}{1,000 \text{ g}} = 113 \text{ g}$$

11. **B.** Note that the formula will produce a total of 20 parts of the mixture. Then, by proportions:

$$x \text{ g kaolin} : 500 \text{ g mix}$$
$$= 12 \text{ parts kaolin} : 20 \text{ parts mix}$$

$$x = 500 \text{ g} \times \frac{12 \text{ parts}}{20 \text{ parts}} = 300 \text{ g}$$

12. **E.** Note that this will be a solution of a solid in a liquid; thus, the concentration will be %(w/v).

$$10\% (\text{w/v}) = x \text{ g destrose} \times \frac{100}{500}$$

$$x = 10 \times \frac{500}{100} = 50 \text{ g}$$

13. **C.** By proportions,

    x g hexachlorophene : 20 g ung. = 1 part

    hexachlorophene : 400 parts ung.

    $$x = 20 \text{ g} \times \frac{1 \text{ part}}{400 \text{ parts}} = 0.05 \text{ g} = 50 \text{ mg}$$

14. **B.** A 1.0 molar solution will contain 95.3 g in 1,000 mL. A 5.0 molar solution will contain 95.3 g $\times$ 5 = 477 g in 1,000 mL. A 5.0 millimolar solution will contain 477 mg in 1,000 mL. Thus, 200 mL of a 5 millimolar solution will contain 477 mg/5 = 95.3 mg in 200 mL.

15. **A.** Because magnesium has a valence of 2, a formula weight of $MgCl_2$ will contain two equivalent weights of magnesium (and chloride, for that matter). Thus, 5 equivalents of magnesium are contained in $5 \times 95.3/2$ g = 238 g $MgCl_2$. Accordingly, 5 mEq of magnesium are contained in 238 mg $MgCl_2$.

16. **E.** Normal saline is 0.90%(w/v), or 0.90 g/100 mL = 9.0 g/1,000 mL.

    $$\text{milliosmolarity} = \left(\frac{9 \text{ g}}{58.5}\right) \times 2 \times 1,000$$
    $$= 308 \text{ mOsm/L}$$

17. **B.**

    $$C_1 = 20\%, Q_1 = 250 \text{ mL},$$
    $$C_2 = 15\%, Q_2 = x$$
    $$C_1 \times Q_1 = C_2 \times Q_2$$
    $$Q_2 = C_1 \times \frac{Q_1}{C_2} = 20\% \times \frac{250 \text{ mL}}{15\%}$$
    $$= 333 \text{ mL}$$

    added water = 333 mL − 250 mL = 83 mL

18. **C.**

20% (concentration of stock A)	15 − 5 = 10 = parts of A
15% (desired concentration)	
5% (concentration of stock B)	20 − 15 = 5 = parts of B

Relative volumes are 10:5, or 2:1. Thus, 200 mL of a 20% dextrose solution (A) will require 100 mL of a 5% dextrose solution (B) to produce 300 mL of a 15% dextrose solution.

19. **B.**

    $$20\% \times 200 \text{ mL} = 4,000 \text{ \%mL}$$
    $$5\% \times 100 \text{ mL} = 500 \text{ \%mL}$$
    $$300 \text{ mL} = 4,500 \text{ \%mL}$$
    $$\text{Mixture concentration} = \frac{4,500 \text{ \%mL}}{300 \text{ mL}} = 15\%$$

20. **D.** Each 100 molecules will provide

    80 Mg ions
    160 Cl ions
    20 undissociated molecules
    260 particles total

    Thus, the dissociation factor = 260/100 = 2.6

21. **A.**

    $$\text{sodium chloride equivalent} = \frac{(58.5)(1.0)}{(468)(1.8)} = 0.069$$

22. **C.** Because 900 mg of sodium chloride in 100 mL is isotonic,

    $$x : 900 \text{ mg} = 30 \text{ mL} : 100 \text{ mL}$$
    $$x = 900 \times \frac{30}{100} = 270 \text{ mg},$$

    which is the amount of sodium chloride alone needed to make 30 mL isotonic. But 1 g of ephedrine sulfate is equivalent to 0.23 g of sodium, thus:

    $$y = 0.25 \text{ g} \times 0.23 = 0.058 \text{ g}$$
    $$= 58 \text{ mg of sodium chloride}$$

    Accordingly, the amount of sodium chloride to add ($z = x - y$) is (270 mg − 58 mg) = 212 mg.

23. **D.** The bag contains 2,000 mg in 500 mL, or 4 mg/mL. Therefore, a rate of 2 mg/min corresponds to 0.5 mL/min, which corresponds to 30 mL/h.

24. **E.**

$$pH = pK_a + \log\left(\frac{salt}{acid}\right)$$

$$= 7.21 + \log\left(\frac{0.05}{0.05}\right) = 7.21$$

25. **C.**

$$9°C = 5°F - 160$$

$$9°C = 5 \times 104 - 160 = 520 - 160 = 360$$

$$C = \frac{360}{9} = 40°C$$

26. **C.** Note that 65 %w/w means 65 g in 100 g syrup. The total weight of the 100 mL syrup is 100 mL × 1.313 (density) = 131.3 g. Every 100 g of syrup contains 35 g of water, so

$$\frac{100 \text{ g}}{131.3 \text{ g}} = \frac{35 \text{ g}}{x}$$

$$x = \frac{(131.3 \times 35)}{100}$$

$$= 45.95 \text{ g} \left(\begin{array}{c}\text{amount of water}\\ \text{in the syrup}\end{array}\right)$$

27. **B.** The 1% phenacaine HCl equals 0.6 g, and the 0.5% chlorobutanol equals 0.3 g. Because we know the E value of phenacaine HCl, we can write the ratio:

$$\frac{0.6 \text{ g drug}}{1 \text{ g drug}} = \frac{x \text{ g NaCl}}{0.2 \text{ g NaCl}}$$

$$x = \frac{(0.2 \times 0.6)}{1} = 0.12 \text{ g NaCl (amount of sodium chloride that is equivalent to 0.6 g drug)}$$

Because we know the E value of chlorobutanol, we can write the ratio:

$$\frac{0.3 \text{ g}}{1 \text{ g}} = \frac{x \text{ g NaCl}}{0.24 \text{ g NaCl}}$$

$$x = \frac{(0.3 \times 0.24)}{1} = 0.072 \text{ g NaCl (amount of sodium chloride that is equivalent to 0.3 g chlorobutanol)}$$

The amount of sodium chloride needed to make 60 mL of solution isotonic is calculated as follows:

$$\frac{0.9 \text{ g NaCl}}{x \text{ g NaCl}} = \frac{100 \text{ mL}}{60 \text{ mL}}$$

$$x = \frac{(0.9 \times 60)}{100} = 0.54 \text{ g NaCl (amount of sodium chloride needed to make 60 mL of water isotonic if no drug or preservative were present)}$$

amount of sodium chloride needed
$$= 0.54 \text{ g} - (0.12 \text{ g} + 0.072 \text{ g})$$
$$= 0.348 \text{ g NaCl}$$

Because we know the E value for boric acid, we can write the ratio:

$$\frac{1 \text{ g}}{x \text{ g}} = \frac{0.52 \text{ g NaCl}}{0.348 \text{ g NaCl}}$$

$$x = \frac{(1 \text{ g} \times 0.348 \text{ g})}{0.52 \text{ g}} = 0.67 \text{ g (boric acid needed to make the prescription isotonic)}$$

28. **D.** The weight of 1% of drug equals 0.3 g. The needed change in freezing point depression to make the solution isotonic is 0.52°C − 0.08°C = 0.44°C, so the ratio is as follows:

$$\frac{0.9 \text{ g\%NaCl}}{x \text{\%NaCl}} = \frac{0.52°C}{0.44°C}$$

$$x = \frac{(0.9 \text{ g\%} \times 0.44)}{0.52} = 0.76 \text{ g\% (percentage of sodium chloride needed to make an isotonic solution based on freezing point depression)}$$

The amount of sodium chloride needed to make 30 mL of water isotonic is calculated as follows:

$$\frac{0.76}{x} = \frac{100 \text{ mL}}{30 \text{ mL}}$$

$$x = \frac{(0.76 \text{ g} \times 30 \text{ mL})}{100 \text{ mL}}$$

$$= 0.228 \text{ g (amount of sodium chloride needed)}$$

29. **A.**

    1 mEq of disodium hydrogen phosphate $= \dfrac{268 \text{ mg}}{2} = 134$ mg

    1 mEq of disodium biphosphate

    $= \dfrac{138 \text{ mg}}{1} = 138$ mg

    We can write the ratio as follows:

    $\dfrac{1 \text{ mEq}}{x \text{ mEq}} = \dfrac{134 \text{ mg}}{18{,}000 \text{ mg}}$

    $x = \dfrac{(18{,}000 \times 1)}{134} = 134.33$ mEq disodium hydrogen phosphate

    We can also write the ratio as follows:

    $\dfrac{1 \text{ mEq}}{x} = \dfrac{138 \text{ mg}}{48{,}000 \text{ mg}}$

    $x = \dfrac{(1 \times 48{,}000)}{138} = 347.83$ mEq sodium biphosphate

    To adjust for volumes, we can write the ratios as follows:

    $\dfrac{134.32 \text{ mEq}}{x_1 \text{ mEq}} = \dfrac{100 \text{ mL}}{30 \text{ mL}}$ and

    $\dfrac{347.82 \text{ mEq}}{x_2 \text{ mEq}} = \dfrac{100 \text{ mL}}{30 \text{ mL}}$

    Thus, $x_1 = 40.29$ mEq disodium hydrogen phosphate, and $x_2 = 104.34$ mEq sodium biphosphate. The total Na^+ mEq $= 104.34 + 40.29 = 144.63$ mEq.

30. **E.** Normality is the number of equivalents in one liter of solvent. The expression "2N normal" means two equivalents dissolved in one liter. Because one equivalent of sulfuric acid equals 49 g, 2N is equivalent to dissolving 98 g of sulfuric acid in 1 L of solvent.

31. **B.**

    1 mEq $= \dfrac{120}{2} = 60$ mg

    $\dfrac{1 \text{ mEq } Mg^{++}}{60 \text{ mg}} = \left(\dfrac{x}{1{,}000 \text{ mg}}\right) x = \dfrac{(1 \times 1{,}000)}{60}$

    $= 16.67$ mEq

32. **D.**

    1 mEq $= \dfrac{147}{2} = 73.5$ mg

    4 mEq $= 4 \times 73.5$ mg $= 294$ mg/mL

    $= 0.294$ g/mL

33. **E.**

    $\dfrac{132}{2.2} = 60$ kg

34. **D.**

    7.5 mg/kg $\times 60$ kg $= 450$ mg

35. **B.**

    52 ml/h $\times 1$ h $\times 24 = 1{,}248$ mL

36. **C.**

    $\dfrac{(52 \times 20)}{60} = \dfrac{x}{1 \text{ min}} = 17$ drops/min

37. **D.**

    $\dfrac{1{,}248 \text{ mL}}{250 \text{ mL/bag}} = 5$ bags

38. **B.**

    $\dfrac{0.05 \text{ g}}{20 \text{ g}} = \dfrac{1}{X}$, so $X = 400$

39. **A.**

    $\dfrac{200{,}000 \text{ units/mL}}{1 \text{ mL}} = \dfrac{5{,}000{,}000}{x}$,

    so $x = 25$ mL, and the volume of powder is $25 - 23 = 2$ mL

40. **B.**

    $\dfrac{5}{100} = \dfrac{20}{x}$, so $x = 400$ g,

    and the amount of ointment

    is $400 - 20 = 380$ g

1-17. References

Ansel HC, Stoklosa MJ. *Pharmaceutical Calculations.* 12th ed. Philadelphia: Lippincott Williams & Wilkins; 2006.

Khan MA, Reddy IK. *Pharmaceutical and Clinical Calculations.* 2nd ed. Lancaster, Pa.: Technomic Publishing Co; 2000.

O'Sullivan TA. *Understanding Pharmacy Calculations.* Washington, D.C.: American Pharmaceutical Association; 2002.

Federal Pharmacy Law

Walter L. Fitzgerald, Jr, BPharm, MS, JD

2

This study guide was developed for the purpose of assisting candidates for the National Association of Boards of Pharmacy (NABP) Multistate Pharmacy Jurisprudence Examination (MPJE). Because candidates will have been exposed, through the academic pharmacy degree program, to the federal and state laws subject to inquiry on the MPJE, this study guide is not intended to be a comprehensive collection or compilation of the text of those laws. Rather, it is a general overview of the relevant federal laws with which the candidate should be familiar.

2-1. Resources to Assist in Preparing for the MPJE

Information from NABP

The body of federal and state law, which the MPJE candidate must be knowledgeable about, is quite extensive. The candidate should begin the process of preparing for the MPJE by reviewing the MPJE competency statements provided in the *NABP Registration Bulletin* for the NAPLEX and MPJE exams. The bulletin is available on the NABP Web site at www.nabp.net. The MPJE statements are very valuable in focusing the candidate on the body of federal law to be reviewed and understood.

As to the body of state law, NABP offers two resources that may be beneficial to the MPJE candidate. More about each of these resources is available on the NABP Web site.

The first resource is the *Survey of Pharmacy Law*, published in CD-ROM format and available for purchase from NABP. The *Survey* is revised annually and provides summary information for individual states on various pharmacy law topics, including prescriptions (issuing, transmitting, and dispensing requirements); patient counseling; and pharmacy technicians. The *Survey* is composed of the following four sections.

- Organization
- Licensing law
- Drug law
- Census data

The second resource is NABPLAW Online. This resource is a searchable, electronic database of the pharmacy practice act and board of pharmacy rules for each of the 50 states. A free NABPLAW demo is available at the NABP Web site.

Candidates can purchase short-term access, varying from 1 day to 6 months. Time periods and prices can be viewed at the NABP Web site.

Information from Electronic Databases of Federal Law

Of great assistance to the MPJE candidate are online, electronic databases of federal law. The candidate is encouraged to use these databases as necessary during the review process. One of the greatest advantages (in addition to being no cost) of these electronic databases is the ability, through active links contained in the databases, to quickly retrieve and review cross-references to individual sections of the laws as well as to other relevant laws.

Because the "pharmacy law course" is taught at different times at colleges and schools of pharmacy, these electronic databases can be very beneficial. If the pharmacy law course was taught, for example, during the first year of the 4-year PharmD curriculum, the candidate may not have been exposed to all of the changes in federal pharmacy law that occurred over the following 3 years.

Because these databases are quite current, the candidate can achieve two objectives by reviewing the federal law databases:

- First, the candidate will be refreshed on laws studied previously in the pharmacy law course.
- Second, the candidate will be exposed to changes that have occurred since completing the pharmacy law course.

Accessing the Federal Food, Drug, and Cosmetic Act and the Federal Controlled Substances Act

Go to the U.S. Code Collection maintained by the Legal Information Institute of the Cornell University Law School. The Web site address for this collection is www4.law.cornell.edu/uscode.

When the Web page appears, scroll down and select Title 21. From the Web page that will next appear, you can access both the federal Food, Drug, and Cosmetic Act (FDCA) and the federal Controlled Substances Act (CSA).

Federal Food, Drug, and Cosmetic Act

On the Web page that appears, select Chapter 9, which is titled "Federal Food, Drug, and Cosmetic Act."

When the next Web page appears, you will see all nine subchapters that constitute the FDCA.

When you select a subchapter, you will then see on the next Web page the individual sections of the act contained in that subchapter or, in some cases, the individual parts contained in that subchapter.

Where the subchapter contains individual parts, selecting one part leads to a Web page with the individual sections contained in that part.

Federal Controlled Substances Act

The same Web page used to access the FDCA should be used to access the CSA, which is located at Chapter 13 instead of Chapter 9.

After selecting Chapter 13, use the same process as described for the FDCA.

Accessing the Regulations of the U.S. Food and Drug Administration and the U.S. Drug Enforcement Administration

Go to the electronic *Code of Federal Regulations* (CFR) maintained by the U.S. Government Printing Office. The Web site address for this collection is www.gpoaccess.gov.

When the Web page appears, in the middle column under Executive Resources select "Code of Federal Regulations."

When the next Web page appears, select "Browse and/or search the CFR," which will take you to the CFR Titles. Scroll down and select "Title 21" and then select the most current date available. This will take you to a Web page that lists the individual parts of Title 21. Parts 1–99 through 800–1299 contain the regulations of the U.S. Food and Drug Administration (FDA). Beginning at Parts 1300–1399, you will find the regulations of the U.S. Drug Enforcement Administration (DEA).

The FDA regulations

The scope of the FDA regulations is significantly large, constituting literally thousands of pages. Therefore, the sections of FDA regulations have not been included in this guide, and the MPJE candidate should go to the GPO's CFR Web site, as described previously, for review.

The FDA regulations governing drugs begin at Part 200, which is found on the Web site at Parts 200–299. Thus, the candidate should select Parts 200–299 in the column with the heading "Browse Parts."

When the next Web page appears, the individual parts will appear. When you select any of the parts, the individual sections in that part will appear on the next Web page. FDA's regulations governing drugs continue into the next set of parts, specifically, Parts 300–499.

The set of parts that follow (500–599) contains FDA's regulations governing animal drugs and should be reviewed. The next set of parts (600–799) concerns two items, biologicals and cosmetics, and also should be reviewed. The final set of parts (800–1299) contains FDA's regulations governing medical devices and should be reviewed.

In reviewing these parts, the candidate need not read each word of every FDA regulation. To do so would require an unreasonable and unnecessary time commitment. It is anticipated that the candidate can recognize whether he or she needs to review the text of the section or move on to the next one.

The MPJE candidate can begin by opening Part 200 of the FDA regulations, as directed previously, and open the first section of Part 200. Then the candidate should recognize from the section title whether it contains (a) information about which the candidate is knowledgeable and does not require review or (b) information that is not subject to inquiry on the MPJE. In the presence of either of these, the candidate should move forward to the next section.

The DEA regulations

As with the FDA regulations, the scope of the DEA regulations is quite extensive, but fortunately the DEA regulations are more manageable than the FDA regulations.

In addition, if the candidate has worked in pharmacy practice to any degree, the DEA regulations likely will be more familiar to him or her than the FDA regulations, because the FDA regulations are not as directly related to daily pharmacy practice as are the DEA regulations.

The MPJE candidate can review each section of the relevant DEA regulations using the process described for the FDA regulations, beginning by opening Part 1300 and then each section in each part.

Information from Electronic Databases of State Law

Candidates for the MPJE are anticipated to have at least two resources for their study of relevant state law. The first of these is the textbook or other compilation of state law that was used in the pharmacy law course taught in the academic degree program. This first resource will, of course, be of value only if the candidate is taking the MPJE and seeking licensure as a pharmacist in the same state where the candidate completed the academic degree program.

The second is what is commonly referred to as the "state board of pharmacy law book." In many states, on submission of an application for examination for licensure as a pharmacist, the applicant will be provided a copy of the state board's pharmacy law book. The candidate may also have received as a final-year pharmacy student the *Survey of Pharmacy Law* described in the section on resources available from NABP.

In addition to these resources, as with federal law, a number of electronic databases are available for ac-

cessing state law. Most directly related to preparing for the MPJE is NABPLAW, described in the section on resources available from NABP. In addition to NABPLAW are various databases that are accessible free of charge.

The candidate should first look to his or her state's Internet home page for resources on state law. Although it is not possible to describe here how to find the relevant state law on each state's home page, the candidate will likely be able to successfully navigate through the state's Web pages.

As an example, the candidate can search to see if the state's secretary of state has an individual home page and, if it does, look on that home page for a link to state agency rules and regulations, such as those of the state board of pharmacy.

Beyond the state home page are legal resource Web sites that the candidate can use for accessing state law, again at no cost. The following Web sites may be useful to the candidate seeking additional information on not only state law, but also federal and other law:

- Rominger Legal: www.romingerlegal.com
- FindLaw: www.findlaw.com
- Law.com: www.law.com
- AllLaw.com: www.alllaw.com
- Georgia State University Law School Meta-Index: http://gsulaw.gsu.edu/metaindex

Publications

At many colleges and schools of pharmacy, a textbook or other compilation of federal and state drug and pharmacy law may have been used in the pharmacy law course. Thus, the MPJE candidate may already have a resource that covers the laws subject to inquiry on the MPJE.

If not, other resources may be of assistance, including those from the reference list that follows. The first two references provide a practical, easy-to-understand explanation of the federal law subject to inquiry on the MPJE. The third reference provides a variety of state-specific (not all states are available) study guides in comprehensive and condensed versions. Resources from this reference will be particularly valuable to a candidate who earned the PharmD degree in a state different from the state in which he or she seeks licensure.

All of these references contain sample questions that will help the MPJE candidate gain experience in answering questions related to federal law and obtain a measure of knowledge prior to the MPJE.

References

Reiss BS, Hall GD. *Guide to Federal Pharmacy Law.* 6th ed. Boynton Beach, FL: Apothecary Press; 2009. Contact information: (888) 609-2665 or www.apothecarypress.com.

Strauss, S. *Strauss' Federal Drug Laws and Examination Review.* 5th ed. Boca Raton, FL: CRC Press; 2000. Contact information: (800) 272-7737 or www.crcpress.com.

State and federal pharmacy law study guides. Contact information: http://rxlaw.org.

Information from Federal Agencies

The value of information available online from federal agencies should not be overlooked in preparing for the MPJE. Primary among these agencies are the FDA, the DEA, and the Consumer Product Safety Commission (CPSC).

The FDA Web site (www.fda.gov) contains many guides on pharmacy compounding, risk evaluation and mitigation strategies, and many other topics. The MPJE candidate should look specifically at the FDA Center for Drug Evaluation and Research Web site at www.fda.gov/cder.

The DEA Web site (www.dea.gov) offers a variety of materials, but the DEA Office of Diversion Control Web site (www.deadiversion.usdoj.gov) provides more information of relevance to the MPJE candidate. Included on the Diversion Control Web site is extensive information about registration requirements and selling of scheduled listed chemical products such as pseudoephedrine.

Requirements for pharmacy with respect to child-resistant packaging may be found on the CPSC Web site at www.cpsc.gov. The MPJE candidate should particularly review the CPSC publication "Poison Prevention Packaging: A Guide for Healthcare Professionals," available at www.cpsc.gov/CPSCPUB/PUBS/384.pdf.

2-2. The Comprehensive Drug Abuse Prevention and Control Act of 1970 and Regulations of the U.S. DEA

The Comprehensive Drug Abuse Prevention and Control Act, enacted by Congress in 1970, has as its primary purpose preventing illicit manufacture, distribution, and use of controlled substances. This purpose is achieved through numerous requirements in the act and DEA regulations.

Introduction

The Comprehensive Drug Abuse Prevention and Control Act, more commonly known as the Controlled Substances Act, establishes a "closed system" for distribution of drugs that are "controlled substances." The term *closed system* means controlled substances can be distributed only by and between persons registered with the DEA.

The DEA, a unit within the U.S. Department of Justice, was established in July 1973 by an executive reorganization plan; it replaced the former Bureau of Narcotics and Dangerous Drugs.

The FDA has also promulgated regulations that affect the distribution of controlled substances. One example is treatment programs for narcotic addicts. The FDA regulations contain medical guidelines for such programs, and the DEA regulations contain requirements for dispensing and recordkeeping activities for such programs.

Note that in 1988, Congress amended existing federal laws, including the CSA, with enactment of the Chemical Diversion and Trafficking Act. This act establishes recordkeeping and reporting requirements for persons who manufacture, distribute, import, or export a listed precursor or essential chemical, as well as tableting and encapsulating machines.

When the MPJE candidate studies the CSA and DEA regulations, the text added as a result of this 1988 act is generally easily recognized. For example, the DEA regulation at 21 CFR 1300.02 is titled "Definitions relating to listed chemicals."

The MPJE candidate needs to be attentive to how the CSA and DEA regulations govern commercially available controlled substances versus chemicals.

Another very important amendment to the CSA occurred in 2005 with enactment of the Combat Methamphetamine Epidemic Act (CMEA). The CMEA introduced a new category of substances (scheduled listed chemical products) and new sale and recordkeeping requirements for those products. Products in this category include ephedrine, pseudoephedrine, and phenylpropanolamine. DEA has promulgated several regulations (see Part 1314 of the DEA regulations) to implement the CMEA.

Also in 2005, the CSA was amended to allow private practice physicians (subject to being certified) to prescribe schedule III, IV, and V narcotic controlled substances for detoxification and maintenance treatment of opioid dependency. Currently two products,

Suboxone and Subutex, may be prescribed for such treatment. For the MPJE candidate unfamiliar with the requirements for prescribing these controlled substances, information is available on the Web site of the Substance Abuse and Mental Health Services Administration at www.samhsa.gov.

Specific information about medication-assisted treatment may be found at www.dpt.samhsa.gov.

Several other developments have occurred in recent years, including DEA's promulgation of regulations to allow practitioners to issue multiple prescriptions for schedule II controlled substances and to allow electronic ordering (but not prescribing) of controlled substances. The MPJE candidate should be familiar with these and other recent developments in the federal laws governing controlled substances.

The CSA and DEA regulations are quite complex and technical, and they affect pharmacy practice significantly; thus, they demand thorough study by the MPJE candidate.

Key Provisions of the CSA

Access the CSA at the Web link (www4.law.cornell. edu/uscode) and follow the process listed earlier. There are two subchapters:

- I. Control and Enforcement
- II. Import and Export

The MPJE candidate should be familiar with both subchapters, particularly the following provisions from Subchapter I of the CSA. In addition, the MPJE candidate should review the sections in Subchapter II on import and export.

Subchapter I. Control and enforcement

Part A—Introductory provisions
§ 801. Congressional findings and declarations: controlled substances
This section sets forth the reasons Congress enacted the CSA. The MPJE candidate should be generally familiar with these findings and declarations.

§ 801a. Congressional findings and declarations: psychotropic substances
This section recognizes the international treaty—the Convention on Psychotropic Substances—that the United States entered into in 1971 and sets forth the reasons Congress implemented the convention. The MPJE candidate should be generally familiar with these findings and declarations.

§ 802. Definitions
The MPJE candidate should be familiar with all terms defined in this section of the CSA, which will aid in understanding the language of the sections that follow. Note the limitation in dispensing that results from the relationship between the definition of *dispense* and the definition of *ultimate user*. Note also that some of the definitions contain important substantive content, such as the definition of a *regulated transaction* and its placing of "thresholds" on the retail sale of ephedrine, pseudoephedrine, and phenylpropanolamine. Finally, note the definition of *anabolic steroid* as amended in 2004.

Part B—Authority to control; standards and schedules
§ 811. Authority and criteria for classification of substances
This section gives the U.S. attorney general the authority to add a drug to a schedule, transfer a drug between schedules, and remove a drug from a schedule. This section also contains the factors to consider when determining whether a drug should be placed in or removed from a schedule. This section also allows exclusion of a nonnarcotic substance from a schedule if the substance may be lawfully sold, under the FDCA, without a prescription. Finally, this section provides that dextromethorphan shall not be included in any schedule by reason of enactment of the CSA unless controlled after October 27, 1970, on the basis of the factors in this section.

§ 812. Schedules of controlled substances
This section establishes the five schedules (I–V) of controlled substances and the findings required for each schedule. The MPJE candidate should be familiar with these findings, such as that a schedule I controlled substance "has no currently accepted medical use in treatment."

§ 813. Treatment of controlled substance analogues
This section provides that a controlled substance analogue, to the extent intended for human use, shall be treated as a controlled substance in schedule I.

§ 814. Removal of exemption of certain drugs
This section, among other things, allows the U.S. attorney general to remove from exemption—see definition (39)(A)(iv) at section 802 concerning ephedrine, pseudoephedrine, and phenylpropanolamine—a drug or group of drugs that is being diverted to obtain a listed chemical for use in illicit production of controlled substances.

Part C—Registration of manufacturers, distributors, and dispensers of controlled substances
§ 821. Rules and regulations
This section authorizes the U.S. attorney general to promulgate rules and regulations and to charge

reasonable fees relating to the registration and control of regulated persons and transactions.

§ 822. Persons required to register

This section sets forth the registration requirements for persons who handle controlled substances. The MPJE candidate should understand who is and who is not required to obtain a registration, that a separate registration is required for separate locations, and that an inspection may be conducted prior to granting a registration.

§ 823. Registration requirements

This section provides specific detail regarding registration of practitioners, including pharmacies but not pharmacists, and the factors to be considered in determining whether to grant a registration.

§ 824. Denial, revocation, or suspension of registration

This section lists the grounds for denying, suspending, or revoking a registration. Note that a suspension or revocation may be limited to a particular schedule or schedules and that the registration can be revoked simultaneously with initiation of proceedings (issuing an "order to show cause") if there is an imminent danger to public health or safety.

§ 825. Labeling and packaging

This section establishes the labeling requirements for commercial containers of controlled substances.

§ 826. Production quotas for controlled substances

This section authorizes the U.S. attorney general to determine and establish production quotas for schedule I and II controlled substances to be manufactured each calendar year to provide for the estimated medical, scientific, research, and industrial needs of the United States, for lawful export requirements, and for the establishment and maintenance of reserve stocks.

§ 827. Records and reports of registrants

This section establishes requirements for the biennial inventory (in relation to May 1, 1971) and for the addition of any newly scheduled drug to the existing inventory. This section requires every registrant to maintain a complete and accurate record of each controlled substance received, sold, delivered, or otherwise disposed of, but it does not require a perpetual inventory. The MPJE candidate should recognize the exceptions to the inventory requirement. Note also the recently added reporting requirements for gamma hydroxybutyric acid.

§ 828. Order forms

This section establishes the requirement that distribution of schedule I and II controlled substances occur only pursuant to a form issued by the U.S. attorney general (the DEA 222 Form). It also lists recordkeeping requirements for the form. As a related item, the MPJE candidate should be sure to review the new DEA regulations on "electronic orders" for controlled substances in Parts 1305 and 1311 of the DEA regulations.

§ 829. Prescriptions

This section sets forth the prescription requirements for each schedule of controlled substances and notes that schedule V controlled substances, when not dispensed pursuant to a prescription, may be sold only for a medical purpose.

§ 830. Regulation of listed chemicals and certain machines

This section establishes the recordkeeping and reporting requirements for those engaged in activities related to listed chemicals and tableting and encapsulating machines.

Part D—Offenses and penalties

§ 841. Prohibited acts A

This section and the next two sections list unlawful acts and the penalties associated with these acts. It is important for the MPJE candidate to recognize that some of the listed unlawful acts apply to all persons, whereas others apply only to registrants. The MPJE candidate should recognize what acts are unlawful and generally be familiar with the associated penalties.

§ 842. Prohibited acts B

See note to section 841.

§ 843. Prohibited acts C

See note to section 841.

§ 844. Penalties for simple possession

This section makes possession by any person (including a registrant) of a controlled substance or listed chemical unlawful unless allowed under the CSA. It also establishes penalties for unlawful possession and defines what is meant by a "drug, narcotic, or chemical offense."

§ 844a. Civil penalty for possession of small amounts of certain controlled substances

This section provides penalties for any person (including a registrant) for unlawful possession of "personal use amounts" as specified by the U.S. attorney general by regulation.

§ 846. Attempt and conspiracy

This section provides that persons who "attempt" or "conspire" to commit a controlled substance offense are subject to the same penalties as prescribed for the offense.

§ 847. Additional penalties

This section provides that any criminal penalties imposed for violation of the CSA do not preclude other civil and administrative penalties, such as monetary fines under the federal Civil Monetary Penalties Law or suspension or revocation of a DEA Certificate of Registration.

§ 848. Continuing criminal enterprise

This section defines a *continuing criminal enterprise* and imposes very severe penalties—including life imprisonment and the death penalty—for those convicted of engaging in such an enterprise. The MPJE candidate should recognize that the text of this section includes other offenses that are not considered a continuing criminal enterprise. For example, this section provides the penalty for any person who during the commission of, in furtherance of, or while attempting to avoid apprehension, prosecution, or service of a prison sentence for a felony violation of the CSA intentionally kills, or counsels, commands, induces, procures, or causes the intentional killing of, any federal, state, or local law enforcement officer engaged in, or on account of, the performance of such officer's official duties. If such killing results, that person may be sentenced to any term of imprisonment, which shall not be less than 20 years and may be up to life imprisonment, or he or she may be sentenced to death.

§ 849. Transportation safety offenses

This section doubles the penalty for the first conviction and triples the penalty for subsequent convictions of certain controlled substance offenses in a *rest area* or *truck stop*, as these terms are defined in this section.

§ 850. Information for sentencing

This section, unless provided otherwise in another federal law, establishes that no limitation be placed on the information concerning the background, character, and conduct of a person convicted of a controlled substance offense that may be received and considered for purposes of imposing an appropriate sentence.

§ 851. Proceedings to establish prior convictions

This section sets forth the process for establishing that a person has prior convictions of a controlled substance offense or offenses.

§ 852. Application of treaties and other international agreements

This section provides that no treaties and other international agreements entered into by the United States shall limit the provision of treatment, education, or rehabilitation as alternatives to conviction or criminal penalty for offenses involving any drug or other substance subject to a treaty or agreement.

§ 853. Criminal forfeitures

This section provides that persons convicted of controlled substance offenses shall forfeit to the United States all real and personal property constituting or derived from any proceeds the person obtained, directly or indirectly, as the result of the offense and any of the person's property used, or intended to be used, in any manner or part, to commit or to facilitate the commission of the offense.

§ 854. Investment of illicit drug profits

This section makes it unlawful for a person to use or invest in certain *enterprises*, as defined in this section, any income derived, directly or indirectly, from a violation of the CSA that is punishable by imprisonment for more than 1 year, provided that the person participated as a principal in the violation. It also provides penalties for making such investments.

§ 855. Alternative fine

This section provides that, in lieu of a fine otherwise authorized by Part D, a defendant who derives profits or other proceeds from an offense may be fined not more than twice the gross profits or other proceeds.

§ 856. Maintaining drug-involved premises

This section makes unlawful knowingly opening or maintaining any place for the purpose of manufacturing, distributing, or using any controlled substance, as well as managing or controlling any building, room, or enclosure, whether as an owner, lessee, agent, employee, or mortgagee, and knowingly and intentionally renting, leasing, or making available for use, with or without compensation, the building, room, or enclosure for the purpose of unlawfully manufacturing, storing, distributing, or using a controlled substance. It also establishes penalties for a violation.

§ 858. Endangering human life while illegally manufacturing controlled substance

This section provides that whoever, while unlawfully manufacturing a controlled substance or attempting to do so, or while transporting or causing to be transported materials, including chemicals, to do so, creates a substantial risk of harm to human life shall be subject to a fine and imprisonment.

§ 859. Distribution to persons under age 21

This section provides enhanced penalties for first and second offenses of a person who is at least 18 years of age unlawfully distributing a controlled substance to a person under 21 years of age.

§ 860. Distribution or manufacturing in or near schools and colleges

This section provides enhanced penalties for first and second offenses of any person who is unlawfully distributing, possessing with intent to distribute, or manufacturing a controlled substance in or on, or within 1,000 feet of, the real property comprising a public or private elementary, vocational, or secondary school; a public or private college, junior college, or university; a playground; or a housing facility owned by a public housing authority. The enhanced penalties also apply if the offense takes place within 100 feet of a public or private youth center, public swimming pool, or video arcade facility. This section also makes it an offense for any person at least 21 years of age to knowingly and intentionally employ, hire, use, persuade, induce, entice, or coerce a person under 18 years of age to violate this section or to knowingly and intentionally employ, hire, use, persuade, induce, entice, or coerce a person under 18 years of age to assist in avoiding detection or apprehension for any offense under this section by any federal, state, or local law enforcement official.

§ 860a. Consecutive sentence for manufacturing or distributing, or possessing with intent to manufacture or distribute, methamphetamine on premises where children are present or reside

This section provides additional penalties for anyone manufacturing or distributing methamphetamine or its salts, isomers, or salts of isomers on premises in which an individual under 18 is present or resides.

§ 861. Employment or use of persons under 18 years of age in drug operations

This section makes it unlawful for any person at least 18 years of age to knowingly and intentionally (a) employ, hire, use, persuade, induce, entice, or coerce a person under 18 years of age to violate any provision of the CSA; (b) employ, hire, use, persuade, induce, entice, or coerce a person under 18 years of age to assist in avoiding detection or apprehension for any offense of the CSA by any federal, state, or local law enforcement official; or (c) receive a controlled substance from a person under 18 years of age, other than an immediate family member, in violation of the CSA. This section also establishes penalties for first and subsequent violations of this section. In addition, this section makes it unlawful to knowingly provide or distribute a controlled substance or a con-

trolled substance analogue to a person under 18 years of age or to a pregnant person.

§ 862. Denial of federal benefits to drug traffickers and possessors

This section provides for denial of federal benefits to drug traffickers and possessors, with differences in denial based on whether the person is a drug trafficker or drug possessor.

§ 862a. Denial of assistance and benefits for certain drug-related convictions

This section provides for denial of federal benefits and assistance to an individual convicted under federal or state law of any offense that is classified as a felony by the law of the jurisdiction involved and that has as an element of the offense the possession, use, or distribution of a controlled substance.

§ 862b. Sanctioning for testing positive for controlled substances

This section provides that the federal government shall not prohibit states from testing welfare recipients for use of controlled substances or from sanctioning welfare recipients who test positive for use of controlled substances.

§ 863. Drug paraphernalia

This section makes unlawful a number of activities with respect to drug paraphernalia, establishes penalties for violations, and defines *drug paraphernalia*.

§ 864. Anhydrous ammonia

This section makes unlawful the stealing of anhydrous ammonia or transporting stolen anhydrous ammonia across state lines, knowing, intending, or having reasonable cause to believe that such anhydrous ammonia will be used to manufacture a controlled substance in violation of this part.

§ 865. Smuggling methamphetamine or methamphetamine precursor chemicals into the United States while using facilitated entry programs

This section provides an enhanced prison sentence for a person convicted of an offense involving methamphetamine when the person convicted was enrolled in, or acting on behalf of a person enrolled in, any dedicated commuter lane, alternative or accelerated inspection system, or other facilitated entry program into the United States, or when the person committed the offense while entering the United States using such a lane, system, or program.

Parts E and F

The last two parts (Part E and Part F) of Subchapter I contain a variety of sections, many of which are not of interest to the MPJE candidate. As directed in the introduction to this study guide, the candidate should open each part and from the titles of the sections in each part determine those that he or she should review.

Subchapter II. Import and export

This subchapter of the CSA contains several sections governing the importation and exportation of controlled substances, including requirements for registration of importers and exporters. The MPJE candidate should review these sections and be generally knowledgeable about the content.

Regulations of the DEA

The DEA regulations may be found in Title 21 of the CFR. The body of DEA regulations is divided into 17 parts.

The MPJE candidate should review relevant DEA regulations on the electronic database as described in the introduction to this study guide. Following is a very basic summary of the content of each part.

Part 1300—Definitions

The DEA regulations begin at Part 1300 of Title 21 of the CFR. Part 1300 has two sections, both of which contain definitions of terms related to controlled substances and to listed chemicals. Because there are many definitions, they are not included here, but as noted previously for definitions contained in the CSA, the MPJE candidate should retrieve and review all of the definitions contained in the two sections of Part 1300. Some of these definitions are quite extensive and contain very important information for the MPJE candidate. For example, restrictions related to the sale of scheduled listed chemical products are found in the definition of *regulated transaction* at 21 CFR 1300.02.

Part 1301—Registration of manufacturers, distributors, and dispensers of controlled substances

Part 1301 governs the many aspects of registration with the DEA. This part includes the sections related to who is required to register, how one applies for registration, what exemptions exist to registration, and what allowances are made for importation for personal use. Also included are specific details about the DEA Certificate of Registration and the number assignment, procedure for suspension or revocation of a registration, and modification or termination of a reg-

istration. A very useful chart listing registration categories, fees, periods, and application form numbers is available at www.deadiversion.usdoj.gov/drugreg/categories.htm. The MPJE candidate should be familiar with each of these aspects of registration.

Very importantly, requirements for security, including the prohibition of employing certain individuals, are included in this part. The MPJE candidate should study this part in detail, paying particular attention to sections 1301.27 and 1301.28, both added in 2005. Although not included specifically in the DEA regulations, the method for determining the legitimacy of a DEA registration number is important for the MPJE candidate and thus is described immediately below.

Before October 1, 1985, DEA Certificate of Registration numbers for practitioners began with the letter "A." Since that date, the DEA Certificate of Registration numbers for practitioners begin with the letter "B." Further, a DEA Certificate of Registration number issued to a midlevel practitioner begins with the letter "M." Following the first letter is a second letter, which is the first letter of the registrant's last name. Following the two letters is a seven-digit computer-generated sequential number. The number is constructed so that it can be tested for verification by using the following formula:

- **Step 1:** Determine the sum of the first, third, and fifth digits.
- **Step 2:** Determine the sum of the second, fourth, and sixth digits, and then multiply the sum by two.
- **Step 3:** Determine the sum of the two numbers determined in steps 1 and 2.
- **Step 4:** The last digit of this third sum should be the same as the last digit of the seven-digit DEA Certificate of Registration number.

Part 1302—Labeling and packaging requirements for controlled substances

Part 1302 contains the requirements for labeling of the "commercial container" of a controlled substance. The MPJE candidate should be generally familiar with these requirements.

Part 1303—Quotas

Part 1303 contains the sections related to the establishment of production and procurement quotas for schedule I and II controlled substances for the estimated medical, scientific, research, and industrial needs. The MPJE candidate should be generally familiar with the sections in this part.

Part 1304—Records and reports of registrants

Part 1304 contains the many requirements associated with recordkeeping in relation to the various aspects of handling controlled substances by practitioners, including narcotic treatment programs. Also included in this part are the requirements associated with inventories of controlled substances, including the "biennial inventory." The MPJE candidate should be very familiar with the sections in this part.

Part 1305—Orders for schedule I and II controlled substances

Part 1305 includes the sections describing the DEA Form 222 for ordering schedule II controlled substances. Also included in this part are the details associated with the granting of a power of attorney to authorize individuals to execute order forms and electronic orders. The MPJE candidate should be very familiar with the sections in this part and should be sure to review the regulations added in 2005 regarding electronic orders for controlled substances.

Part 1306—Prescriptions

Part 1306 contains the sections concerning the many details of issuing, dispensing, and labeling of prescriptions for controlled substances. Also included in this part in relation to prescriptions are the requirements for electronic recordkeeping of prescription refills and for transfer of prescriptions between pharmacies. Finally, this part includes the requirements for the sale of controlled substances that are not "prescription drugs." The MPJE candidate should be very familiar with the sections in this part and should be sure to review the new regulations added in 2005 regarding prescribing of some controlled substances for narcotic treatment, as well as the requirements added more recently at sections 1306.12(b) and 1306.14(e) regarding issuing of multiple prescriptions for a schedule II controlled substance.

Part 1307—Miscellaneous

Part 1307 contains a few sections of interest to the MPJE candidate. Of particular note are the sections on "distribution" by dispensers and disposal of controlled substances.

Part 1308—Schedules of controlled substances

Part 1308 describes the "Administration Controlled Substances Number" and its uses and lists controlled substances in their respective schedules. Part 1308 also provides for "exempt" and "excluded" substances, control of immediate precursors, and emergency scheduling. The MPJE candidate should be generally familiar with controlled substances and the schedule into which they have been placed, as well as those products that are exempt and excluded, as described in Part 1308.

Part 1309—Registration of manufacturers, distributors, importers, and exporters of List I chemicals

Part 1309 includes several provisions related to those engaged in activities with List I chemicals. Although Part 1309 does not generally affect the practice of pharmacy, the MPJE candidate should review these sections for familiarity.

Part 1310—Records and reports of listed chemicals and certain machines

Although some sections of Part 1310 also do not generally affect the practice of pharmacy, some sections in Part 1310 relate to ephedrine, and thus this part deserves review by the MPJE candidate.

Part 1311—Digital certificates

Part 1311 was added in 2005. It governs digital certificates in association with electronic orders for controlled substances, and the MPJE candidate should study it in detail.

Part 1312—Importation and exportation of controlled substances

Part 1312 includes several provisions related to those engaged in importing and exporting controlled substances. Although this part does not generally affect the practice of pharmacy, the MPJE candidate should review these sections for familiarity.

Part 1313—Importation and exportation of list I and list II chemicals

Part 1313 includes several provisions related to those engaged in importing and exporting precursors and essential chemicals. Although this part does not generally affect the practice of pharmacy, the MPJE candidate should review these sections for familiarity.

Part 1314—Retail sale of scheduled listed chemical products

Part 1314 is of importance to pharmacy because it sets forth the many requirements associated with retail sales of scheduled listed chemical products. The MPJE candidate should be very familiar with the details of selling these products at retail, including restrictions on quantity, recordkeeping requirements, staff training requirements, and the annual self-certification process.

Part 1315—Importation and production quotas for ephedrine, pseudoephedrine, and phenylpropanolamine

Part 1315 includes more provisions on scheduled listed chemical products, including a personal use exemption. Although this part does not generally affect the practice of pharmacy, the MPJE candidate should review these sections for familiarity.

Part 1316—Administrative functions, practices, and procedures

Part 1316 contains several sections that address inspections, probable cause, and other issues related to warrants, matters related to research, procedures for hearings, burden of proof, and miscellaneous other matters. The MPJE candidate should be generally familiar with these matters.

2-3. The Food, Drug, and Cosmetic Act of 1938 and Regulations of the U.S. FDA

The Food, Drug, and Cosmetic Act, enacted by Congress in 1938, has as its primary purpose preventing interstate distribution of foods, drugs, cosmetics, and devices that are adulterated or misbranded. This purpose is achieved through numerous requirements in the act and FDA regulations.

Introduction

The MPJE candidate should be familiar with the historical development of the FDCA, and its predecessor, the Pure Food and Drug Act of 1906. The candidate should also be familiar with amendments to the FDCA since 1938, including the following:

- Durham–Humphrey Amendment of 1951
- Kefauver–Harris Amendment of 1962
- Medical Device Amendment of 1976
- Orphan Drug Act of 1983
- Drug Price Competition and Patent Term Restoration Act of 1984

- Prescription Drug Marketing Act of 1987
- Safe Medical Devices Act of 1990
- Dietary Supplement Health and Education Act of 1994
- Food and Drug Administration Modernization Act of 1997
- Best Pharmaceuticals for Children Act of 2002
- Medical Device User Fee and Modernization Act of 2002
- Pediatric Research Equity Act of 2003
- Minor Use and Minor Species Animal Health Act of 2004
- Food Allergen Labeling and Consumer Protection Act of 2004
- Dietary Supplement and Nonprescription Drug Consumer Protection Act of 2006
- Food and Drug Administration Amendments Act of 2007

Key Provisions of the FDCA

The FDCA is located at Chapter 9 of Title 21 of the United States Code. Chapter 9 has the following nine subchapters:

I. Short Title
II. Definitions
III. Prohibited Acts and Penalties
IV. Food
V. Drugs and Devices
VI. Cosmetics
VII. General Authority
VIII. Imports and Exports
IX. Miscellaneous

The MPJE candidate should be particularly familiar with Subchapters II, III, V (which is divided into Subparts A through E), and VI and with the following sections within the subchapters of the FDCA.

Subchapter II. Definitions

§ 321. Definitions; generally
The MPJE candidate should be familiar with all terms defined in this section of the FDCA, which will aid in understanding the language of the sections that follow. The candidate also should be able to distinguish between terms such as *drug, counterfeit drug, new drug, device, dietary supplement, food,* and *cosmetic.*

Subchapter III. Prohibited acts and penalties

§ 331. Prohibited acts
The MPJE candidate should be familiar with conduct that is prohibited by the FDCA, as set forth in this section.

§ 332. Injunction proceedings
This section provides that the U.S. district courts and all courts exercising jurisdiction in U.S. territories have jurisdiction to enjoin violations of section 331, with some exceptions as set forth in this section. Furthermore, an alleged violation of an injunction or restraining order shall, upon demand of the accused, be tried before a jury.

§ 333. Penalties
The penalties for violation of the FDCA range from not very severe to very severe. The MPJE candidate should be familiar with the penalties, and particularly those related to the prescription drug marketing violations (i.e., drug samples) and distribution of human growth hormone. Notice the use of the term *knowingly,* as defined in section 321.

§ 334. Seizure
This section describes the process related to seizure and disposition of adulterated and misbranded foods, drugs, and cosmetics, a process with which the MPJE candidate should be familiar.

§ 335. Hearing before report of criminal violation
This section provides that before any violation of this chapter is reported to a U.S. attorney for criminal proceedings, the person against whom the proceeding is contemplated shall be given appropriate notice and an opportunity to present his or her views, either orally or in writing.

§ 335a. Debarment, temporary denial of approval, and suspension
This section describes the "debarment" from submitting or assisting in the submission of applications for drug approvals of businesses and individuals based on prior misconduct related to the drug approval process. The MPJE candidate should be able to distinguish the various characteristics of mandatory and permissive debarments.

§ 335b. Civil penalties
This section continues the matter of misconduct in the drug approval process. The MPJE candidate should be familiar with the conduct prohibited and the associated penalties, together with the provision concerning informants.

§ 335c. Authority to withdraw approval of abbreviated drug applications
This section authorizes the withdrawal of approval of abbreviated drug applications if the approval was obtained, expedited, or otherwise facilitated through bribery, payment of an illegal gratuity, or fraud or material false statement. Withdrawal is also authorized if

the manufacturer has repeatedly demonstrated a lack of ability to produce the drug for which the application was submitted in accordance with the formulations and manufacturing processes set forth in the application and has introduced, or attempted to introduce, such adulterated or misbranded drug into commerce. This section also provides procedures for withdrawals.

§ 336. Report of minor violations
This section provides that the secretary of Health and Human Services (HHS) is not required to report for prosecution, or for the institution of libel or injunction proceedings, minor violations of this chapter whenever he or she believes that the public interest will be adequately served by a suitable written notice or warning.

§ 337. Proceedings in the name of United States; provision as to subpoenas
This section requires that legal proceedings for enforcement or restraint of violations be in the name of the United States. However, this section also allows states to bring actions under the act, but only upon notice being given to the HHS secretary as set forth in this section.

Subchapter IV. Food

Although this subchapter is titled "Food," the MPJE candidate should review select sections because they contain requirements related to dietary supplements. The MPJE candidate should review the portions addressing dietary supplements in the following sections: 341, 342, 343, 343-1, 343-2, and 350-b. In addition, the MPJE candidate should review section 350 on vitamins and minerals.

Subchapter V. Drugs and devices

Part A—Drugs and devices
§ 351. Adulterated drugs and devices
A drug or device can be "adulterated" for several reasons, as listed in this section. The MPJE candidate should be familiar with these reasons.

§ 352. Misbranded drugs and devices
A drug or device can be "misbranded" for several reasons, as listed in this section. The MPJE candidate should be familiar with these reasons.

§ 353. Exemptions and consideration for certain drugs, devices, and biological products
A key section of the FDCA, this section, among other things, exempts legend drugs from the general labeling requirements of the FDCA, including when sold when

a prescription is presented. (Note the label requirement of the "Rx Only symbol," which replaces the labeling requirement of "Caution: Federal law prohibits dispensing without a prescription," a change created by the Food and Drug Administration Modernization Act of 1997.) Also included in this section are the sales restrictions imposed by the Prescription Drug Marketing Act of 1987 with respect to legend drug samples and coupons for legend drugs, together with the wholesaler licensing requirements. Finally, this section addresses drugs for veterinary use.

§ 353a. Pharmacy compounding

This section was added to the FDCA by the Food and Drug Administration Modernization Act of 1997. However, in an April 29, 2002, opinion, the U.S. Supreme Court ruled the section unconstitutional in the case of *Thompson et al. v. Western States Medical Center et al.*, 535 U.S. 357. Other sections of the FDCA address pharmacy compounding, however. The MPJE candidate should be very familiar with the federal law on pharmacy compounding. A good source for the U.S. Supreme Court opinion and other materials, particularly the FDA Compliance Policy Guidance on pharmacy compounding, is the FDA's Center for Drug Evaluation and Research at www.fda.gov/Drugs/GuidanceComplianceRegulatory Information/PharmacyCompounding/default.htm. The MPJE candidate should be certain to review the FDA compliance guide on pharmacy compounding, available at www.fda.gov/downloads/AboutFDA/CentersOffices/CDER/UCM118050.pdf.

§ 354. Veterinary feed directive drugs

This section defines what is meant by a veterinary feed directive drug and sets forth requirements in relation to use and labeling of such drugs.

§ 355. New drugs

This quite lengthy section sets forth the requirements and process for approval of a "new drug" through filing of a new drug application or abbreviated new drug application. The MPJE candidate should be familiar with the process for approval of drugs and note particularly in this section the definition and use of the terms *bioavailability* and *bioequivalent*. The references listed in the introduction to this study guide provide a good overview of the drug approval process.

§ 355a. Pediatric studies of drugs

This section authorizes the HHS secretary to request pediatric studies, which are defined in this section, from the holder of an approved application for a new or previously approved drug, where the drug may produce health benefits in the pediatric population. If the holder of the approved application completes the studies, the holder will be granted additional "market exclusivity," through extension of patent life for the periods described in this section, for the drug. Finally, this section establishes requirements relative to the conducting of pediatric studies.

§ 355b. Adverse-event reporting

This section requires that the label of a prescription drug contain a toll-free number maintained by HHS to receive reports of adverse events regarding drugs.

§ 355c. Research into pediatric uses for drugs and biological products

This section contains several requirements in relation to assessing the safety and effectiveness of drugs and biological products in pediatric patients and to support dosing and administration of drugs and biological products in pediatric patients.

§ 356. Fast-track products

This section authorizes the HHS secretary, at the request of the sponsor of a new drug, to facilitate the development and expedite the review of the drug if it is intended for the treatment of a serious or life-threatening condition and if it demonstrates the potential to address unmet medical needs for such a condition, which serves as the definition of a *fast-track product*.

§ 356a. Manufacturing changes

This section describes manufacturing changes and sets forth those changes that require filing of a supplemental application and those that do not.

§ 356b. Reports of postmarketing studies

This section establishes the requirements for postmarketing studies where the sponsor of a drug has entered into an agreement with the HHS secretary to conduct such a study.

§ 356c. Discontinuance of life-saving drug

This section creates the requirement that the sole manufacturer of a drug that has an approved application and that was not originally derived from human tissue and was replaced with recombinant product, and that is life supporting, life sustaining, or intended for use in the prevention of a debilitating disease or condition, notify the HHS secretary of discontinuance of manufacture of the product at least 6 months prior to the discontinuance date. Reduction in the 6-month notice requirement is authorized in certain circumstances, as described in this section.

§ 358. Authority to designate official names

This section authorizes the HHS secretary to designate an official name for a drug or device, except where the official name infringes a valid trademark. It also contains a requirement that the HHS secretary review official names in the *United States Pharmacopoeia,* the *Homoeopathic Pharmacopoeia,* and the *National Formulary* to determine whether revision of those names is necessary or desirable. Finally, in such reviews, the HHS secretary is required to make determinations in relation to the designation of an official name on the basis of complexity, usefulness, multiplicity, or lack of a name.

§ 359. Nonapplicability of subchapter to cosmetics

As the title of this section states, nothing in this subchapter applies to cosmetics, unless the cosmetic is also a drug or device or component of a drug or device.

§ 360. Registration of producers of drugs or devices

This section establishes the registration and drug listing and National Drug Code requirements for drug manufacturers. The MPJE candidate should be familiar with the National Drug Code system. Significantly, this section, at (g)(1), exempts pharmacies and certain others from the registration and drug listing requirements under the conditions stated.

§ 360b. New animal drugs

As with drugs for human use, the MPJE candidate should be familiar with new animal drugs under the FDCA, as described in this lengthy section.

§ 360c. Classification of devices intended for human use

The MPJE candidate should be familiar with the FDCA provisions related to devices. This section establishes three classes of devices, as follows.

- Class I: General controls
- Class II: Special controls
- Class III: Premarket approval

This section also sets forth the standards for determination of the safety and effectiveness of a device and provides for classification panel organization and operation.

§ 360d. Performance standards

This section establishes performance standards for class II—and in some cases class III—devices and the procedures for establishing and recognizing the standards.

§ 360e. Premarket approval

This section establishes the requirements and procedures for an application for premarket approval of a class III device.

§ 360f. Banned devices

This section authorizes the HHS secretary to promulgate regulations to ban certain devices, as described in this section.

§ 360g. Judicial review

This section sets forth the procedures for judicial review of decisions of the HHS secretary with regard to devices.

§ 360h. Notification and other remedies

This section provides that when a device presents an unreasonable risk of substantial harm and notification is necessary to eliminate the risk of harm, the HHS secretary may issue an order to ensure that adequate notification is provided, in an appropriate form, by the persons and means best suited under the circumstances involved to all health professionals who prescribe or use the device and to any other person (including manufacturers, importers, distributors, retailers, and device users) who should properly receive such a notification to eliminate such a risk. This section also authorizes the HHS secretary to order the manufacturer of a device to repair, replace, or make refund for the device. Finally, this section gives the HHS secretary authority to order a recall of a device.

§ 360i. Records and reports on devices

This section requires reports, as described in the section, from device manufacturers and device-user facilities, such as hospitals. It also authorizes the HHS secretary to order a device manufacturer to adopt a method for tracking certain class II and III devices.

§ 360j. General provisions respecting control of devices intended for human use

This section contains a variety of requirements, including provisions for custom devices, restricted devices, good manufacturing practice requirements, and exemption of devices for investigational use.

§ 360k. State and local requirements respecting devices

This section establishes the relationship between the FDCA provisions on devices and any state laws that may exist in relation to devices.

§ 360l. Postmarket surveillance

This section authorizes the HHS secretary to impose on manufacturers of certain devices various postmarketing surveillance requirements related to devices.

§ 360m. Accredited persons

This section requires the HHS secretary to establish an accreditation program as described in the section, for persons who review reports related to devices.

Part B—Drugs for rare diseases or conditions

§ 360aa. Recommendations for investigations of drugs for rare diseases or conditions

This section provides that a sponsor of a drug for a disease or condition that is rare may request the HHS secretary to provide written recommendations for the nonclinical and clinical investigations that must be conducted with the drug before it may be approved for treatment of such a disease or condition or, if the drug is a biological product, before it may be licensed for such disease or condition.

§ 360bb. Designation of drugs for rare diseases or conditions

This section allows a manufacturer or sponsor of a drug to request, prior to submission of an application for approval, the HHS secretary to designate the drug as a drug for a rare disease or condition. This section defines a *rare disease or condition* as any disease or condition that affects (a) fewer than 200,000 persons in the United States or (b) more than 200,000 persons in the United States provided that there is no reasonable expectation that the cost of developing and making available in the United States a drug for such a disease or condition will be recovered from sales in the United States. It also contains a requirement for notice to the HHS secretary for discontinuance of production of the drug.

§ 360cc. Protection for drugs for rare diseases or conditions

This section provides that if the HHS secretary approves an application for a drug designated for a rare disease or condition, the HHS secretary may not approve another application for such a drug for such a disease or condition for a person who is not the holder of the approved application until the expiration of 7 years from the date of approval, unless (a) the holder of the approved application cannot ensure the availability of sufficient quantities of the drug to meet the needs of people with the disease or condition for which the drug was designated or (b) the holder provides the HHS secretary written consent for the approval of other applications before the expiration of the 7-year period.

§ 360dd. Open protocols for investigations of drugs for rare diseases or conditions

This section provides, under certain circumstances, for the HHS secretary to encourage the sponsor of a drug designated for a rare disease or condition to design protocols for clinical investigations of the drug that may be conducted to permit the addition to the investigations of people with the disease or condition who need the drug to treat the disease or condition and who cannot be satisfactorily treated by available alternative drugs.

§ 360ee. Grants and contracts for development of drugs for rare diseases and conditions

This section authorizes the HHS secretary to make grants to and enter into contracts with public and private entities and individuals to assist in defraying the costs of qualified testing expenses incurred in connection with the development of drugs for rare diseases and conditions, of development of medical devices for rare diseases or conditions, and of development of medical foods (a food formulated to be consumed or administered enterally under the supervision of a physician) for rare diseases or conditions.

Part D—Dissemination of treatment information

When sections 360aaa–360aaa-6 were enacted, Congress provided that they were to sunset (cease effectiveness) in 2006. Related to this, the FDA has published a "guidance for industry" on good reprint practices. The guidance is available at www.fda.gov/oc/op/goodreprint.html. Although the text of the sections remains in the U.S. Code, rather than review the sections, the MPJE candidate should review the FDA guidance to gain general understanding of requirements and limitations associated with dissemination of treatment information.

Part E—General provisions relating to drugs and devices

§ 360bbb. Expanded access to unapproved therapies and diagnostics

This section authorizes the HHS secretary to allow shipment of investigational drugs or investigational devices for the diagnosis, monitoring, or treatment of a serious disease or condition in emergency situations. Furthermore, an individual patient, acting through a physician, may request from a manufacturer or distributor an investigational drug or device for the diagnosis, monitoring, or treatment of a serious disease or condition if a number of conditions, as set forth in this section, are fulfilled.

§ 360bbb-1. Dispute resolution

This section requires the HHS secretary to establish a procedure for a sponsor, applicant, or manufacturer to obtain a review, including by a scientific advisory panel, in situations in which there is a scientific controversy with the HHS secretary.

§ 360bbb-2. Classification of products

This section provides that a person submitting an application for a product may submit a request to the HHS secretary with respect to the classification of the product as a drug, biological product, device, or a combination or with respect to the component of the

FDA that will regulate the product. In submitting the request, the person shall recommend a classification for the product or a component to regulate the product, as appropriate. This section also describes what action the HHS secretary shall take in response to filing of such a request.

§ 360bbb-3. Authorization for medical products for use in emergencies
This section provides for the use of unapproved drugs, devices, and biological products and for the use of approved drugs, devices, and biological products for unapproved uses in the event of an emergency.

Part F—New animal drugs for minor use and minor species
§ 360ccc. Conditional approval of new animal drugs for minor use and minor species
This section authorizes conditional approval of a new animal drug for a minor use or a minor species. Included are the requirements associated with application for approval and limitations on seeking approval.

§ 360ccc-1. Index of legally marketed unapproved new animal drugs for minor species
This section requires the secretary of HHS to establish a list of (a) new animal drugs intended for use in a minor species for which there is a reasonable certainty that the animal or edible products from the animal will not be consumed by humans or food-producing animals and (b) new animal drugs intended for use only in a hatchery, tank, pond, or other similar contained human-made structure in an early, nonfood life stage of a food-producing minor species, where safety for humans is demonstrated.

§ 360ccc-2. Designated new animal drugs for minor use or minor species
This section provides that the manufacturer or sponsor of a new animal drug for a minor use or use in a minor species may request the secretary of HHS to declare that drug a *designated new animal drug.*

Subchapter VI. Cosmetics

The MPJE candidate should review the three sections (361–363) contained in this subchapter on cosmetics.

The last three subchapters of Chapter 9 contain a variety of sections, many of which are not of interest to the MPJE candidate. As directed in the explanation to the study guide, the candidate should open each subchapter and from the titles of the parts and sections determine those that the MPJE candidate should review.

Regulations of the U.S. FDA

The FDA regulations may be found in Title 21 of the CFR. The body of FDA regulations is divided into subchapters as follows:

- Subchapter A—General (21 CFR Parts 1–99)
- Subchapter B—Food for Human Consumption (21 CFR Parts 100–199)
- Subchapter C—Drugs: General (21 CFR 200–299)
- Subchapter D—Drugs for Human Use (21 CFR Parts 300–499)
- Subchapter E—Animal Drugs, Feeds, and Related Products (21 CFR Parts 500–599)
- Subchapter F—Biologics (21 CFR Parts 600–699)
- Subchapter G—Cosmetics (21 CFR Parts 700–799)
- Subchapter H—Medical Devices (21 CFR Parts 800–899)
- Subchapter I—Mammography Quality Standards Act (21 CFR Parts 900–999)
- Subchapter J—Radiological Health (21 CFR Parts 1000–1099)
- Subchapter K—Reserved
- Subchapter L—Regulations under Certain Other Acts (21 CFR Parts 1200–1299)

The MPJE candidate should review relevant FDA regulations on the electronic database as described in the introduction to this study guide.

2-4. The Poison Prevention Packaging Act of 1970 and Regulations of the U.S. CPSC

The Poison Prevention Packaging Act (PPPA), enacted by Congress in 1970, has as its purpose preventing poisonings in children under 5 years of age. This purpose is achieved through numerous requirements in the act and CPSC regulations.

The PPPA establishes packaging requirements for certain household products. Included among these products are both prescription and nonprescription drug products.

Key Provisions of the PPPA

The MPJE candidate should be familiar with the packaging requirements contained in the PPPA and the regulations of the CPSC. The PPPA is located at Chapter 39A of Title 15 of the United States Code.

The MPJE candidate should retrieve and review the sections contained in Chapter 39A as described in the introduction to this study guide.

Regulations of the U.S. CPSC

The CPSC regulations may be found at Part 1700 of Title 16 of the CFR. The MPJE candidate should retrieve and review the sections contained in Part 1700 as described in the explanation to this study guide.

As mentioned earlier, the MPJE candidate is encouraged to review the CPSC publication "Poison Prevention Packaging: A Guide for Healthcare Professionals," available at www.cpsc.gov/CPSCPUB/PUBS/384.pdf.

2-5. Miscellaneous Federal Laws

Omnibus Budget Reconciliation Act of 1990

The Omnibus Budget Reconciliation Act of 1990 (more commonly referred to as OBRA '90) required the states to enact laws to require patient profiling, prospective drug use review, and patient counseling by pharmacies. Although the federal mandate applied only to the provision of pharmacy services to Medicaid beneficiaries, the states extended application of the requirements to all pharmacy patients. The MPJE candidate should review state law on these requirements, and the federal regulations may be found beginning at section 45 CFR 456.700.

Anti-Tampering Act of 1982

This act makes tampering with consumer products a federal offense and was passed as a result of a series of incidents of intentional contamination of Tylenol capsules while held for sale in retail establishments. Regulatory authority resides with the Federal Bureau of Investigation, U.S. Department of Agriculture, and FDA. Regulations for specific types of products may be retrieved (as described in the introduction to this study guide) and reviewed as follows:

- Over-the-counter drug products (21 CFR 211.132)
- Medical devices (21 CFR 800.12)
- Cosmetics (21 CFR 700.25)

Federal Law on Medicinal Use of Alcohol

Under federal law, retailers that sell alcohol are subject to an annual tax, and to handle any type of alcohol, a license from the U.S. Bureau of Alcohol, Tobacco, and Firearms is required. Retailers selling take-home liquors are required to obtain a federal retail liquor dealer's stamp. In a community pharmacy, if the alcohol is sold only for medicinal purposes, a federal medicinal spirits dealer's stamp may be obtained instead of the retail liquor dealer's stamp. Some pharmacies require much larger volumes (usually obtained in 10- or 55-gallon drums) of alcohol, and the alcohol can be purchased tax free. However, the use of tax-free alcohol is subject to a number of federal law restrictions.

- The alcohol must be used for medicinal or scientific purposes or for patient treatment.
- The alcohol must not be sold or loaned to other pharmacies or other practitioners.
- The alcohol, whether in pure form or in combination with other substances, must not be sold to outpatients, with the exception of nonprofit clinics, as long as the patient is not charged.
- The alcohol must be kept in a secure, fire-resistant room.
- A perpetual inventory of the alcohol stock must be maintained.

For additional information, the MPJE candidate can review the sections beginning at 27 CFR 22.1, as described in the explanation to this study guide.

2-6. Questions

1. Pharmacist Betty Jones decides to open her own community pharmacy. Which of the following DEA forms will she use to apply for a DEA Certificate of Registration for the new pharmacy?

   A. DEA Form 106
   B. DEA Form 222
   C. DEA Form 223
   D. DEA Form 224
   E. DEA Form 224a

2. You arrive at your community pharmacy one morning and discover that during the night someone broke into the pharmacy and stole several commercial containers of controlled substances. Within how many business day(s) must this theft of controlled substances be reported to the field division office of the DEA in your area?

   A. 1
   B. 3

C. 7

D. 10

E. 30

3. As the owner of a community pharmacy, you recently employed a staff pharmacist and granted the pharmacist a power of attorney to order controlled substances. In addition to physically signing the DEA order form for schedule II controlled substances, the staff pharmacist completed the steps necessary to obtain authority from the DEA to place electronic orders for all schedules of controlled substances. Today, this pharmacist resigned from your employment. The pharmacist's resignation must be communicated to the DEA Certification Authority within what period?

A. 6 hours

B. 24 hours

C. 3 days

D. 7 days

E. 30 days

4. Which of the following is the federal agency that certifies private practice physicians to prescribe schedule III, IV, or V narcotic controlled substances for detoxification and maintenance treatment of opioid dependency?

A. DEA

B. FDA

C. OIG

D. SAMHSA

E. FTC

5. Frank Wilson, a U.S. citizen, recently traveled outside the United States on business. While outside the country, he became very ill with a gastrointestinal infection and suffered severe nausea, vomiting, diarrhea, and dehydration. A physician in the town where he was located prescribed medications, consisting of an antibiotic and two controlled substances. A local pharmacy dispensed the prescriptions, which were packaged, labeled, and dispensed in much the same manner as if dispensed in the United States. On returning to the United States 2 days after receiving the prescriptions, he proceeded to U.S. Customs, where he was asked if he was bringing any drugs into the country. He responded yes and handed the Customs officer the prescriptions. As to the controlled substance prescriptions, which of the following is true?

A. If either or both of the prescriptions are for a schedule II controlled substance, they will be seized by the Customs officer because federal law prohibits importation of a schedule II controlled substance.

B. Mr. Wilson can legally bring a maximum of 50 dosage units of each of the two controlled substances into the United States.

C. Mr. Wilson can legally bring a maximum total of 50 dosage units combined of the two controlled substances into the United States.

D. Mr. Wilson can bring the antibiotic prescription into the United States but not the prescriptions for controlled substances.

E. Both A and C.

6. A life-supporting or life-sustaining device that requires FDA approval before it can be marketed in interstate commerce in the United States is a

A. class I device.

B. class II device.

C. class III device.

D. class IV device.

E. class V device.

7. For purposes of classifying a drug as an *orphan drug*, a rare disease or condition is defined as follows: a disease or condition that affects (a) fewer than _____ persons in the United States or (b) more than _____ persons in the United States provided that there is no reasonable expectation that the cost of developing and making the drug available will be recovered.

A. 100,000

B. 200,000

C. 250,000

D. 500,000

E. 1,000,000

8. Which of the following is *not* one of the recognized "Official Compendia" in the federal Food, Drug, and Cosmetic Act?

A. *United States Pharmacopeia*

B. *Homeopathic Pharmacopeia of the United States*

C. *National Formulary*

D. *Approved Drug Products with Therapeutic Equivalence Ratings*

9. When a pharmacy orders schedule II controlled substances using the DEA official triplicate order form, which copy (copies) of the form is (are) sent by the pharmacy to the supplier?

    A. Copy 1
    B. Copy 2
    C. Copy 3
    D. Copies 1 and 2
    E. Copies 2 and 3

10. A quality control manager at Widget Pharmaceuticals has just discovered that a batch sample of a Widget Pharmaceuticals brand of an intravenous solution has tested positive for the presence of a bacterium toxin. If, in fact, the intravenous solution contains a bacterium toxin that is harmful to humans, the solution would be

    A. adulterated.
    B. misbranded.

11. Pharmacies registered under the federal Controlled Substances Act are required to take a complete inventory of all controlled substances every _____ months.

    A. 6
    B. 12
    C. 18
    D. 24
    E. 36

12. Dr. Marcia Wilson is a neurologist treating attention deficit disorder (ADD) and attention deficit hyperactivity disorder (ADHD) patients. Among her treatments for these patients, she prescribes Ritalin, Concerta, and Adderall. Her general policy is that patients using these medications must be seen in her office every 3 months for evaluation. Because most of her patients prefer to obtain their prescriptions locally and third-party prescription drug plans will reimburse for a 30-day supply only, Dr. Wilson is forced to issue 3 prescriptions to provide adequate medication between office visits. According to the applicable DEA regulation on issuing multiple prescriptions for a schedule II controlled substance, for how many total days' supply of a schedule II controlled substance may Dr. Wilson issue multiple prescriptions to a patient?

    A. 60
    B. 90
    C. 120
    D. 150
    E. 180

13. According to the federal Food, Drug, and Cosmetic Act, which of the following may *not* legally receive and possess prescription drug samples from a manufacturer or authorized distributor of record?

    A. Free-standing retail pharmacies
    B. Pharmacies located within a hospital or other health care entity, at the written request of a licensed practitioner
    C. Osteopathic doctors
    D. Dentists

14. One of your regular patients comes into your pharmacy and reports that he developed a dry, hacking cough 2 days ago, and although he has been taking a nonprescription liquid cough suppressant, it has been ineffective in controlling the cough. He says that not too long ago another pharmacy sold him a nonprescription cough suppressant containing codeine that was very effective. He asks if you have such a product, and you reply that you do and agree to sell him the product. Assuming that state law permits selling such a product without a prescription, you may sell not more than 240 cc (8 oz) of a controlled substance containing opium, nor more than 120 cc (4 oz) of any other controlled substance, nor more than 48 dosage units of a controlled substance containing opium, nor more than 24 dosage units of any other controlled substance in any given period of how many hours?

    A. 24
    B. 36
    C. 48
    D. 60
    E. 72

15. According to the federal Food, Drug and Cosmetic Act, which of the following is exempt from registration with the Food and Drug Administration as a manufacturer?

    A. A manufacturer of generic drug products
    B. A manufacturer of brand-name drug products

C. A pharmacy compounding a product pursuant to a lawful prescription order

D. A pharmacy compounding a product to supply a physician for that physician to use in dispensing prescription orders

16. "The rate and extent to which the active ingredient or therapeutic ingredient is absorbed from a drug and becomes available at the site of drug action" is the federal Food, Drug, and Cosmetic Act definition of which of the following?

A. Bioavailability
B. Bioequivalency
C. Dissolution
D. Area under the curve

17. Under federal law, the daily sales limit of ephedrine base, pseudoephedrine base, or phenylpropanolamine base is _____ grams per purchaser, regardless of the number of transactions.

A. 1.8
B. 3.6
C. 7.2
D. 9.0
E. 14.4

18. At least how many days before introducing or delivering for introduction into interstate commerce a dietary supplement that contains a new dietary ingredient that has not been present in the food supply as an article used for food in a form in which the food has not been chemically altered must the manufacturer or distributor of that supplement, or of the new dietary ingredient, submit to the U.S. Food and Drug Administration information, including any citation to published articles, on which basis the manufacturer or distributor has concluded that the dietary supplement can reasonably be expected to be safe?

A. 30
B. 60
C. 75
D. 90
E. 120

19. With respect to pharmacy compounding of pharmaceutical products, which of the following is *not* one of the factors considered by the U.S. Food and Drug Administration in determining whether a pharmacy is "compounding" versus "manufacturing" pharmaceutical products?

A. Compounding drugs in anticipation of receiving prescriptions, except in very limited quantities in relation to the amounts of drugs compounded after receiving valid prescriptions

B. Using commercial-scale manufacturing or testing equipment for compounding drug products

C. Offering compounded drugs at wholesale to other state-licensed persons or commercial entities for resale

D. Setting prices for compounded drugs that are far higher than the prices for the same or similar commercially available drugs

E. Compounding drugs that are commercially available in the marketplace or that are essentially copies of commercially available drugs

20. The federal Food, Drug, and Cosmetic Act prohibits the selling, purchasing, or trading of a prescription drug that was purchased by a public or private hospital or other health care entity or donated or supplied at a reduced price to a charitable organization. Which of the following is *not* one of the exceptions to this prohibition?

A. The purchase or other acquisition by a hospital or other health care entity that is a member of a group-purchasing organization of a drug for its own use from the group-purchasing organization or from other hospitals or health care entities that are members of such an organization

B. A sale, purchase, or trade of a drug or an offer to sell, purchase, or trade a drug among hospitals or other health care entities that are under common control

C. A sale, purchase, or trade of a drug; an offer to sell, purchase, or trade a drug; or the dispensing of a drug pursuant to a prescription

D. The sale, purchase, or trade of a drug or an offer to sell, purchase, or trade a drug by a charitable organization to a nonprofit affiliate of the organization

E. A sale to a community pharmacy for non-emergency dispensing needs

21. A maximum of how many times may a prescription for a schedule III, IV, or V controlled substance may be refilled?

    A. 1
    B. 2
    C. 3
    D. 4
    E. 5

22. Approximately 30 minutes ago, your community pharmacy received a prescription for a schedule II controlled substance by facsimile transmission. The patient for whom the prescription was issued has just arrived for the prescription. You may dispense the prescription solely on the basis of the facsimile prescription and use the facsimile prescription as the original prescription for purposes of recordkeeping.

    A. True
    B. False

23. With respect to a prescription for a controlled substance, which of the following may be maintained in an electronic database used for prescription dispensing rather than having to be placed on the actual prescription form maintained in the pharmacy's prescription files?

    A. Physician's DEA number
    B. Record of refills
    C. Patient address
    D. The word *void* or the word *transfer* required on issuing or receiving, respectively, a transferred prescription for a controlled substance
    E. A and B
    F. B and C
    G. B and D

24. William Wilson has just presented you two empty prescription vials and requests that each be refilled. Both of the prescriptions are for solid, oral dosage formulations. When dispensing the refills (and assuming neither Mr. Wilson nor the prescriber has requested non-child-resistant packaging), you may reuse the prescription vials and closures when dispensing the refills.

    A. True
    B. False

25. The U.S. Food and Drug Administration regulations regarding medication guides provide that where a medication guide is required for a particular prescription drug product, the medication guide must be provided to the patient on the initial dispensing of the drug but not on any refills thereafter.

    A. True
    B. False

2-7. Answers

1. **D.** DEA Form 224 is the application form for a new DEA Certificate of Registration. DEA Form 224a is the renewal application form that DEA mails to registrants approximately 60 days before the expiration of a DEA Certificate of Registration. DEA Form 106 is used to report theft or loss of controlled substances. DEA Form 222 is used to order schedule II controlled substances. DEA Form 223 is the number of the DEA Certificate of Registration that is displayed at the registrant's location. The applicable DEA regulation is 21 CFR 1301.13.

2. **A.** Although notification is required within 1 business day, completion and submission of DEA Form 106 is not required within 1 business day, but the form should be completed and submitted promptly. The applicable DEA regulation is 21 CFR 1301.76.

3. **A.** Recognize that before electronic ordering of controlled substances was permitted, notifying the DEA if a pharmacist with a power of attorney resigned or was terminated was not necessary. The power of attorney was useless without physical access to DEA Form 222. But with electronic ordering of controlled substances, a DEA Form 222 is not needed, so notification must be provided if the pharmacist had obtained the authority from DEA to submit electronic orders. The applicable DEA regulation is 21 CFR 1311.45.

4. **D.** SAMHSA, not the DEA, certifies physicians to prescribe schedule III, IV, and V narcotic controlled substances for detoxification and maintenance treatment of opioid dependency. Prescriptions for the currently approved products Suboxone and Subutex for treatment of opioid dependency must include the physician's DEA number and the physician's "X" number signifying certification to treat opioid depen-

dency. Also, only physicians may be approved to treat opioid dependency. Information about the medication-assisted treatment of opioid dependency is available on the SAMHSA Web site at www.dpt.samhsa.gov. The applicable DEA regulation is 21 CFR 1301.28.

5. **C.** The limitation associated with the exemption from import and export requirements for personal medical use is a combined 50 dosage units and not 50 dosage units of each controlled substance. The applicable DEA regulation is 21 CFR 1301.26.

6. **C.** The federal FDCA provides for three classes of medical devices: class I, class II, and class III. Generally class I devices are not subject to premarket approval, and class II devices are subject to performance standards. Class III devices are life-supporting or life-sustaining devices and require premarket approval by FDA. The applicable section of the federal FDCA is 21 USC 360c.

7. **B.** The applicable section of the federal FDCA is 21 USC 360bb.

8. **D.** Although the *Approved Drug Products with Therapeutic Equivalence Ratings* (FDA Orange Book) is an important publication for pharmacy, it is not one of the official compendia. The official compendia are established by the federal FDCA at 21 USC 321.

9. **D.** The pharmacy keeps copy 3 and sends copies 1 and 2 to the supplier. The applicable DEA regulation is 21 CFR 1305.12.

10. **A.** The applicable section of the federal FDCA is 21 USC 351.

11. **D.** Pharmacies are required to conduct a "biennial" inventory of all controlled substances. The applicable DEA regulation is 21 CFR 1304.11.

12. **B.** The applicable DEA regulation is 21 CFR 1306.12.

13. **A.** The applicable section of the federal FDCA is 21 USC 353.

14. **C.** The applicable DEA regulation is 21 CFR 1306.26.

15. **C.** Pharmacies are exempt from registration, provided that the compounding is "in the regular course of their business of dispensing or selling drugs or devices at retail." The applicable section of the federal FDCA is 21 USC 360.

16. **A.** The applicable section of the federal FDCA is 21 USC 355.

17. **B.** The applicable DEA regulation is 21 CFR 1314.20.

18. **C.** The applicable section of the federal FDCA is 21 USC 3650b.

19. **D.** The other answer choices are contained in the FDA compliance guide on pharmacy compounding, which is available at www.fda.gov/downloads/AboutFDA/CentersOffices/CDER/UCM118050.pdf.

20. **E.** The applicable section of the federal FDCA is 21 USC 353.

21. **E.** As provided in the DEA regulations, "No prescription for a controlled substance listed in Schedule III or IV shall be filled or refilled more than 6 months after the date on which such prescription was issued and no such prescription authorized to be refilled may be refilled more than five times." The applicable DEA regulation is 21 CFR 1306.22.

22. **B.** Although in some situations a facsimile prescription for a Schedule II controlled substance can be dispensed and can be used as the original prescription for recordkeeping, it cannot be in this situation of an ambulatory patient. The applicable DEA regulation is 21 CFR 1306.11.

23. **B.** All information required to be placed on a prescription for a controlled substance by either the CSA or the DEA regulations must be placed on the prescription. The only exemption is the record of refills. The applicable DEA regulation is 21 CFR 1306.22.

24. **B.** As stated by the CPSC in response to whether pharmacists may reuse prescription vials, "As a general rule, no. This prohibition is based on the wear associated with a plastic vial, which could compromise the package's effectiveness. Since such wear or undetected damage with a glass container is negligible, the CPSC staff has indicated that it would have no objection to the reuse of a glass container, provided a new closure is used. This same consideration would be given to any other package type that is not prone to wear." See the CPSC publication "Poison Prevention Packaging: A Guide for Healthcare Professionals" available at www.cpsc.gov/CPSCPUB/PUBS/384.pdf.

25. **B.** Medication guides must be provided on each dispensing. The applicable FDA regulation is 21 CFR 208.24.

Dosage Forms and Drug Delivery Systems

Ram I. Mahato, PhD

3

3-1. Introduction

A pharmaceutical *dosage form* is the entity administered to patients so that they receive an effective dose of a drug. Some common examples are tablets, capsules, suppositories, injections, suspensions, and transdermal patches. Achieving an optimum response from any dosage form requires delivery of a drug to its site of action at a rate and a concentration that both minimize its side effects and maximize its therapeutic effects. The development of safe and effective pharmaceutical dosage forms and delivery systems requires a thorough understanding of physicochemical principles that allow a drug to be formulated into a pharmaceutical dosage form. Design of the appropriate dosage form or delivery system depends on the

- Physicochemical properties of the drug, such as solubility, oil-to-water partition coefficient ($K_{o/w}$), pK$_a$ value, molecular weight, and polymorphism
- Dose of the drug
- Route of administration
- Type of drug delivery systems desired
- Pathologic condition to be treated
- Desired therapeutic effect
- Drug release from the delivery system
- Bioavailability of the drug at the absorption site
- Pharmacokinetics and pharmacodynamics of the drug

How Drug Molecules Move across Barriers in the Body

Most drugs are absorbed from the site of their application by simple diffusion. Drug diffusion through a barrier may occur by simple molecular permeation known as *molecular diffusion* or by movement through pores and channels known as *pore diffusion*. In pore diffusion, drug release rate is affected by degree of crystallinity and crystal size, degree of swelling, porous structure, and tortuosity of polymers.

In passive molecular diffusion, a drug travels by passive transport (which does not require an external energy source) from a region of high concentration to a region of low concentration. However, other transport processes occur in the body as well. For example, active transport of drugs can proceed from regions of low concentration to regions of high concentration through the pumping action of one or more biologic transport systems. These active transport systems require an energy source such as an enzyme or biochemical carrier to ferry the drug across the membrane.

Fick's law of diffusion is a mathematical expression that describes passive diffusion. Fick's first law states that the amount of material (M) flowing through a unit cross-section (S) of a barrier in a unit of time (t), which is known as the flux (J), is proportional to the concentration gradient (dc/dx).

$$J = \frac{dM}{S \cdot dt}$$

where J = flux in g/cm^2 × s; S = cross section of barrier in cm^2; dM/dt = rate of diffusion in g/s; M = mass in grams; and t = time in seconds.

The flux is proportional to the concentration gradient, dC/dx:

$$J = -D\frac{dC}{dx}$$

where D = diffusion coefficient of a penetrant in cm²/s; C = concentration in g/cm³ or g/mL; and x = distance in centimeters of movement perpendicular to the surface of the barrier.

The diffusion coefficient, D, is a physicochemical property of the drug molecule. It is not constant and can vary with changes in concentration, temperature, pressure, solvent properties, molecular weight, and chemical nature of the diffusant. The larger the molecular weight is, the lower the diffusion coefficient will be.

Fick's first law of diffusion describes the diffusion process under the condition of steady state when the concentration gradient (dC/dx) does not change with time. Figure 3-1 shows the diaphragm of thickness h and cross-sectional area S that separate the two compartments of the diffusion cell. Equating both equations for flux, Fick's first law of diffusion may be written as

$$J = \frac{dM}{S \cdot dt} = \frac{D(C_1 - C_2)}{h}$$

in which $(C_1 - C_2)/h$ approximates dC/dx. Concentrations C_1 and C_2 within the membrane can be replaced by the partition coefficient multiplied by the concentration C_d in the donor compartment or C_r in the receptor compartment. The partition coefficient, K, is given by $K = C_1/C_d = C_2/C_r$. Hence,

$$\frac{dM}{dt} = \frac{DSK(C_d - C_r)}{h}$$

Under sink conditions, the drug concentration in the receptor compartment is much lower than the drug concentration in the donor compartment.

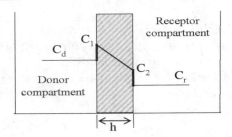

Figure 3-1. Concentration Gradient of Diffusant across a Diaphragm of a Diffusion Cell

Therefore, $C_r \to 0$. The preceding equation can be simplified as

$$\frac{dM}{dt} = \frac{DSKC_d}{h} = PSC_d$$

where D is the diffusion coefficient (in cm²/s); S is the surface area of the cross-section of the barrier (in cm²); K is the partition coefficient; C_d is the concentration of drug in the donor compartment (in g/mL); h is the barrier thickness (in cm); and P is the permeability coefficient (in cm/s), where $P = DK/h$.

Transport of a drug by passive diffusion across a membrane such as the gastrointestinal (GI) mucosa is represented by Fick's law:

$$-\frac{dM}{dt} = \frac{D_m SK}{h}\left(C_g - C_p\right)$$

where M is the amount of drug in the gut compartment at time t, D_m is drug diffusivity in the intestinal membrane, S is the surface area of GI membrane available for absorption, K is the partition coefficient between the membrane and aqueous medium in the intestine, h is the thickness of the GI membrane, C_g is the drug concentration in the intestinal compartment, and C_p is the drug concentration in the plasma compartment.

Because the gut compartment usually has a high drug concentration compared with the plasma compartment, C_p may be omitted. Therefore, the preceding equation then becomes

$$-\frac{dM}{dt} = \frac{D_m SK \cdot C_g}{h}$$

This suggests that the rate of GI absorption of a drug by passive diffusion depends on the surface area of the membrane available for drug absorption. The small intestine is the major site for drug absorption because of the presence of villi and microvilli, which provide an enormous surface area for absorption.

pH Partition Theory and Its Limitation

The *pH partition theory* states that drugs are absorbed from the biological membranes by passive diffusion, depending on the fraction of the un-ionized form of the drug at the pH of the fluids close to that biological membrane. The degree of ionization of the drug depends on both the pK_a and the pH of the drug solution. The GI tract acts as a lipophilic barrier, and thus ionized drugs are more hydrophilic than un-ionized ones and have minimal membrane transport. The solution pH affects the overall partition coefficient of an ionizable substance. The pK_a of the molecule is the pH at which there is a 50:50 mixture of conjugate acid–base forms. The conjugate acid form predominates at a pH lower than the pK_a, and the conjugate base form is present at a pH higher than the pK_a. The extent of ionization of a drug molecule is given by the following Henderson–Hasselbalch equations, which describe a relationship between ionized and nonionized species of a weak electrolyte:

Weakly acidic drugs	Weakly basic drugs
$pH = pK_a + \log\dfrac{[A^-]}{[HA]}$	$pH = pK_a + \log\dfrac{[B]}{[BH]}$

where [HA] is the concentration of un-ionized acid, [A$^-$] is the concentration of ionized base, [B] is the concentration of un-ionized base, and [BH] is the concentration of ionized base. Although pH partition theory is useful, it often does not hold true for certain experimental observations. For example, most weak acids are well absorbed from the small intestine, which is contrary to the prediction of the pH partition hypothesis. Similarly, quaternary ammonium compounds are ionized at all pHs but are readily absorbed from the GI tract. These discrepancies arise because pH partition theory does not take into consideration the following factors, among others:

- Large epithelial surface areas of the small intestine compensate for ionization effects.
- Long residence time in the small intestine also compensates for ionization effects.
- Charged drugs, such as quaternary ammonium compounds and tetracyclines, may interact with opposite-charged organic ions, resulting in a neutral species that is absorbable.
- Some drugs are absorbed by means of active transport.

The Noyes–Whitney Equation of Dissolution

For most drugs, the rate at which the solid drug dissolves in a solvent (dissolution) is often the rate-limiting step in the drug's bioavailability. The rate at which a solid drug of limited water solubility dissolves

in a solvent can be determined using the Noyes–Whitney equation:

$$\frac{dM}{dt} = k \cdot S \cdot (C_s - C)$$

where dM/dt is the rate of dissolution (in mass/time), k is the dissolution rate constant (in cm/s) ($k = D/h$), S is the surface area of exposed solid (in cm^2), D is the diffusion coefficient of solute in solution (in cm^2/s), h is the thickness of the diffusion layer (in cm), C_s is the drug solubility (in g/mL), and C is the drug concentration in bulk solution at time t (in g/mL).

Under sink conditions, when C is much less than C_s, the Noyes–Whitney equation can be simplified as follows:

$$\frac{dM}{dt} = k\,S\,C_s \text{ or } \frac{dC}{dt} = \frac{kSC_s}{V}$$

where dC/dt is the dissolution rate (in concentration/time) and V is the volume of the dissolution medium (in mL).

The following factors influence the dissolution rate:

- The physicochemical conditions in the GI tract affect the dissolution rate. For example, the presence of foods that increase the viscosity of GI fluids decreases the diffusion coefficient, D, of a drug and its dissolution rate.
- The thickness of the diffusion layer, h, is influenced by the degree of agitation experienced by each drug particle in the GI tract. Hence, an increase in gastric or intestinal motility may increase the dissolution rate of poorly soluble drugs.
- The removal rate of dissolved drugs attributable to absorption through the gastrointestinal–blood barrier and the GI fluid volume affects drug concentration in the GI tract and thus also affects the dissolution rate.
- The dissolution rate of a weakly acidic drug in GI fluids is influenced by the drug solubility in the diffusion layer surrounding each dissolving drug particle. The pH of the diffusion layer significantly affects the solubility of a weak electrolyte drug and its subsequent dissolution rate. The dissolution rate of a weakly acidic drug in GI fluid (pH 1–3) is relatively low because of its low solubility in the diffusion layer. If the pH in the diffusion layer could be increased, the solubility (C_s) exhibited by the weak acidic drug in this layer (and hence the dissolution rate of the drug in GI

fluids) could be increased. The potassium or sodium salt form of the weakly acidic drug has a relatively high solubility at the elevated pH in the diffusion layer. Thus, the dissolution of the drug particles takes place at a faster rate.

- Particle size and the surface area of the drug significantly influence the drug dissolution rate. An increase in the total effective surface area of drug in contact with GI fluids causes an increase in its dissolution rate. The smaller the particle size is, the greater will be the effective surface area exhibited by a given mass of drug and the higher the dissolution rate. However, particle size reduction is not always helpful and may fail to increase the bioavailability of a drug. In the case of certain hydrophobic drugs, excessive particle size reduction tends to cause reaggregation into larger particles. Preventing formation of aggregates requires dispersion of small drug particles in polyethylene glycol (PEG), polyvinylpyrrolidone (PVP), dextrose, or other agents. For example, a dispersion of griseofulvin in PEG 4,000 enhances its dissolution rate and bioavailability. Certain drugs, such as penicillin G and erythromycin, are unstable in gastric fluids and do not dissolve readily in them. For such drugs, particle size reduction yields an increased rate of drug dissolution in gastric fluid and also increases the extent of drug degradation.
- Amorphous or noncrystalline forms of a drug may have faster dissolution rates than crystalline forms.
- Temperature also affects solubility. An increase in temperature will increase the solubility of a solid with a positive heat of solution. The solid will therefore dissolve at a more rapid rate on heating the system.
- Surface-active agents will increase dissolution rates by lowering interfacial tension, which allows better wetting and penetration by the solvent. Weakly acidic and basic drugs may be brought into solution by the solubilizing action of surfactants.

Interfacial Electrical Properties

Most dispersed substances in a solvent such as water acquire a surface electric charge by ionization, ion adsorption, and ion dissolution.

- *Ionization:* Surface charge arising from ionization on the particles is the function of the pH of the environment and the pK_a of the drug. Proteins acquire charge through the ionization of carboxyl and amino groups to obtain COO^- and NH_3^+ ions. Ionization of these groups, as well as the net molecular charge, depends on the pH of

the medium. At a pH below its isoelectric point (PI), a protein molecule is positively charged, $^-NH_2 \rightarrow NH_3^+$, and at a pH above its PI, the protein is negatively charged, $^-COOH \rightarrow COO^-$. At the PI of a protein, the total number of positive charges equals the total number of negative charges, and the net charge is zero. This state may be represented as follows:

$R\text{-}NH_2\text{-}COO^-$	Alkaline solution
⇅	
$R\text{-}NH_3\text{-}COO^-$	Isoelectric point (Zwitterion)
⇅	
$R\text{-}NH_3\text{-}COOH$	Acidic solution

Often a protein is least soluble at its isoelectric point and is readily dissolved by water-soluble salts such as ammonium sulfate.

- *Ion adsorption:* A net surface charge can result from the unequal adsorption of oppositely charged ions. Surfaces that are already charged usually show a tendency to adsorb counterions. Counterion adsorption can cause a reversal of charge. Surfactants strongly adsorb by hydrophobic effect and thus will determine the surface charge when adsorbed.
- *Ion dissolution:* Ionic substances can acquire a surface charge by virtue of unequal dissolution of the oppositely charged ions of which they are composed. For example, in a solution of silver iodide with excess [I⁻], the silver iodide particles carry a negative charge; however, the charge is positive if excess [Ag⁺] is present. The silver and iodide ions are referred to as *potential-determining ions* because their concentrations determine the electric potential at the particle surface.

Adsorption at solid interfaces

Adsorption of materials at solid interfaces may take place from either an adjacent liquid or a gas phase. *Adsorption* is different from *absorption*: the process of absorption implies the penetration of an entity through the organs and tissues. The degree of adsorption depends on the chemical nature of the adsorbent (a material that is being adsorbed onto a substrate, called *adsorbate*), the chemical nature of the adsorbate, the surface area of the adsorbent, the temperature, and the partial pressure of the adsorbed gas. Adsorption can be physical or chemical in nature:

- *Physical adsorption:* Physical adsorption is rapid, nonspecific, and relatively weak. Furthermore, it is associated with van der Waals attractive forces and is reversible. Removal of the adsorbate from the adsorbent is known as *desorption.* A physically adsorbed gas may be desorbed from a solid by increasing the temperature and reducing the pressure. Physical adsorption is an exothermic process, and thus the amount of adsorption decreases with rise in temperature

■ *Chemical adsorption:* Chemical adsorption or chemisorption is an irreversible process in which the adsorbent is attached to the adsorbate by primary chemical bonds. Chemisorption is specific and may require activation energy; therefore, the process is slow and only a monomolecular chemisorbed layer is possible.

Factors affecting adsorption from solution

■ *Solubility of adsorbate:* The extent of adsorption of a solute is inversely proportional to its solubility in the solvent from which adsorption occurs.
■ *Solute concentration:* An increase in the solute concentration causes an increase in the amount of adsorption that occurs at equilibrium until a limiting value is reached.
■ *Temperature:* An increase in temperature leads to decreased adsorption.
■ *pH:* The influence of pH is through a change in the ionization and solubility of the adsorbate drug molecule. For many simple small molecules, adsorption increases as the ionization of the drug is suppressed; that is, the extent of adsorption reaches a maximum when the drug is completely un-ionized. For amphoteric compounds, adsorption is at a maximum at the isoelectric point. Because the un-ionized form of most drugs in aqueous solution has a low solubility, pH and solubility effects act in concert.
■ *Surface area of adsorbent:* An increased surface area, achieved by a reduction in particle size or by the use of a porous adsorbing material, increases the extent of adsorption.

Rheology

Rheology is the study of flow properties of liquids and the deformation of solids under the influence of stress. The flow of simple liquids can be described by viscosity, an expression of the resistance to flow; however, other complex dispersions cannot be expressed simply by viscosity. Materials are divided into two general categories, Newtonian and non-Newtonian, depending on their characteristics. Rheological properties are useful for the formulation and analysis of emulsions, suspensions, pastes, lotions, and suppositories. Poura-

bility, spreadability, and syringeability of an emulsion are determined by its rheological properties.

According to Newton's law of viscous flow, the rate of flow (*D*) is directly proportional to the applied stress (τ). That is, $\tau = \eta \cdot D$, where η is the viscosity. Fluids that obey Newton's law of flow are referred to as *Newtonian fluids,* and fluids that deviate are known as *non-Newtonian fluids.* The force per unit area (*F'/A*) required to bring about flow is called the shearing stress (*F*):

$$F = \frac{F'}{A} = \eta \frac{dv}{dr}$$

where η is the viscosity, *dv/dr* is the rate of shear = *G* (s^{-1}), and *F'/A* units are in dynes per cm^2. For simple Newtonian fluids, a plot of the rate of shear against shearing stress gives a straight line (Figure 3-2A); thus, η is a constant. In the case of Newtonian fluids, viscosity does not change with increasing shear rate. Various types of water and pharmaceutical dosage forms that contain a high percentage of water are examples of liquid dosage forms that have Newtonian flow properties.

Most pharmaceutical fluids (including colloidal dispersions, emulsions, and liquid suspensions) do not follow Newton's law of flow, and the viscosity of the fluid varies with the rate of shear. There are three types of non-Newtonian flow: plastic, pseudo-plastic, and dilatant (Figure 3-2B, C, and D).

Plastic flow

Substances that undergo plastic flow are called *Bingham bodies,* which are defined as substances that exhibit a yield value (Figure 3-2B). Plastic flow is associated with the presence of flocculated particles in concentrated suspensions. *Flocculated solids* are light, fluffy conglomerates of adjacent particles held together by weak van der Waals forces. The yield value exists because a certain shearing stress must be exceeded to break up van der Waals forces. A plastic system resembles a Newtonian system at shear stresses above the yield value. Yield value, *f*, is an indicator of flocculation (the higher the yield value, the greater the degree of flocculation). The characteristics of plastic flow materials can be summarized as follows:

■ Plastic flow does not begin until a shearing stress, corresponding to a *yield value, f,* is exceeded.
■ The curve intersects the shearing stress axis but does not cross through the origin.
■ The materials are said to be "elastic" at shear stresses below the yield value.
■ Viscosity decreases with increasing shear rate at shear stress below the yield value.

Figure 3-2. Plots of Rate of Shear as a Function of Shearing Stress for (A) Newtonian, (B) Plastic, (C) Pseudoplastic, (D) Dilatant, and (E) Thixotropic flow

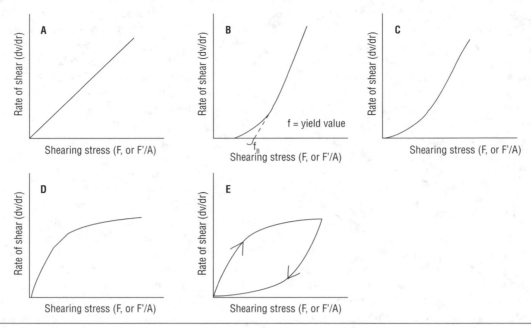

Pseudoplastic flow

Pseudoplastic flow is exhibited by polymers in solution. A large number of pharmaceutical products, including natural and synthetic gums (e.g., liquid dispersions of tragacanth, sodium alginate, methyl cellulose, and sodium carboxymethylcellulose), exhibit pseudoplastic flow properties. The characteristics of pseudoplastic flow materials can be summarized as follows:

- Pseudoplastic substances begin flow when a shearing stress is applied: that is, there is no yield value (it does cross the origin).
- The viscosity of a pseudoplastic substance decreases with increasing shear rate.
- With increasing shearing stress, the rate of shear increases; these materials are called *shear-thinning* systems.
- Shear thinning occurs when molecules (polymers) align themselves along their long axes and slip and slide past each other.

Dilatant flow

Certain suspensions with a high percentage of dispersed solids exhibit an increase in resistance to flow with increasing rates of shear. Dilatant systems are usually suspensions with a high percentage of dis-

persed solids that exhibit an increase in resistance to flow with increasing rates of shear. Dispersions containing a high percentage ($\geq 50\%$) of small, deflocculated particles may exhibit this type of behavior. The characteristics of dilatant flow materials can be summarized as follows:

- Dilatant materials increase in volume when sheared.
- They are also known as *shear-thickening systems* (the opposite of pseudoplastic systems).
- When the stress is removed, the dilatant system returns to its original state of fluidity.
- Viscosity increases with increasing shear rate.
- Dilatant materials may solidify under conditions of high shear.

Thixotropy

Thixotropy is a nonchemical isothermal gel–sol–gel transformation. If a thixotropic gel is sheared (by simple shaking), the weak bonds are broken and a lyophobic solution is formed. On standing, the particles collide, flocculation occurs, and the gel is reformed. The advantage that thixotropic preparations have is that the particles remain in suspension during storage, but when required for use, the pastes are readily made fluid by tapping or shaking. The shearing force on the injection as it is pushed through the needle ensures that it is fluid when injected; however, the rapid resumption of the gel structure prevents excessive spreading in the tissues, and consequently a more compact depot is produced than with non-thixotropic suspensions. Thixotropy is a desirable property in liquid pharmaceutical preparations. A well-formulated thixotropic suspension will not settle out readily in the container and will become fluid on shaking. Flow curves (rheograms) for thixotropic materials are highly dependent on the rate at which shear is increased or decreased and the length of time a sample is subjected to any one rate of shear.

Negative thixotropy

Negative thixotropy is also known as *antithixotropy,* which represents an increase rather than a decrease in consistency on the down curve (an increase in thickness or resistance to flow with an increased time of shear). It may result from an increased collision frequency of dispersed particles (or polymer molecules) in suspension, which causes increased interparticle bonding with time.

Shelf-Life Stability of a Drug Product

The *shelf life* of a drug in a dosage form is the amount of time the product can be stored before it becomes unfit for use because of chemical decomposition, physical deterioration, or both. Shelf-life stability of a dosage form can be determined by the Arrhenius equation $k = A \times e^{-Ea/RT}$, which can be rewritten as

$$k = A \cdot e^{-Ea/RT},\text{ which can be written as}$$

$$\log k = -\frac{Ea}{2.303}\frac{1}{R}$$

$$\log\frac{k_2}{k_1} = \frac{Ea(T_2 - T_1)}{2.303RT_2T_1}$$

where k_2 and k_1 are the reaction rates at the absolute temperatures T_2 and T_1, respectively; R is the gas constant (1.987 cal/kmol), Ea is the activation energy (in cal/mol), and A is the constant (based on molecular weight and molar volume of liquid).

3-2. Surfactants and Micelles

Surface-active agents, or *surfactants,* are substances that absorb to surfaces or interfaces to reduce surface or interfacial tension. They may be used as emulsifying agents, solubilizing agents, detergents, and wetting agents. Surfactants have two distinct regions in one chemical structure. One area is hydrophilic (water liking); another is hydrophobic (water hating). The existence of two such moieties in a molecule is known as *amphipathy,* and the molecules are consequently referred to as *amphipathic molecules* or *amphiphiles.* Depending on the number and nature of the polar and nonpolar groups present, the amphiphile may be predominantly hydrophilic, lipophilic, or somewhere in between. For example, straight chain alcohols, amines, and acids are amphiphiles that change from being predominantly hydrophilic to lipophilic as the number of carbon atoms in the alkyl chain is increased. The hydrophobic portions are usually saturated or unsaturated hydrocarbon chains or, less commonly, heterocyclic or aromatic ring systems.

Surfactants are classified according to the nature of the hydrophilic or hydrophobic groups. In addition, some surfactants possess both positively and negatively charged groups and can exist as either anionic or cationic, depending on the pH of the solution. These surfactants are known as *ampholytic compounds.*

At low concentrations in solutions, amphiphiles exist as monomers. As the concentration is increased, aggregation occurs over a narrow concentration range. These aggregates, which may contain 50 or more monomers, are called *micelles.* Therefore, micelles are small spherical structures composed of both hydrophilic and hydrophobic regions. The concentration of monomer at which micelles are formed is called the *critical micellization concentration,* or CMC. Surface tension decreases up to the CMC but remains constant above the CMC. The longer the hydrophobic chain or the lower the polarity of the polar group, the greater the tendency for monomers to "escape" from the water to form micelles and hence lower the CMC.

Types of Micelles

In the case of amphiphiles in water, in dilute solution (still above but close to the CMC), the micelles are considered to be spherical in shape. At higher concentrations, they become more asymmetric and eventually assume cylindrical or lamellar structures. Oil-soluble surfactants have a tendency to self-associate into *reverse micelles* in nonpolar solvents, with their polar groups oriented away from the solvent.

Factors Affecting CMC and Micellar Size

■ *Structure of hydrophobic group:* An increase in the hydrocarbon chain length causes a logarithmic decrease in the CMC.

- *Nature of hydrophilic group:* An increase in chain length increases hydrophilicity and the CMC. In general, nonionic surfactants have very low CMC values and high aggregation numbers compared with their ionic counterparts with similar hydrocarbon chains.
- *Nature of counterions:* Note that $Cl^- < Br^- < I^-$ for cationic surfactants, and $Na^+ < K^+$ for anionic surfactants.
- *Electrolytes:* The addition of electrolytes to ionic surfactants decreases the CMC and increases the micellar size. In contrast, micellar properties of nonionic surfactants are affected only minimally by the addition of electrolytes.
- *Temperature:* At temperatures up to the cloud point, an increase in micellar size and a decrease in CMC is noted for many nonionic surfactants but has little effect on that of ionic surfactants.
- *Alcohol:* CMCs are increased by the addition of alcohols.

Hydrophilic–Lipophilic Balance Systems

Griffin's method of selecting emulsifying agents is based on the balance between the hydrophilic and lipophilic portions of the emulsifying agent, now widely known as the *hydrophilic–lipophilic balance (HLB) system*. The higher the HLB value of an emulsifying agent, the more hydrophilic it is. The emulsifying agents with lower HLB values are less polar and more lipophilic. The Spans (i.e., sorbitan esters) are lipophilic and have low HLB values (1.8–8.6); the Tweens (polyoxyethylene derivatives of the Spans) are hydrophilic and have high HLB values (9.6–16.7). Surfactants with the proper balance of hydrophilic and lipophilic affinities are effective emulsifying agents because they concentrate at the oil-in-water (o/w) interface. The type of an emulsion that is produced depends primarily on the property of the emulsifying agent. The HLB of an emulsifier or a combination of emulsifiers determines whether an o/w or water-in-oil (w/o) emulsion results. In general, o/w emulsions are formed when the HLB of the emulsifier is within the range of about 9 to 12; w/o emulsions are formed when the range is about 3 to 6. The type of emulsion is a function of the relative solubility of the supernatant. An emulsifying agent with high HLB is preferentially soluble in water and results in the formation of an o/w emulsion. The reverse situation is true with surfactants of low HLB value, which tend to form w/o emulsions.

Micellar Solubilization

Micelles can be used to increase the solubility of materials that are normally insoluble or poorly soluble in the dispersion medium used. For example, surfactants are often used to increase the solubility of poorly soluble steroids. The factors affecting micellar solubilization are the nature of surfactants, the nature of solubilizates, and the temperature.

3-3. Dispersed Systems

Dispersed systems consist of particulate matter, known as the *dispersed phase*, distributed throughout a continuous or dispersion medium. The particulate matter, or dispersed phase, consists of particles that range from 1 nanometer (nm) to 0.5 micrometer (10^{-9} m to 5×10^{-7} m). Depending on the dispersed phase, dispersed systems are classified as follows:

- *Molecular dispersions:* Less than 1 nm, invisible under electron microscopy. Examples are oxygen molecules, ions, and glucose.
- *Coloidal dispersions:* From 1 nm to 0.5 micrometer, visible under electron microscopy. Examples are colloidal silver sols and natural and synthetic polymers.
- *Coarse dispersions:* Greater than 0.5 micrometer, visible under light microscopy. Examples are grains of sand, emulsions, suspensions, and red blood cells.

Types of Colloidal Systems

On the basis of the interaction of the particles, molecules, or ions of the dispersed phase with the molecules of dispersion medium, colloidal systems are classified into three groups: lyophilic, lyophobic, and association colloids.

Lyophilic or hydrophilic colloids

Systems containing colloidal particles that interact with the dispersion medium are referred to as *lyophilic colloids*. In the case of lipophilic colloids, organic solvent is the dispersion medium, whereas water is used as the dispersion medium for hydrophilic colloids. Because of their affinity for the dispersion medium, such materials form colloidal dispersions with relative ease. For example, the dissolution of acacia or gelatin in water, or celluloid in amyl acetate, leads to the formation of a solution. Most lyophilic colloids are polymers (e.g., gelatin, acacia, povidone, albumin, rubber, and polystyrene).

Lyophobic or hydrophobic colloids

Lyophobic colloids are composed of materials that have little attraction for the dispersion medium. Lyophobic colloids are intrinsically unstable and irreversible. Hydrophobic colloids are generally composed of inorganic particles dispersed in water.

Association colloids

Association colloids (referring to amphiphilic colloids) are formed by the grouping or association of amphiphiles (i.e., molecules that exhibit both lyophilic and lyophobic properties). At low concentrations, amphiphiles exist separately and do not form a colloid. At higher concentrations, aggregation occurs at around 50 or more monomers, leading to micelle formation. As with lyophilic colloids, formation of association colloids is spontaneous if the concentration of the amphiphile in solution exceeds the CMC.

Zeta Potential and Its Effect on Colloidal Stability

Zeta (ζ) potential is defined as the difference in potential between the surface of the tightly bound layer (shear plane) and the electroneutral region of the solution. The ζ potential governs the degree of repulsion between adjacent, similarly charged, dispersed particles. If ζ potential is reduced below a certain value, the attractive forces exceed the repulsive forces, and the particles come together. This phenomenon is known as *flocculation.*

Stabilization is accomplished by providing the dispersed particles with an electric charge and a protective solvent sheath surrounding each particle to prevent mutual adherence attributable to collision. This second effect is significant only in the case of lyophilic colloids. Lyophilic and association colloids are thermodynamically stable and exist in a true solution so that the system constitutes a single phase. In contrast, lyophobic colloids are thermodynamically unstable but can be stabilized by preventing aggregation or coagulation by providing the dispersed particles with an electric charge, which can prevent coagulation through repulsion of like particles.

3-4. Pharmaceutical Ingredients

Turning a drug substance into a pharmaceutical dosage form or a drug delivery system requires pharmaceutical ingredients. For example, in the preparation of tablets, diluents or fillers are commonly added to increase the bulk of the formulation. Binders are added to promote adhesion of the powdered drug to other ingredients. Lubricants assist the smooth tabletting process. Disintegrants promote tablet breakup after administration. Coatings improve stability, control disintegration, or enhance appearance. Similarly, in the preparation of pharmaceutical solutions, preservatives are added to prevent microbial growth, stabilizers are added to prevent drug decomposition, and colorants and flavorants are added to ensure product appeal. Thus, for each dosage form, the pharmaceutical ingredients establish the primary features of the product and control the physicochemical properties, drug-release profiles, and bioavailability of the product. Table 3-1 lists some typical pharmaceutical ingredients used in different dosage forms.

3-5. Types of Commonly Used Dosage Forms

Solutions

Solutions are homogeneous mixtures of one or more solutes dispersed in a dissolving medium (solvent). Aqueous solutions containing a sugar or sugar substitute with or without added flavoring agents and drugs are classified as *syrups.* Sweetened hydroalcoholic (combinations of water and ethanol) solutions are termed *elixirs.* Hydroalcoholic solutions of aromatic materials are termed *spirits. Tinctures* are alcoholic or hydroalcoholic solutions of chemical or soluble constituents of vegetable drugs. Most tinctures are prepared by an extraction process. *Mouthwashes* are solutions used to cleanse the mouth or treat diseases of the oral membrane. *Antibacterial topical solutions* (e.g., benzalkonium chloride and strong iodine) will kill bacteria when applied to the skin or mucous membrane.

Solutions intended for oral administration usually contain flavorants and colorants to make the medication more attractive and palatable to the patient. They may contain stabilizers to maintain the physicochemical stability of the drug and preservatives to prevent the growth of microorganisms in the solution. A drug dissolved in an aqueous solution is in the most bioavailable form. Because the drug is already in solution, no dissolution step is necessary before systemic absorption occurs. Solutions that are prepared to be sterile, that are pyrogen free, and that are intended for parenteral administration are classified as *injectables.*

Table 3-1. Typical Pharmaceutical Ingredients

Ingredient type	Definition	Examples
Antifungal preservative	Used in liquid and semisolid formulations to prevent growth of fungi	Benzoic acid, butylparaben, ethylparaben, sodium benzoate, sodium propionate
Antimicrobial preservative	Used in liquid and semisolid formulations to prevent growth of microorganisms	Benzalkonium chloride, benzyl alcohol, cetylpyridinium chloride, phenyl ethyl alcohol
Antioxidant	Used to prevent oxidation	Ascorbic acid, ascorbyl palmitate, sodium ascorbate, sodium bisulfate, sodium metabisulfite
Binder	Used to cause adhesion of powder particles in tablet granulations	Acacia, alginic acid, ethylcellulose, starch, povidone
Diluent	Used as fillers to create desired bulk, flow properties, and compression characteristics in tablet and capsule preparations	Kaolin, lactose, mannitol, cellulose, sorbitol, starch
Disintegrant	Used to promote disruption of solid mass into small particles	Microcrystalline cellulose, carboxymethylcellulose calcium, sodium alginate, sodium starch glycolate, alginic acid
Emulsifying agent	Used to promote and maintain dispersion of finely divided droplets of a liquid in a vehicle in which it is immiscible	Acacia, cetyl alcohol, glyceryl monostearate, sorbitan monostearate
Glidant	Used to improve flow properties of powder mixture	Colloidal silica, cornstarch, talc
Humectant	Used for prevention of dryness of ointments and creams	Glycerin, propylene glycol, sorbitol
Lubricant	Used to reduce friction during tablet compression and to facilitate ejection of tablets from the die cavity	Calcium stearate, magnesium stearate, mineral oil, stearic acid, zinc stearate
Plasticizer	Used to enhance coat spread over tablets, beads, and granules	Glycerin, diethyl palmitate
Surfactant	Used to reduce surface or interfacial tension	Polysorbate 80, sodium lauryl sulfate, sorbitan monopalmitate
Suspending agent	Used to reduce sedimentation rate of drug particles dispersed throughout a vehicle in which they are not soluble	Carbopol, hydroxymethylcellulose, hydroxypropyl cellulose, methylcellulose, tragacanth

Some drugs, particularly certain antibiotics, have insufficient stability in aqueous solution to withstand long shelf lives. These drugs are formulated as dry powder or granule dosage forms for reconstitution with purified water immediately before dispensing to the patient. The dry powder mixture contains all of the formulation components—that is, drug, flavorant, colorant, buffers, and others—except for the solvent. Examples of dry powder mixtures intended for reconstitution to make oral solutions include cloxacillin sodium, nafcillin sodium, oxacillin sodium, and penicillin V potassium.

Sucrose is the sugar most frequently used in syrups; in special circumstances, it may be replaced in whole or in part by other sugars (e.g., dextrose) or nonsugars (e.g., sorbitol, glycerin, and propylene glycol). Most syrups consist of between 60% and 80% su-crose. Sucrose not only provides sweetness and viscosity to the solution, but also renders the solution inherently stable (unlike dilute sucrose solutions, which are unstable).

Compared with syrups, elixirs are usually less sweet and less viscous because they contain a lower proportion of sugar, and they are consequently less effective than syrups in masking the taste of drugs. In contrast to aqueous syrups, elixirs are better able to maintain both water-soluble and alcohol-soluble components in solution because of their hydroalcoholic properties. These stable characteristics often make elixirs preferable to syrups. All elixirs contain flavoring and coloring agents to enhance their palatability and appearance. Elixirs containing over 10% to 12% alcohol are usually self-preserving and do not require the addition of antimicrobial agents for preservation. Alcohols precipitate tragacanth, acacia, agar, and inorganic salts from aqueous solutions; therefore, such substances should either be absent from the aqueous phase or be present in such low concentrations as not to promote precipitation on standing. Examples of some commonly used elixirs include dexamethasone elixir USP, pentobarbital elixir USP, diphenhydramine hydrochloride elixir, and digoxin elixir.

Tablets

Depending on the physicochemical properties of the drug, site and extent of drug absorption in the GI tract, stability to heat or moisture, biocompatibility with other ingredients, solubility, and dose, the following types of tablets are commonly formulated:

- *Swallowable tablets* are intended to be swallowed whole and then disintegrate and release their medicaments in the GI tract.
- *Effervescent tablets* are dissolved in water before administration. In addition to the drug substance, these tablets contain sodium bicarbonate and an organic acid such as tartaric acid. These additives react in the presence of water, liberating carbon dioxide, which acts as a disintegrator and produces effervescence.
- *Chewable tablets* are used when a faster rate of dissolution or buccal absorption is desired. Chewable tablets consist of a mild effervescent drug complex dispersed throughout a gum base. The drug is released from the dosage form by physical disruption associated with chewing, chemical disruption caused by the interaction with the fluids in the oral cavity, and the presence of effervescent material. For example, antacid tablets should be chewed to obtain quick indigestion relief.
- *Buccal* and *sublingual tablets* dissolve slowly in the mouth, cheek pouch (buccal), or under the tongue (sublingual). Buccal or sublingual absorption is often desirable for drugs subject to extensive hepatic metabolism, often referred to as the *first-pass effect*. Examples are isoprenaline sulfate (a bronchodilator), glyceryl trinitrate (a vasodilator), nitroglycerin, and testosterone tablets. These tablets do not contain a disintegrant and are compressed lightly to produce a fairly soft tablet.
- *Lozenges* are compressed tablets that do not contain a disintegrant. Some lozenges contain antiseptics (e.g., benzalkonium) or antibiotics for local effects in the mouth.

- *Controlled-release tablets* are used to improve patient compliance and to reduce side effects. Some water-soluble drugs are formulated as sustained-release tablets so that their release and dissolution are controlled over a long period. A hydrophobic matrix composed of carnauba wax and partially hydrogenated cottonseed oil were used to prepare sustained-release tablets of a highly water-soluble drug, ABT-089, a cholinergic channel modulator for the treatment of cognitive disorders. Theo-Dur is a controlled-release tablet of theophylline and consists of two components: a matrix of compressed theophylline crystals and coated theophylline granules embedded in the matrix. In contact with fluid, theophylline diffuses slowly through the wall of the free granules, which dissolves with time. After oral administration of Theo-Dur 300 mg tablets to human subjects, serum theophylline concentrations over 1 mg/mL were maintained over 24 hours. Core-in-cup tablets, which provide a zero-order release of ibuprofen, were developed by compressing the mixture of ethyl cellulose and carnauba wax, followed by compression with core tablets containing ibuprofen. The combination of high- and low-viscosity grades of hydroxypropyl methylcellulose (HPMC) was used as the matrix base to prepare diclofenac sodium and zileuton sustained-release tablets. A ternary polymeric matrix system composed of protein, HPMC, and highly water-soluble drugs such as diltiazem hydrochloride was developed by the direct compression method. Xanthan gum was used for a hydrophilic matrix for sustained-release ibuprofen tablets. Sustained-release tablets can also be prepared by formulating inert polymers, such as polyvinyl chloride, polyvinyl acetate, and methyl methacrylate. These polymers protect the tablet from disintegration and reduce the dissolution rate of the drug inside the tablet. Examples of commonly used sustained-release drug delivery products are listed in Table 3-2.
- *Coated tablets* are used to prevent decomposition or to minimize the unpleasant taste of certain drugs. Several types of coated tablets are made: film coated, sugar coated, gelatin coated (gel caps), or enteric coated. Enteric coatings are resistant to gastric juices but readily dissolve in the small intestine. These enteric coatings can protect drugs against decomposition in the acidic environment of the stomach. Commonly used polymers for enteric coating are acid-impermeable polymers, such as cellulose acetate trimellitate, HPMC

Table 3-2. Examples of Sustained-Release Drug Delivery Products

Dosage forms	Manufacturer	Active ingredients	Indications
Controlled-release tablets			
Theo-Dur	ALZA Corp.	Theophylline	Asthma
Abacavir (Ziagen)	GlaxoSmithKline	Nucleoside reverse transcriptase inhibitor	HIV-1 infection
Sinemet	Bristol-Myers Squibb	Carbidopa + levodopa	Parkinson's disease
Volmax	ALZA Corp.	Albuterol	Bronchospasm
Voltaren	Novartis	Diclofenac sodium	Osteoarthritis and rheumatoid arthritis
Efidac 24	ALZA Corp.	Chlorpheniramine	Allergy symptoms and nasal congestion
DynaCirc CR	Novartis	Isradipine	Hypertension
Capsules			
Dexedrine Spansules	GlaxoSmithKline	Dextroamphetamine	Narcolepsy
Adderall XL	Shire Pharmaceuticals	Amphetamine + dextroamphetamine	Attention-deficit/hyperactivity disorder (ADHD)
Ritalin LA	Novartis	Methylphenidate hydrochloride	ADHD
Videx EC	Bristol-Myers Squibb	Didanosine	HIV-1 infection
Aerosols			
Ventolin HFA	GlaxoSmithKline	Albuterol sulfate	Bronchodilator
Azmacort	Kos	Triamcinolone acetonide	Asthma
Serevent	GlaxoSmithKline	Salmeterol	Bronchodilator
Osmotic systems			
Oros System	ALZA Corp.	Oral delivery of different drugs	
Ditropan XL	ALZA Corp.	Oxybutynin chloride	Overreacting bladder
Covera-HS	Pfizer	Verapamil	Antihypertensive
Concerta	ALZA Corp.	Methylphenidate HCl	ADHD
DUROS implant systems			
Viadur	ALZA Corp.	Leuprolide	Prostate cancer
Inserts			
Pilocarpine Ocusert	ALZA Corp.	Pilocarpine	Glaucoma
Lacrisert	ALZA Corp.	Hydroxypropyl cellulose	Ophthalmic moisturizer
Progestasert	CollaGenex	Progesterone	Contraceptive
Atridox	ALZA Corp.	Doxycycline	Periodontal disease
Transdermal patches			
Alora	Watson Pharma	Estradiol	Menopausal symptoms
CombiPatch	Novartis	Estradiol/norethindrone acetate	Vasomotor symptoms associated with menopause
Androderm	Watson Pharmaceuticals	Testosterone	Testosterone deficiency
Nicotine transdermal system	Watson Pharmaceuticals	Nicotine	Smoking cessation

Table 3-2. Examples of Sustained-Release Drug Delivery Products *(Continued)*

Dosage forms	Manufacturer	Active ingredients	Indications
PEGylated proteins			
PEGIntron	Schering Corp.	PEGylated interferon	Hepatitis C
PEGASYS	Roche	PEGylated interferon + ribavirin	Hepatitis B, hepatitis C
Liposomes			
Doxil	Ortho Biotech	Doxorubicin HCl	Kaposi's sarcoma
DaunoXome	NeXstar Pharmaceuticals	Daunorubicin	Kaposi's sarcoma
Poly(lactic-co-glycolic acid)/polylactic acid microspheres			
Lupron Depot	TAP Pharmaceuticals	Luteinizing hormone-releasing hormone agonist	Prostate cancer, endometriosis
Zoladex Depot	AstraZeneca	Goserelin acetate	Prostate cancer, endometriosis
Nutropin Depot	Genentech	Recombinant human growth hormone	Growth deficiencies

phthalate, polyvinyl acetate phthalate, cellulose acetate phthalate, and EUDRAGIT. Aspirin formulated as enteric-coated sustained-release tablets has been shown to produce less gastric bleeding than do conventional aspirin preparations. Film-coated tablets are compressed tablets coated with a thin layer of a water-insoluble or water-soluble polymer, such as methylcellulose phthalate, ethylcellulose, povidone, or polyethylene glycol. Abacavir is a capsule-shaped film-coated tablet containing a nucleoside reverse transcriptase inhibitor, which is a potent antiviral agent for the treatment of HIV infection.

Tablet formulation

In addition to the drug, the following materials are added to make the powder system compatible with tablet formulation by the compression or granulation methods:

- *Diluents* or bulking agents are invariably added to very-low-dose drugs to bring overall tablet weight to at least 50 mg, which is the minimum desirable tablet weight. Commonly used diluents are lactose, dicalcium phosphate, starches, microcrystalline cellulose, dextrose, sucrose, mannitol, and sodium chloride. Dicalcium phosphate absorbs less moisture than lactose and is therefore used with hygroscopic drugs such as pethidine hydrochloride.
- *Adsorbents* are substances capable of holding quantities of fluids in an apparently dry state.

Oil-soluble drugs or fluid extracts can be mixed with adsorbents and then granulated and compressed into tablets. Examples are fumed silica, microcrystalline cellulose, magnesium carbonate, kaolin, and bentonite.

- *Moistening agents* are liquids that are used for wet granulation. Examples include water, industrial methylated spirits, and isopropanol.
- *Binding agents (adhesives)* bind powders together in the wet granulation process. They also help bind granules together during compression. Examples include starches, gelatin, PVP, alginic acid derivatives, cellulose derivatives, glucose, and sucrose. Choice of binders affects the dissolution rate. For example, the tablet formulation of furosemide with PVP as the binder has a t_{50} (time required for 50% of the drug to be released during an in vitro dissolution study) of 3.65 minutes, but with starch mucilage as the binder, the t_{50} of the tablets was 117 minutes.
- *Glidants* are added to tablet formulations to improve the flow properties of the granulations. They act by reducing interparticle friction. Commonly used glidants are fumed (colloidal) silica, starch, and talc.
- *Lubricants* have a number of functions in tablet manufacture. They prevent adherence of the tablet material to the surfaces of the punch faces and dies, reduce interparticle friction, and facilitate the smooth ejection of the tablet from the die cavity. Many lubricants also enhance the flow properties of the granules. Commonly used lubricants are magnesium stearate, talc, stearic acid and its

derivatives, PEG, paraffin, and sodium or magnesium lauryl sulfate. Among these lubricants, magnesium stearate is the most popular, because it is effective as both a die and a punch lubricant. However, for many drugs (e.g., aspirin), magnesium stearate is chemically incompatible; therefore, talc or stearic acid is often used. Most lubricants, with the exception of talc, are used in concentrations below 1%.

■ *Disintegrating agents* are added to the tablets to promote breakup or disintegration after administration, which increases the effective surface area and promotes rapid release of the drug. Disintegrants act either by bursting open the tablet or by promoting the rapid ingress of water into the center of the tablet or capsule. Examples include starches, cationic exchange resins, cross-linked PVP, celluloses, modified starches, alginic acid and alginates, magnesium aluminum silicate, and cross-linked sodium carboxymethylcellulose. Among these agents, starch is the most popular disintegrant because it has a great affinity for water and swells when moistened, thus facilitating the rupture of the tablet matrix.

Disintegration, dissolution, and absorption

A solid drug product has to disintegrate into small particles and release the drug before absorption can take place. Tablets that are intended for chewing or sustained release do not have to undergo disintegration. The various excipients for tablet formulation affect the rates of disintegration, dissolution, and absorption. Systemic absorption of most products consists of a succession of rate processes, such as

■ Disintegration of the drug product and subsequent release of drug
■ Dissolution of the drug in an aqueous environment
■ Absorption across cell membranes into the systemic circulation

In the process of tablet disintegration, dissolution, and absorption, the rate at which the drug reaches the circulatory system is determined by the slowest step in the sequence. Disintegration of a tablet is usually more rapid than drug dissolution and absorption. For the drug that has poor aqueous solubility, the rate at which the drug dissolves (dissolution) is often the slowest step, and it therefore exerts a rate-limiting effect on drug bioavailability. In contrast, for the drug that has a high aqueous solubility, the dissolution rate is rapid, and the rate at which the drug

crosses or permeates cell membranes is the slowest or rate-limiting step.

Capsules

Capsules are the dosage forms in which unit doses or powder, semisolid, or liquid drugs are enclosed in a hard or soft, water-soluble container or shell of gelatin. Coating of the capsule shell or drug particles within the capsule can affect bioavailability. There are two types of capsules: hard and soft capsules; hard gelatin capsules are more versatile for controlled drug delivery.

Hard gelatin capsules

A hard gelatin capsule consists of two pieces, a cap and a body, that fit one inside the other. They are produced empty and are then filled in a separate operation. Hard gelatin capsules are usually filled with powders, granules, or pellets containing the drug. After ingestion, the gelatin shell softens, swells, and begins to dissolve in the GI tract. Encapsulated drugs are released rapidly and dispersed easily, leading to high bioavailability. Capsules are supplied in a variety of sizes, and high-speed filling machinery capable of filling approximately 1,500 capsules per minute is available. The hard gelatin empty capsules are numbered from 000, the largest size, to 5, which is the smallest. The approximate filling capacity of capsules ranges from 6,000 to 30 mg, depending on the types and bulk densities of powdered drug materials.

Powder formulations for encapsulation into hard gelatin capsules require careful consideration of the filling process, such as lubricity, compactibility, and fluidity. Additives present in the capsule formulations, such as the amount and choice of fillers and lubricants, the inclusion of disintegrants and surfactants, and the degree of plug compaction, can influence drug release from the capsule. Formulation factors influencing drug release and bioavailability are as follows:

■ *Fillers (or diluents):* Active ingredient is mixed with a sufficient volume of a diluent—usually lactose, mannitol, starch, and dicalcium phosphate—to yield the desired amount of the drug in the capsule when the base is filled with the powder mixture.
■ *Glidants:* The flow properties of the powder blend should be adequate to ensure a uniform flow rate from the hopper. Glidants such as silica, starch, talc, and magnesium stearate are used

to improve the fluidity. The optimal concentration of the glidant used to improve the flow of a powder mixture is generally less than 1%.

- *Lubricants:* These ease the ejection of plugs by reducing adhesion of powder to metal surfaces and friction between sliding surfaces in contact with the powder. Typical lubricants for capsule formulations include magnesium stearate and stearic acid.
- *Surfactants:* These may be included in capsule formulations to increase wetting of the powder mass and to enhance drug dissolution. The most commonly used surfactants in capsule formulations are 0.1% to 0.5% sodium lauryl sulfate and sodium docusate.
- *Wetting agents:* Hydrophilic polymer is used as a wetting agent for improving the wettability of poorly soluble drugs. Powder wettability and dissolution rate of several drugs, including hexobarbital and phenytoin, from hard gelatin capsules have been shown to be enhanced if the drug is treated with methylcellulose or hydroxyethylcellulose.

Vancomycin hydrochloride is a highly hygroscopic antibiotic. To achieve acceptable stability, Eli Lilly has developed a hard gelatin capsule filled with a PEG 6,000 matrix of vancomycin hydrochloride, which produces plasma and urine levels of the antibiotic similar to those obtained with the solution of vancomycin hydrochloride. Controlled-release beads and minitablets are often filled into gelatin capsules for convenient administration of an oral controlled-release dosage form. For example, sustained-release antihistamines, antitussives, and analgesics are first preformulated into extended-release microcapsules or microspheres and then placed inside a gelatin capsule. Another example is enteric-coated lipase minitablets, which are placed in a gelatin capsule for more effective protection and dosing of these enzymes.

Soft gelatin capsules

Soft gelatin capsules are prepared from plasticized gelatin by a rotary die process. They are formed, filled, and sealed in a single operation. Soft gelatin capsules may contain a nonaqueous solution, a powder, or a drug suspension, none of which solubilize the gelatin shell. In contrast to hard gelatin capsules, soft gelatin capsules contain about 30% glycerol as a plasticizer in addition to gelatin and water. The moisture uptake of soft gelatin capsules plasticized with glycerol is considerably higher than that of hard gelatin capsules. Therefore, oxygen-sensitive drugs should not be inserted into soft gelatin capsules, nor should emulsions, because they are unstable and crack the shell of the capsule when water is lost in the manufacturing process. Extreme acidic and basic pH must also be avoided, because a pH below 2.5 hydrolyzes gelatin, while a pH above 9.0 has a tanning effect on the gelatin. Insoluble drugs should be dispersed with an agent such as beeswax, paraffin, or ethylcellulose. Surfactants are also often added to promote wetting of the ingredients. Drugs that are commercially prepared in soft capsules include declomycin, chlorotrianisene, digoxin, vitamin A, vitamin E, and chloral hydrate.

Formulation of soft gelatin capsules involves liquid, rather than powder, technology. It requires careful consideration of the composition of the gelatin shell and filling materials. The composition of the soft capsule shell consists of two main ingredients: gelatin and a plasticizer. Water is used to form the capsule, and other additives are often added as follows:

- *Gelatin:* Properties of gelatin shells are controlled by choice of gelatin grade and by adjustment of the concentration of plasticizer in the shell.
- *Plasticizers:* The main plasticizer used for soft gelatin capsules is glycerol. Sorbitol and polypropylene glycol are also used in combination with glycerol. Compared to hard gelatin capsules and tablet film coatings, a relatively large amount (~30%) of plasticizers is added in soft gelatin capsule formulation to ensure adequate flexibility.
- *Water:* The desirable water content of the gelatin solution used to produce a soft gelatin capsule shell depends on the viscosity of the gelatin used and ranges between 0.7 and 1.3 parts of water to each part of dry gelatin.
- *Other additives:* Preservatives are added to prevent mold growth in the gelatin shell. Potassium sorbate and methyl, ethyl, and propyl hydroxybenzoate are commonly used as preservatives.

Emulsions

An *emulsion* is a thermodynamically unstable system that consists of at least two immiscible liquid phases—one of which is dispersed as globules (dispersed phase) in the other, a liquid phase (continuous phase)—that are stabilized by the presence of an emulsifying agent. Emulsified systems range from lotions of relatively low viscosity to ointments and creams, which are semisolid in nature.

Types of emulsions

One liquid phase in an emulsion is essentially polar (e.g., aqueous), whereas the other is relatively nonpolar (e.g., an oil).

- *Oil-in-water emulsion:* When the oil phase is dispersed as globules throughout an aqueous continuous phase, the system is referred to as an *oil-in-water emulsion.*
- *Water-in-oil emulsion:* When the oil phase serves as the continuous phase, the emulsion is termed a *water-in-oil emulsion.*
- *Multiple (w/o/w or o/w/o) emulsions:* These are emulsions whose dispersed phase contains droplets of another phase. Multiple emulsions are of interest as delayed-action drug delivery systems.
- *Microemulsions:* These consist of homogeneous transparent systems of low viscosity that contain a high percentage of both oil and water and high concentrations of emulsifier mixture. Microemulsions form spontaneously when the components are mixed in the appropriate ratios and are thermodynamically stable.

Externally applied emulsions may be o/w or w/o. The o/w emulsions use the following emulsifiers: sodium lauryl sulfate, triethanolamine stearate, sodium oleate, and glyceryl monostearate. The w/o emulsions are used mainly for external applications and may contain one or several of the following emulsifiers: calcium palmitate, sorbitan esters (Spans), cholesterol, and wool fats.

Interfacial free energy and emulsification

Two immiscible liquids in emulsions often fail to remain mixed because of the greater cohesive force between the molecules of each separate liquid, rather than the adhesive force between the two liquids. These forces lead to phase separation, which is the state of minimum surface free energy. When one liquid is broken into small particles, the interfacial area of the globules constitutes a surface area that is enormous compared with that of the original liquid. The adsorption of a surfactant or other emulsifying agent at the globule interface lowers the oil-to-water or water-to-oil interfacial tension. In addition, the process of emulsification is made easier, and the drug's stability may be enhanced.

Emulsifying agents

Preventing coalescence requires the introduction of an emulsifying agent that forms a film around the dispersed globules. Emulsifying agents may be divided into three groups:

- *Surface-active agents:* Surfactants are adsorbed at oil–water interfaces to form monomolecular films and to reduce interfacial tensions. Unless the interfacial tension is zero, the oil droplets have a natural tendency to coalesce to reduce the area of oil–water contact. The presence of the surfactant monolayer at the surface of the droplet reduces the possibility of collisions leading to coalescence. To retain a high surface area for the dispersed phase, surface-active agents must be used to decrease the surface free energy. Often a mixture of surfactants is used: one with hydrophilic character and the other with hydrophobic character. A hydrophilic emulsifying agent is needed for the aqueous phase, and a hydrophobic emulsifying agent is needed for the oil phase. A complex film results that produces an excellent emulsion. Nonionic surfactants are widely used in the production of stable emulsions. They are less toxic than ionic surfactants and are less sensitive to electrolytes and pH variation. Examples include sorbitan esters and polysorbates.
- *Hydrophilic colloids:* A number of hydrophilic colloids are used as emulsifying agents. They include gelatin, casein, acacia, cellulose derivatives, and alginates. These materials adsorb at the oil–water interface and form multilayer films around the dispersed droplets of oil in an o/w emulsion. Hydrated lyophilic colloids differ from surfactants because they do not appreciably lower interfacial tension. Their action is caused by the strong multimolecular film's resistance to coalescence. Additionally, they increase the viscosity of the dispersion medium. Hydrophilic colloids are used for formation of o/w emulsions because the films are hydrophilic. Most cellulose derivatives are not charged but can sterically stabilize the systems.
- *Finely divided solid particles:* These particles are adsorbed at the interface between two immiscible liquid phases and form a film of particles around the dispersed globules. Finely divided solid particles that are wetted to some degree by both oil and water can act as emulsifying agents. They are concentrated at the interface, where they produce a film of particles around the dispersed droplets that prevents coalescence. Finely divided solid particles that are wetted by water form o/w emulsions; those that are wetted by oil form w/o emulsions. Examples include bentonite, magnesium hydroxide, and aluminum hydroxide.

Types of instability in emulsions

The stability of an emulsion is characterized by the absence of coalescence of the internal phase, the absence of creaming, and the maintenance of elegance with respect to appearance, odor, color, and other physical properties. An emulsion becomes unstable because of creaming, breaking, coalescence, phase inversion, and some other factors.

Creaming and sedimentation

Creaming is the upward movement of dispersed droplets relative to the continuous phase, whereas *sedimentation,* the reverse process, is the downward movement of particles. Density differences in the two phases cause these processes, which can be reversed by shaking. Creaming is undesirable, however, because a creamed emulsion increases the likelihood of coalescence because of the proximity of the globules in the cream. Factors that influence the rate of creaming are similar to those involved in the sedimentation rate of suspension particles and are indicated by Stokes's Law as follows:

$$v = \frac{d^2 (\rho_s - \rho_o) g}{18\eta_o}$$

where v is the velocity of creaming; d is the globule diameter; ρ_s and ρ_o are the densities of dispersed phase and dispersion medium, respectively; η_o is the viscosity of the dispersion medium (poise); and g is the acceleration of gravity (981 cm/s^2). According to this equation, the rate of creaming is decreased by

- A reduction in the globule size
- A decrease in the density difference between the two phases
- An increase in the viscosity of the continuous phase

This decrease may be achieved by homogenizing the emulsion to reduce the globule size and increasing the viscosity of the continuous phase by the use of thickening agents such as tragacanth or methylcellulose.

Creaming, breaking, coalescence, and aggregation

Creaming is a reversible process, whereas breaking is irreversible. When breaking occurs, simple mixing fails to resuspend the globules in a stable emulsified form. Because the film surrounding the particles has been destroyed, the oil tends to coalesce. *Coalescence* is the process by which emulsified particles merge with each other to form large particles. The major factor preventing coalescence is the mechanical strength of the interfacial barrier. Formation of a thick interfacial film is essential for minimal coalescence. In aggregation, the dispersed droplets come together but do not fuse. Aggregation is to some extent reversible.

Phase inversion

An emulsion is said to invert when it changes from an o/w to a w/o emulsion or vice versa. Inversion can be caused by adding an electrolyte or by changing the phase-to-volume ratio. For example, an o/w emulsion stabilized with sodium stearate can be inverted to a w/o emulsion by adding calcium chloride to form calcium stearate.

Microbial growth

Growth of microorganisms in an emulsion can cause physical separation of the phases. Because bacteria can degrade nonionic and anionic emulsifying agents, preservatives must be added to the product in adequate concentrations to prevent bacterial growth.

Suspensions

Suspensions are dispersions of finely divided solid particles of a drug in a liquid medium in which the drug is not readily soluble. Suspending agents are often hydrophilic colloids (e.g., cellulose derivatives, acacia, or xanthan gum) added to suspensions to increase viscosity, inhibit agglomeration, and decrease sedimentation. Highly viscous suspensions may prolong gastric emptying time, slow drug dissolution, and decrease the absorption rate. A suspension that is thixotropic as well as pseudoplastic should prove useful because it forms a gel on standing and becomes fluid when disturbed.

Desired characteristics of suspensions

- Suspended material should settle slowly and should readily disperse on gentle shaking of the container.
- Particle size of the suspension should remain fairly constant.
- The suspension should pour readily and evenly from its container.

Flocculation

The large surface area of the particles is associated with a surface free energy that makes the system thermodynamically unstable. This instability makes particles highly energetic; they tend to regroup, resulting in the decrease in total surface area and surface free energy. The particles in a liquid suspension, therefore, tend to flocculate. *Flocculation* is the formation of light, fluffy conglomerates held together by weak van der Waals forces. *Aggregation* occurs when crystals come together to form a compact cake (growth and fusing together of crystals in the precipitate to form a solid aggregate). Flocculating agents can prevent caking, whereas deflocculating agents increase the tendency to cake. Surfactants can reduce interfacial tension, but they cannot reduce it to zero, so suspensions of insoluble particles tend to have a positive finite interfacial tension, and particles tend to flocculate.

Forces at the surface of a particle affect the degree of flocculation and agglomeration in a suspension. Forces of attraction are of the London–van der Waals type, whereas repulsive forces arise from the interaction of the electric double layers surrounding each particle. When the repulsion energy is high, collision of the particles is opposed. The system remains deflocculated, and when sedimentation is complete, the particles form a close-packed arrangement with the smaller particles filling the voids between the larger ones. Those particles that are lowest in the sediment are gradually pressed together by the weight of the ones above; the energy barrier is thus overcome, allowing the particles to come into close contact with each other. Resuspending and redispersing these particles requires that the high-energy barrier be overcome. Because agitation does not easily achieve this, the particles tend to remain strongly attracted to each other and form a hard cake. When the particles are flocculated, the energy barrier is still too large to be surmounted, and so the approaching particles in the second energy minimum, which are at a distance of separation of perhaps 1,000 to 2,000 Å, are sufficient to form the loosely structural flocs.

Sedimentation of flocculated particles

Flocs tend to fall together, producing a distinct boundary between the sediment and the supernatant liquid. The liquid above the sediment is clear because even the small particles present in the system are associated with flocs. In deflocculated systems with variable particle sizes, by contrast, the large particles settle more rapidly than the smaller particles, and no clear boundary is formed. The supernatant remains turbid for a longer time.

Flocculation or deflocculation?

Whether a suspension is flocculated or deflocculated depends on the relative magnitudes of the electrostatic forces of repulsion and the forces of attraction between the particles. Flocculated systems form loose sediments that are easily redispersible, but the sedimentation rate is usually fast. In contrast, a suspension is deflocculated when the dispersed particles remain as discrete units and will settle slowly. This condition prevents the entrapment of liquid within the sediment, which leads to caking—a serious stability problem encountered in suspension formulation.

Flocculating agents

If the charge on the particle is neutralized, flocculation will occur. If a high charge density is imparted to the suspension particles, then deflocculation will be the result. The following flocculating agents are often used to convert the suspension from a deflocculated to a flocculated state:

- *Electrolytes:* The addition of an inorganic electrolyte to an aqueous suspension will alter the ζ potential of the dispersed particles. If this value is lowered sufficiently, then flocculation may occur. The most widely used electrolytes include sodium salts of acetates, phosphates, and citrates.
- *Surfactants:* Ionic surfactants may also cause flocculation by neutralizing the charge on each particle.
- *Polymeric flocculating agents:* Starches, alginates, cellulose derivatives, tragacanth, carbomers, and silicates are examples of polymeric flocculating agents that can be used to control the degree of flocculation. Their linear branched-chain molecules form a gel-like network within the system and become adsorbed on the surfaces of the dispersed particles, thus holding them in a flocculated state.

Formulation of suspensions

Physically stable suspensions can be formulated in two ways. One is to use a structured vehicle to maintain deflocculated particles in suspension. However, the major disadvantage of deflocculated systems is that when the particles eventually settle, they form a compact cake. The other is by production of flocs, which may settle rapidly but are easily resuspended with a minimum of agitation. Optimum physical stability is obtained when the suspension is formulated with flocculated particles in a structured vehicle of hydrophilic colloid type.

Ointments, Creams, and Gels

Ointments, creams, and gels are semisolid preparations intended for topical applications. These semisolid formulations are designed for local or systemic drug absorption.

Ointments are typically used as

- Emollients to make the skin more pliable
- Protective barriers to prevent harmful substances from coming in contact with the skin
- Vehicles in which to incorporate medication

Ointment bases are classified into four general groups: (1) hydrocarbon bases, (2) absorption bases, (3) water-removable bases, and (4) water-soluble bases.

Hydrocarbon bases

Hydrocarbon (oleaginous) bases are anhydrous and insoluble in water. They cannot absorb or contain water and are not washable in water.

Petrolatum is a good base for oil-insoluble ingredients. It forms an occlusive film on the skin and absorbs less than 5% water under normal conditions. Wax can be incorporated to stiffen the base. Synthetic esters are used as constituents of oleaginous bases. These esters include glycerol monostearate, isopropyl myristate, isopropyl palmitate, butyl stearate, and butyl palmitate.

Absorption bases

Absorption bases are of two types: (1) those that permit the incorporation of aqueous solutions, resulting in the formation of w/o emulsions (e.g., hydrophilic petrolatum and anhydrous lanolin), and (2) those that are already w/o emulsions (emulsion bases) and thus permit the incorporation of small additional quantities of aqueous solutions (e.g., lanolin and cold cream). These bases are useful as emollients although they do not provide the degree of occlusion afforded by the oleaginous bases. Absorption bases are also not easily removed from the skin with water. An aqueous solution may be first incorporated into the absorption base, and then this mixture added to the oleaginous base.

Water-removable bases

Emulsion, water-washable, or water-removable bases, commonly referred to as creams, represent the most commonly used type of ointment base. The majority of dermatologic drug products are formulated in an emulsion or cream base. Emulsion bases are washable and removed easily from skin or clothing. An emulsion base can be subdivided into three component parts: the oil phase, the emulsifier, and the aqueous phase. Drugs can be included in one of these phases or

added to the formed emulsion. The oil phase, also known as the *internal phase*, is typically made up of petrolatum or liquid petrolatum together with cetyl or stearyl alcohol. Following are types of emulsion bases:

- *Hydrophilic ointment* is an o/w emulsion that uses sodium lauryl sulfate as an emulsifying agent. It is readily miscible with water and is removed from the skin easily. The aqueous phase of an emulsion base contains the preservatives that are included to control microbial growth. The preservatives in the emulsion include methylparaben, propylparaben, benzyl alcohol, sorbic acid, or quaternary ammonium compounds. The aqueous phase also contains the water-soluble components of the emulsion system, together with any additional stabilizers, antioxidants, and buffers that may be necessary for stability and pH control.
- *Cold cream* is a semisolid white w/o emulsion prepared with cetyl ester wax, white wax, mineral oil, sodium borate, and purified water. Sodium borate combines with free fatty acids present in the waxes to form sodium soaps that act as the emulsifiers. Cold cream is used as an emollient and ointment base. Eucerin cream is a w/o emulsion of petrolatum, mineral oil, mineral wax, wool wax, alcohol, and Bronopol. It is frequently prescribed as a vehicle for delivery of lactic acid and glycerin to treat dry skin.
- *Lanolin* is a w/o emulsion that contains approximately 25% water and acts as an emollient and occlusive film on the skin, effectively preventing epidermal water loss.
- *Vanishing cream* is an o/w emulsion that contains a large percentage of water as well as a humectant (e.g., glycerin or propylene glycol) that retards surface evaporation. An excess of stearic acid in the formula helps to form a thin film when the water evaporates.

Water-soluble bases

Water-soluble bases may be anhydrous or may contain some water. They are washable in water and absorb water to the point of solubility. Polyethylene glycol ointment is a blend of water-soluble PEG that forms a semisolid base. This base can solubilize water-soluble drugs and some water-insoluble drugs. It is compatible with a wide variety of drugs. It contains 40% PEG 4,000 and 60% PEG 400. Another water-soluble base is the ointment prepared with propylene glycol and ethanol, which form a clear gel when mixed with 2% hydroxypropyl cellulose. This base is a commonly used dermatologic vehicle.

Incorporation of drugs into an ointment

Drugs may be incorporated into an ointment base by levigation and fusion. Normally, drug substances are in fine powdered forms before being dispersed in the vehicle. Levigation of powders into a small portion of base is facilitated by the use of a melted base or a small quantity of compatible levigation aid, such as mineral oil or glycerin. Water-soluble salts are incorporated by dissolving them in a small volume of water and incorporating the aqueous solution into a compatible base. Fusion is used when the base contains solids that have higher melting points (e.g., waxes, cetyl alcohol, or glyceryl monostearate).

Suppositories

A *suppository* is a solid dosage form intended for insertion into body orifices (e.g., rectum, vagina, or urethra). Once inserted, the suppository base melts, softens, or dissolves at body temperature, distributing its medications to the tissues of the region. Suppositories are used for local or systemic effects. Rectal suppositories intended for local action are often used to relieve the pain, irritation, itching, and inflammation associated with hemorrhoids. Vaginal suppositories intended for local effects are used mainly as contraceptives, as antiseptics in feminine hygiene, and to combat invading pathogens. The suppository base has a marked influence on the release of active constituents. Two main classes of suppository bases are in use: the glyceride-type fatty bases and the water-soluble ones. The main water-soluble and water-miscible suppository bases are glycerinated gelatin and polyethylene glycols. Polyethylene glycol suppositories do not melt at body temperature but rather dissolve slowly in the body's fluids. Examples of rectal suppositories include Thorazine (chlorpromazine) and Phenergan (promethazine).

Inserts, Implants, and Devices

Inserts, implants, and devices are used to control drug delivery for localized or systemic drug effects. In these systems, drugs are embedded into biodegradable or nonbiodegradable materials to allow slow release of the drug. The inserts, implants, and devices are inserted into a variety of cavities (e.g., vagina, buccal cavity, cul de sac of the eye, or subcutaneous tissue).

Degradable inserts consist of polyvinyl alcohol, hydroxypropyl cellulose, PVP, and hyaluronic acid. Nondegradable inserts are prepared from insoluble materials such as ethylene vinyl acetate copolymers and styrene–isoprene–styrene block copolymers. The initial use of contact lenses was for vision correction; however, they are becoming more useful as potential drug delivery devices by presoaking them in drug solutions. The use of contact lenses can simultaneously correct vision and release the drug.

A number of degradable and nondegradable inserts are currently available for ophthalmic delivery. These ophthalmic inserts can be insoluble, soluble, or bioerodible. Insoluble inserts are further classified as diffusional, osmotic, and contact lens (Figure 3-3). Ocular inserts are no more affected by nasolacrimal drainage and tear flow than conventional dosage forms; they can provide slow drug release and longer residence times in the conjunctival cul de sac. Ocusert is an interesting device consisting of a drug reservoir (pilocarpine hydrochloride in an alginate gel) enclosed by two release-controlling membranes made of ethylene vinyl acetate copolymer and enclosed by a white ring, allowing positioning of the system in the eye. Pilocarpine Ocusert has demonstrated slow release of pilocarpine, which can effectively control the increased intraocular pressure in glaucoma. Other inserts (e.g., medicated contact lenses, collagen shields, and mini-discs) have been shown to diminish the systemic absorption of ocularly applied drugs as a result of decreased drainage into the nasal cavity. Lacrisert is a soluble insert composed of hydroxypropyl cellulose and is useful in the treatment of dry eye syndrome. The device is placed in the lower fornix, where it slowly dissolves over 6–8 hours to stabilize and thicken the tear film.

In addition to ophthalmic delivery, inserts are used for localized delivery of drugs to various other tissues. For example, the Progestasert device is designed for implantation into the uterine cavity, where it releases 65 mg progesterone per day to provide contraception for 1 year. Similarly, Transderm relies on the rate-limiting polymeric membranes to control

Figure 3-3. Different Types of Ophthalmic inserts

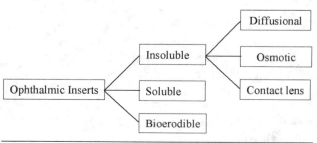

drug release. Atridox, approved by the U.S. Food and Drug Administration (FDA), is a product designed for controlled-release delivery of the antibiotic doxycycline for the treatment of periodontal disease. When injected into the periodontal cavity, the formulation sets, forming a drug delivery depot that delivers the antibiotic to the cavity.

An *implant* is a drug delivery system designed to deliver a drug moiety at a desired rate over a prolonged period. Implants are available in many forms, including polymeric implants and minipumps. Diffusional and osmotic symptoms contain a reservoir that is in contact with the inner surface of a controller, to which it supplies the drug. The reservoir contains a liquid, a gel, a colloid, a semisolid, a solid matrix, or a carrier that contains drug. Carriers consist of hydrophilic or hydrophobic polymers.

ALZA Corporation (acquired by Johnson & Johnson in May 2001) developed ALZET miniosmotic pumps, which permit easy manipulation of drug release rate over a range of periods (from 1 day to 4 weeks). ALZA Corporation also developed DUROS implants for continuous therapy for up to 1 year. The nondegradable, osmotically driven system is intended to enable delivery of small drugs, peptides, proteins, and DNA (deoxyribonucleic acid) for systemic or tissue-specific therapy. Viadur is a once-yearly implant for the palliative treatment of advanced prostate cancer.

One of the more commonly used devices is the oral osmotic pump, composed of a core tablet and a semipermeable coating with a 0.3–4.0 mm diameter hole, produced by a laser beam, for drug exit. This system requires only osmotic pressure to be effective, but the drug release rate depends on the surface area, the nature of the membrane, and the diameter of the hole. When the dosage form comes in contact with water, water is imbibed because of the resultant osmotic pressure of the core, and the drug is released from the orifice at a controlled rate.

Transdermal Drug Delivery Systems

Transdermal drug delivery systems (often called *transdermal patches*) deliver drugs directly through the skin and into the bloodstream. Percutaneous absorption of a drug generally results from direct penetration of the drug through the stratum corneum. Once through the stratum corneum, drug molecules may pass through the deeper epidermal tissues and into the dermis. When the drug reaches the vascularized dermal area, it becomes available for absorption into the general circulation. Among the factors influencing percuta-

neous absorption are the physicochemical properties of the drug, including its molecular weight, solubility, and partition coefficient; the nature of the vehicle; and the condition of the skin. Chemical permeation enhancers or iontophoresis are often used to enhance the percutaneous absorption of a drug.

In general, patches are composed of three key compartments: a protective seal that forms the external surface and protects it from damage, a compartment that holds the medication itself and has an adhesive backing to hold the entire patch on the skin surface, and a release liner that protects the adhesive layer during storage and is removed just prior to application. Examples of transdermal patches include Estraderm (estradiol), Nicoderm (nicotine), Testoderm (testosterone), Alora (estradiol), and Androderm (testosterone).

Aerosol Products

Aerosols are pressurized dosage forms designed to deliver drugs with the aid of a liquefied or propelled gas (propellant). Aerosol products consist of a pressurizable container, a valve that allows the pressurized product to be expelled from the container when the actuator is pressed, and a dip tube that conveys the formulation from the bottom of the container to the valve assembly. Inhalation devices broadly fall into three categories: pressurized metered dose inhalers (MDIs), nebulizers, and dry powder inhalers. The most commonly used inhalers on the market are MDIs. They contain active ingredient as a solution or as a suspension of fine particles in a liquefied propellant held under high pressure. MDIs use special metering valves to regulate the amount of formulation dispensed with each dose. Nebulizers do not require propellants and can generate large quantities of small droplets capable of penetrating into the lung. Sustained release of drugs, such as bronchodilators and corticosteroids for the treatment of asthma and chronic obstructive pulmonary diseases, involves encapsulation of the drugs in slowly degrading particles that can be inhaled. For accumulation in the alveolar zone of the lungs, which has a very large surface area, inhaled liquid or dry powder aerosols should have particle sizes in the range of 1–5 micrometers. Inhaled drugs play a prominent role in the treatment of asthma, because this route has significant advantages over oral or parenteral administration. Azmacort (triamcinolone acetamide), Ventolin HFA (albuterol sulfate), and Serevent (salmeterol) are examples of commercially available aerosols for the treatment of asthma.

3-6. Targeted Drug Delivery Systems

Targeted drug delivery systems are drug carrier systems that deliver the drug to the target or receptor site in a manner that provides maximum therapeutic activity, prevents degradation or inactivation during transit to the target sites, and protects the body from adverse reactions because of inappropriate disposition. Design of an effective delivery system requires a thorough understanding of the drug, the disease, and the target site (Figure 3-4). Examples include macromolecular drug carriers (protein drug carriers); particulate drug delivery systems (e.g., microspheres, nanospheres, and liposomes); monoclonal antibodies; and cells. Plasma clearance kinetics, tissue distribution, metabolism, and cellular interactions of a drug can be controlled by the use of a site-specific delivery system. Targeting of drugs to specific sites in the body can be achieved by linking particulate systems or macromolecular carriers to monoclonal antibodies or to cell-specific ligands (e.g., asialofetuin, glycoproteins, or immunoglobulins) or by altering the surface characteristics so that they are not recognized by the reticuloendothelial systems.

Macromolecular Carrier Systems

Both natural and synthetic water-soluble polymers have been used as macromolecular drug carriers. The drug can be attached to the polymer chain either directly or via a spacer. Attachment of PEG to proteins can protect them from rapid hydrolysis or degradation within the body, increase blood circulation time, and lower the immunogenicity of proteins. PEGylated forms of interferons; PegIntron and PEGASYS (for treatment of hepatitis C, to reduce dosing frequency from daily injections to once-weekly injection dosing); adenosine deaminase; and L-asparaginase are currently on the market. PEGylation improves macromole solubility and stability by minimizing the uptake by the cells of the reticuloendothelial system. Because PEG drug conjugates are not well absorbed from the gut, they are mainly used as injectables. The drug–polymer conjugate may also contain a receptor-specific ligand to achieve selective access to, and interaction with, the target cells.

Particulate Drug Delivery Systems

Many particulate carriers have been designed for drug delivery and targeting. They include liposomes, micelles, microspheres, and nanoparticles.

Liposomes

Liposomes are microscopic phospholipid vesicles composed of uni- or multilamellar lipid bilayers surrounding compartments. Multilamellar vesicles have diameters in the range of 1.0–5.0 micrometers. Sonication of multilamellar vesicles results in the production of small unilamellar vesicles with diameters in the range of 0.02–0.08 micrometers. Large unilamellar vesicles can be made by evaporation under reduced pressure, resulting in liposomes with a diameter of 0.1–1.0 micrometer. The bilayer-forming lipid is the essential part of the lamellar structure, while the other compounds are added to impart certain characteristics to the vesicles. Water-soluble drugs can be entrapped in liposomes by intercalation in the aqueous bilayers, whereas lipid-soluble drugs can be entrapped within the hydrocarbon interiors of the lipid bilayers. Liposomes can encapsulate low-molecular-weight drugs, proteins, peptides, oligonucleotides, and genes. The use of the antifungal agent amphotericin B formulated in liposomes has been approved by the FDA. Because conventional liposomes are recognized by the immune system as foreign bodies, ALZA Corporation developed STEALTH liposomes, which evade recognition by the immune system because of their unique polyethylene glycol coating. Doxil is a STEALTH liposome formulation of doxorubicin, used for the treatment of AIDS-related Kaposi's sarcoma.

Microparticles and nanoparticles

Microencapsulation is a technique that involves the encapsulation of small particles or the solution of drugs in a polymer film or coat. Different methods of microencapsulation result in either microcapsules or microspheres. For example, interfacial polymerization of a monomer usually produces microcapsules,

---

Figure 3-4. Essential Components of Drug Delivery

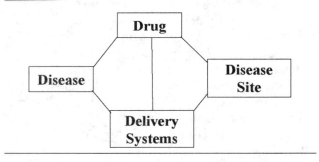

whereas solvent evaporation may result in microspheres or microcapsules, depending on the amount of drug loading. A microcapsule is a reservoir-type system in which the drug is located centrally within the particle, whereas a microsphere is a matrix-type system in which the drug is dispersed throughout the particle. Microcapsules usually release their drug at a constant rate (zero-order release), whereas microspheres typically give a first-order release of drugs. Low-molecular-weight drugs, proteins, oligonucleotides, and genes can be encapsulated into microparticles to provide their sustained release at disease sites.

The most commonly used method of microencapsulation is coacervation, which involves addition of a hydrophilic substance to a colloidal drug dispersion. The hydrophilic substance, which acts as a coating material, may be selected from a variety of natural and synthetic polymers, including shellacs, waxes, gelatin, starches, cellulose acetate phthalate, and ethylcellulose, among others. Following dissolution of the coating materials, the drug inside the microcapsule is available for dissolution and absorption.

Biodegradable polylactide and its copolymers with glycolide [poly(lactic-co-glycolic acid), or PLGA] are commonly used for preparation of microparticles from which the drug can be released slowly over a period of a month or so. Microspheres can be used in a wide variety of dosage forms, including tablets, capsules, and suspensions. Lupron Depot from TAP Pharmaceuticals is an FDA-approved preparation of PLGA microspheres for sustained release of a small peptide luteinizing hormone-releasing hormone agonist. More recently, PLGA microspheres of recombinant human growth hormone have been developed and marketed successfully by Genentech under the trade name Nutropin Depot.

3-7. Key Points

■ Fick's first law of diffusion describes the diffusion process under steady-state conditions when the drug concentration gradient does not change with time.

■ Drug absorption depends not only on the fraction of un-ionized form of the drug but also on the surface area available for absorption.

■ The Noyes–Whitney equation can be used for determining the dissolution rate of a drug from its dosage form, whereas the Arrhenius equation can be used for determining the shelf life of a drug dosage form.

■ Surfactants consist of hydrophilic and hydrophobic groups and can be used as emulsifying agents to reduce interfacial tensions.

■ The pharmaceutical dosage form contains the active drug ingredient in association with non-drug (usually inert) ingredients (excipients). Together they form the vehicle, or formulation matrix.

■ Water-soluble drugs are often formulated as sustained-release tablets so that their release and dissolution rates can be controlled, whereas enteric-coated tablets are used to protect drugs from gastric degradation.

■ Capsules are solid dosage forms with hard or soft gelatin shells that contain drugs and excipients.

■ Aerosols are pressurized dosage forms designed to deliver drugs to pulmonary tissues with the aid of a liquefied or propelled gas.

■ Inserts, implants, and devices allow slow release of the drug into a variety of cavities (e.g., vagina, buccal cavity, cul de sac of the eye, and skin).

■ Transdermal patches deliver drugs directly through the skin and into the bloodstream.

■ The drug delivery system deals with the pharmaceutical formulation and the dynamic interactions among the drug, its formulation matrix, its container, and the physiologic milieu of the patient. These dynamic interactions are the subject of pharmaceutics.

■ Macromolecular drug carriers, such as protein–polymer conjugates, and particulate delivery systems, such as microspheres and liposomes, are commonly used for delivery of drugs with low molecular weight, such as peptides and proteins, to different disease targets.

■ Targeted (or site-specific) drug delivery systems are used for drug delivery to the target or receptor site in a manner that provides maximum therapeutic activity, by preventing degradation during transit to the target site while avoiding delivery to nontarget sites.

3-8. Questions

1. Which of the following is true for Fick's first law of diffusion?

   A. It refers to the non-steady-state flow.
   B. The amount of material flowing through a unit cross-section of a barrier in unit time is known as the concentration gradient.

C. Flux of material is proportional to the concentration gradient.

D. Diffusion occurs in the direction of increasing concentration.

E. All of the above are true.

2. Which equation describes the rate of drug dissolution from a tablet?

A. Fick's law

B. Henderson–Hasselbalch equation

C. Michaelis–Menten equation

D. Noyes–Whitney equation

E. All of the above

3. The pH of a buffer system can be calculated with

A. the Henderson–Hasselbalch equation.

B. the Noyes–Whitney equation.

C. the Michaelis–Menten equation.

D. Yong's equation.

E. all of the above.

4. Which of the following is *not* true for gas adsorption on a solid?

A. Chemical adsorption is reversible.

B. Physical adsorption is based on weak van der Waals forces.

C. Chemical adsorption may require activation energy.

D. Chemical adsorption is specific to the substrate.

E. All of the above.

5. What is bioavailability?

A. Bioavailability is the measurement of the rate and extent of active drug that reaches the systemic circulation.

B. It is the relationship between the physical and chemical properties of a drug and its systemic absorption.

C. It is the movement of the drug into body tissues over time.

D. It is dissolution of the drug in the GI tract.

E. All of the above describe bioavailability.

6. Which of the following may be used to assess the relative bioavailability of two chemically equivalent drug products in a crossover study?

A. Dissolution test

B. Peak concentration

C. Time-to-peak concentration

D. Area under the plasma-level time curve

E. All of the above

7. What condition usually increases the rate of drug dissolution for a tablet?

A. Increase in the particle size of the drug

B. Decrease in the surface area of the drug

C. Use of the ionized, or salt, form of the drug

D. Use of the free acid or free base form of the drug

E. Use of sugar coating around the tablet

8. The characteristics of an active transport process include all of the following *except*

A. active transport moves drug molecules against a concentration gradient.

B. active transport follows Fick's law of diffusion.

C. active transport is a carrier-mediated transport system.

D. active transport requires energy.

E. active transport of drug molecules may be saturated at high drug concentrations.

9. Which of the following dosage forms may use surface-active agents in their formulations?

A. Emulsions

B. Suspensions

C. Colloidal dosage forms

D. Creams

E. All of the above

10. Which of the following statements about lyophilic colloidal dispersions is true?

A. They tend to be more sensitive to the addition of electrolytes than do lyophobic systems.

B. They tend to be more viscous than lyophobic systems.

C. They can be precipitated by prolonged dialysis.

D. They separate rapidly.

E. All of the above.

11. Which of the following is *not* true for tablet formulations?

A. A disintegrating agent promotes granule flow.

B. Lubricants prevent adherence of granules to the punch faces of the tabletting machine.

C. Glidants promote flow of the granules.
D. Binding agents are used for adhesion of powder into granules.
E. All of the above.

12. The absorption rate of a drug is most rapid when the drug is formulated as

A. a controlled-release product.
B. a hard gelatin capsule.
C. a compressed tablet.
D. a solution.
E. a suspension.

13. The passage of drug molecules from a region of high drug concentration to a region of low drug concentration is known as

A. active transport.
B. simple diffusion or passive transport.
C. pinocytosis.
D. bioavailability.
E. biopharmaceutics.

14. Which equation is used to predict the stability of a drug product at room temperature from experiments at increased temperatures?

A. Stokes's equation
B. Arrhenius equation
C. Michaelis–Menten equation
D. Fick's equation
E. Noyes–Whitney equation

15. Choose which of the following statements is true.

A. Flocculation is desirable for pharmaceutical suspensions.
B. The diffusion rate of molecules of a smaller particle size is less than that of molecules of a larger particle size.
C. Particle size of molecular dispersions is larger than a coarse dispersion.
D. Pseudoplastic flow is shear-thickening type, and dilatant is shear-thinning type.
E. All of the above.

16. Choose which of the following statements is false.

A. The Henderson–Hasselbalch equation describes the effect of physical parameters on the stability of pharmaceutical suspensions.

B. The passive diffusion rate of hydrophobic drugs across biological membranes is higher than that of hydrophilic compounds.
C. When the dispersed phase in an emulsion formulation is heavier than the dispersion medium, creaming can still occur.
D. Targeted drug delivery systems deliver the drug to the target or receptor site in a manner that provides maximum therapeutic activity.
E. All of the above.

17. Which of the following is an emulsifying agent?

A. Sorbitan mono-oleate (Span 80)
B. Polyoxyethylene sorbitan mono-oleate (Tween 80)
C. Sodium lauryl sulfate
D. Gum acacia
E. All of the above

18. Which of the following surfactants is incompatible with bile salts?

A. Polysorbate 80
B. Potassium stearate
C. Sodium lauryl sulfate
D. Benzalkonium chloride
E. All of the above

19. Which of the following statements is false?

A The partition coefficient is the ratio of drug solubility in n-octanol to that in water.
B. Absorption of a weak electrolyte drug does not depend on the extent to which the drug exists in its un-ionized form at the absorption site.
C. The drug dissolution rate can be determined using the Noyes–Whitney equation.
D. Amorphous forms of drug have faster dissolution rates than do crystalline forms.
E. All of the above.

20. Which of the following statements is true?

A. Most substances acquire a surface charge by ionization, ion adsorption, and ion dissolution.
B. The term *surface tension* is used for liquid-vapor and solid-vapor tensions
C. At the isoelectric point, the total number of positive charges is equal to the total number of negative charges.
D. All of the above.
E. None of the above.

21. Agents that may be used in the enteric coating of tablets include

    A. hydroxypropyl methylcellulose.
    B. carboxymethylcellulose.
    C. cellulose acetate phthalate.
    D. all of the above.
    E. none of the above.

3-9. Answers

1. **C.** Fick's first law of diffusion states that the amount of material flow through a unit cross-section of a barrier in unit time, which is known as the *flux*, is proportional to the concentration gradient. Fick's first law of diffusion describes the diffusion process under steady-state conditions where the concentration gradient does not change with time.

2. **D.** The Noyes–Whitney equation describes the rate of drug dissolution from a tablet. Fick's first law of diffusion is similar to the Noyes–Whitney equation in that both equations describe drug movement attributable to a concentration gradient. The Michaelis–Menten equation involves enzyme kinetics, whereas Henderson–Hasselbalch equations are used for determination of pH of the buffer and the extent of ionization of a drug molecule.

3. **A.** The Henderson–Hasselbalch equation for a weak acid and its salt is represented as $pH = pK_a + \log [salt]/[acid]$, where pK_a is the negative log of the dissolution constant of a weak acid, as [salt]/[acid] is the ratio of the molar concentration of salt and acid used to prepare a buffer.

4. **A.** Chemical absorption is an irreversible process that is specific and may require activation energy, whereas physical adsorption is reversible and associated with van der Waals forces.

5. **A.** Bioavailability is the measurement of the rate and extent of systemic circulation of an active drug.

6. **D.** The plasma drug concentration versus time curve measures the bioavailability of a drug from a product. The peak plasma drug concentration (C_{max}) relates to the intensity of the pharmacologic response, while the time for peak plasma drug concentration (T_{max}) relates to the rate of systemic absorption.

7. **C.** The ionized, or salt, form of a drug is generally more water soluble and therefore dissolves more rapidly than the nonionized (free acid or free base) form of the drug. According to the Noyes-Whitney equation, the dissolution rate is directly proportional to the surface area and inversely proportional to the particle size. Therefore, an increase in the particle size or a decrease in the surface area slows the dissolution rate.

8. **B.** In passive transport, a drug travels from a high concentration to a low concentration, whereas active transport moves drug molecules against a concentration gradient and requires energy.

9. **E.** Surface-active agents facilitate emulsion formation by lowering the interfacial tension between the oil and water phases. Adsorption of surfactants on insoluble particles enables these particles to be dispersed in the form of a suspension.

10. **B.** Most lyophilic colloids are organic molecules (including gelatin and acacia); they spontaneously form colloidal solutions and tend to be viscous. Dispersion of lyophilic colloids is stable in the presence of electrolytes.

11. **A.** Disintegrating agents are added to the tablets to promote breakup of the tablets when placed in the aqueous environment. Lubricants are required to prevent adherence of the granules to the punch faces and dies. Glidants are added to tablet formulations to improve the flow properties of the granulations. Binding agents are added to bind powders together in the granulation process.

12. **D.** For a drug in solution, no dissolution is required before absorption. Consequently, compared with other drug formulations, a drug in aqueous solution has the highest bioavailability rate and is often used as the reference preparation for other formulations.

13. **B.** In simple diffusion or passive transport, a drug travels from a high concentration to a low concentration, whereas active transport moves drug molecules against a concentration gradient and requires energy. Pinocytosis is a vesicular transport process of engulfment of small particles or fluid volumes.

14. **B.** Stability at room temperature can be predicted from accelerated testing data by the Arrhenius equation: $\log (k_2/k_1) = E_a(T_2 - T_1)/(2.303\ RT_2T_1)$, where k_2 and k_1 are the rate constants at the absolute temperatures T_2 and

T_1, respectively; R is the gas constant; and E_a is the energy of activation. Stokes's equation is used to determine the sedimentation rate of a suspension, whereas the Noyes–Whitney equation is used to determine the dissolution rate.

15. **A.** Flocculation is the formation of light, fluffy conglomerates held together by weak van der Waals forces and is a reversible process. Pseudoplastic flow is a shear-thinning process, whereas dilatant is a shear-thickening type process.

16. **A.** The Henderson–Hasselbalch equation describes the relationship between ionized and nonionized species of a weak electrolyte.

17. **E.** Sorbitan mono-oleate (Span 80), polyoxyethylene sorbitan monooleate (Tween 80), sodium lauryl sulfate, and gum acacia are surfactants used as emulsifiers.

18. **D.** Benzalkonium chloride is a cationic surfactant and can interact with bile salts.

19. **B.** According to pH partition theory, absorption of a weak electrolyte drug depends on the extent to which the drug exists in its unionized form at the absorption site. However, pH partition theory often does not hold true, because most weakly acidic drugs are well absorbed from the small intestine, possibly because of the large epithelial surface areas of the organ.

20. **D.** Most substances acquire a surface charge by ionization, ion adsorption, and ion dissolution. At the isoelectric point, the total number of positive charges is equal to the total number of negative charges.

21. **C.** An enteric-coated tablet has a coating that remains intact in the stomach, but dissolves in the intestine when the pH exceeds 6. Enteric-coating materials include cellulose acetate trimellitate, polyvinyl acetate phthalate, and hydroxypropyl methylcellulose phthalate.

3-10. References

Ansel HC, Popovich NG, Allen LV, eds. *Pharmaceutical Dosage Forms and Drug Delivery Systems*. 6th ed. Malvern, Pa.: Williams & Wilkins; 1995.

Aulton ME, ed. *Pharmaceutics: The Science of Dosage Form Design*. New York: Churchill Livingstone; 1988.

Banker GS, Rhodes CT, eds. *Modern Pharmaceutics*. 3rd ed. New York: Marcel Dekker; 1995.

Block LH, Collins CC. Biopharmaceutics and drug delivery systems. In: Shargel L, Mutnick AH, Souney PH, Swanson LN, eds. *Comprehensive Pharmacy Review*. New York: Lippincott Williams & Wilkins; 2001:78–91.

Block LH, Yu ABC. Pharmaceutical principles and drug dosage forms. In: Shargel L, Mutnick AH, Souney PH, Swanson LN, eds. *Comprehensive Pharmacy Review*. New York: Lippincott Williams & Wilkins; 2001:28–77.

Florence AT, Attwood D. *Physicochemical Principles of Pharmacy*. 3rd ed. Palgrave, N.Y.: Macmillan; 1998.

Gennaro AR, Gennaro AL, eds. *Remington: The Science and Practice of Pharmacy*. Baltimore: Lippincott, Williams & Wilkins; 2000.

Hillery AM. Advanced drug delivery and targeting: An introduction. In: Hillery AM, Lloyd AW, Swarbrick J, eds. *Drug Delivery and Targeting: For Pharmacists and Pharmaceutical Scientists*. New York: Taylor & Francis; 2001:63–82.

Mahato RI. *Pharmaceutical Dosage Forms and Drug Delivery*. New York: Taylor & Francis; 2007.

Martin A. *Physical Pharmacy*. 4th ed. Baltimore: Lippincott Williams & Wilkins; 1993.

Mathiowitz E, Kretz MR, Bannon-Peppas L. Microencapsulation. In: Mathiowitz E, ed. *Encyclopedia of Controlled Drug Delivery*. New York: John Wiley & Sons; 1999:493–546.

Washington N, Washington C, Wilson CG. *Physiological Pharmaceutics: Barriers to Drug Absorption*. 2nd ed. New York: Taylor & Francis; 2001.

Compounding

Charles N. May, BSPh, MSHP

4

4-1. Introduction

Pharmacists extemporaneously compound medications to provide patients and prescribers more options for treatment and therapy than are provided by commercially available products. Patients need individualized custom-prepared medications for many reasons, including the following: (1) some therapeutic agents are not commercially manufactured; (2) some therapeutic agents are not manufactured in the form or size needed; (3) some manufactured therapeutic agents contain offending ingredients, such as dyes, preservatives, fillers, and binders; (4) some manufactured therapeutic agents contain offending flavors, fragrances, or colors; and (5) some patients do not fit into the standard categories that manufactured products treat. In addition, from time to time commercially manufactured products are unavailable for a variety of reasons, such as (1) the drug is recalled, (2) the manufacturing facility is closed down, (3) a strike or disaster occurs, (4) the product is no longer commercially profitable, or (5) the manufacturer no longer supplies the product for other corporate reasons. Several segments of the population are not properly served by pharmaceutical manufacturers, including pediatric patients, geriatric patients, veterinary patients, and patients with rare or very complicated disease states. Prescribers and pharmacists working very closely with patients improve the quality of life for those patients as no other practice can.

4-2. Philosophy of Compounding

- Compounding is extemporaneous per patient.
- It fulfills needs for unique dosage forms and sizes.

- The pharmacist works as part of a three-member team—the patient, the pharmacist, and the prescriber—to satisfy a patient's unique needs that cannot be satisfied by commercially available products.
- The pharmacist follows up with the patient, the prescriber, or both to determine if the compounded preparation needs further adjustment or refinement to completely satisfy the patient's needs.

4-3. Compounding versus Manufacturing

Compounding

- Compounded preparations are patient specific in conjunction with the prescriber.
- They are regulated by the state board of pharmacy.
- Compounded preparations are not advertised.
- Compounded preparations have beyond-use dates.
- Compounded preparations are not prepared in advance except in the case of documented usage or demand.
- Compounded preparations have no National Drug Code (NDC) number.

Manufacturing

- Products are subject to an approved New Drug Application (NDA).
- Products are subject to U.S. Food and Drug Administration (FDA)–approved labeling.
- Products are manufactured in FDA-approved plants in accordance with good manufacturing practices.

- Products may be advertised.
- Products carry an expiration date.
- Products carry an NDC number.
- Products are regulated by the FDA.

4-4. Guidelines for Compounding

The following are published guidelines pharmacists use in designing and carrying out their compounding activities. Pharmacists' compounding practices are regulated by the laws of the state board of pharmacy of the state in which the pharmacist practices.

Allen LV Jr. Extemporaneous prescription compounding. In: *Remington: The Science and Practice of Pharmacy*, 21st ed. Baltimore: Lippincott Williams & Wilkins; 2006:1903–12.

National Association of Boards of Pharmacy. *Good Compounding Practices Applicable to State Licensed Pharmacies*. Park Ridge, Ill.: National Association of Boards of Pharmacy; 1993.

U.S. Food and Drug Administration. Pharmacy compounding. In: *Compliance Policy Guide, Compliance Policy Guidance for FDA Staff and Industry*. Washington, D.C.; 2002. Section 460. 200.

U.S. Pharmacopeial Convention. Good compounding practices: chapter 1075. In: *U.S. Pharmacopeia 32/National Formulary 27*. Rockville, Md.: U.S. Pharmacopeial Convention; 2009:523–26.

U.S. Pharmacopeial Convention. Pharmaceutical calculations in prescription compounding: chapter 1160. In: *U.S. Pharmacopeia 32/National Formulary 27*. Rockville, Md.: U.S. Pharmacopeial Convention; 2009:674–83.

U.S. Pharmacopeial Convention. Pharmaceutical compounding–nonsterile preparations: chapter 795. In: *U.S. Pharmacopeia 32/National Formulary 27*. Rockville, Md.: U.S. Pharmacopeial Convention; 2009:314–18.

U.S. Pharmacopeial Convention. Prescription balances and volumetric apparatus: chapter 1176. *U.S. Pharmacopeia 32/National Formulary 27*. Rockville, Md.: U.S. Pharmacopeial Convention; 2009:691–92.

U.S. Pharmacopeial Convention. Quality assurance in pharmaceutical compounding: chapter 1163. In: *U.S. Pharmacopeia 32/National Formulary 27*. Rockville, Md.: U.S. Pharmacopeial Convention; 2009:684–86.

4-5. Requirements

Pharmacy

Space

- An appropriate amount is required; a dedicated area is ideal.
- Space should be properly arranged and maintained, with ingredients and equipment close at hand.
- A controlled atmosphere is necessary, with limited traffic flow and air flow away from operator.
- Separate areas are needed for sterile and nonsterile compounding.
- A source of potable water and purified water (i.e., sink) should be readily available.
- Facility should be constructed of materials that are as nonporous and seamless as possible; a well lit space with bright fixtures, walls, and floors gives a clean, professional appearance.

Equipment

- Appropriate measuring devices are required (e.g., graduated cylinders, pharmacy graduates, pipettes).
- Appropriate balances for weighing are necessary (e.g., an electronic balance or class A prescription balance).
- Appropriate mixing devices are required (e.g., Wedgwood, porcelain, and glass mortars and pestles, blenders).
- Appropriate counters and shelves are needed; sufficient countertop space must be available so that compounding will not be cramped, and shelving must be sufficient and appropriately located so that ingredients can be convenient and properly stored.
- Appropriate processing equipment is necessary (e.g., hot plates and magnetic stirrers, ointment mills, electronic mortar and pestle, tablet pulverizers).
- Appropriate safety equipment must be available (e.g., rubber gloves, face masks, hair covers, gowns, and goggles for personnel; devices that gently exhaust the air from the work area to keep the air free of contamination with ingredients; and containment areas for personnel who are working with light, fine, fluffy ingredients or ingredients that are irritating or foul smelling).

- Appropriate packaging equipment is required (e.g., capsule-filling machines, tube-sealing equipment, calibrated measuring and filling devices)
- Appropriate computer equipment should be available (e.g., for processing labels, profiles, and formulas and for maintaining required records regarding ingredients)

Formulas

Ingredient classification and quality

- USP/NF: United States Pharmacopeia/National Formulary (ingredients meet official standards and are suitable for human use)
- FCC: Food Chemicals Codex (food grade)
- ACS: American Chemical Society (reagent grade)
- AR: analytical reagent (high purity)
- CP: chemically pure (uncertain quality)
- Tech: technical (industrial quality)

Supplies

- Supplies include weigh boats, weighing paper (parchment and glassine), filter paper, ointment paper, spatulas (stainless steel and hard rubber), stirring rods (glass and polypropylene), rubber scrapers, beakers, flasks, funnels, casseroles, and containers of all types and sizes to properly package all the unique dosage forms and sizes patients require.
- Supplies also include all sizes of prescription bottles, powder jars, capsule vials, and ointment jars as well as ointment tubes, troche molds, plastic suppository molds, powder paper boxes, suppository boxes, "ride-up" tubes, and so forth.

Records

- An exact record of each compounded prescription must be made and maintained.
- A chronological record of each day's compounding activity should be made and kept for future reference and use.
- A Master Formula card must be in place for each preparation compounded, and it must be approved by and signed and dated by the pharmacist in charge.

Policies and procedures

- Standard operating procedures (SOPs)
- Material safety data sheets (MSDSs)

- Certificates of analysis (COAs)
- Quality assurance checks
- Other policies and procedures

The Pharmacist

- *Interest:* A distinct interest in being creative, solving difficult patient problems, working closely with prescribers and patients, and formulating and compounding special customized medications is very important.
- *Education:* The emphasis on compounding varies among colleges of pharmacy. Even graduates of programs that require students to compound a wide variety of formulations may find that they need more training.
- *Training:* Additional training is often obtained through continuing education courses, seminars, professional development programs, or professional associations.
- *Experience:* Experience in compounding is perhaps the key to how effective a pharmacist can be in creating special formulations that make a significant difference in a patient's life when everything else up to that point has failed. It enables the pharmacist to suggest to the prescriber a therapeutic agent in a unique dosage form that has a better chance of solving the patient's problem. Conversely, a pharmacist with less-than-optimal experience and interest may compound a medication that is not effective and thus not satisfy the patient's need—and perhaps may even undermine the prescriber's confidence in all compounded medications. Pharmacists who compound must be certain that they possess the appropriate requisites for the level of compounding they perform.
- *Compounding support:* Compounding pharmacists should join professional organizations that support compounding such as the International Academy of Compounding Pharmacists. They should subscribe to journals that focus on compounding such as the *International Journal of Pharmaceutical Compounding* or the *U.S. Pharmacist.* They should also use the professional resources of the companies that fulfill their compounding needs.

Professional Considerations

- Is there a commercially available product in the exact dosage, size, form, and package needed?

- Is there an alternative product that will completely satisfy the patient's requirements?
- Can I do the required pharmaceutical calculations to make and package the preparation?

Quality Control Requirements

- Accurate calculations
- Accurate weights
- Accurate measurements
- Proper processing techniques
- Proper packaging
- Proper records
- Proper labeling, including beyond-use date

Beyond-Use Dates

- Pharmacists assign beyond-use dates to compounded preparations to provide patients with guidance in the proper use of the preparation.
- The goal is to provide a beyond-use date that will allow the patient enough time to fully use the amount of preparation dispensed, but not enough time to allow the preparation to degrade or lose potency or be stored for future use.
- If the pharmacist does not have a reference on stability of the specific dosage form or if experience with it is insufficient, the USP guidelines are followed.

4-6. Compounded Preparations

Solutions

- *Definition:* Solutions are chemically and physically homogenous mixtures of two or more substances.
- *Types:* Solutions can be syrups, elixirs, aromatic waters, tinctures, spirits, nonaqueous, and so forth.
- *Properties:* Solutions are hypertonic, isotonic, hypotonic, osmolar, osmolal, and so forth.
- *Stability:* Stability of solutions is enhanced by adjusting pH or adding preservatives, antioxidants, and so forth.
- *Rate of dissolution:* The rate of dissolution is enhanced by stirring, heat, particle-size reduction, and so forth.
- *Beyond-use dates:* Aqueous solutions have short beyond-use dates.

- *Testing:* Organoleptic, pH, and other testing is performed.

An example of an isotonic *aqueous* solution follows:

Ephedrine sulfate	1%
Sodium chloride	qs
Purified water, qs ad	30 mL
M.ft. isotonic solution	

Steps in compounding are as follows:

1. Calculate the required quantity of each ingredient (NaCl equivalent of ephedrine sulfate is 0.2).
2. Accurately weigh or measure each ingredient.
3. Dissolve the solid ingredients in about 25 mL of purified water.
4. Add sufficient purified water to measure 30 mL.

The following is an example of a *nonaqueous* solution:

Urea	10 g
Salicylic acid	5 g
Coal tar solution	5 mL
Propylene glycol, qs ad	100 mL

Steps in compounding are as follows:

1. Accurately weigh or measure each ingredient.
2. Dissolve the urea and salicylic acid in about 75 mL of propylene glycol.
3. Add the coal tar solution and mix well.
4. Add sufficient propylene glycol to measure 100 mL.

Note: If using a mechanical stirrer, it may take significant time to dissolve the urea and salicylic acid.

Suspensions

- *Definition:* A suspension is a two-phased system containing a finely divided solid in a vehicle.
- *Requirement:* Drug is uniformly dispersed throughout vehicle.
- *Concentration:* Suspending agents are typically used in a concentration of 0.5–6.0%.
- *Viscosity:* The vehicle has enough viscosity to keep drug particles suspended separately.
- *Insolubility:* The active ingredient is insoluble in vehicle.
- *Tip:* Wet insoluble powder with vehicle-miscible liquid.
- *Advantage:* A suspension allows the preparation of a liquid form of an insoluble drug.
- *Stability:* Stability is enhanced by adding a preservative.
- *Testing:* Organoleptic, pH, and other testing is performed.

Categories of suspending agents

- *Natural hydrocolloids:* Acacia, alginic acid, gelatin, guar gum, sodium alginate, tragacanth, xanthan gum
- *Semisynthetic hydrocolloids:* Ethylcellulose, methylcellulose, sodium carboxymethylcellulose
- *Synthetic hydrocolloids:* Carbomers (Carbopol), poloxamers (Pluronic), polyvinyl alcohol, polyvinylpyrrolidone
- *Clays:* Bentonite, magnesium aluminum silicate (Veegum)

An example of an oral suspension follows:

Progesterone, micronized	1.2 g
Glycerin	3 mL
Methylcellulose 2% solution	30 mL
Flavored syrup, qs ad	60 mL

Steps in compounding are as follows:

1. Accurately weigh or measure each ingredient.
2. In a glass mortar, wet the progesterone with the glycerin, making a thick paste.
3. Slowly add the methylcellulose solution while triturating.
4. When mixed thoroughly, pour into a graduate.
5. Add small amounts of syrup in mortar, mix, and add to graduate until the desired volume is reached.

Emulsions

- *Definition:* An emulsion is a two-phase system of two immiscible liquids, one of which is dispersed throughout the other as small droplets.
- *Components:* An emulsion has a dispersion medium or external or continuous phase, an internal or discontinuous or dispersed phase, and an emulsifying agent.
- *Type:* Types are oil in water (o/w) and water in oil (w/o), depending on which is the internal and which is the external phase
- *Emulsifying agents:* Emulsifying agents can be natural gums (acacia, agar, chondrus, pectin, tragacanth) or hydrophilic or lipophilic agents (the esters of sorbitan)
- *Lipophilic agents:* Trade names for lipophilic agents include Arlacel and Span
- *Hydrophilic agents:* Trade names for hydrophilic agents include Myrj and Tween
- *Hydrophilic–lipophilic balance:* A lower hydrophilic–lipophilic balance (HLB) value favors a w/o emulsion; a higher HLB value favors an o/w emulsion. Agents with an HLB value of 1–9 are considered to be lipophilic; agents with an HLB value of 10 and above are considered to be hydrophilic.
- *Other agents:* Other agents include bentonite, cholesterol, gelatin, lecithin, methylcellulose, soaps of fatty acids, sodium docusate, sodium lauryl sulfate, and triethanolamine.
- *Equipment:* Equipment includes mortar and pestle, homogenizers, colloid mill, mechanical mixers, agitators, and ultrasonic vibrators.
- *Solids:* Solid ingredients should be dissolved before they are incorporated into the emulsion, or if a sizable quantity is added, a levigating or wetting agent may be needed.
- *Flavors:* Flavors should be incorporated into the external phase.
- *Preservatives:* Preservatives should be added in the aqueous phase; they may also be added in the oily phase, if necessary.
- *Stability:* Emulsions either cream or crack.
- *Continental method:* The Continental or dry gum method of preparing an emulsion nucleus involves using the oil:water:dry gum emulsifier in a 4:2:1 ratio.
- *Advantages:* An emulsion can be used to mask taste, improve palatability, increase absorption, and enhance bioavailability.
- *Testing:* Organoleptic testing is performed.

An example of preparing an emulsion by the Continental or dry gum or 4:2:1 method follows:

Cod liver oil	50 mL
Acacia	12.5 g
Syrup	10 mL
Flavor oil	0.4 mL
Purified water, qs ad	100 mL

Steps in compounding are as follows:

1. Accurately weigh or measure each ingredient.
2. Place the cod liver oil in a dry mortar.
3. Add the acacia and give it a very quick mix.
4. Add 25 mL of purified water and immediately triturate rapidly to form the thick, white, homogenous emulsion nucleus.
5. Add the flavor and mix thoroughly.
6. Add the syrup and mix thoroughly.
7. Add sufficient purified water to measure 100 mL.

Capsules

- *Definition:* This dosage form incorporates ingredients into a shell called a *capsule.*

- *Procedure:* Triturate powders to reduce particle size, mix powders by geometric dilution, incorporate diluent by geometric dilution, calculate total weight to fit a certain size capsule, and clean the outside of the filled capsules.
- *Advantages:* Capsules mask unpleasant taste; allow the mixture of ingredients that could not be mixed in other vehicles; alter the release rate of ingredients; incorporate several ingredients into one dosage form; provide an accurate dosage size for liquids, semisolids, and powders; and provide a dosage form that is easier to swallow and more acceptable to the patient.
- *Methods of filling:* Hand punch from powder on pill tile; use a capsule-filling machine.
- *Sizing:* Determining the size of capsule to use for a particular dosage size involves assessing the density or fluffiness of the powder, comparing it to known weights of various reference powders with published capsule size capacities, and then actually weighing the capsule. If the requested dosage does not fill a specific size capsule, a filler should be added.
- *Testing:* Organoleptic, weight percent error, weight variance, and other testing is performed.

An example of an altered-release capsule follows:

Progesterone, micronized	25 mg
Methocel E4M	50%
Lactose, qs ad	
M.ft. capsules	Make 15 doses

Steps in compounding are as follows:

1. Select capsule size and calculate the required quantity of each ingredient.
2. Accurately weigh each ingredient.
3. If necessary, reduce particle size, and mix thoroughly.
4. Fill capsules.
5. Weigh capsules, calculate average weight, and determine percentage of error.

Tablet Triturates (Sublingual or Molded Tablets)

- *Definition:* A tablet triturate is a small tablet that is made in a mold and intended for sublingual administration. It usually weighs about 30–250 mg.
- *Advantages:* A tablet triturate rapidly dissolves under the tongue, is rapidly absorbed, avoids first pass through liver, and provides a rapid therapeutic response.

- *Components:* Tablet triturates consist of an active ingredient and a base, which may consist of lactose, sucrose, dextrose, mannitol, and so forth.
- *Formulation:* On the basis of the size of the mold cavities, mix the active ingredient with the base, which often consists of four parts lactose and one part sucrose. Thoroughly triturate powders, mix by geometric dilution, and then moisten with a solution containing four parts alcohol and one part purified water until the powder mixture is adhesive. Press into mold.
- *Testing:* Organoleptic, weight percent error, weight variance, and other testing is performed.
- *Tip:* Tablets may be flavored and colored by adding flavor and color to the wetting solution.

An example of a tablet triturate follows:

Testosterone	3 mg
Base, qs ad	
M.ft. tabs	

Steps in compounding are as follows:

1. The base may consist of a 1:4 mixture of sucrose and lactose.
2. The wetting solution may consist of a 1:4 mixture of water and alcohol.
3. On the basis of the size mold and the number of tablets it makes, calculate the required quantity of each ingredient.
4. Accurately weigh or measure each ingredient.
5. Reduce particle size and mix ingredients by geometric dilution.
6. In a glass mortar, gradually moisten the powder mixture until it becomes adhesive. *Note:* Drop the wetting solution onto the powder a few drops at a time and triturate after each addition until powder becomes moist and adhesive.
7. Press moist powder evenly into all holes in the tablet triturate mold plate.
8. Place the mold plate on the base plate and press down until the tablets rest on top of the pegs.
9. Let tablets air dry.
10. Very gently remove dried tablets from pegs.

Troches, Lozenges, and Lollipops (Suckers)

- *Definition:* Troches, lozenges, and lollipops are solid dosage forms intended to be slowly dissolved in the mouth for local or systemic effects.
- *Formulation:* Troches, lozenges, and lollipops are composed of an active ingredient and a base that may consist of (1) sugar and other carbohydrates

that produce a hard candy troche, (2) polyethylene glycols and other ingredients that produce a softer troche, or (3) a glycerin–gelatin combination that produces a chewable troche.

- Formulations made in a sucker mold complete with sticks are called *lollipops* or *suckers*.
- Formulations must be calculated to fit the size mold that will be used.
- Flavors and colors are added just before the molds are filled.

■ *Advantages:* Troches, lozenges, and lollipops are easy to administer, are convenient for patients who cannot swallow oral dosage forms, maintain a constant level of drug in the oral cavity and throat, and have a pleasant taste.

■ *Testing:* Organoleptic, weight percent error, weight variance, and other testing is performed.

An example of a troche follows:

Gelatin	4.68 g
Glycerin	16.70 mL
Purified water	2.30 mL
Acacia	0.50 g
Bentonite	0.50 g
Benzocaine	0.30 g
Citric acid	0.66 g
Saccharin sodium	0.17 g
Flavor and color	qs

Steps in compounding are as follows:

1. Depending on the size of the mold to be used and the number of troches to be made, calculate the required quantity of each ingredient.
2. Accurately weigh or measure each ingredient.
3. Heat the glycerin in a boiling water bath for several minutes.
4. Add the water and heat for a few more minutes.
5. While stirring, *very slowly* add the gelatin. *Note:* Gelatin must be lump free; the mixture must be homogeneous.
6. Triturate and thoroughly mix the powders.
7. Add the powders to the warm liquid and mix thoroughly.
8. Add flavor and color, mix, pour into the mold, and let cool.

Transdermal Gels

■ *Definition:* Transdermal gels move medications through the skin in quantities sufficient to produce a therapeutic effect.

■ *Components:* Transdermal gels have the following components:

- Active ingredient or ingredients
- Gelling agents: the carbomers (e.g., Carbopol 934P); methylcellulose; the poloxamers (e.g., Pluronic F-127); sodium carboxymethylcellulose; and so forth
- Wetting or levigating agents: propylene glycol, glycerin, and so forth
- Penetration-enhancing agents: water, alcohol, lecithin, dimethyl sulfoxide, isopropyl myristate, isopropyl palmitate, propylene glycol, polyethylene glycol, and so forth
- Suspending or dispersing agents: bentonite, silica gel, and so forth

■ *Testing:* Organoleptic testing is performed.

■ *Advantages:* Transdermal gels are convenient and effective, have great acceptability to patients, and avoid problems other dosage forms have such as gastrointestinal irritation from oral dosages, pain from injections, and undesirability of suppositories

■ *Formulation:* Use proper techniques for creating the gel, adjust the pH for carbomer gels, respect the temperature for poloxamer gels, use small amounts of nonaqueous solvents, and if possible keep electrolyte ingredients to a minimum.

■ *Tip:* Do not use transdermal gels for the systemic use of antibiotics, and do not try to get large molecules such as proteins through the skin via transdermal gels.

An example of a transdermal gel using carbomer as the base follows:

Ketoprofen	5%
Carbomer 934P	2%
Alcohol	qs
Trolamine	2 mL
Purified water, qs ad	30 mL

Steps in compounding are as follows:

1. Calculate the required quantity of each ingredient.
2. Accurately weigh or measure each ingredient.
3. Triturate the carbomer 934P in a glass mortar.
4. While triturating, gradually add about 18 mL of purified water.
5. Be sure the carbomer and water are thoroughly mixed and the mixture is homogenous.
6. Dissolve the ketoprofen in about 10 mL of alcohol.
7. While triturating, add this solution to the carbomer–water mixture, and mix thoroughly.
8. If necessary, add purified water to make about 28 mL and pour into the ointment jar.
9. Add trolamine and stir quickly with a stirring rod until the gel is thoroughly formed.

Note: A trade name for carbomer 934P is Carbopol 934P.

An example of a transdermal gel using organogel (PLO) as the base follows:

Ketoprofen	5%
Propylene glycol	10%
Lecithin isopropyl palmitate liquid	20%
Poloxamer 407 20% gel, qs ad	100 mL

Steps in compounding are as follows:

1. Calculate the required quantity of each ingredient.
2. Accurately weigh or measure each ingredient.
3. In a glass mortar, triturate the ketoprofen with the propylene glycol.
4. Make a smooth uniform paste.
5. Add the lecithin isopropyl palmitate liquid and mix well.
6. Add sufficient poloxamer 407 20% gel to measure 100 mL.
7. Triturate until a high-quality gel is produced.
8. Package in a light-resistant container.

Note: The lecithin isopropyl palmitate liquid and the poloxamer 407 20% gel should be prepared ahead of time so that they are ready for use.

The lecithin isopropyl palmitate liquid may be prepared as follows:

Soy lecithin, granular	10.0 g
Isopropyl palmitate	10.0 g
Sorbic acid	0.2 g

1. Accurately weigh or measure each ingredient.
2. Add the soy lecithin granules and the sorbic acid to the isopropyl palmitate, mix well, and allow to set overnight at room temperature.
3. The next morning, very gently stir to ensure complete mixing.

Note: Isopropyl myristate may be used in place of isopropyl palmitate.

The poloxamer 407 20% gel may be prepared as follows:

Poloxamer 407	20.0 g
Potassium sorbate	0.2 g
Purified water, qs ad	100 mL

1. Accurately weigh or measure each ingredient.
2. Add the poloxamer 407 and the potassium sorbate to a portion of the purified water, mix well, and add purified water to make 100 mL.
3. Mix thoroughly, ensuring that the poloxamer 407 is completely wet.

4. Allow to set overnight in the refrigerator.
5. The next morning, stir slowly to be sure mixing is complete.
6. Store in the refrigerator.

Note: A trade name for poloxamer 407 is Pluronic F-127.

Suppositories

- **Definition:** Suppositories are solid dosage forms for insertion into the rectum, vagina, or urethra to provide localized therapy or systemic therapy.
- **Sizes:** Rectal suppositories are approximately 2 g, vaginal suppositories are 3–5 g; and urethral suppositories are 2 g (female) or 4 g (male). *Note:* Urethral suppositories were formerly called *bougies.*
- **Formulation:** Suppositories are usually made by fusion with either a fatty or water-miscible base. They can also be hand molded or made by compression.
  - Suppositories are usually made in a metal or plastic mold.
  - The active ingredients in powder form should be triturated (comminuted) to reduce particle size and should be levigated with a levigating or wetting agent before incorporation into the melted base.
  - The melted formulation should be poured continuously into the mold to prevent layering.
- **Calculations:** The capacity in grams of the suppository mold must be known to determine the quantity of base needed. (If this capacity is not known, the capacity must be determined by filling the mold with the suppository base and weighing the resulting suppositories.) The space in the suppository occupied by the active ingredient or ingredients must calculated using the density factor of each active ingredient. (If the density factor is not known, it can be calculated by making a suppository containing a known amount of the active ingredient.)
- **Advantages:** Suppositories deliver medication for local or systemic effects. (The systemically absorbed medication avoids the first pass through the liver.) They can be used when patients cannot take medication orally or by injection.
- **Testing:** Organoleptic, weight percent error, weight variance, and other testing is performed.

An example of a rectal suppository follows:

Progesterone, micronized	25 mg
Polyethylene glycol base	qs
M.ft. supp	dtd #12

Use the following formula for the polyethylene glycol base:

Polyethylene glycol 300	50%
Polyethylene glycol 6000	50%

Steps in compounding are as follows:

1. On the basis of the size of the mold, calculate the required amount of each ingredient.
2. Accurately weigh or measure each ingredient.
3. Carefully heat the polyethylene glycol 6000 until it melts.
4. Add the polyethylene glycol 300 and mix well.
5. Very slowly add the micronized progesterone and mix thoroughly.
6. Pour the mixture into the suppository mold.

Note: When using the plastic molds (shells), the liquid mixture must not be too hot.

Powders

- *Definition:* Powders are fine particles that result from the comminution of dry substances. Particle sizes are usually determined by the size sieve they will pass through and may be described as very coarse, coarse, moderately coarse, fine, and very fine.
- *Mixtures:* Mixtures of powders should have the same size or similar size particles, and mixing should be accomplished by geometric dilution.
- *Preparation: Comminution* is the process of reducing particle size in powders. It is accomplished manually by trituration, levigation, or pulverization by intervention and mechanically by grinders and various types of mills.
- *Uses:* Powders taken by mouth may provide systemic effects. Powders are applied topically for local effects. Powders that contain mucoadhesive ingredients, when insufflated into body cavities, will adhere to moist body surfaces.
- *Advantages:* Because they are dry, powders often have greater stability, and they may not react with ingredients with which they are otherwise incompatible (except explosive mixtures). Once in the gastrointestinal tract, they are ready to be absorbed, and they tend to have longer beyond-use dates.
- *Testing:* Organoleptic testing is performed.

An example of a powder for external use follows:

Calamine	
Zinc oxide, of each	8%
Red mercuric oxide	1%
Magnesium oxide, heavy, qs ad	60 g
M.ft. powder	

Steps in compounding are as follows:

1. Calculate the required amount of each ingredient.
2. Accurately weigh each ingredient.
3. Thoroughly mix the powders by geometric dilution.
4. If using a mortar and pestle, use a porcelain mortar and begin with the ingredient having the smallest weight.
5. Use the "spread test" to determine when the mixture is totally homogeneous.

Powder Papers (Charts)

- *Definition:* Powders or mixtures of powders are enfolded in papers containing one dose each and dispensed in an appropriate box or container.
- *Preparation:* Powders are finely subdivided (comminuted) and mixed by geometric dilution, and a dose of the appropriate size is placed on a powder paper and properly folded. The appropriate size can be obtained by weighing. An alternate method is to place all the powder on a pill tile and to "block and divide" the powder into the proper number of doses, placing one dose on each powder paper.
- *Advantages:* For patients who cannot swallow, those who have difficulty swallowing certain tablets or capsules, and those who have indwelling nasogastric tubes, powder papers provide an ideal dosage form. Several medications can be given as one dose. The medication is in powder form and ready to be absorbed once it is in the gastrointestinal tract. For patients who have many medications to take each day, they may be combined into a smaller number of powder papers. Powder papers have longer beyond-use dates than many other compounded dosage forms.
- *Testing:* Organoleptic, weight percent error, weight variance, and other testing is performed.

An example of a powder paper (chart) follows:

Aspirin	3.5 grains
Acetaminophen	2.5 grains
Caffeine	0.5 grains
M.ft. chart	dtd #12

Steps in compounding are as follows:

1. Calculate the required quantity of each ingredient.
2. Accurately weigh each ingredient.
3. Triturate each ingredient separately to reduce particle size.
4. Thoroughly mix the ingredients by geometric dilution.
5. Weigh the correct amount for each chart on a separate paper.
6. Properly fold each paper and place it in the powder box.

Ointments and Creams

■ *Definition:* Ointments and creams are semisolid dosage forms for external application. Properties are typically characteristic of the base selected (e.g., white petrolatum, hydrophilic petrolatum, cold cream, hydrophilic ointment, polyethylene glycol ointment). Ointments and creams protect the skin and mucous membranes, moisturize the skin, and provide a vehicle for various types of medications. Types and classifications include oleaginous or hydrocarbon, absorption, emulsion, and water soluble.

■ *Characteristics of an oleaginous or hydrocarbon ointment base:* Such a base
  • Is occlusive—white petrolatum
  • Is greasy—white ointment
  • Is an emollient—vegetable shortening
  • Is not water washable
  • Will not absorb water
  • Is insoluble in water

■ *Characteristics of an absorption ointment base:* Such a base
  • Is occlusive—hydrophilic petrolatum
  • Is greasy—lanolin, USP (anhydrous)
  • Is an emollient—Aquaphor
  • Is not water washable—Aquabase
  • Can absorb water
  • Is insoluble in water

■ *Characteristics of an emulsion, w/o ointment base:* Such a base
  • Is occlusive—cold cream
  • Is greasy—rose water ointment
  • Is an emollient—Eucerin
  • Is not water washable—hydrous lanolin
  • Will absorb water—hydrocream
  • Is insoluble in water—Nivea

■ *Characteristics of an emulsion, o/w ointment base:* Such a base
  • Is nonocclusive—hydrophilic ointment
  • Is nongreasy—acid mantle cream

  • Is water washable—Cetaphil
  • Will absorb water—Dermabase
  • Is insoluble in water—Keri lotion, Lubriderm, Neobase, Unibase, vanishing cream, Velvachol

■ *Characteristics of water-soluble ointment bases:*
  • Is nonocclusive—polyethylene glycol ointment
  • Is nongreasy—Polybase
  • Is water washable
  • Will absorb water
  • Is water soluble

■ *Preparation:* Ointments are typically prepared by fusion or levigation. Powders should be comminuted to fine particles; some powders may be dissolved. If using the fusion method, use only enough heat to melt the ingredient with the highest melting point. For the levigation method, an ointment slab and metal spatula usually work well. Levigating agents should be carefully selected, considering both the ingredient or ingredients to be incorporated and the base. Table 4-1 shows commonly used levigating agents grouped by type and matched with the appropriate group of ointment base classifications.

■ *Uses:* Ointments or creams are an effective dosage form for treating skin and mucous membranes. On occasion, an ointment or cream will move sufficient quantities of medication through the skin to produce a systemic effect. Some formulations provide effective protection for the skin and mucous membranes.

Table 4-1. Levigating Agents by Type and Ointment Base Classification

Type of agent	Ointment base classification
Aqueous	
Glycerin	Oil-in-water emulsion
Propylene glycol	Water soluble
Polyethylene glycol 400	Water washable
Oily	
Mineral oil	Oleaginous or hydrocarbon
Castor oil	Absorption
Cottonseed oil	Water-in-oil emulsion

Note: Other agents may be useful for certain preparations, such as Tween 80 for incorporating coal tar. Castor oil is useful for incorporating ichthammol and peru balsam.

- *Packaging:* Typically, ointments and creams are packaged in ointment jars. The tube is often an ideal alternative package because it protects the preparation until it is squeezed out and used.
- *Testing:* Organoleptic, homogenicity, and other testing is performed.

An example of a nongreasy ointment follows:

Benzoyl peroxide	10%
Sulfur	1%
Polyethylene glycol base, qs ad	30 g

Steps in compounding are as follows:

1. Calculate the required quantity of each ingredient. Benzoyl peroxide, hydrous, USP contains about 26% water. The polyethylene glycol base consists of

Polyethylene glycol 400	65%
Polyethylene glycol 3350	35%

2. Accurately weigh or measure each ingredient.
3. Triturate each powder to a fine particle size.
4. Melt the polyethylene glycol 3350 and remove it from the heat source.
5. Add the polyethylene glycol 400 and mix thoroughly.
6. Add the powders and mix thoroughly.
7. Before the preparation begins to harden, stir thoroughly and pour into the ointment jar.

An example of a greasy ointment follows:

Salicylic acid	3%
White petrolatum, qs ad	30 g

Steps in compounding are as follows:

1. Calculate the required quantity of each ingredient.
2. Accurately weigh each ingredient.
3. Triturate the salicylic acid to reduce particle size.
4. Levigate with a small quantity of mineral oil.
5. By geometric dilution, incorporate the levigated salicylic acid into the white petrolatum.

The following is an example of a cream:

Almond oil	56.0 g
White wax	12.0 g
Light mineral oil	10.0 g
Cetyl esters wax	2.5 g
Sodium borate	0.5 g
Purified water	19.0 g
Total	100.0 g

M.ft. cream, S.A.

Steps in compounding are as follows:

1. Accurately weigh or measure each ingredient.
2. Melt the white wax.
3. Add the cetyl esters wax, almond oil, and light mineral oil.
4. Bring to a temperature of 70°C.
5. Dissolve the sodium borate in the purified water.
6. Bring to a temperature of 70°C.
7. With both liquids at 70°C, mix and stir.
8. Stir until the cream is completely formed.
9. Package in a tube or jar.

Sticks

- *Definition:* This topical dosage form is made in the shape of a rod or stick or variation thereof and packaged in a container that allows it to be advanced upward as it is used or consumed.
- *Advantages:* Sticks are an effective, convenient method of applying a topical agent exactly in the location desired. They can deliver a variety of agents—including those that are therapeutic, protective, and cosmetic—and they are very portable.
- *Preparation:* Select a semisolid vehicle from a variety of polyethylene glycols, waxes, and oils that will produce the consistency desired. Triturate solid ingredients, wet them with an appropriate wetting or levigating agent, and add them along with any liquid ingredients to the melted vehicle. Mix thoroughly. Pour into an appropriate "ride-up" container.
- *Testing:* Organoleptic testing is performed.
- *Tip:* Sticks can usually be considered a stable dosage form and assigned a corresponding beyond-use date.

An example of a stick follows:

Menthol	1.00%
Camphor	0.50%
Phenol	0.25%
Flavor	qs
Color	qs
Polyethylene glycol 400	7 g
Polyethylene glycol 4500	3 g

Steps in compounding:

1. Calculate the required quantity of each ingredient.
2. Accurately weigh or measure each ingredient.
3. Melt the polyethylene glycol 4500.
4. Remove from heat source.
5. Add the polyethylene glycol 400 and mix thoroughly.

6. Mix the menthol, camphor, and phenol together; they will liquefy, forming a eutectic mixture.
7. Add the eutectic mixture and the other ingredients and mix thoroughly.
8. Pour into a "ride-up" lip balm tube and let cool.

4-7. Quality Assurance and Preparation Testing

The assurance of high quality influences every facet of compounding. The atmosphere, the area design, the fixtures, the equipment and apparatus, the components, the containers, the expertise and experience of the personnel, the policies and procedures, and many other factors play important roles for achieving the highest quality possible in the compounding of individualized, customized preparations. Perhaps the most important element is commitment—the commitment of each individual who plays any role in the compounding process. This commitment must be of such intensity that the individual will not vary from the correct way of performing every function every time in everything.

Preparation testing must be in place for every compounded preparation. Chapter 1163 in the *U.S. Pharmacopeia 32/National Formulary 27* has a table that shows what types of tests can be performed on every type of compounded preparation. The compounding process of each type of dosage form should include all applicable tests that must be performed each time the dosage form is compounded.

The ultimate test of quality for a compounded preparation consists of having the preparation analyzed by a competent analytical laboratory. The typical goal is to have the contents of the preparation vary no more than plus or minus 5% of the potency stated on the label.

An indicator that the compounding pharmacy is committed to a high-quality practice is accreditation by the Pharmacy Compounding Accreditation Board (PCAB). The PCAB is national in scope, and it very carefully evaluates all aspects of the pharmacy operation and ensures that policies and procedures are in place and operational for a very high-quality practice.

PCAB accreditation is currently the only benchmark available to attest to the quality of a compounding pharmacy. PCAB accreditation should be the goal of every pharmacy that provides compounded preparations.

4-8. Key Points

- Each extemporaneously compounded prescription is for a specific patient.
- Three parties are involved in extemporaneous compounding: the prescriber, the patient, and the pharmacist.
- A thorough knowledge of and proficiency in pharmacy math is required for the extemporaneous compounding of prescriptions.
- The sensitivity of the pharmacy balance must be determined, and the minimum weighable quantity calculated for that particular balance.
- All weighing and measuring must be accurate. Avoid errors of 5% or more.
- Once an ingredient is removed from the stock container, it may not be returned to the stock container.
- Trituration is used to reduce the particle size of powders so that a greater surface area will be available, to uniformly mix powders using geometric dilution, and to dissolve solutes in solvents.
- Levigation is the process of mixing or triturating a powder with a liquid in which it is insoluble to reduce particle size and aid in incorporating the powder into the ointment base.
- The pharmacist must choose a levigating agent that is miscible with the ointment base.
- Mineral oil is an appropriate levigating agent for a hydrophobic ointment base such as white petrolatum.
- Up to 5% of levigating agent is usually sufficient unless the amount of powder is large.
- Heat should be used sparingly in compounding. Use only enough heat to melt ingredients, effect solution, enhance a reaction, and so forth—never any extra.
- Use of a water bath normally prevents overheating ingredients when compounding.
- Care must be taken to never lose or waste any ingredients in the preparation process because doing so can alter the concentration of active ingredients in the finished preparation and produce a subpotent or superpotent preparation.
- To promote accuracy in the compounding process, place all unused stock containers on the left side of the workstation. As each one is used, place it on the right side.
- The dry gum (or Continental) method of preparing an emulsion uses oil, purified water, and gum (e.g., acacia) in a ratio of 4:2:1, respectively.
- The extemporaneously compounded preparation has no NDC number.

4-9. Questions

1. When water is an ingredient in a nonsterile compounded preparation and the type of water is not specified, the pharmacist is correct to use

   A. tap water.
   B. potable water.
   C. purified water.
   D. water for injection.
   E. sterile water for injection.

2. When alcohol is an ingredient in a nonsterile compounded preparation and the type and percent alcohol is not specified, the pharmacist is correct to use

   A. ethyl alcohol 100%.
   B. ethyl alcohol 95%.
   C. ethyl alcohol 70%.
   D. ethyl alcohol 50%.
   E. isopropyl alcohol 70%.

3. Ingredients that soften the skin and make it more flexible when applied topically are called

   A. keratolytics.
   B. emollients.
   C. rubefacients.
   D. counterirritants.
   E. astringents.

4. To increase the stability of potassium iodide oral solution (SSKI),_____ may be used as an antioxidant to prevent the release of free iodine.

   A. sodium alginate
   B. sodium borate
   C. sodium glycinate
   D. sodium succinate
   E. sodium thiosulfate

5. In preparing diluted hydrochloric acid, the pharmacist notes a temperature change. The reaction is called

   A. hypothermic.
   B. hyperthermic.
   C. endothermic.
   D. exothermic.
   E. isothermic.

6. Ingredients that tend to tighten or shrink tissues when applied topically are called

   A. astringents.
   B. emollients.
   C. keratolytic agents.
   D. occlusive agents.
   E. suspending agents.

7. A solution expressed as 35% w/w has the following:

   A. 35 mg of solute dissolved in 100 mL of solution
   B. 35 g of solute dissolved in 100 g of solvent
   C. 35 mg of solute dissolved in 100 g of solvent
   D. 35 g of solute dissolved in 100 g of solution
   E. 35 mL of solute dissolved in 100 mL of solution

8. When dissolving potassium iodide in purified water, the pharmacist notes a temperature change. The reaction is called

   A. hypothermic.
   B. hyperthermic.
   C. endothermic.
   D. exothermic.
   E. isothermic.

9. A solution expressed as 35% w/v has the following:

   A. 35 mg of solute dissolved in 100 mL of solvent
   B. 35 g of solute dissolved in 100 mL of solution
   C. 35 mg of solute dissolved in 100 mL of solution
   D. 35 g of solute dissolved in 100 mL of solvent
   E. 35 mL of solute dissolved in 100 g of solution

10. Hydrophilic ointment, USP, is an o/w type of ointment base; therefore, it possesses the property of being

    A. emollient.
    B. greasy.
    C. occlusive.
    D. water washable.
    E. anhydrous.

11. When compounding an emulsion that contains a flavoring agent, the flavoring agent should be in

    A. the continuous (external) phase.
    B. the discontinuous (internal) phase.
    C. the aqueous phase.
    D. the oil phase.
    E. the emulsifier.

The next four questions pertain to the following compounded prescription:

Mineral oil	60 mL
Acacia	qs
Syrup	12 mL
Flavor	qs
Purified water, qs ad	120 mL

M.ft. emulsion using dry gum method

12. Mineral oil is in the

    I. internal phase.
    II. external phase.
    III. discontinuous phase.

    A. I only
    B. II only
    C. I and III only
    D. II and III only
    E. I, II, and III

13. Acacia is the

    A. primary active ingredient.
    B. preservative.
    C. emulsifying agent.
    D. wetting agent.
    E. coloring agent.

14. How much acacia is needed for this preparation?

    A. 5 g
    B. 10 g
    C. 15 g
    D. 30 g
    E. 35 g

15. How much purified water is needed to make the initial emulsion?

    A. 5 mL
    B. 10 mL
    C. 15 mL
    D. 30 mL
    E. 48 mL

16. When cocoa butter is used as a suppository base, its melting point can pose a problem. To overcome this problem, the compounding pharmacist can replace _____ of the cocoa butter with white wax.

    A. 5%
    B. 10%
    C. 15%
    D. 20–25%
    E. 30%

17. When cocoa butter is used as a suppository base, its melting point can pose a problem. To overcome this problem, the compounding pharmacist can replace _____ of the cocoa butter with cetyl esters wax.

    A. 5%
    B. 10%
    C. 15%
    D. 20–25%
    E. 30%

18. Hydrophilic petrolatum, USP, is used as an ointment base. It possesses the characteristic or characteristics of being

    I. emollient.
    II. occlusive.
    III. greasy.

    A. I only
    B. II only
    C. I and III only
    D. II and III only
    E. I, II, and III

19. When lime water and olive oil are processed together to form an emulsion, a reaction occurs that produces the emulsifying agent, which is

    A. lime oil.
    B. lime oxide.
    C. calcium oxide.
    D. calcium oleate.
    E. olive oxide.

20. The advantage or advantages of sublingual tablets as a dosage form are

    I. quick absorption into the bloodstream.
    II. rapid onset of action.
    III. avoidance of the first pass through the liver.

A. I only
B. II only
C. I and III only
D. II and III only
E. I, II, and III

The next question pertains to the following compounded prescription:

Camphor	1.0%
Menthol	1.0%
Thymol	0.5%
White petrolatum, qs ad	30 g
M.ft. oint	

21. To prepare this compounded prescription, the pharmacist should

   A. dissolve the camphor, menthol, and thymol in alcohol and incorporate them into the white petrolatum by geometric dilution.
   B. dissolve the camphor, menthol, and thymol in glycerin and incorporate them into the white petrolatum by geometric dilution.
   C. dissolve the camphor, menthol, and thymol in propylene glycol and incorporate them into the white petrolatum by geometric dilution.
   D. form a eutectic mixture and incorporate it into the white petrolatum by geometric dilution.
   E. alter the formula to avoid incompatibilities.

22. The advantage or advantages of capsules as a dosage form are that they

   I. provide an accurate dose.
   II. mask unpleasant tastes.
   III. provide an immediate therapeutic response.

   A. I only
   B. II only
   C. I and II only
   D. II and III only
   E. I, II, and III

The next question pertains to the following compounded prescription:

Salicylic acid	5%
White petrolatum, qs ad	30 g

23. The pharmacist has on hand 2% salicylic acid ointment to use in preparing this prescription. When using it, the pharmacist should

   A. weigh 0.5 g of salicylic acid powder and qs to 30 g with 2% salicylic acid ointment, incorporating the salicylic acid powder by geometric dilution.
   B. weigh 0.5 g of salicylic acid powder, levigate it with 5 mL of alcohol, and qs to 30 g with 2% salicylic acid ointment, incorporating the salicylic acid by geometric dilution.
   C. weigh 1.5 g of salicylic acid powder, levigate it with 6 mL of mineral oil, and qs to 30 g with 2% salicylic acid ointment, incorporating the salicylic acid by geometric dilution.
   D. weigh 1.5 g of salicylic acid powder and qs to 30 g with 2% salicylic acid ointment, incorporating the salicylic acid powder by geometric dilution.
   E. weigh 1 g of salicylic acid powder, levigate it with 4.5 mL of mineral oil (SpGr 0.89), and incorporate it into 25 g of 2% salicylic acid ointment by geometric dilution.

24. The advantage or advantages of a transdermal gel as a dosage form is/are

   I. convenience of administration or application.
   II. quick therapeutic response.
   III. patient acceptance.

   A. I only
   B. II only
   C. I and II only
   D. II and III only
   E. I, II, and III

25. One gram of iodine is soluble in 3,000 mL of water. In Lugol's solution (strong iodine solution), 1 g of iodine is dissolved in 20 mL of solution. Lugol's solution contains 5% iodine and 10% potassium iodide. The phenomenon by which the potassium iodide increases the solubility of iodine is known as

   A. alligation.
   B. coalescence.
   C. comminution.
   D. complexation.
   E. diffusion.

4-10. Answers

1. C. For nonsterile compounding, the USP specifies that purified water be used.

2. **B.** When type or percentage of alcohol is not specified, alcohol, USP, is used, and it is 95% ethyl alcohol.

3. **B.** Ingredients that make the skin soft and pliable when applied locally are called *emollients.*

4. **E.** Sodium thiosulfate is the antioxidant that prevents the iodide ion from oxidizing to form free iodine.

5. **D.** When diluted hydrochloric acid is prepared, heat is generated, and the reaction is called *exothermic.*

6. **A.** Ingredients that shrink or tighten the skin when applied locally are called *astringents.*

7. **D.** W/w means weight in weight. Consequently, 35 g of solute must be contained in 100 g of solution to have a 35% w/w solution.

8. **C.** When potassium iodide is dissolved in purified water, the solution becomes distinctively cold and the reaction is called endothermic.

9. **B.** W/v means weight in volume. Consequently, 35 g of solute must be contained in 100 mL of solution to have a 35% w/v solution.

10. **D.** Hydrophilic ointment is water washable but does not possess the other properties listed.

11. **A.** For the flavoring agent to be tasted, it must be in the external or continuous phase.

12. **C.** Mineral oil is in the internal or discontinuous phase and should not be tasted.

13. **C.** Acacia is the emulsifying agent forming an oil-in-water emulsion.

14. **C.** Given the 4:2:1 ratio, the 1 part or 15 g is the acacia.

15. **D.** Given the 4:2:1 ratio, the 2 parts or 30 mL is the water for the initial emulsion.

16. **A.** Five percent cocoa butter replaced by white wax will overcome the low melting point problem.

17. **D.** Twenty to twenty-five percent cocoa butter replaced by cetyl esters wax will overcome the low melting point problem.

18. **E.** Hydrophilic petrolatum is greasy, occlusive, and emollient.

19. **D.** The lime water is calcium hydroxide solution and the olive oil contains oleic acid. The two react together to form calcium oleate, which is the emulsifying agent that forms a water-in-oil emulsion.

20. **E.** All three items are advantages of sublingual tablets as dosage forms.

21. **D.** Camphor, menthol, and thymol are three ingredients that, when mixed together, will liquefy, forming what is called a *eutectic mixture.* This liquid mixture is then gradually incorporated into the white petrolatum by geometric dilution.

22. **C.** Capsules do not provide an immediate therapeutic response; the other two choices are correct.

23. **E.** Your compounded preparation must contain 1.5 g of salicylic acid. Twenty-five grams of your 2% ointment contain 500 mg. You must weigh out 1 g of salicylic acid powder. The remaining ingredients must not contain any salicylic acid. The remaining weight can be made up with the levigating agent or a combination of the levigating agent and white petrolatum.

24. **E.** All three choices are correct.

25. **D.** In solution, potassium iodide ionizes into potassium and the iodide ion. The iodide ion complexes with elemental iodine to form the soluble I^3 complex.

4-11. References

The following are references that should be available in the compounding pharmacy to provide assistance as the pharmacist formulates the variety of dosage forms that customized medications require:

Allen LV Jr. *The Art, Science, and Technology of Pharmaceutical Compounding.* 3rd ed. Washington, D.C.: American Pharmacists Association; 2008.

Ansel HC, Allen LV Jr, Popovich NG. *Ansel's Pharmaceutical Dosage Forms and Drug Delivery Systems.* 8th ed. Baltimore: Lippincott Williams & Wilkins; 2005.

Ansel HC, Stoklosa MJ. *Pharmaceutical Calculations.* 11th ed. Baltimore: Lippincott Williams & Wilkins; 2001.

Hendrickson R, ed. *Remington: The Science and Practice of Pharmacy.* 21st ed. Baltimore: Lippincott Williams & Wilkins; 2006.

O'Neil MJ, ed. *The Merck Index.* 14th ed. Whitehouse Station, N.J.: Merck & Co.; 2006.

Shrewsbury R. *Applied Pharmaceutics in Contemporary Compounding.* Englewood, Colo.: Morton; 2001.

Sweetman SC, ed. *Martindale: The Complete Drug Reference*. 36th ed. London: Pharmaceutical Press; 2009.

Thompson JE, Davidow LW. *A Practical Guide to Contemporary Pharmacy Practice*. 2nd ed. Baltimore: Lippincott Williams & Wilkins; 2004.

Trissel LA. *Stability of Compounded Formulations*. 4th ed. Washington, D.C.: American Pharmacists Association; 2009.

U.S. Pharmacopeial Convention. *U.S. Pharmacopeia 32/National Formulary 73*. Rockville, Md.: U.S. Pharmacopeial Convention; 2009.

U.S. Pharmacopeial Convention. *USP Pharmacists' Pharmacopeia*. 2nd ed. Rockville, Md.: U.S. Pharmacopeial Convention; 2008.

Sterile Products

5

Laura A. Thoma, PharmD

5-1. Parenteral Products

Parenteral products are products that are administered by injection and that, therefore, bypass the gastrointestinal tract. Parenteral products must be sterile and free of pyrogens and particulate matter. Drugs that are destroyed, are inactivated in the gastrointestinal tract, or are poorly absorbed can be given by a parenteral route. Parenteral routes of administration may also be used when the patient is uncooperative, unconscious, or unable to swallow. This route is also used when rapid drug absorption is essential, such as in emergency situations.

Parenteral Routes of Administration

Intravenous route

An intravenous (IV) medication is administered directly into the vein. The IV route gives a rapid effect with a predictable response. It is used for irritating medications because the medication is rapidly diluted. This route does not have as much volume restriction as other parenteral routes.

A *bolus* is an injection of solution into the vein over a short period of time. A bolus is used to administer a relatively small volume of solution and is often written as "IV push" (IVP).

An *infusion* refers to the introduction of larger volumes of solution given over a longer period of time. A continuous infusion is used to administer a large volume of solution at a constant rate. Intermittent infusions are used to administer a relatively small volume of solution over a specified amount of time at specific intervals.

Intramuscular route

An intramuscular (IM) medication is injected deep into a large muscle mass, such as the upper arm, thigh, or buttocks. The medication is absorbed from the muscle tissue, acting more quickly than when given by the oral route, but not as quickly as when given by the IV route. Up to 2 mL may be administered intramuscularly as a solution or suspension given in the upper arm, and 5 mL may be given in the gluteal medial muscle of each buttock. A sustained-release-type action can be achieved with certain drugs that have low solubility because they are released from muscle tissue at a slow rate. IM injections are often painful, and reversing adverse effects from medications given by this route is very difficult. Antibiotics are often given by this route.

Subcutaneous route

Subcutaneous (SC) injections of solution or suspension are given beneath the surface of the skin. Medications administered by this route are not absorbed as well as and have a slower onset of action than medications given by the IV or IM route. The volume of solution or suspension that can be injected subcutaneously is 2 mL or less. Drugs often given by this route include epinephrine, heparin, insulin, and vaccines.

Intradermal route

An intradermal injection is injected into the top layer of the skin. The injection is not as deep as an SC injection. Medications used for diagnostic purposes, such as a tuberculin test or an allergy test, are often administered by this route. The volume of solution that can be administered intradermally is limited to 0.1 mL. The onset of action and the rate of absorption of medication from this route are slow.

Intra-arterial route

An intra-arterial injection is injected directly into an artery. It delivers a high drug concentration to the target site with little dilution by the circulation. Generally, this route is used only for radiopaque materials and some antineoplastic agents.

Other routes

- *Intracardiac:* An injection is made directly into the heart.
- *Intra-articular:* Administration by injection is made into a joint space. Corticosteroids are often administered by this route for the treatment of arthritis.
- *Intrathecal:* An injection is made into the lumbar intraspinal fluid sacs. Local anesthetics are frequently administered by this route during surgical procedures. Preservative-free drugs should be used for intrathecal administration.

5-2. Definitions for Compounding of Sterile Preparations

- *Admixture:* Parenteral dosage forms that are combined for administration as a single entity.
- *Antearea:* An International Organization for Standardization (ISO) Class 8 or better area where personnel hand hygiene and garbing procedures, sanitizing of supplies, and other particulate-generating activities are performed. The area contains a line of demarcation separating the clean side from the dirty side.
- *Aseptic processing:* The separate sterilization of a product and its components, containers, and closures, which are then brought together and assembled in an aseptic environment. The primary objective of aseptic processing is to create a sterile preparation.
- *Aseptic technique:* Performance of a procedure or procedures under controlled conditions in a manner that will minimize the chance of contamination. Contaminants can be introduced from the environment, equipment and supplies, or personnel (see the section on ISO classification).

- *Buffer area:* The area where the primary engineering control is located.
- *Compounding aseptic containment isolator (CACI):* An isolator that protects workers from exposure to undesirable levels of airborne drugs while providing an aseptic environment during the compounding of sterile preparations.
- *Compounding aseptic isolator (CAI):* An isolator that maintains an aseptic compounding environment within the isolator throughout the compounding and material transfer process during the compounding of sterile preparations.
- *Critical site:* Any opening or surface that can provide a pathway between the sterile product and the environment.
- *Hypertonic:* A solution that contains a higher concentration of dissolved substances than the red blood cell, thereby causing the red blood cell to shrink.
- *Hypotonic:* A solution that contains a lower concentration of dissolved substances than the red blood cell, thereby causing the red blood cell to swell and possibly burst.
- *Isotonic:* A solution that has an osmotic pressure close to that of bodily fluids, thus minimizing patient discomfort and damage to red blood cells. Dextrose 5% in water and sodium chloride 0.9% solutions are approximately isotonic.
- *Primary engineering control (PEC):* A device or room that provides an ISO Class 5 environment for the exposure of critical sites when producing compounded sterile preparations (CSPs). These devices could include a laminar airflow workbench, a biological safety cabinet, CAIs, and CACIs.
- *Sterilizing filter:* A filter that, when challenged with the microorganism *Brevundimonas diminuta* at a minimum concentration of 10^7 organisms per cm^2 of filter surface, will produce a sterile effluent. A sterilizing filter has a nominal pore size rating of 0.20 or 0.22 micron.
- *Tonicity:* Osmotic pressure exerted by a solution from the solutes or dissolved solids present.
- *Validation:* Establishment of documented evidence providing a high degree of assurance that a specific process will consistently produce a product meeting predetermined specifications and quality attributes.

ISO Classification

The ISO Classification of Particulate Matter in Room Air is the standard for clean rooms and associated environments. Limits are expressed in particles 0.5 micron and larger per cubic meter. In contrast, the limits from Federal Standard 209E are expressed in particles 0.5 micron and larger per cubic foot (1 cubic meter = 35.31 cubic feet).

ISO class 5 area

The air in an ISO class 5 area has a count of no more than 3,520 particles 0.5 micron or larger per cubic meter of air. This area is equivalent to a class 100 area under Federal Standard 209E, where the air has a count of no more than 100 particles 0.5 micron or larger per cubic foot of air. This class is the quality of air provided by the PEC and required for sterile product preparation.

ISO class 7 area

The air in an ISO class 7 area has a count of no more than 352,000 particles 0.5 micron or larger per cubic meter. This area is equivalent to a class 10,000 area under Federal Standard 209E, where the air has a count of no more than 10,000 particles 0.5 micron or larger per cubic foot of air. This class is the quality of air usually required in the buffer area.

ISO class 8 area

The air in an ISO class 8 area has a count of no more than 3,520,000 particles 0.5 micron or larger per cubic meter. This area is equivalent to a class 100,000 area under Federal Standard 209E, where the air has a count of no more than 100,000 particles 0.5 micron or larger per cubic foot of air. The antearea should have ISO class 8 air or better.

5-3. Sterile Product Preparation Area

The following are examples of PECs that provide the ISO class 5 area for compounding of CSPs.

Horizontal Laminar Flow Workbench

The horizontal laminar flow workbench (HLFW) works by drawing air in through a prefilter. The prefiltered air is pressurized in the plenum for consistent distribution of air to the high-efficiency particulate air (HEPA) filter (Figure 5-1).

The prefilter protects the HEPA filter from prematurely clogging. Prefilters should be checked regu-

Figure 5-1. Horizontal Laminar Flow Workbench

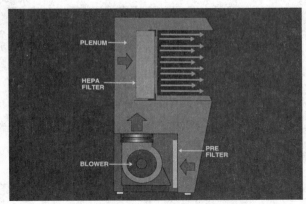

Illustration courtesy of the University of Tennessee Parenteral Medications Lab.

larly and changed as needed. A record of these checks and changes of the prefilter must be kept.

The plenum of the hood is the space between the prefilter and the HEPA filter. Air is pressurized here and distributed over the HEPA filter.

Laminar flow is the air in a confined space moving with uniform velocity along parallel lines. The term *unidirectional flow* has taken the place of laminar flow in more recent publications. Unidirectional flow is airflow moving in a single direction in a robust and uniform manner and at sufficient speed to sweep particles away from the critical processing area. Inside the HLFW is an ISO class 5 area (class 100 area).

Vertical Laminar Flow Workbench

The vertical laminar flow workbench (VLFW) works like a HLFW in that the air is drawn in through the prefilter and is pressurized in the plenum for distribution over the HEPA filter. However, the air is blown down from the top of the workstation onto the work surface, not across it (Figure 5-2).

Working in vertical laminar flow requires different techniques than does working in horizontal laminar flow. In vertical laminar flow, an object or the hands of the operator must not be above an object in the hood. In horizontal laminar flow, an object or the hands of the operator must not be in back of another object. The hands of the operator must never come between the HEPA filter and the object.

A biological safety cabinet, CAI, and CACI also use vertical unidirectional airflow to provide an ISO class 5 environment and are other examples of PECs.

Figure 5-2. Vertical Laminar Flow Workbench

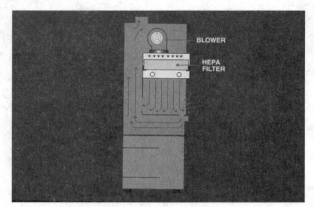

Illustration courtesy of the University of Tennessee Parenteral Medications Lab.

The HEPA Filter

The HEPA filter consists of a bank of filter media separated by corrugated pleats of aluminum. These pleats act as baffles to direct the air into laminar sheets. The HEPA filter is 99.97% efficient at removing particles 0.3 micron and larger.

Certification of the HEPA filter

The velocity of air from the HEPA filter is checked with a velometer or hot wire anemometer. ISO 14644 recommends that the average air velocity should be > 0.2 m/second.

Integrity of the HEPA filter: The dioctyl phthalate (DOP) test

The integrity of the HEPA filter is checked by introducing a high concentration of aerosolized Emery 3004 (a synthetic hydrocarbon) upstream of the filter on a continuous basis, while monitoring the penetration on the downstream side of the HEPA filter.

The aerosol has an average particle size of 0.3 micron. An aerosol photometer is used to check for leaks by passing the wand slowly over the filter and the gasket. None of the surfaces shall yield greater than 0.01% of the upstream smoke concentration. Any value greater than 0.01% indicates that a serious leak is present and must be sealed. All repaired areas must be retested for compliance. At one time, DOP was used to generate the aerosol. However, because DOP is a carcinogen, Emery 3004 is now used. An electronic particle counter cannot be used to certify the integrity of the HEPA filter. The particle counter is used to determine room classification.

Buffer Area (Controlled Area)

The PEC is the cleanest area and provides an ISO class 5 (class 100) area. It must be located in a controlled environment, away from excess traffic, doors, air vents, or anything that could produce air currents greater than the velocity of the airflow from the HEPA filter. Air currents greater than the velocity of the airflow from the HEPA filter may introduce contaminants into the hood. It is very easy to overcome air flowing at 90 feet per minute.

The buffer area should be enclosed from other pharmacy operations. Floors, walls, ceiling, shelving, counters, and cabinets of the controlled area must be of nonshedding, smooth, and nonporous material to allow for easy cleaning and disinfecting. All surfaces shall be resistant to sanitizing agents. Cracks, crevices, and seams shall be avoided, as should ledges or other places that could collect dust. The floor of the buffer area shall be smooth and seamless with coved edges up the wall.

The walls of the buffer area can be sealed panels caulked with silicone or, if drywall is used, painted with epoxy paint, which is nonshedding. The corners of the ceiling and the walls shall be sealed to avoid cracks. A solid ceiling may be painted with epoxy paint, or nonshedding washable ceiling tiles that are caulked into place may be used.

Light fixtures shall be mounted flush with the ceiling and sealed. Anything that penetrates the ceiling or walls shall be sealed.

Air entering the room shall be fresh, HEPA filtered, and air conditioned. The room must be maintained in positive pressure (0.02–0.05 inches of water column) in relation to the adjoining rooms or corridors. If the buffer area is used for compounding of cytotoxic drugs, 0.01 inches of water column negative pressure is required. At least 30 air changes per hour shall occur, with the PECs allowed to provide up to 15 of the 30 required air changes per hour.

People entering the buffer area shall be properly scrubbed and gowned. Access to the buffer area shall be restricted to qualified personnel only.

Controlling the traffic in the buffer area is a critical factor in keeping the area clean. Only items required for compounding shall be brought into the buffer area. These items must be cleaned and sanitized before being taken into the buffer area. Items may be stored in the buffer area for a limited time. However, the number of items stored in the buffer area shall be kept to a minimum. All equipment used in the buffer area should remain in the room except during calibration or repair.

Because they can harbor many organisms, refrigerators and freezers should be located out of the buffer area. Computers and printers should be located outside of the buffer area because they generate many particles. However, if they are required to be in the buffer area, monitor the environment and evaluate their effect on the environment. Cardboard boxes shall not be stored in the buffer area. The items shall be removed from the boxes on the dirty side of the antearea and sanitized and transferred to the clean side of the antearea or to the buffer area for storage. Vials stored in laminated cardboard may be stored in the buffer area. Sinks or floor drains shall not be in the buffer area because potable water contains many organisms and endotoxins.

Preparation of Operators

An operator must be trained and evaluated to be capable of properly scrubbing and garbing before entering the buffer area. This requirement is critical to the maintenance of asepsis. The greatest source of contamination in a clean room is the people in the area. A seated or standing person without movement releases an average of 100,000 particles greater than 0.3 micron in diameter per minute. A person standing with full body movement releases an average of 2,000,000 particles per minute greater than 0.3 micron in diameter, and if moving at a slow walk, he or she releases an average of 5,000,000 particles. The garb is designed to help contain the particles that are being shed.

Before entering the antearea, an operator must remove all cosmetics and all hand, wrist, and other visible jewelry or piercings. Artificial nails or extenders are prohibited while working in the sterile compounding environment, and natural nails must be kept neat and trimmed. Garb is donned in an order proceeding from that considered dirtiest to that considered cleanest. Shoe covers, head and facial hair covers, and facemask or eye shields are donned before performing hand hygiene. Hands and forearms are then washed for 30 seconds with soap and water in the antearea, and hands and forearms are dried using a lint-free disposable towel or an electric hand dryer. While still in the antearea, an operator must don a nonshedding gown that zips or buttons up to the neck, falls below the knees, and has sleeves that fit snugly around the wrists. After entering the buffer area, an operator must use a waterless alcohol-based surgical hand

scrub with persistent activity to again cleanse the hands before putting on sterile gloves. Sterile contact agar plates must be used to sample the gloved finger tips of compounding personnel after garbing to assess garbing competency. For successful completion of this competency, no colony-forming units can be found on any of the agar plate samples. Three consecutive, successful garbing and gloving exercises must be completed before sterile compounding is allowed. Routine application of sterile 70% isopropyl alcohol (IPA) must occur throughout the compounding process and whenever nonsterile surfaces are touched. After this initial evaluation, the entire process is repeated at least once a year for low- and medium-risk compounding and semiannually for high-risk compounding during any media-fill test procedure. The colony-forming unit action level for gloved hands will be based on the total number of colony-forming units on both gloves, not per hand.

Validation of the Operator

A *media fill* or *media transfer* is when a growth promotion media is used instead of the drug product, and all the normal compounding manipulations are done. It is critical that the process mimic the actual compounding process as closely as possible and represent worst-case conditions. Usually, the medium used is soybean-casein digest, which is also known as trypticase soy broth. This medium will support the growth of organisms that are likely to be transmitted to CSPs from the compounding personnel and environment. A media fill is used to check the quality of the compounding personnel's aseptic technique. It is also used to verify that the compounding process and the compounding environment is capable of producing sterile preparations.

Initially, before an operator can compound low- or medium-risk sterile injectable products, he or she must successfully complete one media fill using sterile fluid culture media such as soybean-casein digest medium. Media fill units must be incubated at 20–25°C for a minimum of 14 days or at 20–25°C for a minimum of 7 days and then at 30–35°C for a minimum of 7 days. A successful media fill is indicated by no growth in any of the media fill units. The media fill shall closely simulate the most challenging or stressful conditions encountered during the compounding of low- and medium-risk preparation. The compounding personnel shall perform a revalidation at a minimum of once a year by successfully completing one media fill. The media fills shall be designed to mimic the most challenging techniques the operator will use during a normal day. Validation for high-risk compounding focuses on ensuring that both the process and the compounding personnel are capable of producing a sterile preparation with all its purported quality attributes. Revalidation must be done on at least a semiannual basis. An example of a high-risk operation is the compounding of a sterile preparation from nonsterile drug powder. To mimic this operation, the compounder must use commercially available soybean-casein digest medium made up to a 3% concentration and perform normal processing steps, including filter sterilization. All media fills must occur in an ISO class 5 environment and must be completed without interruption.

5-4. Working in the Laminar Flow Workbench

Items not in a protective overwrap shall be wiped with a lint-free wipe soaked with sterile 70% IPA before being placed in the hood. Containers and packages should be inspected for cracks, tears, or particles as they are decontaminated and placed in the hood. Items in a protective overwrap, such as bags, should be taken from the overwrap at the edge of the hood (within the first 6 inches of the hood) and placed in the hood with the injection port facing the HEPA filter. The overwrap should not be placed in the hood, because doing so would introduce particles and organisms into the hood.

When working in the HLFW, an operator shall arrange supplies to the left or right of the direct compounding area (DCA). The critical site must be in uninterrupted unidirectional airflow at all times. The compounder must be careful not to place an object or hand between the HEPA filter and the critical site because doing so would interrupt the airflow to the critical site. and potentially cause particles to be washed from the hand or object onto the critical site.

All work performed in the HLFW must be done at least 6 inches inside the hood. The unidirectional airflow is blowing toward the operator, who acts as a barrier to the airflow, causing it to pass around the body and create backflow. This turbulence can cause room air to be carried into the front of the hood.

Items placed in the HFLW disturb the unidirectional airflow. The unidirectional airflow is disturbed downstream of the item for approximately three times the diameter of the object. If the item is placed next to the sidewall of the hood, the unidirectional airflow is disturbed approximately six times the diameter of the

object. Air downstream from the nonsterile objects is no longer bathed in unidirectional airflow and may become contaminated with particles. For these reasons, it is very important that a direct path exists between the HEPA filter and the area where the manipulations will occur.

With the VLFW, supplies in the hood should be placed so that the operator may work without placing a hand or object above the critical site. An operator can place many more items in the VLFW and still work without compromising the unidirectional airflow. One must remember that within 1 inch of the work surface the air is turbulent. The unidirectional air, which is coming down from the HEPA filter, strikes the work surface and changes direction to move horizontally across the work surface. Therefore, all work in the VLFW should be done at least 1 inch above the work surface. During the compounding of sterile preparations, all movements into and out of the hood must be minimized to decrease the risk of carrying contaminants into the DCA. This can be achieved by introducing all items needed for the aseptic manipulation into the work area at one time and by waiting until the procedure is completed before removing used syringes, vials, and other supplies from the PEC.

5-5. Syringes, Needles, Ampuls, and Vials

Syringes

The basic parts of the syringe are the barrel, plunger, collar, rubber tip of the plunger, and tip of the syringe. Syringes are sterile and free of pyrogens. They are packaged either in paper or in a rigid plastic container. Syringe packages must be inspected to ensure that the wrap is intact and the syringe is still sterile. Syringes have either a Luer-Lok tip, in which the needle is screwed tightly onto the threaded tip, or a slip tip, in which the needle is held on by friction (Figure 5-3). Syringes are supplied with and without needles attached and are available in a variety of sizes. Care must be taken not to let the syringe tip touch the surface of the hood.

Calibration marks are on the barrel of the syringe. These marks are accurate to one-half the interval marked on the syringe. The critical sites on the syringe are the tip of the syringe and the ribs of the plunger. The ribs of the plunger go back inside the syringe on injection of the fluid from the syringe and could potentially contaminate the syringe.

Figure 5-3. Types of Syringes

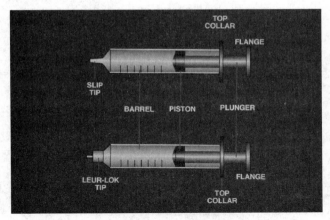

Illustration courtesy of the University of Tennessee Parenteral Medications Lab.

Needles

The basic parts of a needle include the hub, needle shaft, bevel, bevel heel, and tip of the needle (Figure 5-4).

Needles are sterile and are wrapped either in plastic with a twist-off top or in paper. This wrap must be inspected for integrity before the needle is used. The gauge of the needle refers to its outer diameter. The larger the number, the smaller the bore of the needle. The smallest is 27 gauge, and the largest is 13 gauge. The length of the needle is measured in inches, and some common lengths are 1.0–1.5 inches.

The critical sites on the needle are the hub of the needle, the entire needle shaft, and the tip of the needle.

Figure 5-4. Needle

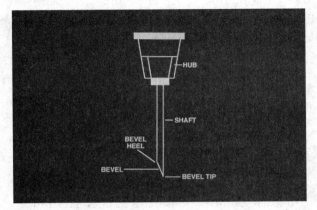

Illustration courtesy of the University of Tennessee Parenteral Medications Lab.

Ampuls

Ampuls are single-dose containers. Once ampuls are broken, they are an open-system container; air can pass freely in and out of the ampul. Any solution taken from an ampul must be filtered with a 5-micron filter needle or filter straw, because glass particles fall into the ampul when it is broken. Before breaking the ampul, one shall wipe the neck of the ampul with a sterile 70% IPA prep pad.

Vials

A vial is a molded glass or plastic container with a rubber closure secured in place with an aluminum seal. It may contain sterile solutions, dry-filled powders, or lyophilized drugs, or it may be an empty evacuated container. Vials may be single-dose or multiple-dose containers.

A single-dose container usually contains no preservative system to prevent the growth of microorganisms if they are accidentally introduced into the container. A single-dose vial punctured in an environment worse than ISO class 5 air must be used within 1 hour. A single-dose vial continuously exposed to ISO class 5 air may be used up to 6 hours after initial needle puncture. When the vial is first used, it should be labeled with the date, time, and initials of the person using the vial so the length of time that the vial has been in the hood can be determined.

A multidose vial contains preservatives, and these vials can be entered more than once. The pharmaceutical manufacturer has done studies to prove that the preservative system will remain effective and the closure will reseal after penetration by the needle. Therefore, the beyond-use date for opened or entered multidose containers is 28 days, unless otherwise specified by the manufacturer.

5-6. Biological Safety Cabinets

A class II biological safety cabinet (BSC) should be used to prepare cytotoxic and other hazardous drugs. Four different types of class II BSCs exist. Types A1 and A2 exhaust 30% of HEPA-filtered air either into the room or to the outside through a canopy connection. Type A1 mixes the supply air in a common plenum and may have ducts and plenum under positive pressure. Type A2 has all contaminated ducts and plenum under negative pressure or surrounded by negative pressure. Type B1 exhausts 70% of total air through a dedicated exhaust duct and must be hard ducted. Type B2 exhausts 100% of total air to the outside without any recirculation and must be hard ducted also. With types B1 and B2, all the ducts and the plenum are under negative pressure and are surrounded by negative pressure.

Preparation of Hazardous Drugs

When working with hazardous drugs, personnel must wear appropriate protective equipment, including gowns, face masks, eye protection, hair and shoe covers, and double sterile chemotherapy-type gloves. Personnel must handle all hazardous drugs with caution at all times, using appropriate chemotherapy gloves, not only during preparation, but also during receiving, distribution, stocking, inventorying, and disposal.

It is imperative that positive pressure not be allowed to build up in the vial. Proper training on the use of a chemotherapy-venting device, which uses a 0.2 micron hydrophobic filter or the negative pressure technique to prevent the build up of positive pressure within the vial, must be done before preparing hazardous drugs and on an annual basis. When a closed system transfer device (one that allows no venting or exposure of hazardous substance to the environment) is used, it shall be used within the ISO class 5 environment of a BSC or CACI.

When compounding, syringes and IV sets with Luer-Lok fittings must be used if possible. Use a large enough syringe so that the plunger does not separate from the barrel of the syringe when filled with solution. Syringes should be filled with no more than 75% of their total volume. When possible, attach IV sets and prime them before adding the hazardous drug. Wipe the outside of the bag or bottle to remove any inadvertent contamination. The use of nonshedding plastic-backed absorbent pads is also conducive to keeping the BSC as clean as possible.

The PEC shall be located in an ISO class 7 area physically separated from other preparation areas and maintained under negative pressure of not less than 0.01 inch water column to the surrounding area.

5-7. Overview of the Standard of Practice Related to Sterile Preparations: The United States Pharmacopeia (USP) 32/National Formulary (NF) 27

Chapter 797, *Pharmaceutical Compounding—Sterile Preparations* in USP 32/NF 27, became official June 2008. Chapter 797 has three microbial risk levels of compounded sterile preparations. The risk levels are determined on the basis of the potential for the introduction of microbial, chemical, or physical contamination into the product. The chapter covers topics such as validation of sterilization and of the aseptic process, environmental control and sampling, end-product testing, bacterial endotoxins, training, and a quality assurance program.

Low-Risk Compounding

Compounding is classified as *low risk* when all of the following conditions prevail:

- Commercially available sterile products, components, and devices are used in compounding within air quality of ISO class 5 or better.
- Compounding involves few aseptic manipulations, using not more than three commercially manufactured sterile products and not more than two entries into any one sterile container.
- Closed-system transfers are used. Withdrawal from an open ampul is classified as a closed system.
- In the absence of passing a sterility test, the storage periods for the compounded sterile preparations cannot exceed the following time periods before administration:
  - Storage for not more than 48 hours at controlled room temperature
  - Storage for not more than 14 days at a cold temperature of 2–8°C
  - Storage for not more than 45 days in a solid frozen state between −25°C and −10°C.

Medium-Risk Compounding

Medium-risk CSPs are those compounded under low-risk conditions when one or more of the following conditions exist:

- Compounding involves pooling of additives for the administration to either multiple patients or to one patient on multiple occasions.
- Compounding involves complex manipulations other than a single volume transfer.
- The compounding process requires a long time period to complete dissolution or homogeneous mixing.
- In the absence of passing a sterility test, the storage periods for the CSPs cannot exceed the following time periods before administration:
  - Exposure for not more than 30 hours at controlled room temperature

- Storage for not more than 9 days at a cold temperature
- Storage for not more than 45 days in a solid frozen state between −25°C and −10°C.

High-Risk Compounding

High-risk compounds are compounded under any of the following conditions and are either contaminated or at high risk to become contaminated with infectious microorganisms:

- A sterile preparation is compounded from nonsterile ingredients.
- Sterile ingredients or components are exposed to air quality inferior to ISO class 5 for more than 1 hour, including storage in environments inferior to ISO class 5 of opened or partially used packages of manufactured sterile products with no antimicrobial preservative system.
- Nonsterile water containing preparations are exposed for more than 6 hours before being sterilized.
- No examination of labeling and documentation from suppliers or direct determination that the chemical purity and content strength of ingredients meet their original or compendia specification occurs.
- Compounding personnel are improperly garbed and gloved.
- In the absence of passing a sterility test, the storage periods for the CSPs cannot exceed the following time periods before administration:
  - Storage for not more than 24 hours at controlled room temperature
  - Storage for not more than 3 days at a cold temperature
  - Storage for not more than 45 days in a solid frozen state between −25°C and −10°C.

5-8. Sterilization Methods

Filtration

Filtration works by a combination of sieving, adsorption, and entrapment. Care must be taken to choose the correct filter to sterilize the preparation. Membrane filters generally are compatible with most pharmaceutical solutions, but interactions do occur—often because of sorption or leaching. *Sorption* is the binding of drug or other formulation components to the filter, which can occur with peptide or protein formulations. There are filters that have little or no affinity for peptides or proteins. Leaching is the extracting of components of the filter into the solution. Surfactants are often added to the filter to make it hydrophilic, and they may leach into the product. Large-molecular-weight peptides may be affected by filtration. Their passage through a filter with a small pore size may cause shear stress and alter the three dimensional structure of the peptide. Solvents in the parenteral formulation may also affect filters. All filter manufacturers have compatibility data on their membrane type and can be a great source of information when choosing a membrane.

Filter choice

Choose the appropriate size and configuration of filtration device to accommodate the volume being filtered and permit complete filtration without clogging of the membrane. A 25 mm syringe disk filter should filter no more than 100 mL of solution. If the solution being filtered has a heavy particulate load, a 5 micron filter should be used before the 0.2 micron filter to decrease the particulate load to the 0.2 micron filter. The filter membrane and housing must be physically and chemically compatible with the product to be filtered and capable of withstanding the temperature, pressures, and hydrostatic stress imposed on the system.

A pharmacy may rely on the certificate of quality provided by the vendor. Certification shall include microbial retention testing with *Brevundimonas diminuta* at a minimum concentration of 10^7 organisms per cm^2, as well as testing for membrane and housing integrity, nonpyrogenicity, and extractables.

Hydrophobic and hydrophilic filters

Hydrophilic membranes wet spontaneously with water. They are used for filtration of aqueous solutions and aqueous solutions containing water-miscible solvents. *Hydrophobic filters* do not wet spontaneously with water. They are used for filtering gases and solvents.

Filter integrity

A sterilizing filter assembly should be tested for integrity after filtration has occurred. The *bubble point* is a simple, nondestructive check of the integrity of the filtration assembly, including the filter membrane. The basis for the test is that liquid is held in the capillary structure of the membrane by surface tension. The minimum pressure required to force the liquid out of the capillary space is a measure of the largest pores in the membrane.

A bubble point test is performed by wetting the filter with water, increasing the pressure of air upstream of the filter, and watching for air bubbles downstream to indicate passage of air through the filter capillaries. The typical water bubble point pressure of a sterilizing filter with a pore size rating of 0.2 micron is > 50 pounds per square inch gauge (psig). As pore size decreases, the bubble point increases. Remember that the bubble point given on the certificate of quality from the filter manufacturer is usually the water bubble point. Many drug formulations have a lower surface tension than water and will have a lower bubble point. Bubble points are also often given for 70% IPA and water. Use the alcohol test for a hydrophobic filter.

After the solution is filtered and before the integrity of the filter membrane is checked, the filter should be flushed with water to wash as much of the product off the membrane as possible. The integrity test may then be performed.

Heat Sterilization

Moist-heat sterilization (autoclave)

Moist-heat sterilization is one of the most widely used methods of sterilization. Saturation of steam at high pressure is the foundation for the effectiveness of moist-heat sterilization. When steam makes contact with a cooler object, it condenses and loses latent heat to the object. The amount of energy released is ~524 kcal/g at 121°C. Most sterilization cycles are at 121°C at 15 psig for a minimum of 15 minutes. Moist-heat sterilization is faster and does not require as high a temperature as dry-heat sterilization. Biological indicators of *Bacillus stearothermophilus* and temperature-sensing devices shall be used to verify the effectiveness of the steam sterilization cycle.

Dry-heat sterilization

Dry-heat sterilization is usually done as a batch process in an oven designed for sterilization. It provides heated filtered air that is evenly distributed throughout the chamber by a blower. The oven is equipped with a system to control the temperature and exposure period. Dry-heat sterilization requires higher temperatures and longer exposure times than does moist-heat sterilization. Typical sterilization cycles are 120–180 minutes at 160°C or 90–120 minutes at 170°C. Biological indicators of *Bacillus subtilis* and temperature-sensing devices shall be used to verify the effectiveness of the dry-heat sterilization cycle.

Depyrogenation by dry heat

Dry heat can also be used for depyrogenation of glass and stainless steel equipment and of vials. The pyrogens are destroyed when the equipment is kept at 250°C for 30 minutes. The effectiveness of the dry-heat depyrogenation cycle shall be verified by using endotoxin challenge vials to determine whether the cycle is adequate to achieve a 3-log reduction in endotoxins.

Beyond-Use Date

Each compounded sterile preparation must have a label that specifies the correct names and amount of ingredients, the total volume, the storage requirements, route of administration, and beyond-use date (BUD). The BUD is the date after which a compounded preparation is not to be used and is determined from the date the preparation is compounded. In the absence of passing the sterility test, the CSPs must comply with the microbial BUD. If the lot of CSP has met the requirements of the sterility test, then the BUD may be based on chemical and physical stability. When assigning a BUD, compounding personnel should consult and apply drug-specific and general stability documentation and literature where available. They should consider the nature of the drug, its degradation mechanism, the container in which it is packaged, the expected storage conditions, and the intended duration of therapy.

5-9. Stability

Stability refers to physical, chemical, and microbial stability.

Instability usually refers to chemical reactions that are incessant and irreversible and result in distinctly different chemical entities. These new chemical entities can be therapeutically inactive and possibly exhibit greater toxicity.

Incompatibility usually refers to physicochemical phenomena such as concentration-dependent precipitation and acid–base reactions that occur when one drug is mixed with others to produce a product unsuitable for administration to the patient. An incompatibility could cause the patient not to receive the full therapeutic effect, or it could cause toxic decomposition products to form. A precipitated incompatibility may irritate the vein or cause occlusion of vessels.

There are three categories of incompatibilities: *therapeutic incompatibility, physical incompatibility,* and *chemical incompatibility.*

Therapeutic Incompatibility

Therapeutic incompatibility occurs when two or more drugs administered at the same time result in undesirable antagonistic or synergistic pharmacologic action.

Physical Incompatibility

Physical incompatibility is the combination of two or more drugs in solution, resulting in a change in the appearance of the solution, a change in color, the formation of turbidity or a precipitate, or the evolution of a gas. Physical incompatibilities are related to solubility changes or container interactions rather than to molecular change to the drug entity itself.

Six major areas of concern about physical incompatibility

Compatibility or incompatibility of two or more drugs mixed in the same syringe
For example, preoperative medications—a combination of a narcotic, an analgesic, an antiemetic, and an anticholinergic—are mixed in the same syringe to save the patient from multiple IM injections.

Compatibility of two or more drugs given through the same IV administration line
This concern is common in intensive care units, where patients are often on a number of IV medications and could also be fluid restricted. For example, dopamine HCl 800 mg in 500 mL D_5W (5% dextrose in water) is prescribed. The nurse wants to push 2 amps of sodium bicarbonate through the IV line. The pH of dopamine is 3.0–4.5, and that of $NaHCO_3$ is approximately 8.0. If this push is done, a color change occurs because of decomposition of the product. The pH of the bicarbonate is too high for dopamine stability.

Compatibility of two or more drugs placed in the same bottle or bag of IV fluid
KCl, the most common additive, is a neutral salt composed of monovalent ions that are not likely to produce compatibility problems. Therefore, if a drug is compatible in a neutral salt, it is probably compatible in KCl.

Parenteral nutrition solutions can be especially difficult. The number of components, the long duration of contact time, and exposure to ambient temperature and light enhance the potential for an adverse compatibility interaction to occur. The interaction of Ca and PO_4 to form $CaPO_4$, which appears as fine white particles that create a milky solution, is a problem.

Some ways to decrease the risk of injury follow:

- Calculate the solubility of the added calcium from the volume at the time when calcium is added. Flush the line in between the addition of any potentially incompatible components.
- Add the calcium before the lipid emulsion. Therefore, if a precipitate forms, the lipid will not obscure its presence.
- Periodically agitate the admixture, and check for precipitates. Train patients and caregivers to visually inspect for signs of precipitation and to stop the infusion if precipitation is noted.

The following factors enhance formation of precipitate of calcium and phosphate:

- High concentrations of calcium and phosphate
- Increases in solution pH
- Decreases in amino acid concentrations
- Increases in temperature
- Addition of calcium before phosphate
- Lengthy time delay or slow infusion rates
- Use of the chloride salt of calcium.

Do not exceed 15 mEq of Ca with up to 15 mL PO_4 per 1000 mL of solution.

Compatibility of the additive with the composition of the IV container itself
Nitroglycerin readily migrates into many plastics, especially polyvinylchloride (PVC). Insulin adsorbs to IV tubing, filters, and both glass and plastic containers.

Compatibility of the additive with the additional equipment used to prepare or administer the IV admixture
Cisplatin interacts with aluminum by forming a black precipitate when coming in contact with it.

Stability of the drug after admixture
Ampicillin sodium is stable for 72 hours when refrigerated and 24 hours at room temperature in normal saline. However, if it is added to D_5W, it is stable for only 4 hours when refrigerated and 2 hours at room temperature.

Other potential sources of physical incompatibilities

Concentration
A drug will remain in aqueous solution as long as its concentration is less than its saturation solubility.

Cosolvent system

Drugs that are poorly water soluble are often formulated using water-miscible cosolvents. Examples of water-miscible cosolvents include ethanol, propylene glycol, and polyethylene glycol. Dilution of drugs that are in a cosolvent system often causes precipitation of the drug. A good example is diazepam injection. Dilution of the drug results in precipitation in some concentrations, but sufficient dilution to a point below diazepam's saturation solubility results in a physically stable admixture.

pH

The greatest single factor in causing an incompatibility is a change in acid–base environment. Solubility of drugs that are weak acids or bases is a direct function of solution pH. The drug's dissociation constant and pH control the portion of drug in its ionized form and the solubility of the un-ionized form. A drug that is a weak acid may be formulated at a pH sufficient to yield the desired solubility. Sodium salts of barbiturates, phenytoin, and methotrexate are formulated at high pH values to achieve adequate solubility.

Sodium salts of weak acids precipitate as free acids when added to IV fluids having an acidic pH. If the pH of these drugs is lowered, the drug's solubility at the final pH may be exceeded, resulting in possible precipitation. Drugs that are salts of weak bases may precipitate in an alkaline solution.

Ionic interactions

Large organic anions and cations may also form precipitates, such as the precipitation that occurs when heparin (anionic) and aminoglycoside antibiotics (cationic) are mixed. These heparin salts of the cationic drug are relatively insoluble in water.

Sorption phenomena

The intact drug is lost from the solution by adsorption to the surface or absorption into the matrix of container material, administration set, or filter.

Adsorption to the surface can result from interactions of functional groups within the drug's molecule to binding sites on the surfaces.

Absorption of lipid-soluble drugs into the matrix of plastic containers and administration sets, especially those made from PVC, does occur. The substantial amount of phthalate plasticizer used to make the PVC bag pliable and flexible allows the lipid-soluble drugs to diffuse from the solution into the plasticizer in the plastic matrix. Plastics such as polyethylene and polypropylene, which contain little or no phthalate plasticizer, do not readily absorb lipid-soluble drugs into the polymer core. Leaching of the phthalate plasticizer into the solution may also occur, especially if surface-active agents or a large amount of organic cosolvent is present in the formulation.

Chemical Incompatibility

Chemical incompatibilities are interactions resulting in molecular changes or rearrangements to different chemical entities. Most chemical interactions are not observable by the unaided eye.

Chemical degradation pathways

Hydrolysis is a common mode of chemical decomposition. Water attacks labile bonds in dissolved drug molecules. Functional groups labile to hydrolysis are carboxylic acid and phosphate esters, amides, lactams, and imines.

Oxidation is an electron loss that causes a positive increase in valence. Many drugs are in the reduced form, and oxygen creates stability problems. Steroids, epinephrine, and tricyclic compounds are sensitive to oxygen. For control of the stability problem, oxygen can be excluded, pH can be adjusted, and chelating agents or antioxidants can be added.

Reduction is when an electron is gained, causing a decrease in valence and the addition of halogen or hydrogen to the double bond. β-lactam antibiotics can produce reducing aldehydes on hydrolysis.

Photolysis is the catalysis by light of degradation reactions such as oxidation or hydrolysis. Examples of drugs that are light sensitive are amphotericin B, furosemide, and sodium nitroprusside. The reaction rate depends on the intensity and wavelength of light. Sodium nitroprusside in D_5W has a faint brownish cast, but exposure to light causes deterioration, which is evident by a change in color to blue caused by the reduction of the ferric to ferrous ion.

Extreme pH can be a catalysis of drug degradation. Drug reaction rates are generally less at intermediate pH values than at high or low ranges. A buffer system is often used to ensure the maintenance of the proper pH.

Effects of temperature may be evident. Usually, but not always, an elevation in temperature may increase reaction rates.

An increase in drug concentration will usually increase the degradation rate exponentially. However, this rule does not always apply. Some drugs appear to have a lower rate of decomposition at a high concentration, such as the reduced hydrolysis of nafcillin in the presence of aminophylline. Greater buffer concentration at higher nafcillin concentrations protects the drug from aminophylline's high pH and slows the hydrolysis.

Expiration dates and removal of the IV bag overwrap are important. The overwrap protects against evaporation of the solution, desiccation of the container, drug oxidation, and photochemical inactivation of the drug. Substantial moisture loss may occur, increasing drug concentration. With ready-to-use dopamine or dobutamine injections, removal of the overwrap can allow oxygen to enter the container, thereby reducing drug stability. After removal of the overwrap, the expiration date should be changed at once.

5-10. Sterile Products Compounded from Nonsterile Drugs

When a sterile preparation is compounded from a nonsterile component, several concerns arise: how to sterilize the drug, how to sterilize the container and closure, and how to ensure that the drug and components are sterile. Every sterilization process must be verified, whether it is terminal sterilization of the CSP in the final container or aseptic processing of the CSP. Sterility testing must be done on all high-risk compounded sterile preparations if they are prepared in groups of more than 25 single-dose packages or in multidose vials for administration to multiple patients. Such testing must also be done if prior to sterilization the preparations are exposed longer than 12 hours to temperatures of 2–8°C or longer than 6 hours to temperatures warmer than 8°C. If the high-risk CSPs are dispensed before the results of the sterility test are known, a method must be in place requiring daily observation of the test specimens and immediate recall of the CSP if there is evidence of microbial growth in the test sample.

Sterility Testing

There are two methods of sterility testing: *direct inoculation* and *membrane filtration*. The USP states that, when possible, membrane filtration should be performed and that two culture media are required: fluid thioglycollate medium (FTM) and trypticase soy broth (TSB), which is also known as soybean-casein digest medium.

Media suitability test

Before beginning the test, one must confirm that the medium being used is sterile and will support the growth of microorganisms.

Sterility
Confirm the sterility of each sterilized batch of medium (1) by incubating a portion of the batch at the specified incubation temperature (TSB, 20–25°C; FTM, 30–35°C) for 14 days or (2) by incubating uninoculated containers as negative controls during a sterility test procedure. When purchasing a new batch of sterile media from a vendor, one should incubate a portion for several days to ensure that it did not become contaminated during shipment.

Growth promotion test
Each lot of ready-prepared medium and each batch of dehydrated medium bearing the manufacturer's lot number must be tested for its growth-promoting qualities. Separately inoculate, in duplicate, containers of each medium with fewer than 100 viable microorganisms of each of the strains listed in the next paragraph. If visual evidence of growth appears in all inoculated media containers within 3 days of incubation in the case of bacteria and 5 days of incubation in the case of fungi, the test media is satisfactory. The test may be conducted simultaneously with testing of the media for sterility.

The organisms to be used for the growth promotion test of FTM are *Staphylococcus aureus* (*Bacillus subtilis* may be used instead), *Pseudomonas aeruginosa* (*Micrococcus luteus* may be used instead), and *Clostridium sporogenes* (*Bacteroides vulgatus* may be used instead). The test organisms for soybean-casein digest media are *Bacillus subtilis*, *Candida albicans*, and *Aspergillus niger*. Soybean-casein digest media are incubated at 20–25°C, and FTM are incubated at 30–35°C, both under aerobic conditions for a minimum of 14 days.

Validation test: Bacteriostasis and fungistasis test
The bacteriostasis and fungistasis test must be done on each product to determine if the product itself will inhibit the growth of microorganisms. This test needs to be done only once for each product tested. The organisms used are the same as those used for growth promotion. The test uses two sets of containers. One set is inoculated with the drug product and microorganisms, and the other set is inoculated with just the microorganisms. Both sets will be incubated at the appropriate temperature for no more than 5 days.

The same amount of growth should be seen in both sets. If the drug is inhibiting the growth of the microorganisms, the conditions of the test must be modified so the drug will not inhibit growth. The modifications made will now become the method for performing the sterility test on the drug preparation.

Number of articles to test

The minimum number of articles to be tested in relation to the number of articles in the batch are as follows:

- For up to 100 articles, test 10% or 4 articles, whichever is greater.
- For more than 100 but not more than 500 articles, test 10 articles.

Interpretation of results

No growth

At days 3, 5, 7, 10, and 14, examine the media visually for growth. If no microbial growth is seen, the article complies with the test for sterility. Lack of growth of the media does not prove that all units in the lot are sterile.

Observed growth

When microbial growth is observed and confirmed microscopically, the article does not meet the requirements of the test for sterility. If there is no doubt that the microbial growth can be ascribed to faulty aseptic techniques or materials used in conducting the testing procedure, the test is invalid and must be repeated.

An investigation must occur, and the organism must be identified down to the species. All records must be reviewed, including all employee training procedures and records, aseptic gowning practices, equipment maintenance records, component sterilization data, and environmental monitoring data.

Visual inspection

Every unit compounded in the pharmacy should be subjected to a physical inspection against a white background and a black background. Any container whose contents show evidence of contamination with visible foreign material must be rejected.

Pyrogens

A pyrogen is a substance that produces fever. An endotoxin is a type of pyrogen.

Gram-negative bacteria produce more potent endotoxins than do Gram-positive bacteria and fungi. The lipopolysaccharide (LPS) portion of the cell wall causes the pyrogenic response. The LPS can be sloughed off, and the bacteria do not have to be living for the LPS to be pyrogenic.

Some of the effects caused by pyrogens in the body are an increase in body temperature, chills, cutaneous vasoconstriction, a decrease in respiration, an increase in arterial blood pressure, nausea and malaise, and severe diarrhea.

The official endotoxin limits are 5 endotoxin units (EU)/kg per hour or 350 EU/total body per hour for drugs and biologicals. Drugs for intrathecal use have a much lower endotoxin limit of 0.2 EU/kg.

Water is the primary source of endotoxins because *Pseudomonas,* a Gram-negative bacterium, grows readily in water. Other sources of endotoxins or pyrogens are raw material, equipment, processing, and human contamination. It is very important to use good-quality raw materials and request a certificate of analysis with each lot of material when compounding. Endotoxins can be destroyed by dry heat. Three to five hours at 200°C will depyrogenate glass vials and beakers. The endotoxin concentration can be reduced by rinsing with sterile water for injection. When a sterile preparation is compounded from a nonsterile product, any equipment that can withstand the heat of 200°C should be depyrogenated. An article that is depyrogenated is also sterile. Endotoxins are not completely removed by filtration, and steam sterilization reduces endotoxin levels by only a small amount.

Pyrogen test (rabbit test)

The pyrogen test is designed to limit, to an acceptable level, the patient's risk of febrile reaction in the administration—by injection—of the product concerned. The test involves measuring the rise in temperature of rabbits following the IV injection of a test solution, and it is designed for products that can be tolerated by the test rabbit in a dose—not to exceed 10 mL/kg—injected intravenously within a period of no more than 10 minutes.

The rabbit test has several limitations. It is an in vivo method, it is an expensive and time-consuming test, and it is not a very sensitive test. Drugs that have pyretic side effects or that are antipyretics cannot be tested using the rabbit test. The test is not quantitative, and the pyrogenic response is dose dependent, not concentration dependent.

Bacterial endotoxin test (limulus amebocyte lysate test)

The bacterial endotoxin test (BET) provides a method for estimating the concentration of bacterial endotoxins that may be present in, or on the sample of, the article to which the test is applied using limulus amebocyte lysate (LAL) reagent. Because the blood cells of the horseshoe crab are sensitive to endotoxin and form a gel in its presence, LAL reagent is made from the lysate of amebocytes from the horseshoe crab.

There are two types of techniques for this test: the *gel-clot technique,* which is based on the formation of the gel, and the *photometric technique,* which is based on either the development of turbidity or the development of color in the test sample.

The routine gel-clot test requires 0.1 mL of test sample to be mixed with 0.1 mL of LAL reagent. This mixture is incubated for 1 hour at 37°C. A positive reaction is confirmed by formation of a firm gel that remains intact when the tube is slowly inverted 180 degrees.

The BET is 5–50 times more sensitive, more simple and rapid, and less expensive than the pyrogen test. However, the clotting enzyme is heat sensitive, pH sensitive, and chemically related to trypsin. It is dependable for detection of only pyrogens originating from Gram-negative bacteria. Also, some drugs can inhibit the reaction, and other drugs can enhance the reaction. The BET does not determine the fever-producing potential of the bacterial endotoxins.

The photometric technique requires the establishment of a standard regression curve. The endotoxin content of the test material is determined by interpolation from the curve. The test can be either an end-point determination, in which the reading is made immediately at the end of the incubation period, or a kinetic test, in which the absorbance is measured throughout the reaction period.

All high-risk CSPs (except those for inhalation and ophthalmic use) that are prepared in groups of 25 or more individual single-dose units or in multidose vials for administration to multiple patients, or that are exposed longer than 12 hours to temperatures of 2–8°C and longer than 6 hours to temperatures warmer than 8°C before sterilization, must comply with the BET.

5-11. Key Points

- A sterilizing filter (0.2 micron) is required to filter sterilize a CSP. The integrity of the filter must be tested before the preparation may be released. The test is often referred to as the *bubble point test.*

- The high-efficiency particulate air filter is 99.97% efficient at filtering out particles 0.3 micron and larger. Certification of the HEPA filter involves testing the velocity of airflow from the filter and the integrity of the filter.

- The air in an ISO class 5 area has no more than 3,520 particles 0.5 micron and larger per cubic meter of air. The laminar flow workbench provides an ISO class 5 area.

- The critical site is any opening or pathway between the CSP and the environment. The larger the critical site is and the longer it is exposed to the environment, the greater the risk of contamination of the preparation.

- The bacterial endotoxin test is designed to detect the level of bacterial endotoxin from Gram-negative organisms in the CSP. All bacterial endotoxins are pyrogens, but not all pyrogens are bacterial endotoxins.

- The sterility test and the BET should be performed on all high-risk compounded sterile preparations intended for administration by injection into the vascular or central nervous system that are prepared in groups of more than 25 identical individual single-dose packages or in multidose vials for administration to multiple patients. The BET must be performed before the CSP can be dispensed.

- Any pharmacist preparing CSPs must have training in aseptic technique. One way to validate aseptic technique is by performing media fills. The growth medium most often used is trypticase soy broth, also known as soybean-casein digest medium in the USP.

- The laminar airflow in a horizontal laminar flow workbench flows toward the operator. The operator must never put his or her hands in back of an object, between the HEPA filter and the critical site. Never break first air.

- The laminar airflow in a vertical laminar flow workbench flows down onto the work surface.

- A biological safety cabinet should always be used for preparing cytotoxic drugs. All biological safety cabinets have vertical laminar airflow.

- The hot air oven is used to depyrogenate items used in compounding and to sterilize compounded preparations that cannot be sterilized by steam.

- Moist-heat sterilization is a common way to sterilize equipment used in the compounding process. Only items that can be moistened by steam can be sterilized by autoclaving.

5-12. Questions

1. Which of the following tests does *not* have to be completed on a high-risk compounded sterile preparation that will be administered by intravascular injection and is prepared in a lot size of 30 single-dose vials before release to a patient?

   A. Bacterial endotoxin test
   B. Visual inspection
   C. Sterility test
   D. Verification of the sterilizing filter integrity
   E. LAL test

2. Which of the following is correct concerning certification of a laminar flow workbench?

   A. The particles introduced into the plenum of the hood must be approximately 0.5 micron.
   B. Airflow from the HEPA filter must be 120 ft/min.
   C. A leak greater than 0.01% of the upstream smoke concentration through the filter is considered a serious leak.
   D. A total particle counter can be used to check the integrity of the HEPA filter.
   E. If a HEPA filter leaks, it cannot be patched; it must be replaced.

3. The bacterial endotoxin test is used to determine

   A. the amount of pyrogens.
   B. the level of pyrogens from Gram-negative bacteria.
   C. the fever-producing potential of bacterial endotoxins from Gram-negative bacteria.
   D. the level of bacterial endotoxin from Gram-positive bacteria.
   E. the amount of live bacteria present in the drug solution.

4. Which of the following is correct concerning USP media transfers?

   A. An operator must successfully complete one media fill before compounding any CSPs.
   B. An operator who passes a written exam may compound sterile preparations until the chief pharmacist finds time to watch his or her aseptic technique.

   C. An operator who has successfully completed a media fill must requalify semiannually if he or she is preparing low-risk CSPs.
   D. When an operator successfully completes one media fill for high-risk compounding, he or she needs to revalidate quarterly by completing one media fill.
   E. Fluid thioglycollate media are used for media transfers.

5. For a transfer of product into the controlled area,

   A. bottles, bags, and syringes must be removed from brown cardboard boxes before being brought into the buffer area.
   B. vials stored in laminated cardboard may not be brought into the controlled area.
   C. stainless steel carts may be used to transfer items into the controlled area directly from the storage area.
   D. large-volume parenteral bags of IV solution must be removed from their protective overwrap before being brought into the controlled area.
   E. the refrigerator should be placed next to the laminar flow hood for easy access.

6. Which of the following is correct concerning a vertical laminar flow hood?

   A. It is always a biological safety cabinet.
   B. In vertical laminar flow, the hands of the operator must not be behind an object.
   C. A vertical laminar flow hood has turbulent airflow within 1 inch of the work surface.
   D. A vertical laminar flow hood has the laminar airflow blowing at the operator.
   E. The operator works in a vertical flow hood and a horizontal flow hood in the same manner.

7. Certain factors may increase the risk of microbial contamination of a CSP. Which of the following would *not* be a risk factor?

   A. Very complex compounding steps
   B. Lengthy exposure of a critical site during compounding
   C. Use of appropriate aseptic technique
   D. Batch compounding without preservatives for multiple patients
   E. Preparation of a CSP from nonsterile powders

8. Which of the following is correct concerning the USP risk levels of compounded sterile preparations?

    A. Preparations intended for administration over 3 days would be classified as low risk.
    B. A high-risk sterile preparation that has met the requirements of the sterility test can be stored for not more than 24 hours at a controlled room temperature.
    C. The storage time for a medium-risk preparation under refrigeration is no longer than 9 days.
    D. A CSP that will be administered to multiple patients or to a single patient multiple times is classified as a high-risk CSP.
    E. After meeting the requirements of the sterility test, a sterile preparation can be stored indefinitely.

9. Which of the following is correct?

    A. For work done in a horizontal laminar flow workbench, arrange items in the hood so that your hand is never between the HEPA filter and an object.
    B. For work done in a horizontal laminar flow workbench, vials that are not being used should be stacked up along the side of the hood to increase workspace in the hood.
    C. Before each shift, 70% isopropyl alcohol is used to sterilize the laminar flow workbench.
    D. An object placed in the horizontal laminar flow workbench disturbs the airflow downstream of the object equal to two times the diameter of the object.
    E. Syringes and IV bags are placed in the hood in their protective overwrap.

10. Which of the following is correct concerning the necessity that operators in the buffer area be properly gowned?

    A. Operators don gowns because they shed particles, and the nonshedding gowns keep them sterile.
    B. Sterile gloves are used to avoid contamination of the CSP in case the operator accidentally touches a critical site during compounding of the preparation.
    C. Frequent sanitization with sterile 70% isopropyl alcohol is essential to keep the operators' hands sterile during the compounding process.
    D. Nonshedding garb and sterile gloves help to contain the particles shed from the operators.
    E. Operators must don gowns before working at the laminar flow workbench but not before entering the buffer area.

11. Which of the following is correct concerning placement of items and work performed in the laminar flow workstation?

    A. Items should be placed in a horizontal flow hood to the right or left of the work area.
    B. Items in a vertical laminar flow hood should be placed so that an operator's hand never goes over the top of a critical site while the operator is working in the hood.
    C. An object placed in a horizontal laminar flow hood disturbs the airflow downstream of the object equal to three times the diameter of the object.
    D. When working in a horizontal laminar flow workstation, an operator must perform all work at least 6 inches inside the hood.
    E. All of the above are correct.

12. Which parts of the syringe are considered critical sites?

    I.   The ribs of the plunger
    II. The collar of the syringe
    III. The tip of the syringe

    A. I only
    B. II only
    C. I and III only
    D. II and III only
    E. I, II, and III

13. Which parts of the needle are considered critical sites?

    I.   The hub
    II. The needle shaft
    III. The bevel and bevel tip of the needle

    A. I only
    B. II only
    C. I and III only
    D. II and III only
    E. I, II, and III

14. Which of the following are correct concerning ampuls?

    I.   Ampuls are single-dose containers.
    II. Ampuls must have the neck wiped with a sterile alcohol pad before being broken.
    III. Ampuls can be left in the hood and used for several days once opened.

    A. II only
    B. I and III only
    C. I and II only
    D. I, II, and III
    E. None of the above

15. Which of the following are correct concerning the steps taken to protect an operator when working with cytotoxic agents?

    I.   Preparation of cytotoxic drugs must occur in a biological safety cabinet.
    II. Syringes with Luer-Lok tips should be used when compounding cytotoxic CSPs.
    III. It is very important that positive pressure not be allowed to build up inside the vial when one is working with cytotoxic preparations.

    A. I only
    B. II only
    C. I and III only
    D. II and III only
    E. I, II, and III

16. Which of the following is correct?

    A. Filter integrity testing of the filter membrane is done to determine at what pressure the filter will break.
    B. The manufacturer of the filter membrane determines the bubble point of the membrane; this value is always the same, no matter what solution has been filtered.
    C. As the pore size of the filter membrane decreases, the pressure at which the air can be pushed from the largest pore increases.
    D. The bubble point test is a destructive test.
    E. It is not necessary to perform the bubble point test if a certificate of quality from the filter manufacturer is provided.

17. Which of the following factors should be considered when choosing a sterilizing filter?

    A. The volume of solution to be filtered
    B. The compatibility of the membrane with the solution to be filtered

    C. Whether the solution to be filtered is hydrophobic or hydrophilic
    D. The compatibility of the filter housing with the product to be filtered
    E. All of the above

18. Which of the following is correct concerning the USP sterility test?

    A. The validation test must be done on each CSP to determine if the article to be tested adversely affects the reliability of the test.
    B. The growth promotion test does not require that the test organisms listed in the USP be used.
    C. After inoculation, the media must be incubated for 14 days or fewer at the appropriate temperature.
    D. No growth on the sterility test proves that the aseptically produced product is sterile.
    E. Trypticase soy broth is incubated at 30–35°C, and fluid thioglycollate is incubated at 20–25°C.

19. Which of the following is correct?

    A. Gram-negative bacteria must be alive to cause a pyrogenic response.
    B. The lipopolysaccharide portion of the cell wall of Gram-negative bacteria causes the pyrogenic response.
    C. Endotoxin can be removed by a 0.2 micron filter.
    D. Steam sterilization will depyrogenate an object just as well as the hot air oven.
    E. An article that is depyrogenated is not necessarily sterile.

20. Which of the following is correct?

    A. The rabbit test and the LAL test are the same test.
    B. LAL reagent will determine the fever-producing potential of the pyrogens.
    C. There are two types of techniques for the BET: the gel-clot technique and the photometric technique.
    D. The CSP being tested has no effect on the test.
    E. All CSPs may be tested using the rabbit test.

21. Which of the following is correct?

    A. The rabbit test is the most sensitive because it can detect pyrogens from all sources.
    B. The rabbit test is an in vitro test.
    C. Some drugs may inhibit the formation of a gel in the BET.

D. No drug will enhance the formation of the gel in the BET.

E. The pyrogen test is a quantitative test.

22. The plenum in a laminar flow workbench is the area

    A. where the air is prefiltered.

    B. where air is pressurized for distribution over the HEPA filter.

    C. where compounding takes place.

    D. that serves no purpose.

    E. directly above the HEPA filter in a horizontal laminar flow hood.

23. Calcium and phosphate can interact to form a precipitate in parenteral nutrition solutions. Of the following situations that could enhance precipitate formation, which one would *not* do so?

    A. High concentration of calcium and phosphate

    B. Increase in solution pH

    C. Decrease in temperature

    D. Use of the chloride salt of calcium

    E. A slow infusion rate

24. Of the following potential sources of physical or chemical incompatibilities, which is *not* a source?

    A. Dilution of a drug in a cosolvent system into an aqueous system

    B. Addition of a drug solution with a high pH into a solution with a low pH

    C. Adsorption of a lipid-soluble drug into the matrix of a polypropylene container

    D. A photosensitive drug such as sodium nitroprusside in 5% dextrose in water exposed to light

    E. Leaching of phthalate plasticizer into the solution from a polyvinyl chloride container

5-13. Answers

1. C. The bacterial endotoxin test (LAL test), visual inspection test, and bubble point test should all be completed before the CSP is dispensed. Because the sterility test takes 14 days, the preparation may be dispensed before the results are known. However, a system to recall the CSP must be in place if it does not meet the test's requirement.

2. C. Any leak greater than 0.01% of upstream smoke concentration is a serious leak. The smoke particles are 0.3 microns. The airflow from the HEPA filter should be 90 ft/min, plus or minus 20%. A total particle counter is used to classify the environment, not to certify the integrity of the HEPA filter. The HEPA filter can be patched.

3. B. The BET determines the level of bacterial endotoxin from Gram-negative bacteria only. The BET cannot determine fever-producing potential of the endotoxins. The Gram-negative bacteria do not have to be alive for the endotoxin to produce an effect.

4. A. The operator must successfully complete one media fill before compounding a sterile preparation. Once validated for low- or medium-risk compounding, the operator must revalidate annually. For high-risk compounding, the operator must revalidate semiannually. Passing only a written exam does not allow the operator to compound a CSP. Trypticase soy broth is the medium most often used in media fills.

5. A. Cardboard must be kept out of the buffer area. Vials stored in laminated cardboard may be stored in the buffer area. No items should be brought into the buffer area without being sanitized. Large-volume parenteral bags should be removed from their overwrap just before being used. The refrigerator should not be in the buffer room because it is a source of contamination.

6. C. There are several types of vertical laminar flow hoods, of which the biological safety cabinet is one. The operator must never work over the top of items in the hood, and all work should be done at least 1 inch above the work surface.

7. C. Use of good aseptic technique is one way to ensure a good preparation.

8. C. A medium-risk CSP may not be stored longer than 9 days at cold temperature. USP 797 does not address administration at all; it applies only up to the time of administration. Once a CSP has met the requirement of the sterility test, the storage periods specified under the risk levels no longer apply. However, the beyond-use date based on chemical stability always applies. A CSP that will be administered to multiple patients or to a single patient multiple times is a medium-risk CSP.

9. A. In an HLFW, never put your hand behind an object, and in a VLFW, never put your hand above an object. In an HLFW, a vial disturbs the laminar airflow equal to three times the diameter of the object. If the vial is next to the side wall, the airflow is disturbed equal to six times the diameter of the object. Syringes and IV bags

should be taken from their overwrap at the edge of the hood.

10. **D.** Operators in the buffer area should wear clean, nonshedding gowns and gloves to help contain the particles that they shed. The sterile gloves are no longer sterile once they are out of the package. Proper aseptic technique must always be used.

11. **E.** All of the statements are correct concerning placement of items and work performed in the laminar flow workstation.

12. **C.** The ribs of the plunger and the tip of the syringe are critical sites of the syringe.

13. **E.** The hub, the needle shaft, and the bevel and bevel tip of the needle are all critical sites.

14. **C.** Once an ampul is opened, it must be used immediately.

15. **E.** When working with cytotoxic agents, an operator must take the following steps for protection: (1) preparation must occur in a biological safety cabinet, (2) syringes with Luer-Lok tips must be used, and (3) positive pressure must not be allowed to build up inside the vial.

16. **C.** The bubble point test is not a destructive test, and the value depends on the solution being filtered. When a CSP is filter sterilized, the bubble point test must be done before the preparation may be dispensed.

17. **E.** All of the factors should be considered.

18. **A.** The validation (bacteriostasis and fungistasis test) must be completed one time for each CSP. The growth promotion organisms listed in the USP are used for the validation test and for the growth promotion test.

19. **B.** Endotoxin will pass through a 0.2 micron filter. Steam sterilization will not depyrogenate an article. Bacteria do not have to be alive to be pyrogenic.

20. **C.** The pyrogen test, also known as the rabbit test, determines the fever-producing potential of the pyrogens. The BET is also known as the LAL test. The drug product can inhibit or enhance the gel formation in the BET.

21. **C.** The pyrogen (rabbit) test is an in vivo test and is not as sensitive as the BET. It is not a quantitative test.

22. **B.** The plenum is the area behind the HEPA filter in an HFLW that allows air to be pressurized for even distribution over the filter.

23. **C.** An increase in temperature could enhance precipitate formation.

24. **C.** Absorption of a lipid-soluble drug into the matrix of polyvinylchloride containers does occur. Polypropylene and polyethylene contain little or no phthalate plasticizer.

5-14. References

Akers MJ, Larrimore D, Guazzo D. *Parenteral Quality Control: Sterility, Pyrogen, Particulate and Package Integrity Testing.* 3rd ed. New York: Marcel Dekker; 2003.

American Society of Health-System Pharmacists. ASHP guidelines on quality assurance for pharmacy-prepared sterile products. *Am J Hosp Pharm.* 2000;57:1150–69.

Anderson RA. The status of environmental control: Practical approaches to the safe handling of anticancer products. Proceedings of a symposium in Mayaguez, Puerto Rico, November 2–5, 1983.

Buchanan C, McKinnon B, Scheckelhoff D, Schneider P. *Principles of Sterile Product Preparation.* Bethesda, Md.: American Society of Health-System Pharmacists; 2002:50.

General Services Administration. Federal standard 209e: Clean room and work station requirements, controlled environments. Washington, D.C.: U.S. Government Printing Office; 1992.

McKinnon B, Avis K. Membrane filtration of pharmaceutical solutions. *Am J Hosp Pharm.* 1993; 50:1021–36.

Trissel LA. *Handbook on Injectable Drugs.* 15th ed. Bethesda, Md.: American Society of Health-System Pharmacists; 2009.

United States Pharmacopeial Convention. Bacterial endotoxin test. In: *United States Pharmacopeia, 32nd Revision: National Formulary.* 27th ed. Rockville, Md.: United States Pharmacopeial Convention; 2009:93–96.

United States Pharmacopeial Convention. Compounded sterile preparations. In: *United States Pharmacopeia, 32nd Revision: National Formulary.* 27th ed. Rockville, Md.: United States Pharmacopeial Convention; 2009: 318–41.

United States Pharmacopeial Convention. Pyrogen test. In: *United States Pharmacopeia, 32nd Revision: National Formulary.* 27th ed. Rockville, Md.: United States Pharmacopeial Convention; 2009: 124–25.

United States Pharmacopeial Convention. Sterility tests. In: *United States Pharmacopeia, 32nd Revision: National Formulary.* 27th ed. Rockville, Md.: United States Pharmacopeial Convention; 2009: 80–86.

Pharmacokinetics, Drug Metabolism, and Drug Disposition

6

Bernd Meibohm, PhD
Charles R. Yates, PharmD, PhD

6-1. Introduction

Pharmacokinetics is the science of a drug's fate in the body. A drug's therapeutic potential is intimately linked to its pharmacokinetic profile. For example, a drug's pharmacologic response may be severely diminished by poor absorption, rapid elimination from the body, or both. The most important factors contributing to drug disposition include absorption, distribution, metabolism, and excretion.

Absorption

The rate and extent of drug absorption is referred to as *bioavailability*. The fraction of drug absorbed (f_a), an important determinant of the extent of bioavailability (represented by F), is affected not only by the drug's physicochemical properties but also by physiologic barriers at the site of absorption. For example, intestinal expression of the drug efflux transporter P-glycoprotein is known to limit oral drugs.

Distribution

Many drugs circulate in the body bound to plasma proteins (e.g., human serum albumin). The fraction of drug not bound to protein (f_{up}) is responsible for the pharmacologic effect. A drug may also bind significantly to tissue proteins (f_{ut}). Drugs with a large f_{up}-to-f_{ut} ratio have a large volume of distribution, whereas drugs with a small f_{up}-to-f_{ut} ratio are largely confined to the vascular space. Volume of distribution is directly related to *half-life* ($t_{1/2}$), the time required to eliminate half the drug from the body.

Metabolism

Approximately 50% of drugs undergo some form of hepatic metabolism. The cytochrome P450 (CYP450) family of drug-metabolizing enzymes is primarily responsible for drug inactivation in the liver. Hepatic clearance depends on liver blood flow and the extraction ratio (ER). Hepatic ER can be used to estimate the fraction of drug escaping first-pass metabolism (F^*), which is an important determinant of oral bioavailability. Intestinal inactivation of drugs by CYP450 enzymes in the gut is responsible for reduced F of a number of drugs.

Excretion

The primary purpose of hepatic metabolism is to increase a drug's water solubility to facilitate its renal elimination. The kidneys also serve as the primary eliminating organ for drugs that do not undergo hepatic metabolism. Renal clearance comprises three main physiologic processes: glomerular filtration, reabsorption, and secretion. *Filtration clearance* is the product of f_{up} and glomerular filtration rate (a physiologic parameter that diminishes with age). Renal reabsorption is a predominantly passive process dependent on physicochemical drug properties and on urine drug concentration and pH, whereas secretion is an active process facilitated by various transport mechanisms. The net of filtration, reabsorption, and secretion determines a drug's total renal clearance.

Interindividual differences in drug pharmacokinetics can at least partially explain variability in drug response. Thus, a thorough understanding of the physiologic processes affecting drug disposition is essential to drug individualization and optimization.

6-2. Absorption and Disposition

Drug Input

Drugs are administered to the body by one of two routes, intravascular or extravascular. For intravascular administration, drugs are usually administered as in intravenous (IV) infusion (continuous, short term, or bolus). The concentration C is given by the following expressions.

IV bolus

$$C = \frac{Dose}{V} \times e^{-K \times t}$$

$\frac{dC}{dt}$ (rate of change in plasma concentration)

= (rate of drug elimination, or output rate)

K = elimination rate constant = CL/V

CL = clearance = $Dose/AUC$

V = Volume

IV infusion

For drugs that are administered extravascularly (by mouth, intramuscularly, or subcutaneously) and act systemically, absorption must occur. See section 6-4.

First-order absorption

$$C = \frac{k_a \times F \times Dose}{V \times (k_a - K)} \times \left(e^{-K \times t} - e^{-k_a \times t}\right)$$

where k_a = first-order rate constant for drug absorption; absorption half-life = $0.693/k_a$; K = first-order rate constant for drug elimination (CL/V); CL = $F \times Dose/AUC$, oral clearance = CL/F = $Dose/AUC$; and F = bioavailability, or fraction of drug absorbed. F refers to the rate *and* extent of absorption.

6-3. Constant Rate Regimens

For many drugs to be therapeutically effective, drug concentrations of a certain level have to be maintained at the site of action for a prolonged period (e.g., β-lactam antibiotics, antiarrhythmics), whereas for others, alternating plasma concentrations are more preferable (e.g., aminoglycoside antibiotics such as gentamicin).

Two basic approaches to administering the drug can be applied to continuously maintain drug concentrations in a certain therapeutic range over a prolonged period:

- Drug administration at a constant input rate
- Sequential administration of discrete single doses (multiple dosing)

Drug Administration as Constant Rate Regimens

At any time during the infusion, the rate of change in drug concentration is the difference between the input rate (infusion rate R_0/volume of distribution V) and the output rate (elimination rate constant $K \times$ concentration C):

Rate of change = input rate – output rate

In concentrations:

$$\frac{dC}{dt} = \frac{R_0}{V} - K \times C$$

In amounts:

$$V \times \frac{dC}{dt} = R_0 - CL \times C$$

R_0 = infusion rate (in amount/time, e.g., mg/h)
V = volume of distribution
CL = clearance
K = first-order rate constant for drug elimination (CL/V)

$$\frac{dC}{dt} = 0, \quad \frac{R_0}{V} = K \times C_{ss}, \text{ or } R_0 = CL \times C_{ss}$$

Hence, the steady-state concentration C_{ss} is determined only by the infusion rate R_0 and the clearance CL.

Drug concentration at steady state:

$$C_{ss} = \frac{R_0}{CL}$$

Drug concentration before steady state:

$$C = \frac{R_0}{CL} \times \left(1 - e^{-K \times t}\right)$$

Time to Reach Steady State

For therapeutic purposes, knowing how long after initiation of an infusion reaching the targeted steady-state concentration C_{ss} will take is often of critical.

Concentration during an infusion before steady state:

$$C = \frac{R_0}{CL} \times \left(1 - e^{-K \times t}\right)$$

Concentration during an infusion at steady state:

$$C_{ss} = \frac{R_0}{CL}$$

The fraction of steady-state f is then

$$f = \frac{C}{C_{ss}} = \left(1 - e^{-K \times t}\right).$$

After a duration of infusion of

$1.0\ t_{1/2} \rightarrow 50\%$ of steady state is reached
$2.0\ t_{1/2} \rightarrow 75\%$ of steady state is reached
$3.0\ t_{1/2} \rightarrow 87.5\%$ of steady state is reached
$3.3\ t_{1/2} \rightarrow 90\%$ of steady state is reached
$4.0\ t_{1/2} \rightarrow 93.8\%$ of steady state is reached
$5.0\ t_{1/2} \rightarrow 96.9\%$ of steady state is reached

The following conclusions can be drawn:

- The approach to the steady-state concentration C_{ss} is exponential in nature and is controlled by the elimination process (elimination rate constant K), *not* the infusion rate R_0.
- Only the value of the steady-state concentration C_{ss} is controlled by the infusion rate R_0 (and of course by the clearance CL).
- Assuming for clinical purposes that a concentration of $> 95\%$ of steady state is therapeutically equivalent to the final steady-state concentration C_{ss}, approximately five elimination half-lives $t_{1/2}$ are necessary to reach steady state after initiation of an infusion.

Concentration-Time Profiles Postinfusion

The plasma concentration postinfusion cannot be distinguished from giving an IV bolus dose. Because the drug input has been discontinued, the rate of change in drug concentration is determined only by the output rate. If the drug follows one-compartment

characteristics, then the plasma concentration profile can be described by

$$C = C' \times e^{-K \times t_{pi}}$$

where C' is concentration at the end of the infusion and t_{pi} is time postinfusion (i.e., time after the infusion has stopped).

Thus, a general expression can be used to calculate the plasma concentration during and after a constant rate infusion:

$$C = \frac{R_0}{CL} \times \left(1 - e^{-K \times t}\right) \times e^{-K \times t_{pi}}$$

where t is the elapsed time after the beginning of the infusion and t_{pi} is the postinfusion time—that is, the difference between the duration of the infusion (infusion time T_{inf}) and t: $t_{pi} = t - T_{inf}$. For describing concentrations during the infusion, t_{pi} is set to zero. For describing concentrations postinfusion, t is set to T_{inf}.

Four different cases can be distinguished:

1. During the infusion, but before steady state is reached:

$$t = t,\ t_{pi} = 0 \Rightarrow C = \frac{R_0}{CL} \times \left(1 - e^{-K \times t}\right)$$

2. During the infusion at steady state:

$$t \rightarrow \infty,\ t_{pi} = 0 \Rightarrow C = \frac{R_0}{CL}$$

3. After cessation of the infusion before steady state:

$$t = T_{inf},\ t_{pi} = t - T_{inf}$$

$$\Rightarrow C = \frac{R_0}{CL} \times \left(1 - e^{-K \times T_{inf}}\right) \times e^{-K \times (t - T_{inf})}$$

4. After cessation of the infusion at steady state:

$$t \rightarrow \infty,\ t_{pi} = t - T_{inf} \Rightarrow C = \frac{R_0}{CL} \times e^{-K \times (t - T_{inf})}$$

Determination of Pharmacokinetic Parameters

The elimination rate constant K and the elimination half-life $t_{1/2}$ can be determined from

- The terminal slope after the infusion has been stopped
- The time to reach half of C_{ss}

■ The slope of the relationship of $\ln(C_{ss} - C)$ vs. t, based on

$$C = C_{ss} \times \left(1 - e^{-K \times t}\right)$$

and the resulting $\ln(C_{ss} - C) = \ln C_{ss} - K \times t$

The clearance CL from the relationship can be determined from

$$CL = \frac{R_0}{C_{ss}}$$

The volume of distribution from the relationship can be determined from

$$V = \frac{CL}{K}$$

Loading Dose and Maintenance Dose

The loading dose LD is supposed to immediately ($t = 0$) reach the desired target concentration C_{target}. It is administered as an IV bolus injection or, more frequently, as a short-term infusion. Following is an expression of target concentration calculated for a drug with one-compartment characteristics:

$$C_{target} = \frac{LD}{V} \rightarrow LD = C_{target} \times V$$

The maintenance dose MD is intended to sustain C_{target}. It is administered as a constant rate infusion. The maintenance dose is the infusion rate necessary to sustain the target concentration:

$$C_{target} = \frac{MD}{CL} \rightarrow MD = R_0 = C_{target} \times CL$$

6-4. Multiple Dosing

Continuous drug concentrations for a prolonged therapy can be maintained either by administering the drug at a constant input rate or by sequentially administering discrete single doses of the drug. The latter is the approach more frequently used and can be applied for extravascular as well as intravascular routes of administration.

Multiple-dose regimens are defined by two components, the dose D that is administered at each dosing occasion, and the dosing interval τ, which is the time between the administrations of two subsequent doses. Dose and dosing interval can be summarized in the dosing rate DR:

$$DR = \frac{D}{\tau}$$

Concentration-Time Profiles during Multiple Dosing

The multiple-dose function MDF can be used for calculating drug concentrations before steady state has been reached during a multiple-dose regimen:

$$MDF = \frac{1 - e^{n \times K \times \tau}}{1 - e^{-K \times \tau}}$$

where K is the respective rate constant of the drug, τ is the dosing interval, and n is the number of the dose.

Once steady state has been reached, n approaches infinity, and MDF simplifies to the accumulation factor AF:

$$AF = \frac{1}{1 - e^{-K \times \tau}}$$

Multiple-Dosing Regimens: Instantaneous Input (IV Bolus)

For an IV bolus multiple-dose regimen, the concentrations during the first dosing interval, the nth dosing interval, and at steady state are described by the relationships shown in Table 6-1.

The peak and trough concentrations at steady state can thus be expressed as the peak and trough after the first dose multiplied by the accumulation factor AF:

$$C_{ss,max} = \frac{C_{1,max}}{1 - e^{-K \times \tau}}$$

$$C_{ss,min} = \frac{C_{1,min}}{1 - e^{-K \times \tau}} = \frac{C_{1,max} \times e^{-K \times \tau}}{1 - e^{-K \times \tau}}.$$

Average steady-state concentration

By definition, the average drug input rate is equal to the average drug output rate at steady state. Whereas the *average input rate* is the drug amount entering the systemic circulation per dosing interval, the *average output rate* is equal to the product of clearance

Table 6-1. IV Bolus Multiple Dose Regimen

Dose number	Equation	Maximum or peak concentration	Minimum or trough concentration at the end of the dosing interval
1	$C = \dfrac{D}{V} \times e^{-K \times t}$	$C_{1,max} = \dfrac{D}{V}$	$C_{1,min} = \dfrac{D}{V} \times e^{-K \times \tau}$
n	$C = \dfrac{D}{V} \times e^{-K \times t} \times \dfrac{1 - e^{-n \times K \times \tau}}{1 - e^{-K \times \tau}}$	$C_{n,max} = \dfrac{D}{V} \times \dfrac{1 - e^{-n \times K \times \tau}}{1 - e^{-K \times \tau}}$	$C_{n,min} = \dfrac{D}{V} \times e^{-K \times \tau} \times \dfrac{1 - e^{-n \times K \times \tau}}{1 - e^{-K \times \tau}}$
Steady state	$C = \dfrac{D}{V} \times \dfrac{e^{-K \times t}}{1 - e^{-K \times \tau}}$	$C_{ss,max} = \dfrac{D}{V} \times \dfrac{1}{1 - e^{-K \times \tau}}$	$C_{ss,min} = \dfrac{D}{V} \times \dfrac{e^{-K \times \tau}}{1 - e^{-K \times \tau}}$

CL and the average plasma concentration within one dosing interval $C_{ss,av}$:

$$\frac{D}{\tau} = CL \times C_{ss,av}$$

Thus, the average steady-state concentration $C_{ss,av}$ during multiple dosing is determined only by the dose, the dosing interval τ (or both together as dosing rate $DR = D/\tau$), and the clearance CL:

$$C_{ss,av} = \frac{D}{\tau \times CL}$$

The area under the curve resulting from administration of a single dose AUC_{single} is equal to the area under the curve during one dosing interval at steady state AUC_{ss} if the same dose is given per dosing interval τ:

$$C_{ss,av} = \frac{AUC_{ss}}{\tau} = \frac{D}{\tau \times CL} = \frac{AUC_{single}}{\tau}$$

Thus,

$$AUC_{single} = AUC_{ss}$$

Extent of accumulation

The extent of accumulation during multiple dosing at steady state is determined by the dosing interval τ and the half-life of the drug $t_{1/2}$ (or the elimination rate constant K):

$$AF = \frac{1}{1 - e^{-K \times \tau}}$$

Thus, the extent of accumulation is dependent not only on the pharmacokinetic properties of a drug but also on the multiple-dosing regimen chosen.

Fluctuation

The degree of fluctuation between peak and trough concentrations during one dosing interval—that is, $C_{ss,max}$ and $C_{ss,min}$—is determined by the relationship between elimination half-life $t_{1/2}$ and dosing interval τ.

$$Fluctuation = \frac{C_{ss,max} - C_{ss,min}}{C_{ss,min}}$$

Multiple-Dosing Regimens: First-Order Input (Oral Dosing)

The average steady-state concentration $C_{ss,av}$ is now determined by the bioavailable fraction F of the dose D administered per dosing interval τ and the clearance CL:

$$C_{ss,av} = \frac{F \times D}{\tau \times CL}$$

The concentration-time profile after a single oral dose is given by

$$C = \frac{F \times D \times k_a}{V \times (k_a - K)} \times \left(e^{-K \times t} - e^{-k_a \times t} \right)$$

Hence, the concentration at any time within a dosing interval during multiple dosing at steady state is determined by

$$C = \frac{F \times D \times k_a}{V \times (k_a - K)} \times \left(\frac{e^{-K \times t}}{1 - e^{-K \times \tau}} - \frac{e^{-k_a \times t}}{1 - e^{-k_a \times \tau}} \right)$$

Thus, the trough concentration is readily available, assuming that the absorption is completed:

$$C_{ss,min} = \frac{F \times D \times k_a}{V \times (k_a - K)} \times \left(\frac{e^{-K \times \tau}}{1 - e^{-K \times \tau}} \right)$$

The peak concentration is assessable via the time-to-peak t_{max}, which is dependent on the rate of absorption and has to be determined through

$$t_{max} = \frac{\ln \left(\frac{k_a \times (1 - e^{-k_e \times \tau})}{K \times (1 - e^{-K \times \tau})} \right)}{(k_a - K)}$$

6-5. Volumes of Distribution and Protein Binding

Drug distribution means the reversible transfer of drug from one location to another within the body. After the drug has entered the vascular system, it becomes distributed throughout the various tissues and body fluids. However, most drugs do not distribute uniformly and in a similar manner throughout the body, as reflected by the difference in their volumes of distribution. Thus, the following material focuses on the factors and processes determining the rate and extent of distribution and the resulting consequences for pharmacotherapy.

Factors affecting distribution are

- Binding to blood or tissue elements
- Blood flow (i.e., the delivery of drug to the tissues)
- Ability to cross biomembranes
- Physicochemical properties of the drug (lipophilicity, extent of ionization) that determine partitioning into tissues

Protein Binding

The fraction unbound in plasma varies widely among drugs. Drugs are classified as follows:

- Highly protein bound:

$$f_u \leq 0.1 (\leq 10\% \text{ unbound}, \geq 90\% \text{ bound})$$

- Moderately protein bound:

$$f_u = 0.1 - 0.4 (10 - 40\% \text{ unbound}, 60 - 90\% \text{ bound})$$

- Low protein bound:

$$f_u = 0.4 (\geq 40\% \text{ unbound}, \leq 60\% \text{ bound})$$

Factors Determining the Degree of Protein Binding

The reversible binding of a drug to proteins obeys the law of mass action,

$$[\text{Drug}] + [\text{Protein}] \underset{k_1}{\overset{k_2}{\rightleftharpoons}} [\text{Drug-Protein-Complex}]$$

where the expressions in brackets represent the molar concentrations of the components, and k_1 and k_2 are rate constants for the forward and reverse reactions, respectively. The equilibrium association constant K_a is defined as k_1/k_2.

This reaction results in the following relationship for the fraction unbound:

$$f_u = \frac{1}{1 + \dfrac{N}{(1/K_a) + C_u}}$$

where N is the number of available binding sites and C_u is the unbound concentration.

Binding Proteins

Human plasma contains more than 60 proteins. Of these, three proteins account for the binding of most drugs. Albumin, which comprises approximately 60% of total plasma protein, fully accounts for the plasma binding of most anionic drugs and many endogenous anions (high-capacity, low-affinity binding site). Many cationic and neutral drugs bind appreciably to α_1-acid glycoprotein (high-affinity, low-capacity binding site) or lipoproteins in addition to albumin. Other proteins, such as transcortin, thyroid-binding globulin, and certain antibodies have specific affinities for a small number of drugs.

Volumes of Distribution

Volume of distribution at steady-state V_{ss}

The volume of distribution at steady state is by definition the sum of the pharmacokinetic volumes of distribution for the different pharmacokinetic compartments. It is the theoretical

$$V_{ss} = V_p + \frac{f_u}{f_{u,t}} \times V_t$$

where V_p is the volume of plasma (3 L); V_t is the volume of tissue water (total body water minus plasma volume: $42 - 3 = 39$ L based on a "standard" person); and f_u and $f_{u,t}$ are the fraction unbound for the drug in plasma and in tissue, respectively.

Besides physicochemical properties of the drug, the relationship for V_{ss} shows that the extent of distribution is largely determined by the differences in protein binding in plasma and tissue, respectively:

$$V_{ss} = 3L + \frac{f_u}{f_{u,t}} \times 39L$$

Unbound steady-state concentrations

The average steady-state concentration during a multiple-dose regimen or during a constant rate infusion is determined by

$$C_{ss} = \frac{Dose\ rate}{CL} = \frac{Dose\ rate}{f_u \times CL_u}$$

The free steady-state concentration $C_{ss,u}$ is given by

$$C_{ss,u} = f_u \times C_{ss}$$

Thus, the unbound steady-state concentration $C_{ss,u}$ is determined by

$$\frac{C_{ss,u}}{f_u} = \frac{Dose\ rate}{f_u \times CL_u} \Rightarrow C_{ss,u} = \frac{Dose\ rate}{CL_u}$$

6-6. Bioavailability and Bioequivalence

The FDA (21 Code of Federal Regulations 320) defines *bioavailability* as "the rate and extent to which the active ingredient or active moiety is absorbed from a drug product and becomes available at the site of action." Because, in practice, drug concentrations can rarely be determined at the site of action (e.g., at a receptor site), bioavailability is more commonly defined as "the rate and extent that the active drug is absorbed from a dosage form and becomes available in the systemic circulation."

Following are factors affecting bioavailability:

- Drug product formulation
- Properties of the drug (salt form, crystalline structure, formation of solvates, and solubility)
- Composition of the finished dosage form (presence or absence of excipients and special coatings)
- Manufacturing variables (tablet compression force, processing variables, particle size of drug or excipients, and environmental conditions)
- Rate and site of dissolution in the gastrointestinal tract
- Physiology

With respect to physiology, the following factors affect bioavailability:

- Contents of the gastrointestinal tract (fluid volume and pH, diet, presence or absence of food, bacterial activity, and presence of other drugs)
- Rate of gastrointestinal tract transit (influenced by disease, physical activity, drugs, emotional status of subject, and composition of the gastrointestinal tract contents)
- Presystemic drug metabolism or degradation (influenced by local blood flow; condition of the gastrointestinal tract membranes; and drug transport, metabolism, or degradation in the gastrointestinal tract or during the first pass of the drug through the liver)

Absolute Bioavailability

Absolute bioavailability is the fraction (or percentage) of a dose administered nonintravenously (or extravascularly) that is systemically available as compared to an intravenous dose. If given orally, absolute bioavailability (F) is

$$F = \frac{AUC_{PO}}{AUC_{IV}} \times \frac{D_{IV}}{D_{PO}}$$

Relative Bioavailability

Relative bioavailability refers to a comparison of two or more dosage forms in terms of their relative rate and extent of absorption:

$$F = \frac{AUC_{test\ formulation}}{AUC_{reference}} \times \frac{D_{reference}}{D_{test\ formulation}}$$

Bioequivalence

Two dosage forms that do not differ significantly in their rate and extent of absorption are termed *bioequivalent.* In general, bioequivalence evaluations involve comparisons of dosage forms that are

■ *Pharmaceutical equivalents:* Drug products that contain identical amounts of the identical active drug ingredient (i.e., the same salt or ester of the same therapeutic moiety, in identical dosage forms)
■ *Pharmaceutical alternatives:* Drug products that contain the identical therapeutic moiety, or its precursor, but not necessarily in the same amount or dosage form or as the same salt or ester

Biopharmaceutics Classification System

With minor exceptions, the FDA requires that bioavailability and bioequivalence of a drug product be demonstrated through in vivo studies. However, the Biopharmaceutics Classification System (BCS) can be used to justify the waiver of the requirement for in vivo studies for rapidly dissolving drug products containing active moieties or active ingredients that are highly soluble and highly permeable (Class 1 drugs).

The BCS divides drugs into classes on the basis of their solubility and permeability:

■ Class 1: high solubility and high permeability
■ Class 2: low solubility and high permeability
■ Class 3: high solubility and low permeability
■ Class 4: low solubility and low permeability

6-7. Elimination and Clearance Concepts

Clearance is defined as the irreversible removal of drug from the body by an organ of elimination. Because the units of CL are flow (e.g., mL/minute or L/h), CL is often defined as the volume of blood irreversibly cleared of drug per unit of time.

CL by the eliminating organ (CL_{organ}) is defined as the product of blood flow (Q) to the organ and the extraction ratio (ER) of that organ:

$$CL_{organ} = Q \times ER$$

Individual organ clearances are additive. For the majority of drugs used clinically, the liver is the major—and sometimes only—site of metabolism; the kidneys are the major site of excretion for drugs and metabolites. Thus, the equation for total clearance can be written to include renal clearance (CL_R) and hepatic clearance (CL_H):

$$CL = CL_R + CL_H$$

The fraction of drug excreted unchanged by the kidneys (f_e) indicates what fraction of the drug administered will be excreted into the urine:

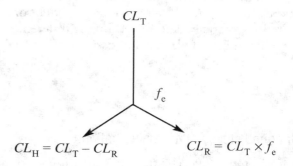

6-8. Renal Clearance

Drugs may undergo three processes in the kidney. Two act to remove drug from the body: *filtration* and *secretion.* The other acts to return drug to the body: *reabsorption.* Thus, one may express renal clearance of a drug as follows:

$$CL_R = \left[CL_{filtration} + CL_{secretion} \right] \times \left(1 - f_{reabsorbed} \right)$$

Calculating Filtration Clearance of Creatinine

Normal serum concentrations of creatinine are 0.8–1.3 mg/dL for men and 0.6–1.0 mg/dL for women.

Creatinine is a useful marker of renal function because it is an endogenous by-product of muscle breakdown. The kidney eliminates creatinine at a rate approximately equal to the glomerular filtration rate (GFR). A number of formulas have been developed that allow creatinine clearance (CL_{cr}) to be estimated from serum creatinine concentrations. The most widely used clinically is the Cockroft–Gault equation:

$$CL_{cr} = \frac{(140 - age) \times IBM}{S_{cr} \times 72}$$

$$(\text{multiply by } 0.85 \text{ if patient is female})$$

where S_{cr} is the serum creatinine concentration in mg/dL, and IBW is the ideal body weight.

$$IBW_{males}(kg) = 50 + (2.3 \times \text{height in inches} > 5\,ft)$$
$$IBW_{females}(kg) = 45.5 + (2.3 \times \text{height in inches} > 5\,ft)$$

Secretion Clearance

Drug in blood may also be secreted into the kidney tubule. This process occurs against a concentration gradient (concentration of drug in kidney tubule is very high because of water reabsorption) and therefore is an active process.

Cellular processes (e.g., presence of active transporters) exist to facilitate tubular secretion. The two most well characterized of these processes include transporters responsible for the secretion of basic (anionic) and acidic (anionic) drugs.

Reabsorption

Passive reabsorption of many drugs also occurs in the kidneys. Because reabsorption is a passive process (i.e., diffusion), reabsorption will depend on the physicochemical properties of the drug (e.g., molecular weight, polarity, and acid disassociation content pK_a).

Weak bases: $B + H^+ \Leftrightarrow BH^+$
Low urine pH = more ionized, less reabsorption
High urine pH = less ionized, more reabsorption

Thus, only weak bases with pK_a between 6 and 12 show changes in the extent of reabsorption (and thus CLR) with changes in urine pH.

Weak acids: $HA \Leftrightarrow A^- + H^+$
Low urine pH = less ionized, more reabsorption
High urine pH = more ionized, less reabsorption

Thus, only weak acids with pK_a in the range of 3.0 to 7.5 show changes in the extent of reabsorption (and thus CL_R) with changes in urine pH.

All drugs that are not bound to plasma proteins are filtered; therefore, filtration clearance is

$$CL_{\text{filtration}} = f_{\text{up}} \times GFR = 125\,\text{mL/minute}$$

Some drugs are secreted or reabsorbed, or both. One can determine the net process a drug undergoes by calculating the excretion ratio (E_{ratio}):

$$E_{\text{ratio}} = \frac{CL_R}{CL_{\text{filtration}}} = \frac{CL_R}{f_{\text{up}} \times 125\,\text{mL/minute}}$$

6-9. Hepatic Clearance

The fraction of drug escaping first-pass metabolism (F^*) can be described in terms of the hepatic extraction ratio:

$$F^* = 1 - ER$$

The overall oral bioavailability (F) of a drug is dependent on the fraction absorbed (f_a), the fraction escaping metabolism in the intestinal wall (f_g), and the fraction escaping hepatic first-pass metabolism (F^*).

$$F = f_a \times f_g \times F^*$$

Venous Equilibrium Model for Hepatic Clearance

The venous equilibrium model relates hepatic extraction ratio ER to its determinants as follows:

$$ER = \frac{f_{\text{up}} \times CL_{\text{int}}}{Q + f_{\text{up}} \times CL_{\text{int}}}$$

and (remembering that $CL_H = Q_H \times ER_H$)

$$CL_H = \frac{Q \times f_{\text{up}} \times CL_{\text{int}}}{Q + f_{\text{up}} \times CL_{\text{int}}}$$

The fraction of drug escaping hepatic first-pass metabolism using the venous equilibrium model is

$$F^* = \frac{Q}{Q + f_{\text{up}} \times CL_{\text{int}}}$$

Drugs undergoing hepatic metabolism can be divided into three broad categories:

1. Low-extraction drugs: $ER < 0.3$ and thus $F^* > 0.7$
2. Intermediate-extraction drugs: $0.3 < ER < 0.7$ and thus $0.3 < F^* < 0.7$
3. High-extraction drugs: $ER > 0.7$ and thus $F^* < 0.3$

Determinants of Hepatic Clearance

Thus, the determinants of hepatic extraction ratio, hepatic clearance, and the fraction escaping hepatic first-pass metabolism are liver blood flow (Q), protein binding (f_{up}), and CL_{int}.

For some drugs, hepatic clearance is limited or restricted to the unbound or free drug ($ER < f_{\text{up}}$). This is known as *restrictive clearance*. Because clearance is limited to unbound drug, changes in protein binding will alter the concentration of drug that is available for elimination.

Some drugs defy this principle so that the hepatic extraction ratio is greater than the fraction of drug unbound in plasma ($ER > f_{up}$). When this occurs, it suggests that drug clearance is not restricted to unbound drug. Drugs behaving in this manner are said to undergo *nonrestrictive clearance*. Because nonrestrictive clearance is not limited to the fraction unbound in plasma, changes in protein binding will *not* alter the concentration of drug that is available for elimination (i.e., all drug is available for elimination regardless of whether it is bound or unbound).

Intrinsic clearance (CL_{int}) is defined as the intrinsic ability of the hepatic enzymes to eliminate drug when blood flow or protein binding causes no limitations. CL_{int} is a measure of the capacity and affinity of drug-metabolizing enzymes (e.g., CYP450s) for the drug. The determinants of CL_{int} can be explained using the Michaelis–Menten equation:

$$\upsilon = \frac{V_{max} \times C_u}{K_m + C_u} \text{ and } CL_u = \frac{V_{max}}{K_m + C_u}$$

where υ is the rate of drug metabolism (amount/time), V_{max} is the maximal rate of metabolism for a given metabolic pathway (amount/time), K_m is the concentration of the drug at which the rate of metabolism is half-maximal (amount/volume), and C_u is the unbound drug concentration (amount/volume).

Physiologically, V_{max} describes the quantity (capacity) of a drug-metabolizing enzyme to metabolize drug. K_m describes the interaction between the drug-metabolizing enzyme and the drug.

Factors that affect CL_{int} are

- *Enzyme induction:* Enzyme induction refers to an increased number (capacity) of drug-metabolizing enzymes, which results in an increase in clearance. An increased number (capacity) of drug-metabolizing enzymes results in an increase in V_{max} and CL_{int}.
- *Enzyme inhibitors:* Competitive inhibition of the drug-metabolizing enzyme by another drug increases the apparent K_m (i.e., a higher concentration of drug will be required to achieve a half-maximal rate of metabolism). Increase in apparent K_m results in decrease in CL_{int}.

An extensive list of potential P450 inducers and inhibitors can be found at www.drug-interactions.com.

6-10. Drug, Disease, and Dietary Influences on Absorption, Distribution, Metabolism, and Excretion

Pharmacokinetics is the science of a drug's fate in the body. Typical reported pharmacokinetic parameters are determined in healthy individuals. However, drugs are prescribed to individuals with one or more altered physiological or pathological conditions. *Clinical pharmacokinetics* focuses on tailoring therapeutic dosing regimens to individuals on the basis of these altered physiological and pathological states. Thus, it is important to consider patient-specific factors that potentially contribute to drug interactions: drug–drug, drug–disease, and drug–dietary factors.

Drug interactions alter the effects of a drug by reaction with another drug or drugs, with foods or beverages, or with a preexisting medical condition. Drug interactions can be broadly classified as

- Drug–drug
- Drug–disease
- Drug–dietary

Drug–Drug Interactions

- Induction of CYP450 enzymes
  - An increased number (V_{max}) of drug-metabolizing enzymes leads to increased clearance.
  - Example: Rifampin increases clearance of warfarin.
- Inhibition of cytochrome P450 enzymes
  - Competitive inhibition of the drug-metabolizing enzyme by another drug leads to increase in apparent K_m, which leads to decreased clearance.
  - Example: Cimetidine decreases the clearance of warfarin.
- Inhibition of drug efflux transporter P-glycoprotein
  - Competitive inhibition of P-glycoprotein occurs.
- Decreased renal clearance for drugs undergoing net secretion
  - Example: Quinidine inhibits the renal secretion of digoxin.
- Increased f_a and F
  - Example: Ketoconazole increases the oral absorption of cyclosporine.
- Protein-binding displacement
  - A drug or drugs is displaced from major binding proteins.

- Increased f_{up}
- Increased volume of distribution
- Increased clearance for restrictively cleared drugs
  - Example: Aspirin displaces warfarin from albumin, leading to an increased distribution and clearance for warfarin.

Drug–Disease Interactions

Cardiovascular disease

Reduced cardiac output associated with congestive heart failure leads to reduced perfusion of key eliminating organs such as the liver and kidney. The following pharmacokinetic effects have been reported:

- Decreased absorption rate (e.g, digoxin, hydrochlorothiazide, procainamide, and quinidine)
- Prolonged hepatic clearance for high extraction ($E > 0.7$) drugs (e.g., lidocaine and theophylline)
- Reduced volume of distribution (e.g., digoxin)

Renal disease

Creatinine clearance is commonly used to assess renal function, and the CL_R of many drugs is known to vary in proportion to CL_{cr}. Thus, renal impairment can be inferred from changes in CL_{cr}.

CL_{cr} is most often estimated by measuring serum creatinine concentration, using the Cockroft–Gault equation, as discussed previously.

Serum creatinine concentrations remain relatively constant (about 1 mg/dL) in adults over age 20. However, patients with compromised renal function may exhibit higher concentrations.

Renal function RF in a patient may be estimated by comparing the patient's creatinine clearance to what CL_{cr} would be in a normal individual (i.e., $f_{up} \times GFR$ or 125 mL/minute).

$$RF = \frac{CL_{cr}^{patient}}{CL_{cr}^{normal}} = \frac{CL_{cr}^{patient}}{125 \text{ mL/minute}}$$

Use of this equation to estimate RF assumes the intact nephron hypothesis (i.e., that renal disease results in the dysfunction of a certain fraction of nephrons but allows the remaining nephrons to remain intact).

To individualize drug treatment in patients with renal impairment, you need to know the drug clearance *in your patient*. This knowledge will allow you to calculate the dose rate of the drug that will maintain an individualized C_{target}. Clearance in your patient with renal impairment will be designated CL^*. Three parameters are needed to calculate CL^*:

- CL of the drug and f_e in normal subjects. These values can be found in textbooks, primary literature, or package inserts.
- RF in your patient is usually estimated using a recent serum creatinine concentration and the equations presented above.

You can then calculate clearance in your patient with renal impairment using the following equation:

$$CL^* = CL \times \left[1 - f_e \times \left(1 - RF \right) \right]$$

CL^* represents *total* clearance in the renally impaired individual.

Liver disease

Hepatic disease results in numerous pathophysiologic changes in the liver that may influence drug pharmacokinetics, including the following:

- Reduction in liver blood flow
  - Decreased clearance for high-extraction drugs
- Reduction in number and activity of hepatocytes
  - Decreased first-pass metabolism for high-extraction drugs
  - Decreased clearance for low-extraction drugs
- Impaired production of human serum albumin
  - Increased distribution of drugs

Drug–Diet Interactions

- Drug–food interactions
  - Type I: Ex vivo bioinactivation
  - Type II: Interactions affecting oral absorption
  - Type III: Interactions affecting systemic disposition
  - Type IV: Interactions affecting either renal or hepatic clearance
- Ex vivo bioinactivation
  - It typically occurs in the delivery device before drugs enter body.
  - Interaction occurs between the drug and the nutritional element or formulation through biochemical or physical reactions.
  - Interaction examples include hydrolysis, oxidation, neutralization, precipitation, and complexation.
  - High ethanol content may precipitate inorganic salts present in enteral feeding formulas.
  - Syrups are acidic solvents and may cause precipitation of inorganic salts.

■ Interactions affecting absorption
  • This type of interaction affects drugs and nutrients delivered by mouth only.
  • It may result in either an increase or a decrease in oral bioavailability.
  • The interacting agent may alter function of either the metabolizing enzyme (e.g., CYP3A4) or the active transport protein (e.g., P-glycoprotein).
  • Meal intake alters oral absorption through mechanisms involving altered (1) gastric pH, (2) gastrointestinal transit time, and (3) dissolution of solid dosage forms.
  • Grapefruit juice inactivates gut CYP3A4, enhancing oral absorption of CYP3A4 substrates (e.g., cyclosporine, midazolam, and nifedipine).
■ Interactions affecting systemic disposition
  • These interactions occur after drug or nutrient has entered the systemic circulation.
  • They involve alteration in tissue disposition or response.
  • Example: Foods high in vitamin K (e.g., broccoli) can alter systemic clotting factors, reducing effectiveness of warfarin.
■ Interactions affecting either renal or hepatic clearance
  • These interactions arise from modification of drug elimination mechanisms in liver, kidney, or both.
  • Acute ethanol ingestion may potentiate central nervous system effects of benzodiazepines (e.g., alprazolam).

6-11. The Pharmacokinetic–Pharmacodynamic Interface

Pharmacokinetics (PK) establishes the relationship between dose and concentration. *Pharmacodynamics* (PD) establishes the relationship between concentration and effect. When individualizing pharmacotherapy, it is important to account for both PK and PD variability. For a number of drugs, the PK variability is much larger than the PD variability. Thus, concentration-based therapeutic drug monitoring is useful for a number of drugs (e.g., theophylline). However, for some drugs, PD variability exceeds PK variability.

Linking the PK and PD allows a more thorough understanding of the effect of dosage adjustments on pharmacologic response.

The simple E_{max} model represents the most widely used model to describe the relationship between drug concentration and effect:

$$Intensity\ of\ effect = E = \frac{E_{max} \times C}{EC_{50} + C}$$

where E_{max} is the maximum effect possible (intrinsic activity) and EC_{50} is the concentration achieving 50% maximal effect (potency).

Figure 6-1 illustrates the three concentration-dependent phases as follows:

■ Linear phase (1)
  • Drug concentration is much smaller than EC_{50} ($C << EC_{50}$).
  • A linear relationship exists between concentration C and effect E:

$$E = \frac{E_{max} \times C}{EC_{50}}$$

■ Constant phase (3)
  • Drug concentration much larger than EC_{50} ($C >> EC_{50}$).
  • Effect E is independent of concentration:

$$E = E_{max}$$

■ Log-linear phase (2)
  • A log-linear relationship exists between C and E when E is between 20% and 80% of E_{max}. $E_{max}/4$ is the slope describing this relationship:

$$E = \frac{E_{max}}{4} \times \ln C + \frac{E_{max}}{4} \times \left(\ln EC_{50} + 2\right)$$

6-12. Hysteresis

Response is linked to concentration and time. In other words, a given concentration may have a different effect depending on time. Therefore, the concentration–effect relationship is described by a *hysteresis loop*, which may be either clockwise or counterclockwise.

■ Counterclockwise hysteresis
  • Distributional delay to effect site
  • Indirect response mechanism
  • Active metabolite (agonism)
  • Sensitization

Figure 6-1. The Three Concentration-Dependent Phases

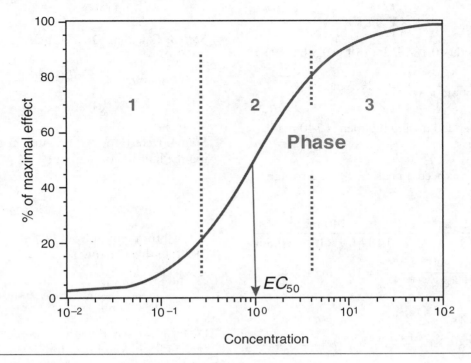

- Clockwise hysteresis
  - Functional tolerance
  - Active metabolite (antagonism)

6-13. Clinical Examples

Clinical Example 1

A patient (55 years old, weighing 73 kg) was started on a multiple-dose regimen with gentamicin 80 mg every 8 hours given as IV short-term infusion over 30 minutes. Because his infection is serious, it is decided to target for a peak concentration of 10 mg/L and a trough concentration of 1 mg/L. Three blood samples were drawn 30 minutes prior to the third dose and 30 minutes and 7 hours after the end of the infusion of the third dose, respectively. The measured plasma concentrations are 1.73, 5.96, and 1.80 mg/L, respectively.

Optimize the gentamicin dosing regimen on the basis of the individual pharmacokinetic parameters of the patient to achieve the therapeutically targeted concentrations.

- **Step 1:** Calculate the elimination rate constant K:

$$K = \frac{\ln\left(\dfrac{C^*_{max}}{C^*_{min}}\right)}{\Delta t} = \frac{\ln\left(\dfrac{5.96}{1.80}\right)}{(8-1-0.5)\text{h}} = 0.184 \text{ h}^{-1}$$

- **Step 2:** Calculate volume of distribution V:

$$C_{max} = \frac{C^*_{max}}{e^{-K \times t^*}} = \frac{5.96 \text{ mg/L}}{e^{-0.184 \text{ h}^{-1} \times 0.5 \text{ h}}} = 6.53 \text{ mg/L}$$

$$C_{min} = C^*_{min} \times e^{-K \times t^*}$$
$$= 1.73 \text{ mg/L} \times e^{-0.184 \text{ h}^{-1} \times 0.5 \text{ h}} = 1.58 \text{ mg/L}$$

$$V = \frac{R_0}{K} \times \frac{1 - e^{-K \times T_{inf}}}{C_{max} - C_{min} \times e^{-K \times T_{inf}}}$$

$$= \frac{80 \text{ mg}}{0.184 \text{ h}^{-1} \times 0.5 \text{ h}}$$

$$\times \frac{1 - e^{-0.184 \text{ h}^{-1} \times 0.5 \text{ h}}}{6.53 \text{ mg/L} - 1.58 \times e^{-0.184 \text{ h}^{-1} \times 0.5 \text{ h}}}$$

$$= 15.0 \text{ L}$$

- **Step 3:** Calculate recommended dosing interval τ:

$$\tau = \frac{\ln\left(\dfrac{C_{ss,max(desired)}}{C_{ss,min(desired)}}\right)}{K} + T_{inf} = \frac{\ln\left(\dfrac{10}{1}\right)}{0.184 \text{ h}^{-1}} + 0.5 \text{ h}$$

$$= 13.0 \text{ h}$$

The practically reasonable, recommended dosing interval is 12 hours.

■ *Step 4:* Calculate recommended dose *D*:

$$D = C_{ss,\max(desired)} \times K \times V \times T_{inf} \times \frac{1 - e^{-K \times \tau}}{1 - e^{-K \times T_{inf}}}$$

$$D = 10 \text{ mg/L} \times 0.184 \text{ h}^{-1} \times 15 \text{ L} \times 0.5 \text{ h}$$

$$\times \frac{1 - e^{-0.184 \text{ h}^{-1} \times 12 \text{ h}}}{1 - e^{-0.184 \text{ h}^{-1} \times 0.5 \text{ h}}} = 139.7 \text{ mg}$$

The recommended dosing regimen is 140 mg every 12 hours.

■ *Step 5:* Check expected peak $C_{ss,\max}$ and trough $C_{ss,\min}$:

$$C_{ss,\max} \frac{R_0}{K \times V} \times \frac{1 - e^{-K \times T_{inf}}}{1 - e^{-K \times \tau}} = \frac{140 \text{ mg}}{0.184 \text{ h}^{-1} \times 15 \text{ L} \times 0.5 \text{ h}}$$

$$\times \frac{1 - e^{-0.184 \text{ h}^{-1} \times 0.5 \text{ h}}}{1 - e^{-0.184 \text{ h}^{-1} \times 12 \text{ h}}} = 10.0 \text{ mg/L}$$

$$C_{ss,\min} = C_{ss,\max} \times e^{-K \times (\tau - T_{inf})}$$

$$= 10.0 \text{ mg/L} \times e^{-0.184 \text{ h}^{-1} \times (12 \text{ h} - 0.5 \text{ h})} = 1.21 \text{ mg/L}$$

Clinical Example 2

A 70-year-old white male weighing 95 lbs is 5 feet tall and has a serum creatinine of 1.1 mg/dL. He is admitted to the hospital complaining of shortness of breath; he denies chest pain. Digoxin is prescribed for him. You are asked to design a dosage regimen using tablets for him to achieve and maintain a $C_{target,ss}$ of 1 ng/mL. The PK parameters for digoxin are as follows: $CL = 2.7$ mL/minute/kg (total body weight, or TBW); $f_e = 0.68$; $V_{ss} = 6.7$ L/kg (IBW); F of tablet = 0.75.

■ *Step 1:* Estimate *CL*, CL_{cr}, *RF*, and *CL** of digoxin in this patient.

IBW = 45.5 kg; TBW = 43 kg. Therefore, use TBW for all calculations.
CL for a normal 43 kg patient = 116 mL/minute. CL_{cr} and *RF* are

$$CL_{cr} = \frac{(140 - 70) \times 43}{1.1 \times 72} = 38 \text{ mL/minute}$$

$$RF = \frac{38 \text{ mL/minute}}{125 \text{ mL/minute}} = 0.304$$

■ *Step 2:* Estimate *CL**, clearance of digoxin in this patient with renal impairment:

$$CL^* = 116 \text{ mL/minute} \times \left[1 - 0.68(1 - 0.304)\right]$$

$$= 61.1 \text{ mL/minute}$$

■ *Step 3:* Calculate Dose Rate*:

$$\text{Dose Rate}^* = \frac{1 \text{ ng/mL} \times 61.1 \text{ mL/minute}}{0.75}$$

$$= 81.5 \text{ ng/minute}$$

■ *Step 4:* Determine dosing interval τ^* by estimating the half-life of digoxin:

$$\tau^*_{1/2} = \frac{0.693 \times V_{ss}}{CL^*}$$

V_{ss} (V_d) for digoxin from PK tables is 6.7 L/kg, or 289 L in this patient. Thus,

$$\tau^*_{1/2} = \frac{0.693 \times 289 \text{ L}}{0.061 \text{ L/minute}} = 3,283 \text{ minutes} \cong 55 \text{ hours}$$

Digoxin is normally administered every 24 hours ($\tau = 24$ h); it could be administered 0.25 mg every 48 hours ($\tau = 48$ h). Here, however, changing the dosing interval is not recommended, because 24 hours is very convenient, and the resultant peak:trough ratio would be lower with $\tau = 24$ h as compared with $\tau = 48$ h.

Clinical Example 3

A. M. is a 61-year-old white male, 6 feet tall, weighing 195 lbs. He has a diagnosis of pneumonia. His serum creatinine is 2.3 mg/dL. Design a dosage regimen of gentamicin to achieve C_{peak} and C_{trough} values of 8 mg/L and 1 mg/L, respectively. $V_d = 0.2$ L/kg IBW.

■ *Step 1:* The *CL* of gentamicin is 85 mL/minute and the $f_e = 1.0$. Calculate the degree of renal impairment:

$$CL = CL_{cr} = \frac{(140 - 61) \times 77.6}{2.3(72)} = 37 \text{ mL/minute}$$

$$RF = \frac{37 \text{ mL/minute}}{125 \text{ mL/minute}} = 0.296$$

■ *Step 2:* Calculate the *CL* of gentamicin in this patient:

$$CL^* = 85 \text{ mL/minute} \times \left[1 - 1 \times (1 - 0.296)\right]$$

$$= 25.2 \text{ mL/minute} = 1.5 \text{ L/h}$$

■ *Step 3:* Calculate the elimination rate constant in this patient:

$$k = \frac{CL}{V_{ss}} = \frac{1.5 \text{ L/h}}{0.2 \text{ L/kg} \times 77.6 \text{ kg}} = 0.097 \text{ h}^{-1}$$

■ *Step 4:* Calculate the infusion rate and dosing interval:

$$\tau = \frac{\ln\left(\dfrac{C_{ss,max(desired)}}{C_{ss,min(desired)}}\right)}{K} + T_{inf} = \frac{\ln\left(\dfrac{8 \text{ mg/L}}{1 \text{ mg/L}}\right)}{0.097 \text{ h}^{-1}} + 0.5 \text{ h}$$

$$= 22 \text{ hours} \cong 24 \text{ hours}$$

$$D = C_{ss,max} \times K \times V \times T_{inf} \times \frac{1 - e^{-K \times \tau}}{1 - e^{-K \times T_{inf}}}$$

$$= 8 \text{ mg/L} \times 0.097 \text{ h}^{-1} \times (0.2 \times 77.6) \times 0.5$$

$$\times \frac{1 - e^{-0.097 \text{h}^{-1} \times 24}}{1 - e^{-0.097 \text{h}^{-1} \times 0.5}}$$

$$= 115 \text{ mg} \cong 120 \text{ mg}$$

Clinical Example 4

Patient D. M. is a 50-year-old white male (74.1 kg) who is being treated for seizure control with phenytoin ($V_d = 0.6$ L/kg), 300 mg/d, using the capsule formulation. He has been taking phenytoin for 2 weeks. He experienced a seizure on day 14 of treatment. His blood level was 5.2 mg/L. His dose rate was increased to 400 mg/d of the capsule formulation. Three weeks later his blood level was 11.8 mg/L.

■ Phenytoin capsules and parenteral solution = sodium phenytoin
■ Phenytoin tablets and suspension = phenytoin acid
■ 100 mg phenytoin sodium = 92 mg phenytoin acid
■ *Step 1:* The V_{max} (mg/d) for phenytoin in patient D. M. is

a. 491
b. 499
c. 542
d. 590
e. 614

Because D. M. is using capsules, you need to multiply the original dose rate by 0.92.

Dose rate (mg/day)	C_{ss} (mg/L)	Dose rate/C_{ss} (L/day)
$300 \times 0.92 = 276$	5.2	53.08
$400 \times 0.92 = 368$	11.8	31.19

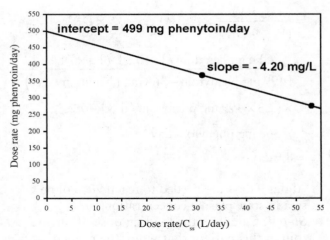

$$DR = V_{max} - \left(\frac{DR}{C_{ss}}\right) \times K_m$$

$$Y = \text{intercept} + X \times (-\text{slope})$$

$$\text{Plot } DR \text{ vs } DR/C_{ss}$$

Y-intercept = V_{max} = 499 mg/d phenytoin
slope = $-K_m$ = -4.2 mg/L; therefore
$\quad K_m = 4.2$ mg/L

■ *Step 2:* What dosage regimen would you recommend to achieve an average steady-state phenytoin concentration of 15 mg/L in patient D. M. using the capsule formulation?

a. 100 mg q6h
b. 100 mg q8h
c. 200 mg q6h
d. 200 mg q8h

$$DR = CL \times C_{ss,target} = \frac{V_{max} \times C_{ss,target}}{K_m + C_{ss,target}}$$

$$= \frac{499 \text{ mg/day} \times 15 \text{ mg/L}}{4.2 \text{ mg/L} + 15 \text{ mg/L}} = 390 \text{ mg phenytoin/day}$$

390 mg/d phenytoin = 424 mg/d sodium phenytoin
Recommend 400 mg Dilantin Kapseals in three or four divided doses (e.g., 100 mg q6h).

■ *Step 3:* Estimate the time required to achieve steady-state levels of phenytoin in patient D. M. at the dosage regimen if it were changed to 100 mg capsule q6h.

a. 1 day
b. 5 days
c. 9 days
d. 13 days
e. 17 days

$$t_{90} = \frac{K_m \times V_{ss}}{\left(V_{max} - DR\right)^2} \times \left(2.3 \times V_{max} - 0.9 \times DR\right)$$

$$t_{90} = \frac{4.2 \text{ mg phenytoin / L} \times 0.6 \text{ L / kg} \times 74.1 \text{ kg}}{\left(499 \text{ mg phenytoin} - 368 \text{ mg phenytoin / day}\right)^2}$$

$$\times \left(2.3 \times 499 \text{ mg phenytoin / day}\right) - 0.9$$

$$\times 368 \text{ mg phenytoin/day}$$

$$t_{90} = 8.9 \text{ days}$$

About 9 days are needed to reach 90% of new steady-state plasma concentration.

■ *Step 4:* Calculate the loading dose of phenytoin in this patient that would be needed to achieve a phenytoin blood level of 12 mg/L. (Assume that blood levels of phenytoin = 0 at time of administration of the loading dose.)

a. 491 mg
b. 535 mg
c. 580 mg
d. 603 mg

$$LD = C_{ss,target} \times V_{ss} = 12 \text{ mg/L phenytoin} \times 0.6 \text{ L/kg}$$

$$\times 74.1 \text{ kg} = 534 \text{ mg of phenytoin}$$

$$= 580 \text{ mg of phenytoin sodium (parenteral)}$$

Clinical Example 5

To treat her asthma exacerbation, L. Y., a 68-year-old woman who weighs 55 kg, has received a continuous infusion of aminophylline (infusion rate 0.45 mg/kg/h) for 5 days. This morning, she suffers from theophylline toxicity indicated by tachycardia, headache, and dizziness. A blood sample is drawn, and the theophylline plasma concentration is 24.3 mg/L. The therapeutic range is 10–20 mg/L; the population average of the volume of distribution is 0.5 L/kg.

■ *Step 1:* What is the theophylline clearance in this patient under the assumption that steady state had already been reached at the time the blood sample was obtained?

a. 0.81 L/h
b. 0.95 L/h
c. 1.35 L/h
d. 2.15 L/h
e. 2.80 L/h

$$CL = \frac{R_0}{C_{ss}} = \frac{0.45 \text{ mg/kg/h} \times 0.8 \times 55 \text{ kg}}{24.3 \text{ mg/L}} = 0.81 \text{ L/h}$$

■ *Step 2:* To what aminophylline infusion rate should the infusion be reduced to achieve a steady-state concentration in the middle of the therapeutic range, that is, 15 mg/L?

a. 0.17 mg/kg/h
b. 0.18 mg//kg/h
c. 0.20 mg/kg/h
d. 0.22 mg/kg/h
e. 0.28 mg/kg/h

$$MD = C_{target} \times CL = 15 \text{ mg/L} \times 0.81 \text{ L/h}$$

$$= 12.15 \text{ mg/h theophylline}$$

$$= 15.2 \text{ mg/h aminophylline}$$

Because the patient weighs 55kg, $MD =$ 0.28 mg/kg/h.

■ *Step 3:* How long does it take approximately to achieve the new steady state after the infusion rate has been changed?

a. 26 hours
b. 68 hours
c. 118 hours
d. 156 hours
e. 192 hours

Estimated $V = 55 \text{ kg} \times 0.5 \text{ L/kg} = 27.5 \text{ L}$

$$t_{1/2} = \frac{\ln 2}{K} = \frac{\ln 2 \times V}{CL} = \frac{0.693 \times 27.5 \text{ L}}{0.81 \text{ L/h}} = 23.5 \text{ h}$$

Time to new steady state approximately $5\ t_{1/2} \approx 118$ hour

■ *Step 4:* The pharmacist suggests that the new target concentration can be achieved faster if the first infusion with the higher infusion rate is completely stopped and the second infusion with the lower infusion rate is not initiated until the plasma concentration has decreased to 15 mg/L, the target concentration. Calculate the time the therapy has to pause (i.e., the time one waits after cessation of the first infusion before the second infusion is started).

a. 14.7 hours
b. 16.4 hours
c. 20.7 hours
d. 36.1 hours
e. 55.1 hours

$$C_{target} = C_{ss,old} \times e^{-K \times t_{pause}}$$

$$t_{pause} = \frac{\ln\left(\dfrac{C_{target}}{C_{ss,old}}\right)}{-K} = \frac{\ln\left(\dfrac{15 \text{ mg/L}}{24.3 \text{ mg/L}}\right) \times 27.5 \text{ L}}{-0.81 \text{ L/h}} = 16.4 \text{ h}$$

6-14. Key Points

■ The clearance CL can be determined from the relationship

$$CL = \frac{DR}{C_{ss,avg}} \text{ or } CL = \frac{D}{AUC}$$

■ The volume of distribution can be determined from the relationship

$$V = \frac{CL}{K}$$

■ The average steady-state concentration $C_{ss,av}$ during multiple dosing is determined only by the dose, the dosing interval τ (or both together as dosing rate $DR = D/\tau$) and the clearance CL:

$$C_{ss,av} = \frac{D}{\tau \times CL}$$

■ The area under the curve resulting from administration of a single dose AUC_{single} is equal to the area under the curve during one dosing interval at steady-state AUC_{ss}, provided that the same dose is given per dosing interval τ:

$$C_{ss,av} = \frac{AUC_{ss}}{\tau} = \frac{D}{\tau \times CL} = \frac{AUC_{single}}{\tau}$$

■ The volume of distribution at steady state is by definition the sum of the pharmacokinetic volumes of distribution for the different pharmacokinetic compartments. It is the theoretical

$$V_{ss} = V_p + \frac{f_u}{f_{u,t}} \times V_t$$

where V_p is the volume of plasma (3 L), V_t is the volume of tissue water (total body water minus plasma volume: $42 - 3 = 39$ L based on a "standard" person), and f_u and $f_{u,t}$ are the fraction unbound for the drug in plasma and tissue, respectively.

■ *Clearance* is defined as the irreversible removal of drug from the body by an organ of elimination. CL by the eliminating organ (CL_{organ}) is defined as the product of blood flow to the organ (Q) and the extraction ratio of that organ (ER). The fraction of drug escaping first-pass metabolism (F^*) can be described in terms of the hepatic ER ($F^* = 1 - ER$).

■ The venous equilibrium model relates hepatic ER to hepatic blood flow Q, unbound drug fraction f_{up}, intrinsic clearance CL_{int}:

$$CL_H = \frac{Q \times f_{up} \times CL_{int}}{Q + f_{up} \times CL_{int}}$$

■ The venous equilibrium model can be simplified for drugs with low ER (< 0.3) and high ER (> 0.7). For low-ER drugs, $CL_H \approx f_{up} * CL_{int}$. For high-$ER$ drugs, $CL_H \approx Q$.

■ Bioavailability is the fraction (or percentage) of a dose administered nonintravenously (or extravascularly) that is systemically available as compared to an intravenous dose. The overall oral bioavailability (F) of a drug is dependent on the fraction absorbed (f_a), the fraction escaping metabolism in the intestinal wall (f_g), and the fraction escaping hepatic first-pass metabolism (F^*).

■ Drugs may undergo three processes in the kidney. Two act to remove drug from the body: filtration and secretion. The other acts to return drug to the body: reabsorption. The net process a drug undergoes can be determined by calculating the excretion ratio (E_{ratio}) using total renal clearance (CL_R) and filtration clearance (CL_F):

$$E_{ratio} = \frac{CL_R}{CL_F} = \frac{CL_R}{f_{up} \times 125 \text{ mL/min}}$$

6-15. Questions

1. A pediatric patient receives an immuno-suppressive therapy with oral cyclosporine solution. His concentration-adjusted dosing regimen is 85 mg every 12 hours. Because of a recent change in his insurance coverage, he needs to be switched from the drug product he is currently using to a generic solution dosage form of cyclosporine that is covered by his insurance. The bioavailability of the dosage form he previously used is 43%; the bioavailability of the generic dosage form is

28%. What is the appropriate dosage regimen for the generic dosage form to maintain the same systemic exposure as obtained from the previously used dosage form?

A. 25 mg every 12 hours
B. 55 mg every 12 hours
C. 184 mg every 12 hours
D. 130 mg every 12 hours
E. 305 mg every 12 hours

2. A drug is administered via continuous infusion at a rate of 60 mg/h, resulting in a steady-state plasma concentration of 5 mcg/mL. If the plasma concentration is intended to be doubled to 10 mcg/mL, the infusion rate must be

A. left the same.
B. increased by 30 mg/h.
C. increased by 60 mg/h.
D. increased by 120 mg/h.
E. decreased by 30 mg/h.

3. Jonathan R. (72 kg, 23 years old) has been admitted to the emergency room with acute asthma symptoms. He will be started on a continuous infusion of aminophylline with a target theophylline concentration of 12 mg/L (therapeutic range 10–20 mg/L). To achieve the target concentration more rapidly, medical personnel will administer an additional loading dose as a short-term infusion over 30 minutes. The population mean values for clearance and volume of distribution of theophylline are 2.7 L/h and 34 L, respectively. What aminophylline loading and maintenance dose should be given? (Select practically useful doses. Remember that aminophylline contains 80% theophylline.)

3a. Loading dose:

A. 400 mg
B. 450 mg
C. 500 mg
D. 550 mg
E. 600 mg

3b. Maintenance dose:

A. 35 mg/h
B. 40 mg/h
C. 45 mg/h
D. 50 mg/h
E. 55 mg/h

4. Lidocaine will be given as a constant rate infusion for the treatment of ventricular arrhythmia. A plasma concentration of 3 mcg/mL was decided on as the therapeutic target concentration. The concentration of the infusion solution is 20 mg/mL lidocaine. The average volume of distribution of lidocaine is 90 L; the elimination half-life is 1.1 hours. What infusion rate (in mL/minute) has to be set on the infusion pump to achieve the desired target concentration?

A. 5 mL/h
B. 8.5 mL/h
C. 14 mL/h
D. 23.5 mL/h
E. 194 mL/h

5. After termination of an intravenous constant rate infusion, the plasma concentration of a drug declines monoexponentially ($C = C_0 \times e^{-k \times t}$). Concentrations measured at 2 hours and 12 hours after the end of the infusion are 12.9 mcg/mL and 6.0 mcg/mL, respectively. Calculate the initial concentration at the end of the infusion, and predict the concentration 24 hours after termination of the infusion.

A. 13.5 and 2.9 mcg/mL
B. 16.5 and 3.8 mcg/mL
C. 16.5 and 1.3 mcg/mL
D. 15 and 2.4 mcg/mL
E. 15 and 1.3 mcg/mL

6. Margaret Q. (100 kg, 26 years old) presents to the emergency room with acute symptoms of asthma. She recently started smoking again and has been taking oral theophylline for several years. The immediate determination of her theophylline plasma concentration results in a level of 4 mg/L.

Theophylline population pharmacokinetic parameters: CL 0.04 L/h/kg; V 0.5 L/kg
Therapeutic range: 10–20 mg/L

What is the appropriate intravenous loading dose of aminophylline for Margaret to achieve a target concentration of 12 mg/L?

A. 300 mg
B. 400 mg
C. 500 mg
D. 600 mg
E. 750 mg

7. For a drug product in clinical drug development, an oral dosing regimen needs to be established for a phase III study that maintains an average steady-state concentration of 50 ng/mL. In single-dose studies, an oral dose of 80 mg resulted in an *AUC* of 962 ng h/mL and an elimination half-life of 10.3 hours. What dosing regimen should be used?

   A. 35 mg every 12 hours
   B. 50 mg every 12 hours
   C. 72 mg every 12 hours
   D. 95 mg every 12 hours
   E. 125 mg every 12 hours

8. Mary D. (47 years old, 68 kg) has recently received her first 0.25 mg dose of digoxin. Plasma digoxin concentrations 12 and 24 hours following oral administration of this dose are 0.72 and 0.33 mcg/L, respectively. The therapeutic plasma concentration range is 0.8–2.0 mcg/L. Predict Mary's digoxin trough concentration at steady state, assuming that oral digoxin therapy is continued at a dose rate of 0.25 mg once daily.

   A. 0.62 mcg/L
   B. 0.93 mcg/L
   C. 1.32 mcg/L
   D. 1.57 mcg/L
   E. 1.95 mcg/L

9. The population average values for the clearance and volume of distribution of nifedipine have been reported as 0.41 L/h/kg and 1.2 L/kg. What would be the maximum dosing interval you can use for a multiple-dose regimen with an immediate-release oral dosage form of nifedipine if peak-to-trough fluctuation should not exceed 100%?

   A. 2 hours
   B. 4 hours
   C. 6 hours
   D. 8 hours
   E. 12 hours

10. Beth R. (63 years old, 58 kg) is suffering from symptomatic ventricular arrhythmia. She will be started on an oral multiple-dose regimen with the antiarrhythmic mexiletine. The population average values of mexiletine for clearance and volume of distribution are $CL = 0.5$ L/h/kg and $V = 6$ L/kg, respectively. Although a therapeutic range of 0.5–2.0 mg/L has been described, avoiding large peak-to-trough fluctuations is recommended. The available oral dosage forms are 150, 200, and 250 mg capsules with an oral bioavailability of $F = 0.9$. Design an appropriate and practically reasonable oral dosing regimen that keeps the plasma concentrations at an average concentration of approximately 1 mg/L, with a peak-to-trough fluctuation $\leq 100\%$ (e.g. with concentrations within the limits of 0.75 and 1.5 mg/L).

    A. 150 mg q6h
    B. 200 mg q6h
    C. 200 mg q8h
    D. 250 mg q8h
    E. 375 mg q12h

11. Edgar W. (20 years old, 58 kg) is receiving 80 mg of gentamicin as IV infusion over a 30-minute period q8h. Two plasma samples are obtained to monitor serum gentamicin concentrations as follows: one sample 30 minutes after the end of the short-term infusion and one sample 30 minutes before the administration of the next dose. The serum gentamicin concentrations at these times are 4.9 and 1.7 mg/L, respectively. Assume steady state. Develop a practically reasonable dosing regimen that will produce peak and trough concentrations of approximately 8 and 1 mg/L, respectively.

    A. 120 mg q8h
    B. 160 mg q8h
    C. 140 mg q12h
    D. 180 mg q12h
    E. 280 mg q24h

12. A patient who is receiving chronic phenytoin therapy is hospitalized for an elective surgical procedure. Admission labs note that the patient has a phenytoin concentration of 8 mcg/mL (therapeutic range: 10–20 mcg/mL) and an albumin concentration of 3.0 g/dL. Phenytoin: $F = 0.2$–0.9, CL-variable, < 1% excreted unchanged in the urine, 88–93% bound to plasma proteins (primarily albumin). Given

this information and the therapeutic range of phenytoin, you would recommend that the physician

A. decrease the dose of phenytoin, because high-extraction drugs (e.g., phenytoin) exhibit increased unbound concentrations with increases in fraction unbound in the plasma.
B. increase the dose rate of phenytoin, because low-extraction drugs (e.g., phenytoin) exhibit increased CL with increases in fraction unbound in the plasma.
C. not change the dose rate of phenytoin because low-extraction drugs (e.g., phenytoin) do not exhibit changes in unbound concentrations with increases in fraction unbound in the plasma.
D. not change the dose rate of phenytoin because low-extraction drugs (e.g., phenytoin) exhibit equal and offsetting changes in CL and F with increases in fraction unbound in plasma.

13. Which of the following conditions indicate the possibility of renal clearance of a weakly acidic drug being sensitive to changes in urine pH?

I.   It is secreted and not reabsorbed.
II. It has a pK_a value of 5.0.
III. It has a small volume of distribution.
IV. All of the drug is excreted unchanged by the kidneys (i.e., $f_e = 1$).

A. Only item I is correct.
B. Only item II is correct.
C. Only item III is correct.
D. Items II and III are correct.
E. Items II and IV are correct.

14. A young man (age 28, 73 kg, creatinine clearance 124 mL/minute) receives a single 200 mg oral dose of an antibiotic. The following pharmacokinetic parameters of the antibiotic are reported in the literature:

- $F = 90\%$
- $V_d = 0.31$ L/kg
- $t_{1/2} = 2.1$ h
- $f_{up} = 0.77$
- 67% of the antibiotic's absorbed dose is excreted unchanged in the urine.

Determine the renal clearance of the antibiotic. What is the probable mechanism for renal clearance of this drug?

A. 84 mL/minute, glomerular filtration and tubular reabsorption
B. 98 mL/minute, glomerular filtration and tubular reabsorption
C. 112 mL/minute, glomerular filtration
D. 167 mL/minute, glomerular filtration and tubular reabsorption
E. 236 mL/minute, glomerular filtration and tubular secretion

15. The pharmacokinetic parameters for captopril in healthy adults are

- Clearance: 800 mL/minute
- $f_e = 0.5$
- V_{ss}: 0.81 L/kg
- Plasma protein binding: 75%

15a. Captopril is a weakly basic drug that is used in the treatment of hypertension. Assume a glomerular filtration rate of 125 mL/minute. What is (are) the mechanism(s) for renal clearance of captopril?

A. Filtration only
B. Reabsorption only
C. Secretion only
D. Filtration and net secretion
E. Filtration and net reabsorption

15b. When cimetidine (a highly lipid soluble weak base that is highly secreted in the renal proximal tubules) and captopril are coadministered, the renal clearance of captopril is reduced to approximately 125 mL/minute. What is the most likely mechanism to account for this reduction in renal clearance?

A. Cimetidine reduces the filtration clearance of captopril.
B. Cimetidine enhances the reabsorption of captopril.
C. Cimetidine increases the unbound fraction of captopril.
D. Cimetidine blocks the renal secretion of captopril.

16. One of the most severe drug interactions is that between digoxin and quinidine. Administration of quinidine to patients taking digoxin results in a two- to threefold increase in digoxin C_{ss}

and AUC after oral and intravenous administration of digoxin. Digoxin and quinidine are substrates for the multidrug resistance transporter, P-glycoprotein. According to the following pharmacokinetic data for digoxin, what is the most likely mechanism to explain this drug–drug interaction?

CL: 125 mL/minute
V_{ss}: 1.2 L/kg (IBW)
f_e: > 0.99
f_{up}: 0.25

A. Quinidine reduces the digoxin fraction escaping first-pass metabolism.
B. Quinidine inhibits renal secretion of digoxin by blocking P-glycoprotein.
C. Quinidine decreases digoxin fraction reabsorbed in the kidney tubule.
D. Quinidine reduces the fraction of digoxin absorbed.

17. The drug transporter P-glycoprotein is involved in numerous processes in drug disposition. P-glycoprotein activity is directly responsible for the following processes:

I. Glomerular filtration
II. Transport of drug from hepatocytes into the bile
III. Transport of drug from the small intestine into the systemic circulation (i.e., bloodstream)
IV. Degradation of drug in the lumen of the duodenum
V. Maintenance of the integrity of the blood–brain barrier by transport of drug out of the brain

A. Only V
B. II and V
C. II and III
D. I, II, and V
E. All of the above

18. A 59-year-old white female is hospitalized for a ruptured duodenal diverticulum. She is 5 feet 6 inches, weighs 65 kg, and has a serum creatinine of 1.5 mg/dL. Design a dosage regimen to achieve C_{peak} and C_{trough} values of 8.0 and 0.5 mg/L with an infusion time = 30 minutes. Assume V_d of gentamicin of 0.2 L/kg IBW in this patient. The typical population value of CL for gentamicin is 85 mL/minute/70 kg.

Which of the following dosage regimens would you recommend for this patient?

A. 100 mg q8h
B. 100 mg q18h
C. 100 mg q24h
D. 160 mg q12h
E. 160 mg q24h

19. J. D. is a 47-year-old white male who has been prescribed codeine for lower back pain. The pharmacist dispensing the medication remembers reading a study in which patients who took codeine with grapefruit juice experienced an enhanced analgesic effect. The study found that grapefruit juice enhanced oral bioavailability (F) of codeine. Interestingly, there was no effect on codeine hepatic clearance or volume of distribution. Thus, the pharmacist counseled the patient not to take his codeine with grapefruit juice. Based on the pharmacokinetic data for codeine (listed below), what is the most likely explanation for the enhanced oral bioavailability of codeine?

CL: 1,350 mL/minute
f_e: 0.10
V_{ss}: 3.3 L/kg
Plasma protein binding: 35%

A. Grapefruit juice increases the absorption (f_a) of codeine.
B. Grapefruit juice decreases the fraction escaping first-pass metabolism (F^*).
C. Grapefruit juice increases renal secretion of codeine.
D. Grapefruit juice increases the fraction escaping first-pass metabolism (F^*).

20. The pharmacokinetic parameters for codeine in healthy adults are as follows:

Oral F: 50%
f_e < 0.01
V_{ss}: 2.6 L/kg
Plasma protein binding: 7%

Codeine is well absorbed ($f_a = 1$, $f_g = 0.8$). You may assume that hepatic blood flow in a 70 kg adult is 1,350 mL/minute. The hepatic clearance of codeine is

A. 851 mL/minute.
B. 1,350 mL/minute.
C. 500 mL/minute.
D. 675 mL/minute.

6-16. Answers

1. **D.** The systemic exposure or average steady-state concentration for an oral dosing regimen is given by

$$C_{ss,av} = \frac{F \times DR}{CL}$$

where DR is the dose rate and F the oral bioavailability of the respective dosing regimens. If $C_{ss,av}$ should be maintained constant, if follows that

$$C_{ss,av} = \frac{F_1 \times DR_1}{CL} = \frac{F_2 \times DR_2}{CL}$$
$$\text{or } F_1 \times DR_1 = F_2 \times DR_2$$

where the subscript denotes the different dosing regimens. Thus DR_2, the dose rate for the generic dosage form, can be calculated as

$$DR_2 = \frac{F_1 \times DR_1}{F_2} = \frac{43\% \times 85 \text{ mg}/12 \text{ h}}{28\%}$$
$$= 130.5 \text{ mg}/12 \text{ h}$$

2. **C.** Steady-state plasma concentration of a constant-rate infusion is directly proportional to the infusion rate R_0 through

$$C_{ss} = \frac{R_0}{CL}$$

Thus, R_0 has to be doubled from 60 mg/h to 120 mg/h to increase C_{ss} from 5 to 10 mcg/mL, that is, an increase of infusion rate by 60 mg/h.

3a. **C.** 500 mg for the loading dose.

3b. **B.** 40 mg/h for the maintenance dose.

The loading dose and maintenance dose can be calculated from target concentration and volume of distribution or clearance:

$$LD = C_{target} \times V = 12 \text{ mg/L} \times 34 \text{ L}$$
$$= 408 \text{ mg theophylline}$$
$$= 510 \text{ mg aminophylline}$$

$$MD = C_{target} \times CL = 12 \text{ mg/L} \times 2.7 \text{ L/h}$$
$$= 32.4 \text{ mg/h theophylline}$$
$$= 40.5 \text{ mg/h aminophylline}$$

4. **B.** The infusion rate R_0 or maintenance dose MD needed to achieve and maintain a steady-sate concentration of 3 mcg/mL is given by

$$MD = R_0 = C_{ss} \times CL = C_{ss} \times V \times \frac{0.693}{t_{1/2}}$$
$$= 3 \text{ mcg/mL} \times 90 \text{ L} \times \frac{0.693}{1.1 \text{ h}} = 170 \text{ mg/hr}$$

The infusion pump setting can then be calculated as

$$\text{Infusion volume/time} = \frac{170 \text{ mg/h}}{20 \text{ mg/mL}} = 8.5 \text{ mL/h}$$

5. **D.** The first step is to calculate the elimination rate constant k from the measured plasma concentrations:

$$k = \frac{\ln\left(\frac{C_{12\text{ h}}}{C_{2\text{ h}}}\right)}{12 \text{ h} - 2 \text{ h}} = \frac{\ln\left(\frac{12.9 \text{ mcg/mL}}{6.0 \text{ mcg/mL}}\right)}{12 \text{ h} - 2 \text{ h}} = 0.077 \text{ h}^{-1}$$

The initial concentration C_0 at the end of the infusion can then be back-extrapolated by solving the following relationship for C_0:

$$C = C_0 \times e^{-k \times t}$$
$$C_0 = \frac{12.9 \text{ mcg/mL}}{e^{-0.077 \text{ h}^{-1} \times 2 \text{ h}}} = 15 \text{ mcg/mL}$$

The concentration 24 hours after termination of the infusion can be predicted by

$$C_{24\text{ h}} = 15 \text{ mcg/mL} \times e^{-0.077 \text{ h}^{-1} \times 24 \text{ h}} = 2.4 \text{ mcg/mL}$$

6. **C.** The loading dose can be determined on the basis of the target concentration to be achieved and the volume of distribution. The predose level of 4 mg/L needs to be subtracted from the target concentration, because the loading dose only has to account for the concentration difference. The calculated theophylline dose needs to be converted to aminophylline:

$$LD = \left(C_{target} - C_{predose}\right) \times V_d$$
$$= \left(12 - 4\right) \text{ mg/L} \times 0.5 \text{ L/kg}$$
$$\times 100 \text{ kg} = 400 \text{ mg theophylline}$$

A loading dose of 400 mg theophylline is equivalent to 500 mg aminophylline.

7. **B.** The maintenance dose *MD* required to achieve an average steady-state concentration of 50 ng/mL for an oral dosing regimen is given by

$$MD = C_{ss,av} \times CL/F$$

The oral clearance *CL/F* can be determined from the relationship between dose and area under the plasma concentration-time curve *AUC*:

$$CL/F = \frac{D}{AUC}$$

Thus, the required *MD* can be calculated as

$$MD = C_{ss,av} \times \frac{D}{AUC} = 50 \text{ ng/mL} \times \frac{80 \text{ mg}}{962 \text{ ng h/mL}}$$
$$= 4.16 \text{ mg/h}$$

This corresponds to a dosing regimen of 50 mg (4.16 mg/hour × 12 hours) given every 12 hours.

8. **D.** Because trough concentrations after the first dose are known (0.33 mcg/L), trough concentrations during multiple dose at steady state can be predicted by multiplying the trough after the first dose with the accumulation factor

$$C_{ss,min} = C_{ss,1} \times \frac{1}{e^{-k \times \tau}}$$

The dosing interval τ is 24 hours; *k* can be calculated from

$$k = \frac{\ln\left(\frac{C_1}{C_2}\right)}{\Delta t} = \frac{\ln\left(\frac{0.72}{0.33}\right)}{(24-12)\text{h}} = 0.065 \text{ h}^{-1}$$

Thus,

$$C_{ss,min} = 0.33 \text{ mcg/L} \times \frac{1}{e^{-0.065 \text{ h}^{-1} \times 24 \text{ h}}} = 1.57 \text{ mcg/L}$$

9. **A.** For immediate-release formulations, upper limits for peak concentrations ($C_{ss,max}$) and lower limits for trough concentrations ($C_{ss,min}$) can be estimated by assuming immediate drug absorption. If fluctuation is equal to 100%, $C_{ss,min}$ is exactly one-half of $C_{ss,max}$. This is the case when the dosing interval τ is equal to the elimination half-life $t_{1/2}$ of the drug. A population average half-life for nifedipine can be calculated as

$$k = \frac{CL}{V} = \frac{0.41 \text{ L/h/kg}}{1.2 \text{ L/kg}} = 0.34 \text{ h}^{-1}$$

$$t_{1/2} = \frac{0.693}{0.34 \text{ h}^{-1}} = \frac{0.41 \text{ L/h/kg}}{1.2 \text{ L/kg}} = 2.03 \text{ h}$$

Thus, τ has to be smaller than 2.03 hours to avoid peak-to-trough fluctuation exceeding 100%.

10. **D.** Calculate necessary dose rate *DR* to maintain $C_{ss,avg} = 1$ mg/L:

$$DR_{necessary} = \frac{D}{\tau} = \frac{C_{ss,av} \times CL}{F}$$
$$= \frac{1 \text{ mg/L} \times 0.5 \text{ L/h/kg} \times 58 \text{ kg}}{0.90}$$
$$= 32.22 \text{ mg/h}$$
$$= 773.3 \text{ mg/day}$$

Determine the maximum dosing interval:

$$\tau_{max} = \frac{\ln\left(\frac{C_{ss,max}}{C_{ss,min}}\right)}{K} = \frac{\ln\left(\frac{C_{ss,max}}{C_{ss,min}}\right) \times V}{CL}$$
$$= \frac{\ln\left(\frac{1.5}{0.75}\right) \times 6 \text{ L/kg}}{0.5 \text{ L/h/kg}} = 8.3 \text{ h}$$

Practical dosing interval: 8 hours

$$D = DR_{necessary} \times \tau = 32.22 \text{ mg/h} \times 8 \text{ h}$$
$$= 257.8 \text{ mg}$$

Recommended dosing regimen: 250 mg every 8 hours

11. **C.** Calculate the elimination rate constant *k*:

$$k = \frac{\ln\left(\frac{C_1}{C_2}\right)}{\Delta t} = \frac{\ln\left(\frac{4.9}{1.7}\right)}{6.5 \text{ h}} = 0.163 \text{ h}^{-1}$$

Calculate the volume of distribution assuming steady state:

$$C_{ss,max} = \frac{C_{measured\ peak}}{e^{-k \times t}} = \frac{4.9\ mg/L}{e^{-0.163\ h^{-1} \times 0.5\ h}} = 5.32\ mg/L$$

$$C_{ss,min} = C_{measured\ trough} \times e^{-k \times t}$$
$$= 1.7\ mg/L \times e^{-0.163\ h^{-1} \times 0.5}$$
$$= 1.57\ mg/h$$

$$V = \frac{R_0}{k} \times \frac{1 - e^{-k \times T_{inf}}}{C_{max} - C_{min} \times e^{-k \times T_{inf}}}$$

$$= \frac{80\ mg}{0.163\ h^{-1} \times 0.5\ h}$$

$$\times \frac{1 - e^{-1.163\ h^{-1} \times 0.5\ h}}{5.32\ mg/h - 1.57\ mg/h \times e^{-0.163\ h^{-1} \times 0.5\ h}}$$

$$= 19.8\ L$$

Calculate the recommended dosing interval:

$$\tau = \frac{\ln\left(\dfrac{C_{ss,max(desired)}}{C_{ss,min(desired)}}\right)}{k} + T_{inf}$$

$$= \frac{\ln\left(\dfrac{8}{1}\right)}{0.163\ h^{-1}} + .5\ h = 13.3\ h$$

Recommended dosing interval: 12 hours

Calculate the recommended dose:

$$D = C_{ss,max(desired)} \times K \times V \times T_{inf} \times \frac{1 - e^{-K \times \tau}}{1 - e^{-K \times T_{inf}}}$$

$$= 8\ mg/L$$
$$\times 0.163\ h^{-1} \times 19.8\ L \times 0.5\ h$$
$$\times \frac{1 - e^{-0.163\ h^{-1} \times 12\ h}}{1 - e^{-0.163\ h^{-1} \times 0.5\ h}}$$
$$D = 142\ mg$$

Recommended dosing regimen: 140 mg every 12 hours

12. **C.** Phenytoin has to be a low-extraction drug because its bioavailability is as high as 90%. The large range in *F* is due to variability in the absorption of the drug. You know it is not high extraction because if it were, you could never get an *F* of 90%. Assume $ER < 0.1$, $f_{up} = 0.07–0.12$. Low-extraction drug and restrictively cleared (assume all low-*ER* drugs are restrictively cleared for the purposes of this course). Normal albumin range: 3.5–5 gm/dL. Thus, patient probably has increased f_{up} because of decreased albumin. F_{up} (according to the following equation) would be 0.14 (slightly elevated).

$$f_{up} = \frac{1}{1 + 2.1 \times Albumin}$$

Because phenytoin is a low-extraction drug, *CL* is dependent on f_{up} and CL_{int}. Increased f_{up} would lead to increased *CL* and decreased total plasma concentrations (thus C_p of 8, which is below therapeutic range). However, unbound concentrations would be predicted to be normal (therapeutic) even though total concentration is low. You would not recommend an increase in patient's phenytoin dose because it may result in toxic concentrations. Obtaining free phenytoin plasma concentration, if available from the hospital's lab, may be reasonable to document therapeutic concentrations.

13. **B.** Only item II is correct. Item I is incorrect. No pH sensitivity in CL_R is expected unless the drug is reabsorbed (i.e., $E_{ratio} \ll 1$). Item II is possible. Weakly acidic drugs with pK_a values between 3.0 and 7.5 can be highly un-ionized in the range of urine pH (5–8) and can thus undergo significant reabsorption if the un-ionized form is nonpolar. Item III is incorrect. Clearance and volume have nothing to do with a drug's likelihood of being affected by changes in urine pH. Item IV is incorrect. The fraction excreted unchanged says nothing about the mechanisms of renal elimination. However, it is important to note that for drugs with high f_e values that are susceptible to changes in urine pH, large changes in the PK of the drug (i.e., CL_R) may be observed.

14. **A.** The antibiotic's total clearance can be determined from the reported V_d and $t_{1/2}$:

$$CL = Vd \times \frac{\ln 2}{t_{1/2}} = 0.31 \text{ L/kg} \times 73 \text{ kg} \times \frac{0.693}{2.1 \text{ h}}$$

$$= 7.47 \text{ L/h}$$

Renal clearance CL_R is then given by total clearance and the fraction excreted f_e:

$$CL_R = f_e \times CL = 0.67 \times 7.47 \text{ L/h} = 5.00 \text{ L/h}$$

$$= 83.3 \text{ mL/minute}$$

The predominant renal clearance mechanism can be estimated by determining the E_{ratio}:

$$E_{ratio} = \frac{CL_R}{f_{up} \times GFR} = \frac{83.3 \text{ mL/minute}}{0.77 \times 124 \text{ mL/minute}}$$

$$= 0.87$$

The $E_{ratio} < 1$ indicates that glomerular filtration and net reabsorption are the probable renal clearance mechanisms.

15a. D.

$$CL_R = CL_T \times f_e$$

$$CL_R = 800 \text{ mL/minute} \times 0.5 = 400 \text{ mL/minute}$$

$$E_{ratio} = \frac{CL_R}{f_{up} \times GFR} = \frac{400 \text{ mL/minute}}{0.25 \times 125 \text{ mL/minute}}$$

$$= 12.8 = \text{filtration and net secretion}$$

15b. D. The most likely mechanism to account for this reduction in renal clearance is that cimetidine blocks the renal secretion of captopril.

16. B.

$$CL_R = CL_T \times f_e$$

$$CL_R = 125 \text{ mL/minute} \times 1.0 = 125 \text{ mL/minute}$$

$$E_{ratio} = \frac{CL_R}{f_{up} \times GFR} = \frac{125 \text{ mL/minute}}{0.25 \times 125 \text{ mL/minute}}$$

$$= 4.0 = \text{filtration and net secretion}$$

17. B. The drug transporter P-glycoprotein is directly responsible for the transport of drug from hepatocytes into the bile and maintenance of the integrity of the blood–brain barrier by transport of drug out of the brain.

18. C. Calculation of CL: IBW = 59.3 kg:

$$CL_{cr} = \frac{(140 - \text{age}) \times \text{IBW}}{72 \times S_{cr}} \times 0.85$$

$$= \frac{(140 - 59) \times 59.3}{72 \times 1.5}$$

$$\times 0.85 = 37.8 \text{ mL/minute}$$

$$RF = \frac{37.8}{125} = 0.30$$

CL of gentamicin is 85 mL/minute/70 kg TBW (1.2 mL/minute/kg). CL of gentamicin in this patient if she did not have renal impairment would be

$$CL = 1.21 \text{ mL/minute/kg} \times 65 \text{ kg}$$

$$= 79 \text{ mL/minute}$$

$$CL^* = CL \times [1 - f_e \times (1 - RF)]$$

$$= 79 \times [1 - 1 \times (1 - 0.30)]$$

$$= 23.7 \text{ mL/minute}$$

$$= 1.42 \text{ L/h}$$

$$K^* = \frac{CL^*}{V_{ss}} = \frac{1.42 \text{ L/h}}{0.2 \text{ L/kg} \times 59.3 \text{ kg}}$$

$$= 0.12 \text{ h}^{-1}$$

Calculate the dosing interval (τ) that you would recommend:

$$\tau = \frac{\ln\left(\frac{8}{0.5}\right)}{0.12 \text{ h}^{-1}} + 0.5 \text{ h} = 23.1 \text{ h}$$

Calculate the dose of gentamicin that will maintain C_{peak} and C_{trough} of 8 and 0.5 mg/L:

$$\text{Dose} = C_{ss,max} \times K \times V \times t_{inf} \times \frac{1 - e^{-K \times \tau}}{1 - e^{-K \times t_{inf}}}$$

$$\text{Dose} = 8 \text{ mg/L} \times 0.12 \text{ h}^{-1} \times 11.86 \text{ L} \times 0.5 \text{ h}$$

$$\times \frac{1 - e^{-0.12 \times 24}}{1 - e^{-0.12 \times .05}} = 92.3 \text{ mg}$$

Administration of 100 mg of gentamicin infused over 30 minutes given every 24 hours will provide C_{peak} and C_{trough} of approximately 8.0 and 0.5 mg/L.

19. **A.**

$$CL_H = 1,350 \times 0.9 = 1,215 \text{ mL/minute}$$

$$ER = \frac{1,215 \text{ mL/minute}}{1,350 \text{ mL/minute}} \approx 1$$

$$F = f_a \times f_g \times F^*$$

No effect on CL_H. No effect on F^*

20. **C.**

$$F = f_a \times f_g \times F^*$$

$$F^* = \frac{F}{F_a \times f_g} = \frac{0.5}{1 \times 0.8} = 0.63$$

$$ER = 1 - F^* = 1 - 0.63 = 0.37$$

$$CL_H = Q \times ER = 1,350 \text{ mL/minute} \times 0.37$$
$$= 500 \text{ mL/minute}$$

6-17. References

Atkinson A, Daniels C, Dedrick R, et al. *Principles of Clinical Pharmacology*. Academic Press, San Diego, Calif.; 2001.

Ensom MH, Davis GA, Cropp CD, Ensom RJ. Clinical pharmacokinetics in the 21st century: Does the evidence support definitive outcomes? *Clin Pharmacokinet*. 1998;34:265–79.

Levy RH, Bauer LA. Basic pharmacokinetics. *Ther Drug Monit*. 1986;8(1):47–58.

Meibohm B, Derendorf H: Basic concepts of pharma-cokinetic/pharmacodynamic (PK/PD) modelling. *Int J Clin Pharmacol Ther*. 1997;35:401–13.

Rolan, PE. Plasma protein binding displacement interactions: Why are they still regarded as clin-ically important? *Br J Clin Pharmacol*. 1994;37: 125–8.

Rowland M, Tozer T. *Clinical Pharmacokinetics*. 3rd ed. Media, Pa.: Williams & Wilkins; 1995.

Saitoh A, Jinbayashi H, Saitoh AK, et al. Parameter estimation and dosage adjustment in the treatment with vancomycin of methicillin-resistant *Staphylo-coccus aureus* ocular infections. *Ophthalmologica*. 1997;211(4):232–35.

Sawchuk RJ, Zaske DE, Cipolle RJ, et al. Kinetic model for gentamicin dosing with the use of indi-vidual patient parameters. *Clin Pharmacol Ther*. 1977;21:362–69.

Tod MM, Padoin C, Petitjean O. Individualising aminoglycoside dosage regimens after therapeu-tic drug monitoring: Simple or complex phar-macokinetic methods? *Clin Pharmacokinet*. 2001; 40:803–14.

Wilkinson, GR, Shand, DG. Commentary: A physio-logical approach to hepatic drug clearance. *Clin Pharmacol Ther*. 1975;18:377–90.

Biotechnology and Pharmacogenomics

Stephanie A. Flowers, PharmD
P. David Rogers, PharmD, PhD, FCCP

7

7-1. Introduction

Since the discovery of the DNA (deoxyribonucleic acid) double helix half a century ago, significant use of biotechnology has been made for the improvement of human health (Table 7-1). Accompanying these advances is a number of biological products with therapeutic applications. With the arrival of the post-genomic era, the field of pharmacogenomics has emerged and shows great promise to revolutionize the way in which pharmacy and medicine are practiced. This chapter highlights key concepts relevant to the practicing pharmacist in the areas of biotechnology and pharmacogenomics.

Biotechnology has revolutionized the pharmaceutical industry by imparting the ability to mass produce safe and pure versions of chemicals produced naturally in the body. A multitude of disease states have been affected by therapeutic agents derived through biotechnology, including AIDS (acquired immune deficiency syndrome), anemia, cancer, congestive heart failure, cystic fibrosis, diabetes, growth hormone deficiency, hemophilia, hepatitis B and C, and multiple sclerosis, to name a few.

Biotechnology is defined by the Merriam-Webster's Dictionary as "the manipulation (as through genetic engineering) of living organisms or their components to produce useful usually commercial products (as pest resistant crops, new bacterial strains, or novel pharmaceuticals)."

Key Terms

- *Antibody (immunoglobulin):* A protein produced by β-lymphocytes in response to antigen molecules determined to be nonself. Antibodies recognize and bind to antigens, resulting in their inactivation or opsonization for phagocytosis or complement-mediated destruction. A number of immunoglobulin (Ig) G products have been developed for therapeutic use in various immune disorders.
- *Antigen:* A molecule that elicits an antibody-mediated immune response.
- *Bioinformatics:* The application of computer sciences and information technology to the management and analysis of biological information.
- *Biotherapy:* Any treatment involving the administration of a microorganism or other biologic material.
- *Clotting factor (blood factor):* Chemical blood constituents that interact to cause blood coagulation.
- *Combinatorial chemistry:* A drug development strategy that uses nucleic acids and amino acids in various combinations to synthesize vast libraries of oligonucleotide or peptide compounds for high-throughput lead compound screening.
- *Cytokine:* An extracellular signaling protein that mediates communication between cells.
- *DNA (deoxyribonucleic acid):* A polynucleotide molecule consisting of covalently linked nucleic acids. DNA serves as the genetic material.
- *Enzyme:* A protein that catalyzes a chemical reaction.
- *Gene:* A region of DNA that encodes a specific RNA (ribonucleic acid) or protein responsible for a specific hereditary characteristic.
- *Gene therapy:* Therapeutic technologies that directly target human genes responsible for disease.
- *Genome:* The complete set of genetic information for a given organism.

Table 7-1. Milestones in Biotechnology

Event	Year
Identification of DNA as a genetic material	1940
Discovery of DNA double helix by James Watson and Francis Crick	1953
Elucidation of the genetic code (64 nucleic acid triplets, or codons, encode 20 amino acids)	1961
Cloning of DNA and the production of the first recombinant DNA–derived protein	1973
Introduction of monoclonal antibodies	1975
Production of the first human protein (somatostatin) from recombinant DNA technology	1977
Cloning of the human insulin gene	1978
Licensing in the United States of technology to derive human insulin from recombinant DNA	1982
Conception of the polymerase chain reaction for amplification of DNA	1983
Initiation of the Human Genome Project	1990
Sequencing of the human genome	2001

- *Genomics:* The scientific discipline of mapping, sequencing, and analyzing genomes. It encompasses structural genomics, functional genomics, and pharmacogenomics.
- *Hormone:* A chemical substance imparting specific cellular effects that is transmitted by the bloodstream to cells distant from its physiologic source.
- *Hybridoma:* A cell line generated by the fusion of antibody-producing β-lymphocytes with lymphocyte tumor cells for the production of monoclonal antibodies.
- *Interferon:* A member of a group of cytokines that prevents viral replication and slows the growth and replication of cancer cells.
- *Interleukin:* A member of a group of cytokines involved in orchestration and regulation of the immune response.
- *Liposome:* A microscopic, sphere-like lipid droplet that functions as a therapeutic carrier.
- *Monoclonal antibody:* An antibody derived from a hybridoma cell line.
- *Pharmacogenomics:* The scientific discipline of using genomewide approaches to understand the inherited basis of differences between individuals in the response to drugs. This field is an expansion of the field of pharmacogenetics, which traditionally considered such inherited differences on a gene-by-gene basis.
- *Plasmid:* A small, circular, extrachromosomal DNA molecule capable of replication independent of that of the genome.
- *Polymerase chain reaction (PCR):* A molecular biologic technique for amplification of specific DNA molecules.
- *Protein:* A functional product of a specific gene consisting of amino acids linked together through peptide bonds in a specific sequence.
- *Proteomics:* The scientific field of the study of sequencing and analyzing the expression, modification, and function of proteins on a genomewide or global scale.
- *Recombinant DNA (rDNA) technology:* The application of DNA molecules derived by joining two DNA molecules from different sources.
- *Restriction endonucleases:* An enzyme capable of cleaving a DNA molecule in a site-specific manner.
- *Ribozymes:* RNA molecules with intrinsic enzymatic activity.
- *RNA (ribonucleic acid):* A polynucleotide molecule consisting of covalently linked ribonucleic acids. Messenger RNA (mRNA) serves as the template for protein synthesis. Transfer RNA (tRNA) serves as the adaptor molecules between amino acids and mRNA during protein synthesis. Ribosomal RNA serves as a component of the ribosome and participates in protein synthesis.
- *Small molecule chemistry:* The field of drug development focusing on small organic nucleotide- or peptide-based molecules derived through either combinatorial chemistry or rational drug design.

- *Single nucleotide polymorphism:* Common DNA sequence variations among individuals involving a single nucleotide substitution.
- *Vaccine:* A preparation of antigenic material administered to stimulate the development of antibodies conferring active immunity against a particular pathogen or disease.

Biological Products

Many FDA-approved biological products are currently on the market, including blood factors, cytokines, enzymes, growth factors, hormones, interferons, monoclonal antibodies, and vaccines. A list of such biological products is provided in Table 7-2.

Table 7-2. Approved Biological Products

Generic name	Brand name (manufacturer)	Indications
Blood factors		
Factor VII	NovoSeven (Novo Nordisk)	Hemophilia
Factor VIII	Bioclate, Recombinate, Advate (Baxter); Kogenate, Helixate (Bayer); ReFacto (Genetics Institute); Xyntha (Wyeth Pharmaceuticals)	Hemophilia A
Factor IX	BeneFIX (Genetics Institute)	Hemophilia B
Cytokines		
Aldesleukin (IL-2)	Proleukin (Chiron)	Metastatic renal cell carcinoma and melanoma
Denileukin diftitox	Ontak (Ligand)	Cutaneous T-cell lymphoma
Interferon alfacon-1	Infergen (InterMune)	Hepatitis C
Interferon alfa-n1	Wellferon (GlaxoSK)	Chronic hepatitis C
Interferon alfa-2a	Roferon-A (Roche)	Hairy cell leukemia; AIDS-related Kaposi's sarcoma; chronic myelogenous leukemia
Interferon alfa-2b	Intron-A (Schering)	Hairy cell leukemia; AIDS-related Kaposi's sarcoma; chronic hepatitis B and C; condylomata acuminata; malignant melanoma
Interferon alfa-n3	Alferon-N (InterMune)	Condylomata acuminata
Interferon beta-1b	Betaseron (Berlex)	Acute relapsing–remitting multiple sclerosis
Interferon beta-1a	Avonex (Biogen); Rebif (Serono)	Acute relapsing–remitting multiple sclerosis
Interferon gamma-1b	Actimmune (InterMune)	Chronic granulomatous disease; osteoporosis
Oprelvekin (IL-11)	Neumega (Genetics Institute)	Thrombocytopenia from chemotherapy
Peginterferon alfa-2a	Pegasys (Roche)	Hepatitis C
Peginterferon alfa-2b	PegIntron (Schering)	Hepatitis C
Enzymes		
Agalsidase beta	Fabrazyme (Genzyme)	Fabry disease
Alglucosidase alfa	Myozyme (Genzyme)	Lysosomal alpha-1,4-glucosidase deficiency
Alpha-1-proteinase inhibitor	Zemaira (Aventis)	Alpha-1-proteinase inhibitor deficiency
Alteplase	Activase (Genentech)	Acute myocardial infarction; pulmonary embolism; stroke
Bivalirudin	Angiomax (Medicines Co.)	Coronary angioplasty (PTCA); unstable angina
Dornase alfa	Pulmozyme (Genentech)	Respiratory complication from cystic fibrosis
Eptifibatide	Integrelin (Millennium)	Acute coronary syndromes; angioplasties
Galsulfase	Naglazyme (Biomarin Pharmaceutical Inc.)	Mucopolysaccharidosis
Idursulfase	Elaprase (Shire Human Genetic Therapies)	Mucopolysaccharidosis
Imiglucerase	Cerezyme (Genzyme)	Type 1 Gaucher's disease

(continued)

Table 7-2. Approved Biological Products *(Continued)*

Generic name	Brand name (manufacturer)	Indications
Laronidase	Aldurazyme (Biomarin)	Mucopolysaccharidosis
Lepirudin	Refludan (Berlex)	Heparin-induced thrombocytopenia
Rasburicase	Elitek (Sanofi-Synthelabo)	Elevated plasma uric acid in pediatric malignancy
Reteplase	Retavase (Centocor/J&J)	Acute myocardial infarction
Tenecteplase	TNKase (Genentech)	Acute myocardial infarction
Tirobifan	Aggrastat (Merck)	Acute coronary syndromes
Growth factors		
Becaplermin (PDGF)	Regranex (Ortho-McNeil)	Diabetic foot ulcer
Darbepoetin alfa	Aranesp (Amgen)	Anemia associated with end-stage renal disease and chronic renal insufficiency
Epoetin alfa	EPOGEN (Amgen); Procrit (Ortho Biotech)	Anemia attributable to chronic renal disease; zidovudine-induced anemia; anemia due to chemotherapy; surgery patients
Filgrastim	Neupogen (Amgen)	Neutropenia attributable to myelosuppressive chemotherapy; myeloid reconstitution after bone marrow transplant; severe chronic neutropenia; peripheral blood progenitor cell transplant; induction and consolidation therapy in acute myelogenous leukemia
Methoxy polyethylene glycol-epoetin beta	Mircera (Roche)	Anemia attributable to chronic renal failure
Palifermin	Kepivance (Biovitrum)	Oral mucositis; mucositis following chemotherapy
Pegfilgrastim	Neulasta (Amgen)	Febrile neutropenia attributable to myelosuppressive chemotherapy
Sargramostim	Leukine (Berlex)	Myeloid reconstitution after bone marrow transplant; bone marrow transplant failure; adjunct to chemotherapy in acute myelogenous leukemia; peripheral blood progenitor cell transplant
Hormones		
Choriogonadotropin alfa	Ovidrel (Serono)	Fertility
Follitropin alfa	Gonal-F (Serono)	Ovulatory failure
Follitropin beta	Follistim (Organon)	Ovulatory failure
Human growth hormone	Protopin, Nutropin (Genentech)	Growth hormone deficiency in pediatric patients
	Humatrope (Eli Lilly)	Growth retardation in chronic renal disease
	Saizen, Serostim (Serono)	AIDS wasting
	Norditropin (Novo Nordisk)	Turner's syndrome
	Genotropin (Pharmacia); Biotropin (Sol Source Technologies)	Growth hormone deficiency in adults
Human insulin	Humulin; Humalog (Eli Lilly); Novolin (Novo Nordisk); Lantus (Aventis)	Insulin-dependent diabetes mellitus
Ganirelix	Antagon (Organon)	Luteinizing hormone surge during fertility therapy
Glucagon	GlucaGen (Novo Nordisk)	Hypoglycemia
Growth hormone-releasing hormone	Geref (Serono)	Growth hormone deficiency in pediatric patients
Thyrotropin	Thyrogen (Genzyme)	Thyroid cancer
Monoclonal antibodies		
Abciximab	ReoPro (Centocor)	Prevention of blood clots following percutaneous coronary intervention; unstable angina prior to percutaneous coronary intervention
Adalimumab	Humira (Abbott)	Acute rheumatoid arthritis
Alemtuzumab	Campath (Berlex)	Chronic lymphocytic leukemia
Basiliximab	Simulect (Novartis)	Acute organ transplant rejection

Table 7-2. Approved Biological Products *(Continued)*

Generic name	Brand name (manufacturer)	Indications
Bevacizumab	Avastin (Genentech)	Colorectal cancer
Certolizumab pegol	Cimzia (UCB)	Crohn's disease
Cetuximab	Erbitux (ImClone Systems)	Colorectal cancer
Daclizumab	Zenapax (Roche)	Kidney transplant; acute rejection
Eculizumab	Soliris (Alexion)	Paroxysmal nocturnal hemoglobinuria
Efalizumab	Raptiva (Genentech)	Psoriasis
Gemtuzumab (ozogamicin)	Mylotarg (Wyeth/PDL)	Acute myeloid leukemia (CD33+)
Ibritumomab (tiuxetan)	Zevalin (IDEC)	B-cell non-Hodgkin's lymphoma
Infliximab	Remicade (Centocor)	Crohn's disease; rheumatoid arthritis
Natalizumab	Tysabri (Amgen)	Crohn's disease; multiple sclerosis
Omalizumab	Xolair (Genentech)	Asthma
Palivizumab	Synagis (MedImmune)	Prevention of respiratory syncytial virus and fatal pneumonia in pediatrics
Panitumumab	Vectibix (Amgen)	Metastatic colorectal cancer
Ranibizumab	Lucentis (Genentech)	Exudative age-related macular degeneration
Rituximab	Rituxan (IDEC/Genentech)	Low-grade non-Hodgkin's lymphoma
Tositumomab	Bexxar (Corixa)	CD20+ non-Hodgkin's lymphoma
Trastuzumab	Herceptin (Genentech/PDL)	Metastatic breast cancer (Her 2 Neu+)
Vaccines		
Haemophilus b/ hepatitis B	Comvax (Merck)	Prevention of *Haemophilus influenzae* and hepatitis B
Hepatitis B vaccine	Engerix-B (GlaxoSK); Recombivax HB (Merck)	Prevention of hepatitis B
Others		
Abatacept	Orencia (BMS)	Rheumatoid arthritis
Anakinra	Kineret (Amgen)	Rheumatoid arthritis
BCNU polymer	Gliadel (Guilford)	Recurrent glioblastoma multiforme
Daunorubicin-liposomal	DaunoXome (Gilead)	Kaposi's sarcoma
Doxorubicin-liposomal	DOXIL (Alza)	Kaposi's sarcoma; ovarian cancer
Drotrecogin alfa	Xigris (Eli Lilly)	Sepsis
Etanercept	Enbrel (Amgen)	Rheumatoid arthritis; psoriatic arthritis
Fomivirsen	Vitravene (Isis)	Cytomegalovirus retinitis
Glatiramer	Copaxone (Teva)	Relapsing multiple sclerosis
Lipid-based amphotericin B	Abelcet (Elan); Amphotec (Sequus); AmBisome (Fujisawa/Gilead)	Aspergillosis; cryptococcal meningitis in HIV; systemic fungal infections
Nesiritide	Natrecor (Scios/Innovex)	Congestive heart failure
Rilonacept	Arcalyst (Regeneron)	Cryopyrin-associated periodic syndromes
Romiplostim	Nplate (Amgen)	Idiopathic thrombocytopenic purpura

AIDS, acquired immunodeficiency syndrome; BCNU, bis-chlorethylnitrosourea; HIV, human immunodeficiency virus; IL, interleukin; PDGF, platelet-derived growth factor; PCI, percutaneous coronary intervention; PTCA, percutaneous transluminal coronary angioplasty.

Gene Expression and Protein Synthesis

Proteins are the major macromolecular component of the cell and are responsible for conducting most of a cell's biological activity. Proteins consist of a linear polymer of amino acids linked together in a specific sequence. This specific sequence is responsible for a protein's structure and function. The initial code for the synthesis of a given protein is stored in a gene on a sequence of DNA that is part of a chromosome within the nucleus of a cell.

The central dogma of molecular biology is that DNA encodes RNA, which, in turn, encodes protein. A given amino acid within a protein is encoded by a triplet of nucleic acid base pairs within the gene encoding the protein. This triplet is called a *codon*. There are 64 codons encoding 20 different amino acids as dictated by the genetic code.

An overview of transcription, translation, and post-translational modification is shown in Figure 7-1.

Recombinant DNA Technology

Recombinant DNA (rDNA) technology uses several molecular biological tools to insert a desired DNA fragment with a specific purpose in proximity to other DNA fragments within a DNA molecule. Most often, a gene encoding a desired protein is isolated through screening of the genomic library or by use of the viral enzyme reverse transcriptase to generate complementary DNA (cDNA) from the mRNA transcript of the gene. Enzymes called *restriction endonucleases* allow

Figure 7-1. Gene Expression: The Synthesis of Proteins

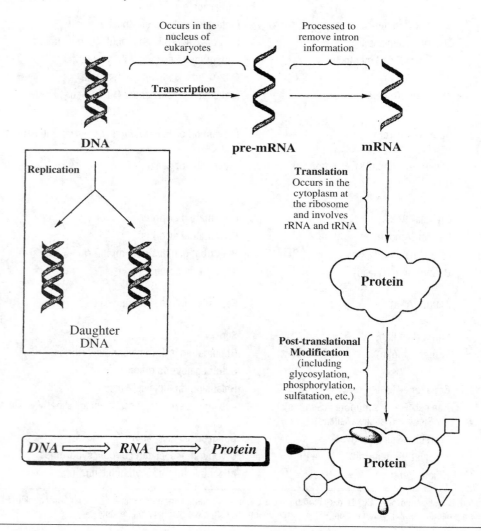

the cleavage of DNA in the plasmid at very specific locations. The gene is then ligated into a vector, such as a plasmid, for gene cloning or for control of the expression of the encoded protein.

An *expression vector* is a plasmid designed to allow inducible expression of the inserted gene within a host cell (such as the bacterium *Escherichia coli* or the yeast *Saccharomyces cerevisiae*). This mechanism permits production of large quantities of the desired protein. The protein must then be isolated and purified for further use. Such techniques, used on an industrial scale, mass produce therapeutically useful biological products such as cytokines, enzymes, hormones, blood factors, and vaccines (Figure 7-2).

Figure 7-2. Summary of Typical rDNA Production of a Protein from Either Genomic DNA or cDNA

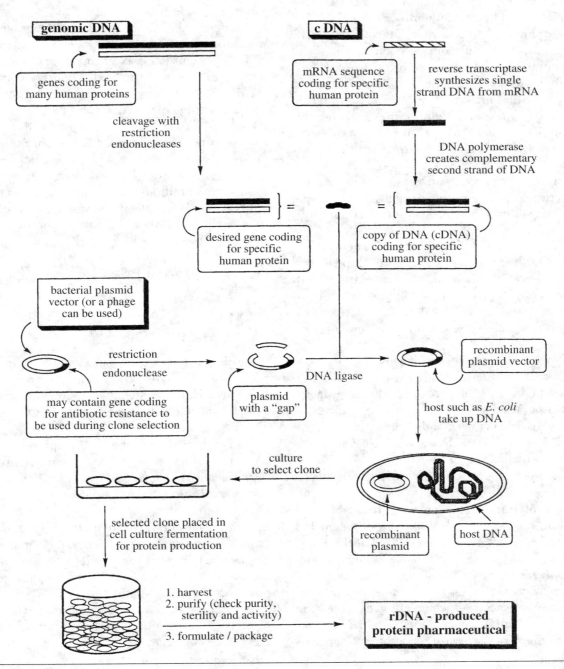

Cytokines (i.e., molecules secreted by cells) orchestrate the immune response and activate immune cells such as lymphocytes, monocytes, macrophages, and neutrophils. Therapeutically useful recombinant cytokines include interferons, interleukins, and colony-stimulating factors. Examples of these include interferon beta-1b (Betaseron), which is used to treat acute relapsing–remitting multiple sclerosis; aldesleukin (IL-2) (Proleukin), which aids in the management of metastatic renal cell carcinoma and melanoma; and oprelvekin (IL-11) (Neumega), which treats thrombocytopenia caused by chemotherapy.

An enzyme is a protein that catalyzes a specific chemical reaction. Numerous different enzymes with therapeutic use have been produced using rDNA technology. Alteplase (Activase), for example, treats acute myocardial infarction, pulmonary embolism, and stroke. Dornase alfa (Pulmozyme) treats respiratory complications that develop in cystic fibrosis. Eptifibatide (Integrelin) is used to treat acute coronary syndromes.

Hormones—chemical substances transmitted through the bloodstream—are designed to impart specific cellular effects to cells distant from their physiologic source. Since the introduction and success of recombinant human insulin in 1982, many other recombinant hormones have been developed, such as human growth hormone, which treats growth hormone deficiency in pediatric patients, and follitropin alfa and beta (Gonal-F and Follistim, respectively), which are used to remedy ovulatory failure.

Clotting or blood factors are chemical blood constituents that interact to cause blood coagulation. Patients suffering from hemophilia A (caused by factor VIII deficiency) and hemophilia B (caused by factor IX deficiency) have benefited greatly from rDNA technology. Factors VII, VIII, and IX are available in recombinant forms for clinical use.

Vaccines—preparations of antigenic material administered to stimulate the development of antibodies—confer active immunity against a particular pathogen or disease. Vaccine development has also benefited from advances in rDNA technology. Traditional vaccine production used killed or non-virulent organisms, microbial toxins, or actual microbial components to elicit long-term immune protection. Safer and more specific vaccine antigens have been devised as recombinant proteins. This technology has led to the very successful recombinant hepatitis B vaccine.

Monoclonal Antibodies

Antibodies, proteins produced by the immune system's β-lymphocytes, use specific methods to recognize foreign molecules within the body. Subsets of β-lymphocyte clones produce identical antibodies that recognize the same antigen. These identical antibodies are *monoclonal*. Fusing β-lymphocytes with lymphocyte tumor cells produces a hybridoma. This fused cell type is immortal and can be cultured in large quantities for the mass production of a given monoclonal antibody.

Monoclonal antibodies that bind to and inactivate their targets can be developed and have great therapeutic utility (Figure 7-3). Nomenclature of monoclonal antibodies is highly structured. The first component of the name is product specific. The second component indicates its therapeutic use: *ci* for cardiovascular use, *li* for use in inflammation, and *tu* for use in cancer. The third component indicates the type of monoclonal antibody: *mo* for murine, *xi* for chimeric, and *zu* for humanized. The fourth component, *mab*, represents monoclonal antibody. An example of a monoclonal antibody used clinically is abciximab (ReoPro), which prevents blood clots following percutaneous transluminal coronary angioplasty (PTCA) and prevents unstable angina prior to PTCA. Another example, infliximab (Remicade), is used to treat Crohn's disease and rheumatoid arthritis.

Gene Therapy

Gene therapy is an excellent example of the therapeutic application of biotechnology. This technology holds promise for the treatment of inherited disorders, as well as acquired illnesses such as infectious diseases and cancer.

The molecular goal of gene therapy is to repair or correct a dysfunctional gene by selectively introducing recombinant DNA into cells or tissues, thereby allowing the expression of a functional gene product.

Novel drug delivery strategies must be used to introduce exogenous DNA into the cell to treat retroviruses, lentiviruses, and adeno-associated viruses. These novel drug delivery strategies also have applications for nonviral delivery systems (e.g., liposomes or uncomplexed plasmid DNA).

Alternative approaches using ribozymes (e.g., RNA repair) may prove effective. The enzymatic activity of these RNA molecules can be used to repair defective mRNAs.

Figure 7-3. Production of Monoclonal Antibodies

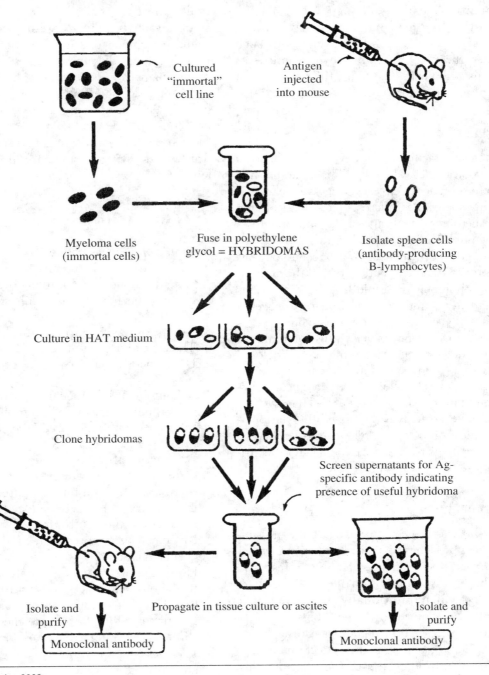

Cultured "immortal" cell line

Antigen injected into mouse

Myeloma cells (immortal cells)

Fuse in polyethylene glycol = HYBRIDOMAS

Isolate spleen cells (antibody-producing B-lymphocytes)

Culture in HAT medium

Clone hybridomas

Screen supernatants for Ag-specific antibody indicating presence of useful hybridoma

Isolate and purify

Propagate in tissue culture or ascites

Isolate and purify

Monoclonal antibody

Monoclonal antibody

Chimeric RNA and DNA oligonucleotides make use of the cell's DNA mismatch repair apparatus to correct mutations at the genomic level. Antisense oligonucleotides for gene inactivation have proved clinically useful. Fomivirsen (Vitravene), one such agent, targets the mRNA of human cytomegalovirus (CMV). This agent is indicated for the treatment of CMV retinitis in patients with AIDS.

Drug Delivery

Biotechnology has facilitated the development of novel drug delivery strategies. The use of liposomes has had a positive effect on drug delivery. Drugs can be formulated into liposomes (i.e., microscopic, spherical lipid droplets). The outer membrane of the liposome fuses with the membrane of the target cell, thereby facilitating highly targeted drug delivery. Such technology has greatly improved the therapeutic index of the antifungal drug amphotericin B. Lipid-based formulations now allow greater quantities of the drug to be delivered with substantially less toxicity to the patient.

Another promising approach is the use of immunotoxins. These delivery agents combine a monoclonal antibody with a toxin such as an anticancer or antimicrobial agent, thereby allowing targeted drug delivery with minimal toxicity.

Another novel strategy is the use of PEGylation—that is, the addition of polyethylene glycol (PEG) to therapeutic proteins to minimize the deleterious immune response to an individual protein.

Pharmacogenomics

Pharmacogenomics is the scientific discipline of using genomewide approaches to understand the inherited basis of differences between individuals in the response to drugs. This field is an expansion of the field of pharmacogenetics, which traditionally considered such inherited differences on a gene-by-gene basis.

Genetic differences in drug metabolism, drug disposition, and drug targets have a large effect on efficacy and toxicity. Comprehension of the relationships between specific genetic factors and drug response can be used to predict drug response and optimize drug therapy in any given individual.

Of particular significance are single nucleotide polymorphisms (SNPs). SNPs are differences in a single nucleotide base that occur at a significant frequency (usually > 5%) within the population. An SNP may or may not promote change in the encoded amino acid of a codon, or it may change the encoded amino acid but

yield no change in the function of the encoded protein. When a SNP causes amino acid substitution, a phenotypic difference that carries clinical relevance may result. Even when the SNP results in no change in the encoded amino acid, it may be associated with a phenotypic change, thereby serving as a predictive marker of that change.

Examples of significant genetic polymorphisms that can influence drug response are shown in Tables 7-3 and 7-4.

Examples of significant genetic polymorphisms in drug-metabolizing enzymes are shown in Tables 7-5 and 7-6.

7-2. Key Points

- *Biotechnology,* as defined by Merriam-Webster's Dictionary, is "the manipulation (as through genetic engineering) of living organisms or their components to produce useful usually commercial products (as pest resistant crops, new bacterial strains, or novel pharmaceuticals)."
- The central dogma of molecular biology is that DNA encodes RNA, which, in turn, encodes protein.
- Recombinant DNA technology makes use of several molecular biological tools that allow for the placement of a desired DNA fragment in proximity to other DNA fragments within a DNA molecule for a specific purpose.
- Cytokines are molecules secreted by cells that orchestrate the immune response. They activate immune cells such as lymphocytes, macrophages, monocytes, and neutrophils.
- An enzyme is a protein that catalyzes a specific chemical reaction.
- Hormones are chemical substances transmitted by the bloodstream to cells distant from their physiologic source that impart specific cellular effects.
- Clotting or blood factors are chemical blood constituents that interact to cause blood coagulation.
- Vaccines are preparations of antigenic material administered to stimulate the development of antibodies for the purpose of conferring active immunity against a particular pathogen or disease.
- Subsets of β-lymphocyte clones produce identical antibodies that recognize the same antigen. These identical antibodies are said to be monoclonal. Fusing β-lymphocytes with lymphocyte tumor cells produces a hybridoma that can be cultured in large quantities for the mass production of a given monoclonal antibody.

Table 7-3. Genetic Polymorphisms in Drug Target Genes That Can Influence Drug Response[a]

Gene or gene product	Medication	Drug effect associated with polymorphism
Angiotensin-converting enzyme (ACE)	ACE inhibitors (e.g., enalapril)	Renoprotective effects; blood pressure reduction; reduction in left ventricular mass; endothelial function
	Fluvastatin	Lipid changes (reductions in low-density lipoprotein cholesterol and apolipoprotein B); progression or regression in coronary atherosclerosis
Arachidonate 5-lipoxygenase	Leukotriene inhibitors	Improvement of FEV_1
β_2-adrenergic receptor	β_2-agonists	Bronchodilatation; susceptibility to agonist-induced desensitization; cardiovascular effects
Bradykinin B_2 receptor	ACE inhibitors	ACE inhibitor–induced cough
Dopamine receptors (D_2, D_3, D_4)	Antipsychotics (e.g., haloperidol and clozapine)	Antipsychotic response (D_2, D_3, D_4); antipsychotic-induced tardive dyskinesia (D_3); antipsychotic-induced acute akathisia (D_3)
Estrogen receptor-α	Conjugated estrogens	Increase in bone mineral density
	Hormone replacement therapy	Increase in high-density lipoprotein cholesterol
Glycoprotein IIIa subunit of glycoprotein IIb/IIIa	Aspirin or glycoprotein IIb/IIIa inhibitors	Antiplatelet effect
Serotonin (5-hydroxytryptamine transporter)	Antidepressants (e.g., clomipramine, fluoxetine, and paroxetine)	Serotonin neurotransmission; antidepressant response

FEV_1, forced expiratory volume in 1 second.
a. The examples shown are illustrative and are not representative of all published studies. Reprinted by permission from Evans, McLeod, 2003.

Table 7-4. Genetic Polymorphisms in Disease-Modifying or Treatment-Modifying Genes That Can Influence Drug Response[a]

Gene or gene product	Disease or response association	Medication	Influence of polymorphism on drug effect or toxicity
Adducin	Hypertension	Diuretics	Myocardial infarction or strokes
Apolipoprotein E	Progression of atherosclerosis; ischemic cardiovascular events	Statins (e.g., simvastatin)	Enhanced survival
	Alzheimer's disease	Tacrine	Clinical improvement
Human leukocyte antigen	Toxicity	Abacavir	Hypersensitivity reaction
Cholesterol ester transfer protein	Progression of atherosclerosis	Statins (e.g., pravastatin)	Slowing of progression of atherosclerosis
Ion channels (HERG, KvLQT1, Mink, and MiRP1)	Congenital long-QT syndrome	Erythromycin; terfenadine; cisapride; clarithromycin; and quinidine	Increased risk of drug-induced torsade de pointes
Methylguanine methyltransferase	Glioma	Carmustine	Response of glioma to carmustine
Parkin	Parkinson's disease	Levodopa	Clinical improvement and levodopa-induced dyskinesias
Prothrombin and factor V	Deep-vein thrombosis; cerebral-vein thrombosis	Oral contraceptives	Increased risk of deep-vein thrombosis and cerebral-vein thrombosis with oral contraceptives
Stromelysin-1	Atherosclerosis progression	Statins (e.g., pravastatin)	Reduction in cardiovascular events by pravastatin (death, myocardial infarction, stroke, angina, and others); reduction in risk of repeated angioplasty

a. The examples shown are illustrative and are not representative of all published studies. Reproduced with permission from Evans, McLeod, 2003.

Table 7-5. Pharmacogenomics of Phase I Drug Metabolism[a]

Drug-metabolizing enzyme	Frequency of variant poor-metabolism phenotype	Representative drugs metabolized	Effect of polymorphism
Butyrylcholinesterase (pseudocholinesterase)	Approximately 1 in 3,500 Europeans	Succinylcholine	Enhanced drug effect
Cytochrome P-450 2D6 (CYP2D6)	6.8% of Swedes	Debrisoquin	Enhanced drug effect
	1% of Chinese	Sparteine	Enhanced drug effect
		Nortriptyline	Enhanced drug effect
		Codeine	Decreased drug effect
Cytochrome P-450 2C9 (CYP2C9)	Approximately 3% of English (those homozygous for the *2 and *3 alleles)	Warfarin	Enhanced drug effect
		Phenytoin	Enhanced drug effect
Cytochrome P-450 2C19 (CYP2C19)	2.7% of white Americans; 3.3% of Swedes; 14.6% of Chinese; 18% of Japanese	Omeprazole	Enhanced drug effect
Dihydropyrimidine dehydrogenase	Approximately 1% of population is heterozygous	Fluorouracil	Enhanced drug effect

a. Examples of genetically polymorphic phase I enzymes that catalyze drug metabolism are listed, including selected examples of drugs that have clinically relevant variations in their effect.
Reproduced with permission from Weinshilboum, 2003.

- Gene therapy, an application of biotechnology, has great potential therapeutic benefit.
- Biotechnology has facilitated the development of novel drug delivery strategies, including liposomal technology, immunotoxins, and PEGylation.
- Pharmacogenomics is the scientific discipline of using genomewide approaches to understand the inherited basis of differences between individual responses to drugs.

- Single nucleotide polymorphisms are differences in a single nucleotide base occurring at a significant frequency (usually > 5%) within the population. They may result in no change in the encoded amino acid of a codon or a change in the encoded amino acid with no change in the function of the encoded protein. However, when the amino acid substitution attributable to a SNP results in a phenotypic difference, it may carry clinical relevance.

Table 7-6. Pharmacogenomics of Phase II Drug Metabolism[a]

Drug-metabolizing enzyme	Frequency of variant poor-metabolism phenotype	Representative drugs metabolized	Effect of polymorphism
N-acetyltransferase 2	52% of white Americans	Isoniazid	Enhanced drug effect
	17% of Japanese	Hydralazine	Enhanced drug effect
Uridine diphosphate-glucuronosyltransferase 1A1 (TATA box polymorphism)	10.9% of whites	Procainamide	Enhanced drug effect
	4% of Chinese	Irinotecan	Enhanced drug effect
	1% of Japanese	Bilirubin	Gilbert's syndrome
Thiopurine S-methyltransferase	Approximately 1 in 300 whites	Mercaptopurine	Enhanced drug effect (toxicity)
	Approximately 1 in 2,500 Asians	Azathioprine	Enhanced drug effect (toxicity)
Catechol O-methyltransferase	Approximately 25% of whites	Levodopa	Enhanced drug effect

a. Examples of genetically polymorphic phase II (conjugating) enzymes that catalyze drug metabolism are listed, including selected examples of drugs that have clinically relevant variations in their effects.
Reproduced with permission from Weinshilboum, 2003.

7-3. Questions

1. The process whereby the ribosome in the cytoplasm reads mRNA codons and matches them with the appropriate tRNAs (which, in turn, carry amino acids responsible for protein synthesis) is referred to as

    A. transcription.
    B. translation.
    C. transformation.
    D. transfection.
    E. transduction.

2. How many nucleotide triplets (or codons) exist for the encoding of the 20 possible amino acids specified by the genetic code?

    A. 4
    B. 12
    C. 20
    D. 61
    E. 64

3. Which of the following refers to a plasmid designed to allow for the expression of an inserted gene within a host cell for the production of the specified protein?

    A. Cloning vector
    B. Expression vector
    C. Transcription factor
    D. Translation initiation factor
    E. Transposable genetic element

4. Which of the following is an example of a recombinant DNA–generated cytokine used for the management of acute relapsing–remitting multiple sclerosis?

    A. Interferon beta-1b (Betaseron)
    B. Aldesleukin (IL-2) (Proleukin)
    C. Eptifibatide (Integrelin)
    D. Bivalirudin (Angiomax)
    E. Abciximab (ReoPro)

5. Alteplase (Activase) is a recombinant DNA protein of which of the following types?

    A. Hormone
    B. Enzyme
    C. Clotting factor
    D. Chemokine
    E. Cytokine

6. Which of the following biological agents is indicated for treatment of ovulatory failure?

    A. Ganirelix (Antagon)
    B. Glucagon (GlucaGen)
    C. Follitropin alfa (Gonal-F)
    D. Eptifibatide (Integrelin)
    E. Thyrotropin (Thyrogen)

7. Which of the following recombinant blood factors is available in recombinant form for clinical therapeutic use?

    A. Factor III
    B. Factor V
    C. Factor VI
    D. Factor VII
    E. Factor X

8. Recombinant DNA technology has led to the development of vaccines for which of the following diseases?

    A. Hepatitis B
    B. Hepatitis A
    C. *Haemophilus influenzae* type B infection
    D. Malaria
    E. AIDS

9. As dictated by the nomenclature for monoclonal antibodies, which of the following is a chimeric monoclonal antibody therapeutically used for inflammatory disease?

    A. Abciximab
    B. Infliximab
    C. Palivizumab
    D. Rituximab
    E. Trastuzumab

10. Which of the following is best described as the repair or correction of a dysfunctional gene by selectively introducing recombinant DNA into cells or tissues (ultimately leading to the expression of a functional gene product)?

    A. Monoclonal antibody therapy
    B. Gene therapy
    C. Antiviral therapy
    D. Cell therapy
    E. Recombinant DNA therapy

11. Fomivirsen (Vitravene) is an example of which of the following biological products?

    A. A liposomal formulation
    B. An antisense oligonucleotide
    C. An siRNA molecule
    D. A recombinant DNA–produced protein
    E. A monoclonal antibody

12. The use of liposomal technology has favorably affected the therapeutic index of which of the following drugs?

    A. Cyclosporine
    B. Itraconazole
    C. Amphotericin B
    D. Cisplatin
    E. Propofol

13. Which of the following is best described as the scientific discipline of using genomewide approaches to understand the inherited basis of differences between individuals in their response to drugs?

    A. Pharmacogenomics
    B. Functional genomics
    C. Comparative genomics
    D. Pharmacodynamics
    E. Molecular genetics

14. A single nucleotide polymorphism (SNP) always results in a change in which of the following?

    A. The nucleotide sequence in the genome
    B. The nucleotide sequence of a codon
    C. The encoded amino acid of the codon
    D. The encoded amino acid of the codon, with no change in function of the encoded protein
    E. The encoded amino acid of the codon, with a clinically relevant change in the function of the encoded protein

15. Which of the following is best described as "the manipulation (as through genetic engineering) of living organisms or their components to produce useful usually commercial products (as pest resistant crops, new bacterial strains, or novel pharmaceuticals)"?

    A. Biology
    B. Biotechnology

    C. Biotherapy
    D. Bioinformatics
    E. Nanotechnology

16. Which of the following is a drug discovery strategy that uses nucleic acids and amino acids in various combinations to synthesize vast libraries of oligonucleotide or peptide compounds for high-throughput lead compound screening?

    A. Whole cell screening
    B. Natural product screening
    C. Gene therapy
    D. Combinatorial chemistry
    E. rDNA technology

17. Which of the following is best defined as the application of computer sciences and information technology to the management and analysis of biological information?

    A. Biometrics
    B. Biotherapy
    C. Bioinformatics
    D. Biostatistics
    E. Biotechnology

18. Which of the following best outlines the central dogma of molecular biology?

    A. RNA→DNA→Protein
    B. DNA→RNA→Protein
    C. Protein→RNA→DNA
    D. DNA→Protein→RNA
    E. Protein→DNA→RNA

19. Which of the following biotechnology agents is indicated for treating anemia caused by chronic renal disease?

    A. Epoetin alfa
    B. Becaplermin
    C. Filgrastim
    D. Alemtuzumab
    E. Sargramostim

20. Which of the following products is indicated for prevention of blood clots post-PTCA?

    A. Abciximab
    B. Basiliximab
    C. Infliximab
    D. Trastuzumab
    E. Becaplermin

7-4. Answers

1. **B.** *Transcription* is the process by which RNA polymerase copies a strand of DNA into complementary RNA. *Transformation* refers to the alteration of the heritable properties of a eukaryotic cell. *Transfection* is the introduction of foreign DNA into a eukaryotic cell. *Transduction* can refer to the transfer of DNA from one bacterium to another through a bacteriophage.

2. **D.** There is degeneracy in the genetic code. Some amino acids may be encoded by as many as six codons, whereas others may be encoded by only one. Of the 64 possible codons, three are stop codons (UAA, UGA, and UAG).

3. **B.** A *cloning vector* is used to carry a fragment of DNA into a cell for cloning. A *transcription factor* is a protein that regulates transcription in eukaryotic cells. A *translation initiation factor,* as its name implies, is involved in the initiation of translation. A *transposable genetic element,* or *transposon,* is a portion of DNA that can move from one part of the genome to another.

4. **A.** Aldesleukin (IL-2) (Proleukin) is a recombinant cytokine indicated for the treatment of metastatic renal cell carcinoma and melanoma. Eptifibatide (Integrelin) is a recombinant enzyme indicated for treatment of acute coronary syndromes. Bivalirudin (Angiomax) is an enzyme indicated for use in coronary angioplasty and unstable angina. Abciximab (ReoPro) is a monoclonal antibody indicated for prevention of blood clots post-PTCA and unstable angina prior to PTCA.

5. **B.** Alteplase (Activase) is a recombinant DNA protein of the enzyme type.

6. **C.** Ganirelix (Antagon) is a recombinant hormone indicated for the treatment of luteinizing hormone surge during fertility therapy. Glucagon (GlucaGen) is a recombinant hormone indicated for treatment of hypoglycemia. Eptifibatide (Integrelin) is a recombinant enzyme indicated for the treatment of acute coronary syndromes. Thyrotropin (Thyrogen) is a recombinant hormone indicated for the treatment of thyroid cancer.

7. **D.** The other factors listed are not clinically available in recombinant form.

8. **A.** Although promising, this technology has not yet yielded vaccines for hepatitis A, malaria, AIDS, or infections caused by *Haemophilus influenzae* type B.

9. **B.** Nomenclature of monoclonal antibodies is highly structured. The first component of the name is product specific; the second component indicates its therapeutic use (*ci* for cardiovascular use, *li* for use in inflammation, *tu* for use in cancer); the third component indicates the type of monoclonal antibody (*mo* for murine, *xi* for chimeric, *zu* for humanized); and the fourth component (*mab*) represents monoclonal antibody.

10. **B.** The repair or correction of a dysfunctional gene by selectively introducing recombinant DNA into cells or tissues, ultimately leading to the expression of a functional gene product, is called *gene therapy.*

11. **B.** Fomivirsen (Vitravene) is the first product based on this technology to come to market.

12. **C.** Formulation of this antifungal agent as a liposomal preparation (Ambisome) has significantly reduced the nephrotoxicity and other adverse effects associated with this drug.

13. **A.** The scientific discipline of using genomewide approaches to understand the inherited basis of differences between individuals in their response to drugs best describes pharmacogenomics.

14. **A.** An SNP may occur outside of an open reading frame (coding region), it may induce a mutation where no change in encoded amino acid occurs, and it may or may not cause a functional change in an encoded protein.

15. **B.** This definition by the Merriam-Webster's Dictionary best describes *biotechnology.*

16. **D.** A drug discovery strategy that uses nucleic acids and amino acids in various combinations to synthesize vast libraries of oligonucleotide or peptide compounds for high-throughput lead compound screening is called *combinatorial chemistry.*

17. **C.** The application of computer sciences and information technology to the management and analysis of biological information best defines *bioinformatics.*

18. **B.** DNA is transcribed into mRNA, which is translated ultimately to protein.

19. **A.** Becaplermin is indicated for the management of diabetic foot ulcers. Filgrastim is indicated for treatment of neutropenia. Alemtuzumab is indicated for treatment of chronic lymphocytic leukemia. Sargramostim is indicated for myeloid reconstitution after bone marrow transplant;

after bone marrow transplant failure, as an adjunct to chemotherapy in acute myelogenous leukemia; and in peripheral blood progenitor cell transplant.

20. **A.** Basiliximab is indicated for management of acute organ transplant rejection. Infliximab is indicated for the treatment of Crohn's disease and rheumatoid arthritis. Trastuzumab is indicated for the management of metastatic breast cancer. Becaplermin is indicated for the treatment of diabetic foot ulcers.

7-5. References

Adams VR, Karlix JL. Monoclonal antibodies. In: Koeller J, Tami J, eds. *Concepts in Immunology and Immunotherapeutics.* 3rd ed. Bethesda, Md.: American Society of Health-System Pharmacists' Production Office; 1997:269–99.

Alberts B, Bray D, Lewis J, et al., eds. *Molecular Biology of the Cell.* 3rd ed. New York: Garland; 1994.

Carrico JM. Human Genome Project and pharmacogenomics—implications for pharmacy. *J Am Pharm Assoc.* 2000;40:115–16.

Evans WE, McLeod HL. Pharmacogenomics: Drug disposition, drug targets, and side effects. *N Engl J Med.* 2003;348:538–49.

Glick BR, Pasternak JJ, eds. *Molecular Biotechnology: Principles and Applications of Recombinant DNA.* 2nd ed. Washington, D.C.: ASM Press; 1998.

Hollinger P, Hoogenboom H. Antibodies come back from the brink. *Nature Biotech.* 1998;16:1015–16.

Regan JW. Biotechnology and drug discovery. In: Delgado JN, Remers WA, eds. *Textbook of Organic Medicinal and Pharmaceutical Chemistry.* 10th ed. Philadelphia: Lippincott-Raven; 1998:139–52.

Rogers CS, Sullenger BA, George AL Jr. Gene therapy. In: Hardman JG, Limbird LE, eds. *Goodman and Gilman's The Pharmacological Basis of Therapeutics.* 10th ed. New York: McGraw-Hill; 2001: 81–112.

Sindelar RD. Pharmaceutical biotechnology. In: Williams DA, Lemke TL, eds. *Foye's Principles of Medicinal Chemistry.* 5th ed. Philadelphia: Lippincott Williams & Wilkins; 2002:982–1015.

U.S. Food and Drug Administration (FDA). Center for Biologics Evaluation and Research Web page: www.fda.gov/cber.

U.S. Food and Drug Administration (FDA). Center for Drug Evaluation and Research Web page: www.fda.gov/cder/.

Vaughan TJ, Osbourn JK, Tempest PR. Human antibodies by design. *Nature Biotech.* 1998;16:535–39.

Weinshilboum R. Inheritance and drug response. *N Engl J Med.* 2003;348:529–37.

Hypertension

8

Benjamin Gross, PharmD, BCPS
L. Brian Cross, PharmD, CDE

8-1. Disease Overview

- Hypertension is defined as a systolic blood pressure >140 mm Hg, a diastolic blood pressure > 90 mm Hg, or a condition in any patient requiring antihypertensive therapy.
- In the United States, 65 million people are affected by hypertension. In approximately 64% of those affected, it is controlled (Table 8-1).
- Incidence increases with age.
- Its onset most commonly occurs in the third to fifth decades of life, and the lifetime risk of hypertension is 90% for those surviving to age 80.
- Prevalence differs by ethnic group (Table 8-2), socioeconomic group, and geographic region.

Classification

Classification of hypertension is based on the Seventh Report of the Joint National Committee on Detection, Evaluation, and Treatment of High Blood Pressure (JNC-VII). Table 8-3 shows the JNC-VII classification.

Clinical Presentation and Complications

Cardiovascular effects

- Left ventricular hypertrophy
- Congestive heart failure (CHF)
- Peripheral arterial disease
- Angina pectoris
- Myocardial infarction
- Sudden death

Renal effects

- Nephropathy
- Renal failure
- Requirements for dialysis

Cerebrovascular effects

- Transient ischemic attacks
- Stroke

Ophthalmologic effects

- Retinal hemorrhage
- Retinopathy
- Blindness

Pathophysiology and Etiology

- Blood pressure = (stroke volume × heart rate) × peripheral resistance (Figure 8-1)

Sympathetic nervous system activation

Central activation

- Presynaptic α_2 stimulation is a negative feedback mechanism, leading to decreased norepinephrine release.
- Presynaptic β stimulation leads to increased norepinephrine release.

Table 8-1. Trends in Awareness, Treatment, and Control of High Blood Pressure in Adults Ages 18–74

	National Health and Nutrition Examination Survey				
Aspect	II, 1976–80 (%)	III, phase 1, 1988–91 (%)	III, phase 2 1991–94 (%)	1999–2000 (%)	2005–06 (%)
Awareness	51	73	68	70	78
Treatment	31	55	54	59	68
Control[a]	10	29	27	34	64

Unpublished data for 1999–2000 computed by M. Woltz, National Heart, Lung, and Blood Institute; adapted from JNC-7 Express, National Heart, Lung, and Blood Institute. Information for 2005–06 comes from the most recent Nhanes data available.
High blood pressure is systolic blood pressure ≥ 140 mm Hg or diastolic blood pressure ≥ 90 mm Hg, or it is evidenced by the taking of antihypertensive medication.
a. Those adults surveyed have systolic blood pressure < 140 mm Hg and diastolic blood pressure < 90 mm Hg.

Peripheral activation
- β_1 Stimulation leads to increased heart rate and contractility, causing increased cardiac output.
- β_2 Stimulation leads to arterial vasodilation.
- β Stimulation also causes increased renin release, causing increased angiotensin II production.
- α_1 Stimulation leads to arterial and venous vaso-constriction.

Renin–angiotensin–aldosterone system

- Decreased renal perfusion pressure causes increases in renin levels.
- Renin reacts with angiotensinogen to produce angiotensin I (AT-I).
- Angiotensin-converting enzyme (ACE) causes AT-I to become angiotensin II (AT-II).
- AT-II is a potent vasoconstrictor and stimulates aldosterone release, which increases sodium and fluid retention.

Table 8-2. Prevalence of Hypertension by Ethnic Group for Adults Ages 20–74 (percent)

Ethnic group	Male	Female
Caucasians	24	19
African Americans	35	34
Mexican Americans	25	22
Asian Americans	13	13

Water and sodium retention

- Acute: Increased fluid volume causes increased cardiac output, which causes increased blood pressure (BP).
- Chronic: Excess intracellular sodium causes vascular hypertrophy, which increases vascular resistance and response to vasoconstriction and, in turn, increases BP.

Etiology

Primary (essential) hypertension
- Unknown cause
- Found in 85–95% of all hypertension cases

Secondary hypertension
- **Renovascular disease:** This condition is suggested by increased blood urea nitrogen (BUN) and creatinine and by abdominal bruits.
- **Primary aldosteronism:** This condition is suggested by unprovoked hypokalemia.
- **Cushing's syndrome:** This condition is suggested by unprovoked hypokalemia and truncal obesity with purple striae.
- **Pheochromocytoma:** This condition is suggested by increased urinary catecholamine excretion (i.e., vanillylmandelic acid and metanephrine) accompanied by headache, palpitations, and perspiration
- **Aortic coarctation:** This condition is suggested by delayed or absent femoral pulses and decreased BP in the lower extremities.

Table 8-3. Classification and Management of Blood Pressure for Adults

Blood pressure classification	SBP[a] (mm Hg)	DBP (mm Hg)	Lifestyle modification	Initial drug therapy Without compelling indication	Initial drug therapy With compelling indications[b]
Normal	< 120	and < 80	Encouraged		
Prehypertension	120–139	or 80–89	Yes	No antihypertensive drug indicated	Drug(s) for compelling indications.[c]
Stage 1 hypertension	140–159	or 90–99	Yes	Thiazide-type diuretics for most; may consider ACEI, ARB, BB, CCB, or combination	Drug(s) for compelling indications;[c] other antihypertensive drugs (diuretics, ACEI, ARB, BB, or CCB) as needed
Stage 2 hypertension	≥ 160	or ≥ 100	Yes	Two-drug combination for most[d] (usually thiazide-type diuretic and ACEI or ARB or BB or CCB)	

Adapted from JNC-7 Express, National Heart, Lung, and Blood Institute.
ACEI, angiotensin-converting enzyme inhibitor; ARB, angiotensin receptor blocker; BB, β-blocker; CCB, calcium channel blocker; DBP, diastolic blood pressure; SBP, systolic blood pressure
a. Treatment is determined by highest blood pressure category.
b. See Table 8-12.
c. Initial combined therapy should be used cautiously in those at risk for orthostatic hypotension.
d. Treat patients with chronic kidney disease or diabetes to blood pressure goal of < 130/80 mm Hg.

Figure 8-1. Sympathetic Nervous System Activation

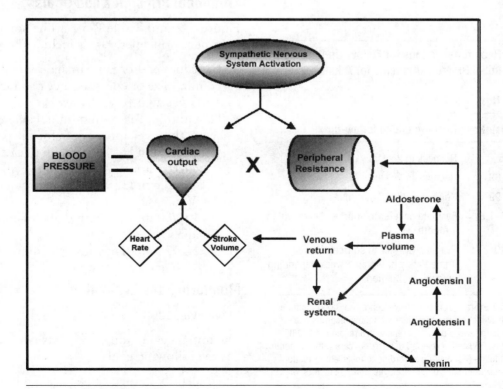

Source: Carter, BL, Saseen, JL, 2002.

■ *Drug-induced hypertension:* The following drugs may induce hypertension:
  - Steroids and estrogens (including oral contraceptives)
  - Alcohol
  - Cocaine
  - Cyclosporine and tacrolimus
  - Sympathomimetics
  - Erythropoietin
  - Licorice (in chewing tobacco)
  - Monoamine oxidase (MAO) inhibitors
  - Tricyclic antidepressants
  - Nonsteroidal anti-inflammatory drugs (NSAIDs)

Diagnostic Criteria

Diagnosis and treatment begin with proper BP measurement, assessment, and follow-up planning (Table 8-4). The patient should avoid ingesting caffeine and smoking for 30 minutes prior to BP measurement and should be resting for 5 minutes prior to BP measurement. BP is measured as follows:

■ Position arm (brachial artery) at heart level.
■ Uncover arm; do not put cuff over clothes.
■ Determine proper size cuff.

Table 8-4. Recommendations for Follow-Up Based on Initial BP Measurements for Adults

Initial BP (mm Hg)[a]

Systolic	Diastolic	Recommended follow-up[b]
< 130	< 85	Recheck in 2 years.
130–139	85–89	Recheck in 1 year.[c]
140–159	90–99	Confirm within 2 months.[c]
160–179	100–109	Evaluate or refer to source of care within 1 month.
~180	~110	Evaluate or refer to source of care immediately or within 1 week depending on clinical situation.

Adapted from JNC-7 Express, National Heart, Lung, and Blood Institute.
a. If systolic and diastolic readings are different, follow recommendations for shorter time to follow-up (e.g., a person with a reading of 160/86 mm Hg should be evaluated or referred to source of care within 1 month).
b. Modify the scheduling of follow-up according to reliable information about past BP measurements, other cardiovascular risk factors, or target organ disease.
c. Provide advice about lifestyle modifications.

Upper arm circumference	Cuff size required
16.0–22.5 cm	Pediatric cuff
22.6–30.0 cm	Regular adult cuff
30.1–37.5 cm	Large adult cuff
37.6–43.7 cm	Thigh cuff

■ Position cuff 1 inch above antecubital crease.
■ Ask patient about previous readings.
■ Place stethoscope over brachial artery (medial to the center).
■ Inflate cuff rapidly to approximately 30 mm Hg above previous readings.
■ Deflate cuff slowly.
■ Remember to deflate cuff completely when done.
■ Wait 1–2 minutes before repeating.
■ Take pressure in both arms.
■ If orthostatic hypotension is suspected, take BP while patient is sitting, standing, and supine.
■ If two readings are taken at least 2 minutes apart, average the readings.
■ If readings differ by > 5 mm Hg, take additional readings.

Treatment Principles and Goals

Figure 8-2 and Table 8-5 outline some important treatment principles. Goals include the following:

■ To reduce end-organ damage
■ To minimize or control other risk factors for cardiovascular (CV) disease
■ To maintain BP, with minimal side effects, at or below the level appropriate for the patient's risk:
  - 140/90 mm Hg with uncomplicated hypertension
  - 140/90 mm Hg with target organ damage or CV disease
  - <130/80 mm Hg with diabetes and chronic kidney disease
  - <125/75 mm Hg with proteinuria > 1 g/24 h

Monitoring and Evaluation

Initial evaluation

The initial evaluation of patients with hypertension has the following goals:

■ To identify known causes of high blood pressure (Table 8-6)

Figure 8-2. Algorithm for the Treatment of Hypertension

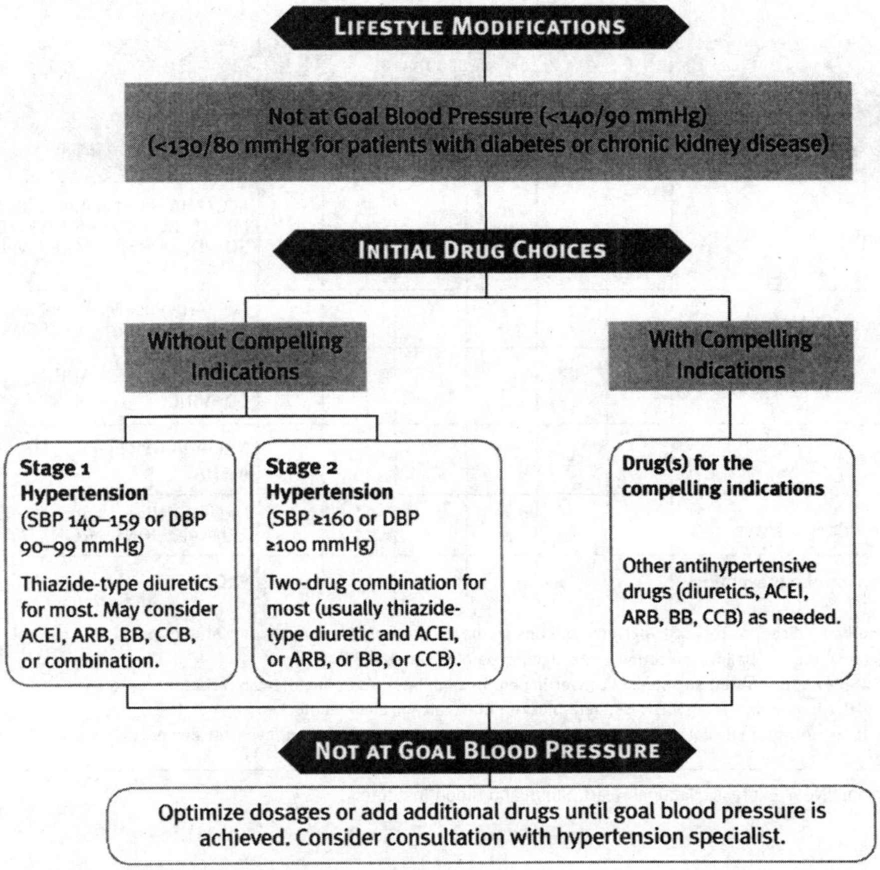

LIFESTYLE MODIFICATIONS

Not at Goal Blood Pressure (<140/90 mmHg)
(<130/80 mmHg for patients with diabetes or chronic kidney disease)

INITIAL DRUG CHOICES

Without Compelling Indications

With Compelling Indications

Stage 1 Hypertension
(SBP 140–159 or DBP 90–99 mmHg)

Thiazide-type diuretics for most. May consider ACEI, ARB, BB, CCB, or combination.

Stage 2 Hypertension
(SBP ≥160 or DBP ≥100 mmHg)

Two-drug combination for most (usually thiazide-type diuretic and ACEI, or ARB, or BB, or CCB).

Drug(s) for the compelling indications

Other antihypertensive drugs (diuretics, ACEI, ARB, BB, CCB) as needed.

NOT AT GOAL BLOOD PRESSURE

Optimize dosages or add additional drugs until goal blood pressure is achieved. Consider consultation with hypertension specialist.

DBP, diastolic blood pressure; SBP, systolic blood pressure.
Drug abbreviations: ACEI, angiotensin converting enzyme inhibitor; ARB, angiotensin receptor blocker; BB, beta-blocker; CCB, calcium channel blocker.

Adapted from JNC-7 Express, National Heart, Lung, and Blood Institute.

Table 8-5. Identifiable Causes, Diagnostic Tests, and Clinical Findings for Secondary Hypertension

Cause or diagnosis	Diagnostic test (clinical finding)
Chronic kidney disease	Estimated GFR (abdominal or flank mass for polycystic kidney disease)
Coarctation of the aorta	CT angiography (delayed or absent femoral pulse)
Cushing's syndrome and other glucocorticoid excess states, including chronic steroid therapy	History; dexamethasone suppression test (truncal obesity, moon facies, buffalo hump, abdominal striae, and hirsutism)
Drug-induced or drug-related condition	History; drug screening
Pheochromocytoma	24-hour urinary metanephrine and normetanephrine (headache, palpitations, and sweating)
Primary aldosteronism and other mineralocorticoid excess states	24-hour urinary aldosterone level or specific measurements of other mineralocorticoids (hypokalemia)
Renovascular hypertension	Doppler flow study; magnetic resonance angiography (abdominal bruit)
Sleep apnea	Sleep study with oxygen saturation (obesity, snoring, and tired during wake time)
Thyroid or parathyroid disease	Thyroid-stimulating hormone; serum parathyroid hormone (goiter; hypercalcemia)

CT, computed tomography; GFR, glomerular filtration rate.

Table 8-6. Clinical Trial and Guideline Basis for Compelling Indications for Individual Drug Classes

COMPELLING INDICATION*	RECOMMENDED DRUGS†						CLINICAL TRIAL BASIS‡
	DIURETIC	BB	ACEI	ARB	CCB	ALDO ANT	
Heart failure	•	•	•	•		•	ACC/AHA Heart Failure Guideline, MERIT-HF, COPERNICUS, CIBIS, SOLVD, AIRE, TRACE, ValHEFT, RALES
Postmyocardial infarction		•	•			•	ACC/AHA Post-MI Guideline, BHAT, SAVE, Capricorn, EPHESUS
High coronary disease risk	•	•	•		•		ALLHAT, HOPE, ANBP2, LIFE, CONVINCE
Diabetes	•	•	•	•	•		NKF-ADA Guideline, UKPDS, ALLHAT
Chronic kidney disease			•	•			NKF Guideline, Captopril Trial, RENAAL, IDNT, REIN, AASK
Recurrent stroke prevention	•		•				PROGRESS

* Compelling indications for antihypertensive drugs are based on benefits from outcome studies or existing clinical guidelines; the compelling indication is managed in parallel with the BP.
† Drug abbreviations: ACEI, angiotensin converting enzyme inhibitor; ARB, angiotensin receptor blocker; Aldo ANT, aldosterone antagonist; BB, beta-blocker; CCB, calcium channel blocker.
‡ Conditions for which clinical trials demonstrate benefit of specific classes of antihypertensive drugs.

Adapted from JNC-7 Express, National Heart, Lung, and Blood Institute.

- To assess presence or absence of target organ damage and CV disease, extent of the disease, and the response to therapies (Box 8-1)
- To identify other CV risk factors or concomitant disorders that may affect prognosis and guide therapy (Box 8-1)

The patient's history should be looked at in the initial evaluation:

- Duration and levels of elevated blood pressure
- History or symptoms of coronary heart disease (CHD), heart failure, cerebrovascular disease, pulmonary vascular disease, diabetes mellitus, renal disease, or dyslipidemia
- Family history of hypertension, premature CHD, stroke, diabetes, dyslipidemia, or renal disease
- Symptoms suggesting the cause of hypertension
- Recent weight changes, physical activity levels, or smoking or other tobacco use
- Dietary assessment of intake of sodium, alcohol, saturated fat, and caffeine

- Complete medication history, including prescription, over-the-counter, and herbal or natural products that may increase BP or decrease effectiveness of antihypertensive agents
- Results and adverse effects of previous antihypertensive therapy
- Psychosocial and environmental factors that may influence hypertension control

An examination should also be done:

- Two or more blood pressure measurements separated by at least 2 minutes
- Measurement of height, weight, and waist circumference
- Funduscopic exam for hypertensive retinopathy
- Exam of neck for carotid bruits, distended veins, or an enlarged thyroid gland
- Exam of heart for abnormalities in rate and rhythm, increased size, precordial heave, clicks, murmurs, and third and fourth heart sounds
- Exam of lungs for rales and evidence of bronchospasm

Box 8-1. Cardiovascular Risk Factors

Major Risk Factors

- Hypertension[a]
- Cigarette smoking
- Obesity[a] (body mass index $\geq$ 30 kg/m²)
- Physical inactivity
- Dyslipidemia[a]
- Diabetes mellitus[a]
- Microalbuminuria or estimated GFR < 60 mL/min
- Age (> 55 for men, > 65 for women)
- Family history of premature cardiovascular disease (men under age 55, women under age 45)

Target Organ Damage

Heart
- Left ventricular hypertrophy
- Angina or prior myocardial infarction
- Prior coronary revascularization
- Heart failure

Brain
- Stroke or transient ischemic attack

Kidney
- Chronic kidney disease
- End stage renal disease

Vascular System
- Peripheral arterial disease

Eyes
- Retinopathy

Adapted from JNC-7 Express, National Heart, Lung, and Blood Institute.
GFR, glomerular filtration rate.
a. Components of the metabolic syndrome.

- Exam of abdomen for bruits, enlarged kidneys, masses, and abnormal aortic pulsation
- Exam of extremities for decreased or absent peripheral arterial pulsations, bruits, and edema
- Neurologic assessment

Routine laboratory are necessary:

- Urinalysis
- Complete blood cell count
- Blood chemistries (sodium, potassium, creatinine, BUN, and glucose)
- Fasting lipid profile: total cholesterol, triglycerides, HDL (high-density lipoprotein), and LDL (low-density lipoprotein)
- Electrocardiogram (ECG)

The following laboratory tests are optional:

- Creatinine clearance
- Microalbuminuria
- 24-hour urinary protein
- Blood calcium
- Uric acid
- Glycosylated hemoglobin
- Thyroid-stimulating hormone
- Limited echocardiography
- Ankle-brachial index
- Plasma renin activity and urinary sodium determination

Follow-up evaluation

Follow-up evaluation includes any of the previous exams completed during the initial evaluation that are required to monitor both response to and possible adverse effects from prescribed antihypertensive therapies, in addition to the assessment of any new symptoms of target organ damage and the assessment of patient adherence to therapy (Box 8-2).

Box 8-2. General Guidelines to Improve Patient Adherence to Antihypertensive Therapy

- Be aware of signs of patient nonadherence to antihypertensive therapy.
- Establish the goal of therapy: to reduce blood pressure to nonhypertensive levels with minimal or no adverse effects.
- Educate patients about the disease, and involve them and their families in its treatment. Have them measure blood pressure at home.
- Maintain contact with patients; consider telecommunication.
- Keep care inexpensive and simple.
- Encourage lifestyle modifications.
- Integrate pill taking into routine activities of daily living.
- Prescribe medications according to pharmacologic principles, favoring long-acting formulations.
- Be willing to stop unsuccessful therapy and try a different approach.
- Anticipate adverse effects. Adjust therapy to prevent, minimize, or ameliorate side effects.
- Continue to add effective and tolerated drugs, stepwise, in sufficient doses to achieve the goal of therapy.
- Encourage a positive attitude about achieving therapeutic goals.
- Consider using nurse case management.

Adapted from JNC-7 Express, National Heart, Lung, and Blood Institute.

8-2. Nondrug Therapy

Lifestyle modifications are recommended to improve both BP and overall cardiovascular health (Table 8-7).

Research has shown that diets rich in fruits, vegetables, and low-fat dairy foods, and with reduced saturated and total fats, significantly lower blood pressure (Tables 8-8 and 8-9).

8-3. Drug Therapy

All patient factors (severity of blood pressure elevation, presence of target organ damage, and presence of CV disease or other risk factors) must be considered when initiating therapy.

Initial Therapy

- For candidates for therapy, see Figure 8-2 and Table 8-5.
- Use of lifestyle modifications (Table 8-7) should continue to be stressed to patients after the decision to initiate drug therapy has been made to further decrease the risk of complications from cardiovascular disease.
- Prehypertension represents a new classification in JNC-VII (Table 8-3) and represents a significant risk for future development of stage 1 hypertension. Lifestyle modifications should be stressed for this classification, and medication therapy should be used only for patients with compelling indications.
- JNC-VII recommends the use of thiazide diuretics as initial therapy in most patients alone or in

Table 8-7. Lifestyle Modifications to Manage Hypertension

MODIFICATION	RECOMMENDATION	APPROXIMATE SBP REDUCTION (RANGE)
Weight reduction	Maintain normal body weight (body mass index 18.5–24.9 kg/m^2).	5–20 mmHg/10 kg weight loss
Adopt DASH eating plan	Consume a diet rich in fruits, vegetables, and lowfat dairy products with a reduced content of saturated and total fat.	8–14 mmHg
Dietary sodium reduction	Reduce dietary sodium intake to no more than 100 mmol per day (2.4 g sodium or 6 g sodium chloride).	2–8 mmHg
Physical activity	Engage in regular aerobic physical activity such as brisk walking (at least 30 min per day, most days of the week).	4–9 mmHg
Moderation of alcohol consumption	Limit consumption to no more than 2 drinks (1 oz or 30 mL ethanol; e.g., 24 oz beer, 10 oz wine, or 3 oz 80-proof whiskey) per day in most men and to no more than 1 drink per day in women and lighter weight persons.	2–4 mmHg[30]

Adapted from JNC-7 Express, National Heart, Lung, and Blood Institute.
DASH, Dietary Approaches to Stop Hypertension. For overall cardiovascular risk reduction, stop smoking. The effects of implementing these modifications are dose and time dependent, and could be greater for some individuals.

Table 8-8. Dietary Suggestions for Hypertensive Patients

Food group	Daily servings	Serving sizes	Examples and notes	Significance of each food group to the DASH diet pattern
Grains and grain products	7–8	1 slice bread; ½ c dry cereal; ½ c cooked rice, pasta, or cereal	Whole wheat bread, english muffins, pita bread, bagel, cereals, grits, and oatmeal	Major sources of energy and fiber
Vegetables	4–5	1 c raw leafy vegetable; ½ c cooked vegetable; 6 oz vegetable juice	Tomatoes, potatoes, carrots, peas, squash, broccoli, turnip greens, collards, kale, spinach, artichokes, beans, and sweet potatoes	Rich sources of potassium, magnesium, and fiber
Fruits	4–5	6 oz fruit juice; 1 medium fruit; ¼ c dried fruit; ¼ c fresh, frozen or canned fruit	Apricots, bananas, dates, grapes, oranges, orange juice, grapefruit, grapefruit juice, mangoes, melons, peaches, pineapple, prunes, raisins, strawberries, and tangerines	Important sources of potassium, magnesium, and fiber
Low-fat or nonfat dairy foods	2–3	8 oz milk; 1 c yogurt; 1.5 oz cheese	Skim or 1% milk, skim or low-fat buttermilk, nonfat or low-fat yogurt, part-skim mozzarella cheese, and nonfat cheese	Major sources of calcium and protein
Meats, poultry, and fish	2 or fewer	3 oz cooked meats, poultry, or fish	Select only lean cuts; trim away visible fats; broil, roast, or boil, instead of frying; and remove skin from poultry	Rich sources of protein and magnesium
Nuts, seeds, and legumes	4–5 per week	1.5 oz or ⅓ c nuts; ½ oz or 2 T seeds; ½ c cooked legumes	Almonds, filberts, mixed nuts, peanuts, walnuts, sunflower seeds, kidney beans, and lentils	Rich sources of energy, magnesium, potassium, protein, and fiber

Adapted from JNC-7 Express, National Heart, Lung, and Blood Institute.
DASH, Dietary Approaches to Stop Hypertension.

Table 8-9. The DASH Diet Sample Menu Based on 2000 Calories per Day

Food	Amount	Servings provided
Breakfast		
Orange juice	6 oz	1 fruit
1% lowfat milk	8 oz (1 c)	1 dairy
Cornflakes (with 1 tsp sugar)	1 c	2 grains
Banana	1 medium	1 fruit
Whole wheat bread (with 1 T jelly)	1 slice	1 grain
Soft margarine	1 t	1 fat
Lunch		
Chicken salad	¾ c	1 poultry
Pita bread	½ large	1 grain
Raw vegetable medley		
Carrot and celery sticks	3–4 sticks each	1 vegetable
Radishes	2	1 vegetable
Loose-leaf lettuce	2 leaves	1 vegetable

(continued)

Table 8-9. The DASH Diet Sample Menu Based on 2000 Calories per Day *(Continued)*

Food	Amount	Servings provided
Lunch		
Part-skim mozzarella cheese	1.5 slices (1.5 oz)	1 dairy
1% lowfat milk	8 oz (1 c)	1 dairy
Fruit cocktail in light syrup	½ c	1 fruit
Dinner		
Herbed baked cod	3 oz	1 fish
Scallion rice	1 c	2 grains
Steamed broccoli	½ c	1 vegetable
Stewed tomatoes	½ c	1 vegetable
Spinach salad:		
Raw spinach	½ c	1 vegetable
Cherry tomatoes	2	1 vegetable
Cucumber	2 slices	1 vegetable
Light Italian salad dressing	1 T	½ fat
Whole wheat dinner roll	1 small	1 grain
Soft margarine	1 t	1 fat
Melon balls	½ c	1 fruit
Snacks		
Dried apricots	1 oz (¼ c)	1 fruit
Minipretzels	1 oz (¾ c)	1 grain
Mixed nuts	1.5 oz (⅓ c)	1 nuts
Diet ginger ale	12 oz	0

Total number of servings in 2000-calorie per day menu

Food group	Servings
Grains	8
Vegetables	4
Fruits	5
Dairy foods	3
Meats, poultry, and fish	2
Nuts, seeds, and legumes	1
Fats and oils	2.5

Tips on eating the DASH way

• Start small. Make gradual changes in your eating habits.

• Center your meal around carbohydrates, such as pasta, rice, beans, or vegetables.

• Treat meat as one part of the whole meal, instead of the focus.

• Use fruits or low-fat, low-calorie foods such as sugar-free gelatin for desserts and snacks.

Remember: If you use the DASH diet to help prevent or control high blood pressure, make it part of a lifestyle that includes choosing foods lower in salt and sodium; keeping a healthy weight; being physically active; and if you drink alcohol, doing so in moderation.

Adapted from JNC-7 Express, National Heart, Lung, and Blood Institute.
DASH, Dietary Approaches to Stop Hypertension.

combination with other agents (angiotensin-converting enzyme inhibitors, angiotensin II receptor blockers, β-blockers, and calcium channel blockers) unless compelling indications for the use of other medication classes exist or if the patient has comorbid conditions that would suggest the use of classes other than thiazide diuretics (Figure 8-2, and Tables 8-5 and 8-10).

- Current data also suggest that angiotensin-converting enzyme inhibitors (ACEIs), calcium channel blockers (CCBs), and angiotensin II receptor blockers (ARBs) can also be considered as initial agents for the treatment of hypertension. European hypertension guidelines do not recommend one particular class of antihypertensive over another for first-line therapy but instead emphasize the importance of selecting a therapy for each individual on the basis of the comorbidities he or she may have.
- For patients who are 20/10 mm Hg greater than their goal blood pressure, two-drug combination therapy (one drug is a diuretic) should be strongly considered.
- If a patient requires a second agent for treatment of hypertension, it is strongly recommended that it be a diuretic if one is not chosen as the initial agent.
- All causes for inadequate response should be addressed before additional agents are added to a patient's antihypertensive regimen (Box 8-3).
- Vasodilators, α_1-receptor antagonists, α_2-receptor agonists, and postganglionic adrenergic neuron blockers should be avoided as initial agents for hypertension.

Diuretics

Thiazide and thiazide-like diuretics

See Table 8-11 for a list of thiazide and thiazide-like diuretics, their usual dose range, and adverse effects associated with these medications.

Mechanism of action
- Direct arteriole dilation
- Reduction of total fluid volume through the inhibition of sodium reabsorption in the distal tubules, which causes increased excretion of sodium, water, potassium, and hydrogen
- Increase in the effectiveness of other antihypertensive agents by preventing reexpansion of plasma volume

- Significant decrease in efficacy in renal failure: serum creatinine > 2 mg/dL or glomerular filtration rate (GFR) < 30 mL/min
- Diuretics are also available in combination with other drugs (Table 8-12).

Patient instructions and counseling
- Medication may be taken with food or milk.
- Take early in the day to avoid nocturia.
- Medication may increase sensitivity to sunlight. Consider using sunscreen with SPF (sun protection factor) > 15.
- Medication may increase blood glucose in diabetics.
- Report problems with muscle cramps, which may indicate decreased potassium level.

Drug–drug and drug–disease interactions
- Steroids cause salt retention and antagonize thiazide action.
- NSAIDs blunt thiazide response.
- Class IA or III antiarrhythmics (that prolong the QT interval) may cause torsades de pointes with diuretic-induced hypokalemia.
- Probenecid and lithium block thiazide effects by interfering with thiazide excretion into the urine.
- Thiazides decrease lithium renal clearance and increase risk of lithium toxicity.

Parameters to monitor
- Blood pressure
- Weight
- Serum electrolytes and uric acid
- BUN and creatinine
- Cholesterol levels

Loop diuretics

See Table 8-11 for a list of loop diuretics, their usual dose range, and adverse effects associated with these medications.

Mechanism of action
- Reduction of total fluid volume occurs through the inhibition of sodium and chloride reabsorption in the ascending loop of Henle, which causes increased excretion of water, sodium, chloride, magnesium, and calcium.
- Loop diuretics are more effective than thiazides in patients with renal failure: serum creatinine > 2 mg/dL or GFR < 30 mL/min.

Patient instructions and counseling
- Medication may be taken with food or milk.
- Take early in the day to avoid nocturia.

Table 8-10. Considerations for Individualizing Antihypertensive Drug Therapy

Indication	Drug therapy
Compelling indications unless contraindicated	
Diabetes mellitus (type 1) with proteinuria	ACEI
Heart failure	ACEI, diuretics
Isolated systolic hypertension (older patients)	Diuretics (preferred), calcium antagonists (long-acting dihydropyridine)
Myocardial infarction	β-blockers (nonintrinsic sympathomimetic activity), ACEI (with systolic dysfunction)
Possible favorable effects on comorbid conditions[b]	
Angina	β-blockers, calcium antagonists
Atrial tachycardia and fibrillation	β-blockers, calcium antagonists (nondihydropyridine)
Cyclosporine-induced hypertension (use caution with the dose of cyclosporine)	Calcium antagonists
Diabetes mellitus (types 1 and 2) with proteinuria	ACEI (preferred), calcium antagonists
Diabetes mellitus (type 2)	Low-dose diuretics
Dyslipidemia	α-blockers
Essential tremor	β-blockers (noncardioselective)
Heart failure	Carvedilol, losartan potassium
Hyperthyroidism	β-blockers
Migraine	β-blockers (noncardioselective), calcium antagonists (nondihydropyridine)
Myocardial infarction	Diltiazem hydrochloride, verapamil hydrochloride
Osteoporosis	Thiazides
Preoperative hypertension	β-blockers
Prostatism (benign prostatic hyperplasia)	α-blockers
Renal insufficiency (use caution in renovascular hypertension and if creatinine ≥ 265.2 micromole/L [3 mg/dL])	ACEI
Possible unfavorable effects on comorbid conditions[a]	
Bronchospastic disease	β-blockers[b]
Depression	β-blockers, central α-agonist, reserpine[b]
Diabetes mellitus (types 1 and 2)	β-blockers, high-dose diuretics
Dyslipidemia	β-blockers (nonintrinsic sympathomimetic activity), diuretics (high-dose)
Gout	Diuretics
Heart block (second- or third-degree)	β-blockers,[b] calcium antagonists (nondihydropyridine)[b]
Heart failure	β-blockers (except carvedilol), calcium antagonists (except amlodipine besylate and felodipine)
Liver disease	Labetalol hydrochloride, methyldopa[b]
Peripheral vascular disease	β-Blockers
Pregnancy	ACEI,[b] angiotensin II receptor blockers[b]
Renal insufficiency	Potassium-sparing agents
Renovascular disease	ACEI, angiotensin II receptor blockers

Adapted from JNC-7 Express, National Heart, Lung, and Blood Institute.
ACEI, angiotensin-converting enzyme inhibitors.
For initial drug therapy recommendations, see Tables 8-11 through 8-19.
a. These drugs may be used with special monitoring unless contraindicated.
b. Contraindicated.

Box 8-3. Causes of Inadequate Responsiveness to Therapy

Pseudoresistance
- "White-coat hypertension" or office elevations
- Pseudohypertension in older patients
- Use of regular adult cuff on a very obese arm

Nonadherence to therapy

Volume overload
- Excess salt intake
- Progressive renal damage (nephrosclerosis)
- Fluid retention from reduction of blood pressure
- Inadequate diuretic therapy

Drug-related causes
- Doses too low
- Wrong type of diuretic
- Inappropriate combinations
- Rapid inactivation (e.g., hydralazine)
- Drug actions and interactions
- Sympathomimetics
- Nasal decongestants
- Appetite suppressants
- Cocaine and other illicit drugs
- Caffeine
- Oral contraceptives
- Adrenal steroids
- Licorice (as may be found in chewing tobacco)
- Cyclosporine or tacrolimus
- Erythropoietin
- Antidepressants
- Nonsteroidal anti-inflammatory drugs

Associated conditions
- Smoking
- Increasing obesity
- Sleep apnea
- Insulin resistance or hyperinsulinemia
- Ethanol intake of more than 1 oz (30 mL) per day
- Anxiety-induced hyperventilation or panic attacks
- Chronic pain
- Intense vasoconstriction (arteritis)
- Organic brain syndrome (e.g., memory deficit)

Identifiable causes of hypertension

Adapted from JNC-7 Express, National Heart, Lung, and Blood Institute.

- Medication may increase sensitivity to sunlight. Consider using sunscreen with SPF > 15.
- Medication may increase blood glucose in diabetics.
- Report problems with muscle cramps, which may indicate decreased potassium level.
- Rise slowly from a lying or sitting position.

Drug–drug and drug–disease interactions
- Aminoglycosides can precipitate ototoxicity when combined with loop diuretics.
- NSAIDs blunt diuretic response.
- Class IA or III antiarrhythmics (that prolong the QT interval) may cause torsades de pointes with diuretic-induced hypokalemia.
- Probenecid blocks loop diuretic effects by interfering with excretion into the urine.

Parameters to monitor
- Weight
- Serum electrolytes
- BUN and creatinine
- Uric acid
- Hearing (in high doses)

Potassium-sparing diuretics

See Table 8-11 for a list of potassium-sparing diuretics, their usual dose range, and adverse effects associated with these medications.

Mechanism of action
- Potassium-sparring diuretics interfere with potassium and sodium exchange in the distal tubule, decrease calcium excretion, and increase magnesium loss.

Patient instructions and counseling
- Take early in day to avoid nocturia.
- Take after meals.
- Avoid excessive ingestion of foods high in potassium and use of salt substitutes.
- Medication may increase blood glucose in diabetics.
- Report problems with muscle cramps, which may indicate decreased potassium levels.
- Sexual dysfunction is possible.

Drug–drug and drug–disease interactions
- ACE inhibitors may increase risk of hyperkalemia.
- Indomethacin can cause decrease in renal function when combined with triamterene.
- Cimetidine increases bioavailability and decreases clearance of triamterene.

Parameters to monitor
- Weight
- Serum electrolytes (especially potassium)
- BUN and creatinine

Table 8-11. Thiazide Diuretics, Thiazide-Like Diuretics, Loop Diuretics, Potassium-Sparing Agents, and Aldosterone-Receptor Blocker

Drug	Trade name	Usual dose range, total mg/d (frequency per day)	Adverse events and comments[a]
Thiazide diuretics			
Bendroflumethiazide	Naturetin	2.5–5 (1)	**Short-term:** increased cholesterol and glucose
Benzthiazide	Aquatag, Exna	12.5–50 (1)	**Biochemical:** decreased potassium, sodium, and magnesium; increased uric acid and calcium
Chlorothiazide	Diuril	125–500 (1)	
Chlorthalidone	Hygroton, Hylidone	12.5–25 (1)	**Rare:** blood dyscrasias, photosensitivity, pancreatitis, hyponatremia, and sulfonamide-type immune reactions
Hydrochlorothiazide	HydroDIURIL, Microzide	12.5–50 (1)	
Hydroflumethiazide	Saluron, Diucardin	25–50 (1)	**Other:** impotence, fatigue, headache, rash, and vertigo
Methyclothiazide	Renese	2.5–5 (1)	
Polythiazide	Metahydrin, Naqua	2–4 (1)	
Trichlormethiazide		2–4 (1)	
Thiazide-like diuretics			
Metolazone	Mykrox	2.5–10 (1)	(Less or no hypercholesterolemia compared to other thiazides; decreased microalbuminuria in diabetes)
Metolazone	Zaroxolyn	2.5–5 (1)	(Less or no hypercholesterolemia compared to other thiazides; decreased microalbuminuria in diabetes)
Indapamide	Lozol	2.5–5 (1)	
Loop diuretics			
Bumetanide	Bumex	0.5–2 (2)	Ototoxicity at high doses
Furosemide	Lasix	20–80 (2)	(Short duration and no hypercalcemia)
Torsemide	Demadex	2.5–10 (1)	(Short duration and no hypercalcemia)
Potassium-sparing agents[b]			
Amiloride	Midamor	5–10 (1–2)	Hyperkalemia
Triamterene	Dyrenium	50–100 (1–2)	(Avoid with history of kidney stones or hepatic disease)
Aldosterone-receptor blocker			
Spironolactone	Aldactone	25–50 (1–2)	

Adapted from JNC-7 Express, National Heart, Lung, and Blood Institute.
a. Adverse events, or side effects, listed are for the class of drugs, except where noted for individual drugs (in parentheses).
b. See Table 8-12 for combination products.

Adrenergic Inhibitors

Postganglionic adrenergic neuron blockers

This medication class is best avoided unless necessary to treat refractory hypertension that is unresponsive to all other agents, because the medications are poorly tolerated. See Table 8-13 for a list of postganglionic adrenergic neuron blockers, their usual dose range, and adverse effects associated with these medications.

Mechanism of action
Postganglionic adrenergic neuron blockers cause presynaptic inhibition of the release of the neurotransmitter from peripheral neurons by agonistic activity on the α_2 receptor and depletion of the neurotransmitter

Table 8-12. Combination Drugs for Hypertension

Fixed-dose combination (mg)[a]	Trade name
ACEIs and CCBs	
Amlodipine/benazepril hydrochloride (2.5/10, 5/10, 5/20, 10/20)	Lotrel
Enalapril maleate/felodipine (5/5)	Lexxel
Trandolapril/verapamil (2/180, 1/240, 2/240, 4/240)	Tarka
ACEIs and diuretics	
Benazepril/hydrochlorothiazide (5/6.25, 10/12.5, 20/12.5, 20/25)	Lotensin HCT
Captopril/hydrochlorothiazide (25/15, 25/25, 50/15, 50/25)	Capozide
Enalapril maleate/hydrochlorothiazide (5/12.5, 10/25)	Vaseretic
Lisinopril/hydrochlorothiazide (10/12.5, 20/12.5, 20/25)	Prinzide
Moexipril HCL/hydrochlorothiazide (7.5/12.5, 15/25)	Uniretic
Quinapril HCL/hydrochlorothiazide (10/12.5, 20/12.5, 20/25)	Accuretic
ARBs and CCBs	
Amlodipine/valsartan (5/160, 5/320, 10/160, 10/320)	Exforge
Amlodipine/olmesartan (5/20, 5/40, 10/20, 10/40)	Azor
ARBs and diuretics	
Candesartan cilexetil/hydrochlorothiazide (16/12.5, 32/12.5)	Atacand HCT
Eprosartan mesylate/hydrochlorothiazide (600/12.5, 600/25)	Teveten/HCT
Irbesartan/hydrochlorothiazide (150/12.5, 300/12.5)	Avalide
Losartan potassium/hydrochlorothiazide (50/12.5, 100/25)	Hyzaar
Telmisartan/hydrochlorothiazide (40/12.5, 80/12.5)	Micardis/HCT
Valsartan/hydrochlorothiazide (80/12.5, 160/12.5)	Diovan/HCT
BBs and diuretics	
Atenolol/chlorothalidone (50/25, 100/25)	Tenoretic
Bisoprolol fumarate/hydrochlorothiazide (2.5/6.25, 5/6.25, 10/6.25)	Ziac
Propranolol LA/hydrochlorothiazide (50/25, 80/25)	Inderide
Metoprolol tartrate/hydrochlorothiazide (50/25, 100/25)	Lopressor HCT
Nadolol/bendrofluthiazide (40/5, 80/5)	Corzide
Timolol maleate/hydrochlorothiazide (10/25)	Timolide
Centrally acting drug and diuretics	
Methyldopa/hydrochlorothiazide (250/15, 250/25, 500/30, 500/50)	Aldoril
Reserpine/chlorothiazide (0.125/250, 0.25/500)	Diupres
Reserpine/hydrochlorothiazide (0.125/25, 0.25/50)	Hydropres
RIs and diuretics	
Aliskiren/hydrochlorothiazide (150/12.5, 150/25, 300/12.5, 300/25)	Tekturna HCT
Other combinations	
Amiloride HCL/hydrochlorothiazide (5/50)	Moduretic
Spironolactone/hydrochlorothiazide (25/25, 50/50)	Aldactazide
Triamterene/hydrochlorothiazide (37.5/25, 50/25, 75/50)	Dyazide, Maxzide

Adapted from JNC-7 Express, National Heart, Lung, and Blood Institute.
Abbreviations: BB, β-blocker; RI, renin inhibitor.
a. Some drug combinations are available in multiple fixed doses. Each drug dose is reported in milligrams.

Table 8-13. Postganglionic Adrenergic Neuron Blockers

Drug	Trade name	Usual dose range, total mg/d (frequency per day)	Adverse events and comments
Guanadrel	Hylorel	10–75 (2)	Postural hypotension and diarrhea
Guanethidine monosulfate	Ismelin	10–150 (1)	Postural hypotension and diarrhea
Reserpine[a]	Serpasil	0.05–0.25 (1)	Nasal congestion, sedation, depression, activation of peptic ulcer, dizziness, lethargy, memory impairment, sleep disturbances, and weight gain

Adapted from JNC-7 Express, National Heart, Lung, and Blood Institute.
a. Reserpine also acts centrally.

through competitive uptake into the neurosecretory vesicles.

Patient instructions and counseling
- Report symptoms of dizziness or hypotension.
- Do not take over-the-counter (OTC) cold products without first asking the doctor or pharmacist.
- Rise slowly from a lying or sitting position.
- Report new fluid retention.
- Sexual dysfunction is possible.

Drug–drug and drug–disease interactions
- OTC sympathomimetics may potentiate an acute hypertensive effect.
- Tricyclic antidepressants and chlorpromazine antagonize therapeutic effects of guanethidine.
- Pheochromocytoma is a contraindication to this class of medications.
- This medication class should be avoided in patients with CHF, angina, and cerebrovascular disease.

Parameters to monitor
- History of depression (reserpine)
- Sleep disturbances, drowsiness, and lethargy (reserpine)
- Symptoms of peptic ulcer (reserpine)

Centrally active α_2-agonists

See Table 8-14 for a list of centrally active α_2-agonists, their usual dose range, and adverse effects associated with these medications.

Mechanism of action
These medications cause decreased sympathetic outflow to the cardiovascular system by agonistic activity on central α_2 receptors.

Patient instructions and counseling
- Report symptoms of dizziness or hypotension.
- Exercise sedation precautions.
- Fever and flu-like symptoms may represent hepatic dysfunction (methyldopa).
- Report new fluid retention.
- Sexual dysfunction is possible.

Drug–drug and drug–disease interactions
- Use cautiously with other sedating medications.
- Use cautiously in patients with angina, recent myocardial infarction (MI), cerebrovascular accident (CVA), and hepatic or renal disease (guanabenz and guanfacine).

Table 8-14. Centrally Active α_2-Agonists

Drug	Trade name	Usual dose range, total mg/d (frequency per day)	Adverse events and comments[a]
Clonidine HCl[b]	Catapres	0.1–0.8 (2)	Sedation, dry mouth, bradycardia, withdrawal hypertension, orthostatic hypotension, depression, impotence, and sleep disturbances
Guanabenz acetate	Wytensin	8–32 (2)	(More withdrawal)
Guanfacine HCl	Tenex	1–3 (1)	(Less withdrawal)
Methyldopa	Aldomet	250–1,000 (2)	(Hepatic and "autoimmune" disorders)

Adapted from JNC-7 Express, National Heart, Lung, and Blood Institute.
a. Adverse events, or side effects, listed are for the class of drugs, except where noted for individual drugs (in parentheses).
b. Clonidine HCl is also available as a once-weekly transdermal patch.

Parameters to monitor

- Complete blood count (CBC)—positive Coombs test in 25% of those tested; less than 1% develop hemolytic anemia (methyldopa)
- Sleep disturbances, drowsiness, or dry mouth
- Symptoms of depression
- Impotence
- Pulse
- Rebound hypertension

Peripherally acting α_1-adrenergic blockers

See Table 8-15 for a list of peripherally acting α_1-adrenergic blockers, their usual dose range, and adverse effects associated with these medications.

Mechanism of action

- Blocks peripheral α_1 postsynaptic receptors, which causes vasodilation of both arteries and veins (indirect vasodilators)
- Causes less reflex tachycardia than do direct vasodilators (hydralazine and minoxidil)

Patient instructions and counseling

- Take first dose of no more than 1 mg of any agent, and take at bedtime.
- Rise slowly from a lying or sitting position.
- Medication may cause dizziness.
- Priapism is possible.

Table 8-15. Peripherally Acting α_1-Adrenergic Blockers

Drug	Trade name	Usual dose range, total mg/d (frequency per day)	Adverse events and comments
Doxazosin mesylate	Cardura	1–16 (1)	Postural hypotension, syncopal episode with first dose, postural hypotension, diarrhea, weight gain, peripheral edema, dry mouth, urinary urgency, constipation, priapism, nausea, dizziness, headache, palpitations, and sweating; no effects on glucose or cholesterol
Prazosin HCl	Minipress	2–20 (2–3)	
Terazosin HCl	Hytrin	1–20 (1–2)	

Reprinted with permission from JNC-VII.

Drug–drug and drug–disease interactions

- NSAIDs decrease antihypertensive effects of α_1 blockers.
- Increased antihypertensive effects occur with diuretics and β-blockers.

Parameters to monitor

- BP and pulse
- Peripheral edema

β-blockers

See Table 8-16 for a list of β-blockers, their usual dose range, and adverse effects associated with these medications.

Mechanism of action

These medications competitively block response to β-adrenergic stimulation:

- Block secretion of renin
- Decrease cardiac contractility, thereby decreasing cardiac output
- Decrease central sympathetic output
- Decrease heart rate, thereby decreasing cardiac output

Patient instructions and counseling

- Report symptoms of dizziness or hypotension.
- Exercise sedation precautions (with lipid-soluble compounds).
- Abrupt withdrawal of the drug should be avoided.
- Sexual dysfunction is possible.

Drug–drug and drug–disease interactions

- Use with caution in patients with diabetes.
- Use with caution in patients with Raynaud's phenomenon or peripheral vascular disease.
- β-blockers may decrease effectiveness of sulfonylureas.
- Nondihydropyridines may increase effect and toxicity of β-blockers.

Parameters to monitor

- ECG
- Rebound hypertension
- Cholesterol levels
- Pulse (apical and radial)
- Glucose levels

Table 8-16. β-Blockers and Combination α- and β-Blockers

Drug	Trade name	Lipid solubility/primary (secondary) routes of elimination	Usual dose range, total mg/d (frequency per day)	Adverse events and comments[a]
β-blockers				
Acebutolol[b,c]	Sectral	Low/H (R)	200–800 (1)	Bronchospasm, bradycardia, and heart failure; may mask insulin-induced hypoglycemia; *less serious:* impaired peripheral circulation, insomnia, fatigue, decreased exercise tolerance, and hypertriglyceridemia, except agents with intrinsic sympathomimetic activity
Atenolol[b]	Tenormin	Low/R (H)	25–100 (1)	
Betaxolol[b]	Kerlone	Low/H (R)	5–20 (1)	
Bisoprolol fumarate[b]	Zebeta	Low/R (H)	2.5–10 (1)	
Carteolol HCl[c]	Cartrol	Low/R	2.5–10 (1)	
Metoprolol tartrate[b]	Lopressor	Moderate/H (R)	50–100 (2)	
Metoprolol succinate[b]	Toprol-XL	Moderate/H (R)	50–100 (1)	
Nadolol	Corgard	Low/R	40–120 (1)	
Penbutolol sulfate[c]	Levatol	High/H (R)	10–20 (1)	
Pindolol[c]	Visken	Moderate/H (R)	10–60 (2)	
Propranolol HCl	Inderal	High/H	40–160 (2)	
	Inderal LA	High/H	60–180 (1)	
Timolol maleate	Blocadren	Low–moderate/H (R)	20–40 (2)	
Combined α- and β-blockers				
Carvedilol	Coreg	Moderate/bile into feces	12.5–50 (2)	Postural hypotension, bronchospasm
Labetalol	Normodyne, Trandate	Moderate/R (H)	200–800 (2)	

Reprinted with permission from JNC-VII.
H, hepatic; R, renal.
a. Adverse events, or side effects, listed are for the class of drugs.
b. Cardioselective.
c. Intrinsic sympathomimetic activity.

Direct Vasodilators

This medication class is best avoided (second-line agents) unless necessary to treat refractory hypertension that is unresponsive to all other agents.

These agents should *not* be used alone secondary to increases in plasma renin activity, cardiac output, and heart rate and should therefore be used only when β-blockers and diuretics are part of the antihypertensive regimen.

See Table 8-17 for a list of direct vasodilators, their usual dose range, and adverse effects associated with these medications.

Mechanism of action

These agents cause direct relaxation of peripheral arterial smooth muscle and thereby significantly decrease peripheral resistance.

Table 8-17. Direct Vasodilators

Drug	Trade name	Usual dose range, total mg/d (frequency per day)	Adverse events and comments[a]
			Headaches, fluid retention, tachycardia, peripheral neuropathy, and postural hypotension
Hydralazine HCl	Apresoline	25–100 (2)	(Lupus syndrome)
Minoxidil	Loniten	2.5–80 (1–2)	(Hirsutism)

Adapted from JNC-7 Express, National Heart, Lung, and Blood Institute.
a. Adverse events, or side effects, listed are for the class of drugs, except where noted for individual drugs (in parentheses).

Patient instructions and counseling

- Report symptoms of dizziness or hypotension.
- Hirsutism is possible (minoxidil).
- Report any new symptoms of fatigue, malaise, low-grade fever, and joint aches.
- Report rapid weight gain (> 5 pounds), unusual swelling, and pulse increases of > 20 beats per minute above normal.
- Rise slowly from a lying or sitting position.

Drug–drug and drug–disease interactions

- Use with caution in patients with pulmonary hypertension.
- Use with caution in patients with significant renal failure or CHF.
- Use with caution in patients with coronary artery disease or a recent MI.

Parameters to monitor

- Weight (fluid status)
- BP and pulse
- CBC with antinuclear antibody test (hydralazine)

Calcium Antagonists

Low-renin hypertensive, African American, and elderly patients respond well to this class of medications. See Table 8-18 for a list of calcium antagonists, their usual dose range, and adverse effects associated with these medications.

Mechanism of action

- Inhibits the influx of calcium ions through slow channels in vascular smooth muscle and causes relaxation of both coronary and peripheral arteries
- Causes sinoatrial (SA) and atrioventricular (AV) nodal depression and a decrease in myocardial contractility (nondihydropyridines)

Patient instructions and counseling

- Report symptoms of dizziness or hypotension.
- Constipation is possible (verapamil).
- Report any new symptoms of shortness of breath, fatigue, or increased swelling of the extremities.
- Rise slowly from a lying or sitting position.

Table 8-18. Calcium Antagonists

Drug	Trade name	Usual dose range, total mg/d (frequency per day)	Adverse events and comments[a]
Nondihydropyridines			
Diltiazem HCl	Cardizem SR, Cardizem CD, Dilacor XR, Tiazac	180–420 (1) 120–360 (1)	Conduction defects, worsening of systolic dysfunction, and gingival hyperplasia
Verapamil immediate-release	Calan, Isoptin	80–320 (2)	(Nausea and headache)
Verapamil long-acting	Calan SR, Isoptin SR	120–360 (1–2)	(Constipation)
Verapamil COER	Covera HS, Verelan PM	120–360 (1)	
Dihydropyridines			
Amlodipine besylate	Norvasc	2.5–10 (1)	Edema of the ankle, flushing, headache, and gingival hyperplasia
Felodipine	Plendil	2.5–20 (1)	
Isradipine	DynaCirc	2.5–10 (2)	
	DynaCirc CR	5–20 (1)	
Nicardipine	Cardene SR	60–120 (1)	
Nifedipine	Procardia XL, Adalat CC	30–60 (1)	
Nisoldipine	Sular	10–40 (1)	

Adapted from JNC-7 Express, National Heart, Lung, and Blood Institute.
a. Adverse events, or side effects, listed are for the class of drugs, except where noted for individual drugs (in parentheses).

Drug–drug and drug–disease interactions

- Use with caution in patients on β-blockers (nondihydropyridines), which may increase CHF and bradycardia. This combination can also cause conduction abnormalities to the AV node.
- Use with extreme caution in patients with conduction disturbances in the SA or AV node.
- Grapefruit juice may increase the levels of some dihydropyridines.

Parameters to monitor

- ECG
- Peripheral edema
- BP and pulse
- Bowel habits
- Symptoms of conduction disturbances

Angiotensin-Converting Enzyme Inhibitors and Angiotensin II Receptor Blockers

Ethnic differences exist in the response to these classes of medications. These agents are relatively ineffective as monotherapy in African American patients. However, the addition of diuretic therapy has been shown to sensitize African American patients to these agents to obtain similar responses as in non–African American patients.

See Table 8-19 for a list of ACEIs and ARBs, their usual dose range, and adverse effects associated with these medications.

Mechanism of action

ACEIs

- Inhibit the conversion of angiotensin I to angiotensin II (a potent vasoconstrictor; see Figure 8-1)

Table 8-19. Angiotensin-Converting Enzyme Inhibitors and Angiotensin II Receptor Blockers

Drug	Trade name	Usual dose range, total mg/d (frequency per day)	Adverse events and comments[a]
ACEIs			
Benazepril HCl	Lotensin	10–40 (1–2)	**Common:** cough
Captopril	Capoten	25–100 (2–3)	**Rare:** angioedema, hyperkalemia, rash, loss of taste, and leucopenia
Enalapril maleate	Vasote	2.5–40 (1–2)	**Other:** vertigo; headache; fatigue; first-dose hypotension; minor GI disturbances; acute renal insufficiency in patients with predisposing factors such as renal stenosis and coadministration with thiazide diuretics; and proteinuria (especially in patients with history of renal disease)
Fosinopril	Monopril	10–40 (1–2)	
Lisinopril	Prinivil, Zestril	10–40 (1)	
Moexipril	Univasc	7.5–30 (1)	
Perindopril	Aceon	4–8 (1–2)	
Quinapril HCl	Accupril	10–40 (1–2)	
Ramipril	Altace	1.25–20 (1)	
Trandolapril	Mavik	1–4 (1)	
ARBs			
Candesartan	Atacand	8–32 (1)	Angioedema and hyperkalemia
Eprosartan	Teveten	400–800 (1–2)	
Irbesartan	Avapro	150–300 (1)	
Losartan	Cozaar	25–100 (1–2)	
Olmesartan	Benicar	20 (1)	
Telmisartan	Micardis	40–80 (1)	
Valsartan	Diovan	80–320 (1)	

Reprinted with permission from JNC-VII.

■ Indirectly inhibit fluid volume increases by inhibiting angiotensin II–stimulated release of aldosterone

ARBs

■ Inhibit the binding of angiotensin II to the angiotensin II receptor, thereby inhibiting the vasoconstrictive properties of angiotensin II as well as its ability to stimulate release of aldosterone
■ Currently considered as alternative therapy in patients not able to tolerate ACEIs because of cough

Patient instructions and counseling

■ Report symptoms of dizziness or hypotension.
■ Symptoms of swelling of the lips, mouth, or face should be considered an emergency. Report immediately to a doctor's office or emergency department.
■ Report new rashes (especially with captopril).
■ Do not use salt substitutes containing potassium, and do not take OTC potassium supplements.
■ Rise slowly from a lying or sitting position.

Drug–drug and drug–disease interactions

■ NSAIDs will decrease the effectiveness of ACEIs and ARBs.
■ Potassium-sparing diuretics, potassium supplements, and salt substitutes will increase the risk of hyperkalemia when used in combination with ACEIs and ARBs.
■ ACEIs and ARBs should be avoided in patients with bilateral renal artery stenosis or stenosis in a single kidney.
■ ACEIs and ARBs should be avoided in pregnant patients.

Parameters to monitor

■ Serum electrolytes (especially creatinine and potassium)
■ Symptoms of angioedema
■ BP
■ Symptoms of hypotension
■ CBC (especially with captopril and enalapril) for neutropenia, which is more common in patients with preexisting renal impairment
■ Cough
■ Urinary proteins

Direct Renin Inhibitor

■ See Table 8-20 for a list of direct renin inhibitors, their usual dose range, and adverse effects associated with these medications.

Mechanism of action

Direct renin inhibitors competitively inhibit human renin, which decreases plasma renin activity and inhibits the conversion of angiotensinogen to angiotensin I.

Patient instructions and counseling

■ Medicine can be taken with or without food.
■ Establish a routine pattern for taking aliskiren with regard to meals. High-fat meals decrease absorption significantly.
■ Store the medicine in a closed container at room temperature, away from heat, moisture, and direct light.
■ Report symptoms of dizziness or hypotension.
■ Diarrhea is possible.
■ Symptoms of swelling of the lips, mouth, or face should be considered an emergency. Report immediately to a doctor's office or emergency department.

Drug–drug and drug–disease interactions

■ Concomitant use of aliskiren with cyclosporine is not recommended.

Table 8-20. Direct Renin Inhibitors

Drug	Trade name	Usual dose range, total mg/d (frequency per day)	Adverse events and comments
Aliskiren	Tekturna	150–300 mg (1)	**Common:** diarrhea **Rare:** elevated uric acid, gout, renal stone, angioedema, and rash **Other:** headache, nasopharyngitis, dizziness, fatigue, upper respiratory tract infection, back pain, and cough

Drug product package insert.

- Potassium-sparing diuretics, potassium supplements, and salt substitutes will increase risk of hyperkalemia when used in combination with aliskiren.
- Blood concentrations of furosemide are significantly reduced when given with aliskiren.
- Ketoconazole significantly increases aliskiren plasma levels.
- Aliskiren should be avoided in pregnant patients.

Parameters to monitor

- Symptoms of angioedema
- BP
- Symptoms of hypotension
- Serum electrolytes (especially creatinine and potassium)

8-4. Hypertensive Urgencies and Emergencies

The classification of hypertensive urgencies and emergencies is determined by the presence or absence of acute target-organ damage, not by BP, and determines the appropriate treatment approach.

The relative rise and rate of increase in BP is more important than the actual BP.

Hypertensive Emergencies

Acute elevations of BP (> 180 mm Hg systolic or > 120 mm Hg diastolic) with the presence of acute or ongoing target organ damage constitute a hypertensive emergency (Box 8-4). This situation requires immediate lowering of BP to prevent or minimize target organ damage.

Table 8-21 shows details of parenteral drugs used for treatment of hypertensive emergencies. Such emergencies should be treated as follows:

- As an initial goal, reduce mean arterial pressure (MAP) by no more than 25% within minutes to hours. Reach BP of 160/100 mm Hg within 2–6 hours.
- Measure BP every 5–10 minutes until goal MAP is reached and life-threatening target organ damage resolves.
- Maintain goal BP for 1–2 days, and further reduce BP toward normal over several weeks.
- Excessive falls in BP may precipitate renal, cerebral, or coronary ischemia.

Box 8-4. Clinical Findings of Target Organ Damage

Target Organ Damage
Hypertensive encephalopathy
Intracranial hemorrhage
Unstable angina
Acute myocardial infarction
Acute left ventricular failure with pulmonary edema
Dissecting aortic aneurysm
Eclampsia

Clinical Findings
Funduscopic: papilledema, hemorrhage, exudates
Neurologic: somnolence, confusion, seizures, coma, visual deficits or blindness
Cardiac: S_4 gallop, ischemic changes on ECG, chest x-ray consistent with pulmonary edema, chest pain
Renal: oliguria, progressive azotemia, hematuria, proteinuria
Other: dyspnea

Reprinted with permission from JNC-VII.

- Intravenous agents are preferred because of the ability to titrate dosages on the basis of BP response; however, specific agents should be chosen on the basis of patient findings (Table 8-22).

Hypertensive Urgencies

Hypertensive urgencies are accelerated, malignant, or perioperative elevations in blood pressure in the absence of new or progressive target organ damage; therefore, immediate lowering of BP is not required.

Table 8-23 shows the agents used to treat hypertensive urgencies. Such situations require the following considerations:

- There is no agent of choice; medications should be selected on the basis of patient characteristics.
- Oral therapy is preferred.
- Onset of action should be in 15–30 minutes, and peak effects should be seen in 2–3 hours.
- Check BP every 15–30 minutes to ensure response.
- Use of immediate-release nifedipine is inappropriate to lower BP in patients with hypertensive urgencies.

8-5. Key Points

- *Hypertension* is defined as a systolic blood pressure exceeding 140 mm Hg, a diastolic blood pressure exceeding 90 mm Hg, or any condition in a patient that requires antihypertensive therapy.

Table 8-21. Parenteral Drugs for Treatment of Hypertensive Emergencies

Drug	Dose	Onset of action	Duration of action	Adverse effects[a]	Special indications
Vasodilators					
Sodium nitroprusside	0.25–10 mcg/kg/min IV infusion[b] (maximal dose for 10 min only)	Immediate	1–2 min	Nausea, vomiting, muscle twitching, sweating, and thiocyanate and cyanide intoxication	Most hypertensive emergencies; caution with high intracranial pressure or azotemia
Nicardipine hydrochloride	5–15 mg/h IV	5–10 min	1–4 h	Tachycardia, headache, flushing, and local phlebitis	Most hypertensive emergencies, except acute heart failure; caution with coronary ischemia
Fenoldopam mesylate	0.1–0.3 mcg/kg/min IV infusion	< 5 min	30 min	Tachycardia, headache, nausea, and flushing	
Nitroglycerin	5–100 mcg/min IV infusion[c]	2–5 min	3–5 min	Headache, vomiting, methemoglobinemia, and tolerance with prolonged use	Coronary ischemia
Enalaprilat	1.25–5 mg every 6 h IV	15–30 min	6 h	Precipitous fall in pressure in high-renin states; response variable	Acute left ventricular failure; avoid in acute myocardial infarction
Hydralazine hydrochloride	10–20 mg IV; 10–50 mg IM	10–20 min; 20–30 min	3–8 h	Tachycardia, flushing, headache, vomiting, and aggravation of angina	Eclampsia
Diazoxide	50–100 mg IV bolus repeated, or 15–30 mg/min IV infusion	2–4 min	6–12 h	Nausea, flushing, tachycardia, and chest pain	Now obsolete; when no intensive monitoring available
Adrenergic inhibitors					
Labetalol hydrochloride	20–80 mg IV bolus every 10 min; 0.5–2.0 mg/min IV infusion	5–10 min	3–6 h	Vomiting, scalp tingling, burning in throat, dizziness, nausea, heart block, and orthostatic hypotension	Most hypertensive emergencies, except acute heart failure
Esmolol hydrochloride	250–500 mcg/kg/min for 1 min, then 50–100 mcg/kg/min for 4 min; may repeat sequence	1–2 min	10–20 min	Hypotension and nausea	Aortic dissection, perioperative
Phentolamine	5–15 mg IV	1–2 min	3–10 min	Tachycardia, flushing, and headache	Catecholamine excess

Reprinted with permission from JNC-VII.
a. Hypotension may occur with all agents.
b. Requires special delivery system.

- Prehypertension (120–139/80–89 mm Hg) represents a new classification in JNC-VII that significantly increases the risk of developing stage 1 hypertension. Lifestyle modifications should be stressed for this classification, and medication therapy should be used only for patients with compelling indications.
- Secondary causes of hypertension include renovascular disease, primary aldosteronism, Cushing's syndrome, pheochromocytoma,

Table 8-22. Selected Agents for Specific Hypertensive Emergencies

Emergency	Recommended therapy	Comments
Encephalopathy	Labetalol, nicardipine, and nitroprusside	Avoid methyldopa (sedation), diazoxide (reduces cerebral blood flow), reserpine (sedation), and hydralazine (increases intracranial pressure).
Myocardial infarction or unstable angina	Nitroglycerin and esmolol	Reduce BP until pain is relieved, and use in conjunction with conventional therapy for MI/angina.
		Avoid diazoxide and hydralazine (increases oxygen demand), dihydropyridines (may worsen angina), and nitroprusside (coronary steal).
Congestive heart failure	Nitroprusside, nitroglycerin, and enalaprilat	Avoid labetalol, esmolol, and other β-blockers (reduces cardiac output).
Subarachnoid hemorrhage, intracerebral hemorrhage, and stroke	Nitroprusside	BP reduction is controversial because it may cause hypoperfusion; generally recommended for severe hypertension (systolic blood pressure > 220 or diastolic blood pressure > 120 mm Hg).
Dissecting aortic aneurysm	Trimethaphan, esmolol, and nitroprusside	Avoid diazoxide and hydralazine (increase shear force).
Pheochromocytoma and cocaine overdose	Phentolamine and labetalol	Anecdotal reports suggest increased BP with labetalol; unopposed β blockade may worsen crisis.
Renal insufficiency	Nitroprusside, calcium channel blocker, and labetalol	Monitor cyanide and thiocyanate levels.
Postoperative hypertension	Nitroprusside, nicardipine, and labetalol	Blood pressure levels of >180/110 should be controlled before surgery. Contributing factors to postoperative hypertension may include pain and increased intravascular volume, which may require parenteral loop diuretics.

aortic coarctation, and drugs (steroids and estrogens, alcohol, cocaine, cyclosporine and tacrolimus, sympathomimetics, erythropoietin, licorice, MAO inhibitors, tricyclic antidepressants, and NSAIDs).

■ Recommended lifestyle modifications to improve both BP and overall cardiovascular health include losing weight; limiting alcohol intake; increasing aerobic physical activity; reducing sodium intake; maintaining adequate dietary intake of potassium, magnesium, and calcium; stopping smoking; and reducing dietary cholesterol and saturated fat intake.

■ Diuretics are considered by JNC-VII to be the initial agent for treatment of hypertension in most patients unless compelling indications for the use of other medication classes exist or the patient has comorbid conditions that would suggest the use of classes other than diuretics.

■ JNC-VII considers ACEIs, ARBs, β-blockers, and CCBs equivalent choices as initial therapy for hypertension.

■ Vasodilators, α_1-receptor antagonists, α_2-receptor agonists, and postganglionic adrenergic neuron blockers should be avoided as initial agents for hypertension.

■ Antihypertensive drug therapy should be individualized. There are classifications of recommendations from JNC-VII based on the level of evidence, which include compelling indica-

Table 8-23. Agents Used to Treat Hypertensive Urgencies

Drug	Dose	Onset	Duration	Adverse effects
Captopril	25 mg, repeat in 1–2 hours as needed	5–15 min	4–6 h	Hypotension, acute renal failure, and angioedema
Clonidine	0.1–0.2 mg, repeat in 1–2 hours as needed (up to 0.6 mg)	5–15 min	6–12 h	Hypotension, drowsiness, sedation, and dry mouth
Labetalol	100–400 mg, repeat in 2–3 hours as needed	15–30 min	4–6 h	Hypotension, heart block, and bronchoconstriction

tion unless contraindicated, possibility of favorable effects on comorbid conditions, and possibility of unfavorable effects on comorbid conditions.

■ The classification and treatment of hypertensive urgencies and emergencies is determined by the presence or absence of acute target organ damage and not by blood pressure.

■ All causes for inadequate response should be addressed before additional agents are added to a patient's antihypertensive regimen (i.e., pseudoresistance, nonadherence, volume overload, drug-related causes, associated conditions, and secondary causes of hypertension).

8-6. Questions

1. According to the Seventh Report of the Joint National Committee on Detection, Evaluation, and Treatment of High Blood Pressure (JNC-VII), all of the following agents are suitable as initial therapy for the treatment of uncomplicated hypertension *except*

   A. hydrochlorothiazide.
   B. chlorthalidone.
   C. indapamide.
   D. hydralazine.
   E. atenolol.

2. Hyperkalemia is a possible adverse effect of all the following medications *except*

   A. trandolapril.
   B. Teveten.
   C. doxazosin.
   D. amiloride.
   E. captopril.

3. A 48-year-old patient presents with a new diagnosis of hypertension. The patient is also noted to have congestive heart failure with an ejection fraction of 28%. Which agent would be an appropriate choice as initial therapy in this patient based on JNC-VII?

   A. Clonidine
   B. Guanethidine
   C. Diltiazem
   D. Perindopril
   E. Nisoldipine

4. A 62-year-old patient with a history of hypertension and gout presents to begin pharmacotherapy for hypertension. Which agent is the most appropriate choice as initial therapy based on JNC-VII?

   A. Chlorothiazide
   B. Torsemide
   C. Tenormin
   D. Chlorthalidone
   E. Metolazone

5. All of the following medications can cause bradycardia *except*

   A. terazosin.
   B. verapamil.
   C. diltiazem.
   D. Ziac.
   E. clonidine.

6. A patient requires a cardioselective β-blocker in his or her outpatient medication regimen after recent discharge from the hospital with a new myocardial infarction. You suggest he or she take

   A. labetalol.
   B. esmolol.
   C. propranolol.
   D. atenolol.
   E. carvedilol.

7. A patient presents to your ambulatory clinic with a blood pressure of 210/125 mm Hg. Past medical history is significant for type 2 diabetes, congestive heart failure, and renal insufficiency. Which of the following would cause the patient to be classified as a hypertensive emergency?

   A. Blood glucose levels > 300 mg/dL, which increase the patient's risk for acute renal failure
   B. A serum creatinine of 3 mg/dL
   C. Nausea, vomiting, and diarrhea for 3 days
   D. S_4 gallop and a chest x-ray consistent with pulmonary edema
   E. Polyuria combined with polydipsia

8. What are the treatment goals for the patient with hypertensive emergency described in question 7?

   A. Systolic pressure should be reduced to 120 mm Hg within the first hour of treatment to reduce the risk of further end organ damage.
   B. Diastolic pressure should be reduced to 80 mm Hg within the first hour of treatment to reduce the risk of further end organ damage.

C. Blood pressure should be reduced to 160/100 mm Hg in the first 2–6 hours of therapy.

D. Mean arterial pressure should be reduced by at least 50% within the first minutes to hours of therapy.

E. Blood pressure should be reduced to no lower than 180/110 mm Hg in the first hour, because excessive falls in blood pressure may precipitate coronary ischemia.

9. What would be the recommended treatment for the patient with hypertensive emergency described in question 7?

A. Clonidine orally, 0.1–0.2 mg; repeat in 1–2 hours as needed (up to 0.6 mg)

B. Labetalol orally, 100–400 mg; repeat in 2–3 hours as needed

C. Nifedipine sublingually, 10 mg; repeat in 0.5–1.0 hours as needed (up to 60 mg)

D. Labetalol intravenously, 20- to 80-mg bolus, followed by 0.5–2.0 mg/min infusion

E. Enalaprilat intravenously 1.25–5.0 mg every 6 hours

10. Which of the following antihypertensive agents can cause first-dose syncope, palpitations, peripheral edema, and priapism?

A. Hydralazine
B. Nitroprusside
C. Prazosin
D. Verapamil
E. Moexipril

11. Which of the following antihypertensive agents is most likely to cause lupus syndrome, postural hypotension, and peripheral neuropathy?

A. Atenolol
B. Hydralazine
C. Guanfacine
D. Mibefradil
E. Nitroprusside

12. Which of the following medications is not associated with drug-induced hypertension?

A. Prednisone
B. Indomethacin
C. Rosiglitazone
D. Cocaine
E. Cyclosporine

13. What is the best recommendation for antihypertensive medication in a patient who

has atrial fibrillation, coronary artery disease with angina, and hyperthyroidism?

A. Minoxidil
B. Betaxolol
C. Telmisartan
D. Nicardipine
E. Amiloride

14. What antihypertensive agent should not be used in a patient with essential hypertension and a history of depression with suicidal ideation?

A. Captopril
B. Prazosin
C. Metolazone
D. Reserpine
E. Amlodipine

15. All of the following are secondary causes of hypertension *except*

A. renovascular disease.
B. pheochromocytoma.
C. systemic lupus erythematosus.
D. primary aldosteronism.
E. aortic coarctation.

Answer questions 16–20 on the basis of the patient medication profile provided on the next page.

A. I only is correct.
B. III only is correct.
C. I and II are both correct.
D. II and III are both correct.
E. I, II, and III are correct.

16. Possible complications that the patient is at risk of developing secondary to uncontrolled hypertension include

I. hyperaldosteronism.
II. myocardial infarction.
III. blindness.

17. Education regarding lifestyle modification issues in this patient should include

I. Limit smoking to a half pack per day and alcohol intake to no more than 2 drinks per day.
II. Maintain adequate intake of dietary magnesium, calcium, and sodium.
III. Increase aerobic physical activity, lose weight, and limit dietary saturated fat and cholesterol.

Patient Profile
Date: 4/12/09

Patient name: Buddy Manwich
Phone: 555-8181
Height: 5'11"
Race: African American
Known diseases: DM (15 years), HTN (20 years), Obstructive Sleep Apnea (5 years), Osteoarthritis
OTC use: Aleve, Actron

Address: 61 Heavenly Highway
Date of birth: 4/14/44
Weight: 248 lb
Allergies: NKDA
Pharmacist notes and other patient information: + tobacco—1.5 ppd, 4–5 cups of coffee/day, ETOH—2 drinks/week

Date	Rx No.	Medication/Strength	Route	Quantity	Regimen	Refills	Pharmacist	Prescriber
1/15/09	001	Glipizide 5 mg	PO	30	1 qd	5	BCE	NTE
1/15/09	002	Lisinopril 5 mg	PO	30	1 qd	5	BCE	NTE
1/15/09	003	Hydrodiuril 12.5 mg	PO	30	1 qd	5	BBC	NPR
1/20/09	003	Ibuprofen 800 mg	PO	90	1 tid	5	REM	FTD
2/11/09	001-RF	Glipizide 5 mg	PO	30	1 qd	4	BCE	NTE
2/11/09	003-RF	Hydrodiuril 12.5 mg	PO	30	1 qd	4	BBC	NPR
2/11/09	004-RF	Ibuprofen 800 mg	PO	90	1 td	4	REM	FTD
3/13/09	001-RF	Glipizide 5 mg	PO	30	1 qd	3	BCE	NTE
3/13/09	002-RF	Lisinopril 5 mg	PO	30	1 qd	3	BCE	NTE
3/13/09	004-RF	Ibuprofen 800 mg	PO	90	1 td	3	REM	FTD

18. Possible reasons for the patient's blood pressure being uncontrolled include

    I. Use of NSAIDs, which cause decreased effectiveness of ACE inhibitor therapy
    II. Possible problems with adherence to antihypertensive therapy
    III. Lack of blood pressure response to ACE inhibitor therapy, which should not be used in combination with diuretics in an African American patient

19. The appropriate initial antihypertensive agent in this patient could be

    I. benazepril.
    II. terazosin.
    III. minoxidil.

20. If the patient is not able to tolerate lisinopril because of adverse effects such as cough, an appropriate alternative agent would be

    I. telmisartan.
    II. labetalol.
    III. guanabenz.

8-7. Answers

1. **D.** Appropriate choices for initial agents in the treatment of uncomplicated hypertension include α-blockers and diuretics. Hydralazine is a direct vasodilator, which would never be considered a first-line agent in the treatment of hypertension.
2. **C.** Hyperkalemia is a possible side effect with angiotensin-converting enzyme inhibitors, angiotensin II receptor antagonists, and potassium-sparing diuretics. Doxazosin is a peripherally acting α₁ blocker, which does not cause hyperkalemia.
3. **D.** For patients who have hypertension and congestive heart failure, JNC-VII recommends the use of ACE inhibitors, diuretics, β-blockers, and aldosterone antagonists (see Table 8-10). The only listed ACE inhibitor is perindopril.
4. **C.** For patients who have hypertension and gout, JNC-VII recommends not using diuretic therapy, which increases the risk of gouty attacks (see Table 8-10). The only medication listed that is not a diuretic is atenolol (Tenormin), which is a β-blocker.

5. **A.** Verapamil and diltiazem are nondihydropyridine calcium channel blockers, Ziac (bisoprolol and hydrochlorothiazide) is a β-blocker, and clonidine is a centrally acting α₂ agonist. They all have negative inotropic effects on the myocardium. Terazosin is a peripherally acting α₁ blocker, which does not cause bradycardia.

6. **D.** Labetalol, propranolol, and carvedilol are all nonselective β-blockers. Esmolol is a cardioselective agent available only in injectable form and, therefore, would not be for outpatient use. Atenolol is a cardioselective β-blocker that is available as an oral tablet and, therefore, can be used for outpatient dosing.

7. **D.** The classification of hypertensive urgencies and emergencies is determined by the presence or absence of acute target organ damage and not by the actual blood pressure measurement. Presence of an S₄ gallop and a chest x-ray consistent with pulmonary edema suggests acute left ventricular failure with pulmonary edema, which represents defined target organ damage and, in turn, means the patient should be classified as a hypertensive emergency.

8. **C.** According to JNC-VII, the initial goal of blood pressure lowering in patients with hypertensive emergencies is a drop in mean arterial pressure of no more than 25% within minutes to hours and to 160/100 mm Hg within 2–6 hours.

9. **E.** In a patient with CHF and a hypertensive emergency, recommended treatments include nitroglycerin, nitroprusside, and enalaprilat (Table 8-21). Clonidine and labetalol (PO) are incorrect choices because the patient requires intravenous (IV) therapy. Nifedipine SL is not indicated for immediate reduction of blood pressure. Labetalol IV is not an appropriate choice in this patient with CHF because it could decrease cardiac output.

10. **C.** Possible side effects of peripherally acting α₁ blockers (prazosin) include first-dose syncope, palpitations, peripheral edema, and priapism (Table 8-15).

11. **B.** Possible side effects of direct vasodilators (hydralazine) include postural hypotension and peripheral neuropathy. However, lupus syndrome is unique to hydralazine and does not occur with minoxidil (Table 8-17).

12. **C.** All agents listed are possible causes of drug-induced hypertension through multiple mechanisms except rosiglitazone (Box 8-3).

13. **B.** The diagnoses of atrial fibrillation, coronary artery disease with angina, and hyperthyroidism are all considered comorbid conditions with hypertension in which the use of β-blockers may have favorable effects.

14. **D.** Because of its possible increased risk of depression, reserpine should not be used for patients for whom the risk for depression or suicide already exists.

15. **C.** All listed diseases are possible causes of secondary hypertension through various mechanisms, except systemic lupus erythematosus.

16. **D.** Uncontrolled hypertension causes multiple organ system problems, including cardiovascular (CHF, MI, and peripheral arterial disease); ophthalmologic (retinopathy and blindness); cerebrovascular (transient ischemic attack and CVA); and renovascular (nephropathy, renal failure, and dialysis) issues. Therefore, this patient is at risk for MI and blindness, not for hyperaldosteronism.

17. **B.** Lifestyle modification issues to be considered in hypertensive patients include weight loss; limit of alcohol intake; increased aerobic activity; reduced sodium intake; maintenance of adequate dietary potassium, calcium, and magnesium intake; and smoking cessation.

18. **C.** Possible causes for inadequate responsiveness to therapy are listed in Box 8-3.

19. **A.** In patients with hypertension and comorbid conditions of CHF and diabetes, the initial agent should be an ACE inhibitor (Table 8-10).

20. **A.** In patients who cannot tolerate ACE inhibitor therapy secondary to the adverse effect of cough, angiotensin II receptor antagonists are considered good alternative agents.

8-8. References

Carter BL, Saseen JL. Hypertension. In: DiPiro JT, Talbert RL, eds. *Pharmacotherapy: A Pathophysiologic Approach*. New York: McGraw-Hill; 2002:157–83.

JNC-VII (The Seventh Report of the Joint National Committee on Prevention, Detection, Evaluation and Treatment of High Blood Pressure). *Hypertension*. 2003;42:1206–52.

JNC-7 Express (Joint National Committee on Prevention, Detection, Evaluation, and Treatment of High Blood Pressure [JNC-7] Express). NIH Pub. No. 03-5233, May 2003. Available at www.nhlbi.gov/guidelines/hypertension/express.pdf.

Heart Failure

Robert B. Parker, PharmD, FCCP

9-1. Overview

Heart failure is a clinical syndrome resulting from a variety of cardiac disorders that impair the ventricle's ability to fill with or eject blood. When the ventricle is impaired as such, the heart is unable to pump blood at a sufficient rate to meet the metabolic demands of the body, a condition that is described as heart failure.

- Nearly 6 million people in the United States have heart failure; 670,000 new patients are diagnosed each year.
- Heart failure is the only major cardiovascular disease that is increasing in prevalence.
- Approximately 300,000 patients die from heart failure each year. At the time of heart failure diagnosis, the 5-year mortality rate is nearly 50%.
- A large majority of patients are elderly; approximately 10% of individuals over the age of 75 have heart failure.
- Each year, there are more than 1 million hospital discharges for heart failure, and it is the most common hospital discharge diagnosis for Medicare patients. More Medicare dollars are spent for diagnosis and treatment of heart failure than for any other disorder.
- Current estimates indicate that annual expenditures for heart failure exceed $37 million.

Classification

The New York Heart Association Functional Classification for heart failure has been widely used for many years. The classification scheme primarily reflects the severity of heart failure symptoms based on a subjective assessment by the provider. A patient's functional class can change frequently over a short period because of changes in medications, diet, or intercurrent illnesses. The classification scheme, as follows, does not recognize preventive measures, nor does it recognize the progressive nature of heart failure:

- *Functional class I* includes patients with cardiac disease but without limitations of physical activity. Ordinary physical activity does not cause undue fatigue, dyspnea, or palpitations.
- *Functional class II* includes patients with cardiac disease that results in slight limitations of physical activity. Ordinary physical activity results in fatigue, palpitations, dyspnea, or angina.
- *Functional class III* includes patients with cardiac disease that results in marked limitation of physical activity. Although patients are comfortable at rest, less than ordinary activity will lead to symptoms.
- *Functional class IV* includes patients with cardiac disease that results in an inability to carry on physical activity without discomfort. Symptoms of heart failure are present even at rest. With any physical activity, increased discomfort is experienced.

The most recent guidelines for evaluation and management of heart failure from the American College of Cardiology (ACC) and the American Heart Association (AHA) recommend an additional classification scheme that emphasizes both the evolution and the progression of the disease. That additional classification scheme more objectively identifies patients within the course of the disease and links to treatments that are appropriate for each stage. Patients in stages A and B do not have heart failure but do have risk factors that predispose them to the development of heart failure.

- *Stage A* includes patients at high risk of developing heart failure because of the presence of conditions that are strongly associated with heart failure. Patients in stage A have no known cardiac abnormalities and no heart failure signs or symptoms. Examples include patients with hypertension, coronary artery disease, and diabetes mellitus.
- *Stage B* includes patients with structural heart disease that is strongly associated with the development of heart failure but who have never shown signs or symptoms of heart failure. Examples include patients with previous myocardial infarction, left ventricular hypertrophy, or impaired left ventricular systolic function.
- *Stage C* includes patients who have current or prior symptoms of heart failure associated with underlying structural heart disease. Examples include patients with dyspnea or fatigue attributable to left ventricular systolic dysfunction, as well as asymptomatic patients who are undergoing treatment for prior symptoms of heart failure. Most patients with heart failure are in stage C.
- *Stage D* includes patients who have advanced structural heart disease, who have marked symptoms of heart failure at rest despite maximal medical therapy, and who require specialized interventions. Patients in stage D include those who frequently are hospitalized for heart failure and cannot be discharged from the hospital safely, those who are in the hospital awaiting heart transplantation, and those who are supported with a mechanical circulatory assist device.

Acute Decompensated Heart Failure

Both the growing number of patients with heart failure and the progressive nature of the syndrome have led to substantial increases in hospitalizations for heart failure. *Acute decompensated heart failure* (ADHF) is defined as new or worsening signs or symptoms that are usually caused by (1) volume overload (pulmonary congestion, systemic congestion, or both); (2) hypoperfusion (hypotension, renal insufficiency, shock syndrome, or some combination); or (3) both volume overload and hypoperfusion. ADHF frequently requires hospitalization for acute treatment.

Causes of ADHF include medication and dietary noncompliance, atrial fibrillation, myocardial ischemia, uncorrected high blood pressure, recent addition of negative inotropic drugs, nonsteroidal anti-inflammatory drugs (NSAIDs), excessive alcohol or illicit drug use, and progression of heart failure.

To determine the proper approach to therapy, patients are assigned to one of four hemodynamic profiles:

- *Warm and dry:* Adequate perfusion (i.e., cardiac output) and no signs or symptoms of volume overload
- *Warm and wet:* Adequate perfusion but signs or symptoms of volume overload
- *Cold and dry:* Inadequate perfusion and no signs or symptoms of volume overload
- *Cold and wet:* Inadequate perfusion and signs or symptoms of volume overload

Most patients (about 70%) are assigned to the warm and wet classification.

Clinical Presentation

The primary manifestations of heart failure are (1) dyspnea and fatigue that may limit exercise tolerance and (2) fluid retention that may lead to pulmonary and peripheral edema. Both abnormalities can limit a patient's functional capacity and quality of life, but they do not necessarily occur at the same time. Some patients may have marked exercise intolerance but little evidence of fluid retention, whereas others may have prominent edema with few dyspnea or fatigue symptoms.

Other symptoms may include paroxysmal nocturnal dyspnea, orthopnea, tachypnea, cough, ascites, and nocturia. Other signs include jugular venous distension, hepatojugular reflux, hepatomegaly, bibasilar rales, pleural effusion, tachycardia, pallor, and S_3 gallop. Patients with ADHF experience similar symptoms but they may be more severe.

Pathophysiology

Heart failure can result from any disorder (see "Specific Causes of Heart Failure" next) that impairs the heart's systolic function (i.e., pumping ability) or diastolic function (impaired cardiac relaxation). Many patients have manifestations of both abnormalities. In either case, the initiating event in heart failure is a decrease in cardiac output, which results in the activation of a number of compensatory mechanisms that attempt to maintain an adequate cardiac output.

Recent studies suggest that mutations in certain adrenergic receptors (β_1 and α_{2c}) and β-receptor signaling pathways may play an important role in the development of heart failure and response to therapy.

The beneficial effects of angiotensin-converting enzyme (ACE) inhibitors, β-blockers, and aldosterone antagonists on reducing mortality and slowing heart failure progression have resulted in the neurohormonal model of heart failure pathophysiology. The decrease in cardiac output leads to the activation of compensatory systems that release a number of neurohormones, including angiotensin II, norepinephrine, aldosterone, proinflammatory cytokines, and vasopressin. Those neurohormones can increase renal sodium and water retention, vasoconstriction, and tachycardia and can stimulate ventricular hypertrophy and remodeling. Activation of the compensatory systems results in a systemic disorder that is not confined just to the heart, whose progression is largely mediated by these neurohormones.

Specific Causes of Heart Failure

Coronary artery disease is the cause of heart failure in about 65% of patients with left ventricular systolic dysfunction. Other causes include nonischemic cardiomyopathy (e.g., attributable to hypertension, thyroid disease, or valvular disease). Most of those patients have a reduced left ventricular ejection fraction (usually less than 40%).

Approximately 20%–50% of patients with heart failure have preserved (normal) left ventricular systolic function, and their heart failure is secondary to diastolic dysfunction. This type of heart failure is most often observed in elderly patients.

A number of drugs can precipitate or worsen heart failure:

- Drugs with negative inotropic effects include antiarrhythmics (disopyramide, flecainide, propafenone, and others); β-blockers; calcium channel blockers (verapamil and diltiazem); and oral antifungals (itraconazole and terbinafine).
- Cardiotoxic drugs include doxorubicin, daunorubicin, cyclophosphamide, ethanol, amphetamines (cocaine and methamphetamine), trastuzumab, and imatinib.
- Drugs that cause sodium and water retention can precipitate or worsen heart failure and include NSAIDs (which can also attenuate the efficacy and increase the toxicity of diuretics and ACE inhibitors), glucocorticoids, rosiglitazone, and pioglitazone.

Diagnostic Criteria

No single diagnostic test for heart failure exists; rather, the diagnosis is a clinical one based on history, signs and symptoms, and physical examination. A thorough history and physical examination are important for identifying cardiac and noncardiac disorders or be-

haviors (e.g., diet, adherence to medications) that may cause or hasten the progression of heart failure.

A rapid bedside assay for B-type natriuretic peptide (BNP) often is used in acute care settings (e.g., emergency departments) as an aid in the diagnosis of suspected heart failure. BNP is synthesized and released from the ventricles in response to pressure or volume overload. BNP counteracts increased sympathetic nervous system activity and renin–angiotensin–aldosterone system activity by increasing diuresis, renal sodium excretion, and vasodilation. The degree of elevation of BNP correlates with prognosis. The BNP assay is useful for differentiating between heart failure exacerbations and other causes of dyspnea, such as chronic obstructive pulmonary disease (COPD), asthma, or infection). Patients with dyspnea secondary to heart failure will have elevated plasma BNP concentrations.

The echocardiogram is one of the most useful diagnostic tests in patients with heart failure.

Patients with a left ventricular ejection fraction (LVEF) less than 40% generally are considered to have systolic dysfunction. LVEF can be determined by an echocardiogram, by nuclear imaging scans, or during a cardiac catheterization. Note that, in general, there is a poor correlation between LVEF and symptoms.

Treatment Principles and Goals of Therapy

The goals of therapy include improving the patient's quality of life, reducing symptoms, reducing hospitalizations for heart failure exacerbations, slowing progression of the disease, and improving survival.

ACC–AHA guidelines for heart failure treatment according to stage are shown in Figure 9-1. In stages A and B, therapy primarily is targeted toward prevention of heart failure development; in stages C and D, however, the focus is targeted toward treatment of patients with symptomatic heart failure.

An algorithm for treatment of patients with ADHF is shown in Figure 9-2.

9-2. Drug Therapy of Heart Failure

The following section on drug therapy focuses on treatment of patients with stage C heart failure (i.e., patients with left ventricular dysfunction with current or prior symptoms). This drug therapy commonly is referred to as *outpatient treatment*. Patients with stage C heart failure should be routinely managed with a combination of three drugs: a diuretic (if needed to control volume retention), an ACE inhibitor,

Figure 9-1. American College of Cardiology–American Heart Association Stages of Heart Failure and Recommended Therapy by Stage

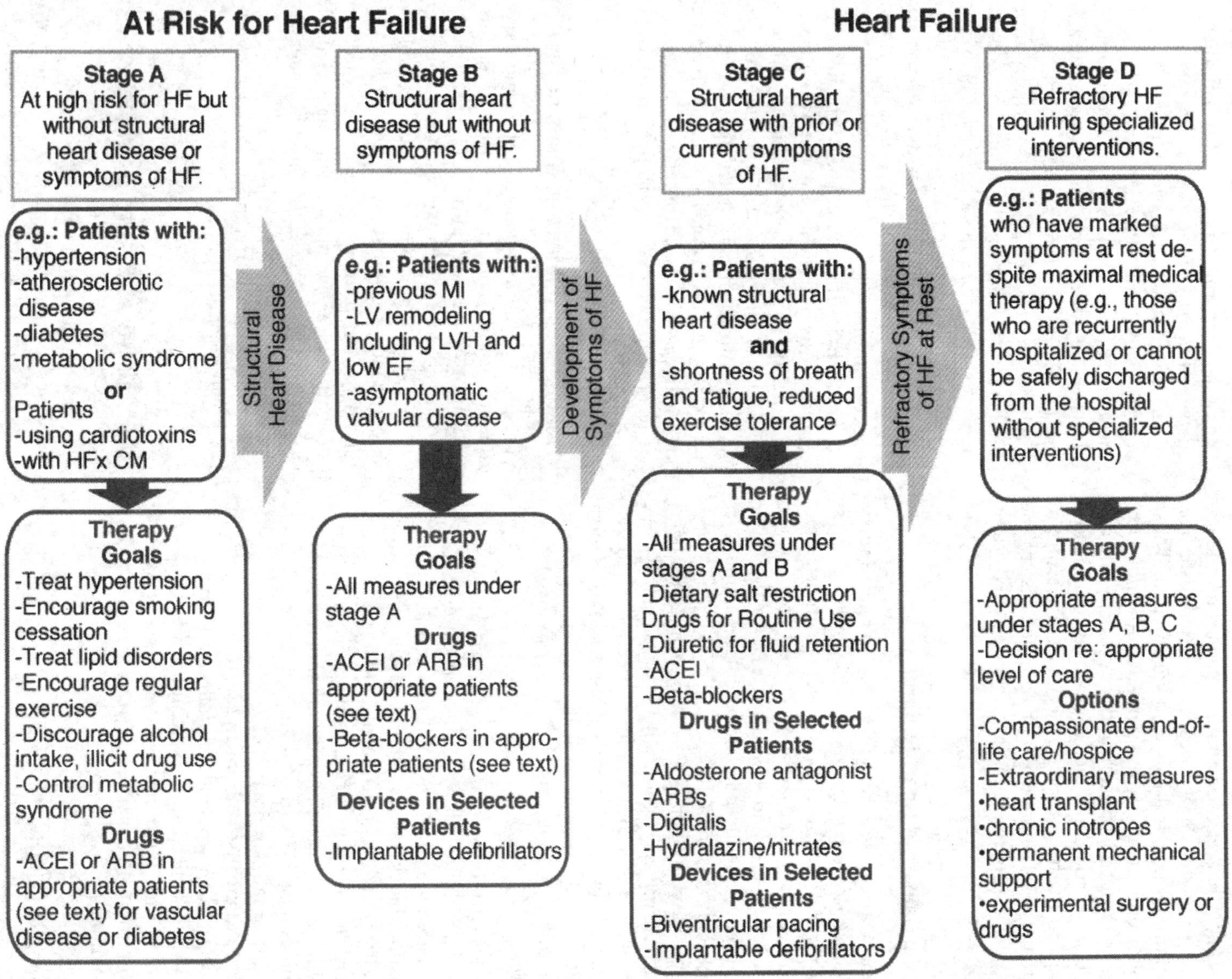

Heart Failure

At Risk for Heart Failure

Stage A
At high risk for HF but without structural heart disease or symptoms of HF.

e.g.: Patients with:
- hypertension
- atherosclerotic disease
- diabetes
- metabolic syndrome

or

Patients
- using cardiotoxins
- with HFx CM

→ **Therapy Goals**
- Treat hypertension
- Encourage smoking cessation
- Treat lipid disorders
- Encourage regular exercise
- Discourage alcohol intake, illicit drug use
- Control metabolic syndrome

Drugs
- ACEI or ARB in appropriate patients (see text) for vascular disease or diabetes

Structural Heart Disease →

Stage B
Structural heart disease but without symptoms of HF.

e.g.: Patients with:
- previous MI
- LV remodeling including LVH and low EF
- asymptomatic valvular disease

→ **Therapy Goals**
- All measures under stage A

Drugs
- ACEI or ARB in appropriate patients (see text)
- Beta-blockers in appropriate patients (see text)

Devices in Selected Patients
- Implantable defibrillators

Development of Symptoms of HF →

Stage C
Structural heart disease with prior or current symptoms of HF.

e.g.: Patients with:
- known structural heart disease

and

- shortness of breath and fatigue, reduced exercise tolerance

→ **Therapy Goals**
- All measures under stages A and B
- Dietary salt restriction

Drugs for Routine Use
- Diuretic for fluid retention
- ACEI
- Beta-blockers

Drugs in Selected Patients
- Aldosterone antagonist
- ARBs
- Digitalis
- Hydralazine/nitrates

Devices in Selected Patients
- Biventricular pacing
- Implantable defibrillators

Refractory Symptoms of HF at Rest →

Stage D
Refractory HF requiring specialized interventions.

e.g.: Patients
who have marked symptoms at rest despite maximal medical therapy (e.g., those who are recurrently hospitalized or cannot be safely discharged from the hospital without specialized interventions)

→ **Therapy Goals**
- Appropriate measures under stages A, B, C
- Decision re: appropriate level of care

Options
- Compassionate end-of-life care/hospice
- Extraordinary measures
  • heart transplant
  • chronic inotropes
  • permanent mechanical support
  • experimental surgery or drugs

Hunt et al., 2005.

Figure 9-2. Acute Decompensated Heart Failure

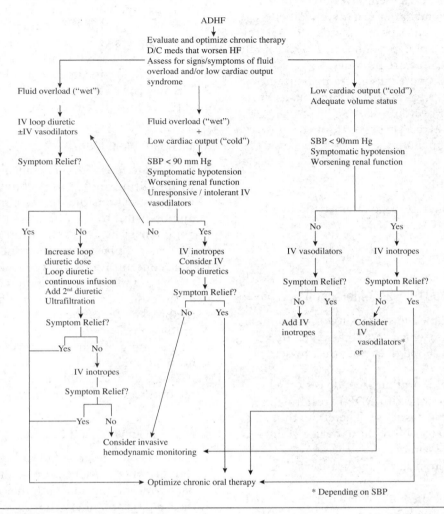

SBP, systolic blood pressure; D/C, discontinue.
Parker et al., 2008.

and a β-blocker. Drug therapies that can be considered in selected patients include angiotensin II receptor blockers (ARBs), digoxin, aldosterone antagonists, and hydralazine-isosorbide dinitrate.

Loop Diuretics

Only patients with signs or symptoms of volume overload will need diuretic therapy. Most heart failure patients require use of the more potent loop diuretics versus thiazide diuretics (Table 9-1).

Mechanism of action

Loop diuretics reduce the sodium and fluid retention associated with heart failure by inhibiting reabsorption of sodium and chloride in the loop of Henle.

Patient instructions and counseling

- Patients allergic to sulfa-containing medications also may be allergic to loop diuretics.
- Patients should take medication once a day in the morning, or, if taking twice daily, take in the morning and afternoon.

Table 9-1. Loop Diuretics

Generic name	Trade name	Dosage form	Dosage range and frequency
Furosemide	Lasix	Oral tablet	20.0–160.0 mg qd bid
Bumetanide	Bumex	Oral tablet	0.5–5.0 mg qd bid
Torsemide	Demadex	Oral tablet	10.0–100.0 mg qd bid

- Loop diuretics can cause frequent urination.
- Patients should weigh themselves daily (preferably in the morning, after urinating). Patients who gain more than 1 pound per day for several consecutive days or 3–5 pounds in a week should contact their health care provider.
- Patients should report muscle cramps, dizziness, excessive thirst, weakness, or confusion, as those may be signs of overdiuresis.
- Patients should avoid sun exposure or use sunscreen when taking loop diuretics.

Adverse drug events

- Electrolyte depletion: hypokalemia and hypomagnesemia
- Hypotension
- Renal insufficiency

Drug–drug and drug–disease interactions

- Food decreases the bioavailability of furosemide and bumetanide, which should be taken on an empty stomach. Food does not affect torsemide absorption.
- The absorption of oral furosemide is slowed significantly in patients with ADHF, resulting in decreased diuretic response. Therefore, those individuals usually will require the use of intravenous (IV) furosemide.
- NSAIDs may diminish the medication's diuretic effect.
- Potassium supplementation may not be required in patients also receiving ACE inhibitors, ARBs, or aldosterone antagonists.

Parameters to monitor

- Serum sodium, potassium, magnesium, creatinine, and blood urea nitrogen (BUN)
- Patient weight (a loss of 0.5–1.0 kg daily is desired until the patient achieves the desired dry weight)
- Urine output
- Blood pressure
- Jugular venous distension
- Improvement in heart failure symptoms (dyspnea and peripheral edema)

Kinetics

Bioavailability of torsemide is not affected by food and is less variable than that of furosemide.

Angiotensin-Converting Enzyme Inhibitors

Angiotensin-converting enzyme inhibitors (ACEIs) are recommended for all patients with current or prior symptoms of heart failure and reduced LVEF, unless contraindicated (Table 9-2). Clinical trials in more than 7,000 patients consistently demonstrate that ACEIs alleviate symptoms, improve clinical status and quality of life, and improve mortality.

Mechanism of action

- ACEIs interfere with the renin–angiotensin system by inhibiting angiotensin-converting enzyme, which is responsible for the conversion of angiotensin I to the potent vasoconstrictor angiotensin II. That inhibition results in a decrease in plasma angiotensin II and aldosterone concentrations, thus reducing the adverse effects of those neurohormones. Inhibition of angiotensin-converting enzyme also prevents the breakdown of the endogenous vasodilator bradykinin.
- ACEIs improve heart failure symptoms and reduce hospitalizations for heart failure.
- ACEIs reduce mortality by 20%–30% and slow the progression of heart failure.

Patient instructions and counseling

- Patients who are pregnant or breast-feeding should not take ACEIs. If patients become pregnant while taking an ACEI, they should contact their physician immediately.
- Captopril should be taken on an empty stomach, either 1 hour before or 2 hours after meals.

Table 9-2. Angiotensin-Converting Enzyme Inhibitors

Generic name	Trade name	Dosage form	Dosage range and frequency
Captopril	Capoten	Oral tablet	6.25–50.0 mg tid
Enalapril	Vasotec	Oral tablet	2.5–20.0 mg bid
Fosinopril	Monopril	Oral tablet	5.0–40.0 mg qd
Lisinopril	Zestril, Prinivil	Oral tablet	2.5–40.0 mg qd
Quinapril	Accupril	Oral tablet	10.0–40.0 mg bid
Ramipril	Altace	Oral capsule	2.5–5.0 mg bid
Perindopril	Aceon	Oral tablet	2.0–16.0 mg qd
Trandolapril	Mavik	Oral tablet	0.5–4.0 mg qd

- Salt substitutes that contain potassium should be used cautiously.
- Patients should call their physician immediately if they experience swelling of the face, eyes, lips, tongue, arms, or legs or if they have difficulty breathing or swallowing.
- ACEIs may cause cough.

Adverse drug events

- Hypotension
- Dizziness
- Renal insufficiency
- Cough
- Angioedema
- Hyperkalemia
- Rash
- Taste disturbances

Drug–drug and drug–disease interactions

- NSAIDs can increase the risk of renal insufficiency and attenuate the beneficial effects of ACEIs.
- Potassium supplements or potassium-sparing diuretics should be used with caution.
- Cyclosporine and tacrolimus may increase the risk of nephrotoxicity and hyperkalemia.
- Diuretics increase the risk of hypotension.

Parameters to monitor

- Blood pressure
- Renal function (i.e., serum BUN and creatinine)
- Serum potassium
- Heart failure symptoms
- Dose (initiate therapy at low doses; if lower doses are tolerated well, follow with gradual increases)

Other

ACEIs are pregnancy category C during the first trimester and pregnancy category D during the second and third trimesters. ACEIs can cause fetal and neonatal morbidity and death when administered to pregnant women.

Angiotensin Receptor Blockers

ACEIs remain the drugs of choice for inhibiting the renin–angiotensin–aldosterone system in patients with chronic heart failure. Recent clinical trials confirm the efficacy and safety of candesartan and valsartan in the treatment of heart failure. Whether other ARBs are equally effective in the treatment of heart failure is unknown. Current guidelines recommend candesartan or valsartan for patients that are intolerant to ACEIs—both of those agents are approved for use in patients with heart failure. Intolerance to ACEIs is most often due to cough or angioedema, although caution is advised when using ARBs in patients that have angioedema secondary to an ACEI. Note that ARBs are just as likely as ACEIs to cause impaired renal function, hyperkalemia, or hypotension (Table 9-3).

Mechanism of action

- ARBs interfere with the renin–angiotensin system by blocking the angiotensin-1 receptor, thereby attenuating the detrimental effects of this hormone.
- Unlike ACEIs, ARBs do not affect the kinin system and thus are not associated with cough.
- ARBs reduce hospitalizations and improve survival.

Patient instructions and counseling

- Patients who are pregnant or breast-feeding should not take ARBs. If a patient becomes pregnant while taking an ARB, she should contact her physician immediately.
- Use salt substitutes that contain potassium cautiously.
- Dizziness or light-headedness may occur, especially in patients taking diuretics.

Adverse drug events

- Hypotension
- Dizziness
- Renal insufficiency
- Hyperkalemia

Drug–drug and drug–disease interactions

- Potassium supplements or potassium-sparing diuretics should be used with caution.
- Diuretics increase the risk of hypotension.

Table 9-3. Angiotensin Receptor Blockers

Generic name	Trade name	Dosage form	Dosage range and frequency
Candesartan	Atacand	Oral tablet	4–32 mg qd
Valsartan	Diovan	Oral tablet	20–160 mg bid

Parameters to monitor

- Blood pressure
- Renal function (i.e., serum BUN and creatinine)
- Serum potassium
- Heart failure symptoms
- Dose (initiate therapy at low doses; if lower doses are tolerated well, follow with gradual increases)

Other

- ARBs are pregnancy category C during the first trimester and pregnancy category D during the second and third trimesters. ARBs can cause fetal and neonatal morbidity and death when administered to pregnant women.

β-Blockers

Because of their negative inotropic effects, β-blockers once were considered to be contraindicated in patients with heart failure. However, by inhibiting the deleterious effects of long-term activation of the sympathetic nervous system in heart failure, β-blockers repeatedly have been shown to provide hemodynamic, symptomatic, and survival benefits. Metoprolol succinate (extended-release metoprolol), bisoprolol, and carvedilol all have been shown to be effective, and one of those three agents should be used for the treatment of heart failure (Table 9-4).

Mechanism of action

- Blockade of β-receptors antagonizes the increase in sympathetic nervous system activity that is one of the important mechanisms responsible for the progression of heart failure. Bisoprolol and metoprolol succinate are β_1-selective agents, whereas carvedilol blocks β_1-, β_2-, and α_1-receptors. Whether those differences in pharmacologic actions have any important effects on outcomes for patients with heart failure remains uncertain.
- Treatment with β-blockers reduces symptoms, improves clinical status, and decreases the risk of death and hospitalization.
- One of the three β-blockers that have been shown to reduce mortality (bisoprolol, carvedilol, and extended-release metoprolol succinate) should be used in all stable patients with current or prior heart failure symptoms and reduced LVEF, unless contraindicated.
- In general, β-blockers should be used in combination with ACEIs and diuretics.

Patient instructions and counseling

- β-blockers may cause fluid retention or worsening of heart failure upon initiation of therapy or after an increase in dose. Patients should report any cases of body or leg swelling or increased shortness of breath. Patients should weigh themselves daily; if they gain more than 1 pound per day for several consecutive days or 3–5 pounds in a week, they should contact their health care provider.
- Fatigue or weakness may occur in the first few weeks of treatment but usually will resolve spontaneously.
- Patients should report any cases of dizziness, lightheadedness, or blurred vision, which may be caused by the patient's blood pressure being too low or from bradycardia or heart block.
- Patients should take carvedilol with food.
- It is important not to miss doses or stop taking these medications abruptly.
- In patients with diabetes, β-blockers may cause an increase in blood sugar, possibly masking the signs of hypoglycemia (except for sweating).

Adverse drug events

A list of adverse events most commonly observed in heart failure patients receiving β-blockers follows. For other adverse effects of β-blockers, see the chapters on hypertension and ischemic heart disease.

- Fluid retention and worsening heart failure
- Fatigue
- Bradycardia and heart block
- Hypotension
- Abrupt withdrawal can lead to hypertension, tachycardia, or myocardial ischemia

Table 9-4. β-Blockers

Generic name	Trade name	Dosage form	Dosage range and frequency
Bisoprolol	Zebeta	Oral tablet	1.25–10.0 mg qd bid
Carvedilol	Coreg	Oral tablet	3.125–50.0 mg bid
Carvedilol	Coreg CR	Oral capsule	10.0–80.0 mg qd
Metoprolol succinate extended-release	Toprol-XL	Oral tablet	12.5–200.0 mg qd

Drug–drug and drug–disease interactions

- Amiodarone and calcium channel blockers (verapamil and diltiazem) can increase the risk of bradycardia, heart block, and hypotension.
- Quinidine, fluoxetine, paroxetine, and other inhibitors of cytochrome P4502D6 inhibit hepatic metabolism of metoprolol and carvedilol and may result in increased plasma concentrations and enhanced effects.
- Concomitant use of ophthalmic β-blockers may increase the risk of bradycardia, heart block, and hypotension.
- β-blockers may cause bronchoconstriction in patients with asthma or COPD.
- Do not use β-blockers in patients with symptomatic bradycardia or heart block unless a pacemaker is present.
- β-blockers may worsen blood glucose control in diabetics and mask the signs of hypoglycemia.

Parameters to monitor

- Blood pressure and heart rate
- Heart failure symptoms
- Weight (daily)

Kinetics

- Bisoprolol is eliminated about 50% by the kidneys, so dosage adjustment may be required in patients with renal insufficiency.
- Both metoprolol and carvedilol are metabolized by the liver.

Other

- Patients must be stable (i.e., minimal evidence of fluid overload or volume retention) before β-blocker treatment is initiated.
- Treatment should be initiated with low doses and titrated slowly upward until the target dose is reached. Doses usually are increased no more frequently than every 2 weeks, with close monitoring of symptoms required during the titration period.
- Fluid accumulation during dose titration usually can be managed by adjusting diuretic doses.
- Staggering the schedule of other heart failure medications that lower blood pressure (e.g., ACEIs and diuretics) may help reduce the risk of hypotension.
- A recent study comparing the effects of carvedilol with immediate-release metoprolol (metoprolol tartrate) in patients with heart failure found that survival is improved in patients receiving carvedilol. Whether carvedilol is superior to extended-release metoprolol (metoprolol succinate) is unknown. However, these results strongly suggest that only β-blockers proven to improve survival (carvedilol, metoprolol succinate, and bisoprolol) should be used in patients with heart failure.

Aldosterone Antagonists

Elevated plasma aldosterone plays an important detrimental role in the pathophysiology and progression of heart failure. Although short-term treatment with ACEIs or ARBs lowers circulating aldosterone concentrations, that suppression is not sustained with long-term therapy. In low doses, the aldosterone antagonists spironolactone and eplerenone reduce the risk of death and hospitalization in patients with moderate to severe heart failure. Current guidelines recommend the addition of aldosterone antagonists in patients with moderately severe to severe symptoms of heart failure and reduced LVEF that can be monitored closely for renal function and serum potassium (Table 9-5).

Mechanism of action

Antagonism of aldosterone results in reduced renal potassium excretion.

Patient instructions and counseling

- Potassium-containing salt substitutes should be avoided.
- Patients should call their physician immediately if they experience muscle weakness or cramps; numbness or tingling in hands, feet, or lips; or slow or irregular heartbeat.
- Spironolactone may cause swollen or painful breasts in men.

Adverse drug events

- Hyperkalemia
- Gynecomastia (only with spironolactone)
- Irregular menses

Table 9-5. Aldosterone Antagonists

Generic name	Trade name	Dosage form	Dosage range and frequency
Spironolactone	Aldactone	Oral tablet	12.5–50.0 mg qd or qod
Eplerenone	Inspra	Oral tablet	25.0–50.0 mg qd

Drug–drug and drug–disease interactions

- ACEIs, ARBs, and NSAIDs increase the risk of hyperkalemia.
- Spironolactone can increase digoxin plasma concentrations.
- Potassium supplements increase the risk of hyperkalemia. Supplements should not be used if serum potassium exceeds 3.5 mEq/L.
- Elderly patients and patients with diabetes are at an increased risk of hyperkalemia.
- Erythromycin, clarithromycin, verapamil, ketoconazole, fluconazole, itraconazole, and other inhibitors of cytochrome P450 3A4 inhibit hepatic metabolism of eplerenone and may result in increased plasma concentrations and enhanced effects.

Parameters to monitor

- Serum creatinine should be less than 2.5 mg/dL in men or less than 2.0 mg/dL in women before therapy is initiated.
- Serum potassium should be less than 5.0 mEq/L before therapy is initiated. Potassium should be evaluated three days after therapy is started, again one week after therapy is started, and at least monthly for the first three months of therapy.

Digoxin

Unlike ACEIs or β-blockers, digoxin does not improve mortality but does appear to produce symptomatic benefits (Table 9-6).

Mechanism of action

- Digoxin inhibits the Na^+-K^+-ATPase pump, which results in an increase in intracellular calcium that, in turn, causes a positive inotropic effect.
- Recent evidence indicates that digoxin reduces sympathetic outflow from the central nervous system, thus blunting the excessive sympathetic activation that occurs in heart failure. Those effects occur at low plasma concentrations, where little positive inotropic effect is seen.

Patient instructions and counseling

Patients should report any of the following to their health care provider:

- Dizziness, lightheadedness, or fatigue
- Changes in vision (blurred or yellow vision)
- Irregular heartbeat
- Loss of appetite
- Nausea, vomiting, or diarrhea

Adverse drug events

Major adverse effects involve three systems:

- Cardiovascular (cardiac arrhythmias, bradycardia, and heart block)
- Gastrointestinal (anorexia, abdominal pain, nausea, and vomiting)
- Neurological (visual disturbances, disorientation, confusion, and fatigue)

Toxicity typically is associated with serum digoxin concentrations >2 ng/mL but may occur at lower levels in elderly patients and in patients with hypokalemia or hypomagnesemia.

Drug–drug and drug–disease interactions

The following drugs increase serum digoxin concentrations:

- Quinidine, verapamil, and amiodarone (the dose of digoxin should be decreased by 50% if these medications are added)
- Propafenone
- Flecainide
- Macrolide antibiotics (erythromycin and clarithromycin)
- Itraconazole and ketoconazole
- Spironolactone
- Cyclosporine

Drugs that decrease serum digoxin concentrations include:

- Antacids
- Cholestyramine and colestipol
- Kaolin-pectin
- Metoclopramide

Table 9-6. Digoxin

Generic name	Trade name	Dosage form	Dosage range and frequency
Digoxin	Lanoxin	Oral tablet, IV, elixir	0.125–0.25 mg qd
Digoxin	Lanoxicaps	Oral capsule	0.1–0.2 mg qd

Diuretics increase the risk of digoxin toxicity in the presence of hypokalemia or hypomagnesemia.

Digoxin clearance is reduced in patients with renal insufficiency (see section on kinetics).

Parameters to monitor

- Digoxin serum concentration
  - There is little relationship between serum digoxin concentration and therapeutic effects in heart failure.
  - Current guidelines suggest a target range of 0.5–1.0 ng/mL.
- Heart rate
- Serum potassium and magnesium
- Renal function (serum BUN and creatinine)
- Heart failure symptoms

Kinetics

See Table 9-7 for information about the pharmacokinetics of digoxin. Note the following:

- Approximately 60%–80% of the dose is eliminated unchanged in the kidney; therefore, dosage adjustment is required in patients with renal insufficiency.
- Lower doses (0.125 mg daily or every other day) should be used in the elderly or in patients with a low lean body mass.
- No loading dose is needed in the treatment of heart failure.
- Because of the long distribution phase after either oral or intravenous digoxin administration, blood samples for determination of serum digoxin concentrations should be collected at least 6 and preferably 12 hours or more after the last dose.

Table 9-7. Digoxin Pharmacokinetics

Oral bioavailability

Tablets	0.50–0.90 (average 0.65)
Elixir	0.75–0.85 (average 0.80)
Capsules	0.90–1.00 (average 0.95)

Elimination half-life

Normal renal function	36 hours
Anuric patients	5 days
Volume of distribution	7 L/kg
Fraction excreted unchanged in urine	0.65–0.70

Hydralazine–Isosorbide Dinitrate

Hydralazine and isosorbide dinitrate initially were combined because of complementary hemodynamic actions. An early clinical trial reported reduced mortality with this combination when compared with placebo. A comparison with an ACEI, however, showed that the ACEI was superior to hydralazine–isosorbide dinitrate. Adverse effects with the combination are common (primarily headache, dizziness, and gastrointestinal complaints), and those effects lead many patients to discontinue therapy. Current guidelines indicate that hydralazine-isosorbide dinitrate can be considered as a therapeutic option in patients who cannot be given an ACEI or an ARB because of drug intolerance, hypotension, or renal insufficiency.

A recent clinical trial found that the hydralazine–isosorbide dinitrate combination, when added to standard background therapy (ACEIs or ARBs, β-blockers, diuretics, digoxin), reduced mortality in African Americans with heart failure by 40% compared with placebo. Whether those benefits are specific to African Americans is unclear. The current heart failure treatment guidelines indicate that the addition of hydralazine–isosorbide dinitrate is a reasonable therapy in patients with reduced LVEF and persistent heart failure symptoms despite therapy with ACEIs and β-blockers.

A fixed-dose combination product is now available (BiDil).

9-3. Drug Therapy for Acute Decompensated Heart Failure

Patients with ADHF usually are admitted to the hospital for aggressive treatment with IV diuretics, vasodilators (see Table 9-8), or positive inotropic drugs (see Table 9-9). When such patients have hypotension in addition to low cardiac output, they are said to have cardiogenic shock. In those severe cases, therapy may be guided by invasive hemodynamic monitoring. Treatment goals include reducing volume overload and improving cardiac output. The approach to treatment is dictated by the patient's hemodynamic profile.

Warm and Dry

- No specific therapy is needed.

Warm and Wet

- The goal is to reduce volume overload and minimize congestive symptoms.

Table 9-8. Vasodilators

Generic name	Trade name	Mechanism of action	Dose[a]	Adverse effects and comments
Nitroprusside	Nipride	Arterial and venous dilator	Initial dose 0.1–0.25 mcg/kg/min and titrate to response	Hypotension, headache, tachycardia, cyanide and thiocyanate toxicity, myocardial ischemia
Nitroglycerin	Nitro-Bid, Nitrostat	Venous dilator but also an arterial dilator at higher doses	Initial dose 5–10 mcg/min and titrate to response	Hypotension, headache, tachycardia, tolerance to hemodynamic effects
Nesiritide	Natrecor	B-type natriuretic peptide that increases diuresis and is an arterial and venous dilator	Initially 2 mcg/kg bolus followed by 0.01 mcg/kg/min infusion; can increase to 0.03 mcg/kg/min	Hypotension, headache when used in combination with diuretics

a. All are given by continuous IV infusion.

Table 9-9. Inotropes

Generic name	Trade name	Mechanism of action	Dose[a]	Adverse effects and comments
Dopamine	Intropin	Dose-dependent agonist of dopamine, β-, and α_1-receptors	0–3 mcg/kg/min: stimulates dopamine receptors; may improve urine output. 3–10 mcg/kg/min: stimulates β_1- and β_2-receptors to increase cardiac output. > 10 mcg/kg/min: stimulates α_1-receptors to increase blood pressure	Increases heart rate, contractility, myocardial oxygen demand, myocardial ischemia, arrhythmias, and systemic vascular resistance; should be used only in patients with marked systemic hypotension or cardiogenic shock
Dobutamine	Dobutrex	β_1- and β_2-receptor agonist and weak α_1 agonist; increases cardiac output and vasodilates	2.5–20.0 mcg/kg/min	Increases heart rate, contractility, myocardial oxygen demand, myocardial ischemia, arrhythmias; not useful to increase blood pressure in hypotensive patients
Milrinone	Primacor	Inhibits phosphodiesterase III, resulting in positive inotropic and vasodilating effects	50 mcg/kg loading dose over 10 min, followed by 0.375 mcg/kg/min; can titrate to 0.75 mcg/kg/min on basis of response	Arrhythmias, hypotension, and headache; is an alternative to patients not responding to dobutamine or dopamine; may be useful for patients receiving β-blockers because its positive inotropic effects are not mediated by β-receptors; adjust dose in patients with renal insufficiency; preferred over inamrinone because of decreased risk of thrombocytopenia

a. All are given by continuous IV infusion.

- IV loop diuretics often are used. For patients who are unresponsive to loop diuretics, the addition of supplemental thiazide diuretics (e.g., metolazone) may be helpful.
- The addition of IV vasodilators (nitroglycerin, nitroprusside, and nesiritide) also can reduce symptoms.
- Inotropic therapy usually is not necessary.

Cold and Dry

- Patients may be clinically stable and often do not present with acute symptoms.
- Rule out volume depletion from overdiuresis as the cause of decreased cardiac output.
- Gradual introduction of β-blockers may be helpful.

Cold and Wet

- Improve cardiac output first (i.e., before removing excess volume).
- Cardiac output can be increased by IV vasodilators or inotropes, or both.
- The relative roles of vasodilators and inotropes in this patient population are controversial.

9-4. Nondrug Therapy

Nondrug therapies include the following:

- Ultrafiltration
- Intra-aortic balloon pump
- Left ventricular assist devices
- Biventricular pacing
- Implantable cardioverter-defibrillator
- Cardiac transplantation

9-5. Key Points

- Heart failure is a clinical syndrome caused by the heart's inability to pump sufficient blood to meet the body's needs.
- Although heart failure has many causes, the most common are coronary artery disease and hypertension.

- Several compensatory mechanisms are activated to help maintain adequate cardiac output; activation of those systems is responsible for heart failure symptoms and contributes to disease progression. Medications that improve patient outcomes antagonize those compensatory mechanisms.
- Drugs that can precipitate or worsen heart failure should be avoided (e.g., NSAIDs, verapamil, and diltiazem).
- All patients with stage C (symptomatic) heart failure should be treated with diuretics, ACEIs, and β-blockers.
- The goal of treatment with diuretics is to eliminate signs of fluid retention, thus minimizing symptoms.
- ACEIs are an integral part of heart failure pharmacotherapy. They improve survival and slow disease progression. ARBs are the preferred alternative for patients who are intolerant to ACEIs.
- β-blockers are recommended for all patients with systolic dysfunction and mild to moderate symptoms. β-blockers improve survival, decrease hospitalizations, and slow disease progression. Bisoprolol, carvedilol, and extended-release metoprolol succinate are agents with proven benefits. They should be started at low doses with slow upward titration to the target dose.
- Digoxin does not improve survival in patients with heart failure but does provide symptomatic benefits. The goal plasma concentration is 0.5–1.0 ng/mL.
- Spironolactone and eplerenone improve survival in patients with moderate to severe heart failure.
- Patients with ADHF often require hospitalization and aggressive therapy with IV diuretics, vasodilators, and positive inotropic drugs.

9-6. Questions

1. Which of the following combinations represents optimal pharmacotherapy of chronic heart failure?

    A. Furosemide, clonidine, hydrochlorothiazide, and propranolol

B. Furosemide, lisinopril, and carvedilol
C. Carvedilol, verapamil, amlodipine, and nesiritide
D. Cardizem, hydrochlorothiazide, digoxin, and sotalol
E. Dobutamine, amiodarone, furosemide, and nitroglycerin

2. Which of the following mechanisms most likely contributes to the benefits of β-blockers in the treatment of heart failure?

A. Stimulation of β_2-receptors
B. Increased heart rate and decreased blood pressure
C. Stimulation of β_1-receptors
D. Blockade of increased sympathetic nervous system activity
E. Blockade of angiotensin II receptors

3. Appropriate monitoring parameters for enalapril therapy in the treatment of heart failure include

I.   serum creatinine.
II. serum potassium.
III. hemoglobin A1c.

A. I only
B. III only
C. I and II only
D. II and III only
E. I, II, and III

4. Patients taking eplerenone for heart failure should avoid taking

A. NSAIDs.
B. ACEIs.
C. β-blockers.
D. Demadex.
E. calcium supplements.

5. All of the following are adverse effects of digoxin *except*

A. nausea.
B. anorexia.
C. confusion.
D. arrhythmias.
E. acute renal failure.

6. Heart failure may be exacerbated by which of the following medications?

I.   Naproxen
II. Glipizide
III. Crestor

A. I only
B. III only
C. I and II only
D. II and III only
E. I, II, and III

7. Cough is an adverse effect associated with which of the following medications?

A. Ramipril
B. Valsartan
C. Carvedilol
D. Torsemide
E. Eplerenone

8. Which of the following ACEIs has the shortest duration of action?

A. Ramipril
B. Captopril
C. Lisinopril
D. Monopril
E. Fosinopril

9. Which of the following adverse effects of lisinopril can be avoided by switching to candesartan?

I.   Hypotension
II. Renal insufficiency
III. Hyperkalemia
IV. Cough

A. I, II, and III
B. I and III only
C. II and III only
D. III only
E. IV only

10. A significant interaction can occur if digoxin is administered with

A. Biaxin.
B. fosinopril.
C. glyburide.
D. Lipitor.
E. warfarin.

11. All of the following medications can cause bradycardia *except*

A. carvedilol.
B. amiodarone.

C. digoxin.
D. verapamil.
E. dobutamine.

12. Which of the following is contraindicated in patients with a history of lisinopril-induced angioedema?

    A. Captopril
    B. Torsemide
    C. Spironolactone
    D. Milrinone
    E. Carvedilol

13. Nesiritide would be indicated in

    A. patients with asymptomatic left ventricular dysfunction.
    B. patients with acute decompensated heart failure not responsive to IV diuretics.
    C. patients with stage B heart failure.
    D. patients with type 2 diabetes.
    E. patients intolerant to digoxin.

14. All of the following are true about the use of furosemide in heart failure *except*

    A. the drug reduces mortality and slows heart failure progression.
    B. hypokalemia is a common adverse effect.
    C. response can be evaluated by monitoring patient weight.
    D. oral absorption is slowed in patients with acute decompensated heart failure.
    E. furosemide's bioavailability is reduced by food.

15. Which of the following is an important consideration when using β-blockers for treating heart failure?

    A. They are effective only in post–myocardial infarction patients.
    B. All β-blockers are equally effective for the treatment of heart failure.
    C. Therapy should be initiated at the target dose.
    D. Patients with fluid overload are the optimal candidates for initiating therapy.
    E. Therapy should be initiated at low doses and titrated upward slowly.

16. The dose of which of the following medications should be reduced in patients with renal insufficiency?

    A. Metoprolol
    B. Carvedilol
    C. Digoxin
    D. Nitroglycerin
    E. Dobutamine

17. Which of the following is true regarding digoxin therapy in patients with chronic heart failure?

    A. Digoxin reduces mortality.
    B. Concomitant amiodarone therapy decreases digoxin plasma concentrations.
    C. Digoxin is contraindicated in patients with heart failure and atrial fibrillation.
    D. The target digoxin plasma concentration is 0.5–1.0 ng/mL.
    E. Concomitant glyburide therapy increases digoxin plasma concentrations.

18. Which of the following β-blockers also blocks α_1-receptors and is effective for treating heart failure?

    A. Metoprolol
    B. Carvedilol
    C. Bisoprolol
    D. Propranolol
    E. Atenolol

19. Patients with heart failure who experience fluid retention after β-blocker initiation should have

    A. the β-blocker dose increased.
    B. the digoxin dose increased.
    C. the β-blocker discontinued.
    D. the ACEI discontinued.
    E. their diuretic dose adjusted.

20. Which of the following is correct regarding the treatment of ADHF?

    A. Nesiritide is the agent of choice in patients with ADHF and hypotension.
    B. Milrinone is preferred over dobutamine in patients receiving concomitant β-blocker therapy.
    C. Absorption of oral loop diuretics is increased.
    D. Dobutamine and milrinone improve survival.
    E. Verapamil reduces volume overload and improves cardiac output.

Use Patient Profile 1 to answer questions 21 and 22.

21. Which of the following medications should be added to Mr. Johnson's regimen?

   A. Lisinopril and carvedilol
   B. Valsartan and prazosin
   C. Torsemide and amlodipine
   D. Verapamil and amiodarone
   E. Clonidine and hydrochlorothiazide

22. Mr. Johnson's serum potassium level of 2.0 mEq/L (normal 4.0–5.0 mEq/L) could

   A. increase the risk of Lanoxin toxicity.
   B. be treated by increasing the dose of Lasix.
   C. be considered a side effect of therapy with EC aspirin.
   D. be caused by an interaction between Zocor and Lanoxin.
   E. increase the risk of bleeding from Plavix.

Patient Profile 1

Patient Name	William Johnson		
Age	64	Height	5'11"
Sex	Male	Weight	185 lbs
Allergies	NKA		

DIAGNOSIS   Myocardial infarction 2008

                   Hypertension

                   Heart failure

                   Hyperlipidemia

LABORATORY AND DIAGNOSTIC TESTS

    Echocardiogram in 12/08 showed LVEF 30%

    Blood pressure on 4/1/09: 145/90 mm Hg

    Heart rate on 4/1/09: 88 bpm

    Lipid profile on 4/1/09:

        Total cholesterol, 160 mg/dL

        LDL cholesterol, 95 mg/dL

        HDL cholesterol, 50 mg/dL

        Triglycerides, 100 mg/dL

        Serum potassium, 2.0 mEq/L

MEDICATION RECORD

Date	Rx #	Physician	Drug/Strength	Quantity	Sig	Refills
4/1	1000	Smith	Lanoxin 0.125 mg	90	1 tab qd	2
4/1	1001	Smith	Lasix 40 mg	60	1 tab q am	3
4/1	1002	Smith	KCl 20 mEq	90	1 tab q am	1
4/1	1003	Smith	Zocor 40 mg	90	1 tab qhs	3
4/1	1004	Smith	EC aspirin 325 mg	90	1 tab q am	2
4/1	1005	Smith	Plavix 75 mg	90	1 tab q am	3

Use Hospital Inpatient Profile 2 to answer questions 23 and 24.

23. According to her profile, the recent worsening of Mrs. Smith's heart failure most likely is related to

    A. Zestril.
    B. naproxen.
    C. subtherapeutic serum digoxin concentration.
    D. furosemide.

E. drug interaction between Zestril and furosemide.

24. Toprol-XL is an agent that

    A. is contraindicated in heart failure.
    B. blocks β_1-, β_2-, and α_1-receptors.
    C. blocks only β_1-receptors.
    D. should not be used in combination with Zestril.
    E. increases the serum digoxin concentration.

Hospital Inpatient Profile 2

Patient Name	Ellen Smith		
Age	71	Height	5'4"
Sex	Female	Weight	150 lbs
Allergies	NKA		

DIAGNOSIS   Heart failure exacerbation with 20-lb weight gain over last 3–4 weeks

Hypertension

Osteoarthritis

LABORATORY AND DIAGNOSTIC TESTS

Echocardiogram in 2/09 showed LVEF 25%

Blood pressure on 4/1/09: 130/85 mm Hg

Heart rate on 4/1/09: 80 bpm

Serum digoxin concentration on 4/1/09: 0.8 ng/mL

MEDICATION RECORD

Date	Rx #	Physician	Drug/Strength	Quantity	Sig	Refills
2/1	100	Jones	Lanoxin 0.125 mg	90	1 tab qd	2
3/1	101	Jones	Furosemide 80 mg	60	1 tab q am	3
1/4	102	Jones	Zestril 20 mg	90	1 tab q am	1
1/4	103	Jones	Toprol-XL 50 mg	90	1 tab qd	3
3/1	104	Nelson	Naproxen 500 mg	90	1 tab bid with food	3

9-7. Answers

1. **B.** Furosemide, lisinopril (an ACEI), and carvedilol (a β-blocker) in combination should be used routinely in patients with heart failure.

2. **D.** Activation of the sympathetic nervous system plays an important role in the initiation and progression of heart failure. The benefits of β-blockers are thought to be due to the blockade of the sympathetic nervous system's increased activity.

3. **C.** Enalapril, as well as other ACEIs, can cause renal insufficiency and an increase in serum potassium. Thus, serum creatinine and potassium should be monitored.

4. **A.** Use of eplerenone is associated with renal potassium retention. Concomitant use of NSAIDs significantly increases the risk of hyperkalemia.

5. **E.** Nausea, anorexia, confusion, and arrhythmias all are common signs and symptoms of digoxin toxicity. Digoxin does not affect renal function.

6. **A.** Naproxen, an NSAID, can worsen heart failure (1) by increasing renal sodium and water retention and (2) by attenuating the efficacy and enhancing the toxicity of ACEIs and diuretics. Neither glipizide nor Crestor affects heart failure.

7. **A.** Cough is frequently encountered as an adverse effect of ACEIs.

8. **B.** Captopril must be given three times daily in patients with heart failure. The other agents can be given once daily.

9. **E.** The angiotensin receptor blocker candesartan is just as likely to cause hypotension, hyperkalemia, and renal insufficiency as is lisinopril (or any other ACEI). Candesartan is an alternative agent for patients intolerant to ACEIs because of cough.

10. **A.** The macrolide antibiotic Biaxin (clarithromycin) is associated with a 50%–100% increase in serum digoxin concentrations.

11. **E.** Dobutamine is a β-receptor agonist and is associated with an increase in heart rate. The other choices listed as possible answers all slow heart rate through various mechanisms.

12. **A.** Lisinopril is an ACEI, and angioedema is a known adverse effect of all agents in that class. Thus, captopril, which also is an ACEI, should not be used in this situation.

13. **B.** Nesiritide is indicated for use only in patients with severe or decompensated heart failure. It must be given intravenously.

14. **A.** Although furosemide plays an important role in patients with heart failure by interfering with sodium and water retention, it provides only symptomatic benefits. Furosemide and other diuretics do not improve survival or affect heart failure progression.

15. **E.** When used to treat heart failure, β-blocker therapy should be started at low doses and gradually titrated upward to the target dose that was shown in clinical trials to improve survival. Starting at the target dose or initiating treatment in patients with fluid overload increases the risk of worsening heart failure. Only carvedilol, bisoprolol, and metoprolol succinate extended-release are proven to be effective in heart failure.

16. **C.** Only digoxin is eliminated by the kidneys.

17. **D.** Current guidelines suggest a target digoxin plasma concentration of 0.5–1.0 ng/mL. Digoxin does not improve survival in patients with heart failure—it only improves symptoms. Amiodarone increases digoxin plasma concentrations; glyburide does not affect digoxin concentrations. Digoxin is useful in the management of patients with heart failure who also have atrial fibrillation.

18. **B.** Only carvedilol blocks α_1-receptors and has been shown to be effective in patients with heart failure.

19. **E.** Some patients with heart failure may experience increases in fluid retention after initiation of β-blocker therapy. Fluid retention typically is managed best by adjusting the diuretic dose and closely monitoring the patient's weight.

20. **B.** The positive inotropic effects of milrinone are not mediated through the β-receptor; therefore, its effects are not diminished by concomitant β-blocker therapy. Nesiritide is associated with an increased risk of hypotension. No inotropic agents are shown to improve survival. Absorption of oral loop diuretics is decreased in ADHF. Verapamil has negative inotropic effects and would worsen volume overload.

21. **A.** An ACEI and β-blocker are indicated in this patient with heart failure to improve survival and slow disease progression.

22. **A.** Hypokalemia increases the risk of digoxin toxicity.

23. **B.** The addition of the NSAID naproxen approximately 3–4 weeks before admission likely is the cause of this episode of ADHF. NSAIDs can increase sodium and water retention and negate the effects of diuretics and ACEIs.

24. **C.** Toprol-XL (metoprolol succinate) is a cardioselective β-blocker. It blocks only the β_1-receptor at usual therapeutic doses.

9-8. References

Adams KF, Lindenfeld J, Arnold JMO, et al. Evaluation and management of patients with acute decompensated heart failure. *J Card Fail*. 2006; 12:e86–103.

Brater DC. Pharmacology of diuretics. *Am J Med Sci*. 2000;319:38–50.

Cohn JN, Tognoni G, for the Valsartan Heart Failure Trial Investigators. A randomized trial of the angiotensin receptor blocker valsartan in chronic heart failure. *N Engl J Med*. 2001;345:1667–75.

Digitalis Investigation Group. The effect of digoxin on mortality and morbidity in patients with heart failure. *N Engl J Med*. 1997;336:525–33.

Effect of metoprolol CR/XL in chronic heart failure: Metoprolol CR/XL randomised intervention trial in congestive heart failure (MERIT-HF). *Lancet*. 1999;353:2001–7.

Gislason GH, Rasmussen JN, Abildstrom SZ, et al. Increased mortality and cardiovascular morbidity associated with use of nonsteroidal anti-inflammatory drugs in chronic heart failure. *Arch Int Med*. 2009;169:141–9.

Hunt SA, Abraham WT, Chin MH, et al. ACC/AHA 2005 guideline update for the diagnosis and management of chronic heart failure in the adult: A report of the American College of Cardiology/American Heart Association Task Force on Practice Guidelines (Writing Committee to update the 2001 guidelines for the evaluation and management of heart failure). *Circulation*. 2005;112:e154–235.

Jessup M, Abraham WT, Casey DE, et al., writing on behalf of the 2005 Guideline Update for the Diagnosis and Management of Chronic Heart Failure in the Adult Writing Committee. 2009 focused update: ACC/AHA guidelines for the diagnosis and management of heart failure in adults—A report of the American College of Cardiology/American Heart Association Task Force on Practice Guidelines. *J Am Coll Cardiol*. 2009;53:1–40.

Packer M, Bristow MR, Cohn JN, et al. The effect of carvedilol on morbidity and mortality in patients with chronic heart failure. *N Engl J Med*. 1996; 334:1349–55.

Parker RB, Rodgers JE, Cavallari LH. Heart failure. In: DiPiro JT, Talbert RL, Yee GC, et al., eds. *Pharmacotherapy: A Pathophysiologic Approach*. 7th ed. New York: McGraw-Hill; 2008:173–216.

Petersen JW, Felker GM. Inotropes in the management of acute heart failure. *Crit Care Med*. 2008; 36:S106–11.

Pfeffer MA, Swedberg K, Granger CB, et al. Effects of candesartan on mortality and morbidity in patients with chronic heart failure: The CHARM-Overall programme. *Lancet*. 2003;362:759–66.

Pitt B, Remme W, Zannad F, et al. Eplerenone, a selective aldosterone blocker, in patients with left ventricular dysfunction after myocardial infarction. *N Engl J Med*. 2003;348:1309–21.

Pitt B, Zannad F, Remme WJ, et al. The effect of spironolactone on morbidity and mortality in patients with severe heart failure. *N Engl J Med*. 1999;341:709–17.

Poole-Wilson PA, Swedberg K, Cleland JGF, et al. Comparison of carvedilol and metoprolol on clinical outcomes in patients with chronic heart failure in the Carvedilol or Metoprolol European Trial (COMET): Randomised controlled trial. *Lancet*. 2003;362:7–13.

Schentag J, Bang A, Kozinski-Tober J. Digoxin. In: Burton M, Shaw L, Schentag J, Evans W, eds. *Applied Pharmacokinetics and Pharmacodynamics*. 4th ed. Baltimore: Lippincott Williams and Wilkins; 2006:411–39.

Taylor AL, Ziesche S, Yancy C, et al. Combination of isosorbide dinitrate and hydralazine in blacks with heart failure. *N Engl J Med*. 2004;351:2049–57.

Wong J, Patel RA, Kowey PR. The clinical use of angiotensin-converting enzyme inhibitors. *Prog Cardiovasc Dis*. 2004;47:116–30.

Cardiac Arrhythmias

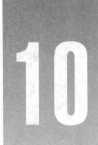

Robert B. Parker, PharmD, FCCP

Cardiac arrhythmias are abnormal heart rhythms resulting from alterations in impulse formation or conduction.

10-1. Electrophysiology

Impulse Generation (Automaticity) and Conduction

- Initiation and propagation of the electrical impulse in cardiac cells is dependent on regulation of the action potential.
- Conduction velocity is determined by regulation of action potential, specifically the slope of phase 0 depolarization (Figure 10-1 and Table 10-1).
- The *absolute refractory period* is the time during which cardiac cells cannot conduct or propagate an action potential (Figure 10-1 and Table 10-1).
- The *relative refractory period* is the time during which cardiac cells may conduct and propagate action potentials secondary to strong electrical stimuli.

Normal Conduction System

The sinoatrial (SA) node, located in the right atrium, initiates an impulse that

- Stimulates the left atrium and atrioventricular (AV) node, which
- Stimulates the left and right bundle branches via the bundle of His, which then

- Stimulates Purkinje fibers and causes ventricular contraction

10-2. Mechanisms of Arrhythmia

Cardiac arrhythmias arise secondary to the following disorders:

- Automaticity (impulse generation)
- Latent pacemaker (non-SA node pacemaker)
- Triggered automaticity (early or late after-depolarizations)
- Reentry
- Impulse conduction
- Automaticity and impulse conduction

10-3. Clinical Manifestations

Symptoms

Symptoms associated with ventricular arrhythmias range from asymptomatic to loss of consciousness and death. Patients with ventricular tachycardia (VT) may be asymptomatic, but VT can result in hypotension, syncope, or death. Ventricular fibrillation (VF) produces no cardiac output and causes most cases of sudden cardiac death.

Symptoms generally related to poor cardiac output include dizziness, syncope, chest pain, fatigue, confusion, and exacerbation of heart failure. Patients with tachyarrhythmias may report palpitations. With atrial fibrillation or flutter, patients may also experience dizziness, palpitations, light-headedness, and dyspnea

Figure 10-1. Action Potential for Atrial and Ventricular Tissue

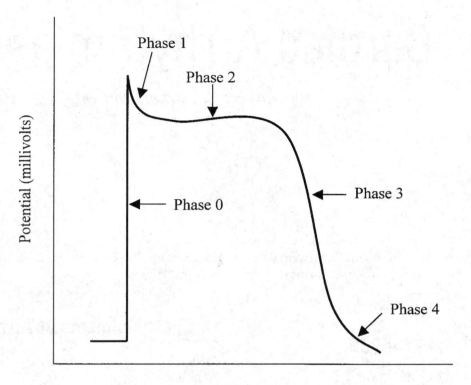

as well as symptoms of transient ischemic attack (TIA) or stroke.

Signs

- Electrocardiogram (ECG) abnormalities may present.
- Ventricular rate can be assessed by documenting the heart rate from the radial artery or by carotid palpation.

10-4. Diagnostic Criteria and Therapy According to Arrhythmia Classification

Arrhythmias are defined by

- Anatomic location
  - Supraventricular arrhythmias arise from abnormalities in the SA node, the atrial tissue, the AV node, or the bundle of His.

Table 10-1. Phases of Atrial and Ventricular Tissue Action Potential

Phase	Process	Ion flow	Corresponding ECG
0	Depolarization	Na+ fast channel opens; Na+ enters cell.	Atrial: P wave; ventricular: QRS
1	Initial repolarization	Na+ channel closes; passive Cl– influx.	
2	Prolongs depolarized state	Predominantly Ca2+ enters cell.	ST segment
3	Repolarization	Rapid efflux of K+ out of cell.	T wave, QT interval
4	Repolarization	Na+ leaks into cell; K+ pumped out of cell.	

- Ventricular arrhythmias originate from below the bundle of His.
- Ventricular rate
  - *Bradyarrhythmias:* Heart rate < 60 beats per minute (bpm).
  - *Tachyarrhythmias:* Heart rate > 100 bpm.

Bradyarrhythmias

Sinus bradycardia

Diagnostic criteria and characteristics
Heart rate is less than 60 bpm; otherwise, the ECG is normal.

Mechanism of arrhythmia
The mechanism of arrhythmia is decreased SA node automaticity.

Clinical etiology
Causes include acute myocardial infarction; hypothyroidism; drug-induced causes (β-blockers including ophthalmic agents, digoxin, calcium channel blockers [diltiazem, verapamil], clonidine, amiodarone, and cholinergic agents); and hyperkalemia

Treatment goals
Restore normal sinus rhythm if the patient is clinically symptomatic.

Drug and nondrug therapy
For intermittent symptomatic episodes: give atropine 0.5–1.0 mg intravenously repeated up to maximum dose of 3.0 mg.

For persistent episodes or if there is no response to atropine: place transvenous or transcutaneous pacemaker.

Atrioventricular block

Diagnostic criteria and characteristics
Criteria are as follows:

- *First-degree:* Prolonged PR interval > 0.20 seconds, 1:1 atrioventricular conduction
- *Second-degree Mobitz type I:* Gradual prolongation of PR interval followed by P wave without ventricular conduction
- *Second-degree Mobitz type II:* Constant PR interval with intermittent P wave without ventricular conduction; may have widened QRS complex

- *Third-degree:* Heart rate 30–60 bpm; no temporal relation between atrial and ventricular contraction; ventricular contraction initiated by AV junction or ventricular tissue

Mechanism of arrhythmia
The mechanism of arrhythmia is prolonged conduction.

Clinical etiology
Causes include AV nodal disease; acute myocardial infarction; myocarditis; increased vagal tone; drug-induced causes (β-blockers, digoxin, calcium channel blockers [diltiazem and verapamil]; clonidine, amiodarone, cholinergic agents); and hyperkalemia.

Treatment goals
Restore sinus rhythm if the patient is symptomatic

Drug and nondrug therapy
If the cause is reversible, treat with a temporary pacemaker or intermittent atropine.

If the condition is chronic, implant a permanent pacemaker.

Supraventricular Arrhythmias

Atrial fibrillation and atrial flutter

Diagnostic criteria and characteristics
Criteria are as follows:

- *Atrial Fibrillation:* No P waves; irregularly irregular QRS pattern
- *Atrial Flutter:* Sawtooth P wave pattern; regular QRS pattern
- *Ventricular response:* Usually fast but can also be slow or normal

Mechanism of arrhythmia
The mechanism of arrhythmia is enhanced automaticity and reentrant circuits.

Clinical etiology
Causes include rheumatic heart disease, heart failure, hypertension, ischemic heart disease, pericarditis, cardiomyopathy, mitral valve prolapse, cardiac surgery, infection, alcohol abuse, hyperthyroidism, chronic obstructive pulmonary disease, pulmonary embolism, and idiopathic causes (lone atrial fibrillation).

Atrial fibrillation and flutter are the most commonly occurring arrhythmia, and risk increases with age.

Complications include stroke, heart failure exacerbation.

Specific treatment goals for atrial fibrillation
Figure 10-2 illustrates the treatment algorithm for atrial fibrillation.

Control the ventricular rate
Digoxin is the drug of first choice in patients with left ventricular systolic dysfunction (e.g., left ventricular ejection fraction < 40%); it slows the ventricular rate but has poor control in hyperadrenergic-induced atrial fibrillation.

The most effective agents are β-blockers (esmolol, metoprolol, propranolol, others).

Calcium channel blockers (diltiazem, verapamil) may be used but should be avoided in patients with left ventricular systolic dysfunction.

For rapid control of ventricular rate, the intravenous (IV) route of administration should be used.

Digoxin, calcium channel blockers, and β-blockers do not restore sinus rhythm.

Restore and maintain sinus rhythm
Acute conversion to sinus rhythm may be required in patients with atrial fibrillation who are hemodynamically unstable (e.g., hypotensive).

Restoration of sinus rhythm is usually accomplished by electrical cardioversion or administration of antiarrhythmic drugs (AADs).

An important area of controversy centers on whether chronic AAD therapy should be administered to maintain sinus rhythm after cardioversion (*rhythm control approach*) or whether patients should simply be treated with agents to control ventricular response and anticoagulants to prevent thromboembolic stroke (*rate control approach*).

Historically, AADs were frequently used to restore and maintain sinus rhythm in patients with atrial fibrillation (rhythm control approach). With chronic therapy, AADs approximately double the chances of a patient remaining in sinus rhythm. However, this approach exposes patients to the large number of adverse effects associated with AADs. The rationale for this approach includes the possibility of fewer symptoms, lower risk of stroke, improved quality of life, and reduced mortality. However, these benefits had never been proven in large clinical trials.

The alternative approach, so called rate control, involves using drugs to control the ventricular response and chronic anticoagulation, usually with warfarin, for stroke prevention.

The rate control and rhythm control approaches have recently been compared in a number of large clinical trials, and the studies demonstrate no advantage for rhythm control over the rate control approach. Regardless of the approach, adequate anticoagulation is needed to prevent stroke.

Even when chronic antiarrhythmic therapy is used to maintain sinus rhythm, it is not 100% effective. Therefore, this approach is usually reserved for patients with recurrent, symptomatic episodes.

Prevent thromboembolism
Prior to use of pharmacologic or direct-current cardioversion: If atrial fibrillation is present for ≥ 48 hours or of unknown duration, anticoagulate with warfarin (INR [international normalized ratio] 2–3) for 3 weeks prior to elective cardioversion, and continue for at least 4 weeks after sinus rhythm has been restored.

If atrial fibrillation is present for ≥ 48 hours or of unknown duration, transesophageal echocardiography (TEE) is often used to determine the presence of atrial thrombus. If no thrombus is seen, cardioversion can be attempted after initiation of IV unfractionated heparin (aPTT [activated partial thromboplastin time] 50–70 seconds) or low molecular weight heparin (full deep vein thrombosis treatment doses). If cardioversion is successful and sinus rhythm is maintained, patients should receive warfarin (INR 2–3) for at least 4 weeks. If atrial thrombus is seen on TEE, anticoagulation should be initiated and repeat TEE performed before attempting later cardioversion.

Risk factors for nonvalvular atrial fibrillation thromboembolism are as follows:

■ Previous ischemic stroke, systemic embolism, or TIA
■ History of hypertension
■ Moderately or severely impaired left ventricular systolic function, heart failure, or both
■ Diabetes mellitus
■ Age over 75 years

Recommended antithrombotic therapy
The following treatments are recommended:

■ Patients with a prior ischemic stroke, systemic embolism, or TIA should receive warfarin INR 2–3.
■ Patients with *two or more* of the following risk factors should receive warfarin (INR 2–3): (1) age exceeding 75 years; (2) history of hypertension; (3) diabetes; and (4) moderately or severely impaired left ventricular systolic function, heart failure, or both. This treatment corresponds to individuals with a CHADS$_2$ (cardiac failure, hypertension, age, diabetes, stroke [doubled]) score ≥ 2.

Figure 10-2. Treatment Algorithm for Atrial Fibrillation

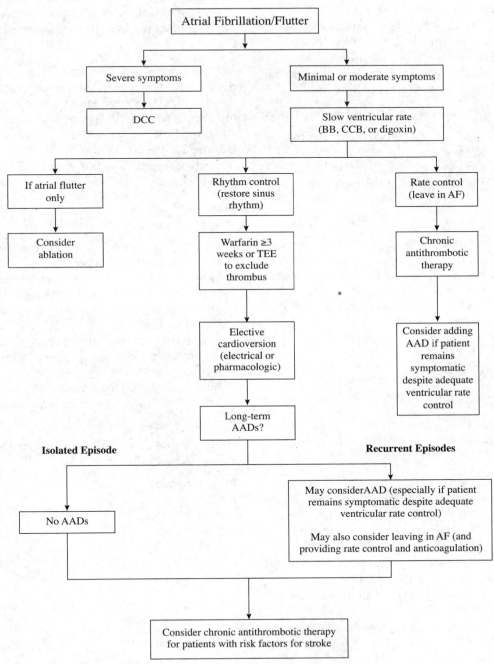

Note: Selection of the most appropriate antithrombotic therapy is based on the presence of risk factors for stroke, regardless of whether the rhythm or rate control approach is selected. AADs = antiarrhythmic drugs; AF = atrial fibrillation; BB = β-blocker; CCB = nondihydropyridine calcium channel blocker; DCC = direct-current cardioversion; TEE = transesophageal echocardiography.

Reproduced with permission from Sanoski CA, Schoen MD, Bauman JL, 2008.

- Patients with *only one* of the following risk factors should receive warfarin (INR 2–3) or aspirin 75–325 mg daily: (1) age exceeding 75 years; (2) history of hypertension; (3) diabetes; (4) moderately or severely impaired left ventricular systolic function, heart failure, or both.
- Patients with *none* of the following risk factors should receive aspirin 75–325 mg daily: (1) age > 75 years; (2) history of hypertension; (3) diabetes; (4) moderately or severely impaired left ventricular systolic function, heart failure, or both.

Dosage forms for warfarin (Coumadin) are as follows:

- Tablets: 1 mg (pink), 2 mg (lavender), 2.5 mg (green), 3 mg (tan), 4 mg (blue), 5 mg (peach), 6 mg (teal), 7.5 mg (yellow), 10 mg (white)
- Injections (IV): 5 mg powder for reconstitution (2 mg/mL)

Mechanism of action

Warfarin inhibits vitamin K epoxide-reductase and vitamin K reductase, preventing the conversion of vitamin K epoxide to vitamin K. It ultimately inhibits formation of vitamin K–dependent coagulation factors II, VII, IX, and X, as well as proteins C and S

Absorption

Bioavailability of warfarin is 80% to 100% following oral administration. It is absorbed in the upper gastrointestinal tract. Food or enteral feedings may decrease rate and extent of absorption.

Distribution

Warfarin is 99.0% to 99.5% protein bound, primarily to albumin.

Metabolism and elimination:

Warfarin is administered as a racemic mixture of S- and R-warfarin; the S-isomer is five times more potent than the R-isomer. The S-isomer is primarily metabolized in the liver via cytochrome P450 2C9 (CYP2C9). The R-isomer is metabolized by several other enzymes of the cytochrome P450 system.

Warfarin has low-extraction pharmacokinetic characteristics.

Clearance decreases with increasing age.

The half-life of the R-isomer is 45 hours; for the S-isomer, it is 33 hours.

Pharmacogenomics

Recent studies show that genetic polymorphisms can markedly influence the metabolism and response to warfarin. Mutations in two genes—CYP2C9, which codes for the hepatic enzyme that metabolizes S-warfarin, and VKORC1, which regulates the vitamin K epoxide-reductase enzyme (VKORC1)—can account for up to 50% of the variability in the dose of warfarin. The current package insert contains information regarding altered responses caused by polymorphisms in the CYP2C9 and VKORC1 genes. However, the use of genetic testing to prospectively determine the dose of warfarin remains controversial.

Pharmacodynamics

The S-isomer is approximately five times more potent than the R-isomer in inhibiting vitamin K reductase. Its pharmacodynamic effect (change in INR) is an indirect effect of the decreased formation of the vitamin K–dependent coagulation factors II, VII, IX, and X. The long half-lives of these factors result in delayed onset of action and delayed response to dosage changes.

Adverse effects

Several adverse effects are possible:

- Bleeding can occur, roughly proportional to the degree of anticoagulation.
- Skin necrosis, related to depletion of or deficiency of protein C, is possible. This effect usually occurs within 10 days of warfarin initiation. Incidence is low.
- Purple-toe syndrome may occur. This syndrome usually occurs 3–8 weeks after warfarin initiation. Incidence is low.
- Birth defects and fetal hemorrhage are possible. Therefore, warfarin is pregnancy category X.

Some common drug interactions

Medications decreasing warfarin anticoagulant response are as follows:

- Barbiturates
- Carbamazepine
- Cholestyramine
- Griseofulvin
- Nafcillin
- Phenytoin (chronic therapy)
- Rifampin

Medications increasing warfarin anticoagulant response are as follows:

- Acetaminophen
- Allopurinol
- Amiodarone
- Azole antifungal agents
- Cimetidine
- Ciprofloxacin, levofloxacin
- Diltiazem
- Erythromycin, clarithromycin
- Fenofibrate

- Fish oil
- Metronidazole
- Omeprazole (R-enantiomer)
- Phenytoin (acute therapy)
- Propafenone
- Simvastatin, fluvastatin
- Sulfinpyrazone
- Trimethoprim-sulfamethoxazole

Dosing management

Patients should take a once-daily dose of 1–10 mg orally. Patient response is highly variable. Management of elevated INR is described in Table 10-2.

Monitoring

The standard for assessing the degree of anticoagulation is the INR = (observed prothrombin ratio)^{ISI}, where ISI is the International Standardized Index, which corrects for variability in thromboplastin sensitivity.

Initially, the INR is monitored every 1–2 days until the desired INR is achieved and has stabilized at a given dose. Periodic INR monitoring (i.e., monthly) is recommended thereafter unless dosage changes are made.

Paroxysmal supraventricular tachycardia

Diagnostic criteria and characteristics

Criteria for paroxysmal supraventricular tachycardia (PSVT) are as follows:

- Heart rate of 160–240 bpm that is abrupt in onset and termination with a normal QRS interval
- 1:1 AV conduction

Mechanism of arrhythmia

The mechanism of arrhythmia is reentry.

Clinical etiology

Causes include idiopathic causes, fever, and drug-induced causes (sympathomimetics, anticholinergics, β-agonists).

Treatment goals

See Figure 10-3 for the treatment algorithm for PSVT. Treatment goals are as follows:

- **Acute:** Terminate reentry circuit by prolonging refractoriness and slowing conduction.
- **Chronic:** Prevent or minimize the number and severity of episodes. Antiarrhythmic drugs are no longer the treatment of choice to prevent recurrences. Most patients undergo radiofrequency catheter ablation of the reentrant substrate, which is curative and is associated with a low complication rate.

Acute nonpharmacologic therapy

Vagal maneuvers may terminate PSVT: carotid massage and Valsalva maneuver (most common), squatting, deep breathing, coughing, inducing eyeball pressure, and diving reflex (less common).

Ventricular Arrhythmias

Major classifications and diagnostic criteria

- Premature ventricular contractions
  - Premature ventricular contractions (PVCs) are extra abnormal heartbeats that originate in the

Table 10-2. Management of Elevated International Normalized Ratio

INR	Significant bleeding	Recommendations
< 5.0 but above therapeutic range	No	Lower dose or omit single dose and restart at lower dose when INR is therapeutic.
≥ 5.0 and < 9.0	No	Omit 1–2 doses and resume at lower dose when INR is therapeutic; if more rapid reversal desired, omit dose and give ≤ 5 mg vitamin K orally; restart warfarin at lower dose when INR is therapeutic or clinically appropriate.
> 9.0	No	Hold warfarin and give 2.5–5.0 mg vitamin K orally; use additional vitamin K if necessary; resume warfarin at lower dose when INR is therapeutic.
Serious bleeding at any elevation of INR	Yes	Hold warfarin; give 10 mg vitamin K IV via slow infusion (over at least 10 minutes); supplement with fresh-frozen plasma, rVIIa, or prothrombin complex concentrate if necessary; repeat vitamin K 10 mg IV q12h if necessary.
Life-threatening bleeding at any elevation of INR	Yes, life threatening	Hold warfarin; give fresh-frozen plasma, prothrombin complex concentrate, or rVIIa with vitamin K 10 mg via IV slow infusion; repeat as necessary

Figure 10-3. Treatment Algorithm for Paroxysmal Supraventricular Tachycardia

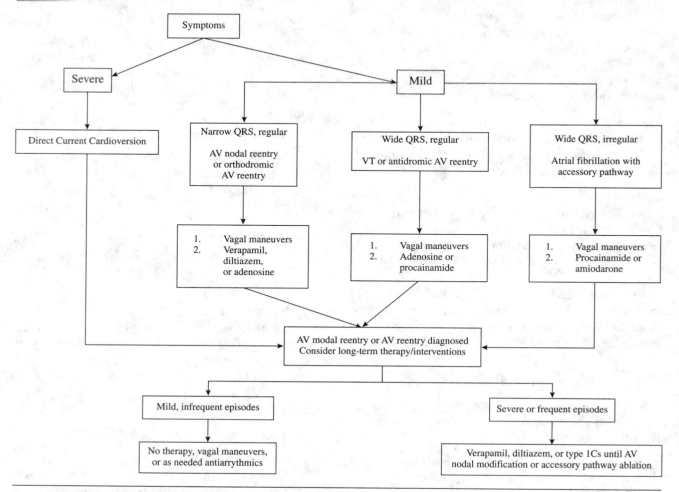

Reproduced with permission from Sanoski CA, Schoen MD, Bauman JL, 2008.

ventricles. They are termed *premature* because they occur before the normal heartbeat.

- PVCs often are asymptomatic or cause only mild palpitations.

Ventricular tachycardia

- Ventricular tachycardia (VT) is defined as three or more consecutive PVCs at a rate exceeding 100 bpm and a wide QRS interval (> 0.12 seconds), usually with a regular pattern.
- Nonsustained VT (NSVT) is defined as an episode that lasts less than 30 seconds.
- Sustained VT is defined as an episode lasts more than 30 seconds.

Ventricular fibrillation

- Ventricular fibrillation is defined as an absence of organized cardiac electrical or mechanical

activity and no recognizable P waves, QRS complexes, or T waves on the ECG.

- Ventricular fibrillation rapidly results in no effective cardiac output, blood pressure, or pulse.

Clinical etiology

Causes include acute myocardial infarction, electrolyte disturbances, catecholamines, and drug-induced causes.

Treatment goals

- Treat acute symptoms precipitating causes
- Restore sinus rhythm
- Prevent/minimize recurrences

10-5. Drug and Nondrug Therapy

Premature Ventricular Contractions

Apparently healthy patients without underlying structural heart disease are not at increased risk for VT or sudden cardiac death; therefore, no drug therapy is necessary.

Patients with PVCs and underlying heart disease (e.g., previous myocardial infarction) are at increased risk for more serious arrhythmias. However, AADs do not reduce this risk, and in fact, their use is associated with increased risk of lethal arrhythmias. All such patients should receive medications proven to improve survival, including β-blockers, antiplatelet agents, statins, ACE inhibitors, and aldosterone antagonists if appropriate. An implantable cardioverter defibrillator (ICD) is indicated in such patients with a left ventricular ejection fraction (LVEF) ≤ 30–40% to reduce mortality.

Nonsustained Ventricular Tachycardia

For patients with heart disease and LVEF > 40%, Maximize other cardiovascular medications with proven effects on survival (see previous paragraph).

For patients with heart disease and LVEF ≤ 30% to 40%, recent studies indicate that they are at increased risk for sudden cardiac death (usually from ventricular fibrillation). Use of an ICD improves survival in this group, whereas amiodarone does not affect survival. Even in the absence of PVCs or NSVT in this patient group, these patients are at increased risk for sudden cardiac death, and an ICD is indicated to improve survival.

Unless contraindicated, these patients should also receive standard background therapy, which includes aspirin, ACE inhibitors, β-blockers, statins, and aldosterone antagonists.

Sustained Ventricular Tachycardia or Ventricular Fibrillation (Postresuscitation)

If the event occurs within 24–48 hours of myocardial infarction or because of other reversible causes, no antiarrhythmic drug therapy is needed except β-blockers.

If the event is not secondary to myocardial infarction or another reversible cause, ICD placement is recommended.

Antiarrhythmic drugs (i.e., amiodarone) may still be required to decrease the number of defibrillator discharges, increase patient comfort, and prolong battery life.

Amiodarone can be considered if the patient refuses ICD placement.

Torsades de Pointes

This is a specific variety of ventricular tachycardia with QRS complexes that appear to twist around the ECG baseline. It is associated with a prolonged QT interval.

Clinical etiology

Causes are as follows:

- Genetic abnormalities in cardiac potassium channels
- Acquired
  - Hypokalemia, hypomagnesemia
  - Myocardial ischemia or infarction
  - Subarachnoid hemorrhage
  - Hypothyroidism
  - Myocarditis or cardiomyopathy
  - Arsenic poisoning
  - Drug-induced causes (known association with torsades de pointes)
    - *Antiarrhythmics:* Quinidine, procainamide, disopyramide, sotalol, ibutilide, dofetilide, amiodarone
    - *Antipsychotics:* Chlorpromazine, haloperidol, mesoridazine, thioridazine, pimozide, atypical antipsychotics (e.g., quetiapine, ziprasidone)
    - *Antidepressants:* amitriptyline, desipramine, doxepin, imipramine, nortriptyline
    - *Antibiotics:* erythromycin, clarithromycin, gatifloxacin, moxifloxacin, sparfloxacin, pentamidine, trimethoprim-sulfamethoxazole
    - *Others:* methadone, droperidol

Treatment

- Stop the offending drug if possible.
- Administer direct-current cardioversion for hemodynamically unstable patients.
- Administer magnesium sulfate 2 g over 1 minute IV.
- Use a pacemaker or isoproterenol infusion to increase heart rate.
- Correct hypokalemia or hypomagnesemia.

Drug therapy

See Tables 10-3, 10-4, and 10-5 for information about antiarrhythmic drugs. Antiarrhythmic drugs terminate or minimize arrhythmias by

Table 10-3. Effects of Antiarrhythmic Drugs on Cardiac Electrophysiology

Drug class	Ion block	Conduction	Refractory period	Automaticity
Ia	Sodium	↓	↑	↓
Ib	Sodium	0/↓	↓	↓
Ic	Sodium	↓↓	↑	↓
II	Calcium (Indirect effect)	↓	↑	↓
III[1]	Potassium	0	↑↑	0
IV	Calcium	↓	↑	↓

↓ Decreases
↑ Increases
[1]Sotalol also possesses β-blocking activity. Amiodarone also possesses sodium and calcium channel blockade.

■ Decreasing automaticity of abnormal pacemaker tissues
■ Altering conduction characteristics of reentry
■ Increasing refractory period
■ Eliminating premature impulses that trigger reentry

Patient counseling

Patients should be counseled to take medication as prescribed. If a dose is missed, have the patient take the dose as soon as it is remembered, unless close to the next scheduled dose. In this case, the patient should skip the missed dose and continue the regular regimen; doses should not be doubled.

Many drug interactions are possible. Patients should inform health care providers of medications prescribed prior to starting new medications, including over-the-counter medications (Table 10-6).

Periodic ECG and laboratory assessments may be required to minimize or prevent adverse effects.

Patients should be educated that complete remission of their arrhythmia is unlikely. However, symptomatic arrhythmias that have increased in frequency or severity should be reported to the physician immediately.

Patients with atrial fibrillation or flutter should be educated about the importance of antithrombotic therapy as well as the signs and symptoms of stroke. Patients with symptoms including sudden onset of slurred speech, facial drooping, or muscle weakness should seek emergent care.

Antiarrhythmic drugs that are administered as extended-release formulations should not be crushed, opened, or chewed. Advise patients to swallow the dose whole.

Drug-specific information

Amiodarone

The U.S. Food and Drug Administration now requires that a medication guide be distributed directly to each patient to whom amiodarone is dispensed.

Visual disturbances are rare but should be reported immediately to the physician.

Difficulty breathing, shortness of breath, wheezing, or persistent cough should be reported immediately to the physician.

If the patient experiences nausea or vomiting, passes brown or dark-colored urine, feels more tired than usual, or experiences stomach pain, or if the patient's skin or whites of the eyes turn yellow, the symptoms should be reported immediately to the physician.

Cardiac symptoms such as pounding heart, skipping a beat, or very rapid or slow heartbeats, as well as lightheadedness or feeling faint, should be reported immediately to the physician.

Periodic laboratory tests to evaluate thyroid function, liver function, and pulmonary function, as well as diagnostic tests such as chest x-ray, ECG, and eye exams may be necessary to assess and prevent adverse events (Table 10-7).

Amiodarone may cause skin photosensitivity. Patients should be advised to wear protective clothing and sunscreen when exposed to sunlight or ultraviolet light.

Prolonged use may cause blue-gray skin discoloration.

Patients should tell their doctor and pharmacist about all other medicines they take, including prescription and nonprescription medicine, vitamins, and herbal supplements.

Frequent administration with grapefruit juice may increase oral absorption. Encourage patients to drink water with amiodarone or separate grapefruit juice consumption by at least 2 hours.

β-blockers (including sotalol)

Patients with asthma and chronic obstructive pulmonary disease should be advised that β-blockers may worsen their symptoms of airway disease. Advise patients to notify physician immediately if this occurs.

Patients with diabetes should be advised that β-blockers may mask symptoms of hypoglycemia.

Patients should avoid abrupt withdrawal of β-blocker therapy. If withdrawal of β-blocker therapy is desired, the patient should contact the physician for the dosage-tapering regimen, if necessary.

Digoxin

Refer to chapter 9.

Table 10-4. Antiarrhythmic Drug Availability and Standard Dosing Regimens

Generic name	Trade name	Dosage forms	Loading dose	Maintenance dose
Class Ia				
Quinidine gluconate	Quinaglute Dura-Tabs, Duraquin, Quinalan, Quinatime	324, 330 mg tablets 80 mg/mL injection	IV: not recommended	328–648 mg PO tid
Quinidine sulfate	Quinidex Extentabs, Cin-Quin, Quinora	100, 200, 300 mg tablets	PO: 200 mg q 2–3 h for 5–8 doses (sulfate salt only)	200–400 mg PO qid
Quinidine polygalacturonate	Cardioquin	275 mg tablets		275 mg PO bid or tid
Procainamide	Pronestyl	100, 500 mg/mL injection Oral procainamide no longer available	IV: 15–18 mg/kg at 20–50 mg/min	IV: 1–6 mg/min
Disopyramide	Norpace, Norpace CR	100, 150 mg capsules 100, 150 mg capsules		150–300 mg q6h 300–600 mg q12h
Moricizine	Ethmozine	200, 250, 300 mg tablets		200–300 mg q8h
Class Ib				
Lidocaine		10 mg/mL (5 mL and 10 mL) 20 mg/mL (5 mL) IV infusion: 2 (500 mL), 4 (250, 500, 1,000 mL), 8 (250, 500 mL) mg/mL in D_5W	IV: 100 mg repeat up to 2 times	IV: 1–4 mg/min
Tocainide	Tonocard	400, 600 mg tablets		400–600 mg q8h
Mexiletine	Mexitil	150, 200, 250 mg capsules		100–300 mg q8h
Class Ic				
Flecainide	Tambocor	50, 100, 150, 200 mg tablets	600 mg PO for conversion of atrial fibrillation to sinus rhythm	50–200 mg q12h
Propafenone	Rythmol, Rythmol-SR	150, 225, 300 mg tablets 225, 325, 425 mg capsules		150–300 mg q8h 225–425 mg q12h
Class II: β-blockers				
Metoprolol	Lopressor, Toprol XL	25, 50, 100 mg tablets 25, 50, 100, 200 mg tablets; 1 mg/mL injection	IV: 2.5–5 mg up to 3 doses	25–450 mg PO daily
Propranolol	Inderal, Inderal LA	10, 20, 40, 60, 80 mg tablets 60, 80, 120, 160 mg capsules 20, 40 mg/mL oral solution 1 mg/mL (5 mL) injection	IV: 0.15 mg/kg IV: 0.5 mg/kg	PO: 80–240 mg daily
Esmolol	Brevibloc	10 and 250 mg/mL injection	0.5 mg/kg/min × 1 min	IV: 0.05–0.2 mg/kg/min

(continued)

Table 10-4. Antiarrhythmic Drug Availability and Standard Dosing Regimens *(Continued)*

Generic name	Trade name	Dosage forms	Loading dose	Maintenance dose
Class III				
Amiodarone	Cordarone, Pacerone	100, 200, 400 mg tablets	800–1,600 mg/d in divided doses × 2–4 weeks	PO: 100–400 mg qd
		5, 50 mg/mL IV solution	IV (VT/VF): 150 mg/10 min or 900 mg in 500 mL D_5W at 1 mg/min × 6 h	IV: 0.5 mg/min
			IV (cardiac arrest): 300 mg	
Sotalol	Betapace, Betapace AF	80, 120, 160, 240 mg tablets		80–160 mg q12h
Ibutilide	Corvert	0.1 mg/mL (10 mL) injection	1.0 mg IV over 10 min; repeat × 1 if needed	Not applicable
Dofetilide	(Tikosyn)	125, 250, 500 mcg capsules		CrCl > 60 mL/min = 500 mcg bid; 40–60 mL/min = 250 mcg bid; 20–39 mL/min = 125 mcg bid; < 20 mL/min = not recommended
Class IV: calcium channel blockers				
Verapamil	Calan, Calan SR, Isoptin SR, Covera-HS, Verelan, Verelan-PM	40, 80, 120 mg tablets	2.5–10 mg IV over 2 min	PO: 120–360 mg/d
		120, 180, 240 mg tablets		IV: 5–15 mg/h
		180, 240 mg tablets		Calan, Isoptin: tid-qid
		120, 180, 240, 360 mg capsules		Calan SR, Isoptin SR, Covera-HS, Verelan: qd
		100, 200, 300 mg capsules		
		2.5 mg/ml injection		
Diltiazem	Cardizem, Cardizem CD, Cardizem Monovial, Cardizem Lyo-Ject, Cardizem SR, Cartia XT, Dilacor XR, Diltia XT, Tiazac, Cardizem LA	30, 60, 90, 120 mg tablets	20 mg IV over 2 min	IV: 5–15 mg/h
		5 mg/mL injection		PO: 120–360 mg/d
		120, 180, 240, 300, 360 mg capsules		Cardizem: qid
		100 mg/mL injection		Cardizem SR: bid
		25 mg injection		Cardizem CD, Cardizem LA, Dilacor XR, Tiazac: qd
		60, 90, 120 mg capsules		
		120, 180, 240, 300 mg capsules		
		120, 180, 240 mg capsules		
		120, 180, 240, 300 mg capsules		
		120, 180, 240, 300, 360, 420 mg tablets		

Table 10-4. Antiarrhythmic Drug Availability and Standard Dosing Regimens *(Continued)*

Generic name	Trade name	Dosage forms	Loading dose	Maintenance dose
Miscellaneous				
Atropine		0.1, 0.3, 0.4, 0.5, 0.6, 0.8, 1.0 mg/mL injection	0.5–1.0 mg q 5 min up to 3 mg total	
Adenosine	Adenocard	3 mg/mL injection		Initial dose: 6 mg IV bolus; if necessary, can be followed by 12 mg q 2 min as IV bolus; flush IV line after each administration
Digoxin	Lanoxin, Lanoxicaps	125, 250, 500 mcg tablets 50 mcg/mL elixir 100, 250 mcg/mL injection 50, 100, 200 mcg capsules	IV and PO: 0.25 mg q 2 h up to 1.5 mg	IV and PO: 0.125–0.375 mg qd

Table 10-5. Pharmacokinetics of Antiarrhythmic Drugs

Drug	Bioavailability (%)	Protein binding (%)	Primary route of elimination	Substrate for	Inhibitor of	Half-life	Therapeutic range (mg/L)
Quinidine	70–80	80–90	Hepatic	CYP3A4	CYP2D6, CYP3A4, P-gp	5–9 h	2–6
Procainamide	75–95	10–20	Hepatic and renal	NAT		2.5–5.0 h	4–15
Disopyramide	70–95	50–80	Hepatic and renal	CYP3A4		4–8 h	2–6
Moricizine	34–38	92–95	Hepatic			1–6 h	
Lidocaine	20–40	65–75	Hepatic	CYP3A4, CYP2D6, CYP1A2	CYP1A2	60–180 min	1.5–5.0
Tocainide	90–95	10–30	Hepatic			12–15 h	4–10
Mexiletine	80–95	60–75	Hepatic	CYP2D6, CYP1A2	CYP1A2	6–12 h	0.8–2.0
Flecainide	90–95	35–45	Hepatic and renal	CYP2D6	CYP2D6	13–20 h	0.2–1.0
Propafenone	11–39	85–95	Hepatic	CYP2D6, CYP 1A2, CYP3A4	CYP2D6	3–25 h	
Amiodarone	22–88	95–99	Hepatic	CYP3A4, CYP1A2, CYP2C19, CYP2D6	CYP1A2, CYP2C9, CYP2D6, CYP3A4, CYP2C19, P-gp	15–100 d	1.0–2.5
Sotalol	90–95	30–40	Renal			12–20 h	
Ibutilide		40	Hepatic			3–6 h	
Dofetilide	> 90	60–70	Renal	CYP3A4		6–10 h	
Digoxin	60–85 (90–100) for Lanoxicaps	20–30	Renal	P-gp		34–44	0.5–2.2 ng/mL
Diltiazem	35–50	70–85	Hepatic	CYP3A4, CYP2C9, CYP2D6	CYP3A4, CYP2C9, CYP2D6, P-gp	4–10 h	
Verapamil	20–40	95–99	Hepatic	CYP3A4, CYP1A2, CYP2C9	CYP3A4, CYP1A2, CYP2C9, CYP2D6, P-gp	4–12 h	

Note: CYP = cytochrome P450 isoenzyme; NAT = N-acetyltransferase; P-gp = P-glycoprotein.

Table 10-6. Antiarrhythmic Drug Interactions and Significant Adverse Effects

Drug	Effect of disease/drugs on antiarrhythmic drug concentrations	Effect of antiarrhythmic on other drug concentrations	Common or severe adverse effects
Quinidine	*Elevated:* cimetidine, amiodarone, verapamil, diltiazem, ketoconazole, urine alkalinization *Reduced:* enzyme inducers	*Elevated:* warfarin, digoxin, β-blockers, disopyramide, procainamide, propafenone, mexiletine, flecainide	QTc prolongation, torsades de pointes, diarrhea, fever, hepatitis, thrombocytopenia
Procainamide	*Elevated:* cimetidine, trimethoprim, amiodarone		Lupus-like syndrome, QTc prolongation, torsades de pointes, hypotension, gastrointestinal (GI) distress, agranulocytosis
Disopyramide	*Reduced:* enzyme inducers *Elevated:* erythromycin, protease inhibitors, cimetidine		Anticholinergic side effects, decreased cardiac contractility, heart failure, QTc prolongation, torsades de pointes, hypoglycemia
Moricizine	*Elevated:* cimetidine	*Elevated:* theophylline	Dizziness, nausea, tremor, ataxia, paresthesias, proarrhythmia
Lidocaine	*Increased:* with decreased cardiac output		Central nervous system (CNS) toxicity: paresthesias, dizziness, muscle twitching, confusion, nausea and vomiting, slurred speech, seizures, sinus arrest
Tocainide	*Decreased:* cimetidine, enzyme inducers		GI distress; CNS: dizziness, paresthesias, confusion, seizures; pulmonary fibrosis or pneumonitis; agranulocytosis
Mexiletine	*Reduced:* enzyme inducers *Elevated:* quinidine, amiodarone, ritonavir	*Elevated:* theophylline	GI distress; CNS: tremor, dizziness, confusion, vertigo, nystagmus, diplopia, tremor, ataxia; hypotension, sinus bradycardia, AV block
Flecainide	*Elevated:* cimetidine, amiodarone	*Elevated:* digoxin	Proarrhythmia, prolonged PR interval and QRS complex; dizziness, blurred vision, headache, tremor, heart failure
Propafenone	*Reduced:* enzyme inducers *Elevated:* cimetidine, quinidine	*Elevated:* warfarin, digoxin, cyclosporine, theophylline	Metallic/bitter taste; CNS: dizziness, paresthesias, fatigue; GI distress; heart failure, liver injury, bradycardia, AV block, proarrhythmia
Amiodarone[a]		*Elevated:* quinidine, procainamide, warfarin, digoxin, phenytoin, cyclosporine, lovastatin, simvastatin, atorvastatin	IV: phlebitis; general: corneal microdeposits, photophobia, increased liver enzymes, photosensitivity, blue-gray skin discoloration, pulmonary fibrosis, hyper- and hypothyroidism, polyneuropathy
Sotalol			β-blocking effects: bradycardia, fatigue, dyspnea, bronchospasm, heart failure; QTc prolongation, torsades de pointes
Ibutilide			QTc prolongation, torsades de pointes
Dofetilide	*Elevated:* verapamil, cimetidine, ketoconazole, trimethoprim, megestrol, prochlorperazine		QTc prolongation, torsades de pointes
Digoxin	*Elevated:* quinidine, amiodarone, verapamil, diltiazem		
Diltiazem	*Elevated:* cimetidine	*Elevated:* cyclosporine, carbamazepine, digoxin	Hypotension, bradycardia, heart failure
Verapamil	*Reduced:* rifampin, phenobarbital	*Elevated:* theophylline, digoxin, carbamazepine, cyclosporine, simvastatin, lovastatin	Hypotension, bradycardia, heart failure, constipation

a. See Table 10-7.

Table 10-7. Suggested Monitoring Guidelines for Amiodarone

Test	Baseline		6 months	12 months
Electrocardiogram	▪		▪	▪
Pulmonary function tests	▪	Routine monitoring is controversial; may repeat tests if patient becomes symptomatic.		
Ophthalmologic examination	▪	Periodic exam is recommended.	▪	▪
Chest x-ray	▪	Repeat earlier if patient becomes symptomatic.	▪	▪
Thyroid function tests	▪		▪	▪
Liver enzymes	▪		▪	▪

Warfarin

Warfarin should be avoided at any time during pregnancy.

To determine the correct dosage, the physician may need to check the patient's INR regularly.

Encourage patients to maintain consistency in their diet. Abrupt changes, particularly in the intake of green leafy vegetables, may alter the effectiveness of warfarin.

Minor cuts may take longer to stop bleeding. If a cut or injury fails to stop bleeding, patients should be advised to contact their health care provider.

Excessive alcohol intake may alter the effectiveness of this medication.

Patients should tell their doctor and pharmacist about all other medicines they take, including prescription and nonprescription medicine, vitamins, and herbal supplements.

10-6. Key Points

▪ All antiarrhythmic drugs are proarrhythmic.
▪ Cardiac arrhythmias range from benign to lethal.
▪ Antiarrhythmic drug therapy should be individualized to patient response while minimizing adverse effects.
▪ Most antiarrhythmic drugs are hepatically eliminated and are associated with significant drug interactions.
▪ Nonpharmacologic therapy is an important treatment modality, particularly for life-threatening ventricular tachycardia and ventricular fibrillation.
▪ Treatment of atrial fibrillation should always include an assessment of antithrombotic therapy.
▪ Direct-current cardioversion is typically the treatment of choice for severely symptomatic arrhythmias.

▪ Anticoagulant response to warfarin therapy is influenced by numerous factors, including diet, drug interactions, genetics, and concomitant diseases.
▪ The treatment of excessive anticoagulation secondary to warfarin should be based on the INR, the presence of active bleeding, and the risk of recurrent thromboembolism.
▪ Patient education and appropriate monitoring are important aspects of successful therapy that can minimize adverse effects.

10-7. Questions

1. Which of the following is (are) adverse effect(s) of orally administered amiodarone?

   I. Photosensitivity
   II. Pulmonary fibrosis
   III. Phlebitis

   A. I only
   B. III only
   C. I and II only
   D. II and III only
   E. I, II, and III

2. Which of the following antiarrhythmic agents' mechanism of action is primarily the result of sodium ion transport blockade?

   A. Propafenone
   B. Ibutilide
   C. Sotalol
   D. Verapamil
   E. Diltiazem

3. First-degree atrioventricular heart block can be categorized as a disorder of

   I.   automaticity.
   II. reentry.
   III. conduction.

   A. I only
   B. III only
   C. I and II only
   D. II and III only
   E. I, II, and III

4. Each of the following can be symptoms of atrial fibrillation *except*

   A. dizziness.
   B. palpitations.
   C. angina.
   D. hypertension.
   E. sudden-onset slurred speech.

5. Each of the following is recommended for monitoring patients requiring chronic amiodarone therapy *except*

   A. electrocardiogram.
   B. coagulation tests.
   C. thyroid function tests.
   D. liver function tests.
   E. chest x-ray.

6. For the treatment of chronic atrial fibrillation, each of the following patients should receive long-term warfarin therapy with a target INR 2.0–3.0 *except* for

   A. patients with heart failure and diabetes.
   B. patients over 75 years old with hypertension.
   C. a 50-year-old male with no risk factors for thromboembolism.
   D. a 77-year-old female with diabetes and hypertension.
   E. a 63-year-old male who has had a previous stroke.

7. Patients with which type of arrhythmia should be educated on performing vagal maneuvers to restore sinus rhythm?

   A. Paroxysmal supraventricular tachycardia
   B. Torsades de pointes
   C. Atrial flutter
   D. Sinus bradycardia
   E. Ventricular fibrillation

8. Which of the following medications would be preferred for control of ventricular response in patients with atrial fibrillation and heart failure?

   A. Digoxin
   B. Verapamil
   C. Diltiazem
   D. Amlodipine
   E. Dofetilide

9. Which of the following medications is (are) associated with torsades de pointes?

   I.   Dofetilide
   II. Droperidol
   III. Erythromycin

   A. I only
   B. III only
   C. I and II only
   D. II and III only
   E. I, II, and III

10. Which of the following are important determinants of the pharmacokinetics and response to warfarin?

    I.   CYP2C9 genotype
    II. CYP2D6 genotype
    III. VKORC1 genotype

    A. I only
    B. II only
    C. I and II only
    D. I, II, and III
    E. I and III only

11. What is the recommended dosage regimen for dofetilide in a patient with a calculated creatinine clearance of 30 mL per minute?

    A. Dofetilide therapy not recommended.
    B. 125 mcg PO bid
    C. 125 mg PO bid
    D. 500 mcg PO bid
    E. 500 mg PO bid

12. Sotalol is metabolized by and inhibits the metabolism of which cytochrome P450 enzymes, respectively?

    A. CYP3A4 and CYP2D6
    B. CYP2D6 and CYP3A4
    C. P-gp and CYP2D6
    D. P-gp and CYP3A4
    E. None of the above

13. Which of the following antiarrhythmic agents does not increase digoxin concentrations when used concomitantly?

    A. Quinidine
    B. Dofetilide
    C. Amiodarone
    D. Diltiazem
    E. Verapamil

14. A 66-year-old male with a past medical history of congestive heart failure and hypertension is receiving lisinopril 10 mg PO qd, digoxin 0.25 mg PO qd, carvedilol 25 mg bid, and spironolactone 25 mg PO qd at home. He now presents to the emergency room with a 1-week history of intermittent palpitations and dizziness. The ECG reveals atrial fibrillation with a ventricular rate of 130 bpm. The decision is made to attempt to restore normal sinus rhythm. Which of the following represents the best therapeutic approach to cardioverting the patient?

    A. Perform transesophageal echocardiography; if no thrombus is present, cardiovert; no need for anticoagulation.
    B. Perform transesophageal echocardiography; if no thrombus is present, cardiovert; anticoagulate for at least 4 weeks postcardioversion.
    C. Anticoagulate for 4 weeks prior to cardioversion; discontinue anticoagulation postcardioversion.
    D. Anticoagulate for 2 weeks prior to cardioversion; continue anticoagulation for at least 4 weeks postcardioversion.
    E. Direct-current cardiovert immediately.

15. After the initial successful cardioversion, the patient in the previous question continues to have recurrent symptomatic atrial fibrillation episodes. Chronic therapy to maintain sinus rhythm is to be initiated. Which of the following antiarrhythmic drugs would be the best choice to maintain sinus rhythm?

    A. Flecainide
    B. Amiodarone
    C. Sotalol
    D. Ibutilide
    E. Digoxin

16. In a patient with mildly symptomatic paroxysmal supraventricular tachycardia, verapamil should be used for which rhythm(s)?

    I.   Narrow QRS complex, regular interval
    II. Wide QRS complex, regular interval
    III. Wide QRS complex, irregular interval

    A. I only
    B. III only
    C. I and II only
    D. II and III only
    E. I, II, and III

17. A 53-year-old male has a past medical history of myocardial infarction and hypertension. He presents to his doctor complaining of short (about 10 seconds in duration), intermittent palpitations during the past 2 days. Tests rule out an acute myocardial infarction, and an echocardiogram shows a left ventricular ejection fraction of 25%. The patient is sent home with a Holter monitor to identify any arrhythmias. The Holter monitor reveals episodes of PVCs and nonsustained ventricular tachycardia. What is the most appropriate intervention for this patient?

    A. No therapy is indicated.
    B. Place an implantable cardioverter defibrillator (ICD).
    C. Start propafenone.
    D. Start verapamil.
    E. Use direct-current cardioversion.

18. Treatment of torsades de pointes may include all of the following *except*

    A. discontinuing any drugs associated with prolonged QT interval.
    B. isoproterenol infusion.
    C. adenosine.
    D. magnesium sulfate.
    E. atrial–ventricular pacing.

19. Which of the following antiarrhythmic agents requires dosage adjustment in patients with impaired renal function?

    A. Digoxin
    B. Amiodarone
    C. Lidocaine
    D. Verapamil
    E. Propafenone

20. Which of the following is not a characteristic of atrial fibrillation?

    A. No discernable P waves
    B. Ventricular rate of 100–130 bpm
    C. Regular QRS pattern
    D. Narrow QRS complex
    E. Chaotic atrial contractions

21. Which of the following would be the best choice for ventricular rate control in atrial fibrillation secondary to hyperthyroidism?

    A. Adenosine
    B. Digoxin
    C. Verapamil
    D. Propranolol
    E. Atropine

22. A dose-limiting adverse effect of sotalol is

    A. bradycardia.
    B. polyneuropathy.
    C. metallic taste.
    D. agranulocytosis.
    E. lupus-like syndrome.

23. Which of the following is not available in both intravenous and oral dosage forms?

    A. Metoprolol
    B. Amiodarone
    C. Verapamil
    D. Digoxin
    E. Ibutilide

24. Dosage adjustment should be considered when warfarin is administered with the following drugs, *except* for

    A. amiodarone.
    B. sotalol.
    C. quinidine.
    D. propafenone.
    E. diltiazem.

10-8. Answers

1. C. Photosensitivity is a common adverse effect of oral amiodarone. Patients should be counseled to limit sun exposure and use sunscreen. Pulmonary fibrosis occurs during prolonged therapy. Phlebitis would be expected to occur only during intravenous amiodarone infusion, particularly through a peripheral intravenous line. A central line is preferred to decrease risk of phlebitis.

2. A. Propafenone blocks sodium entry into the cardiac cell, slowing depolarization. Ibutilide and sotalol act primarily by blocking potassium transport, whereas verapamil and diltiazem inhibit the calcium channel.

3. B. Atrioventricular heart block is caused by slowed conduction through the atrioventricular node.

4. D. Because of loss of functional atrial contraction and rapid ventricular rate (producing palpitations), cardiac output may decrease, resulting in decreased perfusion of major organs, particularly the brain (dizziness, confusion, etc.) and heart (angina and heart failure exacerbation). Depending on the vascular tone, blood pressure may remain stable or fall as a direct result of decreased cardiac output; however, hypertension would not be expected. Patients with atrial fibrillation are at increased risk of thrombosis, particularly stroke, secondary to pooling of blood in the left atrium and subsequent thrombus formation.

5. B. See Table 10-7 for recommended monitoring parameters and schedule. Coagulation tests are not routinely recommended for patients receiving amiodarone therapy. Coagulation tests may be required if a patient develops severe hepatotoxicity secondary to amiodarone or simply requires concomitant warfarin therapy for atrial fibrillation.

6. C. Patients under age 75 with no thromboembolic risk factors are at low risk of stroke and should be treated with aspirin 75–325 mg daily rather than warfarin.

7. A. Vagal maneuvers are effective nonpharmacologic therapy for PSVT because the reentry impulse circuit exists in the atrioventricular node. Although vagal maneuvers will slow the rate in atrial fibrillation or flutter, they will not terminate the arrhythmia because the reentry circuit is in the atrial tissue. Vagal maneuvers will have no effect on ventricular arrhythmia because the impulse arises from below the AV node.

8. A. Digoxin would be the drug of first choice because it will help slow the ventricular rate and it does not have negative inotropic effects. Both verapamil and diltiazem are negative inotropes and should not be used in patients with heart failure and low LVEF. Although it is a calcium

channel blocker, amlodipine does not affect AV nodal conduction. Dofetilide is used for conversion to and maintenance of sinus rhythm, not rate control.

9. **E.** All three medications are associated with torsades de pointes.

10. **E.** S-warfarin is primarily metabolized by CYP2C9. The VKORC1 gene determines the activity of the vitamin K epoxide-reductase enzyme, which is the target for warfarin. Together, the CYP2C9 and VKORC1 genotypes account for nearly 50% of the variability in warfarin dose. Warfarin is not affected by mutations in the CYP2D6 gene.

11. **B.** Dofetilide is renally eliminated and therefore must be adjusted according to creatinine clearance to decrease the significant risk of torsades de pointes. See Table 10-4.

12. **E.** Sotalol is eliminated almost entirely by the kidneys and is not affected by CYP450 enzymes.

13. **B.** Dofetilide does not increase digoxin concentrations when used concomitantly.

14. **B.** Since the patient appears to have been in atrial fibrillation for 1 week by history, there is a significant risk of thromboembolism during conversion to sinus rhythm. Proper treatment would require at least 3–4 weeks of anticoagulation (warfarin INR 2–3) prior to cardioversion, followed by at least 4 weeks of anticoagulation postcardioversion. Alternatively, a transesophageal echocardiogram can be used to rule out an atrial thrombus, allowing immediate cardioversion. Because the atria will require time to recover normal contractile activity, anticoagulation will be required for at least 4 weeks postconversion.

15. **B.** Because the patient has heart failure, the results of the Cardiac Arrhythmia Suppression Trial (CAST) indicate that class Ic agents should be avoided because of increased risk of death. Sotalol may worsen heart failure. Ibutilide is indicated for conversion only, not for maintenance of sinus rhythm. Digoxin will control only the ventricular rate; it will have no effect on maintaining sinus rhythm.

16. **A.** A wide QRS complex signifies conduction via an accessory pathway other than the AV node. Because calcium channel blockers prolong conduction in the AV node and not in the accessory pathways, administration of these agents will block the AV node and force

impulses to be conducted via the accessory pathways, which have shorter refractory periods. Consequently, the ventricular response will significantly increase.

17. **B.** Patients with LVEF ≤ 30–40% and previous myocardial infarction are at increased risk of sudden cardiac death, usually from ventricular fibrillation. Implantation of an ICD in these patients reduces the risk of mortality. Propafenone has negative inotropic effects and may worsen heart failure. The risk of ventricular proarrhythmia is significantly increased if propafenone is used in this patient. Verapamil also would worsen heart failure and not reduce the risk of mortality. Direct-current cardioversion is not indicated because the patient is stable. All standard heart failure medications should be optimized.

18. **C.** Adenosine is typically used only to terminate paroxysmal supraventricular tachycardia. Discontinuation of drugs that prolong the QT interval is essential to terminate torsades de pointes and prevent recurrences. Treatment should consist of intravenous magnesium sulfate and electrical pacing. An isoproterenol infusion can be used while waiting for electrical pacing.

19. **A.** Digoxin requires dosage adjustment in patients with impaired renal function.

20. **C.** Atrial fibrillation represents chaotic atrial activity resulting in no identifiable P wave. Because atrial fibrillation originates above the AV node, the QRS complex is narrow and the ventricular rate is typically greater than 100 bpm.

21. **D.** β-blockers are the preferred rate-controlling agent for hyperthyroidism because they inhibit the adrenergic response and decrease thyroid hormone conversion (especially propranolol). Digoxin is not as effective in controlling the ventricular rate related to a hyperadrenergic state (hyperthyroidism).

22. **A.** Sotalol possesses significant β-blocking activity, and therefore the patient may experience adverse effects similar to traditional β-blockers.

23. **E.** All of these medications except ibutilide are available in both intravenous and oral dosage forms.

24. **B.** Warfarin is metabolized by multiple cytochrome P450 isoenzymes, including CYP2C9, CYP1A2, and CYP3A4. Amiodarone inhibits by CYP2C9, CYP1A2, and CYP3A4, quinidine by unknown mechanisms,

propafenone by CYP1A2 and CYP3A4, and diltiazem by CYP3A4. Sotalol is primarily renally eliminated and does not result in cytochrome P450–mediated drug interactions.

10-9. References

Ansell J, Hirsh J, Hylek E, et al. Pharmacology and management of the vitamin K antagonists. *Chest.* 2008;133:160S–98S.

Antiarrhythmics Versus Implantable Defibrillators (AVID) Investigators. A comparison of antiarrhythmic drug therapy with implantable defibrillators in patients resuscitated from near fatal ventricular arrhythmias. *N Engl J Med.* 1997;337:1576–83.

Atrial Fibrillation Follow-up Investigation of Rhythm Management (AFFIRM) Investigators. A comparison of rate control and rhythm control in patients with atrial fibrillation. *N Engl J Med.* 2002; 347:1825–33.

Bardy GH, Lee KL, Mark, DB, et al. Amiodarone or an implantable cardioverter-defibrillator for congestive heart failure. *N Engl J Med* 2005;352:225–37.

Blomstrom-Lundqvist C, Scheinman MM, Aliot EM, et al. ACC/AHA/ESC guidelines for the management of patients with supraventricular arrhythmias: Executive summary. *J Am Coll Cardiol.* 2003; 42:1493–531.

Cheng JWM, Frank L, Garrett SD, et al. Key articles and guidelines in pharmacotherapeutic management of arrhythmias. *Pharmacotherapy.* 2004;24: 248–79.

Echt DS, Liebson PR, Mitchell LB, et al. Mortality and morbidity in patients receiving encainide, flecainide, or placebo. *N Engl J Med.* 1991; 324:781–88.

Fuster V, Ryden LE, Cannom DS, et al. ACC/AHA/ESC guidelines for the management of patients with atrial fibrillation: A report of the American College of Cardiology/American Heart Association Task Force on Practice Guidelines and the European Society of Cardiology Committee for Practice Guidelines (Writing Committee to Revise the 2001 Guidelines for the Management of Patients with Atrial Fibrillation). *J Am Coll Cardiol.* 2006;48: e149–246.

Josephson M, Wellens HJ. Implantable defibrillators and sudden cardiac death. *Circulation.* 2004; 2685–91.

Klein AL, Grimm RA, Murray RD, et al. Use of transesophageal echocardiography to guide cardioversion in patients with atrial fibrillation. *N Engl J Med.* 2001;344:1411–20.

Limdi NA, Veenstra DL. Warfarin pharmacogenetics. *Pharmacotherapy.* 2008;28:1084–97.

Ommen SR, Odell JA, Stanton MS. Atrial arrhythmias after cardiothoracic surgery. *N Engl J Med.* 1997;336:1429–34.

Sanoski CA, Schoen MD, Bauman JL. The Arrhythmias. In: Dipiro JT, Talbert RL, Yee GC, et al, eds. *Pharmacotherapy: A Pathophysiologic Approach.* 7th ed. New York: McGraw-Hill; 2008:279–314.

Singer DE, Albers GW, Dalen JE, et al. Antithrombotic therapy in atrial fibrillation. *Chest.* 2008;133:546S–92S.

Trujillo TC, Nolan PE. Antiarrhythmic agents: Drug interactions of clinical significance. *Drug Safety.* 2000;23:509–12.

Zipes DP, Camm AJ, Borggrefe M, et al. ACC/AHA/ESC 2006 guidelines for management of patients with ventricular arrhythmias and the prevention of sudden cardiac death: A report of the American College of Cardiology/American Heart Association Task Force and the European Society of Cardiology Committee for Practice Guidelines (Writing Committee to Develop Guidelines for Management of Patients with Ventricular Arrhythmias and the Prevention of Sudden Cardiac Death). *Circulation.* 2006;114:e385–484.

Ischemic Heart Disease

11

Kelly C. Rogers, PharmD
Carrie S. Oliphant, PharmD, BCPS
Shannon Finks, PharmD, BCPS (AQ Cardiology)

11-1. Introduction

Definitions

- *Ischemia:* Lack of oxygen from inadequate perfusion caused by an imbalance between oxygen supply and demand.
- *Ischemic heart disease (IHD):* Disease caused most frequently by atherosclerosis. IHD may present as silent ischemia, chest pain (at rest or on exertion), or myocardial infarction (MI).
- *Angina:* Syndrome classically described as discomfort or pain in the chest, arm, shoulder, back, or jaw. Angina is frequently worsened by physical exertion or emotional stress and usually relieved by sublingual (SL) nitroglycerin (NTG). Patients with angina usually have coronary artery disease (CAD) in at least one large epicardial artery.
- *Atypical angina:* Transient pain or discomfort lacking one or more of the criteria of classic angina. Atypical angina is more common in women, elderly patients, and diabetics.
- *Acute coronary syndrome (ACS):* Syndrome encompassing the following:
  - Unstable angina (UA)
  - Non-ST-segment myocardial infarction (NSTEMI)
  - ST-segment myocardial infarction (STEMI)
- *Coronary artery disease:* Chronic disorder that typically cycles in and out of the clinically defined phases of ACS and asymptomatic, stable, or progressive angina.
- *Percutaneous coronary intervention (PCI):* Procedure to reopen a partially or completely occluded coronary vessel to restore blood flow.
- *Coronary artery bypass graft (CABG):* Surgical procedure in which a vein is harvested from the leg and attached to the heart as a new coronary vessel in order to bypass a diseased vessel.

Epidemiology of IHD

IHD is the leading cause of death in the United States for both men and women. It causes as many deaths as cancer, chronic lower respiratory diseases, accidents, and diabetes combined.

Approximately 80 million adult Americans have some type of cardiovascular disease, which includes high blood pressure, coronary heart disease (CHD), heart failure, stroke, and congenital defects. In 2006, 829,072 Americans died of cardiovascular disease—nearly 2,400 per day, which averages to one death every 37 seconds. Approximately every 25 seconds an American will suffer a coronary event, and every minute someone will die from one. In 2006, there were 4,378,000 visits to emergency departments and 72,151,000 physician office visits with a primary diagnosis of cardiovascular disease.

In 2009, the estimated direct and indirect cost of cardiovascular disease is $475.3 billion. CHD, which includes acute MI, angina, atherosclerotic cardiovascular disease, and all forms of chronic IHD, is the single largest killer of American men and women. CHD caused one of every five deaths in the United States in 2005.

In 2009, an estimated 785,000 people will have a new coronary attack. About 470,000 will have a recurrent attack, and approximately 195,000 silent attacks occur per year.

For adults under 40 years of age, the lifetime risk for developing CHD is 49% for men and 32% for women.

11-2. Normal Physiology versus Pathophysiology

Normal Physiology

The arterioles change their resistance and dilate as needed to enable the heart to receive a fixed amount of O_2. In response to physical exertion, an increase in blood pressure (BP), or an increase in myocardial oxygen demand (MVO_2), the arterioles dilate to maintain O_2 supply to the heart.

Note: In atherosclerosis, plaque narrows the conductance vessel, causing the arterioles to dilate under normal or resting conditions to prevent ischemia. With stress or exercise, the vasodilator response is minimal, which causes ischemia and angina.

Pathophysiology Determinants of MVO_2

- *Heart rate (HR):* Tachycardia will increase MVO_2.
- *Contractility:* Increases in contractility will increase MVO_2.
- *Myocardial wall tension:* It depends on ventricular volume and pressure. Increased pressure or enlargement of the ventricle will increase systolic wall force and increase MVO_2.

Determinants of Myocardial Oxygen Supply and Flow

Myocardial O_2 supply is determined by

- Arterial O_2 saturation and myocardial O_2 extraction, which are relatively fixed under normal circumstances
- Coronary flow, which is dependent on the luminal cross-sectional area of the coronary artery and coronary arteriolar tone

Limits of flow are as follows: thrombi, spasm, congenital abnormalities, severe anemia, and severe ventricular hypertrophy attributable to hypertension or aortic stenosis (abnormally high oxygen demands).

Autoregulation of coronary blood flow occurs as follows:

- Adenosine, a potent vasodilator, is released from myocardial cells in response to decreased O_2 supply (e.g., occlusion); increased sympathetic activity (exercise, mental stress, exposure to cold); increased BP; and increased HR, which leads to increased MVO_2.
- Normal arteries respond to the increased demand with increased blood flow and some vasodilation of the large epicardial vessels.

- Atherosclerotic vessels lose this vasodilator response and develop constriction.

Vascular endothelium and control of arteriolar tone

The endothelium is the protective surface of the artery wall that separates the blood from the vascular smooth muscle of the artery wall and promotes smooth muscle relaxation and inhibits thrombogenesis. It secretes substances such as nitric oxide (NO), which produces vasodilation similar to the therapeutic effects of NTG. Additionally, these substances are antithrombotic and anti-inflammatory and can be thought of as defense mechanisms against noxious stimuli.

It also secretes substances that cause vasoconstriction. Normally, there is a beneficial balance between vasodilation and vasoconstriction.

Things that can damage the endothelium (cigarettes, oxidized low-density lipoprotein, hypertension, and PCI) lead to decreased NO production and loss of the endothelium's protective effects, which leads to an imbalance promoting vasoconstriction as the predominant response to stress.

Diastole

Normally, the distribution of blood flow between the epicardial and endocardial layers is equal during the period when coronary artery filling occurs.

In atherosclerosis, subendocardial blood flow is reduced.

Coronary vasospasm

A coronary vasospasm reduces blood flow, thereby causing ischemia, usually in areas of atherosclerotic plaques.

Atherosclerosis

Atherosclerosis is the most common cause of myocardial ischemia. A decrease in the lumen of coronary arteries attributable to stenosis leads to reduced myocardial perfusion and subsequent ischemia.

Segmental atherosclerotic narrowing is most commonly caused by a plaque, which can fissure, hemorrhage, and cause thrombosis, which then worsens the obstruction, reduces blood flow further, and leads to ACS.

11-3. Diagnostic Procedures

Diagnostic procedures include the following:

- History and physical examination
- Laboratory workup:
  - Complete blood count (CBC) with platelet count

- Serial creatine kinase-myocardial bound and troponin levels (enzyme markers specific for myocardial necrosis)
- Activated partial thromboplastin time (aPTT)
- Prothrombin time (PT) and international normalized ratio (INR)
- Fasting lipid panel within 24 hours of admission
■ Resting electrocardiogram (ECG)

Exercise Tolerance Test

The following drugs can interfere with the exercise tolerance test (ETT, or treadmill test):

■ Digoxin causes abnormal exercise-induced ST depression in about 30% of healthy patients.
■ β-blockers and vasodilators alter hemodynamic response to BP:
  - Hold four or five half-lives before ETT.
  - Withdraw β-blockers gradually to avoid precipitating an attack.
  - In some situations, patient may continue anti-ischemic therapy.
■ Nitrates can attenuate angina.
■ Flecainide may cause exercise-induced ventricular tachycardia.

Stress Imaging

Thallium Stress Test

The thallium stress test is a type of nuclear scanning test.

Pharmacologic stress imaging

In pharmacologic stress imaging, drugs "do the exercise" by increasing MVO_2.

Dobutamine
■ High doses up to 40 mcg/kg per minute cause positive inotropic and chronotropic effects that increase cardiac demand that lead to ischemia.
■ This drug is commonly used with an echocardiogram. Side effects include nausea, anxiety, tremor, arrhythmias, angina, and headache.

Dipyridamole, adenosine, and regadenoson
■ These drugs induce coronary vasodilation; they are used in conjunction with myocardial perfusion scintigraphy.
■ Dipyridamole side effects occur in up to 50% of patients and include angina, headache, nausea, dizziness, flushing, and severe bronchospasm in patients with chronic obstructive pulmonary disease (COPD) or asthma.

■ Adenosine side effects occur in up to 80% of patients and include chest pain, headache, flushing, shortness of breath, first-degree atrioventricular (AV) block, and severe bronchospasm in patients with COPD or asthma.
■ Regadenoson, a newer agent, has fewer side effects than adenosine. The most common are shortness of breath and headache.

Drug interactions
■ Xanthines (theophylline, caffeine) are adenosine receptor antagonists that attenuate the effects of adenosine and dipyridamole.
■ β-blockers interact with dobutamine, but the interaction can be overcome by increasing the dose of dobutamine.

Cardiac Catheterization

Cardiac catheterization (also called *cath* or *angiography*) involves the following procedure:

■ A catheter is inserted into the femoral artery and guided to the heart.
■ Radiocontrast dye is injected directly into the coronary arteries.
■ The dye shows which arteries are involved and the extent of occlusion.

Complications may arise as follows:

■ The patient can have an allergic reaction to iodine in the dye.
■ The dye can be nephrotoxic.
■ Arterial bleeding from access site, stroke, MI, or in rare cases death may occur.

11-4. Chronic Stable Angina, Prinzmetal's or Variant Angina, and Silent Ischemia

Clinical Presentation

Chronic stable angina

Symptoms are caused by decreased O_2 supply secondary to reduced flow.

Angina is considered stable if symptoms have been occurring for several weeks without worsening. Characteristics of stable angina are as follows:

■ Pain located over sternum that may radiate to left shoulder or arm, jaw, back, right arm, or neck
■ Pressure or heavy weight on chest, burning, tightness, deep, squeezing, aching, viselike, suffocating, crushing
■ Duration of 0.5–30.0 minutes

■ Symptoms may be precipitated by exercise, cold weather, postprandial, emotional stress, sexual activity

■ Pain relieved by SL NTG or rest

Prinzmetal's or variant angina

■ This uncommon form of angina is usually caused by spasm without increased MVO_2.

■ Most patients have severe atherosclerosis.

■ Recurrent, prolonged attacks of severe ischemia are characteristic.

■ Patients are often between 30 and 40 years old.

■ Pain usually occurs at rest or awakens the patient from sleep.

■ ECG shows ST-segment elevation, which returns to baseline when the patient is given NTG.

Silent ischemia

■ Ischemia in the absence of symptoms is "silent."

■ About 75% of ischemic episodes in patients with stable angina are undetected.

■ ECG shows ST-segment changes with elevation or depression during activity, but patient experiences no symptoms.

■ Silent ischemia occurs in about 20–30% of post-MI patients.

■ Of patients with stable angina, 50% have silent ischemia; it is common in diabetics.

Pharmacologic Management

Chronic stable angina

Goals of therapy are as follows:

■ To prevent MI and death

■ To reduce symptoms of angina and occurrence of ischemia to improve quality of life

Antiplatelets

■ Aspirin decreases the incidence of MI, adverse cardiovascular events, and sudden death.

■ Clopidogrel (Plavix) has a greater antithrombotic effect than ticlopidine (Ticlid) and has fewer side effects. *Note:* Ticlopidine has not been shown to reduce cardiovascular events in stable angina.

■ Indications for therapy are as follows:
  • Aspirin (75–162 mg daily) is recommended in all patients with chronic IHD (with or without symptoms) in the absence of contraindications.
  • Clopidogrel (75 mg daily) is chosen when aspirin is absolutely contraindicated.

• Ticlopidine is not recommended because of its poor side effect profile.

• The combination of clopidogrel plus aspirin is not indicated in patients with stable disease not undergoing PCI.

Anti-ischemic therapy
β-blockers

■ Effects on MVO_2 are as follows:
  • Inhibit catecholamine effects, thereby decreasing MVO_2
  • Decrease HR (negative chronotrope effects cause a decrease in conduction through the AV node)
  • Decrease contractility (negative inotrope effects cause a decrease in force of contraction)
  • Reduce BP

■ Effects on oxygen supply are as follows:
  • β-blockers cause no direct improvement of oxygen supply.
  • They increase diastolic perfusion time (coronary arteries fill during diastole) secondary to decreased HR, which may enhance left ventricle (LV) perfusion.
  • Ventricular relaxation causes increased sub-endocardial blood flow.
  • Unopposed alpha stimulation may lead to coronary vasoconstriction.

■ Dosing is as follows:
  • Start low, go slow.
  • Titrate to resting HR of 55–60 bpm, maximal exercise HR ≤ 100.
  • Avoid abrupt withdrawal, which can precipitate more severe ischemic episodes and MI; taper over 2 days.

■ Selection of β-blockers is based on the following factors:
  • β-blockers with cardioselectivity have fewer adverse effects; they lose cardioselectivity at higher doses.
  • The intrinsic sympathomimetic activity (ISA) with acebutolol, carteolol, penbutolol, and pindolol may not be as effective because the reduction in HR would be minimal; therefore, there is a small reduction in MVO_2. β-blockers with ISA are generally reserved for patients with low resting HR who experience angina with exercise.
  • Lipophilicity is associated with more central nervous system (CNS) side effects.
  • β-blockers should be avoided in patients with primary vasospastic angina.

- β-blockers are preferred in patients with a history of MI, chronic heart failure, high resting HR, and fixed angina threshold.
- Indications for therapy are as follows:
  - β-blockers are used as first-line therapy if not contraindicated in patients with prior MI, ACS, or history of heart failure.
  - They are often used as initial therapy if not contraindicated in patients without prior MI.
  - They are more effective than nitrates and calcium channel blockers (CCBs) in silent ischemia.
  - They are effective as monotherapy or with nitrates, CCBs, ranolazine, or a combination thereof.
  - They should be avoided in Prinzmetal's angina.
  - They improve symptoms 80% of the time.
  - All β-blockers are effective, but not all are FDA indicated.

Nitrates (endothelium-independent vasodilators)

- Effects on MVO_2 are as follows:
  - Peripheral vasodilation leads to decreased blood return to the heart (preload), which leads to decreased LV volume, decreased wall stress, and decreased O_2 demand.
  - Arterial vasodilation leads to decreased peripheral resistance (afterload), decreased systolic BP, and decreased O_2 demand.
  - Nitrates can cause a reflex increase in sympathetic activity, which may increase HR or contractility and lead to an increase in O_2 demand in some patients. This problem can be overcome with the use of a β-blocker.
- Effects on O_2 supply: Dilation of large epicardial coronary arteries and collateral vessels in areas with or without stenosis leads to increased O_2 supply.
- Indications for therapy are as follows:
  - SL nitroglycerin or NTG spray can be used for the immediate relief of angina.
  - Long-acting nitrates should be used as initial therapy to reduce symptoms only if β-blockers or CCBs are contraindicated.
  - Long-acting nitrates in combination with β-blockers can be used when initial treatment with β-blockers is ineffective.
  - Long-acting nitrates can be used as a substitute for β-blockers if β-blockers cause unacceptable side effects.
  - Nitrates are used in patients with CAD or other vascular disease.
  - Nitrates are preferred agents in the treatment of Prinzmetal's or vasospastic angina.

- Nitrates improve exercise tolerance.
- They produce greater effects in combination with β-blockers or CCBs.

Calcium channel blockers

- Effects on MVO_2 are as follows:
  - CCBs act primarily by decreasing systemic vascular resistance and arterial BP by vasodilation of systemic arteries.
  - They cause decreased contractility and O_2 requirement (all CCBs exert varying degrees of negative inotropic effects): verapamil > diltiazem > nifedipine.
  - Verapamil and diltiazem promote additional decreases in MVO_2 by decreasing conduction through the AV node, thereby decreasing HR.
- Effects on O_2 supply are as follows:
  - Increased diastolic perfusion time secondary to decreased HR, which may enhance LV perfusion
  - Decreased coronary vascular resistance and increased coronary blood flow by vasodilation of coronary arteries
  - Coronary vasodilation at sites of stenosis
  - Prevention or relief of vasospastic angina by dilation of the epicardial coronary arteries
- Indications for therapy are as follows:
- CCBs can be used as initial therapy for reduction of symptoms. They are usually second line when β-blockers are contraindicated.
- They are used in combination with β-blockers when initial treatment with β-blockers is not successful.
- They are used as a substitute for β-blockers if initial treatment with β-blockers causes unacceptable side effects.
- Slow-release, long-acting dihydropyridines and nondihydropyridines are effective in stable angina.
- Avoid using short-acting dihydropyridines.
- Newer-generation dihydropyridines, such as amlodipine or felodipine, can be used safely in patients with depressed LV systolic function and can be used in combination with β-blockers.

Combination therapy: β-blockers and nitrates

- β-blockers can potentially increase LV volume and LV end-diastolic pressure. Nitrates attenuate this effect.
- Nitrates increase sympathetic tone and may cause a reflex tachycardia. β-blockers attenuate this response.

Combination therapy: β-blockers and CCBs

- β-blockers and long-acting dihydropyridine CCBs are usually efficacious and well tolerated.
- CCBs, especially the dihydropyridines, increase sympathetic tone and may cause reflex tachycardia. β-blockers attenuate this effect.
- β-blockers and nondihydropyridine CCBs should be used together cautiously because the combination can lead to excessive bradycardia or AV block. The combination can also precipitate symptoms of heart failure in susceptible patients.

Ranolazine

- Unlike β-blockers and CCBs, ranolazine's antianginal and anti-ischemic effects occur without causing any hemodynamic changes in BP or HR.
- The mechanism of action is not clearly understood, but it appears to inhibit the late Na current (I_{Na}), preventing Ca overload and ultimately blunting the effects of ischemia by improving myocardial function and perfusion.
- Ranolazine is indicated as first-line or add-on therapy in combination with β-blockers, CCBs, or nitrates for management of chronic stable angina.

Angiotensin-converting enzyme inhibitors

- Angiotensin-converting enzyme inhibitors (ACEIs) reduce the incidence of MI, cardiovascular death, and stroke in patients at high risk for vascular disease (data from the Heart Outcomes Prevention Evaluation [HOPE] trial).
- Controversy exists whether all ACEIs are equally effective or whether "tissue ACEIs" provide better protection.
- Low-risk patients with stable CAD and normal or slightly reduced LV function may not benefit from ACEI therapy as greatly as high-risk patients.
- Indications for therapy are as follows:
  - ACEIs are used in all patients with left ventricular ejection fraction (LVEF) ≤ 40% and in those with hypertension, diabetes, or chronic kidney disease unless contraindicated.
  - They are used in all patients with CAD (by angiography or previous MI) or other vascular disease.
  - It is reasonable to consider angiotensin receptor blockers (ARBs) for patients who have hypertension and other indications but who are intolerant of ACEIs, have heart failure, or have had a MI with LVEF ≤ 40%.

Lipid-lowering therapy

- Clinical trials have proved that lipid-lowering therapy should be recommended in patients with established CAD, including chronic stable angina, even if only mild or moderate elevations of LDL (low-density lipoprotein) cholesterol are present.
- Omega-3 fatty acids can be encouraged in either dietary consumption or capsule form (1 g daily) for risk reduction; higher doses are recommended for treatment of elevated triglycerides.
- Therapeutic options to treat triglycerides or non-HDL cholesterol include niacin and fibrates (after LDL-lowering therapy).
- Indications for therapy are as follows:
  - Lipid-lowering therapy is used in patients with documented or suspected CAD or CHD risk equivalents and LDL ≥100 mg/dL: target LDL < 100 mg/dL.
  - It is used in high-risk patients: target LDL < 70 mg/dL may be appropriate.
  - A combination of statins with other lipid-lowering therapy requires careful monitoring for prevention of myopathy, rhabdomyolysis, and elevation of liver enzymes.

Prinzmetal's or variant angina

- β-blockers have no role in management and may increase painful episodes.
- β-blockers may induce coronary vasoconstriction and prolong ischemia.
- Nitrates are often used for acute attacks.
- CCBs may be more effective, may be dosed less frequently, and have fewer side effects than nitrates.
- Nifedipine, diltiazem, or verapamil are all equally effective as single agents.
- Nitrates can be added if there is no response to CCBs.
- Combination therapy with nifedipine + diltiazem or nifedipine + verapamil has been reported to be useful.
- Dose titration is recommended to obtain efficacy without unacceptable side effects.
- Treat acute attacks and provide prophylactic treatment for 6–12 months.

Silent ischemia

- The goal is to decrease the number of episodes, both symptomatic and asymptomatic.

- The initial step is to modify risk factors for IHD (smoking, hypercholesterolemia, hypertension).
- β-blockers have shown improvement in patients with ischemic episodes and are preferred in patients post-MI.
- CCBs are somewhat less effective than β-blockers.

11-5. Unstable Angina or Non-ST-Segment Elevation Myocardial Infarction Pathophysiology

The process of ischemic syndromes involves two essential events:

- Disruption of an atherosclerotic plaque
- Formation of a platelet-rich thrombus

The clinical manifestation depends on the extent and duration of the thrombotic occlusion. In UA or NSTEMI, the thrombus does not completely occlude the vessel.

Pathogenesis and clinical presentations of UA and NSTEMI are similar but differ in severity. Many structural and functional differences in disease pathophysiology exist between men and women. Women present more commonly than men with NSTEMI and are found to have less obstructive coronary disease than men.

Presentation

- Central or substernal or crushing chest pain can radiate to the neck, jaws, back, shoulders, and arms.
- Patients may present with diaphoresis, nausea, vomiting, arm tingling, weakness, shortness of breath, or syncope.
- Pain may be similar to typical angina except that the occurrences are more severe, may occur at rest, and may be caused by less exertion than typical angina.
- UA and NSTEMI may be incorrectly interpreted as dyspepsia or indigestion.
- Pain is not relieved by SL NTG or rest.
- UA and NSTEMI may evolve into STEMI without treatment.

Diagnosis

- Chest pain persisting longer than 5 minutes that is unrelieved by SL NTG or rest
- Cardiac enzymes and ECG changes (Table 11-1)

Table 11-1. Cardiac Enzymes and ECG Changes: UA versus NSTEMI/STEMI

	UA	NSTEMI/STEMI
Cardiac enzymes	Negative	Positive
ECG changes: ST-segment, T-wave changes	If present, are transient	Always present

Goals of Therapy

- Completely restore blood flow to the myocardium
- Prevent MI, arrhythmias, and ischemia

Pharmacologic Management of UA and NSTEMI

Morphine, oxygen, nitrates, and aspirin

Indications for therapy are shown in Table 11-2.

Anti-ischemic therapy

β-adrenergic blockade
- Preference is for an agent without ISA.
- Agents with β$_1$ selectivity are preferred in patients with bronchoconstrictive disease.
- There is no evidence that one agent is superior to another.
- Initial choices include metoprolol, atenolol, and propranolol.
- Indications for therapy are as follows:
  - β-blockers can be used in all patients without contraindications.
  - The first dose should be given orally within the first 24 hours unless contraindications exist, including signs of heart failure, symptoms of low output state, increased risk of cardiogenic shock, or other relative contraindications (e.g., bradycardia, hypotension, heart block, reactive airway disease).

Nitrates
Nitrates are discussed in Table 11-2.

Calcium channel blockers
- There is no mortality benefit from the use of CCBs; therefore, they are not recommended as first-line therapy.
- Indications for therapy are as follows:
  - In patients with contraindications to β-blockers, a nondihydropyridine CCB

Table 11-2. Morphine, Oxygen, Nitrates, and Aspirin Therapy

Medication	Details
Morphine	Vasodilatory properties on both arterial and venous sides decrease both preload and afterload. Pain relief decreases tachycardia, along with decrease in preload and afterload; all work to decrease myocardial O_2 demand.
	Increments of 2–4 mg IV are given every 5–15 minutes until pain is relieved.
	Nausea, vomiting, hypotension, sedation, and respiratory depression may occur.
	Morphine produces a vagotonic effect that may be contraindicated in patients with bradycardia. Watch closely for hypotension, respiratory depression, and allergic reactions.
Meperidine	Meperidine can be used in patients who are intolerant of morphine. It has vagolytic effects, so it is the analgesic of choice in patients who are bradycardic; 25–75 mg IV.
Oxygen	Supplemental O_2 2–4 L/min by nasal cannula is recommended to correct and avoid hypoxia, particularly within the first 2–3 hours. More aggressive ventilatory support should be considered and given as needed.
Nitroglycerin	All patients should receive NTG as a sublingual tablet or spray, followed by IV administration as needed for the relief of ischemia.
	Long-acting nitrates (oral, transdermal) should be used as secondary prevention in patients who do not tolerate β-blockers and CCBs. These nitrates can be used in patients who have continual chest pain despite the use of β-blockers and CCBs.
Aspirin (ASA)	Nonenteric-coated aspirin 162–325 mg should be given at the onset of chest pain unless contraindicated. Chew and swallow the first dose.
	A dose of 75–162 mg should be taken daily for life.
	Poststent, aspirin 162–325 mg is used in combination with clopidogrel for at least 1 month after BMS, 3 months after sirolimus-eluting stents, and 6 months after paclitaxel-eluting stents. With the newer DES, everolimus, and zotarolimus, a minimum of 75 mg of aspirin daily is acceptable immediately after PCI. After this initial period, the dose of aspirin can be reduced to 75–162 mg daily.
	Clopidogrel may be substituted if a true aspirin allergy is present or if the patient is considered unresponsive to ASA.

(verapamil, diltiazem) should be used in the absence of significant LV dysfunction or other contraindications.
- Oral long-acting dihydropyridine CCBs provide additional control of anginal symptoms in patients who are already receiving β-blockers and nitrates.
- Avoid short-acting dihydropyridines.

Inhibition of the renin–angiotensin–aldosterone system

- ACEIs, ARBs, and aldosterone inhibitors are used for inhibition of the renin–angiotensin–aldosterone (RAA) system.
- Indications for therapy are as follows:
  - ACEIs should be started orally within the first 24 hours in all patients with UA, NSTEMI, or STEMI with pulmonary congestion or LVEF ≤ 40% unless contraindicated.
  - It is reasonable to use ACEIs orally within the first 24 hours of STEMI in patients without pulmonary congestion or LVEF ≤ 40% unless contraindicated.

- ACEIs are recommended for life in those patients post UA or post NSTEMI with heart failure, hypertension, or diabetes unless contraindicated.
- On the basis of the results from the HOPE trial, ACEIs may be considered in all patients post UA or NSTEMI who do not have contraindications.
- ACEIs are recommended indefinitely in all patients post STEMI with LVEF ≤ 40% and for those with hypertension, diabetes, or chronic kidney disease, unless contraindicated.
- ARBs should be given to those patients who are intolerant of an ACEI and who have heart failure, LVEF ≤ 40%, or hypertension. Valsartan and candesartan are the only ARBs that have established efficacy for this indication.
- Unless contraindicated, long-term aldosterone blockade should be prescribed for post-UA, NSTEMI, or STEMI patients already receiving therapeutic doses of ACEIs and BBs who have an LVEF ≤ 40% and either symptomatic heart failure or diabetes.

Antiplatelet therapy

Aspirin
Aspirin is discussed in Table 11-2.

Thienopyridines
- Thienopyridines include clopidogrel (Plavix) and ticlopidine (Ticlid).
- Inhibition of platelet aggregation is irreversible and takes 2–5 days to achieve full effect. Often clopidogrel or ticlopidine is given in a loading dose for a more rapid effect (within 2 hours).
- Clopidogrel is the preferred agent in this class. Ticlopidine is rarely used because of severe toxicities.
- The mechanism of platelet aggregation for clopidogrel and aspirin (ASA) differs; therefore, their effects are additive.
- Indications for therapy are as follows:
  - Clopidogrel is an alternative for patients who are allergic to ASA or who have a gastrointestinal intolerance to ASA.
  - Clopidogrel should be combined with ASA in patients undergoing stent implantation for a minimum of 1–12 months, depending on the type of stent used and bleeding risk.
  - In patients who do not undergo a PCI procedure, clopidogrel 75 mg daily should be combined with ASA for at least 1 month and ideally up to 12 months.

Glycoprotein IIb/IIIa receptor inhibitors (GPIs)
Agents
- Abciximab (ReoPro)
- Eptifibatide (Integrilin)
- Tirofiban (Aggrastat)

Uses
- All of the agents can be used as adjunctive therapy in patients undergoing PCI.
- In combination with heparin and ASA, eptifibatide and abciximab have been shown to reduce the incidence of combined death, MI, and recurrent ischemia in patients with UA or NSTEMI who undergo PCI.
- GPIs are alternatives to clopidogrel when the appropriate loading dose was not given prior to PCI.
- Abciximab is used only when PCI will likely be done shortly after starting infusion.
- Eptifibatide and tirofiban are the preferred agents if PCI will be delayed.
- Special attention should be focused on proper dosage adjustments of renally cleared agents,

especially in elderly patients, women, and those with renal insufficiency.
- Indications for therapy are as follows:
  - GPIs can be considered as an adjunct to ASA, clopidogrel, and anticoagulation during PCI.
  - GPIs can be given during the intervention procedure just before stent deployment or angioplasty.
  - GPIs can be given upstream (prior to PCI) with aspirin +/– clopidogrel, depending on risk factors.
  - Upstream eptifibatide and tirofiban are preferred over abciximab.
  - These agents are appropriate to use in patients who are not given a clopidogrel loading dose upstream or in cases where the loading dose was not given more than 2–6 hours prior to PCI.

Anticoagulant therapy

Unfractionated heparin
- Heparin or enoxaparin should be given to all patients in combination with ASA and clopidogrel.
- Heparin is continued for a total of 24–48 hours or until a PCI procedure is completed.
- In patients with a planned CABG within 24 hours, heparin use is preferred to low molecular weight heparin (LMWH).

Low molecular weight heparin and anti-Xa inhibitors
- Enoxaparin (Lovenox) is an LMWH.
- LMWH differs from unfractionated heparin (UFH) in size and affinity for thrombin.
- Advantages of LMWH over UFH include better bioavailability, a more predictable response, ease of administration, fewer side effects, and no recommended routine monitoring.
- Trials comparing UFH to LMWH for the treatment of UA and NSTEMI have shown superiority of enoxaparin over UFH, whereas trials with dalteparin showed equivalence to UFH.
- Fondaparinux (Arixtra) is an anti-Xa inhibitor.
- Fondaparinux has been found to be noninferior to enoxaparin in reducing the risk of ischemic events.
- Fondaparinux significantly lowers major bleeding events compared with enoxaparin.
- Fondaparinux currently does not have FDA approval for this indication.
- Indications for therapy are as follows:
  - Enoxaparin or UFH in combination with aspirin and clopidogrel should be given to all patients unless contraindicated.

- Enoxaparin or fondaparinux is continued for the duration of hospitalization, up to 8 days, or until a PCI procedure is completed.
- Enoxaparin may be superior to heparin in patients with UA or NSTEMI.
- For patients with increased risk of bleeding and not undergoing angiography, fondaparinux is preferred.
- Fondaparinux is not recommended if a patient is going to undergo PCI.

Lipid-lowering therapy

- Lipid-lowering therapy is used in patients with documented or suspected CAD or CHD risk equivalents and LDL ≥ 100 mg/dL: target LDL < 100 mg/dL.
- In high-risk patients, target LDL < 70 mg/dL may be appropriate.
- Lipid-lowering medications should be initiated prior to discharge.

11-6. Acute Myocardial Infarction: STEMI

Pathophysiology

More than 85% of all MIs occur by thrombus formation precipitated by atherosclerotic plaque rupture. Aggregated platelets after plaque rupture can serve as a substrate for thrombus propagation, leading to formation of an occlusive thrombus. This complete occlusion results in abrupt and persistent ischemia that clinically manifests as STEMI. Left untreated, occlusion of the coronary arteries can lead to sudden cardiac death. See Table 11-3 for a comparison of STEMI and NSTEMI.

Location

Patients with right ventricular (RV) wall infarction should be managed similarly to LV infarction except that NTG, diuretics, and other preload reducing agents should be avoided in RV wall MIs because these patients are dependent on preload.

RV MI may require volume loading with IV fluids to maintain preload and cardiac output.

Symptoms differ from an LV wall MI in that an RV wall MI can cause hypotension, elevated jugular venous pressure, and cardiogenic shock because of inadequate filling of the LV.

Table 11-3. STEMI versus UA or NSTEMI

STEMI	NSTEMI
Totally occlusive thrombus is found.	Platelet-rich thrombi, which do not completely block coronary blood flow, are found.
More extensive damage occurs.	Smaller, less extensive damage occurs.
STEMI results in an injury that affects the entire thickness of the myocardial wall.	NSTEMI involves only the subendocardial myocardium.
Occlusion persists long enough to compromise myocardial function and leads to myocardial necrosis.	Unstable angina is ischemia; NSTEMI may still result in necrosis, but not to the extent of STEMI.
ST-segment elevation on ECG is present.	ST depression or no ST elevation on ECG is present.
Lytic therapy or primary reperfusion is a main treatment strategy.	Antiplatelets and anticoagulants are used to target platelet-rich thrombus.

Ventricular remodeling

Ventricular remodeling can occur as a result of myocardial necrosis and may continue for months following MI. It leads to activation of the neurohormonal and renin-angiotensin systems that will ultimately affect ventricular shape, size, and function. It precipitates chronic changes in ventricular volume, ventricular dilation, hypertrophy, and eventually heart failure. ACEIs, ARBs, and β-blockers and the combination of hydralazine plus nitrates reduce the progression of ventricular remodeling. A combination of ACEI plus ARB has been noted to cause more frequent side effects, such as renal dysfunction and hyperkalemia. Aldosterone blockade has been proven beneficial in the post-MI setting with LV dysfunction with eplerenone.

Prognosis

Mortality factors

- The highest risk of death from MI is generally within the first 48 hours.
- Anterior MIs usually involve a larger area of the myocardium than do inferior MIs, and thereby have a higher mortality.
- An important prognostic factor following MI is LV function because heart failure is one of the most serious complications of MI.

- Large anterior wall MIs, LV dysfunction, and complex ventricular ectopy carry the highest mortality rate post-MI.
- Early identification and risk stratification can reduce mortality following MI.

Predictors of death

- High troponin concentration correlates with higher death rates in STEMI and NSTEMI.
- Predictors of death within 30 days post-MI include age greater than 70 years, hypertension, atrial fibrillation, tachycardia, large infarct size, previous MI, and female.
- Lower-risk patients include those younger than 71 years of age with an LVEF ≥ 40%.
- Patients who continue to have frequent ventricular arrhythmias following MI are at high risk of sudden cardiac death.

Presentation

Symptoms are similar to UA/NSTEMI. Atypical presentation is common in women, elderly patients, and those with diabetes.

Diagnosis

Two of the following three criteria must be met:

- Chest pain generally lasting for more than 30 minutes
- ECG changes such that there is ST-segment elevation of 0.1 mV in two contiguous limb leads or 0.1–0.2 mV elevation in at least two contiguous precordial leads
- With respect to cardiac isoenzymes, troponin T or I elevation

Goals of Therapy in Acute MI

- Limit infarct size.
- Reverse myocardial ischemia and thereby salvage myocardium.
- Minimize complications.
- Reduce mortality.

Pharmacologic Management of STEMI

Morphine, oxygen, nitrates, and aspirin

Refer to see Table 11-2 for information about morphine, oxygen, nitrates, and aspirin therapy.

The following points apply to nitrate use in STEMI:

- If chest pain is not relieved by sublingual nitroglycerin, intravenous nitrates may be used for the first 24–48 hours in all patients with acute MI who do not have hypotension, bradycardia, tachycardia, or suspected RV infarctions. Nitrates salvage ischemic myocardium by relaxation of vascular smooth muscles in veins, arteries, and arterioles.
- Nitrates demonstrate insignificant reductions in mortality beyond 48 hours. Use is reserved for those patients with large acute MIs, persistent chest discomfort, heart failure, hypertension, or persistent pulmonary congestion.
- Cautions and contraindications: Carefully titrate in patients with inferior wall MI because of its frequent association with RV infarction. Such patients are especially dependent on adequate RV preload to maintain cardiac output and can experience profound hypotension during nitrate administration.
- Do not administer nitrates to patients who have received a phosphodiesterase inhibitor for erectile dysfunction within the last 24 hours (48 hours for tadalafil).

Reperfusion therapy

Primary PCI
(See Section 11-7 for more information.)

- PCI is an intervention designed to reopen a partially or completely occluded coronary artery to reestablish blood flow.
- The goal is door-to-balloon time of < 90 minutes.
- Mechanical reperfusion (percutaneous transluminal coronary angioplasty, or PTCA, with coronary stenting) has been shown to be more successful than fibrinolysis.
- In patients who receive a stent, dual antiplatelet therapy with aspirin and clopidogrel therapy should be added to the regimen, as in UA and NSTEMI, and continued for at least 12 months.

Fibrinolytic therapy

- Fibrinolytic therapy is also known as *thrombolytic therapy*.
- Fibrinolytic therapy improves myocardial O_2 supply, limits infarct size, and decreases mortality.
- Controversy exists about one lytic agent's superiority over another.
- A door-to-needle time of < 30 minutes is an important goal.

- Signs of successful reperfusion include relief of chest pain, resolution of ST-segment changes, and reperfusion arrhythmias, usually ventricular in nature.
- Fibrinolytic therapy is unsuccessful in approximately 22–30% of patients.
- Indications for therapy are as follows:
  - ST-segment elevation is > 1 mm in two or more contiguous leads or left bundle branch block is present (obscuring ST observational changes).
  - Presentation is within 12 hours of symptom onset.
  - The patient has no contraindications to fibrinolytic therapy and indications for therapy.
  - In patients age > 75 years, fibrinolytic therapy may be useful and appropriate.
  - Fibrinolytic therapy can be used in STEMI when time to therapy is 12–24 hours if chest pain is ongoing.
  - It should not be used if the time to therapy is > 24 hours and the ischemic pain is resolved.
  - It should not be used for ST depression.
- Long-term therapy (e.g., 1 year) with clopidogrel plus aspirin is reasonable in patients who receive fibrinolytic therapy.

Antithrombotic and anticoagulant therapy

- Indications for UFH, enoxaparin, and fondaparinux therapy are as follows:
  - IV UFH is administered with selective fibrinolytics (e.g., alteplase, reteplase, and tenecteplase) for the prevention of recurrent coronary thrombosis for a minimum of 48 hours.
  - IV UFH can be administered with nonselective fibrinolytic agents (e.g., streptokinase) in patients at high risk for systemic emboli (large or anterior MI, atrial fibrillation, previous emboli, or known LV thrombus).
  - Enoxaparin can be used as an alternative to UFH in patients receiving fibrinolytic therapy, with different dosing strategies dependent on age and renal function.
  - Patients not treated with a thrombolytic and without contraindications can be treated with IV UFH or LMWH (enoxaparin 1 mg/kg subcutaneous bid or fondaparinux 2.5 mg IV followed by 2.5 mg subcutaneous daily) for at least 48 hours for UFH and for up to 8–9 days for the latter agents.
  - Two studies support the benefits of clopidogrel 75 mg daily in addition to aspirin in STEMI

patients regardless of whether they receive fibrinolytic therapy or no reperfusion therapy. In patients < 75, it is reasonable to administer a 300 mg loading dose of clopidogrel.

β-adrenergic blockade

- Early β-blocker use post-MI reduces infarct size, cardiovascular mortality, reinfarction rate, and nonfatal cardiac arrests and increases probability of long-term survival.
- Oral β-blocker therapy should be administered within the first 24 hours to patients who do not have contraindications.
- It is reasonable to administer early IV β-blocker therapy to STEMI patients who are hypertensive and without any contraindications (e.g., heart failure, low output state, risk for cardiogenic shock, bradycardia, blocks, hypotension).
- Late administration of a β-blocker (at least 24 hours after MI) improves LV diastolic filling and reduces risk of recurrent MI and death.
- Indications for therapy are as follows:
  - *Early therapy:* β-blockers should be given to all patients with acute MI who can be treated within 12 hours of STEMI, regardless of administration of concomitant thrombolytic therapy. IV or oral treatment should be started as soon as possible in all patients within 12–24 hours after onset of symptoms if no contraindications exist.
  - *Late therapy:* β-blockers should be given to all patients without a clear contraindication to β-blocker therapy. Treatment should begin within a few days of the event (if not initiated earlier) and should be continued indefinitely.

Glycoprotein IIb/IIIa Inhibitors (GPIs)

- Trials evaluating the role of platelet GPI in STEMI in combination with full- and half-dose fibrinolytic agents have shown a more complete reperfusion at the price of higher bleeding rates, especially in elderly patients.
- Abciximab administered early before primary PCI reduces the incidence of combined death, MI, and recurrent ischemia in patients with STEMI.

Inhibition of the RAA system: ACEIs, ARBs, and aldosterone inhibitors

- The primary goal is to limit postinfarction LV dilatation and hypertrophy so that pump function is preserved or improved. ACEIs attenuate the remodeling process and thereby slow the progression to heart failure post-MI.

- Benefits of ACEIs are clearly most pronounced in patients with evidence of ventricular dysfunction (either objective evidence such as LVEF ≤ 40% or subjective evidence such as heart failure symptoms).
- Other high-risk patients (previous MI, heart failure, and anterior MI without thrombolytic therapy) have shown marked benefit from ACEIs.
- Recent studies of ACEI therapy suggest acute treatment should be given to patients considered at higher risk because of a history of hypertension, diabetes, or previous MI and should be continued indefinitely.
- An ARB can be used for those patients who are intolerant of an ACEI and have either clinical or radiological signs of heart failure or an LVEF of ≤ 40%.
- Aldosterone blockade (eplerenone, spironolactone) should be prescribed post-STEMI in those patients already on an ACEI with an LVEF ≤ 40% and with either symptomatic heart failure or diabetes.
- Aldosterone blockers should be avoided in patients with renal dysfunction (serum creatinine ≥ 2.5 mg/dL in men or ≥ 2.0 in women) or hyperkalemia (potassium > 5 mEq/L).
- Indications for therapy are discussed in Section 11-5.

Lipid lowering

Indications for therapy are discussed in Section 11-5.

Calcium channel blockers

- Verapamil or diltiazem should be used only with continuing ischemia when β-blockers are either contraindicated or used at maximum dose with nitrates.
- Verapamil or diltiazem should not be used in patients with left ventricular systolic dysfunction, AV block, hypotension, or bradycardia.

Warfarin

- Warfarin is recommended in patients with indications for anticoagulation (e.g., LV thrombus, atrial fibrillation, extensive wall motion abnormalities).
- In patients requiring triple therapy with aspirin, clopidogrel, and warfarin, an INR range of 2.0–2.5 is recommended with low-dose aspirin (75–81 mg daily).
- Use of warfarin in combination with aspirin, clopidogrel, or both is associated with an increased risk of bleeding and should be carefully monitored.

Treatment of ventricular fibrillation post-MI

- The risk of ventricular fibrillation (VF) is at highest during the first 4 hours post-MI and then declines sharply.
- Prophylactic antiarrhythmic use has been shown to increase all-cause mortality when used to prevent VF; it is not recommended.
- Amiodarone may be used if patients experience VF or hemodynamically compromising ventricular tachycardia following MI.

11-7. Revascularization

Percutaneous Coronary Intervention Procedures

Procedure types include balloon angioplasty (PTCA), coronary stenting, and ablative technologies (laser, atherectomy).

Primary PCI is a very effective method for reestablishing coronary perfusion and is suitable for at least 90% of patients. Primary PCI should be performed as quickly as possible with the goal of a medical contact–to–balloon or door-to-balloon time of 90 minutes or less. Primary PCI is favored over fibrinolytic therapy because PCI-treated patients experience lower short-term mortality rates and fewer nonfatal reinfarctions and hemorrhagic strokes than those treated with fibrinolytic therapy.

Facilitated PCI refers to a strategy of planned immediate PCI after an initial pharmacologic regimen, such as full-dose fibrinolytics, GPIs, or another pharmacologic regimen. *Rescue PCI* refers to the use of PCI when fibrinolytic therapy has failed.

Revascularization is not preferred in women with low-risk features.

Potential complications of invasive PCI include problems with arterial access site, technical complications, acute vessel closure, restenosis, and acute renal failure secondary to nephrotoxic dye.

Bare Metal Stents and Drug-Eluting Stents

Restenosis is the loss of 50% or more of the diameter of the in-stent lumen at the site of an initially successful intervention; it usually occurs within the first 3–6 months.

Drug-eluting stents (DES) were introduced in 2003 and have the principal advantage of reducing restenosis over angioplasty alone and bare metal stents (BMS).

Pharmacologic agents, such as sirolimus, paclitaxel, zotarolimus, and everolimus, are embedded in the steel stent and released over time.

DES have reduced the rate of restenosis to less than 5%.

Anticoagulation during PCI

Anticoagulation is mandatory because the vessel manipulation during PCI is inherently thrombogenic. Possible agents include the following:

- UFH has traditionally been the mainstay of therapy.
- Studies have shown that the direct thrombin inhibitor bivalirudin may be as effective as heparin but with less bleeding. The use of bivalirudin seems to eliminate the need for GPIs when an appropriate clopidogrel loading dose is given.
- Enoxaparin use during PCI can be challenging. Dosing is determined based on the last administered dose of enoxaparin. If the last subcutaneous dose was administered within 8 hours, no additional enoxaparin needed; if the last dose was administered after 8–12 hours, 0.3 mg/kg IV should be given.
- Fondaparinux is not recommended during PCI secondary to catheter thromboses. If PCI is planned, an alternative anticoagulant should be used.

Antiplatelet therapy during PCI

Aspirin and clopidogrel
Clopidogrel in combination with aspirin is used to reduce in-stent thrombosis and is used for at least 1 month with BMS, ideally up to 12 months, and a minimum of 12 months with DES for patients not at high risk for bleeding.

The dose of aspirin is 162–325 mg daily for at least 1 month after BMS, 3 months after sirolimus-eluting stents, and 6 months after paclitaxel-eluting stents. With the newer DES, everolimus, and zotarolimus, a minimum of 75 mg of aspirin daily is acceptable after PCI. After the initial poststent period is complete, the dose of aspirin can be reduced to 75–162 mg daily.

Glycoprotein IIb/IIIa inhibitors
Although similar effects have been noted with each of the GPIs, the timing of PCI should be determined before an agent is selected.

GPIs are administered before or during PCI for patients who are troponin-positive or have other high-risk features.

Use abciximab or eptifibatide if PCI is anticipated soon after presentation (< 4 hours).

GPIs can be omitted if bivalirudin is used in place of UFH and at least 300 mg clopidogrel was administered at least 6 hours prior.

Coronary Artery Bypass Graft Surgery

CABG is indicated in patients with multivessel disease with LV dysfunction or significant disease of a major coronary vessel that is not amenable to PCI.

Clopidogrel should not be used for a minimum of 5 days prior to CABG to reduce the risk of bleeding.

11-8. Primary Prevention: Risk Factor Modification

The majority of the causes of cardiovascular disease are known and modifiable. Therefore, risk factor screening should begin at age 20 with the hope that all adults know the levels and significance of risk factors as routinely assessed by their primary care provider.

Nonmodifiable Risk Factors
Age
- Men > 45
- Women > 55 (or those who had an early hysterectomy regardless of age)

Race
Higher risk in African American males and females than in Caucasian males and females

Family history
- Father or brother with a coronary event before age 55
- Mother or sister with a coronary event before age 65

Modifiable Risk Factors
- Smoking
- Hypertension
- Hyperlipidemia
- Diabetes

- Metabolic syndrome
- Obesity
- Physical inactivity
- Alcohol consumption

Pharmacologic Therapy

Aspirin

The Eighth American College of Clinical Pharmacy Evidence-Based Clinical Practice Guidelines on Antithrombotic and Thrombolytic Therapy (Chest Guidelines) recommends that ASA (75–325 mg/day) be considered for individuals who have at least moderate risk (based on age and cardiac risk factor profile with a > 10% risk of cardiac event over 10 years) for CAD and who are without contraindications.

The American College of Cardiology and American Heart Association (AHA) recommend doses of 75–162 mg/day in persons at higher risk of cardiovascular disease (especially those with a 10-year risk of CHD > 10%).

The American Diabetes Association recommends ASA therapy to prevent cardiovascular events in most patients with diabetes who are > 40 years of age and have no contraindications to ASA.

The recommendation for aspirin use for primary prevention is stronger in men than in women, and aspirin can be prescribed based on risk profile (stroke versus MI) and age:

- For women < 65 years of age who are at risk for ischemic stroke and low bleeding risk, 75–100 mg/day can be preventive.
- For women > 65 years of age who are at risk for ischemic stroke or MI and low bleeding risk, 75–100 mg/day can be preventive.

ACEIs and ARBs

In the HOPE trial, ramipril demonstrated effectiveness in reducing the risk of MI, stroke, and death from cardiovascular causes in patents at high risk of a major cardiovascular event. ACEIs may be used as protective agents.

The European Trial on Reduction of Cardiac Events with Perindopril in Stable Coronary Artery Disease (EUROPA) similarly showed perindopril to be beneficial in patients with evidence of coronary heart disease but without heart failure and has led to the increased use of ACEIs in patients with vascular disease but without heart failure or LV dysfunction.

Results from the Prevention of Events with Angiotensin Converting Enzyme (PEACE) inhibition trial suggest that low-risk patients with CAD who are receiving maximal therapy with β-blockers, aspirin, and lipid-lowering therapies do not gain clinically significant benefit from the addition of trandolapril 4 mg daily.

Chronic ACEI therapy may be most beneficial in high-risk patients (uncontrolled hyperlipidemia, hypertension, smoking, proteinuria, vascular disease).

Lipid lowering

Consider lipid lowering in all patients at risk for a coronary event.

Antioxidants

There is no consistent evidence with vitamin E or other antioxidant therapy to recommend its use for primary prevention of heart disease.

Nonpharmacologic Therapy for IHD

Smoking cessation

Smoking cessation is one of the most important risk-modifying behaviors. Evidence suggests that the best adherence to a cessation program combines pharmacotherapy with behavioral modification.

A wide range of smoking cessation aids (prescription and nonprescription) products is available.

Nicotine replacement alone is not an effective management strategy for smoking cessation. Nicotine combined with bupropion has been the most successful.

Diet

Diets low in saturated fat and high in fruits, vegetables, whole grains, and fiber are associated with a reduced risk of cardiovascular disease. With respect to omega-3 fatty acids: the AHA Dietary Guidelines recommends inclusion of at least two servings of fish per week (particularly fatty fish). Food sources high in alpha-linolenic acid (e.g., soy bean, canola, walnut, and flaxseed oil and walnuts and flaxseeds) are also recommended.

Exercise

Regular aerobic physical activity increases a person's capacity for exercise. Exercise plays a role in both primary and secondary prevention of cardiovascular disease.

Current guidelines from the U.S. Centers for Disease Control and Prevention and National Institutes of

Health recommend that Americans should accumulate at least 30 minutes of moderate-intensity physical activity on most, preferably all, days of the week to prevent risk of chronic disease in the future. The Institute of Medicine recommends 60 minutes of physical activity per day.

Weight loss

Weight loss can reduce blood pressure, lower blood glucose levels, and improve blood lipid abnormalities. A goal of 5% to 10% of body weight loss is associated with decreased morbidity and mortality.

Pharmacotherapy used for weight loss should be reserved for (a) those with a body mass index exceeding 30 and (b) those with a body mass index exceeding 25 plus other risk factors for comorbid diseases.

Alcohol consumption

Lowest cardiovascular mortality occurs in those who consume one or two drinks per day. People with no alcohol consumption have higher total mortality than those drinking one or two drinks per day.

In the absence of alcohol-related illnesses, one or two drinks per day in males and one alcoholic drink per day in females may be considered for high-risk patients. A drink equivalent amounts to a 12-ounce bottle of beer, a 4-ounce glass of wine, or a 1.5-ounce shot of 80 proof spirits.

A general increase in alcohol consumption at the population level is not recommended.

11-9. Pharmacology

Anti-ischemic Drug Therapy

β-blockers

The use of β-blockers in anti-ischemic drug therapy is discussed in Chapter 8.

Nitrates

Mechanism of action
- Organic nitrates are prodrugs that must be transformed to exert pharmacological effect.
- NTG leads to denitration of the nitrate, liberation of NO, guanylyl cyclase stimulation, the conversion of guanosine triphosphate to cGMP, and vasodilation.
- NO also reduces platelet adhesion and aggregation and affects endothelial function and vascular growth.

Properties
- ***Oral:*** Isosorbide dinitrate and NTG undergo extensive first-pass metabolism when given orally. Mononitrate does not; it is completely bioavailable.
- ***IV:*** IV use achieves the highest concentrations. Usually, IVs are used for only 24 hours to avoid developing tolerance.
- ***SL tablet or spray for immediate-release:*** Unlike tablets, spray does not degrade when exposed to air. The half-life is 1–5 minutes regardless of route.

Doses
See Table 11-4 for information about doses.

Monitoring parameters
Blood pressure and heart rate should be monitored.

Adverse drug reactions
Adverse drug reactions to nitrate are described in Table 11-5.

Drug–drug interactions
Nitrate drug–drug interactions are described in Table 11-6.

Drug–disease interactions
- Glaucoma
  - Intraocular pressure may increase.
  - Use with caution in patients with glaucoma.
- Hypertrophic obstructive cardiomyopathy
- Severe aortic stenosis: Can cause hypotension and syncope

Contraindications
- If sildenafil and vardenafil are used within 24 hours.
- If tadalafil is used within 48 hours.
- Hypersensitivity to nitrates can occur.

Patient instructions and counseling
- General instructions:
  - Avoid alcohol consumption.
  - May cause dizziness; use caution when driving or engaging in hazardous activities until drug effect is known.
  - When standing from a sitting position, rise slowly to avoid an abrupt drop in blood pressure.
  - Notify physician of acute headache, dizziness, or blurred vision.
- Instructions for sublingual tablets:
  - Keep tablets in their original container.
  - Dissolve tablet under the tongue. Lack of tingling does not indicate a lack of potency.

Table 11-4. Pharmacologic Properties and Doses of Nitrates

Drug	Route	Onset	Duration of action	Dose
Nitroglycerin sublingual tablet (Nitrostat, Nitroquick)	Sublingual	1–3 min	30–60 min	0.2–0.6 mg every 5 min. Seek emergency treatment if chest pain is unrelieved after 1 dose.
Nitroglycerin spray (Nitrolingual)	Translingual	2 min	30–60 min	0.4 mg every 5 min. Seek emergency treatment if chest pain unrelieved after 1 spray.
Nitroglycerin transmucosal tablets (Nitroguard)	Buccal	1–2 min	3–5 hours	Insert 1 tablet into cheek every 3–5 hours.
Nitroglycerin ointment (Nitrobid, Nitrol)	Topical	30–60 min	2–12 hours	1–2 inches every 8 hours up to 4–5 inches every 4 hours.
Nitroglycerin transdermal patches (Nitro-dur, Transderm Nitro, Nitrek, Nitrodisc, Deponit, Minitran)	Topical	30–60 min	Up to 24 hours	Starting dose: 0.2–0.4 mg/hour. Apply and allow patch to stay in place for 12 hours. Remove the patch after 12 hours to allow a nitrate-free interval.
Nitroglycerin sustained-release tablets or capsules (Nitrong, Nitroglyn, Nitro-Time)	Oral	20–45 min	3–8 hours	Starting dose: 2.5 mg tid-qid. Increase the dose by 2.5 mg two to four times daily to reach effective dose.
Nitroglycerin intravenous (Tridil, Nitro-Bid IV)	IV	1–2 min	3–5 min	Starting dose: 5 mcg/min. Titrate to response.
Isosorbide mononitrate (Ismo, Monoket)	Oral	30–60 min	No data	20 mg bid (given 7 hours apart). May need to start with 5 mg bid for low-weight patients.
Isosorbide mononitrate, extended-release (Imdur, Isotrate ER)	Oral	30–60 min	No data	Starting dose: 30–60 mg daily. Maximum dose: 240 mg daily.
Isosorbide dinitrate (Isordil Titradose, Sorbitrate)	Oral	20–40 min	4–6 hours	Starting dose: 5–20 mg q6h. Maintenance dose: 10–40 mg q6h.
Isosorbide dinitrate, sustained-release tablets or capsules (Isordil Tembids, Dilatrate-SR)	Oral	Up to 4 hours	6–8 hours	Initial dose: 40 mg q8h. Maintenance dose: 40–80 mg q8–12 h.

Table 11-5. Nitrate Adverse Reactions

Type	Reaction
Tolerance	Tolerance to the vasodilatory effects can develop if dosing does not allow for a nitrate-free interval (10–12 hours).
CNS	Headache (up to 50%), dizziness, anxiety, and nervousness can occur.
Cardiovascular	Hypotension, tachycardia, palpitations, and syncope can occur.
Gastrointestinal	Nausea, vomiting, and dyspepsia can occur.
Dermatologic	Rash or dermatitis can occur.
Other	Blurred vision, muscle twitching, perspiration, edema, and arthralgia can occur.

Table 11-6. Nitrate Drug–Drug Interactions

Interacting medication	Effect
Sildenafil (Viagra), vardenafil (Levitra), tadalafil (Cialis)	Significant reduction of systolic and diastolic blood pressure may occur. Do not give sildenafil or vardenafil within 24 hours of nitrate use. Do not give tadalafil within 48 hours of nitrate use.
Calcium channel blockers	Marked symptomatic hypotension may occur.
Alcohol	Severe hypotension may occur.

- Take one tablet at the first sign of chest pain. If chest pain is unrelieved, seek emergency medical attention.
- Instructions for translingual spray:
  - Spray under tongue or onto tongue.
  - Hold spray nozzle as close to the mouth as possible and spray medicine onto or under the tongue.
  - Do not inhale the spray, use near heat or open flame, or use while smoking.
  - Close mouth immediately after spraying.
  - Avoid eating, drinking, or smoking for 5–10 minutes.
  - If the pain does not go away after one spray, seek emergency medical attention.
- Instructions for transmucosal tablets:
  - Place tablet between cheek and gum. Do not chew tablet; allow it to dissolve over a 3- to 5-hour period.
  - Touching the tablet with the tongue or hot liquids may increase release of the medication.
- Instructions for ointment:
  - Measure the correct amount using the papers provided with the product.
  - Use papers for the application, not fingers.
  - Apply to the chest or back.
- Instructions for transdermal patches:
  - Tear the wrapper open carefully. Never cut the wrapper or patch with scissors. Do not use any patch that has been cut by accident.
  - Apply to a hairless area and rotate sites to avoid irritation. Be sure to remove the old patch before applying a new one.
  - Do not put the patch over burns, cuts, or irritated skin.
  - Remove the patch approximately 12–14 hours after placing it on every day. This prevents tolerance to the beneficial effects of NTG.
  - Used patches may still contain residual medication; use caution when disposing around children and pets.
  - Store the patches at room temperature in a closed container, away from heat, moisture, and direct light. Do not refrigerate.
- Instructions for sustained-release tablets:
  - Take at the same time each day as directed.
  - Do not chew or crush tablets or capsules.

Calcium channel blockers

The use of calcium channel blockers in anti-ischemic drug therapy is discussed in Chapter 8.

Ranolazine (Ranexa)

Mechanism of action

The mechanism of action of ranolazine not clearly understood, but appears to inhibit the late Na current (I_{Na}), preventing Ca overload and ultimately blunting the effects of ischemia by improving myocardial function and perfusion.

Dose

- Initiate at 500 mg po bid and titrate to a maximum dose of 1 g po bid as tolerated.
- Take without regard to meals. Do not crush, break, or chew tablet.

Monitoring parameters

- Monitor anginal symptoms.
- Perform baseline and follow-up ECGs to evaluate QT interval.
- Monitor BP regularly in patients with severe renal insufficiency.

Adverse drug reactions

Adverse reactions to ranolazine are described in Table 11-7.

Drug–drug interactions

Drug–drug interactions are described in Table 11-8.

Contraindications

- Use with strong CYP3A inhibitors.
- Use with CYP3A inducers.
- Use in patients with clinically significant hepatic impairment.

Patient instructions and counseling

- Ranolazine is not for acute anginal symptoms.
- Notify physician if you take any other medications, including over-the-counter medications.

Table 11-7. Ranolazine Adverse Drug Reactions

Type	Reaction
CNS	Dizziness, headache, asthenia
Cardiovascular	Bradycardia, palpitations, hypotension, orthostatic hypotension
Gastrointestinal	Nausea, abdominal pain, vomiting, dry mouth, constipation
Other	Tinnitus, vertigo, dyspnea, peripheral edema

Table 11-8. Ranolazine Drug–Drug Interactions

Interacting medication	Effect
Strong CYP3A inhibitors: ketoconazole, itraconazole, clarithromycin, nefazodone, ritonavir, nelfinavir, indinavir, saquinavir	Medication increases average steady-state plasma concentration of ranolazine 3.2-fold, which can precipitate QTc prolongation. Concomitant use is contraindicated.
Moderated CYP3A inhibitors: diltiazem, verapamil, erythromycin, fluconazole, grapefruit juice	Medication increases ranolazine steady-state plasma concentrations about twofold, which can precipitate QTc prolongation. Concomitant use is cautioned.
P-glycoprotein inhibitors: cyclosporine	Increased ranolazine concentrations can occur; use lower doses of ranolazine.
CYP3A and P-glycoprotein inducers: rifampin, rifabutin, phenobarbital, phenytoin, carbamazepine, St. John's Wort	Medication decreases plasma concentrations of ranolazine by up to 95% (rifampin).
Simvastatin	Plasma levels of simvastatin, a CYP3A4 substrate, are increased approximately twofold.

- Notify physician if you have any history or family history of QTc prolongation or congenital long-QT syndrome or if you are receiving drugs that prolong the QTc interval, such as antiarrhythmic agents, erythromycin, and certain antipsychotics (thioridazine, ziprasidone).
- Do not take drugs that are strong CYP3A inhibitors (e.g., ketoconazole, clarithromycin, nefazodone, ritonavir) or strong inducers of CYP3A (e.g., rifampin, carbamazepine, phenytoin).
- Notify physician if you take drugs that are moderate CYP3A inhibitors (e.g., diltiazem, verapamil, erythromycin) or P-glycoprotein inhibitors (e.g., cyclosporine).
- Ranolazine can be taken with or without meals.
- Ranolazine should be swallowed whole; do not crush, break, or chew tablets.
- Ranolazine may cause dizziness or lightheadedness; therefore, notify physician if you experience fainting spells, and know how you react to this drug before operating heavy machinery.

Inhibition of the RAA system

See Chapter 9 for information about angiotensin-converting enzyme inhibitors, angiotensin receptor blockers, and aldosterone blockers.

Antiplatelet Drug Therapy

Aspirin

Mechanism of action

Aspirin blocks prostaglandin synthesis, which prevents the formation of thromboxane A_2.

Dose

- **At the onset of chest pain:** 160–325 mg chewed and swallowed
- **Maintenance dose:** 75–162 mg for life, except immediately post PCI, when a maintenance dose of 75–325 mg daily is appropriate depending on the type of stent received
- **Monitoring parameters:** signs of bleeding, renal function, tinnitus

Adverse drug reactions

Adverse reactions to aspirin are described in Table 11-9.

Drug–drug interactions

Antiplatelet agents, anticoagulants, nonsteroidal anti-inflammatory drugs (NSAIDs), and celecoxib may all increase the risk of bleeding if used in combination with ASA.

Drug–disease interactions

- Peptic ulcer disease (PUD).
- Other active bleeding.
- Aspirin may cause gastric ulceration.
- An enteric-coated tablet is recommended.

Patient instructions and counseling

- Avoid additional over-the-counter products containing ASA, NSAIDs, or salicylate ingredients without the direction of a physician.

Table 11-9. Aspirin Adverse Reactions

Type	Reaction
Cardiovascular	Hypotension, edema, tachycardia
CNS	Fatigue, nervousness, dizziness
Dermatologic	Rash, urticaria, angioedema
Gastrointestinal	Nausea, vomiting, dyspepsia, gastrointestinal ulceration, gastric erosion, duodenal ulcers
Hematologic	Bleeding, anemia
Otic	Hearing loss, tinnitus
Renal	Renal impairment, increased serum creatinine, proteinuria
Respiratory	Asthma, bronchospasm, dyspnea, tachypnea, respiratory alkalosis

- Patients who received a stent or were treated medically after an acute coronary event will need the combination of clopidogrel and aspirin.
- Notify physician of dark, tarry stools, persistent stomach pain, difficulty breathing, unusual bruising or bleeding, or skin rash.
- Do not crush an enteric-coated product.

Thienopyridines

Mechanism of action

Thienopyridines block adenosine diphosphate (ADP)–mediated activation of platelets by selectively and irreversibly blocking ADP activation of the glycoprotein IIb/IIIa complex.

Dose
Clopidogrel
- Loading dose: 300–600 mg orally
- Maintenance dose:
  - 75 mg daily combined with aspirin for at least 1 month and ideally up to 12 months in patients who were treated medically and did not undergo cardiac cath
  - 75 mg daily combined with aspirin for at least 1 month with BMS, ideally up to 12 months, and a minimum of 12 months with DES for patients not at high risk for bleeding
  - 75 mg daily for life in patients who cannot tolerate aspirin

Ticlopidine
- Loading dose: 500 mg orally
- Maintenance dose: 250 mg bid

Monitoring parameters
Clopidogrel
Monitor for signs of bleeding.

Ticlopidine
Monitor CBC with differential every 2 weeks for the first 3 months of therapy, liver function tests periodically, and for signs of bleeding.

Discontinue ticlopidine if the absolute neutrophil count drops to < 1,200 or platelet count drops to < 80,000.

Adverse drug reactions
Adverse reactions to thienopyridine are described in Table 11-10.

Drug–drug interactions
Drug–drug interactions are described in Table 11-11.

Drug–disease interactions
PUD or other active bleeding

Table 11-10. Thienopyridine Adverse Reactions

Type	Reaction
Clopidogrel	Chest pain, headache, dizziness, abdominal pain, vomiting, diarrhea, arthralgia, back pain, upper respiratory infections, flu-like symptoms; < 1% blood dyscrasias, bleeding, rash
Ticlopidine	Rash, nausea, dyspepsia, diarrhea; 2.4% neutropenia; < 1% blood dyscrasias, thrombotic thrombocytopenic purpura, bleeding

Contraindications
- Hypersensitivity to an individual product
- Active bleeding (e.g., gastrointestinal or intracranial hemorrhage)
- Severe liver disease
- Neutropenia, thrombocytopenia

Patient instructions and counseling
- All patients who received a stent or were treated medically after an acute coronary event will need the combination of clopidogrel and aspirin.
- Avoid additional ASA, salicylates, and NSAID products unless under the direction of a physician.
- Notify physician for unusual bleeding or bruising; blood in the urine, stool, or emesis; skin rash; or yellowing of the skin or eyes.
- Do not stop taking without discussing with physician.
- Discontinue clopidogrel at least 5 days prior to CABG.

Glycoprotein IIb/IIIa receptor inhibitors

Mechanism of action
- Blockade of the glycoprotein IIb/IIIa receptor prevents fibrinogen binding, thus inhibiting platelet aggregation, the final common pathway for platelet aggregation.

Properties of individual agents
See Table 11-12 for properties of GPIs.

Table 11-11. Thienopyridine Drug–Drug Interactions

Interacting medication	Effect
Antiplatelet agents, anti-coagulants, NSAIDs, and celecoxib	Combination may increase the risk of bleeding.
CYP4502C9 substrates (phenytoin, fluvastatin, NSAIDs, losartan, irbesartan, valsartan)	Medication may increase serum levels.

Table 11-12. Pharmacologic Properties of Glycoprotein IIb/IIIa Receptor Inhibitors

Drug	Chemical nature	Duration of effect (hours)	Renal elimination	Renal dosing adjustment
Abciximab (ReoPro)	Antibody	>12[a]	No	No
Eptifibatide (Integrilin)	Nonpeptide	4–8	Yes	Yes
Tirofiban (Aggrastat)	Peptide fragment	4	Yes	Yes

a. Action can be reversed by a platelet infusion.

Indications and doses
Table 11-13 provides information about indications and doses.

Monitoring parameters
Hematocrit and hemoglobin, platelet count, PT and aPTT, and activated clotting time (with PCI) should be monitored.

Adverse drug reactions
Adverse drug reactions include bleeding, thrombocytopenia, and allergic reaction from repeated exposure (abciximab).

Drug–drug interactions
Antiplatelet agents, anticoagulants, NSAIDs, and celecoxib may all increase the risk of bleeding if used in combination with GPIs.

Drug–disease interactions
PUD or other active bleeding

Contraindications
- Active bleeding
- Platelet count < 100,000
- History of intracranial hemorrhage, neoplasms, AV malformations, or aneurysm
- History of stroke within the past 30 days or any history of hemorrhage stroke
- Severe hypertension (BP > 180/110 mm Hg)
- Major surgery within past 6 weeks
- Dialysis dependent (eptifibatide only)

Anticoagulants

Heparin

Mechanism of action
Heparin enhances the action of antithrombin III, thereby inactivating thrombin and preventing the conversion of fibrinogen to fibrin.

Dose
- *UA and NSTEMI:* 60–70 units/kg (maximum 5,000 units) IV bolus, 12–15 units/kg/h (maximum 1,000 units/h) infusion titrated to an aPTT range of 50–70 seconds
- *STEMI (in combination with tPA, rPA, or tenecteplase):* 60 units/kg (maximum 4,000 units) IV bolus, 12 units/kg/h (maximum 1,000 units/h)

Table 11-13. Indications and Doses of the Glycoprotein IIb/IIIa Receptor Inhibitors

Drug	Indication	Dose
Abciximab (ReoPro)	Adjunct to PCI or when PCI is planned within 24 hours	0.25 mg/kg IV bolus, 0.125 mg/kg infusion continued for 12 hours post-procedure; maximum length of infusion: 18–24 hours
Eptifibatide (Integrilin)	Adjunct to PCI	180 mcg/kg IV bolus × 2, 10 min apart; 2 mcg/kg/min infusion (creatinine clearance < 50 mL/min; 1 mcg/kg/min) started after the first bolus and continued for 18–24 hours postprocedure (minimum of 12 hours)
	Patients with ACS managed with or without PCI	180 mcg/kg IV bolus, 2 mcg/kg/min infusion (creatinine clearance < 50 mL/min; 1 mcg/kg/min) continued until discharge, up to 72 hours; or if post-PCI for 18–24 hours; maximum length of infusion: 96 hours
Tirofiban (Aggrastat)	Adjunct to PCI	0.4 mcg/kg/min IV bolus for 30 min, 0.1 mcg/kg/min infusion (creatinine clearance < 30mL/min; bolus and infusion are reduced by 50%) for 12–24 hours postprocedure
	Patients with ACS managed with or without PCI	10 mcg/kg IV bolus over 3 min followed by 0.15 mcg/kg/min infusion for 36 hours or 0.4 mcg/kg IV bolus over 30 min, 0.1 mcg/kg/min infusion for 72 hours (creatinine < 30 mL/min, bolus and infusion are reduced by 50%)

infusion titrated to an aPTT range of 50–70 seconds for 48 hours

Monitoring parameters
Monitor aPTT, PT, platelet count, hemoglobin and hematocrit, signs of bleeding, and activated clotting time (with PCI).

Adverse drug reactions
Bleeding, thrombocytopenia, hemorrhage, epistaxis, allergic reactions, and osteoporosis may occur.

Protamine can be used to reverse the effects of heparin; 1 mg of protamine neutralizes 100 units of heparin.

Drug–drug interactions
Antiplatelet agents, anticoagulants, NSAIDs, and celecoxib may all increase the risk of bleeding if used in combination with UFH. Switching from heparin to LMWH may increase the risk of bleeding and has been reported to cause death.

Drug–disease interaction
PUD or other active bleeding

Contraindications
■ History of heparin-induced thrombocytopenia
■ Severe thrombocytopenia
■ Active bleeding
■ Suspected intracranial hemorrhage

LMWH (enoxaparin) and factor Xa inhibitors (fondaparinux)

Mechanism of action
The mechanism of action is similar to that of heparin; however, these drugs are stronger inhibitors of thrombin formation through inhibition of factor Xa.

Properties
Properties are described in Table 11-14.

Dose
■ Enoxaparin (Lovenox):
  • *UA and NSTEMI:* 1 mg/kg SC q12h (creatinine clearance < 30 mL/min: 1 mg/kg SC q24h)
  • *STEMI with fibrinolytic therapy:* 30 mg IV then, 1 mg/kg SC q12h (creatinine clearance < 30 mL/min: 1 mg/kg SC q24h); for patients > 75 years of age, eliminate the IV bolus and give 0.75 mg/kg SQ q12h

Table 11-14. Properties of Low Molecular Weight Heparin versus Unfractionated Heparin

Drug	Half-life (hours)	Molecular weight (daltons)	Anti-Xa: Anti-IIa	Renal elimination
Enoxaparin	4.5	4,500	2.7:1.0	Yes
UFH	1	15,000	1.0:1.0	No

■ Fondaparinux (Arixtra), as an alternative to UFH:
  • *UA and NSTEMI:* For patients in whom a conservative strategy is selected over an invasive strategy, 2.5mg SC daily up to 9 days
  • *STEMI (with or without fibrinolytics):* 2.5 mg IV, then SC daily up to 9 days; not recommended if patient undergoing primary PCI

Monitoring parameters
Serum creatinine, platelet count, hemoglobin and hematocrit, anti-Xa levels (optional), and signs of bleeding should be monitored. It is not necessary to monitor aPTT or PT with LMWH or direct Xa inhibitors.

Adverse drug reactions
Adverse reactions include bleeding, thrombocytopenia, hemorrhage, and epistaxis.

Drug–drug interactions
Antiplatelet agents, anticoagulants, NSAIDs, and celecoxib may all increase the risk of bleeding if used in combination with LMWH.

Switching from LMWH to UFH may increase the risk of bleeding and has been reported to cause death.

Drug–disease interactions
PUD or any active bleeding

Warnings
Patients with recent or anticipated epidural or spinal anesthesia are at risk of hematoma and subsequent paralysis.

Contraindications
■ Severe thrombocytopenia
■ Active bleeding
■ Suspected intracranial hemorrhage

Thrombolytic Therapy

Mechanism of action

Thrombolytic therapy acts either directly or indirectly to activate or convert plasminogen to plasmin to lyse a formed clot. The conversion of plasminogen to plasmin activates the body's natural thrombolytic–fibrinolytic system, which lyses the clot and releases fibrin degradation products.

Dose

Thrombolytic doses are given in Table 11-15.

Monitoring parameters

CBC, ECG, aPTT, signs of bleeding, and signs of reperfusion should be monitored.

Adverse drug reactions

Adverse reactions include bleeding, intracranial hemorrhage (< 1%), stroke (< 2%), and epistaxis.

Drug–drug interactions

Antiplatelet agents, anticoagulants, NSAIDs, and celecoxib may all increase the risk of bleeding if used in combination with thrombolytics.

Contraindications

Contraindications
- Any prior intracranial hemorrhage
- Known structural cerebrovascular lesion

Table 11-15. Thrombolytic Doses

Drug	Dose
Streptokinase (Streptase)	1.5 million units in 50 mL of normal saline or D_5W given over 60 min
Tissue plasminogen activator (Alteplase)	15 mg IV bolus, followed by 0.75 mg/kg IV infusion over 30 min (not to exceed 50 mg); then 0.5 mg/kg IV infusion over 1 hour (not to exceed 35 mg)
Reteplase (Retevase)	10 units IV push over 2 min, followed in 30 min by a repeat 10 units IV bolus over 10 min
Tenecteplase (TNKase)	< 60 kg, give 30 mg IV bolus; 60–69.9 kg, give 35 mg IV bolus; 70–79.9 kg, give 40 mg IV bolus; 80–89.9 kg, give 45 mg IV bolus; > 90 kg, give 50 mg IV bolus; each bolus given over 5 seconds

- Ischemic stroke within 3 months, except acute ischemic stroke within 3 hours
- Known intracranial neoplasm (primary or metastatic)
- Active internal bleeding or bleeding diathesis (does not include menses)
- Suspected aortic dissection
- Significant closed head or facial trauma within 3 months

Relative contraindications
- Severe uncontrolled hypertension (BP > 180/110 mm Hg)
- History of prior ischemic stroke greater than 3 months, dementia, or known intracerebral pathology not covered in contraindications
- Current use of anticoagulants in therapeutic doses (INR > 2–3)
- Traumatic or prolonged (> 10 min) cardiopulmonary resuscitation or major surgery (< 3 weeks)
- Noncompressible vascular punctures
- Recent (within 2–4 weeks) internal bleeding
- For streptokinase, prior exposure (especially within 5 days to 2 years) or prior allergic reaction
- Pregnancy
- Active peptic ulcer
- History of chronic severe hypertension

11-10. Key Points

- Angina is a syndrome described as discomfort or pain in the chest, arm, shoulder, back, or jaw. Angina is frequently worsened by physical exertion or emotional stress and is usually relieved by sublingual NTG. Patients with angina usually have CAD.
- Anginal symptoms are caused by a decrease in O_2 supply because of reduced blood flow.
- The goals for treating stable angina are to prevent death, reduce symptoms, and improve quality of life.
- Aspirin has been shown to decrease the incidence of MI, adverse cardiovascular events, and sudden death in patients with CAD.
- β-blockers are first-line therapy for treatment of angina in patients with or without a history of MI if there are no contraindications.
- Patients prescribed nitrates for treatment of angina need to be counseled on their appropriate use.
- Ranolazine is a novel antianginal medication that does not affect BP or HR. It can be used as initial

therapy or in combination with other antianginal medications.

- Upon hospital presentation with UA, NSTEMI, or STEMI, initial therapy for all patients is morphine, oxygen, nitroglycerin, and aspirin. If there are no contraindications, all patients should be given aspirin therapy for life.
- The first-line anti-ischemic therapy for the treatment of UA and NSTEMI is a β-blocker. If chest pain continues or a β-blocker is contraindicated, a calcium channel blocker or long-acting nitrate should be considered, in that order.
- In addition to aspirin therapy for life, clopidogrel should be administered to all patients who undergo stent replacement for at least 1 month after BMS but ideally up to 12 months and for at least 12 months after DES stents. Long-term treatment with clopidogrel may be beneficial in patients with established vascular disease. Clopidogrel should be withheld for 5–7 days prior to surgery to reduce the risk of major bleeding.
- Any of the available glycoprotein IIb/IIIa agents should be considered in patients undergoing a PCI procedure. In patients without a planned PCI, eptifibatide or tirofiban can be used for medical treatment.
- All patients presenting with UA or NSTEMI should receive anticoagulation with UFH or LMWH.
- STEMI differs from UA and NSTEMI in that a totally occlusive clot causes damage across the entire thickness of the myocardial wall. The damage to the heart is more extensive with STEMI and ECG changes differ.
- Primary reperfusion (either PCI or fibrinolytic therapy) is the main treatment strategy for STEMI, with primary PCI being preferred.
- Ventricular remodeling (post-MI) resulting after myocardial damage can be slowed and possibly reversed by using long-term ACE inhibition and β-blockade (use ARBs as alternative to ACEIs and hydralazine + nitrates in combination with ACEIs in African American patients with LV dysfunction).
- Secondary prevention of MI should include aspirin, β-blockers, ACEIs, and statin therapy (to achieve an LDL goal of < 100 mg/dL; < 70 mg/dL in high-risk patients) in all patients who have no contraindications.
- Aldosterone blockade should be considered post-STEMI in patients with an LVEF ≤ 40% and either symptomatic heart failure or diabetes.

11-11. Questions

Questions 1–3 refer to this case:

Mr. Smith is a 66-year-old white male who presented to his local physician with complaints of chest pain. He described the pain as sharp, aching, and non-radiating. The pain, which he has had for the past few weeks, has occurred mainly during his daily walk and is usually relieved when he stops to rest.

Past medical history: hypertension, PUD, asthma, CAD

Family history: Father died of a stroke at 86; mother died at age 82 with diabetes mellitus and heart failure; sister died of MI at 52

Social history: Smokes 1 pack per day × 40 years; drinks alcohol socially 1–2 times a week

Medications:

- Proventil MDI 2 puffs prn
- Flovent 44 mcg 2 puffs bid
- Prilosec 20 mg daily
- Aspirin 75 mg daily
- HCTZ 25 mg daily

Vital signs: BP 148/92; HR 82; RR 18; height 72″; weight 200 lbs

Labs: (fasting) total cholesterol 226 mg/dL; TG 110 mg/dL; HDL 38 mg/dL; LDL 166 mg/dL; Chem 12-within normal limits

ECG: Normal (patient currently pain free)

Cath 6 years ago: Minimal two-vessel disease

1. How would you classify Mr. Smith's chest pain?

   A. Unstable angina
   B. Stable angina
   C. Variant angina
   D. Silent ischemia
   E. NSTEMI

2. Considering Mr. Smith's situation, which of the following would be the most appropriate therapeutic intervention?

   A. SL NTG prn
   B. Propranolol
   C. Tirofiban
   D. Verapamil and SL NTG prn
   E. Atenolol, amlodipine, and SL NTG

3. What additional medication should be considered for Mr. Smith?

   A. Ticlopidine
   B. Atorvastatin

C. Clopidogrel

D. Eptifibatide

E. Reteplase

4. Which of the following effects on myocardial oxygen demand do β-blockers *not* cause?

A. Decreased HR

B. Decreased BP

C. Decreased contractility

D. Peripheral vasodilation

E. Decreased conduction through the AV node

5. Which of the following statements is true regarding the use of calcium channel blockers in IHD?

A. Amlodipine and felodipine reduce MVO_2 by decreasing conduction through the AV node.

B. Calcium channel blockers should be used as first-line therapy in patients with stable angina.

C. Newer-generation dihydropyridines like nifedipine immediate-release are safe in the treatment of IHD.

D. Calcium channel blockers can be used in combination with β-blockers to attenuate the effect of increased sympathetic tone that some dihydropyridines may cause.

E. The combination of verapamil and metoprolol in a patient with reduced LV systolic function is safe and well tolerated by most patients.

6. Which of the following counseling points should be made to a patient being prescribed SL NTG?

I. Take at the same time each day as directed.

II. Keep tablets in their original container.

III. Take at the first sign of chest pain; if chest pain is unrelieved, seek emergency medical attention.

A. III only

B. I, II, and III

C. I and III only

D. I and II only

E. II and III only

7. Which of the following is *not* considered a potential cardiovascular benefit of ACEIs in IHD?

A. They reduce the incidence of MI.

B. They reduce the incidence of cardiovascular death and stroke in patients at high risk for vascular disease.

C. Agents with high tissue ACE inhibition have been proven to be superior and provide better protection.

D. ACE inhibitors should be used in all stable angina patients with known CAD who also have diabetes.

E. ACE inhibitors have shown greater benefit post-MI in higher-risk patients.

8. Which of the following drugs do *not* appear to interact with an exercise tolerance test (ETT)?

A. Nitrates

B. Digoxin

C. Atenolol

D. Flecainide

E. Clopidogrel

9. Ideal properties for a β-blocker in the treatment of UA or NSTEMI include which of the following?

A. Available as an IV product, cardioselectivity

B. Low lipophilicity, has intrinsic sympathomimetic activity (ISA)

C. Has ISA, cardioselectivity

D. Cardioselectivity, low lipophilicity, does not have ISA

E. Noncardioselective, high lipophilicity

10. Nitrates decrease oxygen demand through the following mechanism(s):

I. Peripheral vasodilation

II. Arterial vasodilation

III. Decreasing contractility

A. I only

B. II only

C. I and II only

D. II and III only

E. I, II, and III

11. The possible benefits of LMWH over UFH include all of the following *except*

A. predictable response.

B. ease of administration.

C. no recommended routine monitoring.

D. stronger affinity for thrombin.

E. no renal adjustment necessary.

12. Which of the following β-blockers has ISA activity?

   A. Tenormin
   B. Sectral
   C. Inderal
   D. Lopressor
   E. Coreg

13. Which of the following medications is contraindicated within 24 hours of a nitrate?

   A. Metoprolol
   B. Quinapril
   C. Verapamil
   D. Sildenafil
   E. Felodipine

14. Which of the following is the preferred narcotic to relieve chest pain after the use of SL NTG?

   A. Meperidine
   B. Oxycodone
   C. Morphine
   D. Hydromorphone
   E. Fentanyl

Questions 15 and 16 refer to this case:

J. O. is a 54-year-old male who presents to the hospital with crushing substernal chest pain and radiation to his left arm. Past medical history is significant for hypertension, COPD, and gout. J. O. has a history of smoking × 30 years and occasionally consumes alcohol. Vital signs on admission include BP 170/85; pulse 72; RR 18; temp 97. Before admission, the patient was taking enteric-coated aspirin 81 mg daily; Combivent inhaler 2 puffs qid; Tiazac 240 mg daily; allopurinol 300 mg daily.

Allergies: sulfa

Lab/diagnostic tests:

- ECG: ST-segment depression, T-wave changes
- Troponin: T-positive × 3
- Ejection fraction: < 35%
- LDL: 135 mg/dL

Diagnosis:

- NSTEMI
- Heart failure

15. What is the preferred β-blocker for this patient?

   A. Propranolol
   B. Carvedilol
   C. Labetalol
   D. Metoprolol
   E. Nadolol

16. All of the following therapies should be considered in this patient *except*

   A. reteplase.
   B. clopidogrel.
   C. enalapril.
   D. simvastatin.
   E. unfractionated heparin.

Questions 17 and 18 refer to this case:

S. D. is a 56-year-old female who presents to the local emergency room complaining of crushing, substernal chest pain × 3 hours, which has been unrelieved by SL NTG. PMH is pertinent for hypertension, T2DM, hypercholesterolemia, and metabolic syndrome. Heart rate and rhythm are regular, and no S_3 or S_4 sounds are present. Vital signs include BP 184/119, HR 100, and RR 32/min. S. D.'s ECG shows ST-segment elevation > 1 mm in leads II, III, and aVF. She is immediately admitted to the chest pain center and started on oxygen.

17. Which of the following criteria for the diagnosis of MI are present in S. D.?

   A. Chest pain symptoms are relieved by SL NTG.
   B. ST-segment elevation is greater than 1 mm in two or more noncontiguous leads.
   C. Chest pain symptoms with ECG changes are consistent with MI or necrosis.
   D. S. D. does not meet the criteria for MI based on the above presentation because myocardial enzymes have not been evaluated.
   E. Negative enzymes rule out MI.

18. Which of the following agents should be administered to S. D.?

   A. tPA 100 mg IV over 90 minutes
   B. IV magnesium
   C. Prophylactic lidocaine
   D. Metoprolol 5 mg IV
   E. Diltiazem 240 mg po

19. What medications should a patient who is post-MI with preserved LVEF receive as discharge therapy?

    A. Aspirin, clopidogrel, diltiazem, and simvastatin
    B. Aspirin, metoprolol, enalapril, atorvastatin, and SL NTG
    C. Clopidogrel, metoprolol, enalapril, and simvastatin
    D. Morphine, aspirin, SL NTG, and clopidogrel
    E. Morphine, SL NTG, aspirin, and oxygen

20. The anticoagulant effect of unfractionated heparin requires the binding to which plasma cofactor?

    A. Thrombospondin
    B. Antithrombin III
    C. Plasminogen
    D. Factor XIIa
    E. Factors II, VII, IX, and X

Question 21 refers to this case:

S. P. is a 45-year-old marathon runner. He presents to the emergency department with complaints of chest pain during his morning run. His father died of a myocardial infarction at age 48. His past medical history is positive for angina, hyperlipidemia, and hypertension. His current medications include aspirin, pravastatin, nifedipine, and clonidine. His electrocardiogram is consistent with acute ischemia. His HR is 52 and BP is 170/100. CBC and Chem-7 are within normal limits.

21. All of the following interventions are appropriate for S. P. *except*

    A. enoxaparin 1 mg/kg SC bid.
    B. IV metoprolol followed by po metoprolol.
    C. nitroglycerin SL prn and IV drip titrated to pain and blood pressure.
    D. continue aspirin.
    E. morphine if NTG does not control the pain.

22. Which one of the following agents is not indicated in the setting of STEMI when pharmacologic reperfusion is the planned strategy?

    A. Eptifibatide
    B. LMWH

C. Aspirin
D. tPA
E. Metoprolol

23. Which of the following agents would not be administered at the same time as heparin?

    A. tPA
    B. Reteplase
    C. Eptifibatide
    D. TNKase
    E. Streptokinase

24. Which of the following statements about the GPIs is *not* true?

    A. Abciximab, eptifibatide, and tirofiban are all administered as a bolus followed by a continuous infusion.
    B. It is possible to experience an allergic reaction after repeated exposure to abciximab.
    C. Eptifibatide, tirofiban, and abciximab can all be reversed by a platelet infusion.
    D. Tirofiban and eptifibatide are renally eliminated; therefore, dosage adjustment is required for patients with renal dysfunction.
    E. Abciximab, eptifibatide, and tirofiban are all indicated as adjuncts to PCI.

11-12. Answers

1. **B.** Angina is considered stable if symptoms have been occurring for several weeks without worsening, it lasts < 30 minutes, and it is relieved by rest or SL NTG.

2. **D.** This regimen will help control his angina without β_2-blocking effects in this asthmatic patient, as well as lower his BP. SL NTG will be useful for acute attacks. A is not the best answer because this patient also needs a medication to lower his BP. B is incorrect because propranolol is not β_1-selective and could worsen his asthma. C is incorrect because GPIs are not indicated in stable angina. E is incorrect; combination therapy is not recommended as first-line therapy and should be considered only when initial treatment with a β-blocker is not successful.

3. **B.** Mr. Smith has an elevated LDL with known heart disease, and he needs to be treated to a goal LDL of < 100 mg/dL (consider LDL

< 70 mg/dL). A and C are incorrect; these antiplatelet agents are not indicated for treating stable angina unless a patient cannot tolerate aspirin. D and E are incorrect because GPIs and thrombolytics are not indicated in stable angina.

4. **D.** Unlike nitrates or calcium channel blockers, β-blockers do not cause peripheral vasodilation.

5. **D.** The increased sympathetic tone caused by some dihydropyridines can lead to a reflex tachycardia, which would be detrimental in an IHD patient. Therefore, using a β-blocker to block this effect would be desirable. A is incorrect; unlike verapamil or diltiazem, the dihydropyridines do not decrease conduction through the AV node. B is incorrect; CCBs are not indicated as first-line therapy unless a patient has a contraindication to a β-blocker. C is incorrect because immediate release nifedipine can lead to increased side effects if not combined with a β-blocker. E is incorrect because both verapamil and metoprolol can lead to worsening systolic function, and used in combination, they would be unsafe.

6. **E.** SL NTG should be kept in the original amber bottle, because exposure to light or extreme temperatures will cause it to lose potency. III is correct, and patients should be counseled to take one tablet and seek medical attention if chest pain is not relieved. I is incorrect; SL NTG is used on a prn basis and should not be taken at the same time each day.

7. **C.** It has not been proven that so-called tissue ACEIs are better than other ACE inhibitors.

8. **E.** Clopidogrel, or Plavix, does not have any pharmacologic interaction with an ETT. Digoxin can cause an abnormal exercise-induced ST depression in approximately 30% of healthy patients. β-blockers and vasodilators can alter hemodynamic response to BP and should be withdrawn gradually 4–5 half-lives before ETT. Nitrates can attenuate angina and flecainide may cause exercise-induced ventricular tachycardia.

9. **D.** Ideally, a β-blocker used for the treatment of UA or NSTEMI would have β_1-receptor selectivity, no ISA, and low lipophilicity. Being available as an intravenous agent is not an advantage because β-blockers should be initiated orally to avoid adverse effects. β_1-receptor selectivity would reduce the chance for bronchospasm, and low lipophilicity would reduce the neurological side effects. β-blockers with ISA reduce heart rate to a lesser degree than non-ISA β-blockers, thus producing a smaller decrease in oxygen demand.

10. **C.** Nitrates are vasodilators acting on both arteries and in the periphery, thereby decreasing preload and afterload. Regarding anti-ischemic therapy, only β-blockers and nondihydropyridine calcium channel blockers reduce contractility.

11. **E.** Renal adjustment is necessary with LMWH. UFH does not require dosage adjustment in renal patients and is preferred to LMWH in patients with a creatinine clearance < 30 mL/min. LMWH does appear to have advantages over UFH in ease of administration, its affinity to thrombin (stronger than UFH), its more predictable response, and the fact that it does not require monitoring.

12. **B.** β-blockers with ISA activity include Sectral (acebutolol), Cartrol (carteolol), Levatol (penbutolol), and Visken (pindolol). Tenormin (atenolol), Inderal (propranolol), Lopressor (metoprolol), and Coreg (carvedilol) do not have ISA activity.

13. **D.** Sildenafil use is contraindicated within 24 hours of a nitrate. β-blockers (metoprolol), ACEIs (quinapril), and calcium channel blockers (verapamil and felodipine) can be safely combined with nitrates.

14. **C.** Morphine has vasodilator properties, thereby decreasing both preload and afterload, which decreases oxygen demand. In addition, morphine lowers heart rate by relieving pain and anxiety. If a true morphine allergy exists, meperidine may be used as an alternate agent. Oxycodone, hydromorphone, and fentanyl are not recommended for the treatment of anginal pain.

15. **D.** With the patient's history of COPD, a β-blocker with β_1-receptor selectivity is preferred. The only agent with β_1-selectivity in this list is metoprolol. All of the remaining agents are nonselective. In addition, metoprolol would be an appropriate β-blocker to use in this patient with heart failure.

16. **A.** Reteplase is a thrombolytic agent, which does not have a role in the treatment of NSTEMI. Thrombolytic therapy is indicated for the treatment of STEMI. Clopidogrel and GPI (eptifibatide) should be considered in all patients with NSTEMI with or without PCI. Eptifibatide and tirofiban can be used in patients who are medically managed; abciximab is reserved for patients with a scheduled PCI procedure. Lipid-lowering therapy with an HMG-CoA reductase inhibitor (e.g., simvastatin) should be initiated in this patient because his LDL is > 130 mg/dL. This patient has a clear indication

for an ACEI (enalapril) because of his ejection fraction of < 40%. An anticoagulant should be started on presentation; options include UFH or LMWH.

17.   **C.** A is incorrect. Although chest pain unrelieved by NTG is a diagnostic criterion for MI, two criteria must be present before the diagnosis can be made. B is incorrect because ST-segment elevation > 1 mm must be found in two or more contiguous leads. S. D. has both chest pain symptoms and ECG changes that are consistent with myocardial infarction. C is correct because she meets two of the three criteria for diagnosing MI. S. D. does not have positive enzymes, which would meet the third diagnostic criteria. D is incorrect because positive enzymes do not have to be present for the diagnosis of MI to be made (as is the case with S. D.).

18.   **D.** One of the relative contraindications to fibrinolytic therapy is severe uncontrolled hypertension (BP > 180/110 mm Hg). A is not appropriate in this patient with BP of 184/119 mm Hg. Routine use of magnesium post-MI is not recommended and should be reserved for patients with hypomagnesemia. No labs were given for S. D., so answer B is not appropriate at this time. Prophylactic lidocaine has been shown to increase all-cause mortality and is not recommended in the early management of STEMI for prevention of VF. Therefore, C is incorrect. β-blockers reduce the incidence of ventricular arrhythmias, recurrent ischemia, reinfarction, infarct size, and mortality in patients with STEMI. Because S. D. does not have any contraindications to β-blockade, D is the correct choice. E, calcium channel blockers, do not have a role in STEMI when a β-blocker can be given.

19.   **B.** ACEIs, β-blockers, aspirin, statin therapy, and SL NTG should be given to all patients without contraindications post-MI. Clopidogrel can be combined with aspirin and can be continued for at least 12 months regardless of whether the patient underwent PCI. Answers A and C, which include clopidogrel, are incorrect, however, because A omits β-blockade, and C omits aspirin therapy. Calcium channel blockers can be given if a patient has contraindications to β-blockade, but it is not recommended as first-line treatment. Answers D and E are incorrect because ACE inhibition and β-blockade are omitted. Answer E would be a correct choice for the immediate treatment of someone who presents with STEMI, but not as discharge therapy.

20.   **B.** Heparin's anticoagulant effect requires binding to antithrombin (previously antithrombin III), and that binding converts antithrombin from a slow, progressive thrombin inhibitor to a very rapid inhibitor of thrombin and factor Xa.

21.   **B.** One of the contraindications to β-blockade is a HR < 55 bpm. Because S. P. has an HR of 52 bpm, the only inappropriate therapy of the choices given would be B. Enoxaparin, NTG, morphine, and aspirin are all therapies that should be continued.

22.   **A.** Glycoprotein IIb/IIIa inhibition is still controversial in the setting of STEMI, especially when a fibrinolytic agent is administered. The role of GPIs in STEMI is rapidly evolving, and trials to date in combination with full- and half-dose fibrinolytic agents have shown a more complete reperfusion at the price of higher bleeding rates. At this point, there is no formal recommendation on using eptifibatide or another GPI in STEMI.

23.   **E.** A GPI should be administered with heparin, and therefore C is not the correct answer. Combination of UFH with streptokinase is less desirable because it is a nonspecific fibrinolytic, and UFH may increase the risk of bleeding because of streptokinase's long half-life. Therefore, answer E is the correct choice. Heparin should be administered for at least 48 hours with the other lytic choices to reduce risk of reocclusion.

24.   **C.** The only GPI that is reversed by a platelet infusion is abciximab. All of the remaining selections are true statements. All of the available GPI agents are administered as a bolus and infusion. Abciximab is a monoclonal antibody; therefore, it is possible to develop an allergic reaction upon rechallenge. Only two GPIs are renally eliminated: eptifibatide and tirofiban. All of the agents are indicated as adjunct to PCI, so E is true.

11-13. References

American Diabetes Association. Aspirin therapy in diabetes. *Diabetes Care.* 2004;27(suppl 1): S72–73.

Anderson JL, Adams CD, Antman EM, et al. ACC/AHA 2007 guidelines update for the management of patients with unstable angina/non-ST-segment elevation myocardial infarction: A report of the American College of Cardiology/American Heart Association Task Force on Practice Guidelines

(Writing Committee to Revise the 2002 Guidelines for the Management of Patients with Unstable Angina/Non-ST-Elevation Myocardial Infarction). *J Am Coll Cardiol.* 2007;50:1–57. Available at: http://content.onlinejacc.org/cgi/content/full/50/7/e1.

Antman EM, Anbe DT, Armstrong PW, et al. *ACC/AHA Guidelines for the Management of Patients with ST-Elevation Myocardial Infarction: A Report of the American College of Cardiology/ American Heart Association Task Force on Practice Guidelines (Committee to Revise the 1999 Guidelines for the Management of Patients with Acute Myocardial Infarction).* 2004. Available at: www.acc.org/qualityandscience/clinical/guidelines/stemi/STEMI%20Full%20Text.pdf.

Antman EM, Hand M, Armstrong PW, et al. 2007 Focused update of the ACC/AHA 2004 guidelines for the management of patients with ST-elevation myocardial infarction: A report of the American College of Cardiology/American Heart Association Task Force on Practice Guidelines. *J Am Coll Cardiol.* 2008;51:210–47. Available at: http://content.onlinejacc.org/cgi/reprint/51/2/210.pdf.

Becker RC, Meade TW, Berger PB, et al. The primary and secondary prevention of coronary artery disease. *Chest.* 2008;133:776S–814S.

Dagenais GR, Yusuf S, Bourassa MG, et al. Effects of ramipril on coronary events in high-risk persons: Results from the Heart Outcomes Prevention Evaluation Study. *Circulation.* 2001;104:522–26.

Deepak LB, Fox KA, Hacke W, et al. Clopidogrel and aspirin versus aspirin alone for the prevention of atherothrombotic events. *N Engl J Med.* 2006;354: 1706–17.

Dobesh PP, Trujillo TC. Ranolazine: A new option in the management of chronic stable angina. *Pharmacotherapy.* 2007;27:1659–76.

Fox KM, European Trial on Reduction of Cardiac Events with Perindopril in Stable Coronary Artery Disease Investigators. Efficacy of perindopril in reduction of cardiovascular events among patients with stable coronary artery disease: Randomised, double-blind, placebo-controlled, multicentre trial (the EUROPA study). *Lancet.* 2003;362:782–8.

Fraker TD Jr, Fihn SD, writing on behalf of the 2002 Chronic Stable Angina Writing Committee. 2007 chronic angina focused update of the ACC/AHA 2002 guidelines for the management of patients with chronic stable angina: A report of the American College of Cardiology/American Heart Association Task Force on Practice Guidelines Writing Group to develop the focused update of the 2002 guidelines for the management of patients with chronic stable angina. *J Am Coll Cardiol.* 2007;50: 2264–74. Available at: http://content.onlinejacc.org/cgi/reprint/50/23/2264.pdf.

Gibbons RJ, Abrams J, Chatterjee K, et al. *ACC/AHA 2002 Guideline Update for the Management of Patients with Chronic Stable Angina: A Report of the American College of Cardiology/American Heart Association Task Force on Practice Guidelines (Committee to Update the 1999 Guidelines for the Management of Patients with Chronic Stable Angina).* 2002. Available at: www.acc.org/qualityandscience/clinical/guidelines/stable/stable_clean.pdf.

Grundy SM, Cleeman JI, Berz NB, et al. Implications of recent clinical trials for the national cholesterol education program adult treatment panel III guidelines. *Circulation.* 2004;110:227–39.

King SB III, Smith SC Jr., Hirshfeld JW Jr, et al. 2007 focused update of the ACC/AHA/SCAI 2005 guideline update for percutaneous coronary intervention: A report of the American College of Cardiology/American Heart Association Task Force on Practice Guidelines: (2007 Writing Group to Review New Evidence and Update the 2005 ACC/AHA/SCAI Guideline Update for Percutaneous Coronary Intervention). *J Am Coll Cardiol.* 2008;51:172–209. Available at: http://content.onlinejacc.org/cgi/content/full/51/2/172.

Lloyd-Jones D, Adams R, Carnethon M, et al. Heart disease and stroke statistics—2009 update: A report from the American Heart Association Statistics Committee and Stroke Statistics Subcommittee. *Circulation.* 2009;119:e21–181.

Mehta SR, Yusuf S, Peter RJ, et al. Effects of pretreatment with clopidogrel and aspirin followed by long-term therapy in patients undergoing percutaneous coronary intervention: The PCI-CURE study. *Lancet.* 2001;358:527–33.

Meister FL, Stringer KA, Spinler SA, et al. Thrombolytic therapy for acute myocardial infarction. *Pharmacotherapy.* 1998;18:686–98.

Mosca L, Banka CL, Benjamin EJ, et al. Evidence-based guidelines for cardiovascular disease prevention in women: 2007 update. *Circulation.* 2007; 115:1481–501.

Patrono C, Baigent C, Hirsh J, Roth G. Antiplatelet drugs: American College of Chest Physicians Evidence-Based Clinical Practice Guidelines (8th edition). *Chest.* 2008;133:199S–233S.

PEACE trial investigators. Angiotensin-converting enzyme inhibition in stable coronary artery disease. *N Engl J Med.* 2004;351:2058–68.

Ridker PM, Cook NR, Lee I-M, et al. A randomized trial of low-dose aspirin in the primary prevention of cardiovascular disease in women. *N Engl J Med.* 2005;352:1293–304.

Smith SC Jr, Allen J, Blair SN, et al. AHA/ACC guidelines for secondary prevention for patients with coronary and other atherosclerotic vascular disease: 2006 update. *Circulation* 2006;113:2363–72.

Smith SC Jr, Feldman TE, Hirshfeld JW Jr, et al. ACC/AHA/SCAI 2005 guideline update for percutaneous coronary intervention: A report of the American College of Cardiology/American Heart Association Task Force on Practice Guidelines (ACC/AHA/SCAI Writing Committee to Update the 2001 Guidelines for Percutaneous Coronary Intervention). *J Am Coll Cardiol.* 2006;47:e1–121.

Spinler SA, de Denus S. Acute coronary syndromes. In: DiPiro JT, Talbert RL, Yee GC, et al., eds. *Pharmacotherapy: A Pathophysiologic Approach.* 7th ed. New York: McGraw-Hill; 2008:249–78.

Steinhubl SR, Berger PB, Mann JT, et al. Early and sustained dual oral antiplatelet therapy following percutaneous coronary intervention: A randomized controlled trial. *JAMA.* 2002;288:2411–20.

Summary of the Second Report of the National Cholesterol Education Program (NCEP). Expert Panel on Detection, Evaluation, and Treatment of High Blood Cholesterol in Adults (Adult Treatment Panel III). *JAMA.* 2001;285:2486–97.

Talbert RL. Ischemic heart disease. In: DiPiro JT, Talbert RL, Yee GC, et al., eds. *Pharmacotherapy: A Pathophysiologic Approach.* 7th ed. New York: McGraw-Hill; 2008:217–47.

Trujillo TC, Dobesh PP. Traditional management of chronic stable angina. *Pharmacotherapy.* 2007;27: 1677–92.

Wong GC, Giugliano RP, Antman EM. Use of low molecular-weight heparins in the management of acute coronary artery syndromes and percutaneous coronary intervention. *JAMA.* 2003;289:331–42.

Hyperlipidemia

Lawrence M. Brown, PharmD, PhD

12-1. Introduction

- *Hyperlipidemia* is an elevation in the blood concentration of a lipid such as cholesterol or triglyceride (in the form of lipoprotein).
- *Dyslipidemia* refers to any lipid disorder.
- *Lipids* include cholesterol, triglycerides (TGs), and phospholipids.
- *Lipoproteins* are apolipoproteins + cholesterol + TGs + phospholipids.
- *Major lipoproteins* are chylomicrons, very-low-density lipoproteins (VLDLs), intermediate-density lipoproteins (IDLs), low-density lipoproteins (LDLs), high-density lipoproteins (HDLs), and lipoprotein (a).
- *Apolipoproteins* are structural components of lipoproteins.
- The *Friederwald equation* is a formula used to calculate LDL:

$$LDL = total\ cholesterol - (HDL + TG/5).$$

Classification of Lipids

Total cholesterol, LDL, HDL, and TG are measured in mg/dL. Adult Treatment Panel III (ATP III) recommendations from the National Cholesterol Education Program (NCEP) are shown in Table 12-1.

Clinical Presentation

Hyperlipidemia can cause atherosclerosis, atheroma formation, atherothrombosis, and the subsequent consequences of the following disease processes:

- Coronary artery disease (angina and myocardial infarction)
- Cerebrovascular disease (transient ischemic attack, stroke, or both)
- Peripheral arterial disease (intermittent claudication)

A state of elevated lipids alone generally promotes no symptoms, except in some familial lipid disorders, in which there may be cutaneous manifestations of lipid deposition (e.g., tendon xanthomas, planar xanthomas, xanthelasmas, and eye manifestations [corneal arcus]).

Pathophysiology of Atherosclerosis

A progressive, systemic disease starting early in life, atherosclerosis has the following pathophysiology:

- Atheroma lesions, called *fatty streaks,* develop in the arterial vascular walls as a result of the accumulation of cholesterol within vessel walls.
- Atheroma lesions may lead to occlusion by thrombus or embolus formation.
- LDL cholesterol accumulates below the intimal surface of the artery. The general guideline is the higher the cholesterol elevation in the blood, the more LDL migration into the artery.
- Endothelial dysfunction occurs, which increases LDL cholesterol's permeability.
- LDL becomes oxidized and recruits monocytes.
- Monocytes are transformed into macrophages and ingest the oxidized LDL.
- This process results in lipid-filled cells called *foam cells.*
- Foam cells are the initial lesion of atherosclerosis. Growth factors are produced by macrophages.
- Other processes are also occurring (e.g., additional endothelial cell injury and inflammatory

Table 12-1. Classification of Lipids

Type	Classification
LDL cholesterol (primary target of therapy)	
< 100 mg/dL	Optimal
100–129 mg/dL	Near optimal or above optimal
130–159 mg/dL	Borderline high
160–189 mg/dL	High
≥ 190 mg/dL	Very high
Total cholesterol	
< 200 mg/dL	Desirable
200–239 mg/dL	Borderline high
≥ 240 mg/dL	High
HDL cholesterol	
< 40 mg/dL	Low
≥ 60 mg/dL	High
Triglycerides (secondary target of therapy)	
< 150 mg/dL	Normal
150–199 mg/dL	Borderline high
200–499 mg/dL	High
> 500 mg/dL	Very high

responses that can further accelerate the development of plaque).

- Elevated cholesterol and hyperlipidemia enhance this process.
- Plaque may continue to develop, may become stable, or may rupture.
- Plaque rupture exposes atherogenic materials in the lesion to blood.
- Platelets are activated, and a clot may form.
- Partial occlusion or obstruction can result in angina; complete occlusion results in myocardial infarction (MI).
- Other vascular beds promote similar outcomes.

Diagnostic Criteria

Lipid disorders (dyslipidemias) are classified as *familial* or *secondary*.

Familial disorders

- Familial disorders usually are caused by a defect in lipid metabolism.

- They are categorized into the *hypercholesterolemias* and the *combined hyperlipidemias*.
- Assessment of fasting lipid panels provides diagnostic information and classification of lipid disorders.
- For familial hypercholesterolemia, LDL = 250–450 mg/dL.
- Familial defective apolipoprotein B-100 may be present.
- Polygenic hypercholesterolemia is the most common form (LDL = 160–250 mg/dL).
- Combined hyperlipidemias are as follows:
  - Familial combined hyperlipidemia (LDL = 160–250 mg/dL and TG = 200–800 mg/dL)
  - Familial hyperapobetalipoproteinemia
  - Hypoalphalipoproteinemia
  - Dysbetalipoproteinemia
  - Elevated lipoprotein (a)
- Familial disorders are characterized by variations in the amounts of HDL, IDL, LDL, and VLDL.

Secondary disorders

The most common secondary causes of lipid disorders are as follows:

- Diabetes mellitus
- Hypothyroidism
- Renal failure
- Obstructive liver disease
- Drugs such as β-blockers, thiazide diuretics, oral contraceptives, oral estrogens, glucocorticosteroids, and cyclosporine

Risk factors are used to assess the potential for an individual to develop coronary heart disease (CHD) or another equivalent atherosclerotic process over the next 10 years. The Framingham Global Risk Score is calculated to provide this information. The major nonlipid risk factors for CHD are counted and used to assess the 10-year risk of developing CHD.

Major nonlipid risk factors for CHD are as follows:

- Cigarette smoking
- Hypertension (patient with blood pressure ≥ 140/90 mm Hg or patient on antihypertensive medication)
- Low HDL cholesterol (< 40 mg/dL)
- Family history of premature CHD (CHD in a male first-degree relative age < 55 years and CHD in a female first-degree relative age < 65 years)
- Age (men ≥ 45 years; women ≥ 55 years)

HDL ≥ 60 mg/dL counts as a negative risk factor and acts to remove one of the other risk factors from the total count.

Treatment Principles

Treatment and target lipid goals are based on the estimation of risk for CHD using the Framingham Global Risk Score.

If a patient has a form of clinical CHD, such as angina, MI, stroke, or transient ischemic attack, he or she is considered to be at high risk for another ischemic event within the next 10 years.

Those at highest risk require the most aggressive therapy (i.e., drug therapy and achievement of the lowest possible LDL level). The major nonlipid risk factors noted previously are used in the risk analysis for those individuals who do not have CHD or a CHD risk equivalent. Table 12-2 identifies risk categories, lipid goals, and risk of event.

Treatment consists of lifestyle changes (i.e., therapeutic lifestyle changes), which are discussed in the nonpharmacologic and pharmacotherapy sections of this chapter.

The algorithm for drug therapy in primary prevention (< 20% risk) is as follows:

- Initiate LDL-lowering drug therapy (statins, niacin, and resin) for 6 weeks.
- If the LDL goal is not met, intensify LDL-lowering therapy (higher dose or combination therapy) for 6 weeks.
- If LDL goal is still not achieved, intensify drug therapy or refer to a lipid specialist for 4–6 months.
- Monitor response and adherence.

Drug therapy in secondary prevention (> 20% risk) requires the most aggressive treatment. A large LDL reduction requires a statin and possibly a statin in combination with another agent. Follow the same algorithm as outlined in the primary prevention (< 20% risk) algorithm just listed.

Monitoring (Clinical Evaluation) of Adults

For screening, the NCEP's ATP III recommends that, starting at age 20, adults receive a fasting lipid pro-

Table 12-2. Risk Categories, Lipid Goals, and Risk of Event

Risk category	LDL goal	Risk of event
CHD and CHD risk equivalent[a]	< 100 mg/dL	> 20% over 10 years
Multiple risk factors (2+)	< 130 mg/dL	10–20% over 10 years
0–1 risk factor	< 160 mg/dL	< 10% over 10 years

a. CHD risk equivalent = clinical CHD, symptomatic carotid artery disease, peripheral arterial disease, abdominal aortic aneurysm, and diabetes.

file (FLP). If the FLP is normal, screening is repeated in 5 years.

Monitoring and Treatment of Children and Adolescents

The American Academy of Pediatrics has historically recommended cholesterol screening of children with a family history of high cholesterol or heart disease. However, the academy now recommends screening of children age 2 to 10 if family history is unknown or if the child has other risk factors for heart disease such as obesity, hypertension, or diabetes. Screenings that result in normal range results should be repeated in 3 to 5 years.

Children age 8 and older (previously age 10 and older) with LDL levels > 190 mg/dL should be considered for medication therapy (> 160 mg/dL for children with family history of heart disease or more than two other risk factors and > 130 mg/dL for children with diabetes). First line medication options include bile acid sequestrants, cholesterol absorption inhibitors, and statins (statins previously not recommended as first-line medication option). Niacin products are not recommended for use, and fibrates should be used with caution and under the supervision of a pediatric lipid specialist.

Children age 2 and older who are overweight or obese and who have a high TG level or low HDL level should receive a recommendation of weight management and increased physical activity as the primary treatment.

Monitoring Tool

The main monitoring tool is a fasting lipid panel. The baseline FLP is done before drug or dietary interventions.

After therapeutic lifestyle changes or drug therapy is started, the patient should be monitored every 6 weeks for 12 weeks initially, again in 4–6 months, and then periodically thereafter (usually annually). Results of the FLP will show the effects of lifestyle and drug therapy interventions and help direct changes in therapy.

12-2. Drug Therapy

See Tables 12-3, 12-4, and 12-5 for details on dosing, efficacy, and drug combinations.

Table 12-3. Drug Products and Dosage

Generic name	Trade name	Dosage range and schedule	Dosage form and strength
Statins			
Atorvastatin	Lipitor	10–80 mg/d qhs	10-, 20-, 40-, and 80-mg tablet
Fluvastatin	Lescol	20–80 mg/d qhs	20- and 40-mg capsule; 80-mg XL tablet
Lovastatin	Mevacor	20–80 mg/d qhs	10-, 20-, 40-mg tablet
Lovastatin extended-release	Altoprev	10–60 mg/d qhs	10-, 20-, 40-, and 60-mg tablet
Pravastatin	Pravachol	20–80 mg/d qhs	10-, 20-, 40-, and 80-mg tablet
Simvastatin	Zocor	20–80 mg/d qhs	5-, 10-, 20-, 40-, and 80-mg tablet
Rosuvastatin	Crestor	5–40 mg/d hs	5-, 10-, 20-, and 40-mg tablet
Bile acid sequestrants			
Cholestyramine	Questran	4–16 g/d divided	Powder
Colestipol	Colestid	5–20 g/d divided	Powder or tablet
Colesevelam	WelChol	2.6–3.8 g/d (once or bid)	625-mg tablet
Nicotinic acid			
Immediate release	Niacor	1.5–3 g/d (divided tid)	500-mg tablet
Sustained release	Slo-Niacin	1–2 g/d qhs	250-, 500-, and 750-mg tablet
Extended release	Niaspan	1–2 g/d qhs	500-, 750-, and 1,000-mg tablet
Fibric acids			
Gemfibrozil	Lopid	600 mg before meals bid	600-mg tablet
Fenofibrate	Tricor	48–145 mg/d	48- and 145-mg tablet
Cholesterol inhibitors			
Ezetimibe (Zetia)		10 mg/d	10-mg tablet
Omega-3 fatty acids			
Omega-3 fatty acid	Lovaza	4 g qd or 2 g bid	1-g capsule
Combinations			
Aspirin + pravastatin[a]	Pravigard PAC	81/20–325/80 mg qhs	81/20-, 81/40-, and 81/80-mg tablets; 325/20-, 325/40-, and 325/80-mg tablets
Ezetimibe + simvastatin	Vytorin	10/10–10/80 mg qhs	10/10-, 10/20-, 10/40-, and 10/80-mg tablets
Lovastatin + Niaspan	Advicor	20/500–40/2,000 mg/d	20/500-, 20/750-, and 20/1,000-mg tablets

a. Aspirin tablets and pravastatin tablets are separate tablets within the PAC.

Statins

- Conduct baseline liver function tests (LFTs) and creatine kinase (CK) before therapy is initiated. LFTs should be repeated again in 4–6 weeks, at 3 months, and then periodically (usually annually).
- CK needs to be monitored only if the patient has suspected muscle damage.
- Assess effectiveness at 6 weeks.

Resins

- Determine baseline FLP to screen for hyper-triglyceridemia:
  - If TG > 200 mg/dL, use resins with caution.
  - If TG > 400 mg/dL, resins are contra-indicated.
- Assess effectiveness at 6 weeks.

Table 12-4. Efficacy of Drugs Used to Treat Hyperlipidemia

Drug class	Lipid and lipoprotein effect
Statins	LDL ↓18–55%
	HDL ↑5–15%
	TG ↓7–30%
Resins	LDL ↓15–30%
	HDL ↑3–5%
	TG (no change)
Nicotinic acid	LDL ↓5–25%
	HDL ↑15–35%
	TG ↓20–50%
Fibric acids	LDL ↓5–20%
	HDL ↑10–20%
	TG ↓20–50%
Cholesterol inhibitors	LDL ↓17%
	HDL ↓1.3%
	TG ↓6%
Omega-3 fatty acid (Lovaza)	LDL ↑25–31%
	HDL ↑4–13%
	TG ↓45%

Nicotinic Acid

- Determine baseline fasting glucose, conduct LFTs, and determine serum uric acid levels before initiating therapy.
- Repeat these tests 4–6 weeks after each dose level is reached.

Table 12-5. Pharmacotherapeutic Options for Treatment of Hyperlipidemia

Lipid target	Pharmacotherapy
LDL	Statin most potent and effective for large LDL reductions
	Niacin and resins effective for moderate LDL reductions
	Combination of statin + niacin
	Combination of statin + ezetimibe
	Combination of statin + resin
LDL + TG	Combination of statin + niacin
	Combination of statin + fibric acid
TG	Fibric acid or niacin

- Sustained-release niacin requires monthly LFT readings while dosage is titrated; subsequent LFT readings should occur every 12 weeks for the first year and then periodically.
- Diabetics require routine fasting glucose tests.
- Monitor serum uric acid after the highest dose level is achieved in patients with a history of hyperuricemia or gout.
- Assess effectiveness at 6 weeks.

Fibric Acids

- Determine baseline FLP (total cholesterol, HDL, LDL, and TG) before therapy and again at 3 and 6 months.
- Monitor changes in TG at 3 months, and assess effectiveness.

Cholesterol Inhibitors

- Determine baseline FLP.
- Assess effectiveness at 6 weeks.

Omega-3 Fatty Acids

- Determine very high baseline TG of ≥ 500 mg/dL.
- Can be used in combination with diet therapy or with diet and statin therapy.
- Assess effectiveness at 2 months. Discontinue use if decrease in TG level is adequate.
- Periodic monitoring of alanine aminotransferase levels is recommended.
- Periodic monitoring is recommended for increase in LDL cholesterol levels.

Mechanisms of Action

HMG-CoA reductase inhibitors (statins)

These agents competitively inhibit HMG-CoA (3-hydroxy-3-methyl-glutaryl-coenzyme A) reductase, which is the enzyme responsible for conversion of HMG-CoA to mevalonate.

Mevalonate is an early precursor to and a rate-limiting step in cholesterol synthesis. This reduction in liver cholesterol synthesis results in upregulation of liver LDL receptors and increased clearance of LDL and VLDL particles in the blood. These actions induce a decrease in total cholesterol and LDL cholesterol, promote a slight increase in HDL cholesterol, and effect a modest decrease in TG.

Bile acid sequestrants (resins)

Nonabsorbable anion exchange resins exchange chloride ions for bile acids and other anions in the intestine. This action inhibits enterohepatic recycling, which results in bile excretion and a decrease in the cholesterol pool in the liver. LDL receptors are upregulated, increased LDL is cleared, and LDL is lowered.

Niacin

Niacin reduces LDL cholesterol and TG and increases HDL. It may decrease VLDL synthesis, thereby leading to decreased LDL cholesterol and TG. It may inhibit metabolism of apolipoprotein A-I, which increases HDL cholesterol.

Fibric acids (fibrates)

Fibrates reduce TG by reduction of apolipoproteins B, C-III, and E. They increase HDL by increasing apolipoproteins A-I and A-II.

Cholesterol inhibitors (ezetimibe)

Cholesterol inhibitors selectively inhibit intestinal absorption of dietary and biliary cholesterol at the brush border of the small intestine, which results in a decrease in the absorption of cholesterol and a decrease in cholesterol in the blood.

Omega-3 fatty acids

The mechanism of action for omega-3 fatty acids is not completely understood. Possible mechanisms of action include the following:

- Inhibition of acyl CoA: 1,2-diacylglycerol acyltransferase
- Increased mitochondrial and peroxisomal β-oxidation in the liver
- Decreased lipogenesis in the liver
- Increased lipoprotein lipase activity

Patient Instructions and Counseling

Statins

Statins are usually administered in the evening because most hepatic cholesterol production occurs during the night. Lovastatin conventional tablets should be given with the evening meal because absorption is better with food; however, the extended-release lovastatin products should be taken at bedtime. The lovastatin plus Niaspan combination product should be taken at bedtime with a low-fat snack.

Non-extended release statins can be dosed once daily. Other regular dosage forms should be divided as the doses are raised above 40 mg/day.

Atorvastatin may be given any time of the day because of its longer half-life.

Rosuvastatin dosage adjustment is required in patients with severe renal impairment. Plasma concentrations of rosuvastatin increased to a clinically significant extent (about threefold) in patients with severe renal impairment (creatinine clearance < 30 mL/min/1.73m²) compared with healthy subjects (creatinine clearance > 80 mL/min/1.73m²). Dosage adjustment is also required in patients with liver disease.

Monitor LFTs and muscle toxicity as described earlier.

Bile acid sequestrants (resins)

Cholestyramine and colestipol should be started with one dose daily with the largest meal. They may be increased (after the patient adjusts to the resin) to two doses daily with the largest meals or divided between breakfast and dinner.

Titrate doses slowly to avoid gastrointestinal side effects.

Powdered doses can be mixed with food, such as soup, oatmeal, nonfat yogurt, applesauce, and so forth. The mixture can also be chilled overnight to improve palatability. Do not mix with carbonated beverages, because they promote increased air swallowing. Counsel the patient that drinking through a straw may also help.

Patients who suffer constipation with the resins may mix them with psyllium; however, this mixture should be ingested immediately after mixing to prevent a gel from forming.

Counsel the patient to rinse the glass and drink remains to ensure ingestion of all resin.

Colesevelam is a tablet formulation, which may be easier for some patients to self-administer. However, the tablets are large, and some patients may not be able to swallow them.

Monitor for adherence and gastrointestinal side effects for all resins.

Nicotinic acid (niacin)

Immediate-release niacin should be started at a low dose and slowly titrated upward:

- Start with 100 mg tid and adjust upward the second week to 200 mg tid; the next week, increase to 350 mg tid; and the following week, raise to 500 mg tid. When 1,500 mg/day is reached and maintained for 4 weeks, assess effectiveness before increasing the dose.

- If further titration is needed, go to 750 mg tid and assess effectiveness after 4 weeks before increasing titration. Maximum dose is 1,000 mg tid.
- Aspirin 325 mg or ibuprofen 200 mg must be given 30 minutes before the morning dose to minimize flushing and itching.
- Caution patients to avoid hot beverages and hot showers so as not to exacerbate the flushing effect.

Extended-release formulation should be taken at bedtime (500 mg) and titrated weekly to a maximum dose of 1,500 mg/day. Aspirin should be taken 30 minutes before the dose.

Sustained-release formulations are started at 250 mg bid and increased at weekly intervals to a maximum dose of 2,000 mg/day. Aspirin should be given 30 minutes before the dose.

Monitor for adherence and side effects. The titration schedule for some patients may have to be gradual because of flushing and itching.

Fibric acids (fibrates)

Gemfibrozil should be taken twice daily 30 minutes before meals.

Tricor can be taken with or without food once daily.

Reduce the dose in patients with renal insufficiency, and monitor for muscle toxicity, especially when used in combination with statins and niacin.

Cholesterol inhibitors

Cholesterol inhibitors are dosed once daily without regard to food. They can be taken simultaneously in combination with statins.

Omega-3 fatty acids

The daily dose (4 g) can be taken in single or divided dose (2 g bid). These agents should be taken with meal(s).

Use of omega-3 fatty acids does not reduce the importance of patient adhering to a diet.

Omega-3 fatty acids are not for use in patients with a history of allergy or sensitivity to fish.

Assess effectiveness at 2 months. Discontinue use if the decrease in TG level is adequate.

Adverse Drug Events

HMG-CoA reductase inhibitors (statins)

- Myopathy owing to muscle damage may occur.
- Myalgia from muscle soreness or tenderness may occur.

- Myositis occurs in 0.2% of patients:

  myalgia + ↑ creatine kinase

  (3 – 10 times upper limit of normal)

- Rhabdomyolysis occurs rarely, but can cause acute renal failure. Stop the drug immediately.

  severe myositis + creatine kinase

  10 × upper limit of normal,

  ↑ serum creatinine and urine myoglobin

- Elevated liver enzymes occur in 0.1–2.3% of patients. Obtain baseline LFTs, and repeat at 4–6 weeks, again at 6 months, and yearly thereafter.
- Flu-like symptoms and headache may occur.
- Patients may have mild gastrointestinal (GI) complaints.
- Contraindication is absolute in active or chronic liver disease.
- Contraindication is relative in combination with certain drugs (see discussion of drug interactions).

Bile acid sequestrants (resins)

- GI distress may occur.
- Patients may experience palatability problems with the resin slurry.
- Constipation may occur that increases with the dose and in the elderly.
- Decreased absorption of other drugs may occur. Dose other drugs 1 hour before or 4 hours after ingestion of resin.
- Contraindication is absolute in dysbetalipoproteinemia (highly elevated VLDL) and TG > 400 mg/dL.
- Contraindication is relative when TG > 200 mg/dL.

Nicotinic acid (niacin)

- Flushing is common. Pretreat with aspirin (325 mg) 30 minutes before the first niacin dose of the day.
- Hyperglycemia is a risk. Use with caution in diabetics.
- Hyperuricemia (or gout) may occur:
  - Upper GI distress
  - Hepatotoxicity
  - Absolute contraindication in chronic liver disease and severe gout
  - Relative contraindication in diabetes, hyperuricemia, or severe gout

Fibric acids (fibrates)

- Dyspepsia may occur.
- Gallstones may occur.
- Myopathy increases when combined with statins.
- Contraindication is absolute in severe renal or severe hepatic disease.

Cholesterol inhibitors

- Elevated liver enzymes (same as placebo) may occur.
- GI distress (less than with resins) may occur.
- Contraindication is absolute in moderate to severe hepatic disease.

Omega-3 fatty acids

- Burping
- Indigestion
- Taste sense alteration
- Backache

Drug–Drug and Drug–Disease Interactions

HMG-CoA reductase inhibitors (statins)

CYP450 (cytochrome P450) mixed-function oxidase enzymes metabolize statins, and drugs that inhibit this process can cause increases in statin concentrations, thus predisposing patients to myopathy and liver toxicity.

Common CYP450 3A4 inhibitors include amiodarone, clarithromycin, cyclosporine, danazol, delavirdine, diltiazem, erythromycin, fluoxetine, fluvoxamine, grapefruit juice, indinavir, itraconazole, ketoconazole, miconazole, nefazodone, nelfinavir, nicardipine, nifedipine, pimozide, propoxyphene, quinidine, ritonavir, saquinavir, sildenafil, tacrolimus, tamoxifen, testosterone, troleandomycin, verapamil, and zafirlukast.

Pravastatin is not metabolized by the CYP450 system; therefore, these drug–drug interactions are avoided.

Contraindication is absolute in active or chronic liver disease.

Bile acid sequestrants (resins)

Avoid concomitant use with all other drugs, especially digoxin, levothyroxine, tetracycline, warfarin, fat-soluble vitamins, and minerals.

Always separate other drugs by 1 hour before use and 4 hours after use.

Colesevelam does not appear to have these drug and nutrient interactions.

Contraindication is absolute in dysbetalipoproteinemia.

Nicotinic acid (niacin)

Use caution in combination with resins. Combination therapy with statins and gemfibrozil may cause an increased risk of myopathy.

Contraindication is absolute in chronic liver disease and severe gout.

Fibric acids (fibrates)

These agents are highly protein bound, and they are metabolized by the CYP450 3A4 enzyme system.

The effect of warfarin may be increased.

Cyclosporine may increase gemfibrozil concentrations.

Fenofibrate may have less interaction potential with warfarin and cyclosporine.

Bile acid sequestrants (resins) decrease fibrate absorption.

Combinations with statins and niacin may increase the risk of myopathy.

Contraindication is absolute in severe renal disease and severe liver disease.

Cholesterol inhibitors

Cyclosporine may increase ezetimibe concentrations.

Combination with a resin may decrease absorption. Combination with a fibric acid may predispose to gallbladder disease.

Contraindication is absolute in moderate to severe hepatic disease.

Omega-3 fatty acids

Possible prolonged bleeding time may occur when used with anticoagulants.

Landmark Clinical Trials with Statins

Primary prevention trials

West of Scotland Study
This trial with pravastatin showed decreased coronary morbidity and mortality in hypercholesterolemic men with no clinical evidence of CHD.

Air Force–Texas Coronary Atherosclerosis Prevention Study
This trial with lovastatin showed reduced incidence of first acute major coronary events in patients who did not have CHD but did have normal to mildly elevated total cholesterol and LDL with low HDL.

Secondary prevention trials

Scandinavian Simvastatin Survival Study

This trial with simvastatin showed decreased cardiac morbidity and mortality in patients with CHD and elevated cholesterol.

Cholesterol and Current Events Study

This trial with pravastatin showed reduced incidence of MI, death from CHD, stroke, and need for revascularization procedures in patients with recent MI and normal cholesterol levels.

Long-Term Intervention with Pravastatin in Ischemic Disease Study

This trial with pravastatin showed reduced mortality and incidence of MI and stroke in patients with CHD and a broad range of cholesterol.

Heart Protection Study

This trial with simvastatin is the largest single cholesterol trial (as of 2002) in patients at high risk of CHD (prior MI, diabetes, or hypertension) and LDL > 135 mg/dL. Antioxidants studied included vitamins E and C and beta-carotene. Simvastatin therapy showed a reduced incidence of CHD regardless of age (also elderly) or preexisting condition. There was no threshold for LDL at 100 mg/dL (i.e., benefits extended below this level). In addition, there was no cardiovascular protective effect from vitamins E and C and beta-carotene.

12-3. Nondrug Therapy

Nonpharmacologic therapy focuses on therapeutic lifestyle changes (TLCs), which incorporate dietary changes, physical activity, and weight reduction. "Heart healthy" nutrition is the foundation for any therapeutic interventions.

General TLC Recommendations

- Decrease the amount of high-fat foods consumed (especially foods high in saturated fat).
- Decrease intake of high-cholesterol foods.
- Replace saturated fats with monounsaturated fats and fish oils.
- Use foods high in complex carbohydrates (fiber, starch, fruits, and vegetables).
- Strive for and maintain an acceptable weight.
- Patients should be instructed on how to read a nutrition label.

- Recommended nutrient makeup of the TLC diet is shown in Table 12-6.

Algorithm for TLCs

Begin lifestyle therapies and continue for 6 weeks. Evaluate LDL response, and if the LDL goal is not achieved, intensify LDL-lowering therapy (diet + weight management + physical activity) for 6 more weeks. Evaluate LDL response, and if LDL goal is still not achieved, consider adding drug therapy (if not already added). Monitor adherence to TLC every 4–6 months thereafter.

Other Nonpharmacologic Therapies

- Soluble fiber and plant sterols and stanols can help lower LDL.
- Viscous or soluble fiber such as psyllium or pectin in the amount of 5–10 g/d or other sources of fiber such as vegetables, fruits, and whole grains can reduce LDL by up to 8%.
- The active ingredient in fish oils is omega-3 fatty acid. Fish oils can reduce TGs as much as 30–60%. Fish oils can be added when niacin or fibrates do not control TGs.
- Recent clinical trials have shown that antioxidants; vitamins A, C, and E; and betacarotene are not protective for cardiovascular disease.
- Light to moderate alcohol use (one drink per day for women, two drinks per day for men) has been associated with reductions in CHD rates. The benefit may be due to a rise in HDL. Use of alcohol should not be encouraged as a means of

Table 12-6. Nutrient Makeup of the TLC Diet

Nutrient	Recommended intake
Saturated fat	< 7% of total calories
Polyunsaturated fat	Up to 10% of total calories
Monounsaturated fat	Up to 20% of total calories
Total fat	25–35% of total calories
Carbohydrate	50–60% of total calories
Fiber	20–30 g/d
Protein	About 15% of total calories
Cholesterol	< 200 mg/d
Total calories	Individualize to balance energy intake and expenditure to maintain desirable weight or prevent weight gain.

lowering cholesterol. Excessive alcohol use can cause elevations of TGs.

■ Alternative therapies such as herbal therapies have not been systematically studied in hyperlipidemia and should not be recommended for treatment of hyperlipidemia or other lipid disorders.

12-4. Key Points

■ Hyperlipidemia is the elevation of the blood concentration of a lipid such as cholesterol or triglyceride (in the form of lipoprotein).

■ There are four major classifications of lipids: total cholesterol, low-density lipoproteins, high-density lipoproteins, and triglycerides.

■ The process of atherosclerosis begins with atheroma lesions in the arterial vascular walls resulting from the accumulation of cholesterol within vessel walls.

■ Polygenic hypercholesterolemia (LDL = 160–250 mg/dL) is the most common form of familial dyslipidemia.

■ Major nonlipid risk factors for coronary heart disease are cigarette smoking, hypertension, family history of premature CHD, and age (men ≥ 45 years, women ≥ 55 years).

■ People with a history of CHD, such as angina, MI, stroke, or transient ischemic attack, are considered at highest risk of having another ischemic event in the next 10 years and require the most aggressive therapy and the lowest target LDL goal (< 100 mg/dL).

■ Monitoring for drug therapy of hyperlipidemia includes laboratory monitoring for adverse effects (e.g., liver function tests, uric acid, and creatine kinase) and fasting lipid profiles for effectiveness.

■ The mechanism of action of statin agents to treat hyperlipidemia is to competitively inhibit HMG-CoA reductase, which is the enzyme responsible for conversion of HMG-CoA into mevalonate—an early precursor to and a rate-limiting step in cholesterol synthesis.

■ The statins are usually administered in the evening (except for atorvastatin, which has a longer half-life than the other agents in this class) because most hepatic cholesterol production occurs during the night.

■ Lovaza is a prescription formulation of omega-3 fatty acid, and its use should be discontinued if an adequate reduction in TGs is not achieved after 2 months of use.

■ The only class of agents to control hyperlipidemia that is not contraindicated in patients with active or chronic liver disease is the bile acid sequestrant (resin) type.

■ Pravastatin is not metabolized by the CYP450 enzyme system and, thus, avoids most of the drug interactions with the other statin agents.

■ Cholesterol screenings are now recommended for children age 2–10 years if they have a family history of high cholesterol or heart disease, if the family history is unknown, or if the child has other risk factors for heart disease such as obesity, hypertension, or diabetes.

■ Advicor should not be substituted for equivalent doses of immediate-release (crystalline) niacin. For patients switching from immediate-release niacin to extended-release niacin, therapy with the latter should be initiated with low doses (i.e., 500 mg once daily at bedtime), and the dose should then be titrated to the desired therapeutic response.

■ The bile acid sequestrants (resins) may decrease the absorption of digoxin, levothyroxine, tetracycline, warfarin, fat-soluble vitamins, and minerals.

■ The new formulation of Tricor can be taken with or without food once daily.

■ Therapeutic lifestyle changes that incorporate dietary changes, increased physical activity, and weight reduction are the first recommended therapy for hyperlipidemia for 6–12 weeks prior to addition of drug therapy.

12-5. Questions

Use the following case study to answer Questions 1–5.

J. B. is a 50-year-old man who comes to your pharmacy for cholesterol and medication monitoring. His medical history is notable for stage 1 hypertension, recent-onset type 2 diabetes, and hypercholesterolemia. Family history is noncontributory. Social history indicates he neither smokes nor uses alcohol. He has no known allergies. His medication history reveals that he occasionally takes acetaminophen for headaches and no other over-the-counter medications or herbal products. Current medications include hydrochlorothiazide 25 mg/d (for 4 years) and a new prescription today for atorvastatin 10 mg/d. Your physical assessment reveals the following: BP 144/90 mm Hg; pulse, 70 and regular; weight, 185 pounds; height, 5'9". An FLP today reveals the following: total cholesterol = 250 mg/dL, HDL = 40 mg/dL, and triglycerides = 145 mg/dL.

1. What is J. B.'s LDL cholesterol?

   A. 130 mg/dL
   B. 153 mg/dL
   C. 162 mg/dL
   D. 178 mg/dL
   E. 181 mg/dL

2. What is J. B.'s LDL goal?

   A. < 100 mg/dL
   B. 130–160 mg/dL
   C. 160–189 mg/dL
   D. < 200 mg/dL
   E. > 40 mg/dL

3. J. B. is started on TLC and atorvastatin because of his high LDL. When should you assess the effectiveness of therapy?

   A. 12 weeks
   B. 6 months
   C. 3 weeks
   D. 6 weeks
   E. Annually

4. J. B. is most likely to have which of the following?

   A. Familial hypercholesterolemia
   B. Polygenic hypercholesterolemia
   C. Familial combined hyperlipidemia
   D. Elevated triglycerides
   E. Isolated low HDL

5. J. B. returns for reassessment at the appropriate time. His FLP shows that his LDL is now 115 mg/dL. What is your recommendation?

   A. Stop the statin because the patient has achieved optimal LDL.
   B. Increase statin dose.
   C. Intensify TLC.
   D. Add gemfibrozil.
   E. Add cholestyramine.

6. The National Cholesterol Education Program Expert Panel identifies which of the following as a positive risk factor for coronary heart disease?

   A. Hypertension
   B. Low HDL (< 40 mg/dL)
   C. Family history of premature CHD
   D. Current cigarette smoking
   E. All of the above

7. Which of the following is *not* a secondary cause of hyperlipidemia?

   A. High LDL
   B. Hypothyroidism
   C. Diabetes
   D. Renal disease
   E. β-blockers

8. Cholesterol biosynthesis can be decreased by which of the following?

   A. Statins
   B. Oat bran
   C. Bile acid sequestrants (resins)
   D. Ezetimibe
   E. Aspirin

9. Choose the medication with the greatest effect on raising HDL.

   A. Lovastatin
   B. Pravastatin
   C. Gemfibrozil
   D. Niaspan
   E. Colesevelam

10. Choose the drug class with the most potent lowering effect on LDL.

    A. Nicotinic acid
    B. Fibric acids
    C. Omega-3 fatty acids
    D. Cholesterol inhibitors
    E. HMG-CoA reductase inhibitors

11. The initial lesion in the development of atherosclerosis is

    A. development of foam cells.
    B. increase in HDL reverse transport.
    C. rupture of a vulnerable plaque.
    D. clot formation in the artery lumen.
    E. development of a thin cap over the lipid pool.

12. Choose the correct statement.

    A. Diabetes is an absolute contraindication to the use of nicotinic acid.
    B. Aspirin is dosed three times per day to prevent flushing from niacin.
    C. Gemfibrozil may reduce triglycerides by as much as 50%.
    D. Colesevelam has similar patient tolerability problems as does cholestyramine.
    E. Ezetimibe frequently causes muscle toxicity.

13. Hyperlipidemia refers to

    A. elevation of apolipoproteins.
    B. hypercholesterolemia.
    C. high levels of white blood cells.
    D. increased ingestion of protein.
    E. endothelial dysfunction.

14. Which of the following indicates an optimal LDL?

    A. > 190 mg/dL
    B. < 40 mg/dL
    C. > 60 mg/dL
    D. < 100 mg/dL
    E. < 150 mg/dL

15. Polygenic hypercholesterolemia is characterized by which of the following?

    A. LDL = 150–450 mg/dL
    B. LDL = 160–250 mg/dL
    C. TG > 400 mg/dL
    D. HDL = 50 mg/dL
    E. LDL = 160–250 mg/dL + TG > 400 mg/dL

16. Identify a baseline laboratory test required before statin treatment.

    A. White blood cell count
    B. Complete blood cell count
    C. Liver function test
    D. Serum creatinine
    E. Creatinine clearance

17. The major troublesome side effect in nicotinic acid therapy is

    A. diarrhea.
    B. vomiting.
    C. hair growth.
    D. flushing.
    E. dizziness.

18. Which of the following medications has this warning: "For patients switching from immediate-release niacin, therapy with this drug should be initiated with a low dose and then titrated to the desired therapeutic response"?

    A. Pravigard
    B. Vytorin
    C. Advicor
    D. Atorvastatin
    E. Ezetimibe

19. Identify the drug interaction that involves the CYP450 system.

    A. Ezetimibe + niacin
    B. Colestipol + simvastatin
    C. Gemfibrozil + cholestyramine
    D. Fenofibrate + ezetimibe
    E. Lovastatin + itraconazole

20. A TLC diet could include

    A. antioxidant therapy such as vitamin E.
    B. < 7% of total calories from saturated fat.
    C. 150–250 g/d of fiber.
    D. 2–4 drinks of alcohol per day.
    E. assessment of the effectiveness of TLC at 12-week intervals.

12-6. Answers

1. E. Use the Friederwald equation to calculate LDL:

$$LDL = total\ cholesterol - (HDL + TG/5)$$

$$LDL = 250 - (40 + 145/5) = 181$$

2. A. J. B. has type 2 diabetes, which is a risk equivalent for coronary heart disease. Therefore, he is at highest risk for an event in the future, and his LDL goal should be optimal or < 100 mg/dL.

3. D. Both TLC and drug therapy measures should be assessed at 6-week intervals.

4. B. J. B.'s LDL is 181 mg/dL, which falls into the range for polygenic hypercholesterolemia (160–250 mg/dL), and he does not have elevated TGs or low HDL.

5. C. Because J. B.'s LDL is still slightly above optimal, intensify TLC. That is, continue to decrease saturated fat in the diet and to intensify weight reduction and physical activity. If the LDL is still above 100 mg/dL at the next assessment in 6 weeks, options would be to increase the statin dose (double it) or add another agent such as niacin or ezetimibe.

6. E. All of the answers are positive risk factors for CHD as defined by the NCEP's Adult Treatment Panel III. The remaining positive risk factors are gender and age (i.e., males 45 years and over and females 55 years and over).

7. A. Causes of hyperlipidemia must be ruled out. The common secondary causes are renal fail-

ure; hypothyroidism; obstructive liver disease; diabetes; and drugs such as β-blockers, thiazide diuretics, oral contraceptives, oral estrogens, glucocorticoids, and cyclosporine.

8. **A.** Statins competitively inhibit HMG-CoA reductase, which is the enzyme responsible for converting HMG-CoA to mevalonate. Inhibition of mevalonate reduces cholesterol synthesis.

9. **D.** Nicotinic acid (Niaspan) has the most efficacy in raising HDL compared with other therapies. HDL may be raised 15–35%.

10. **E.** Statins (HMG-CoA reductase inhibitors) have the most efficacy in lowering LDL. LDL may be lowered 18–55%.

11. **A.** Foam cells represent the initial lesion of atherosclerosis and develop as a result of the ingestion of oxidized LDL by macrophages in the subintimal space of the artery.

12. **C.** Diabetes is a relative contraindication to the use of nicotinic acid. Aspirin is dosed once daily, before the first nicotinic acid dose of the day. Gemfibrozil can reduce TGs 20–50%. Colesevelam is a tablet and avoids most of the palatability problems of other resins. Ezetimibe does not cause muscle toxicity.

13. **B.** *Hyperlipidemia* is defined as an elevation of a lipid in the blood. The lipid can be cholesterol or triglyceride in the form of a lipoprotein.

14. **D.** Level < 100 = optimal; 100–129 = near optimal or above optimal; 130–159 = borderline high; 160–189 = high; and ≥ 190 = very high.

15. **B.** Polygenic hypercholesterolemia is the most common cause of mild to moderately elevated LDL (LDL = 160–250 mg/dL).

16. **C.** Baseline tests before statin use include liver function tests and creatine kinase.

17. **D.** The most common side effect is flushing, which may occur in many patients. To decrease flushing intensity, a patient should take aspirin 325 mg 30 minutes prior to the first dose of nicotinic acid. Itching may also occur with flushing.

18. **C.** Advicor (Niaspan + lovastatin) contains Niaspan, which is not dose equivalent to immediate-release niacin or modified-release (sustained-release or time-release) niacin preparations.

19. **E.** Lovastatin is metabolized by CYP450 3A4 enzymes, and itraconazole will inhibit this enzyme system. Inhibition causes lovastatin blood and tissue concentrations to rise, thus predisposing the patient to muscle or liver toxicity.

20. **B.** A TLC diet includes < 7% saturated fat, 20–30 g/d fiber, avoidance of alcohol, and assessment at 6 weeks. Vitamin E is not recommended for cardiovascular risk reduction.

12-7. References

Beaird SL. HMG-CoA reductase inhibitors: Assessing differences in drug interactions and safety profiles. *J Am Pharm Assoc.* 2000;40:6337–44.

Daniels SR, Greer FR, Committee on Nutrition. Lipid screening and cardiovascular health in childhood. *Pediatrics.* 2008;122:198–208.

Downs JR, Clearfield M, Weis S, et al. Primary prevention of acute coronary events with lovastatin in men and women with average cholesterol levels: Results of AFCAPS/TexCAPS. *JAMA.* 1998;279: 1615–22.

Expert Panel on Detection, Evaluation, and Treatment of High Blood Cholesterol in Adults. Executive summary of the Third Report of the National Cholesterol Education Program (NCEP) Expert Panel on Detection, Evaluation, and Treatment of High Blood Cholesterol in Adults (Adult Treatment Panel III). *JAMA.* 2001;285:2486–97.

Heart Protection Study Collaborative Group. MRC/BHF Heart Protection Study of cholesterol lowering with simvastatin in 20,536 high-risk individuals: A randomised placebo-controlled trial. *Lancet.* 2002;360:7–22.

Knopp RH. Drug treatment of lipid disorders. *N Engl J Med.* 1999;341:498–511.

Long-Term Intervention with Pravastatin in Ischaemic Disease (LIPID) Study Group. Prevention of cardiovascular events and death with pravastatin in patients with coronary heart disease and a broad range of initial cholesterol levels. *N Engl J Med.* 1998;339:1349–57.

McKenney JM, Hawkins DW, eds. *Handbook on the Management of Lipid Disorders.* Springfield, N.J.: Scientific Therapeutics Information/National Pharmacy Cardiovascular Council; 2001.

Pasternak RC, Smith SC Jr, Bairey-Merz CN, et al. ACC/AHA/NHLBI clinical advisory on the use and safety of statins. *J Am Coll Cardiol.* 2002;40: 568–73.

Scandinavian Simvastatin Survival Study Group. Randomised trial of cholesterol lowering in 4,444 patients with coronary heart disease: The

Scandinavian Simvastatin Survival Study (4S). *Lancet*. 1994;344:1383–89.

Sudhop T, Lutjohann D, Kodal A, et al. Inhibition of intestinal cholesterol absorption by ezetimibe in humans. *Circulation*. 2002;106:1943–48.

Talbert RL. Hyperlipidemia. In: DiPiro JT, Talbert RL, Yee GC, et al., eds. *Pharmacotherapy: A Pathophysiologic Approach*. 5th ed. New York: McGraw-Hill; 2002:395–418.

West of Scotland Coronary Prevention Study Group. Influence of pravastatin and plasma levels on clinical events in the West of Scotland Coronary Prevention Study (WOSCOPS). *Circulation*. 1998; 97:1440–45.

Wolf MI, Vartnian SF, Ross JL, et al. Safety and effectiveness of Niaspan when added sequentially to a statin for treatment of dyslipidemia. *Am J Cardiol*. 2001;87:476–79.

Diabetes Mellitus

13

Joni Foard, PharmD, CDE
L. Brian Cross, PharmD, CDE

13-1. Overview

Diabetes mellitus (DM) is a group of chronic metabolic diseases caused by defects in insulin secretion, action, or both that result in hyperglycemia; abnormal metabolism of carbohydrates, fats, and proteins; and long-term macrovascular and microvascular complications.

DM affects 23.6 million people or approximately 8% of the population: 17.9 million diagnosed and 5.7 million undiagnosed.

It is the seventh-leading cause of death. Risk of death is two times that of people without diabetes of similar age.

Classification

Type 1 diabetes

Type 1 diabetes was previously called insulin-dependent diabetes mellitus or juvenile-onset diabetes. It requires exogenous insulin for survival. It comprises 5–10% of all diagnosed cases.

Type 2 diabetes

Type 2 diabetes was previously called *noninsulin-dependent diabetes mellitus* or *adult-onset diabetes*. It comprises 90–95% of all diagnosed cases.

Gestational diabetes mellitus

Gestational diabetes mellitus (GDM) involves glucose intolerance with onset of pregnancy or first recognition during pregnancy (second and third trimesters). Approximately 7% of pregnancies develop GDM: > 200,000 annually. Women with GDM have 40–60% chance of later developing type 2 diabetes; 5–10% of

those are diagnosed in the postpartum period. The primary fetal complication of concern is macrosomia.

Other types: Secondary DM

Secondary DM is attributable to genetic defects of β-cell function (e.g., maturity-onset diabetes of youth), surgery, drugs, malnutrition, infections, and other illnesses. It comprises 1–5% of all diagnosed cases.

Prediabetes

In prediabetes, plasma glucose levels are higher than normal but lower than those diagnostic for diabetes. Prediabetes was formerly characterized as *impaired fasting glucose* (IFG) and *impaired glucose tolerance* (IGT). It is a risk factor for future diabetes and cardiovascular disease.

Clinical Presentation

Classic signs and symptoms include polydipsia, polyuria, and polyphagia. Other common findings include fatigue, blurred vision, and frequent infections.

Type 1 diabetes

Signs include rapid onset and unexplained weight loss. Patients are potentially ketonuric or experience ketoacidosis. They may experience a "honeymoon" period, a phase of erratic insulin secretion lasting months to a year during destruction of β-cells.

Type 2 diabetes

Onset is progressive. Patients may be asymptomatic or experience mild classic signs and symptoms; 80% are obese or have history of obesity. Patients may present with microvascular and macrovascular chronic complications

Pathophysiology and Etiology

Type 1 diabetes

- β-cell destruction leads to absolute insulin deficiency.
- Subgroups are as follows:
  - Immune mediated, in which a strong human leukocyte antigen association indicates genetic predisposition. This subgroup is related to environmental factors; a stimulus (e.g., virus) triggers the immunologic process.
  - Idiopathic, in which there is no evidence of autoimmunity or other known etiology.
- Patients are prone to ketoacidosis.
- Peak onset occurs at the time of puberty but may occur at any age.

Type 2 diabetes

- Insulin resistance and progressive β-cell dysfunction are characteristic.

- Development of type 2 DM often involves a strong genetic predisposition.
- It is also associated with environmental factors such as excessive calorie intake, decreased activity, weight gain, and obesity.
- Insulin resistance may be present years before the onset of diabetes.
- Initially normal glucose levels are maintained by increased insulin secretion by β-cells.
- Increasing insulin resistance or a failure of β-cells to maintain insulin secretion leads to glucose intolerance and development of diabetes.
- Insulin resistance is influenced by age, ethnicity, physical activity, medications, and weight.
- Type 2 DM is usually diagnosed in adulthood but can occur at any age.
- The incidence of type 2 diabetes is higher among certain ethnic populations (Figure 13-1).

Diagnostic Criteria

Box 13-1 shows the criteria for the diagnosis of DM.

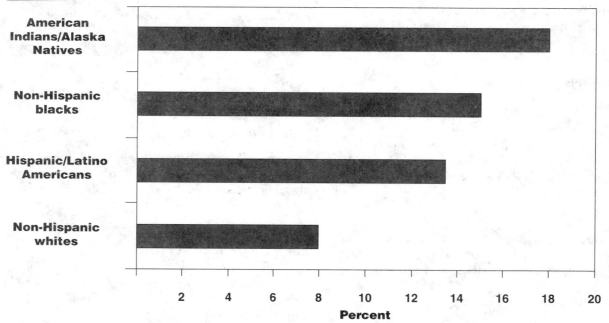

Figure 13-1. Estimated Age-Adjusted Total Prevalence of Diabetes in People 20 Years or Older, by Race and Ethnicity: United States, 2005

Source: *For American Indians/Alaska Natives, the estimate of total prevalence was calculated using the estimate of diagnosed diabetes from the 2003 outpatient database of the Indian Health Service and the estimate of undiagnosed diabetes from the 1999-2002 National Health and Nutrition Examination Survey. For the other groups, 1999-2002 NHANES estimates of total prevalence (both diagnosed and undiagnosed) were projected to year 2006.*

* Graph and information obtained from CDC (Centers for Disease Control and Prevention) website at http://www.cdc.gov/diabetes/pubs/estimatesDS.html#prev4 on December 1, 2006.

Box 13-1. Criteria for the Diagnosis of Diabetes Mellitus

Symptoms of diabetes and a casual plasma glucose ≥ 200 mg/dL (11.1 mmol/L). *Casual* is defined as any time of day without regard to time since last meal. The classic symptoms of diabetes include polyuria, polydipsia, and unexplained weight loss.

OR

FPG ≥ 126 mg/dL (7.0 mmol/L). *Fasting* is defined as no caloric intake for at least 8 hours.

OR

Two-hour plasma glucose ≥ 200 mg/dL (11.1 mmol/L) during an OGTT. The test should be performed as described by the World Health Organization, using a glucose load containing the equivalent of 75 g anhydrous glucose dissolved in water.

Source: Expert Committee on the Diagnosis and Classification of Diabetes Mellitus. Report of the Expert Committee on the Diagnosis and Classification of Diabetes Mellitus. *Diabetes Care* 1997;20:1183–97. Reprinted with permission from the American Diabetes Association.
Note: In the absence of unequivocal hyperglycemia, criteria should be confirmed by repeat testing on a different day.

Type 1 and type 2 DM

Diagnosis can be made on the basis of a fasting plasma glucose (FPG) test, a random plasma glucose test, or an oral glucose tolerance test (OGTT). Diagnosis must be confirmed on a subsequent day using any of the three methods.

The FPG test is the test of choice because of simplicity, lower cost, and reproducibility.

Abnormal results not meeting criteria outlined in Box 13-1 are classified as prediabetes:

- IFG = FPG ≥ 100 mg/dL to 125 mg/dL
- IGT = 2-hour OGTT plasma glucose ≥ 140 mg/dL to 199 mg/dL

Serum C peptide level is diagnostic for functioning of β-cells and may be used for classification.

Gestational diabetes mellitus

OGTT is preferred screening test in pregnancy. For average-risk patients, test at 24–28 weeks of gestation. For high-risk patients (marked obesity, personal history of GDM, glycosuria, diagnosis of polycystic ovarian syndrome, or strong family history of DM), perform a risk assessment at the first prenatal visit and test as soon as possible; if initial screenings are negative, retest between 24 and 28 weeks of gestation.

In average- or high-risk patients use one of two approaches:

- *One-step approach:* diagnostic 100 g OGTT
- *Two-step approach:* 1-hour 50 mg glucose challenge test followed by diagnostic 100 g glucose OGTT if 1-hour level ≥ 140 mg/dL

Diagnosis of GDM with a 100 g glucose load is positive if at least two glucose values meet or exceed the following levels:

- Fasting: ≥ 95 mg/dL
- 1 hour: ≥ 180 mg/dL
- 2 hours: ≥ 155 mg/dL
- 3 hours: ≥ 140 mg/dL

If on the subsequent day FPG ≥ 126 mg/dL or casual plasma glucose ≥ 200 mg/dL, a glucose challenge is not needed. Reevaluation and reclassification should be conducted 6–12 weeks postpartum.

Treatment Principles and Goals

- To achieve and maintain glycemic control (Table 13-1)
- To attain recommended blood pressure and lipid goals (Table 13-1)
- To modify lifestyle to promote general health and achieve weight management goals
- To prevent or slow progression of chronic complications
- To prevent or resolve acute complications
- To achieve an acceptable quality of life and satisfaction with care

Prevention of complications

The following activities can prevent complications from arising:

- Smoking cessation
- Aspirin or antiplatelet therapy
  - Use as secondary prevention with a history of cardiovascular disease.
  - Use as primary prevention if patient is > 40 years of age or has additional risk factors (family history of cardiovascular disease, hypertension, smoking, dyslipidemia, or albuminuria).
  - Prescribe aspirin 75–162 mg/d.
- Immunization
  - Annual influenza vaccine if patient is 6 months of age or older and no contraindications
  - At least one lifetime pneumococcal vaccine for adults with no contraindications

Table 13-1. Summary of Recommendations for Adults with Diabetes

Area	Recommended goal
Glycemic control:	
A_{1c}	< 7.0%[a]
Preprandial capillary plasma glucose	70–130 mg/dL
Peak postprandial capillary plasma glucose[b]	< 180 mg/dL
Blood pressure:	< 130/80 mmHg
Lipids:[c]	
LDL	< 100 mg/dL[d]
Triglycerides	< 150 mg/dL
HDL	> 40 mg/dL[e]

Key concepts in setting glycemic goals:

- A_{1c} is the primary target for glycemic control.
- Goals should be individualized.
- More or less stringent glycemic goals may be appropriate for individual patients.
- Postprandial glucose may be targeted if A_{1c} goals are not met despite reaching preprandial glucose goals.

---

a. Referenced to a nondiabetic range of 4.0–6.0% using a Diabetes Control and Complications Trial–based assay.
b. Postprandial glucose measurements should be made 1–2 hours after the beginning of the meal—generally peak levels in patients with diabetes.
c. Current National Cholesterol Education Program–Adult Treatment Panel III guidelines suggest that in patients with triglycerides ≥ 200 mg/dL, the "non-HDL cholesterol" (total cholesterol – HDL) be used. The goal is 130 mg/dL.
d. In individuals with overt cardiovascular disease, a lower LDL cholesterol goal of < 70 mg/dL is an option.
e. For women, it has been suggested that the HDL goal be increased by 10 mg/dL.
Source: Adapted from American Diabetes Association. Standards of medical care in diabetes—2009. *Diabetes Care.* 2009: 32(suppl 1):S13–61.

- One-time pneumococcal revaccination if patient is > 64 years of age, previously immunized at < 65 years of age, and vaccine administered > 5 years ago
- Foot care: self-inspection daily, visual inspection at each office visit, and an annual comprehensive exam
- Skin care: self-inspection and care daily
- Dental care: annual examination
- Eye care: annual dilated eye examination

Complications of diabetes

Chronic complications

- ***Coronary atherosclerosis:*** Death rate is two to four times higher in adults with DM than in adults without diabetes.

- ***Cerebrovascular atherosclerosis:*** Risk of stroke is two to four times higher among people with diabetes.
- ***Peripheral vascular disease:*** Pain is due to intermittent claudication; insufficient circulation impairs healing and increases risk of gangrene and amputation.

Microvascular disease

- Retinopathy
  - It is the leading cause of new cases of blindness in adults 20–74 years of age.
  - Retinopathy may develop without symptoms; annual dilated eye examination is recommended for detection.
  - Treatment includes glycemic and blood pressure control and laser photocoagulation.
- Nephropathy
  - It occurs in 20–40% of diabetics and is the leading cause of end-stage renal disease.
  - Random spot collection of the albumin-to-creatinine ratio should be performed yearly; a value of > 30 mg/g is considered abnormal.
  - Serum creatinine should be measured at least annually for the estimation of glomerular filtration rate (GFR).
  - Treatment includes glycemic and blood pressure control; angiotensin-converting enzyme (ACE) inhibitors or angiotensin II receptor blockers should be used except during pregnancy.
- Polyneuropathy
  - Sensorimotor nervous system dysfunction occurs.
  - Pain and diminished sensation occur, with potential for poor detection of trauma, which increases risk for ulcers and infection.
- Autonomic neuropathy
  - Gastrointestinal (GI) effects include gastroparesis, constipation, and diarrhea.
  - Genitourinary effects include neurogenic bladder and sexual dysfunction in men.
  - Cardiovascular effects include orthostatic hypotension and resting tachycardia.
- Diabetic foot problems
  - DM accounts for > 60% of nontraumatic amputations in the United States.
  - Prevention, early detection with regular foot exams, and prompt treatment of lesions are essential to avoid complications.

Acute complications

- Hypoglycemia
  - *Hypoglycemia* is defined as plasma glucose < 70 mg/dL.

- Glucose (15–20 g) is the preferred treatment, but other forms of carbohydrates that contain glucose can be used.
- Treatment effects should be seen in 15 minutes.
- Symptoms can range from mild (tremor, palpitations, sweating) to severe (unresponsiveness, unconsciousness, or convulsions).
- Severe hypoglycemia may require assistance from another individual for treatment with glucagon or IV glucose.
- Diabetic ketoacidosis (DKA)
  - DKA is a medical emergency in type 1 diabetes because of absolute or relative insulin deficiency.
  - Omission of insulin, major stress, infection, or trauma may precipitate DKA.
  - DKA is characterized by glucose > 250 mg/dL, elevated ketones, arterial pH < 7.2, plasma bicarbonate < 15 mEq/L.
  - Ketone bodies are formed in excess because of fatty acid metabolism in the liver, leading to ketonuria and ketonemia and ultimately diabetic ketoacidosis.
  - Kussmaul respirations (deep and rapid) are characteristic in an attempt to compensate for metabolic acidosis.
  - DKA requires prompt intervention with insulin, fluids, and electrolytes to prevent coma and death.
- Hyperosmolar hyperglycemic state
  - It is also known as *hyperglycemic hyperosmolar nonketotic coma*.
  - It is a complication of type 2 diabetes.
  - The state is characterized by elevated plasma glucose (typically > 500 mg/dL), dehydration, and hyperosmolality in the absence of significant ketoacidosis.
  - It may be triggered by infection or other stressors such as stroke or myocardial infarction.
  - Treatment includes fluid and electrolyte replacement as well as insulin.

13-2. Drug Therapy

Oral Medications for DM Treatment

Secretagogues

Mechanism of action

The primary mechanism of secretagogues is to cause a reduction in blood glucose by stimulating the release of insulin from the pancreas. This mechanism may in turn cause a decrease in hepatic gluconeogenesis and a slight decrease in insulin resistance at the muscle level. Effectiveness depends on pancreatic β-cell function.

Clinical and counseling considerations

- Medication should be taken before meals: sulfonylureas, qd bid; meglitinides, before each meal.
- Medication causes a 1–2 kg weight gain.
- A positive risk of hypoglycemia exists, which is greater with sulfonylureas than with meglitinides.
- Secretagogues are typically not indicated during pregnancy, when breast-feeding, or in children.
- A fast-acting oral carbohydrate should be carried for emergency use.

A_{1c} reduction

- 1–2% (sulfonylureas)
- 0.5–2% (meglitinides)

Cost

- Medications are generically available.
- For meglitinides, the monthly cost is about $75–200.

Cautions and contraindications

- Use with caution in elderly patients; do *not* use chlorpropamide.
- Use with caution in cases of renal and hepatic insufficiency; glipizide and glimepiride safer.
- Avoid in patients with significant alcohol use.
- Drug interactions (worse with first-generation sulfonylureas) may cause increased risk of hypoglycemia: anticoagulants, fluconazole, salicylates, gemfibrozil, sulfonamides, tricyclic antidepressants, digoxin.
- Use is contraindicated in patients with DKA, severe infection, surgery, or trauma.
- Patients should wear medical identification.
- Store drug in a cool, dry place (not the bathroom or kitchen).
- Syndrome of inappropriate antidiuretic hormone secretion, disulfiram-like reaction with alcohol (ETOH), and sun-sensitivity reactions are more common in first-generation sulfonylureas than in second-generation sulfonylureas.

Dosing

See Table 13-2 for information about dosing.

Biguanides

Mechanism of action

The primary mechanism is seen through decreased hepatic gluconeogenesis as well as improved glucose

Table 13-2. Sulfonylureas

Drug	Trade name	Strength	Daily dose	Duration of action	Comments
First generation					
Acetohexamide	Dymelor	250, 500 mg	250–1,500 mg	Up to 16 hours	Active metabolite excreted by kidney
Chlorpropamide	Diabinese	100, 250 mg	100–500 mg	Up to 72 hours	Contraindicated in renal insufficiency
Tolazamide	Tolinase	100, 250, 500 mg	100–1,000 mg	Up to 10 hours	
Tolbutamide	Orinase	250, 500 mg	500–3,000 mg qd–bid	Up to 10 hours	
Second generation					
Glipizide	Glucotrol, Glucotrol XL	5, 10 mg	5–40 mg qd–bid 5–20 mg qd (XL)	Up to 20 hours	Given with or without meal; do not cut XL tab
Glyburide	DiaBeta, Micronase	1.25, 2.50, 5.00 mg	1.25–20.00 mg qd–bid	Up to 24 hours	3 mg Glynase = 5 mg glyburide
Glyburide micronized	Glynase	1.5, 3.0, 4.5, 6.0 mg	1.5–12.0 mg qd	Up to 24 hours	
Glimepiride	Amaryl	1, 2, 4 mg	1–8 mg qd	24 hours	Begin with 1 mg in renal insufficiency
Meglitinides and phenylalanines					
Repaglinide	Prandin	0.5, 1.0, 2.0 mg	0.5–4.0 mg before each meal; maximum dose = 16 mg/d	Peak effect: ~ 1 hour; duration: ~ 2–3 hours	Skip dose if meal skipped; do not give in combination with sulfonylureas
Nateglinide	Starlix	60, 120 mg	60–120 mg before each meal	Peak effect: ~ 1 hour; duration: ~ 4 hours	Efficacy: Prandin > Starlix

utilization and uptake in peripheral tissues and decreased intestinal absorption of glucose.

Clinical considerations
- Biguanides are considered the first choice when beginning drug treatment in newly diagnosed DM patients unless contraindicated.
- They pose minimal risk of hypoglycemia unless combined with secretagogues or insulin.
- They may decrease weight up to 5 kg.
- They decrease triglycerides, decrease LDL, and increase HDL.
- GI symptoms (nausea, vomiting, bloating, flatulence, anorexia, and diarrhea) are the most common adverse effects.
  - Take doses with or after meals to reduce GI symptoms.
  - GI symptoms are transient and improve in most patients over time.

- Titrate the dose up slowly to minimize GI symptoms: 500 mg qd with the largest meal × 1 week; then increase to 500 mg bid with the two largest meals × 1 week; then increase to 1 g (two 500 mg tablets) with largest meal and 500 mg with the second-largest meal × 1 week; then increase to 1 g bid with the two largest meals of the day.
- Biguanides interfere with vitamin B_{12} absorption.
- They may require as much as 8 weeks of therapy before effectiveness can be assessed.
- Biguanides are generally not indicated during pregnancy or breast-feeding.
- They are indicated for the treatment of type 2 DM in children 10 years and older.
- They may decrease the progression to diabetes from IGT and IFG (prediabetes).
- They have positive cardiovascular benefits when used in obese patients with DM.

A_{1c} reduction
A reduction of 1–2% is expected.

Cost
Biguanides are generically available.

Cautions and contraindications
Most cautions and contraindications are related to the ability of biguanides to increase the risk of lactic acidosis with metformin (less than one case per 100,000 treated patients).

Contraindications
- Renal insufficiency (serum creatinine, or SCr ≥ 1.4 females; SCr ≥ 1.5 males) is a contraindication; recent studies have suggested that metformin is safe unless the estimated GFR falls to < 30ml/min.
- Hepatic dysfunction is a contraindication.
- Excessive alcohol use (binge or chronic use of more than two drinks per day or at one sitting) is a contraindication.
- Medication may be contraindicated in congestive heart failure (New York Heart Association classifications III and IV).

Cautions
- Medication should be held back in situations of increased risk for lactic acidosis, including acute myocardial infarction, congestive heart failure exacerbation, severe respiratory disease, shock, and septicemia.
- Medication should be held back 48 hours after iodinated contrast media and major surgeries.

Dosing
See Table 13-3 for information about dosing.

Thiazolidinediones (glitazones/TZDs)

Mechanism of action
Thiazolidinediones (also called *glitazones* or *TZDs*) are agonists of the PPARγ (peroxisome proliferators-activated receptor-γ) receptor, which, when stimulated, improves peripheral muscle and adipose tissue insulin sensitivity as well as suppresses hepatic glucose output.

Clinical considerations
- Minimal risk of hypoglycemia exists unless combined with secretagogues or insulin.
- TZDs may cause a 5 kg weight gain—more if combined with secretagogues or insulin.
- They decrease triglycerides (pioglitazone > rosiglitazone), increase high-density lipoprotein (HDL) (pioglitazone = rosiglitazone), and increase low-density lipoprotein (LDL) (rosiglitazone)/LDL (pioglitazone).
- They are dosed qd, though rosiglitazone may be slightly more effective when dosed bid.
- As much as 16 weeks of therapy may be required before assessing effectiveness.
- Generally, they are not indicated during breast-feeding or pregnancy.
- They may decrease the progression to diabetes from IGT and IFG.
- Edema may best be treated by aldosterone antagonists.
- They are not indicated by the U.S. Food and Drug Administration for treatment of type 2 DM in children, though they have been used.
- They may be helpful in nonalcoholic fatty liver disease.
- Recent meta-analyses suggest a 30–40% relative increase in risk for myocardial infarction with rosiglitazone, though not with pioglitazone.

Table 13-3. Biguanides

Drug	Trade name	Strength	Daily dose	Duration of action	Comments
Metformin	Glucophage	500, 850, 1,000 mg	1,000–2,550 mg (adult) up to 2,000 mg (10 years and older)	≥ 24 hours	
Metformin extended release	Glucophage XR Glumetza	500, 750 mg 500, 1,000 mg	2,000 mg qpm; may take 1 g bid if qd dosing causes GI symptoms		*Do not* cut, crush, or chew

A1c reduction

A reduction of 1–2% is expected.

Cost

The monthly cost of the medication is approximately $120–200.

Cautions and contraindications:

- Edema—with oral therapies (approximately 5%), with insulin (approximately 15%)—may occur in patients with *no* history of heart problems. (The condition may be dose related.) Recommendation: Discontinue therapy if the problem is significant, decrease the dose if the problem is minor, and consider further cardiac workup.
- Recently, a black box warning was added for congestive heart failure (pioglitazone and rosiglitazone).
- Hepatotoxicity incidence is approximately 0.2% of alanine aminotransferase (ALT) > three times upper limit of normal (ULN) for both agents. Recommendation: Liver function tests (LFTs) every other month for first 12 months and periodically thereafter. If ALT > 2.5 ULN, do not start; if ALT = 1.0–2.5 ULN, monitor closely; if ALT 3× ULN, discontinue medication.
- Medication may cause resumption of ovulation in anovulatory women.
- Medication decreases oral contraceptive effectiveness.

Dosing

See Table 13-4 for information about dosing.

Alpha-glucosidase inhibitors

Mechanism of action

Alpha-glucosidase inhibitors delay the digestion of carbohydrates into simple sugars and their subsequent absorption in the small intestine.

Clinical considerations

- Minimal risk of hypoglycemia exists unless the drug is combined with secretagogues or insulin.
- Alpha-glucosidase inhibitors have minimal effect on weight but can cause possible decrease in weight secondary to side effects.
- Main target of therapy should be postprandial hyperglycemia.
- GI symptoms (flatulence, GI upset, abdominal pain, diarrhea, bloating) are the most common side effects. These side effects tend to dissipate over time with continued treatment. Dosing must be individualized and slowly titrated up as tolerated: 25 mg qd × 1 week; then 25 mg bid × 1 week; then 25 mg tid × 1 week; then continued increased dose as tolerated up to 50 mg tid.
- Patient should be counseled to increase complex carbohydrate intake and decrease intake of simple sugars.
- Treatment of hypoglycemia:
  - Patient should use milk (lactose) or fruit juice (fructose), *not* sucrose.
  - Any carbohydrate can be used if > 2–3 hours since last dose of alpha-glucosidase inhibitor agent.
- Alpha-glucosidase inhibitors are generally not indicated during pregnancy, while breast-feeding, or in children.
- Alpha-glucosidase inhibitors decrease the bioavailability of digoxin, propranolol, and ranitidine.

A1c reduction

A reduction of 0.5–1.0% is expected.

Cost

The monthly cost of the medication is approximately $75–100.

Cautions and contraindications

- Avoid use in patients with GI disorders such as ulcerative colitis, Crohn's disease, possible bowel obstruction, and short bowel syndrome.

Table 13-4. Thiazoladinediones

Drug	Trade name	Strength	Daily dose	Duration of action	Comments
Rosiglitazone	Avandia	2, 4, 8 mg	4–8 mg qd or 2–4 mg bid	24 hours	May be more effective when given bid
Pioglitazone	Actos	15, 30, 45 mg	30–45 mg qd	24 hours	

Table 13-5. Alpha-Glucosidase Inhibitors

Drug	Trade name	Strength	Daily dose	Duration of action	Comments
Acarbose	Precose	50, 100 mg	25–100 mg tid	1–3 hours	Maximum dose: < 60 kg = 50 mg tid; > 60 kg = 100 mg tid
Miglitol	Glyset	25, 50, 100 mg	25–100 mg tid	1–3 hours	

- Avoid use in patients with SCr > 2 mg/dL (acarbose) or creatinine clearance (CrCl) of ≤ 25mL/min (both agents).
- Increased LFTs may be needed (acarbose) depending on the dose (> 300 mg/day) and weight of patient. Avoid use in patients with cirrhosis.

Dosing
See Table 13-5 for information about dosing.

Dipeptidyl peptidase—4 inhibitors

Mechanism of action
Dipeptidyl peptidase—4 (DPP-4) inhibitors inhibit the degradation of endogenous glucagon-like peptide-1 (GLP-1) and glucose-dependent insulinotropic polypeptide (GIP), which in turn causes (1) increased insulin production in a glucose-dependent fashion, (2) decreased production of glucagon, and (3) improved β-cell functioning.

Clinical considerations
- Minimal risk of hypoglycemia exists unless drug is combined with secretagogues or insulin.
- These drugs have minimal or no effect on weight.
- They can be used either as monotherapy or in combination with metformin or thiazolidinediones and possibly with insulin.
- This is the only drug class affecting the GLP-1 system dosed orally.
- Generally, DPP-4 inhibitors are very well tolerated. The most common side effects include nasopharyngitis and upper respiratory tract infections.
- Secondary to newness of the drug, no significant long-term outcome data are yet available.

A_{1c} reduction
A reduction of 0.6–0.9% is expected.

Cost
The monthly cost is about $150.

Cautions and contraindications
- The dose should be adjusted for renal insufficiency.
- The drug may cause adverse immunologic reactions through T-cell inhibition.
- The drug should not be used in patients with DKA or type 1 DM.

Dosing
See Table 13-6 for information about dosing.

Combination oral agents for DM

Figure 13-2 shows the combination oral agents for DM. See individual agents for details.

Injectable Medications for DM Treatment

Insulin products

Mechanism of action
At low levels, insulin causes suppression of endogenous hepatic glucose production. At higher

Table 13-6. Dipeptidyl Peptidase–4 Inhibitors

Drug	Trade name	Strength	Daily dose	Duration of action	Comments
Sitagliptin	Januvia	25, 50, 100 mg	100 mg qd	24 hours	CrCl 30–50: 50 mg qd; CrCl < 30: 25 mg qd

Figure 13-2. Combination Oral Agents

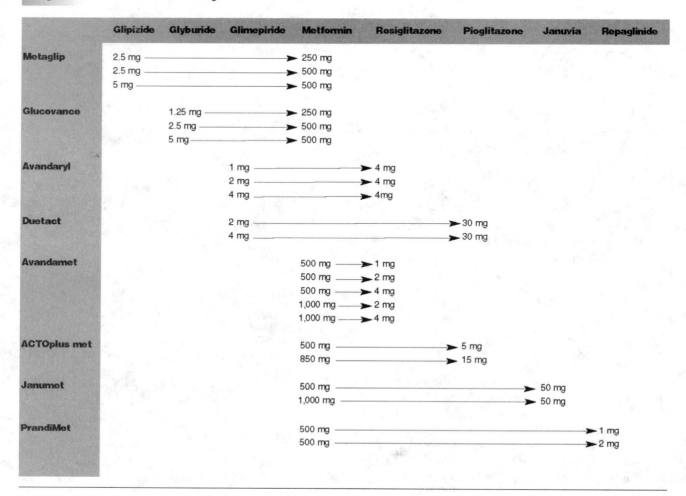

	Glipizide	Glyburide	Glimepiride	Metformin	Rosiglitazone	Pioglitazone	Januvia	Repaglinide
Metaglip	2.5 mg			250 mg				
	2.5 mg			500 mg				
	5 mg			500 mg				
Glucovance		1.25 mg		250 mg				
		2.5 mg		500 mg				
		5 mg		500 mg				
Avandaryl			1 mg		4 mg			
			2 mg		4 mg			
			4 mg		4 mg			
Duetact			2 mg			30 mg		
			4 mg			30 mg		
Avandamet				500 mg	1 mg			
				500 mg	2 mg			
				500 mg	4 mg			
				1,000 mg	2 mg			
				1,000 mg	4 mg			
ACTOplus met				500 mg		5 mg		
				850 mg		15 mg		
Janumet				500 mg			50 mg	
				1,000 mg			50 mg	
PrandiMet				500 mg				1 mg
				500 mg				2 mg

levels, insulin promotes glucose uptake by muscle tissue.

Clinical considerations
- Insulin carries a positive risk of hypoglycemia.
- It causes an increase in weight.
- Insulin should be considered as initial agent if glucose is > 250 mg/dL or A$_{1c}$ is > 10%.
- There is no dosage limit.
- Dosing is often started with a basal insulin (0.1–0.2 units/kg/d) and added to an existing oral regimen of two or more agents.
- Insulin regimen should be individualized to the patient accounting for
  - Glucose readings
  - Patient preferences
  - Patient schedule
  - Patient education and intelligence level
  - Level of intensity needed
  - Cost to patient

- Consider patient for prandial insulin coverage when
  - Patient with fasting blood glucose target (< 100), but A$_{1c}$ ≥ 7%
  - A$_{1c}$ ≥ 7% with evidence of frequent 2-hour postprandial glucose values > 160 mg/dL
  - Nighttime or daytime hypoglycemia with skipped or delayed meals

A$_{1c}$ reduction
A reduction of 2.5% is expected.

Cost
Monthly cost varies, depending on the insulin product prescribed and the device used (i.e., pen versus vial or syringe).

Cautions and contraindications
- Dose cautiously in patients with renal and hepatic insufficiency.
- Dose cautiously in elderly patients.

- Do not mix the following insulins with any others: Lantus, Levemir, Lente, and Ultralente.
- Counsel patients on signs and symptoms of hypoglycemia and how to appropriately treat.
- Most insulin products are stable at room temperature for 30 days, other than premixed insulin products (14 days) and Levemir (45 days).

Dosing

Table 13-7 provides sample titration schedules for basal and prandial insulin. See Table 13-8 for further dosing information.

Incretin mimetics

Mechanism of action

Incretin mimetics are receptor agonists of endogenous GLP-1 that cause (1) increased insulin production in a glucose-dependent fashion, (2) decreased production of glucagon, (3) slowing of gastric emptying, (4) increased satiety and weight loss, and (5) improved β-cell functioning.

Clinical considerations

- Minimal risk of hypoglycemia exists unless the drug is combined with secretagogues (consider initial reduction in secretagogue). There is a minor increase in hypoglycemia risk if the drug is combined with TZDs.
- Moderate weight loss of about 10 pounds is seen after sustained use.
- A dose-limiting side effect is nausea. Approximately 50% of patients report some degree of nausea, but stop the drug secondary to the problem. This problem seems to lessen with time.
- Patients should decrease meal size and carbohydrate content of meals prior to use of exenatide to lessen problem of nausea.
- Dose should be given 10–15 minutes prior to the two largest meals of the day, which should be spaced at least 6 hours apart.
- Drugs can be stored at room temperature for 30 days after first dose is given.
- Drugs can be combined with sulfonylurea, metformin, sulfonylurea + metformin, TZDs, or metformin + TZD. Currently, they are not indicated in combination with insulin.
- Begin with 5 mcg injected bid for 1 month; then increase to 10 mcg bid as tolerated secondary to GI toxicity.
- Drugs are supplied as a pen device that contains 60 doses (1-month supply).
- They are most effective in lowering postprandial glucose elevations.
- Recent reports suggest a possible risk for pancreatitis associated with use of GLP agonists; however, whether the relationship is causal or coincidental is not yet clear.

A_{1c} reduction

A reduction of 0.5–1.0% is expected.

Cost

The monthly cost is approximately $150–200.

Table 13-7. Sample Titration Schedules for Basal and Prandial Insulin

Basal insulin titration		Prandial insulin titration	
Fasting blood glucose levels for 3 consecutive days	Adjust basal insulin dose (units)	Preprandial or bedtime glucose levels for 3 consecutive days	Adjust rapid-acting insulin dose (units)
≥ 180 mg/dL	+8	≥ 180 mg/dL	+3
160–180 mg/dL	+6	140–180 mg/dL	+2
140–160 mg/dL	+4	140–180 mg/dL	+2
120–140 mg/dL	+2	120–140 mg/dL	+1
100–120 mg/dL	+1	100–120 mg/dL	No change
80–100 mg/dL	No change	80–100 mg/dL	−1
60–80 mg/dL	−2	60–80 mg/dL	−2
< 60 mg/dL	−4	< 60 mg/dL	−4

Note: To increase fasting glucose, adjust basal dose *only*. Increase preprandial or bedtime glucose levels as follows: (1) if increase at lunchtime, adjust breakfast prandial insulin; (2) if increase at dinnertime, adjust lunchtime prandial insulin; (3) if increase at bedtime, adjust dinnertime prandial insulin.

Table 13-8. Insulin Products

Insulin type	Trade name	Device availability	Onset of action	Time of peak	Duration of action
Rapid acting:					
Glulisine	Apidra	OptiClick pen, SoloSTAR	15–30 min	30–90 min	1–3 hours
Aspart	Novolog	NovoPen	10–15 min	30–90 min	3–5 hours
Lispro	Humalog	Lilly pen, HumaPen MEMOIR, Luxura HD pen	10–15 min	30–90 min	
Intermediate acting:					
Human NPH	Novolin N	NovoPen, InnoLet	1–3 hours	4–12 hours	10–18 hours
	Humulin N	Lilly pen	1–3 hours	4–12 hours	10–18 hours
Lente human			2–5 hours	7–15 hours	24 hours
Basal:					
Glargine	Lantus	OptiClick pen, SoloSTAR	1–2 hours	Peakless	24 hours
Detemir	Levemir	NovoPen	1–2 hours	6–8 hours	18–24 hours
Premixed:					
NPH + regular	Novolin 70/30	NovoPen, InnoLet			
	Humulin 70/30	Lilly pen			
	Humulin 50/50	Lilly pen			
Insulin protamine + analogs	Novolog 70/30	NovoPen			
	Novolog 50/50	NovoPen			
	Humalog 75/25	Lilly pen			
	Humalog 50/50	Lilly pen			

Note: Most common available concentration = 100 units per mL. Concentration used in severe insulin resistance = 500 units per mL.

Cautions and contraindications

- Medication should *not* be given to patients with GFR ≤ 30 mL/min.
- It should *not* be given to patients with severe gastrointestinal disease, including gastroparesis.
- It should not be used in patients with DKA or type 1 DM.

Dosing
Table 13-9 provides further dosing information.

Amylin mimetics

Mechanism of action
The medication is an analog of endogenous amylin that when dosed at therapeutic levels causes (1) decreased production of glucagon, (2) slowing of

Table 13-9. Incretin Mimetics

Drug	Trade name	Strength	Daily dose	Duration of action
Exenitide	Byetta	5, 10 mcg pen	5–10 mcg bid	~ 8–10 hours

gastric emptying, and (3) increased satiety and weight loss.

Clinical considerations

- Drug can be used in combination with insulin therapy in both type 1 and type 2 DM patients who have failed to achieve desired glucose control.
- Because of significant risk of severe hypoglycemia, prandial insulin dose should be decreased by 50% when starting pramlintide.
- A dose-limiting side effect is nausea, which seems to lessen over time.
- For type 2 DM, start with 60 mcg (10 units) before meals; increase to 120 mcg before meals when no significant nausea has occurred for 3–7 days.
- For type 1 DM, start with 15 mcg (2.5 units) before meals; increase to 30 to 60 mcg before meals when no significant nausea has occurred for 3–7 days.
- Opened vials may be stored at room temperature for 28 days.

A_{1c} reduction

A reduction of 0.5–1.0% is expected.

Cost

The cost per month is about $100–300.

Cautions and contraindications

The medication should *not* be used in patients with

- Severe gastrointestinal disease, including gastroparesis
- Poor adherence with current insulin regimen or self-monitoring of blood glucose
- Recurrent severe hypoglycemia requiring assistance in the past 6 months
- $A_{1c} \geq 9\%$
- Hypoglycemia unawareness

Dosing

Table 13-10 provides further dosing information.

13-3. Nondrug Therapy

Weight loss is recommended for all diabetics who are overweight or obese. Modest weight loss (5%) has been shown to decrease insulin resistance in type 2 diabetes.

Lifestyle changes through diet and exercise should be emphasized. Patient education is an essential component of successful diabetes management.

Medical Nutrition Therapy

Medical nutrition therapy (MNT) should be individualized to achieve treatment goals with consideration of usual dietary habits, metabolic profile, and lifestyle.

Carbohydrate (CHO) should be monitored by exchanges, carbohydrate counting, or experience-based estimation. CHO should be 45–60% of total daily caloric intake. If intensive insulin therapy is used with a premeal bolus dose of insulin, insulin should be adjusted to cover the daily CHO intake. With basal insulin therapy (when the premeal bolus is not used) or oral antidiabetic medications, the CHO intake must be adjusted so that it is consistent with the effects of therapy.

Protein should be 15–20% of total daily caloric intake. Protein intake should be modified if renal function is reduced. Saturated fat should be < 7% of total daily calories. Cholesterol should be < 200 mg/d.

Fiber intake should be encouraged, but there is no reason to recommend a greater amount than that recommended for persons without DM (14 g fiber/1,000 kcal).

Daily alcohol intake should be limited (adult females: one drink or fewer; adult males: two drinks or fewer).

Physical Activity and Exercise

Regular exercise improves blood glucose control, reduces cardiovascular risk factors, and contributes to

Table 13-10. Amylin Mimetics

Drug	Trade name	Strength	Daily dose	Duration of action	Comments
Pramlintide	(Symlin)	0.6 mg/mL–5 mL vial	Type 1 DM: 15–60 mcg tid with meals; type 2 DM: 60–120 mcg tid with meals	4–6 hours	Dosed using an insulin syringe: 30 mcg = 5 units, 60 mcg = 10 units, 120 mcg = 20 units

weight loss. An exercise regimen should be individualized. The patient's preexercise program history and a detailed medical examination are essential.

For most patients, a program of 150 min/week of moderate-intensity aerobic exercise is recommended. The program should be adjusted in the presence of macro- and microvascular complications that may be worsened:

- *Retinopathy:* Vigorous exercise may be contraindicated because of the risk of triggering vitreous hemorrhage or retinal detachment.
- *Peripheral neuropathy:* Non-weight-bearing activities may be best because decreased pain sensation in the extremities increases the risk of skin breakdown and infection.
- *Autonomic neuropathy:* Patients should undergo cardiac investigation before increasing physical activity, which may lead to decreased cardiac responsiveness to exercise, postural hypotension, and so forth.

Blood glucose monitoring may be necessary before and after exercise. Fast-acting oral carbohydrates should be available during and after exercise.

Diabetes Self-Management Education

Diabetes self-management education (DSME) provides a means for persons with DM to become empowered and assist with self-care. Education content includes the disease process; acute and long-term complications; drug and nondrug treatments; monitoring; preventive measures; decision-making skills; specific self-care measures relative to foot, skin, dental, and eye care; goal setting; and psychosocial adjustment.

DSME should be offered in a variety of settings, typically by a multidisciplinary team.

13-4. Key Points

- DM is a group of chronic metabolic diseases exhibiting hyperglycemia resulting from defects in insulin secretion, action, or both.
- Type 1 diabetes results from immune-mediated β-cell destruction, which leads to absolute insulin deficiency.
- Type 2 diabetes is characterized by relative insulin deficiency, insulin resistance, or both.
- See Table 13-11 for a comparison of type 1 and type 2 diabetes.

Table 13-11. Comparison of Type 1 and Type 2 Diabetes Mellitus

	Type 1	Type 2
Previous names	Insulin-dependent diabetes mellitus; juvenile-onset diabetes	Non-insulin-dependent diabetes mellitus; adult-onset diabetes
Percentage of DM cases	5–10	90–95
Age of occurrence	< 30 years (usually childhood or adolescence); at any age following autoimmune stimulus (e.g., virus)	> 30 years; increasing in childhood andadolescence in association with obesity and inactivity
Onset	Rapid	Gradual
Primary etiology	Autoimmune-mediated mechanism with genetic predisposition	Genetic and environmental (e.g., family history, ethnicity, obesity, inactivity)
Pathogenesis	Destruction of β-cells resulting in absolute insulin deficiency and abnormal glucose control	Increasing resistance of tissue (liver and skeletal muscle) to insulin; impaired insulin secretion resulting in relative deficiency of insulin; increased hepatic glucose production
Signs and symptoms	Polyuria, polydipsia, polyphagia, unexplained weight loss, fatigue, blurred vision, possibly ketoacidosis	Polyuria, polydipsia, polyphagia, obesity, fatigue, blurred vision, possibly asymptomatic
Ketoacidosis	Ketosis prone (DKA)	Not ketosis prone because of residual insulin (hyperglycemic hyperosmolar nonketotic syndrome)
Treatment:		
Nondrug therapy	Medical nutrition therapy and physical activity approved by physician	Essential adjunct to oral antidiabetic therapy; may be sufficient as monotherapy to control blood glucose
Drug therapy	Insulin monotherapy *or* rarely oral antidiabetic drugs as adjunct to insulin therapy (if accompanied by insulin resistance)	MNT monotherapy *or* oral antidiabetic drugs *or* oral antidiabetic drugs in combination therapy *or* insulin monotherapy *or* insulin and oral antidiabetic drugs

- The principal treatment goals include maintaining blood glucose levels in the normal or near-normal range and preventing acute and chronic complications.
- Goals of diabetes therapy include achieving and maintaining glycemic control and reaching recommended blood pressure and lipid goals.
- Outcomes of uncontrolled blood glucose include cardiovascular, kidney, eye, and nerve disease.
- Pharmacotherapy treatment of DM should be individualized to each patient considering such factors as glucose control goals; length of time with DM; concomitant diseases; psychosocial issues, including available support for the patient, patient motivation, medication and DM supply costs, and the level of risk for complications secondary to DM control.
- Multiple studies have shown improved glycemic control delays the onset of, slows the progression of, and lowers the risk of long-term microvascular complications.
- Combination therapy of two or more po therapies, po therapies *plus* insulin, or po products *plus* GLP-1 analogs will be required in most patients to maintain continued DM control.
- Metformin
  - Is considered first-line therapy in newly diagnosed type 2 DM
  - Is contraindicated in renal dysfunction patients
  - Has low or minimal risk of hypoglycemia with monotherapy
  - Has GI side effects (flatulence, GI upset, abdominal pain, diarrhea, bloating), which are dose-limiting problems
  - Causes no weight gain
  - May decrease the progression to DM in high-risk patients
- Secretagogues
  - Are helpful in combination with other po agents and injectable products
  - Increase risk of hypoglycemia (sulfonylureas > meglitinides)
  - Increase weight (sulfonylureas > meglitinides)
  - Have high rate of failure over time
  - Must be used with caution in renally impaired and elderly patients
- Thiazolidinediones
  - Help improve peripheral insulin resistance
  - Increase weight and edema
  - Have low or minimal risk of hypoglycemia with monotherapy
  - Are contraindicated in patients with congestive heart failure
  - Have delayed time to see full effects on DM control

- May decrease the progression to DM in high-risk patients
- Alpha-glucosidase inhibitors
  - Block absorption of carbohydrates in the small intestine
  - Have low or minimal risk of hypoglycemia with monotherapy
  - Have GI side effects (flatulence, GI upset, abdominal pain, diarrhea, bloating), which are dose-limiting problems
  - Are more effective for postprandial hyperglycemia
  - Have minimal effect on weight
- GLP-1 and amylin-based medications
  - Include Byetta (GLP-1 analog)
  - Increase insulin production in a glucose-dependent fashion
  - Decrease production of glucagon
  - Improve β-cell functioning
  - Slow gastric emptying
  - Increase satiety and possible weight loss
  - Have a dose-limiting side effect of nausea
  - Are injectable products
  - Are for use in type 2 DM
  - Are high cost
- DPP-IV inhibitor (Januvia)
  - Increases insulin production in a glucose-dependent fashion
  - Decreases production of glucagon
  - Improves β-cell functioning
  - Has no effect on weight
  - Is well tolerated with few side effects
  - Is for use in type 2 DM
  - Is high cost
- Amylin mimetic (Symlin)
  - Decreases production of glucagons
  - Slows gastric emptying
  - Increases satiety and possible weight loss
  - Has significant risk of hypoglycemia in combination with insulin in type 1 DM
  - Has the dose-limiting side effect of nausea
  - Is for use in type 1 and 2 DM
  - Is high cost
- Insulin
  - Is essential for type 1 DM
  - Is often used in type 2 DM in combination with other therapies
  - Should be considered initial agent if glucose is > 250 mg/dL or A_{1c} > 10%
  - Is often started as basal therapy (0.1–0.2 units/kg/d) added to an existing po regimen
  - Should be individualized to the patient's goals and motivation: intensive insulin therapy (> 3 doses/d or use of continuous subcutaneous insulin infusion) is replacing conventional

insulin therapy (split-mix dosing: two-thirds of total daily dose)

- Varies principally by source; appearance; time-activity profiles (onset, peak, and duration); dosing; and route of administration
- May have these adverse events: hypoglycemia, weight gain, and lipodystrophies
- Has the same mechanism of action for all types

- Patient education is essential for the management of DM because it provides a means for persons with this chronic disease to become empowered, cope effectively, and engage in appropriate self-care.
- Recommended lifestyle modifications include weight management, increased physical activity, and smoking cessation.

Patient Profile 1—Institution or Nursing Home Care

Patient Name:	Barbara Evens
Address:	413 Summit Street
Age:	68
Height:	5' 5"
Weight:	190 lb
Sex:	Female
Race:	African American
Allergies:	Penicillin, sulfa drugs

Diagnosis:

Primary 1) Type 2 DM

Secondary 1) Hypertension

2) Asthma

Lab/Diagnostic Tests:

	Date	Test
1)	2/1	LFTs
2)	2/1	Serum K
3)	5/1	LFTs
4)	5/1	Serum K
5)	6/1	A_{1c}
6)	6/1	Serum creatinine
7)	6/1	BUN
8)	6/1	Serum K

Additional Orders:

1) Referral to dietitian for weight reduction diet

2) Low impact exercise 30 mins 3 days per week

Dietary Considerations:

1) Dietary changes per dietitian consult

2) Enteral and parenteral

Pharmacist Notes and Other Patient Information:

	Date	Comment
1)	2/1	Advise patient to continue SMBG and to report any hypoglycemic episodes. Instructed patient to treat hypoglycemia with glucose or lactose products. Instructed patient to take acarbose with first bite of meal. Foot exam negative. Patient reports having 1-2 drinks of bourbon per day.
2)		Informed patient to report any changes in BG.

Medication Orders:

Date	RX No	Physician	Drug & strength	Qty	Sig	Refills
2/1	834924	Jones	Propranolol 20 mg	30	1 PO bid	3
2/1	834925	Jones	Albuterol inhaler	1	1-2 inhalations q4-6h	3
2/1	834926	Jones	Acarbose 25 mg	90	1 tab PO w/meals	2
5/1	834927	Jones	Acarbose 50 mg	90	1 tab PO w/meals	2
6/1	834928	Jones	Prednisone 10 mg	30	1 tab PO daily	0
6/1	834929	Jones	Propranolol 20 mg	30	1 tab PO bid	3
6/1	834930	Jones	Albuterol inhaler	1	1-2 inhalations q4-6h	3
6/1	834931	Jones	ASA 81 mg	30	1 tab PO daily	3

13-5. Questions

Use Patient Profile 1 to answer Questions 1–5.

1. Chlorpropamide would be problematic in this case for which of the following reasons?

    I. Alcohol intake
    II. Sulfa allergy
    III. Asthma
    IV. Hypertension
    V. Drug–drug interaction

    A. I only
    B. III only
    C. I and II only
    D. II, III, and IV
    E. I, II, and V

2. Because of a renal protection mechanism, the drug class of choice for Ms. Even's hypertension is a(n)

    A. β-blocker.
    B. loop diuretic.
    C. thiazide diuretic.
    D. α-adrenergic blocker.
    E. angiotensin-converting enzyme inhibitor.

3. One of the most common adverse drug events caused by Ms. Even's oral antidiabetic agent is

    A. flatulence.
    B. hypoglycemia.
    C. renal failure.
    D. hyperglycemia.
    E. weight gain.

4. Which of the following medications on the medication list in this case can mask the symptoms of hypoglycemia?

    A. Propranolol
    B. Albuterol
    C. Acarbose
    D. Prednisone
    E. Aspirin

5. What change in the following laboratory tests might be observed with the addition of prednisone to Ms. Even's drug regimen?

    A. Increase in LFTs
    B. Decrease in BUN
    C. Decrease in serum creatinine
    D. Increase in serum creatinine
    E. Increase in blood glucose

Use Patient Profile 2 to answer questions 6–10.

6. What is the principal drug-related problem in this patient's medication record?

    A. Insulin therapy not indicated for persons with type 2 DM
    B. Therapeutic duplication of sulfonylurea therapy
    C. Potential decrease of BG because of drug–drug interaction between phenytoin and tolazamide
    D. Potential increase of BG because of drug–drug interaction between glimepiride and itraconazole
    E. Use of an ACE inhibitor for hypertension in type 2 DM

7. All of the following monitoring parameters are necessary for Mr. Right *except*

    A. periodic glycosylated hemoglobin A_{1c}.
    B. SMBG levels.
    C. phenytoin levels.
    D. blood pressure readings.
    E. quarterly serum C-peptide level.

8. Which of the following is an inappropriate treatment for a mild hypoglycemic episode?

    A. ½ cup of diet soda
    B. 6–7 hard candies containing sugar
    C. 3 glucose tablets
    D. ½ cup of regular soda
    E. 5 small sugar cubes

9. Persons on insulin therapy should be advised to rotate their injection sites for which of the following reasons?

    A. It reduces the risk of infection.
    B. It reduces the risk of lipoatrophy.
    C. It reduces the risk of lipohypertrophy.
    D. It reduces the risk of generalized myalgia.
    E. This advice is outdated because of the use of human insulin.

10. Which of the following is the most appropriate treatment for a severe hypoglycemic episode?

    A. ½ cup of diet soda
    B. 3 hard candies containing sugar
    C. 1 glucose tablet
    D. Glucagon injection
    E. 2–3 small sugar cubes

Patient Profile 2—Community

Patient Name:	Tom Right
Address:	20 Blue Ridge Drive
Age:	48
Height:	5' 6"
Weight:	135 lb
Sex:	Male
Race:	Caucasian
Allergies:	NKDA

Diagnosis:

Primary 1) Type 2 DM
2) Epilepsy

Secondary 1) Hypertension
2) Fungal infection under toenails

Pharmacist Notes and Other Patient Information:

	Date	Comment
1)	4/8	Patient should be monitored closely for hypoglycemia. Teach patient signs and symptoms of hypoglycemia and treatment measures.

Medication Orders:

Date	RX No	Physician	Drug & strength	Qty	Sig	Refills
1/6	765321	Smith	Tolazamide 250 mg	90	1 tab PO daily	0
4/8	765323	Smith	Glimepiride 2 mg	90	1 tab PO daily	0
8/6	765324	Smith	Lisinopril 5 mg	90	1 tab PO daily	0
8/6	765325	Thomas	Phenytoin extended	60	300 mg PO daily	0
8/6	765366	Smith	Itraconazole	14	50 mg PO daily	0
8/6	765367	Smith	Regular insulin	Trial	5 units SC before meals	0

11. Commercially available insulin (as of May 2005) may be administered by which of the following routes?

    I. Intravenously
    II. Subcutaneously
    III. Via inhalation
    IV. Transdermally
    V. Sublingually

    A. I only
    B. II only
    C. I and II only
    D. II, III, and IV
    E. I, II, and V

12. Insulin therapy is indicated in all of the following *except*

    A. newly diagnosed type 1 DM.
    B. gestational diabetes mellitus not controlled by diet.
    C. hyperglycemic hyperosmolar nonketotic syndrome (HHNS).
    D. newly diagnosed type 2 DM.
    E. diabetic ketoacidosis (DKA).

13. Insulin dosing is adjusted on the basis of the following parameters:

    I. Liver function test results
    II. Dietary intake
    III. Physical activity and exercise
    IV. Blood glucose levels
    V. Ophthalmic examinations

    A. I only
    B. II only
    C. I and II only
    D. II, III, and IV
    E. I, II, and V

14. Which of the following oral antidiabetic agents is a micronized formulation?

    A. Micronase
    B. Glynase
    C. Glucotrol XL
    D. Amaryl
    E. Orinase

15. Insulin that has been stored in a refrigerator should be allowed to reach room temperature prior to administration to

A. allow for proper mixing.
B. minimize painful injections.
C. prevent frosting or clumping.
D. delay systemic absorption.
E. prevent change in clarity.

16. When mixing rapid- or short-acting insulin with intermediate- or long-acting insulin, which of the following insulins should be drawn up first?

    A. Regular
    B. NPH
    C. Lente
    D. Ultralente
    E. Glargine

17. Uniform dispersion of insulin suspensions can be obtained by

    A. vigorously shaking the vial.
    B. rolling the vial gently between the hands.
    C. warming the vial in a microwave.
    D. packing the vial in dry ice.
    E. keeping the vial at room temperature (68–75°F).

18. Of the following types of insulin, which can be administered intravenously?

    A. Glargine
    B. Lente
    C. Regular
    D. Ultralente
    E. NPH

19. Diabetes mellitus is the leading cause of which of the following complications?

    A. Pancreatitis
    B. Fatty liver
    C. Blindness
    D. Stroke
    E. Deafness

20. Which of the following is an indication that a patient is developing a long-term complication from diabetes mellitus?

    A. Tachycardia
    B. Glucosuria
    C. Leukocytosis
    D. Proteinuria
    E. Tinnitus

21. Which sulfonylurea has been associated with the greatest incidence of prolonged hypoglycemia in the elderly?

    A. Tolazamide
    B. Tolbutamide
    C. Chlorpropamide
    D. Glimepiride
    E. Glipizide

22. Which of the following drugs taken with alcohol is most likely to cause a disulfiram-like reaction?

    A. Chlorpropamide
    B. Acarbose
    C. NPH insulin
    D. Glucagon
    E. Pioglitazone

23. Metformin should be withheld for 48 hours prior to any procedure requiring the use of parenteral iodinated contrast medium because of the potential for this adverse drug event:

    A. Optic neuritis
    B. Metabolic alkalosis
    C. Lactic acidosis
    D. Purple-toe syndrome
    E. Tinnitus

24. The use of insulin in a woman with GDM helps reduce the incidence of which complication in the fetus?

    A. Macrosomia
    B. Cystic fibrosis
    C. Deafness
    D. "Soft bones"
    E. Eczema

25. Metformin would not be an option for a patient with which of the following diagnoses?

    A. Iron deficiency anemia
    B. Impaired renal function
    C. Hypertension
    D. Type 2 DM
    E. Frequent hypoglycemic episodes

26. Nocturnal hypoglycemia resulting in rebound hyperglycemia in type 1 DM is termed

    A. honeymoon period.
    B. Somogyi effect.
    C. dawn phenomenon.
    D. hyperglycemic phase.
    E. insulin resistance syndrome.

27. Which of the following is a potentially fatal adverse drug event of Glucophage?

    A. Weight gain
    B. Frequent urination
    C. Diarrhea
    D. Lactic acidosis
    E. Angioedema

28. All of the following are true of acarbose therapy *except*

    A. it is contraindicated in inflammatory bowel disease.
    B. it should be taken with the first bite of each meal.
    C. it does not cause hypoglycemia or weight gain.
    D. hypoglycemia attributable to combination therapy should be treated with sucrose.
    E. LFTs are given every 3 months during the first year and periodically thereafter (if the dose is > 50 mg tid).

29. Prandin is a nonsulfonylurea secretagogue. Adverse drug events include all of the following *except*

    A. upper respiratory infection.
    B. arthropathy.
    C. hypoglycemia.
    D. back pain.
    E. hyperglycemia.

30. Patient counseling relative to meglitinides should include the following points:

    I. It must be taken 30 minutes before main meals.
    II. If a meal is omitted, do not take.
    III. It enhances preprandial glucose utilization.
    IV. Hyperglycemia is a potential adverse drug event.
    V. Disulfiram-like reaction is possible when ingested with ETOH.

    A. I only
    B. III only
    C. I and II only
    D. II, III, and IV
    E. I, II, and V

31. Which one of the following antidiabetic agents does *not* require liver function tests for monitoring?

    A. Glargine
    B. Miglitol

C. Rosiglitazone
D. Acarbose
E. Metformin

32. Adverse drug events reported for pioglitazone (Actos), a thiazolidinedione, include all of the following *except*

    A. exacerbation of congestive heart failure.
    B. resumption of ovulation.
    C. edema.
    D. upper respiratory infection.
    E. megaloblastic anemia.

33. All of the following drugs have a direct glucogenic effect *except*

    A. thiazide diuretics.
    B. corticosteroids.
    C. nicotinic acid.
    D. sympathomimetics.
    E. acetohexamide.

34. Which of the following is the mechanism of action for the sulfonylureas?

    A. They stimulate pancreatic β-cells to secrete insulin.
    B. They delay carbohydrate metabolism and absorption (owing to inhibition of intestinal and pancreatic enzymes).
    C. They increase hepatic insulin sensitivity and decrease hepatic glucose production.
    D. They increase skeletal muscle and adipose tissue insulin sensitivity and decrease hepatic glucose production.
    E. They decrease blood glucose and assist with blood glucose control by increasing glucose uptake and use by peripheral tissues.

35. All of the following are signs or symptoms of hypoglycemia *except*

    A. tachycardia.
    B. diaphoresis.
    C. shakiness.
    D. polyuria.
    E. pallor.

36. Pramlintide (Symlin)

    A. is a basal insulin.
    B. is an insulin analog.
    C. is an oral insulin.
    D. is an inhaled insulin.
    E. is an injectable synthetic version of the human hormone amylin.

13-6. Answers

1. **E.** Chlorpropamide is contraindicated in persons with a sulfa allergy. Alcohol (ETOH) ingestion with chlorpropamide could lead to a disulfiram-like reaction. Also, acute ingestion of ETOH (especially in the fasting state) includes the risk of severe hypoglycemia. Chlorpropamide and prednisone may produce a drug–drug interaction resulting in hyperglycemia. Items III and IV are nonproblematic in this case in relation to chlorpropamide.

2. **E.** Angiotensin-converting enzyme inhibitors exhibit a renal protective mechanism in people with DM. None of the remaining drugs exhibits such an effect.

3. **A.** The most common adverse drug events for acarbose are flatulence, abdominal pain, and diarrhea. These adverse effects may be decreased by titrating the dose gradually and taking the drug with the first bite of each meal. There may also be an increase in LFTs.

4. **A.** Propranolol (a nonselective β-blocker) can mask the symptoms of hypoglycemia (i.e., tachycardia [palpitations], pallor, shakiness [tremor], paresthesia, hunger, diaphoresis [sweating], dizziness, and blurred vision). None of the remaining drugs listed has this effect.

5. **E.** The increase in LFTs may be due to acarbose, and the increase in serum creatinine may represent the development or progression of nephropathy, a long-term complication of DM. The decrease in the serum creatinine and BUN (blood urea nitrogen) are incorrect answers. Prednisone, a corticosteroid, has a dose-dependent, direct glucogenic and glycosuric effect, and therefore an increase in blood glucose (BG) might be observed.

6. **B.** Although tolazamide and glimepiride are first- and second-generation sulfonylureas, duplication of drug class is inappropriate. These agents are both intermediate acting and therefore might potentiate the adverse drug event of hypoglycemia. Insulin may be indicated in a person with type 2 DM as the disease progresses. The potential drug–drug interaction between phenytoin and tolazamide could result in an increased BG (blood glucose) level, and the potential drug–drug interaction between glimepiride and itraconazole could result in a decreased BG level. An ACE inhibitor for hypertension in type 2 DM is appropriate because this drug is renal protective.

7. **E.** The A_{1c} and self-monitoring of blood glucose (SMBG) tests are essential for monitoring the success of glucose control therapy. The SMBG gives an immediate determination of BG level, and the A_{1c} gives an average reading over the previous 2–3 months (or 120 days, the lifespan of a red blood cell). Phenytoin levels are necessary for monitoring therapeutically appropriate levels, and blood pressure readings are necessary for monitoring the success of antihypertensive therapy. A serum C-peptide might be diagnostic for the determination of functioning β-cells; however, if performed, it is done very infrequently to reduce cost.

8. **A.** One-half cup of diet soda would be inappropriate because a mild hypoglycemic episode requires a fast-acting oral carbohydrate for resolution and diet soda has none. The other options would all be appropriate for resolution of the event.

9. **C.** Lipohypertrophy (a bulging of the injection site) is due to nonrotation of injection sites. The risk of infection may be reduced by using aseptic injecting technique. Lipoatrophy (a pitting of the injection site) may be due to an antigenic response to insulin. The advice regarding rotation of injection site is not outdated.

10. **D.** Glucagon, a pancreatic hormone that is given parenterally, is the most appropriate treatment for a severe hypoglycemic episode (life threatening), because the patient may be unconscious and not able to take a fast-acting carbohydrate by mouth. The other items represent inappropriate treatment for mild to moderate hypoglycemia (the amounts of items B, C, and E are inadequate, and the soda in item A should be regular soda).

11. **C.** Pharmaceutical research has developed inhaled insulin products that are still being tested. At present, the commercially available insulins may be administered only intravenously or subcutaneously. A previously available inhaled insulin product, Exubra, was voluntarily withdrawn from the market by the manufacturer.

12. **D.** Newly diagnosed type 2 DM should first have a trial with MNT and exercise, and if this nondrug therapy fails, oral antidiabetic monotherapy should be added. Combination oral therapy would be indicated next with failure of monotherapy. Then, following the failure of oral therapy, insulin monotherapy or insulin therapy in combination with oral agents is indicated. Insulin is indicated in all the other situations.

13. **D.** Dietary intake, physical activity and exercise, and blood glucose levels are the parameters used

in adjusting insulin dosing (e.g., if the parameters of dietary intake and blood glucose levels are decreased and if physical activity and exercise are increased, the insulin dosing would require reduction to avoid hypoglycemia). Monitoring of these parameters is critical to adjusting the insulin regimen. Items I and V are incorrect.

14. **B.** Glynase is a micronized formulation of glyburide that is significantly absorbed (e.g., a 3 mg tablet provides blood levels similar to a 5 mg conventional tablet). Micronase is a trade name for nonmicronized glyburide. Glucotrol XL is the name of an extended formulation of glipizide. Orinase is the trade name for tolbutamide (the only first-generation sulfonylurea listed here), and Amaryl is the trade name for glimepiride.

15. **B.** Refrigerated insulin is allowed to reach room temperature prior to administration to minimize painful injections. Proper mixing, prevention of frosting or clumping, or maintenance of clarity have nothing to do with reaching room temperature. Systemic absorption would actually be enhanced by increasing to room temperature, not delayed.

16. **A.** Regular or clear insulin is always drawn up first to ensure that all persons mixing insulins will use the same procedure and that no intermediate- or long-acting insulin will be placed in the regular insulin vial, potentially causing contamination and dose variance. Glargine is also a clear insulin; however, it is never to be mixed with other insulins because of the low pH (4.0) of its diluents.

17. **B.** Uniform dispersion of insulin suspensions can be obtained by gently rolling the vial between the hands. Insulin is a fragile molecule, and all the other means listed could cause molecular degradation.

18. **C.** Of these insulins, regular is the only one that can be administered intravenously. Although glargine is clear like regular insulin, its pH is 4.0, and it should never be given intravenously. The remaining insulins are suspensions and also should never be given intravenously.

19. **C.** DM is the leading cause of new cases of blindness among adults 20–74 years of age in the United States. There is also an increased incidence of stroke with DM, but DM is not the leading cause of this problem. The other items are incorrect.

20. **D.** Proteinuria is an indication that a patient is developing the long-term complication of nephropathy. Items A, B, and C could be related to acute complications such as DKA (glucosuria and leukocytosis) and hypoglycemia (tachycardia). Item E is incorrect.

21. **C.** Chlorpropamide has a $t_{1/2}$ of 35 hours and a duration of action of 60 hours; therefore, it has been associated with prolonged hypoglycemia in the elderly (perhaps because of their declining renal function). The other sulfonylureas have reported less hypoglycemia.

22. **A.** Chlorpropamide has had the greatest reporting of this drug interaction relative to the first-generation sulfonylureas. The remaining drugs listed have not had reports of this adverse drug event.

23. **C.** Lactic acidosis can result if metformin (Glucophage) is given in this situation, and it can be potentially fatal. Renal function must be evaluated following such a procedure, and it must be normal before metformin may be resumed. The other items are incorrect.

24. **A.** Macrosomia (abnormally large fetal body size) is one of the fetal complications of concern in GDM. The primary benefit of insulin therapy is reduction in the incidence of macrosomia. The other items are incorrect.

25. **B.** Contraindications for metformin are renal dysfunction for those predisposed to lactic acidosis. Metformin does not cause hypoglycemia, and it is indicated in type 2 DM. Hypertension and iron deficiency anemia are incorrect answers. Metformin may cause megaloblastic anemia.

26. **B.** The Somogyi effect is rebound hyperglycemia or early morning hyperglycemia secondary to nocturnal hypoglycemia. The person with type 1 DM may experience a honeymoon period—a phase of erratic insulin secretion during destruction of β-cells by islet cell antibodies. This short-lived remission lasts months to a year. The dawn phenomenon is fasting hyperglycemia (prebreakfast) caused by decreased plasma insulin during the night or the anti-insulin effect of nocturnal growth hormone. Items D and E are incorrect.

27. **D.** Lactic acidosis is a potentially fatal adverse drug event of Glucophage (metformin). It does not cause weight gain. Modest weight loss is possible, and no hypoglycemia is reported when metformin is used as monotherapy. Diarrhea is an adverse drug event, but with gradual dose titration and administration with food, it decreases over time. Items B and E are incorrect.

28. **D.** Oral glucose instead of carbohydrate sources with sucrose (cane sugar) or fructose is used be-

cause absorption of these is inhibited. The remaining items are true of acarbose therapy.

29. **E.** Prandin may cause hypoglycemia like the sulfonylureas. Hyperglycemia is not one of the adverse drug events reported. Prandin may cause all the other adverse drug events.

30. **C.** Meglitinides should be taken 30 minutes before main meals, and if a meal is omitted, the drug should not be taken. It enhances postprandial glucose utilization; hypoglycemia, not hyperglycemia, may occur; and disulfiram-like reactions are not reported.

31. **A.** The α-glucosidase inhibitors (e.g., acarbose), biguanides (e.g., metformin), and thiazolidinediones (e.g., rosiglitazone) all require LFTs for monitoring. Glargine, a long-acting insulin, does not require LFTs for monitoring; rather it requires blood glucose monitoring.

32. **E.** Megaloblastic anemia is a reported adverse drug effect for metformin, but not for Actos. All the other items listed are reported adverse drug effects. Since troglitazone (Rezulin), a thiazolidinedione, was withdrawn from the market in 2000 because of severe liver toxicity, this adverse drug effect could potentially occur with Actos; therefore, LFTs should be performed periodically.

33. **E.** Acetohexamide has a hypoglycemic effect. All the other drugs listed have a direct glucogenic effect.

34. **A.** The sulfonylureas stimulate pancreatic β-cells to secrete insulin. Item B is the mechanism of action for α-glucosidase inhibitors, item C is the mechanism of action for the biguanide metformin, item D is the mechanism of action for the glitizones, and item E is the mechanism of action for insulin.

35. **D.** Polyuria (excessive urination) is one of the classic signs and symptoms of DM. All of the other answers listed are some of the signs and symptoms of hypoglycemia, which can be life threatening.

36. **E.** Pramlintide (Symlin) was approved in March 2005 as the first new type 1 diabetes treatment in more than 80 years. It is an injectable synthetic version of the human hormone amylin.

13-7. References

American Diabetes Association. Standards of medical care in diabetes—2009. *Diabetes Care.* 2009: 32(suppl 1):S13–61.

Bode BW, ed. *Medical Management of Type 1 Diabetes.* Alexandria, Va. American Diabetes Association; 2008.

Burant CF, ed. *Medical Management of Type 2 Diabetes.* Alexandria, Va. American Diabetes Association; 2008.

Expert Committee on the Diagnosis and Classification of Diabetes Mellitus. Report of the Expert Committee on the Diagnosis and Classification of Diabetes Mellitus. *Diabetes Care.* 1997;20:1183–97.

Expert Committee on the Diagnosis and Classification of Diabetes Mellitus. Follow-up report on the diagnosis of diabetes mellitus. *Diabetes Care.* 2003;26:3160–67.

Funnell MM, Brown TL, Childs BP, et al. National Standards for Diabetes Self-Management Education. *Diabetes Care.* 2007;30:1630–7.

Diabetes Control and Complications Trial Research Group. The effect of intensive treatment on the development and the progress of long-term complications in insulin-dependent diabetes mellitus. *N Engl J Med.* 1993;329:977–86. Available at: http://content.nejm.org/cgi/content/full/329/14/977.

Setter SM, White JR Jr, Campbell RK. Diabetes. In: Helms RA, Quan DJ, Herfindal ET, Gourley DR, eds. *Textbook of Therapeutics.* 8th ed. Philadelphia: Lippincott Williams & Wilkins; 2006:1042–105.

Stoneking K, Farr G. Early use of insulin in type 2 diabetes. *Drug Topics* October 2, 2002. Available at: http://drugtopics.modernmedicine.com/drugtopics/Diabetes/CE--Early-use-of-insulin-in-Type-2-diabetes-mellit/ArticleStandard/Article/detail/117448.

Triplett CL, Reasner CA, Isley WL. Diabetes mellitus. In: Dipiro JT, Talbert RL, Yee GC, et al., eds. *Pharmacotherapy: A Pathophysiologic Approach.* 7th ed. New York: McGraw-Hill; 2008:1205–41.

UK Prospective Diabetes Study (UKPDS) Group. Effect of intensive blood-glucose control with metformin on complications in overweight patients with type 2 diabetes (UKPDS 34). *Lancet.* 1998;352:854–65.

UK Prospective Diabetes Study (UKPDS) Group. Intensive blood-glucose control with sulphonylureas or insulin compared with conventional treatment and risks of complications in patients with type 2 diabetes (UKPDS 33). *Lancet.* 1998;352:837–53.

University Group Diabetes Program. A study of the effects of hypoglycemic agents on vascular complications in patients with adult onset diabetes. *Diabetes.* 1970;19(suppl 2):1–26.

White JR, Campbell RK. Drug/drug and drug/disease interactions and diabetes. *Diabetes Educator.* 1995;21:283–9.

Thyroid, Adrenal, and Miscellaneous Endocrine Drugs

Jeremy Thomas, PharmD, CDE

14

14-1. Thyroid

Hypothyroidism

Disease overview

Definition and epidemiology

- Hypothyroidism is a syndrome resulting from deficient thyroid hormone production that results in a slowing down of all bodily functions.
- Retardation of growth occurs in infants and children.
- Its prevalence is greater in women and increases with age; it affects 1.5% to 2.0% of women and 0.2% of men.

Types

- Most cases are caused by thyroid gland failure (primary hypothyroidism).
- Hashimoto's disease (chronic lymphocytic thyroiditis) is the cause of 90% of primary hypothyroidism.
- Pituitary failure causes secondary hypothyroidism.
- Hypothalamic failure causes tertiary hypothyroidism.
- Iatrogenic hypothyroidism follows exposure to radiation with radioiodine or external radiation.
- Other causes may include thyroidectomy, iodine deficiency, enzymatic defects, iodine, lithium, and interferon-alfa.

Clinical presentation

- Symptoms include cold intolerance, fatigue, somnolence, constipation, menorrhagia, myalgia, and hoarseness.
- Signs include thyroid gland enlargement or atrophy, bradycardia, edema, dry skin, and weight gain.

- Myxedema coma is an end stage of hypothyroidism characterized by weakness, confusion, hypothermia, hypoventilation, hypoglycemia, hyponatremia, coma, and shock.

Pathophysiology

- Thyroxine (T_4) is the major hormone secreted by the thyroid; T_4 is converted to the more potent triiodothyronine (T_3) in tissues.
- Thyroxine secretion is stimulated by thyroid-stimulating hormone (TSH).
- TSH secretion is inhibited by T_4, forming a negative feedback loop.
- Hashimoto's disease is an autoimmune-mediated disease resulting from cell- and antibody-mediated thyroid injury.
- Antimicrosomal antibodies are directed against thyroidal antigens.

Diagnosis

- Plasma TSH assay is the initial test of choice if hypothyroidism is suspected clinically.
- TSH levels are elevated in primary hypothyroidism.
- Low plasma-free T_4 (or T_4 index) confirms the diagnosis of hypothyroidism.

Treatment principles

- Synthetic thyroxine (levothyroxine) is the drug of choice for hypothyroidism because it is chemically stable, inexpensive, and free of antigenicity and because it has uniform potency.
- The typical dose is 100–125 mcg po once daily; the dose is reduced to 50 mcg in the elderly and to 25 mcg in patients with coronary artery disease to decrease the risk of precipitating angina.
- The goal of therapy is to maintain plasma TSH in the normal range.

- Dose changes are made at 6- to 8-week intervals until the TSH is normal.
- Overtreatment is detected by subnormal TSH and is associated with osteoporosis and atrial fibrillation.
- Failure to respond to appropriate doses is most often due to poor compliance.
- Do not use thyroid hormones to facilitate weight loss in euthyroid patients.
- Thyroid hormones have a narrow therapeutic index; careful monitoring of clinical condition and thyroid function is required.

Drug therapy for hypothyroidism

Thyroid preparations for the treatment of hypothyroidism are described in Table 14-1.

Mechanism of action
Thyroid hormones enhance oxygen consumption by most tissues and increase basal metabolic rate and metabolism of carbohydrates, lipids, and proteins.

Patient counseling
- Take once daily, 30 minutes before breakfast, because food may decrease absorption.
- Replacement therapy is usually for life; do not discontinue without advice of the prescriber.
- Notify the prescriber if you experience rapid or irregular heartbeat, chest pain, shortness of breath, nervousness, irritability, tremors, heat intolerance, or weight loss.
- Do not take antacids, calcium, or iron supplements within 4 hours of levothyroxine.

Adverse effects
- *Cardiovascular:* Tachycardia, arrhythmia, angina, myocardial infarction
- *Central nervous system (CNS):* Tremor, headache, nervousness, insomnia, irritability, hyperactivity
- *Gastrointestinal (GI):* Diarrhea, vomiting, cramps
- *Miscellaneous:* Weight loss, fatigue, menstrual irregularities, excessive sweating, heat intolerance, fever, muscle weakness, hair loss, decreased bone mineral density, hypersensitivity

Drug interactions
- Amiodarone may cause hypothyroidism or hyperthyroidism.
- Antacids decrease absorption of levothyroxine. Separate administration by at least 4 hours.
- Antidiabetic agents may be less effective with levothyroxine. An increase in the insulin or oral hypoglycemic dose may be needed.
- Bile acid sequestrants reduce absorption of levothyroxine. Separate administration by at least 4 hours.
- Enzyme-inducing antiepileptic agents increase hepatic degradation of levothyroxine. The thyroxine dosage may need to be increased.
- Estrogens may decrease response to levothyroxine. The levothyroxine dosage may need to be increased.
- Lithium commonly causes hypothyroidism.
- Levothyroxine may enhance warfarin's effect. The warfarin dosage may need to be decreased.
- Levothyroxine supplementation may reduce digoxin levels.
- Sucralfate may decrease levothyroxine absorption. Separate administration by at least 4 hours.

Table 14-1. Thyroid Preparations for the Treatment of Hypothyroidism

Trade name	Generic name	Dosage forms	Usual dosage range
Synthroid, Levothroid, Levoxyl, Unithroid, Thyro-Tabs	Levothyroxine sodium (T_4)	Tablets: 0.025, 0.05, 0.075, 0.088, 0.1, 0.112, 0.125, 0.137, 0.15, 0.175, 0.2, 0.3 mg Injection: 200, 500 mcg	0.1–0.15 mg po qd for hypothyroidism (dosage is individualized); higher doses used in treating thyroid cancer
Armour Thyroid, Nature-Throid, Westhroid	Desiccated thyroid USP	Tablets: 15, 30, 32.4, 60, 64.8, 65, 90, 120, 129.6, 130, 180, 194.4, 195, 240, 300 mg	60–120 mg po qd for hypothyroidism (dosage is individualized); higher doses used in treating thyroid cancer
Cytomel, Triostat	Liothyronine (T_3)	Tablets: 5, 25, 50 mcg Injection: 10 mcg	25 mcg po qd for hypothyroidism
Thyrolar	Liotrix (T_4 and T_3 in a 4:1 ratio)	Tablets: 3.1/12.5 mcg, 6.25/25 mcg, 12.5/50 mcg, 25/100 mcg, 37.5/150 mcg	60–120 mg po qd for hypothyroidism

- Soybean formula decreases levothyroxine absorption.
- Sympathomimetic drugs may potentiate the effects of levothyroxine.
- Levothyroxine may enhance theophylline clearance.

Monitoring parameters

- Plasma TSH should be done every 6–8 weeks until normalization.
- Signs and symptoms of hypothyroidism should improve within a few weeks.
- Once the optimum replacement dose is attained, a physical examination should be made and TSH level should be monitored every 6–12 months.
- Patients at risk for coronary artery disease should be monitored for angina.

Pharmacokinetics

- The U.S. Food and Drug Administration states that all levothyroxine products should be considered therapeutically inequivalent unless equivalence (AB rating) has been established and noted in the "Orange Book."
- Levoxyl, Levothroid, Synthroid, Unithroid, and some generics are bioequivalent.
- Because of the narrow therapeutic index of levothyroxine, many experts recommend rechecking TSH concentrations 6–8 weeks after any change in formulation, even when bioequivalent.
- Oral absorption is improved by fasting but decreased by dietary fiber, drugs, and foods.
- A half-life of 7 days allows once-daily dosing.
- Average bioavailability of levothyroxine products ranges from 40% to 80%. When a switch is made from oral to intravenous levothyroxine, the dosage should be reduced by 25% to 50%.

Other

- Use of natural thyroid hormones such as desiccated thyroid USP is discouraged because their potency and stability are less predictable than synthetic levothyroxine.
- Synthetic T_3 (liothyronine) has a shorter half-life than levothyroxine, has a higher incidence of cardiac side effects, and is more difficult to monitor.

Hyperthyroidism

Disease overview

Definition and epidemiology

- Hyperthyroidism (thyrotoxicosis) is the clinical syndrome that results when tissues are exposed to high levels of thyroid hormone.
- Thyrotoxicosis is more common in women than men, occurring in 3 per 1,000 women.

Types

- Graves' disease is the most common cause of hyperthyroidism.
- Toxic multinodular goiter (MNG), toxic adenoma, and exogenous thyroid hormone ingestion may also cause hyperthyroidism.
- Thyroid storm is a life-threatening, sudden exacerbation of all the symptoms of thyrotoxicosis, characterized by fever, tachycardia, delirium, and coma.
- Hyperthyroidism may be caused by drugs such as amiodarone and iodine.

Clinical presentation

- Symptoms include heat intolerance, weight loss, weakness, palpitations, and anxiety.
- Signs include tremor, tachycardia, weakness and eyelid lag, and warm, moist skin.
- Other manifestations include atrial fibrillation and congestive heart failure.

Pathophysiology

- Graves' disease is an autoimmune disease in which thyroid-stimulating antibodies are produced. These antibodies mimic the action of TSH on thyroid tissue.
- Toxic adenomas and MNGs are masses of thyroid tissue that secrete thyroid hormones independent of pituitary control.

Diagnosis

Elevated T_4 or T_3 in the presence of a decreased TSH confirms the diagnosis of hyperthyroidism.

Treatment principles

- There are three primary methods for controlling hyperthyroidism: surgery, radioactive iodine (RAI), and antithyroid (thioamide) drugs.
- The goal is to minimize symptoms and eliminate excess thyroid hormone.
- RAI is often considered the treatment of choice in Graves' disease, toxic adenomas, and MNGs.
- Propylthiouracil is preferred in pregnancy; RAI is contraindicated.
- Thioamide drugs (propylthiouracil and methimazole) have no permanent effect on thyroid function.
- Adjunctive treatments for hyperthyroidism include β-adrenergic receptor blockers or calcium channel blockers to control tachycardia associated with hyperthyroidism.

Drug therapy of hyperthyroidism

Antithyroid medications are summarized in Table 14-2.

Thioamides
Mechanism of action
- Propylthiouracil and methimazole inhibit the synthesis of thyroid hormones by preventing the incorporation of iodine into iodotyrosines and by inhibiting the coupling of monoiodotyrosine and diiodotyrosine to form T_4 and T_3.
- Propylthiouracil inhibits the peripheral conversion of T_4 to T_3.

Patient counseling
- This medication prevents excessive thyroid hormone production.
- It must be taken regularly to be effective.
- Do not discontinue use without first consulting your physician.
- Notify your physician if fever, sore throat, unusual bleeding, rash, abdominal pain, or yellowing of the skin occurs.

Adverse effects
- *CNS:* Fever, headache, paresthesias
- *General:* Rash, arthralgia, urticaria
- *GI:* Jaundice, hepatitis
- *Hematologic:* Agranulocytosis, leukopenia, bleeding

Drug interactions
Potentiation of warfarin's effect may occur.

Monitoring parameters
- Monitor for improvement in signs and symptoms of hyperthyroidism.
- Perform thyroid function tests; watch for signs and symptoms of agranulocytosis (fever, malaise, sore throat).

Pharmacokinetics
Propylthiouracil has a short half-life, requiring more frequent dosing than methimazole.

Iodides
Mechanism of action
- Medication blocks hormone release and inhibits thyroid hormone synthesis.
- Medication may be used when rapid reduction in thyroid hormone secretion is desired, such as in thyroid storm, or to decrease glandular vascularity prior to thyroidectomy.

Patient instructions
- Dilute with water or fruit juice to improve taste.
- Notify physician if fever, skin rash, metallic taste, swelling of the throat, or burning of the mouth occurs.

Adverse effects
Adverse effects include rash, swelling of salivary glands, metallic taste, burning of the mouth, GI distress, hypersensitivity, and goiter.

Drug interactions
Lithium potentiates antithyroid effect of iodides.

Monitoring parameters
Monitor for improvement in signs and symptoms of hyperthyroidism and for adverse effects.

14-2. Adrenals

Cushing's Syndrome
Disease overview

Definition and epidemiology
- Cushing's syndrome results from chronic glucocorticoid excess.

Table 14-2. Antithyroid Medications

Drug name	Drug contains	Dosage forms	Usual dosage range
PTU	Propylthiouracil	Tablets: 50 mg	150–300 mg po daily at 8-hour intervals
Tapazole	Methimazole	Tablets: 5, 10 mg	5–40 mg po in single daily dose or divided
Lugol's solution	Strong iodine solution	Solution: 5% iodine and 10% potassium iodide; delivers 6.3 mg iodine per drop	0.1–0.3 mL (3–5 drops) po tid
SSKI	Saturated solution of potassium iodide	Solution: 1 g/mL; delivers 38 mg iodine per drop of saturated solution	1–5 drops po tid in water or juice

- The incidence rate is 2–4 persons per million population cases each year.

Types
- Cushing's syndrome is usually iatrogenic, caused by therapy with glucocorticoid drugs.
- Endogenous Cushing's syndrome is usually caused by overproduction of adrenocorticotropic hormone (ACTH) by pituitary gland adenomas (Cushing's disease).

Clinical presentation
Patients may present with obesity involving the face, neck, trunk, and abdomen; hypertension; hirsutism; acne; amenorrhea; depression; thin skin; easy bruising; diabetes; and osteopenia.

Pathophysiology
The hypothalamus produces corticotropin-releasing hormone, which stimulates the anterior pituitary gland to release ACTH. Circulating ACTH stimulates the adrenal cortex to produce cortisol.

Diagnosis
- Diagnosis is usually based on signs and symptoms of hypercortisolism.
- Dexamethasone suppression test or 24-hour urine cortisol measurement may be used.

Treatment principles
- If the syndrome is iatrogenic, minimization of corticosteroid exposure is essential.
- Pharmacotherapy of Cushing's syndrome is aimed at reducing cortisol production or activity with drugs, radiation, or surgery.

Drug therapy of Cushing's syndrome

Drugs for Cushing's syndrome are described in Table 14-3.

Mechanism of action
- Drugs used to treat Cushing's disease suppress synthesis of cortisol.

- Ketoconazole inhibits cytochrome P-450 (CYP450)-dependent enzymes and cortisol synthesis.
- Aminoglutethimide inhibits conversion of cholesterol to pregnenolone.
- Mitotane is a cytotoxic drug that suppresses ACTH secretion and reduces synthesis of cortisol.
- Metyrapone decreases cortisol synthesis by inhibition of 11-hydroxylase activity.

Patient counseling
Ketoconazole should be taken with food. Separate from antacids by at least 2 hours. Notify the physician if abdominal pain, yellow skin, or pale stool occurs.

Adverse effects
- Ketoconazole causes nausea, vomiting, headache, impotence, and hepatotoxicity.
- Aminoglutethimide causes drowsiness, rash, weakness, hypotension, nausea, loss of appetite, hypothyroidism, and blood dyscrasias.
- Metyrapone causes nausea, vomiting, dizziness, and sedation.
- Mitotane may cause nausea, vomiting, diarrhea, and tiredness.

Drug interactions
- Ketoconazole is a CYP450 3A4 enzyme inhibitor and may increase serum concentrations of cyclosporine, warfarin, cisapride, and triazolam. Drugs that lower gastric acidity will decrease ketoconazole absorption. Rifampin decreases ketoconazole levels.
- Aminoglutethimide may induce metabolism of warfarin.

Monitoring parameters
Cortisol monitoring is required with mitotane.

Adrenal Insufficiency
Disease overview

Definition and epidemiology
- Primary adrenocortical deficiency (Addison's disease) is caused by autoimmune-mediated

Table 14-3. Drugs for Cushing's Syndrome

Trade name	Generic name	Dosage forms	Usual dosage range
Nizoral	Ketoconazole	Tablets: 250 mg	800–1,200 mg po qd
Cytadren	Aminoglutethimide	Tablets: 250 mg	250 mg po q6h
Lysodren	Mitotane	Tablets: 500 mg	9–10 g/d po in divided doses
Metopirone	Metyrapone	Capsules: 250 mg	1–6 g/d po in 4–6 divided doses

destruction of the adrenal cortex and results in glucocorticoid and mineralocorticoid deficiency.

- Addison's disease occurs in 5–6 persons per million population per year.

Types

- Primary adrenal insufficiency (Addison's disease) involves autoimmune destruction of the adrenal cortex.
- Secondary insufficiency occurs after cessation of chronic exogenous corticosteroid use.
- Acute adrenal insufficiency, or Addisonian crisis, is an endocrine emergency precipitated by severe stress.

Clinical presentation

- Glucocorticoid deficiency (weight loss, malaise, abdominal pain, and depression)
- Mineralocorticoid deficiency (dehydration, hypotension, hyperkalemia, and salt craving)

Pathophysiology

- Cortisol is synthesized in the adrenal cortex when cholesterol is converted to pregnenolone by ACTH.
- The adrenal cortex secretes aldosterone, cortisol, and androgenic hormones.
- Mineralocorticoids (e.g., aldosterone) enhance reabsorption of sodium and water from the distal tubule of the kidney and increase urinary potassium excretion.
- Glucocorticoids affect glucose, carbohydrate, and fat metabolism; produce anti-inflammatory and immunosuppressive effects; and affect other physiologic processes.
- Chronic administration of corticosteroids produces inhibition of pituitary ACTH secretion and reduced cortisol production (hypothalamic-pituitary-adrenocortical [HPA] axis suppression).
- Abrupt cessation of steroids may precipitate adrenal insufficiency.

Diagnosis

A cosyntropin (ACTH) stimulation test may be used to assess hypocortisolism.

Treatment principles

- Addison's disease requires lifelong glucocorticoid and mineralocorticoid replacement.
- Hydrocortisone 100 mg intravenous (IV) q8h is the drug of choice for acute adrenal crisis.
- "Stress doses" of corticosteroids are given for minor illness, injury, or surgery. If stress is severe, hydrocortisone 100 mg IV q8h is used.

- Gradual tapering of corticosteroids reduces the risk of adrenal insufficiency in patients with HPA axis suppression.
- Nonadrenal uses for corticosteroids are numerous, including allergic reactions; inflammatory conditions; hematologic disorders; rheumatic disorders; neurologic diseases; cancer; immunosuppression; pulmonary, renal, skin and thyroid diseases; and hypercalcemia.
- Fludrocortisone has minimal anti-inflammatory activity and is used only when mineralocorticoid activity is needed, such as when increased blood pressure is desired.

Drug therapy of adrenal insufficiency

Information about corticosteroids is provided in Table 14-4.

Mechanism of action

- Glucocorticoids increase blood glucose by stimulating gluconeogenesis and glycogenolysis; fat deposition is increased.
- Catabolic effects occur in lymphoid, connective tissue, bone, muscle, fat, and skin.
- Inhibition of inflammation and immunosuppression, vasoconstriction, reduction in prostaglandin and leukotriene synthesis, decreased neutrophils at sites of inflammation, and inhibition of macrophage function result.

Patient counseling

- These drugs may cause stomach upset, so take them with food.
- It is preferable to take the dose before 9:00 am.
- Wear or carry identification if on chronic steroid therapy.
- Therapy may mask signs of infection.
- Drugs may increase insulin or oral hypoglycemic requirements if patient is diabetic.
- Notify the physician if weight gain, muscle weakness, sore throat, or infection occurs.
- Report tiredness, stomach pain, weakness, and high or low blood sugar to the physician.
- Do not discontinue abruptly if taking long term.

Adverse effects

- *Cardiac:* Hypertension, sodium and fluid retention, atherosclerosis
- *CNS:* Insomnia, anxiety, depression, psychosis
- *Metabolic:* Obesity, hyperglycemia, hypokalemia, amenorrhea, impotence
- *Ophthalmic:* Cataracts, glaucoma

Table 14-4. Corticosteroids and Dose Equivalents

Trade name	Generic name	Anti-inflammatory potency	Sodium-retaining potency	Equivalent dose (mg)	Half-life
Cortone	Cortisone	0.8	2	25	Short
Cortef, Hydrocortone, Solu-Cortef	Hydrocortisone	1.0	2	20	Short
Deltasone, Liquid Pred	Prednisone	4.0	1	5	Medium
Prelone, Pediapred, Delta-Cortef	Prednisolone	4.0	1	5	Medium
Medrol, Solu-Medrol, Depo-Medrol, A-Methapred	Methylprednisolone	5.0	0	4	Medium
Aristocort, Kenacort, Kenalog	Triamcinolone	5.0	0	4	Medium
Decadron, Dexameth, Dexone, Hexadrol	Dexamethasone	30.0	0	0.75	Long
Celestone	Betamethasone	25.0	0	0.75	Long
Florinef	Fludrocortisone	15.0	150	2	Medium

- *Immune:* Infections, impaired wound healing, leukocytosis
- *Musculoskeletal:* Myopathy, osteoporosis

Drug interactions
- Rifampin and other enzyme-inducing drugs increase metabolism of corticosteroids and decrease their effectiveness.
- Concomitant use of nonsteroidal anti-inflammatory drugs (NSAIDs) and corticosteroids increases risk of peptic ulcer disease.
- Corticosteroids may impair immunologic response to vaccines.
- Estrogens may increase corticosteroid clearance.
- Ketoconazole, macrolides, and other CYP450 3A4 enzyme-inhibiting drugs may decrease clearance of corticosteroids.
- Corticosteroids increase insulin and oral hypoglycemic drug requirements.

Monitoring parameters
Patients should be monitored for weight gain, edema, increased blood pressure, electrolytes, blood glucose, and infection.

Pharmacokinetics
Many dosage forms, doses, and schedules are used, including tablets, topicals, enemas, oral liquids, injections, and depot injection forms for intra-articular or intramuscular use.

14-3. Miscellaneous Endocrine Drugs

ACTH and Cosyntropin

Table 14-5 provides information about ACTH and cosyntropin.

Table 14-5. ACTH and Cosyntropin

Trade name	Generic name	Dosage forms	Usual dosage range
Cortrosyn	Cosyntropin	Injection: 0.25 mg	0.25–0.75 mg for testing
Acthar (ACTH)	Corticotropin	Injection: 25, 40 units	10–25 units for testing
H.P. Acthar Gel		Repository injection: 40, 80 units/mL	40–80 units of repository injection every 1–3 days

Therapeutic uses

ACTH and cosyntropin are used for diagnosis of adrenal insufficiency. Occasionally, ACTH is used as an alternative to corticosteroids.

Mechanism of action

- ACTH stimulates the adrenal cortex to secrete adrenal hormones.
- If ACTH fails to elicit an appropriate cortisol response, adrenal insufficiency is present.
- Cosyntropin is a synthetic peptide that is similar to human ACTH, but less allergenic.

Patient counseling and adverse effects

Patients should receive the same counseling as for corticosteroids. Adverse effects are the same.

Drug interactions

Enzyme-inducing drugs will decrease effects.

Monitoring parameters

Monitoring parameters are the same as for corticosteroids.

Vasopressin and Desmopressin

Table 14-6 describes the dosages for vasopressin and desmopressin.

Therapeutic uses

- *Vasopressin:* Diabetes insipidus, variceal hemorrhage, shock, ventricular fibrillation
- *Desmopressin:* Nocturnal enuresis, diabetes insipidus, hemophilia A, von Willebrand's disease

Mechanism of action

- Vasopressin is also known as antidiuretic hormone (ADH); it increases water resorption.
- Vasopressin causes vasoconstriction in portal and splanchnic vessels (GI tract).
- Desmopressin is a synthetic derivative of vasopressin with ADH activity and only minimal vasoconstrictive properties; it increases clotting factor VIII levels.

Patient counseling

For intranasal desmopressin, the patient should be instructed on proper intranasal use. The following instructions should also be given:

- Discard the bottle after 25 or 50 doses.
- Do not transfer the solution to another bottle.
- The drug may cause nasal irritation.
- Notify the physician if bleeding is not controlled or if headache, shortness of breath, or severe abdominal cramps occur.

Adverse effects

- *Vasopressin:* Angina, myocardial infarction, vasoconstriction, hyponatremia, gangrene, abdominal cramps, tissue necrosis if extravasation occurs, hypersensitivity
- *Desmopressin:* Abdominal pain, headache, flushing, nausea, nasal irritation, vulvar pain, nosebleed, rhinitis, hypersensitivity

Drug interactions

- Drugs may enhance effects of other pressors.
- Carbamazepine and chlorpropamide potentiate the effect of desmopressin on ADH.

Table 14-6. Vasopressin and Desmopressin

Trade name	Generic name	Dosage forms	Usual dosage range
Pitressin	Vasopressin	Injection: 20 units/mL	10–20 units intramuscular, subcutaneous, or IV daily at 3- to 4-hour intervals or as a continuous infusion
Stimate (DDAVP)	Desmopressin	Tablets: 0.1, 0.2 mg	Nocturnal enuresis: 0.2–0.6 mg po qhs
		Nasal solution: 0.1 mg/mL, 1.5 mg/mL	Diabetes insipidus: 0.1–0.2 mg po bid, 0.1–0.4 mL intranasally in single or divided doses
		Injection: 4 mcg/mL	

Monitoring parameters

- With diabetes insipidus, monitor urine volume and plasma osmolality.
- With von Willebrand's disease, monitor factor VIII levels and bleeding time.
- When intravenous vasopressin is used, monitor blood pressure and pulses.

Androgens and Anabolic Steroids

Table 14-7 provides information about androgens and anabolic steroids.

Therapeutic uses

- Androgens and anabolic steroids are used to treat hypogonadism, delayed puberty, metastatic breast cancer, anemia, AIDS wasting in HIV-infected men, corticosteroid-induced hypogonadism and osteoporosis, and moderate to severe vasomotor symptoms associated with menopause (when combined with estrogen).
- They are schedule C-III controlled substances because they are intentionally misused for performance-enhancing effects and enhanced muscular development and endurance.

Mechanism of action

- Androgens promote growth and development of male sex organs and maintenance of secondary sex characteristics.
- Androgens also cause retention of nitrogen, sodium, potassium, and phosphorus; increase protein anabolism; and decrease protein catabolism.
- Androgens are responsible for the growth spurt of adolescence and termination of linear growth by fusion of epiphyseal growth centers.
- Exogenous androgens stimulate production of red blood cells and suppress endogenous testosterone release through feedback inhibition of luteinizing hormone and suppress spermatogenesis through feedback inhibition of follicle-stimulating hormone.

Patient counseling

- Medication may cause stomach upset.
- Notify a physician if swelling of the ankles or persistent erections occur.

Table 14-7. Androgens and Anabolic Steroids

Trade name	Generic name	Dosage forms	Usual dosage range
Testoderm Androderm	Testosterone transdermal system	Patch: 2.5, 4, 5, 6 mg/24 h	Patch: 2.5–6 mg for 24 h
AndroGel 1%, Testim	Testosterone	1% gel	5 grams applied once daily
Depo-Testosterone	Testosterone cypionate (in oil)	Injection in oil: 100 mg/mL, 200 mg/mL	50–400 mg every 2–4 weeks
Delatestryl	Testosterone enanthate (in oil)	Injection in oil: 100 mg/mL, 200 mg/mL	50–400 mg every 2–4 weeks
Testopel	Testosterone	Pellet for subcutaneous implantation: 75 mg	150–450 mg every 3–6 months
Striant	Testosterone	Buccal tablet: 30 mg	30 mg every 12 h
Methitest Testred, Android	Methyltestosterone	Tablets: 10, 25 mg Capsules: 10 mg	10–50 mg once daily
Halotestin, Androxy	Fluoxymesterone	Tablets: 2, 5, 10 mg	5–10 mg once daily
Anadrol-50	Oxymetholone	Tablets: 50 mg	50–100 mg once daily
Winstrol	Stanozolol	Tablets: 2 mg	2 mg qd tid
Oxandrin	Oxandrolone	Tablets: 2.5, 10 mg	2.5–10 mg qd
Deca-Durabolin	Nandrolone decanoate	Injection: 100, 200 mg/mL (in oil)	100–200 mg once weekly

- This product is a controlled substance; do not misuse or abuse it.
- For females, notify physician if deepening of the voice, increased facial hair, or menstrual irregularities occur.
- Patients receiving transdermal testosterone should be provided with the manufacturer's patient instructions and carefully counseled on use and disposal of the system.

Adverse effects

- *General:* Jaundice, hepatitis, edema, high abuse potential in an effort to enhance athletic performance, hypercholesterolemia and atherosclerosis, increased aggression and libido
- *Women:* Hirsutism, voice deepening, acne, decreased menses, clitoral enlargement
- *Men:* Acne, sleep apnea, gynecomastia, azoospermia, prostate enlargement, decreased testicular size

14-4. Key Points

- Levothyroxine is the drug of choice for hypothyroidism.

- Lower doses of levothyroxine are used in elderly and cardiac patients.
- Overtreatment with thyroid hormones causes osteoporosis and atrial fibrillation.
- Antacids, bile acid sequestrants, sucralfate, calcium, and iron supplements decrease absorption of levothyroxine and must be separated by at least 4 hours.
- Propylthiouracil and methimazole are thioamide derivatives used to treat hyperthyroidism.
- Thioamides may cause life-threatening agranulocytosis or hepatitis, so patients must report to their physician if they experience fever, sore throat, abdominal pain, or jaundice.
- Drugs used to treat Cushing's disease inhibit synthesis of cortisol.
- Corticosteroid should be used at the lowest dose for the shortest time to reduce the risk of HPA axis suppression and adrenal insufficiency.
- Patients with adrenal insufficiency must receive supplemental corticosteroids in times of physiologic stress.
- Vasopressin and desmopressin are antidiuretic hormones.
- Androgens and anabolic steroids are abused by athletes seeking to enhance performance.

Patient Profile 1—Corn State Community Pharmacy

Patient name: Jasmine Ricardo

Age: 78

Sex: Female

Race: Hispanic

Diagnosis:

Primary	1. Hypercholesterolemia
	2. Anemia
	3. Coronary artery disease
Secondary	1. Hypertension

Address: 189 Jonesborough Road

Height: 48 inches

Weight: 103 lbs

Allergies: Cats

Pharmacist notes

Date	Comment
2/23	Patient reminded to continue taking aspirin 325 mg for CAD
2/23	Patient to take OTC ferrous sulfate 325 mg daily for 3 months for anemia. Advised patient to begin docusate 100 mg qd if constipation occurs.

Medication orders:

Date	Rx no.	Physician	Drug and strength	Quantity	Sig	Refills
3/21	89995	Stubie	Synthroid 0.025 mg	30	1 po qd	0
2/23	88768	Hooper	Zocor 40 mg	30	1 po qhs	5
2/23	88769	Hooper	Questran 4 g	60	1 packet bid, mix with juice	5
2/23	88770	Hooper	Tenormin 50 mg	30	1 po qd	5
2/23	88771	Hooper	Enalapril 5 mg	60	1 po bid	5

14-5. Questions

Use Patient Profile 1 to answer questions 1 and 2.

1. The Synthroid prescription dispensed to Mrs. Ricardo on 3/21 requires advising her to

    A. take 4 hours before or 4 hours after Questran.
    B. take with food.
    C. watch for signs of infection.
    D. take as needed to keep her desired level of energy.
    E. discontinue if she experiences nausea.

2. Which of the following of Mrs. Ricardo's conditions could the Synthroid exacerbate?

    A. Hypercholesterolemia
    B. Anemia
    C. Coronary artery disease
    D. Hypertension
    E. Constipation

3. Excessive doses of levothyroxine may cause

    A. weight gain.
    B. osteoporosis.
    C. cold intolerance.
    D. bradycardia.
    E. sedation.

4. Which of the following drugs may produce hypothyroidism?

    I.   Amitriptyline
    II. Lithium
    III. Amiodarone

    A. I only
    B. III only
    C. I and II only
    D. II and III only
    E. I, II, and III

5. All of the following may decrease the effect of thyroid hormone supplementation *except*

    A. antacids.
    B. bile acid sequestrants.
    C. estrogens.
    D. sucralfate.
    E. theophylline.

6. A patient who is suffering from heat intolerance, weight loss, tachycardia, tremor, and anxiety may be treated with

    A. acetaminophen.
    B. mitotane.
    C. cyproheptadine.
    D. propylthiouracil.
    E. diazepam.

7. A patient with atrial fibrillation may require a decreased warfarin dosage when which of the following drugs is initiated?

    A. Liothyronine
    B. Rifampin
    C. Methimazole
    D. Phenytoin
    E. Diphenhydramine

8. Which of the following drugs is used to treat Cushing's disease?

    I.   Ketoconazole
    II. Aminoglutethimide
    III. Mitotane

    A. I only
    B. III only
    C. I and II only
    D. II and III only
    E. I, II, and III

9. Which of the following drugs works by decreasing cortisol synthesis?

    A. Cortrosyn
    B. ACTH
    C. Oxandrolone
    D. Prednisone
    E. Metyrapone

10. Decreased ketoconazole absorption may occur if it is administered concomitantly with which of the following?

    A. Antacids
    B. Food
    C. Warfarin
    D. Cyclosporine
    E. CYP450 3A4 inhibitors

11. Close monitoring of adrenal hormone secretion may be required when administering which of the following?

    A. Methyltestosterone
    B. Mitotane
    C. Desmopressin
    D. Iodides
    E. Propylthiouracil

12. Which of the following is used to treat adrenal crisis?

    A. Cosyntropin
    B. Aminoglutethimide
    C. Fluoxymesterone
    D. Vasopressin
    E. Hydrocortisone

13. Which of the following is *not* an effect of glucocorticoids?

    A. Immunosuppression
    B. Decreased prostaglandin synthesis
    C. Inhibition of glycogenolysis
    D. Decreased neutrophils at sites of infection
    E. Inhibition of macrophages

Patient Profile 2—Big Sky Hospital

Patient name: Stuart Big

Address: 440 Mountain Lane

Age: 28

Sex: Male

Race: White

Date of admission: 4/21 at 15:26

Height: 5'8"

Weight: 178 lbs

Allergies: Aspirin

Diagnosis:

Admit diagnosis	1. Anaphylactic reaction to aspirin
Secondary	1. Type 2 diabetes mellitus
	2. Hypertension

Laboratory:

Date	Time	Lab	Result	(Normal range)
4/21	15:29	Glucose	144	(60–110 mg/dL)
4/21	19:20	Glucose	181	(60–110 mg/dL)
4/22	06:00	Glucose	240	(60–110 mg/dL)
4/22	12:21	Glucose	289	(60–110 mg/dL)
4/22	19:15	Glucose	352	(60–110 mg/dL)
4/23	06:20	Glucose	391	(60–110 mg/dL)
4/23	12:32	Glucose	443	(60–110 mg/dL)

Active medication orders:

Date	Time	Name and strength	Route	Frequency or schedule
4/21	15:30	Solu-Medrol 125 mg	IV	q6h
4/21	15:30	Dextrose 5%/NaCl 0.9%	IV	200 mL/h
4/21	15:30	Diphenhydramine 50 mg	IV	q6h
4/21	17:03	Glipizide 5 mg	po	bid
4/21	17:03	Glucophage 850 mg	po	bid
4/21	17:03	Captopril 50 mg	po	tid

Discontinued medication orders:

Date	Time	Name and strength	Route	Frequency or schedule
4/21	15:30	Epinephrine 0.1 mg	Subcutaneous	Stat
4/21	15:30	Diphenhydramine 50 mg	IV	Stat

Dietary:

Date	
4/21	1,800 kcal American Diabetes Association diet

Use Patient Profile 2 to answer questions 14 and 15.

14. Which of the following is *least* likely to contribute to the increased blood glucose seen in this patient?

    A. Dextrose 5%/NaCl 0.9% solution
    B. Captopril
    C. Epinephrine
    D. Methylprednisolone
    E. Anaphylaxis

15. Mr. Big is discharged on a new prescription for Deltasone 40 mg qd for 7 days. He should be instructed to

    A. check feet closely for wounds.
    B. take ibuprofen for musculoskeletal pain.
    C. take on an empty stomach.
    D. take at bedtime.
    E. wear identification for steroid therapy.

16. Chronic administration of glucocorticoids predisposes patients to which of the following?

    A. Arthritis
    B. Obesity
    C. Alzheimer's disease
    D. Osteoporosis
    E. Hepatitis

17. A patient is taking prednisone 40 mg daily for 6 months. On abrupt cessation, which of the following may occur?

    A. Myopathy
    B. Diabetes
    C. Infection
    D. Adrenal crisis
    E. Psychosis

18. An increased risk of peptic ulcer disease occurs when NSAIDs are combined with which of the following?

    A. Ranitidine
    B. Ferrous sulfate
    C. Dexamethasone
    D. Carbamazepine
    E. Acetaminophen

19. Which of the following drugs may be used to diagnose adrenal insufficiency?

    A. Desmopressin
    B. Clemastine

C. Captopril
D. Cosyntropin
E. Aminoglutethimide

20. Decreased urine production is an effect of

    A. carmustine.
    B. propylthiouracil.
    C. ACTH.
    D. desmopressin.
    E. SSKI.

21. Which of the following hormones is secreted by the pituitary gland?

    A. Adrenocorticotropic hormone
    B. Testosterone
    C. Cortisol
    D. Thyroxine
    E. Corticotropin-releasing hormone

22. Chronic administration of Winstrol may produce all of the following complications *except*

    A. prostate enlargement.
    B. increased testicular size.
    C. gynecomastia in men.
    D. accelerated atherosclerosis.
    E. decreased menses in women.

23. Androderm is administered

    A. once daily.
    B. three times per week.
    C. once weekly.
    D. every 2 weeks.
    E. monthly.

24. Which of the following is *not* an acceptable indication for testosterone?

    A. Anemia
    B. Hypogonadism
    C. Delayed puberty
    D. Body building
    E. Metastatic breast cancer

14-6. Answers

1. **A.** Bile acid sequestrants reduce levothyroxine absorption and must be separated from levothyroxine administration by at least 4 hours. Levothyroxine should be administered before a meal on an empty stomach to maximize absorption.

2. **C.** Thyroid hormones enhance oxygen consumption and increase the oxygen demand. Mrs. Ricardo has a past medical history of coronary artery disease (CAD) and is elderly. Thyroid supplementation would actually lower her cholesterol in the long run but may precipitate angina acutely.

3. **B.** Levothyroxine decreases bone mineral density and when given in supratherapeutic doses may cause osteoporosis. For this reason, the lowest possible replacement dose should be administered.

4. **D.** Lithium and amiodarone have both been associated with hypothyroidism. Amiodarone contains iodine and may cause hypo- or hyperthyroidism.

5. **E.** Numerous drugs are known to decrease thyroid hormone absorption, including antacids that contain divalent and trivalent cations, calcium salts, magnesium, sucralfate, and bile-acid sequestrants. Estrogens and enzyme-inducing drugs may decrease circulating thyroid hormone levels and necessitate a dose increase of thyroxine.

6. **D.** Heat intolerance, weight loss, tachycardia, tremor, and anxiety are cardinal features of hyperthyroidism. Propylthiouracil is effective at reducing the excessive thyroxine level.

7. **A.** Liothyronine (Cytomel) is T_3, a potent thyroid hormone. In states of hypothyroidism, metabolism is decreased. However, if thyroid hormone is supplemented, blood clotting factors will be metabolized more quickly, leading to decreased warfarin requirements.

8. **E.** Ketoconazole, aminoglutethimide, and mitotane are all used to treat Cushing's disease. Ketoconazole is most commonly known as an antifungal agent, but it inhibits cortisol synthesis at high doses (800–1,200 mg daily).

9. **E.** Metyrapone (Metopirone) inhibits 11 hydroxylase activity and thus decreases cortisol synthesis.

10. **A.** Ketoconazole requires the presence of stomach acid to be absorbed. Any drug that decreases gastric acidity will decrease the extent of ketoconazole absorption. Food increases ketoconazole absorption because food stimulates release of gastric acid.

11. **B.** Mitotane is cytotoxic to adrenal cells and thus reduces cortisol synthesis and release. ACTH increases cortisol release. Close monitoring of cortisol levels is important when this drug is used.

12. **E.** Hydrocortisone is the drug of choice for adrenal crisis because it possesses both mineralocorticoid and glucocorticoid properties. Although cosyntropin increases cortisol release, patients with adrenal crisis may not have enough adrenal reserve to meet their increased demand.

13. **C.** Glucocorticoids have potent effects on glucose and carbohydrate metabolism. They promote glycogen breakdown, rather than inhibit it.

14. **B.** Captopril increases insulin sensitivity and would not be expected to contribute to increased blood glucose. This patient's blood glucose began rising shortly after admission. His IV fluids contain glucose; epinephrine increases blood glucose by increasing glycogen breakdown, methylprednisolone (Solu-Medrol) promotes glycogenolysis, and anaphylaxis would be expected to increase stress response, thereby leading to increased epinephrine release and increased blood glucose.

15. **A.** The patient has a history of diabetes and will be given prednisone (Deltasone), which would be expected to increase blood glucose. When diabetes is poorly controlled, infections are more likely to occur. For this reason, he should monitor more closely for wounds that may become infected. He will not be taking prednisone long enough to develop adrenal insufficiency, so there is no need for him to wear identification for steroid therapy.

16. **D.** Glucocorticoids have catabolic effects on a number of tissues, including muscle, fat, skin, and bone. Chronic administration leads to osteopenia and osteoporosis.

17. **D.** Chronic administration of glucocorticoids such as prednisone will lead to feedback inhibition of pituitary ACTH release and atrophy of the adrenal cortex. When prednisone is abruptly stopped, the adrenals will not be able to meet the body's demand for cortisol during severe stress, and adrenal crisis may occur.

18. **C.** Corticosteroids such as dexamethasone (Decadron) are known to increase the risk of peptic ulcers when used in combination with NSAIDs.

19. **D.** Cosyntropin (Cortrosyn) is a synthetic analogue of ACTH that is used to diagnose adrenal insufficiency. It works by stimulating the adrenal cortex to secrete cortisol. If cosyntropin administration does not result in an appropriate increase in cortisol release, adrenal insufficiency is present.

20. **D.** Desmopressin (DDAVP) is a synthetic analogue of vasopressin, or antidiuretic hormone. Thus, it decreases urine production by increasing water resorption.

21. **A.** Adrenocorticotropic hormone, or ACTH, is released by the pituitary and acts on the adrenal glands to increase cortisol release. Corticotropin-releasing hormone is released by the hypothalamus and acts on the pituitary to stimulate ACTH release.

22. **B.** Stanozolol (Winstrol) is an androgen that would be expected to promote growth and development of male sex organs. However, chronic administration leads to feedback inhibition of testosterone secretion, which leads to testicular atrophy.

23. **A.** Testosterone transdermal systems (Androderm, Testoderm) are applied once daily for 24 hours. Longer-acting androgens are available, such as nandrolone decanoate (Deca-Durabolin), for once-weekly administration.

24. **D.** Anabolic steroids may be abused by those who are seeking enhanced muscular development and endurance, such as athletes. For this reason, all of these agents are subject to the Controlled Substances Act.

14-7. References

Baskin HJ, Cobin RH, Duick DS. American Association of Clinical Endocrinologists Medical Guidelines for Clinical Practice for the evaluation and treatment of hyperthyroidism and hypothyroidism (AACE Thyroid Task Force). *Endocr Pract.* 2002; 8:457–69.

Chrousos GP. Adrenocorticosteroids and adrenocortical antagonists. In: Katzung BG, ed. *Basic and Clinical Pharmacology.* 11th ed. New York: McGraw-Hill; 2009.

Chrousos GP. The gonadal hormones and inhibitors. In: Katzung BG, ed. *Basic and Clinical Pharmacology.* 11th ed. New York: McGraw-Hill; 2009.

Dayan CM, Daniels GH. Chronic autoimmune thyroiditis. *N Engl J Med.* 1996;335:99–106.

Dong BJ. Thyroid disorders. In: Herfindal ET, Gourley DR, eds. *Textbook of Therapeutics: Drug and Disease Management.* Philadelphia: Lippincott Williams & Wilkins; 2006.

Dong BJ, Greenspan FG. Thyroid and antithyroid drugs. In: Katzung BG, ed. *Basic and Clinical Pharmacology.* 11th ed. New York: McGraw-Hill; 2009.

Dong, BJ, Hauck WW, Gambertoglio JG, et al. Bioequivalence of generic and brand name levothyroxine products in the treatment of hypothyroidism. *JAMA.* 1997;277:1205–13.

Hoffmeister AM, Tietze KJ. Adrenocortical dysfunction and clinical use of steroids. In: Herfindal ET, Gourley DR, eds. *Textbook of Therapeutics: Drug and Disease Management.* Philadelphia: Lippincott Williams & Wilkins; 2006.

Master SB. Hypothalamic and pituitary hormones. In: Katzung BG, ed. *Basic and Clinical Pharmacology.* 11th ed. New York: McGraw-Hill; 2009.

McEvoy GK, ed. *AHFS Drug Information 2009.* Bethesda, Md.: American Society of Health-System Pharmacists; 2009.

U.S. Food and Drug Administration. Orange book: Approved drug products with therapeutic equivalence evaluations. Accessed at: http://www.accessdata.fda.gov/scripts/cder/ob/default.cfm.

Women's Health

Andrea S. Franks, PharmD, BCPS

15-1. Postmenopausal Hormone Replacement Therapy

Menopause is the permanent cessation of menses resulting from diminishing ovarian follicular function. It is defined as 12 consecutive months of amenorrhea. Median age of onset in the United States is 51 years of age (range 40–55). Physiologic changes and symptoms of menopause may present up to 8 years prior to cessation of menses.

Perimenopause, also called the *menopausal transition,* is the time before menopause and the first year following menopause. Ovarian function and production of estrogen decline during this time, and menstrual cycles may be irregular.

Clinical Presentation

- Cessation of menses for at least 12 consecutive months
- Symptoms of perimenopause related to declining estrogen:
  - Anovulation
  - Dysfunctional uterine bleeding
  - Extended menstrual cycle intervals
  - Oligomenorrhea
- Symptoms of menopause directly related to lack of estrogen:
  - Vaginal dryness and vulvar or vaginal atrophy
  - Vasomotor symptoms (night sweats, hot flashes)
- Symptoms associated with menopause, but without a proven link to estrogen deficiency:
  - Arthralgia
  - Depression
  - Insomnia
  - Migraines
  - Mood swings
  - Myalgia
  - Urinary frequency
  - Cognitive changes (memory, concentration)

Pathophysiology

- Loss of ovarian follicular activity results in endocrine, biologic, and clinical changes.
- Ovarian production of estradiol and progesterone diminishes.
- Follicle-stimulating hormone and luteinizing hormone concentrations increase.
- Primary estrogen available is now estrone (which is converted peripherally from androstenedione and is less potent), not estradiol.

Treatment Principles

- Women with an intact uterus must be treated with estrogen plus progestin to reduce the risk of endometrial hyperplasia and endometrial cancer.
- Women who have had a hysterectomy are treated with unopposed estrogen.
- Hormone replacement therapy (HRT) should be initiated on an individual basis with careful consideration of the risks and benefits.
- Contraindications to estrogen replacement therapy (ERT) are
  - Abnormal, undiagnosed genital bleeding
  - Known, suspected, or history of breast cancer
  - History of deep-vein thrombosis or pulmonary embolism
  - Estrogen-dependent neoplasia

- Pregnancy
- Stroke or myocardial infarction in the past year
- Liver dysfunction or disease

Drug Therapy

Table 15-1 provides an overview of selected HRT products.

Estrogen and progestin

Mechanism of action
ERT is used alone (if no uterus) or in combination with progestin to replace diminished levels of endogenous hormones.

Combined estrogen–progestin therapy (EPT) includes progestin to prevent endometrial hyperplasia and cancer.

Patient instructions and counseling
- Side effects of estrogen may be diminished by starting with a low dose and may be alleviated by changing products. Most side effects improve with time.
- Side effects of progestin may be alleviated or diminished by changing products or changing from a continuous to a cyclic regimen.
- Patients should be instructed to immediately report any unusual vaginal bleeding.
- Patients should be instructed to contact their physician promptly if any of the following events occur:
  - Abdominal tenderness, pain, or swelling
  - Coughing up of blood
  - Disturbances of vision or speech
  - Dizziness or fainting
  - Lumps in the breast
  - Numbness or weakness in an arm or leg
  - Severe vomiting or headache
  - Sharp chest pain or shortness of breath
  - Sharp pain in the calves

Adverse drug events
Increased risks for venous thromboembolism, stroke, coronary heart disease, and breast cancer were identified in the Women's Health Initiative (WHI) trial with postmenopausal women receiving estrogen and estrogen plus progestin products. The beneficial effects included reductions in fractures and colorectal cancer. Both ERT and EPT should be used at the lowest doses and for the shortest possible time period for women who are experiencing moderate to severe vasomotor

symptoms or vulvovaginal atrophy. Consider topical estrogen.

The following adverse effects are most common with estrogen:

- Breast tenderness
- Heavy or irregular bleeding
- Headache
- Nausea

The following adverse effects are most common with progestin:

- Depression
- Headache
- Irritability

Drug–drug and drug–disease interactions
Estrogen may exacerbate illness in the following disease states:

- Depression
- Hypertriglyceridemia (avoid by using transdermal product)
- Thyroid disorder (patients may require an increased dose of thyroid supplement)
- Impaired hepatic function (poor metabolism of estrogens)
- Cardiovascular disorders (coronary heart disease and venous thromboembolism risk may be increased with estrogens)
- Cholelithiasis
- Gastroesophageal reflux disease

Interaction may result in decreased pharmacologic effect of estrogens:

- Cytochrome P450 (CYP450) 3A4 inducers:
  - Barbiturates
  - Carbamazepine
  - Rifampin
  - St. John's wort
- Phenytoin

Interaction may result in increased pharmacologic effect of estrogens:

- CYP450 3A4 inhibitors:
  - Azole antifungales
  - Macrolide antibiotics
  - Ritonavir

Parameters to monitor
Laboratory monitoring is not recommended. Patients should be monitored for symptom improvement, adverse effects, and appropriate health maintenance (e.g., through annual mammograms).

Table 15-1. Selected Hormone Replacement Therapy Products

Medication	Available strengths and dosing
Oral estrogen products	
Conjugated equine estrogens (CEE) (Premarin)	0.3, 0.45, 0.625, 0.9, 1.25, 2.5 mg daily
Synthetic conjugated estrogens (Cenestin, Enjuvia)	0.3 mg, 0.45 mg, 0.625 mg, 0.9 mg, 1.25 mg daily
Micronized estradiol (Estradiol, Estrace, Gynodiol)	0.5, 1, 1.5, 2 mg daily
Estrone sulfate (Estropipate, Ortho-Est, Ogen)	0.625, 1.25, 2.5, 5 mg daily
Esterified estrogens (Estratab, Menest)	0.3, 0.625, 1.25, 2.5 mg daily
17-β-Estradiol	2 mg daily
Synthetic conjugated estrogen	0.3, 0.625, 0.9, 1.25 mg daily
Transdermal products	
Estradiol transdermal patch (Estraderm, Esclim, Alora, Vivelle)	Apply twice weekly
Estradiol transdermal patch (Climara, Fempatch, Menostar)	Apply once weekly
Estradiol and levonorgestrel (Climara Pro)	Apply once weekly
Estradiol and norethindrone (CombiPatch)	Apply twice weekly
Estradiol topical emulsion (Estrasorb)	Apply daily
17-β-estradiol micronized gel (Estrogel)	Apply daily
17-β-estradiol transdermal spray (Evamist)	Apply one spray daily
Vaginal estrogen products	
Estrace vaginal cream (local effects)	0.1 mg estradiol/g; dose: 2–4 g daily for 1–2 weeks; maintenance dose: 1 g 1–3 times/week
Premarin vaginal cream (local effects)	0.625 mg conjugated estrogen/g; dose: 0.5–2 g daily for 3 weeks, then 1 week off
Estring vaginal ring, 17-β-estradiol (local effects)	2 mg estradiol ring releases 7.5 mcg/24 hr; ring remains in vagina for 3 months
Vagifem vaginal tablet (local effects)	25 mcg estradiol/tablet; dose: 1 tablet once daily for 2 weeks; maintenance dose: 1 tablet twice/week
Femring vaginal ring, estradiol acetate (systemic absorption)	0.05 mg/d or 0.1 mg/d
Oral combination estrogen–progestin products	
Activella	Estradiol/norethindrone: 1 mg/0.5 mg or 0.5 mg/0.1 mg
Femhrt	2.5 or 5 mcg ethinyl estradiol, 0.5 or 1 mg norethindrone acetate
Prempro	0.3 mg/1.5 mg, 0.45/1/5 mg, 0.625 mg/2.5 mg, or 0.625 mg/5 mg or conjugated estrogen/medroxyprogesterone
Premphase	0.625 mg conjugated estrogen, 5 mg medroxyprogesterone (2 weeks of estrogen alone, 2 weeks of combination)
Combination estrogen–androgen products	
Estratest HS, Covaryx HS	0.625 mg esterified estrogens, 1.25 mg methyltestosterone
Estratest, Covaryx HS	0.625 mg esterified estrogens, 2.5 mg methyltestosterone

Adapted from *Pharmacist's Letter* 2008; Kalantaridou, Davis, Calis 2008.

Androgens (testosterone)

Mechanism of action

Androgens are the precursor hormones to estrogen production by the ovaries and peripheral sites. Ovarian testosterone production declines with menopause.

Androgens act at androgen receptor sites or exhibit action following conversion to estrogen. Androgen replacement improves deficiency-related symptoms (i.e., decreased sexual desire, decreased energy, diminished well-being).

Patient instructions and counseling

■ Testosterone therapy should be administered only to postmenopausal women who are receiving concurrent estrogen therapy.
■ The following are relative contraindications to testosterone therapy:
  • Androgenic alopecia
  • Hirsutism
  • Moderate to severe acne

Adverse drug events

■ Fluid retention
■ Decreased high-density lipoprotein and triglycerides
■ Hepatic dysfunction
■ Hepatocellular carcinoma (prolonged use of high doses)

Parameters to monitor

Laboratory monitoring is not recommended.

Nondrug Therapy

Phytoestrogens

■ Phytoestrogens are plant compounds (isoflavones, lignans, coumestans).
■ Food sources of phytoestrogens include soy (milk, edamame, tofu); flaxseed; and alfalfa sprouts.
■ Some studies have shown improvement in vaginal symptoms.
■ Phytoestrogens may decrease loss of bone mineral density.
■ No evidence supports improvement in other symptoms of menopause (i.e., hot flashes, depression, anxiety, headache, myalgia).
■ Phytoestrogens may have beneficial effects on lipids, weight, blood pressure.

15-2. Contraception

Contraception is the prevention of pregnancy by one of two methods:

■ Preventing implantation of the fertilized ovum in the endometrium
■ Inhibiting contact of sperm with mature ovum

Prescription Contraceptive Options

Oral contraceptives

■ Estrogen plus progestin (combined oral contraceptive)
■ Progestin only (minipill)
  • Appropriate for use in breast-feeding women
  • Less efficacious than combined oral contraceptives
  • Free of cardiovascular risks associated with estrogen-containing products
■ Long-term injectable or implanted products: progestin only
■ Estrogens and progestins used in prescription contraceptives (Table 15-2):
  • Estrogens:
    ▪ Ethinyl estradiol
    ▪ Mestranol
  • Progestins:
    ▪ Desogestrel
    ▪ Norgestrel; levonorgestrel
    ▪ Ethynodiol diacetate
    ▪ Norethindrone, norethindrone acetate, norethynodrel
■ Drospirenone: progestin with progestogenic, antiandrogenic, and antimineralocorticoid activity

Drug Therapy

Mechanism of action

Estrogens prevent development of a dominant follicle by suppression of follicle-stimulating hormone. They do not block ovulation.

Progestin blocks ovulation. It contributes to the production of thick and impermeable cervical mucus. It also contributes to involution and atrophy of the endometrium.

Patient instructions and counseling

■ Efficacy is high but depends on appropriate use and adherence.
■ Oral contraceptives do not prevent the transmission of sexually transmitted diseases.
■ Patients should be educated on warning signs of important complications:
  • Severe abdominal pain
  • Severe chest pain, shortness of breath, coughing up of blood

Table 15-2. Prescription Contraceptive Products		
Product	**Estrogen**	**Progestin**
Progestin-only oral contraceptives		
Micronor, Errin, Nor-QD, Nora-BE, Camila	—	Norethindrone 0.35 mg
Monophasic low-dose estrogen oral contraceptives		
Aviane, Lessina, Levlite	Ethinyl estradiol 20 mcg	Levonorgestrel 0.1 mg
Loestrin 1/20, Loestrin Fe 1/20, Microgestin Fe 1/20	Ethinyl estradiol 20 mcg	Norethindrone 1 mg
Yasmin	Ethinyl estradiol 30 mcg	Drospirenone 3 mg
Levlen, Levora, Nordette, Portia	Ethinyl estradiol 30 mcg	Levonorgestrel 0.15 mg
Cryselle, Lo/Ovral, Low-Ogestrel	Ethinyl estradiol 30 mcg	Norgestrel 0.3 mg
Apri, Desogen, Ortho-Cept	Ethinyl estradiol 30 mcg	Desogestrel 0.15 mg
Ovcon-35	Ethinyl estradiol 30 mcg	Norethindrone 0.4 mg
Brevicon, Modicon, Necon 0.5/35, Nortrel 0.5/35	Ethinyl estradiol 35 mcg	Norethindrone 0.5 mg
Necon 1/35, Norinyl 1+35, Nortrel 1/35, Ortho-Novum 1/35	Ethinyl estradiol 35 mcg	Norethindrone 1 mg
Monophasic high-dose estrogen oral contraceptives		
Ogestrel 0.5/50	Ethinyl estradiol 50 mcg	Norgestrel 0.5 mg
Demulen 1/50, Zovia 1/50	Ethinyl estradiol 50 mcg	Ethynodiol diacetate 1 mg
Ovcon-50	Ethinyl estradiol 50 mcg	Norethindrone 1 mg
Necon 1/50, Norinyl 1+50, Ortho-Novum 1/50	Mestranol 50 mcg	Norethindrone 1 mg
Biphasic oral contraceptives		
Ortho-Novum 10/11, Necon 10/11	Ethinyl estradiol 35 mcg	Norethindrone 0.5 mg × 10 days; 1 mg × 11 days
Mircette, Kariva	Ethinyl estradiol 20 mcg × 10 days, placebo × 2 days, then 10 mcg × 5 days	Desogestrel 0.15 mg × 21 days
Triphasic oral contraceptives		
Enpresse, Tri-Levlen, Triphasil, Trivora	Ethinyl estradiol 30 mcg × 6 days, 40 mcg × 5 days, 30 mcg × 10 days	Levonorgestrel 0.05 mg × 6 days; 0.075 mg × 5 days; 0.125 mg × 10 days.
Tri-Norinyl, Leena, Aranelle	Ethinyl estradiol 35 mcg × 21 days	Norethindrone 0.5 mg × 7 days, 1 mg × 9 days, 0.5 mg × 5 days
Necon 7/7/7, Ortho-Novum 7/7/7, Nortrel 7/7/7	Ethinyl estradiol 35 mcg × 21 days	Norethindrone 0.5 mg × 7 days, 0.75 mg × 7 days, 1 mg × 7 days
Cyclessa, Velivet	Ethinyl estradiol 25 mcg × 21 days	Desogestrel 0.1 mg × 7 days, 0.125 mg × 7 days, 0.15 mg × 7 days
Ortho Tri-Cyclen Lo	Ethinyl estradiol 25 mcg × 21 days	Norgestimate 0.18 mg × 7 days, 0.215 mg × 7 days, 0.25 mg × 7 days
Ortho Tri-Cyclen, Trinessa	Ethinyl estradiol 35 mcg × 21 days	Norgestimate 0.18 mg × 7 days, 0.215 mg × 7 days, 0.25 mg × 7 days
Estrostep Fe	Ethinyl estradiol 20 mcg × 5 days, 30 mcg × 7 days, 35 mcg × 9 days	Norethindrone 1 mg × 21 days

(continued)

Table 15-2. Prescription Contraceptive Products *(Continued)*

Product	Estrogen	Progestin
Extended-cycle oral contraceptives		
Loestrin-24 FE	Ethinyl estradiol 20 mcg	Norethindrone 1 mg
Seasonale, Jolessa, Quasense	Ethinyl estradiol 30 mcg	Levonorgestrel 0.15 mg
Yaz	Ethinyl estradiol 20 mcg	Drospirenone 3 mg
Continuous-cycle oral contraceptives		
Lybrel	Ethinyl estradiol 30 mcg	Levonorgestrel 90 mg
Transdermal contraceptive system		
Ortho Evra	Ethinyl estradiol 20 mcg per 24 hours	Norelgestromin 0.15 mg per 24 hours; applied weekly
Vaginal ring contraceptive system		
NuvaRing	—	Etonogestrel 0.12 mg per 24 hours; insert for 3 weeks, then remove 1 week
Contraceptive implants		
Implanon	—	Etonogestrel subdermal rod; release rate varies over time
Contraceptive injection		
Depo-Provera CI	—	Medroxyprogesterone acetate 150 mg intramuscular q 3 months
Depo-SubQ Provera	—	Medroxyprogesterone acetate 104 mg subcutaneous q 3 months
Intrauterine contraceptive systems		
Mirena	—	Levonorgestrel 20 mcg/day × 5 years

Adapted from Dickerson et al. 2008; *Pharmacist's Letter* 2007.

- Severe headache
- Eye problems (i.e., blurred vision, flashing lights, or blindness)
- Severe leg pain in the calf or thigh
- Patients should be advised to expect changes in characteristics of the menstrual cycle.
- Use of a backup contraceptive method is advised if more than one dose is missed per cycle.

Adverse drug events

The World Health Organization (WHO) suggests refraining from prescribing combined oral contraceptives to women with the following diagnoses:

- Breast cancer
- Deep-vein thrombosis or pulmonary embolism
- Cerebrovascular disease or coronary artery disease
- Diabetes with nephropathy, neuropathy, retinopathy, or other vascular disease
- Migraine headaches
- Uncontrolled hypertension ($\geq$ 160/90 mm Hg)
- Breast-feeding women (< 6 weeks postpartum)
- Liver disease
- Pregnancy
- Surgery with prolonged immobilization or any surgery on the legs
- Age > 35 years and currently smoking ($\geq$ 15 cigarettes a day)
- Hypercoagulable states (e.g., factor V Leiden, protein C or S deficiency)

For these medical conditions, use of progestin-only oral contraceptives, depot medroxyprogesterone acetate, or an intrauterine device may be an appropriate contraceptive choice.

The most common adverse drug events are

- Nausea and vomiting (usually resolves within 3 months)
- Breakthrough bleeding, spotting, amenorrhea, and altered menstrual flow
- Melasma
- Headache or migraine
- Weight change or edema

Serious but less common effects are venous thrombosis, pulmonary embolism, myocardial infarction, coronary thrombosis, arterial thromboembolism, and cerebral thrombosis.

Potential hormonal effects are associated with an imbalance in estrogen and progestin (Table 15-3).

Drug–drug and drug–disease interactions

Interaction with the following drugs may result in decreased pharmacologic effect of oral contraceptives:

- Ampicillin, griseofulvin, sulfonamides, tetracycline
- Anticonvulsants (barbiturates, carbamazepine, felbamate, phenytoin, topiramate)
- Some antiretroviral medications (e.g., nevirapine, lopinavir + ritonavir)
- Rifampin

Interaction with these drugs may result in increased plasma levels of oral contraceptives:

- Atorvastatin
- Vitamin C
- CYP450 3A4 inhibitors

Interaction with the following drugs may result in decreased pharmacologic effect of the interacting drug:

- Anticoagulants (estrogens have a procoagulant effect)
- Some benzodiazepines (e.g., lorazepam, oxazepam, temazepam)
- Methyldopa
- Phenytoin

Interaction with the following may result in increased pharmacologic effect of interacting drug:

- Tricyclic antidepressants
- Benzodiazepine tranquilizers (other than the benzodiazepines previously listed)
- β-blockers
- Theophylline

Parameters to monitor

Patients must monitor themselves for warning signs of serious complications previously listed. Laboratory monitoring is not recommended with use of oral contraceptives.

Nondrug Therapy

Nondrug therapy includes use of the following:

- Condoms
- Diaphragms
- Intrauterine devices
- Spermicides

Table 15-3. Potential Hormonal Effects Associated with an Imbalance in Estrogen or Progestin

Type of imbalance	Effect
Estrogen excess	Breast tenderness, fullness
	Nausea
	Edema and bloating
	Hypertension
	Melasma
	Headache
Progestin excess	Acne or oily scalp
	Breast tenderness
	Depression or irritability
	Hypomenorrhea
	Increased appetite and weight gain
	Fatigue
	Constipation
Estrogen deficiency	Breakthrough bleeding (early or midcycle)
	Hypomenorrhea
	Vasomotor symptoms
Progestin deficiency	Amenorrhea
	Breakthrough bleeding (late)
	Hypermenorrhea

Adapted from Dickerson et al. 2008; *Pharmacist's Letter* 2007.

15-3. Osteoporosis

Osteoporosis is characterized by low bone mineral density and deterioration of bone tissue, increasing fragility of bone, and subsequent risk of fracture.

Types of Osteoporosis

- Primary
  - Type I: Postmenopausal (most common and the focus of this chapter)
  - Type II: Age related
- Secondary
  - Drug induced
  - Medical conditions

Diagnostic Criteria

Dual-energy x-ray absorptiometry (DEXA) scans are used to diagnosis osteoporosis. T scores are used to guide diagnosis and decision to treat osteoporosis. The WHO classification of bone mass is based on T scores:

- *Osteopenia:* T score −1.0 to −2.5 standard deviations below the young adult mean
- *Osteoporosis:* T score *below* −2.5 standard deviations below the young adult mean

Risk factors for osteoporosis are as follows:

- Advanced age
- Amenorrhea
- Cigarette smoking
- Current low bone mass
- Late menarche or early menopause
- Ethnicity (Caucasian or Asian)
- Excessive alcohol use
- Family history of osteoporosis or history of fracture in a primary relative
- Female
- History of fracture over the age of 50
- Inactive lifestyle
- Long-term use of corticosteroids or anti-convulsants
- Low lifetime calcium intake
- Low testosterone levels in men (hypogonadism)
- Thin or small frame
- Vitamin D deficiency

Medical conditions associated with increased risk of osteoporosis are as follows:

- Acquired immune deficiency syndrome (AIDS)
- Cushing's disease
- Eating disorders
- Hyperthyroidism
- Hyperparathyroidism
- Inflammatory bowel disease
- Insulin-dependent diabetes mellitus
- Lymphoma and leukemia
- Malabsorption syndromes
- Rheumatoid arthritis
- Chronic kidney disease
- Chronic obstructive pulmonary disease

The following drugs are associated with an increased risk of osteoporosis:

- Anticonvulsants (phenobarbital, phenytoin)
- Cytotoxic drugs
- Glucocorticoids
- Immunosuppressants
- Lithium
- Long-term heparin use
- Depot medroxyprogesterone
- Supraphysiologic thyroxine doses
- Tamoxifen (premenopausal)
- Aromatase inhibitors

The American Association of Clinical Endocrinologists and the National Osteoporosis Foundation recommend that all women 65 years of age and older be screened for osteoporosis. In addition, postmenopausal women less than 65 years of age with a family history of osteoporosis or clinical risk factors and women with a fracture history unrelated to trauma should be screened.

Clinical Presentation

- Shortened stature
- Vertebra, hip, or forearm fracture
- Kyphosis
- Lordosis
- Bone pain (especially back pain, which could indicate vertebral compression fracture)

Pathophysiology

There are two types of bone: trabecular (i.e., vertebrae, wrist and ankle, and ends of long bones, which are the most susceptible to fracture) and cortical. Osteoblasts (formation) and osteoclasts (destruction) create a constant state of bone remodeling.

Bone formation exceeds destruction during childhood. Peak bone mass is reached around age 25–35; then bone density begins to decline:

- A 3% to 4% decline per decade in men
- A 8% to 12% decline per decade in women 10 years after menopause

Following menopause (postmenopausal osteoporosis), estrogen production declines and osteoclastic activity increases.

Treatment Principles

Adequate calcium and vitamin D intake through diet or supplementation is recommended for everyone (calcium 1,000–1,500 mg daily plus 400–1,000 IU [international units] vitamin D daily) (Table 15-4).

Lifestyle modifications are recommended, including weight-bearing exercise, smoking cessation, limited alcohol intake, dietary calcium, and vitamin D.

Prescription drug therapy should be initiated on an individual basis, considering risk factors, bone mineral density, fracture history, and concomitant diseases and medications.

Initiation of Treatment

The National Osteoporosis Foundation recommends initiation of therapy in the following situations:

- History of vertebral or hip fracture
- T score below −2.5 (osteoporosis)
- T score −1 to −2.5 (osteopenia) with
  - Secondary causes (steroids, immobility)
  - History of other fractures
  - 10-year probability of hip fracture ≥ 3% or 10-year probability of any major fracture ≥ 20%

Table 15-4. Select Calcium Supplement Products

Product	Calcium (mg)
Calcium citrate (24% calcium content)	
Citracal	Tablet: 200; liquitab: 500
Citracal + vitamin D	200–315 plus 200 IU vitamin D
Calcium carbonate (40% calcium content)	
Caltrate 600	600
Titralac	Chewable: 168, 300; liquid: 400/5 mL
Tums	Chewable: 200, 300, 400, 500
Viactiv chews	500 plus 200 IU vitamin D
Mylanta Supreme liquid	160 mg/5 ml
Calcium carbonate + vitamin D	
Caltrate 600 + D	600 plus 200 IU
Calcilyte + vitamin D	500 plus 200 IU
Oscal + vitamin D	500 plus 125 IU
Calcium phosphate tribasic (39% calcium content)	
Posture	600
Posture-D	600 plus 125 IU

Adapted from O'Connell, Vondracek 2008; www.nof.org.

based on the U.S.-adapted WHO algorithm (Fracture Risk Assessment Tool, or FRAX)

Drug Therapy

Calcium and vitamin D

Mechanism of action

Calcium is necessary to improve bone mass. It is absorbed through the gastrointestinal (GI) tract, stored in the bone, and made available when calcium levels become low.

Vitamin D facilitates absorption and regulation of calcium levels.

Patient instructions and counseling

- Approximately 500 mg of calcium can be absorbed from the GI tract at a time; separate doses appropriately to achieve a dose of 1,000–1,500 mg per day.
- Calcium carbonate contains the highest level of elemental calcium; take with food to facilitate absorption.
- Calcium citrate products may be administered without regard to meals.

Adverse drug events

The most common adverse drug events are as follows:

- GI upset (nausea, vomiting, cramping, flatulence, especially with carbonate)
- Headache
- Hypophosphatemia and hypercalcemia
- Nephrolithiasis

Drug–drug and drug–disease interactions

Concomitant administration may decrease the bioavailability of fluoroquinolones, tetracyclines, and levothyroxine.

Parameters to monitor

Laboratory monitoring is not recommended.

Bisphosphonates

Table 15-5 provides summary information about bisphosphonates.

Mechanism of action

Bisphosphonates bind to bone (hydroxyapatite) and incorporate into bone to increase and stabilize bone mass. They inhibit osteoclasts and have a very long half-life in the bone.

Table 15-5. Antiresorptive Agents

Medication	Dosing	FDA indication, availability
Bisphosphonates		
Alendronate (Fosamax)	Prevention: 5 mg daily or 35 mg weekly	Prevention and treatment of post-menopausal osteoporosis
	Treatment: 10 mg daily or 70 mg weekly	Osteoporosis in men and glucocorticoid-induced osteoporosis
		Available as tablet, liquid, and tablet plus vitamin D
Risedronate (Actonel)	Prevention: 5 mg daily	Prevention and treatment of post-menopausal osteoporosis
	Treatment: 5 mg daily or 35 mg po weekly, 75 mg po daily × 2 consecutive days monthly, or 150 mg po monthly	Osteoporosis in men
		Glucocorticoid-induced osteoporosis
		Available as tablets and tablets plus calcium
Ibandronate (Boniva)	2.5 mg po daily, 150 mg po monthly, 3 mg IV Q 3 months	Prevention and treatment of post-menopausal osteoporosis
Zoledronic acid (Reclast)	5 mg IV infusion over 15 minutes once yearly	Treatment of postmenopausal osteoporosis
Selective estrogen receptor modulator		
Raloxifene (Evista)	60 mg daily	Prevention and treatment of post-menopausal osteoporosis
Other agents		
Calcitonin (Miacalcin)	Intranasal: 200 IU daily, alternating nostrils	Treatment of postmenopausal osteoporosis in women at least 5 years postmenopause
	Intramuscular or subcutaneous: 100 IU every other day	
Teriparatide (Forteo)	Injection: 20 mcg daily	Treatment of postmenopausal women with osteoporosis who are at high risk for fractures or who have failed or are intolerant to other therapies
		Treatment of men with primary or hypo-gonadal osteoporosis who are at high risk for fractures

Adapted from O'Connell, Vondracek 2008; www.nof.org; MacLaughlin, Raehl 2008.

Patient instructions and counseling

- Bisphosphonates must be taken with a full glass of water (8 oz) 30–60 minutes prior to the first meal of the day and 30–60 minutes before any other medications.
- Remain in an upright position for at least 30 minutes following ingestion.
- Take medication on a regularly scheduled basis.
- Compliance may be increased by extended dosing intervals (weekly, monthly, quarterly); however, studies demonstrated antifracture benefits with daily dosing.

Adverse drug events

The most common adverse drug events are GI related: abdominal pain, dyspepsia, constipation, diarrhea, flatulence, nausea, gastritis, esophageal ulceration (if not taken appropriately). Rarely, patients experience osteonecrosis of the jaw (mostly in cancer patients on intravenous bisphosphonates) or myalgia, arthralgia, or flu-like symptoms (especially with intravenous [IV] zoledronic acid)

Drug–drug and drug–disease interactions

Interaction may result in decreased pharmacologic effect of bisphosphonates such as calcium supplements and antacids. Separate administration by 1 hour.

Interaction may result in increased pharmacologic effect of bisphosphonates such as ranitidine. IV ranitidine may double bioavailability of alendronate.

Interaction may result in increased toxicity of interacting drugs such as aspirin. Alendronate > 10 mg daily may increase risk of upper GI side effects of aspirin.

Parameters to monitor
Laboratory monitoring is not recommended.

Estrogen replacement therapy

ERT has a beneficial effect on bone mineral density and fracture risk, but the risks of long-term therapy appear to outweigh that benefit. ERT should be used at the lowest effective dose for the shortest duration in women experiencing vasomotor symptoms or vulvovaginal atrophy.

Estrogen agonist–antagonist (selective estrogen receptor modulator): raloxifene (Evista)

Mechanism of action
Raloxifene is an estrogen receptor agonist in the bone. It decreases resorption of bone and overall bone turnover. It acts as an antagonist in breast tissue.

Patient instructions and counseling
- This medication may be taken without regard to food.
- Concomitant use with estrogen therapy is not recommended.
- This medication will not treat symptoms of menopause such as hot flashes and may aggravate them.
- In the event of prolonged immobilization, discontinue raloxifene 3 days prior to and during the immobile period when possible.

Adverse drug events
The most common adverse drug events are as follows:

- *Cardiovascular:* Hot flashes, chest pain, syncope
- *GI:* Nausea, diarrhea, vomiting
- *Musculoskeletal:* Arthralgia, myalgia, nocturnal leg cramps
- *Central nervous system (CNS):* Insomnia, neuralgia
- *Skin:* Rash, sweating
- *Thrombotic:* deep-vein thrombosis, pulmonary embolism

Drug–drug and drug–disease interactions
For the following drugs, interaction may result in decreased pharmacologic effect of raloxifene:

- *Ampicillin:* Peak levels are reduced by 28% and overall absorption is reduced by 14%. Coadministration is not contraindicated because of maintained systemic exposure and elimination.
- *Cholestyramine:* Absorption and enterohepatic cycling are reduced. Do not administer together.

In the case of warfarin, interaction may result in decreased pharmacologic effect of the interacting drug. Prothrombin time may decrease up to 10%. Patients with history of venous thromboembolism should not be on raloxifene.

Parameters to monitor
Laboratory monitoring is not recommended.

Calcitonin (Miacalcin, Fortical)

Mechanism of action
Calcitonin participates in the regulation of calcium and bone metabolism. It inhibits bone resorption by binding to osteoclast receptors.

Patient instructions and counseling
- If this medication is administered as an injection, it should be given in the upper arm, thigh, or buttocks.
- Proper education regarding administration of the injection and the nasal spray preparation is necessary.
- Patient should be advised that if a shot is missed, it should be administered as soon as possible, but not if it is almost time for the next dose.
- Store the nasal spray in the refrigerator until time for use. Warm the spray to room temperature prior to first use and then store at room temperature.

Adverse drug events
The most common adverse drug events are as follows:

- *Skin:* Facial flushing and hand flushing (most common overall)
- *GI:* Nausea, diarrhea, vomiting, abdominal pain
- *Taste disorder:* Salty taste
- *Genitourinary:* Nocturia, urinary frequency
- *Nasal (with nasal spray):* Rhinitis, nasal dryness, irritation, itching, congestion
- *Ophthalmic:* Blurred vision, abnormal lacrimation

Drug–drug and drug–disease interactions

In the case of lithium, interaction may result in decreased pharmacologic effect of interacting drug. Concomitant administration may decrease lithium levels.

Salmon calcitonin should be avoided in patients with a true allergy to seafood.

Parameters to monitor

Laboratory monitoring is not recommended.

Parathyroid hormone: teriparatide (Forteo)

Mechanism of action

Teriparatide increases the rate of bone formation by stimulating osteoblasts, thereby increasing bone mass density and decreasing fracture risk.

Because of limited long-term safety data (< 2 years) and risks of osteosarcoma in animal models, this medication is recommended for use only in men and women at high risk of fracture.

Patient instructions and counseling

Patients should be educated regarding appropriate use of the prefilled pen delivery device, storage (refrigerator), and adverse effects (orthostasis with first dose).

Adverse drug events

The most common adverse drug events are as follows:

- *Musculoskeletal:* Pain, arthralgia
- *CNS:* Paresthesias
- *GI:* Nausea, diarrhea, abdominal cramps
- *Taste disorder:* Metallic taste
- *Skin:* Injection pain, urticaria

Drug–drug and drug–disease interactions

No drug–drug or drug–disease interactions are known; however, teriparatide is contraindicated in patients who are at increased risk of osteosarcoma, including those who have received radiation to the bone, adolescents or young adults with open epiphyses, and individuals with Paget's disease.

Parameters to monitor

Laboratory monitoring is not recommended.

Nondrug Therapy

Nondrug therapies include

- Weight-bearing exercise
- Smoking cessation
- Limited alcohol consumption
- Calcium-rich diet
- Strategies to reduce the risk of falls

15-4. Key Points

Postmenopausal Hormone Replacement Therapy

Postmenopausal HRT must be selected on an individual basis taking into account the risks and benefits, concomitant diseases, and medications. Important patient parameters to consider include menopause symptoms, risk of coronary artery disease, risk of osteoporosis, risk of breast cancer, and risk of thromboembolism.

The primary indication for initiating HRT is to relieve vasomotor and other menopause symptoms to improve quality of life. Hormone replacement therapy is not recommended for use in the primary prevention of any other disease states.

Hormone replacement therapy should be used at the lowest effective dose and for the shortest duration possible. Estrogen plus progestin therapy is indicated in patients with a uterus. Estrogen alone is indicated in women who no longer have a uterus.

Contraceptives

Oral contraceptives are highly effective and safe when used properly according to the manufacturer's recommended dose and administration. Selection of prescription contraceptives requires careful consideration of patient medical history, lifestyle, compliance, and preference.

In addition to the contraceptive benefit of these products, other menstrual-related health problems may be resolved or lessened (e.g., menstrual pain, irregular menses, headache, and spotting).

Changes in dose or product are often necessary to achieve an appropriate balance of estrogen and progestin that minimizes undesirable adverse effects associated with deficiencies or excess amounts of the hormones.

Patients must be educated to report immediately the onset of severe abdominal pain, severe chest pain, shortness of breath, severe headache, visual disturbances, or severe pain in the leg or calf.

Osteoporosis

Women should be counseled about the following preventive measures:

- Adequate calcium consumption, using dietary supplements if dietary sources are not adequate
- Adequate vitamin D consumption (400–1,000 IU daily) and the natural sources of this nutrient
- Regular weight-bearing and muscle-strengthening exercises to reduce falls and prevent fractures
- Smoking cessation
- Moderation of alcohol intake
- Fall prevention strategies

Bone mineral density testing should be recommended to all postmenopausal women 65 years of age or older and for postmenopausal women younger than 65 years who have one or more risk factors for osteoporosis.

Therapy must be selected on an individual basis considering risks and benefits, concomitant diseases, and medications.

Appropriate calcium and vitamin D intake is an important component of prevention and treatment. If they are not obtained in the diet, supplementation is recommended for all individuals, especially patients receiving prescription therapy for osteoporosis.

Bisphosphonates are first-line pharmacologic options for osteoporosis prevention and treatment. They must be taken with a full glass of water 30–60 minutes prior to the first meal of the day or any other medications. The patient must remain upright for at least 30 minutes after taking a dose.

Estrogen replacement therapy is not approved for the treatment of osteoporosis and should not be initiated for this reason. It is approved for prevention of osteoporosis, but should be used only short term for women who are experiencing vasomotor or vaginal atrophy symptoms.

15-5. Questions

1. A. J. is a 35-year-old premenopausal woman who is concerned about her family history of osteoporosis. She does not eat dairy products because she is lactose intolerant. Her recent bone mineral density screening revealed a T score of 1.0. Select the appropriate therapy recommendation from the choices below.

    A. Daily estrogen replacement therapy
    B. Daily calcium and vitamin D supplementation
    C. Daily combined estrogen and progestin replacement therapy
    D. Daily teriparatide injections
    E. Daily calcitonin nasal spray

2. The pharmacist receives a prescription for Fosamax 70 mg daily for prevention of osteoporosis with instructions to the patient to take with food and remain upright for at least 30 minutes following ingestion. From the choices below, identify the errors in this prescription.

    A. The dose of Fosamax should be 35 mg weekly for prevention.
    B. Fosamax should be taken at least 30 minutes prior to a meal; it should not be taken with food.
    C. Patients should lie down for 1 hour following administration of Fosamax.
    D. Choices B and C are correct.
    E. Choices A and B are correct.

3. What is the recommended dosage range of daily calcium intake for an adult?

    A. 200–400 mg
    B. 250–500 mg
    C. 300–600 mg
    D. 500–1,000 mg
    E. 1,000–1,500 mg

4. Which of the following agents is considered first-line therapy for postmenopausal osteoporosis?

    A. Alendronate
    B. Calcitonin
    C. Prempro
    D. Denosumab
    E. Teriparatide

5. Which of the following products is available in an injectable and nasal spray dosage form?

    A. Raloxifene
    B. Alendronate
    C. Teriparatide
    D. Calcitonin
    E. Prempro

6. Which of the following drugs does *not* increase the risk of osteoporosis?

    A. Anticonvulsants
    B. Tamoxifen
    C. Glucocorticoids
    D. Estrogen
    E. Depo-Provera

7. What is the recommended dose of raloxifene in the prevention and treatment of post-menopausal osteoporosis?

 A. 10 mg daily
 B. 15 mg daily
 C. 40 mg daily
 D. 60 mg daily
 E. 120 mg daily

8. S. T. is a 32-year-old woman who wants to begin using a prescription contraceptive product. She is a new mother and would like to know if any products are safe for use during breast-feeding. S. T. states that she is not interested in using a device intravaginally and experiences irritation and inflammation with condom use. Which of the following product(s) would be an appropriate choice for S. T.?

 A. Ortho Tri-Cyclen
 B. Micronor
 C. Depo-Provera
 D. A or B
 E. B or C

9. T. H. is a 27-year-old woman currently taking Nordette oral contraceptive pills. She presents to your pharmacy with a prescription of ampicillin 500 mg qid for 1 week. Which of the following choices describes appropriate action taken by the pharmacist?

 A. Call the physician and request a change to amoxicillin to avoid a drug interaction between Nordette and ampicillin.
 B. Dispense the ampicillin and counsel T. H. on the appropriate administration and duration of therapy for the antibiotic.
 C. Dispense the ampicillin and counsel T. H. regarding the potential for ampicillin to interfere with the efficacy of Nordette. Instruct T. H. to use a backup method of contraception until her next menstrual period begins.
 D. Refuse to fill the ampicillin prescription, and counsel T. H. that she should never take antibiotics while she is on oral contraceptives.

10. Which of the following oral contraceptives is a biphasic product?

 A. Ortho Tri-Cyclen
 B. Ortho-Novum 10/11

 C. Ortho-Novum 1/35
 D. Yasmin
 E. Seasonale

11. Which of the following products is a progestin-only oral contraceptive?

 A. Nordette
 B. Ortho Tri-Cyclen
 C. Nor-QD
 D. Demulen 1/50
 E. Necon 1/35

12. A 26-year-old female who is recently initiated on a combination hormonal oral contraceptive complains of late-cycle breakthrough bleeding. Which of the following is she most likely experiencing?

 A. Too much estrogen
 B. Too little estrogen
 C. Too much progestin
 D. Too little progestin
 E. Too much androgen

13. What is the highest dose of estrogen (ethinyl estradiol) offered in an oral contraceptive?

 A. 25 mcg
 B. 30 mcg
 C. 35 mcg
 D. 40 mcg
 E. 50 mcg

14. A progestin-only oral contraceptive would be preferable over a combination oral contraceptive in all of the following cases *except*

 A. a one pack per day smoker over 35 years old.
 B. a patient with fibrocystic breast changes.
 C. a lactating woman.
 D. a patient with a history of thromboembolic disease.

15. A. J. is a 55-year-old woman who presents to your pharmacy with a prescription for Premarin 0.625 mg daily. She has an intact uterus and has been recently diagnosed with menopause. Which of the following statements describes the appropriate action to be taken by the pharmacist?

 A. Refuse to fill the prescription and recommend a phytoestrogen supplement.

B. Call the physician and confirm that the patient has an intact uterus and recommend a product containing estrogen plus progestin.

C. Fill the prescription and counsel the patient regarding administration instructions and potential adverse effects.

D. None of the above.

16. Which of the following factors is a contraindication to the use of hormone replacement therapy in postmenopausal women?

A. Diabetes
B. Basal cell skin cancer
C. Thromboembolic disease
D. Depression
E. Obesity

17. From the choices below, select the most common side effect(s) associated with estrogen replacement.

A. Breast tenderness
B. Depression
C. Nausea
D. Brittle fingernails
E. A and C

18. The Women's Health Initiative study was terminated because HRT increased the risk of all of the following conditions *except*

A. breast cancer.
B. stroke.
C. cardiovascular disease.
D. uterine cancer.
E. pulmonary embolism.

19. Which of the following product dosing regimens is correct?

A. Climara Transdermal: apply to skin once daily.
B. Vagifem: 1 tablet vaginally once daily for 2 weeks; then 1 tablet vaginally twice weekly.
C. Estring: insert ring intravaginally once daily at bedtime.
D. Premarin tablets: 0.625–2.5 mg tid.
E. Premarin vaginal cream: 20–40 g vaginally once daily.

20. Which of the following drug interactions may result in increased pharmacologic effect of estrogen?

A. Macrolide antibiotics
B. Itraconazole
C. Ketoconazole
D. A and C
E. A, B, and C

15-6. Answers

1. **B.** A. J. has neither osteopenia nor osteoporosis with a T score of 1.0. At this point, preventive therapy is appropriate, with adequate calcium and vitamin D intake. Prescription therapy is not indicated at this time.

2. **E.** The appropriate use of Fosamax (alendronate sodium) for prevention of osteoporosis includes a 35 mg weekly or 5 mg daily dose. The 70 mg weekly dose is for treatment of osteoporosis. The medication should be taken with a full glass of water at least 30 minutes prior to ingesting food or other beverages. Patients should remain in the upright position for at least 30 minutes following ingestion of Fosamax.

3. **E.** According to the National Osteoporosis Foundation, adults < 50 years of age require 1,000 mg daily, and those 50 and older should have 1,200 mg daily. The recommended dosage range of daily calcium intake for an adult is 1,000–1,500 mg.

4. **A.** Bisphosphonates are first-line therapy for osteoporosis because data demonstrates that they reduce the risk of fracture.

5. **D.** Injectable and nasal spray dosage forms of calcitonin are available. Teriparatide is available as an injection only. Prempro, raloxifene, and alendronate are available only in oral dosage forms.

6. **D.** Estrogen decreases rather than increases the risk of osteoporosis.

7. **D.** The approved and recommended dose of raloxifene is 60 mg once daily.

8. **E.** Micronor is a progestin-only (minipill) oral contraceptive and is considered compatible with breast-feeding. Depo-Provera is an injectable progestin-only contraceptive option that is considered safe and appropriate for women who desire to breast-feed because it does not affect milk production or adversely affect infant development. Ortho Tri-Cyclen is a combined oral contraceptive that may decrease the quantity of breast milk available and may adversely affect the infant.

9. **C.** Ampicillin may interact with combined oral contraceptives. Although clinical studies have

not consistently demonstrated an interaction, more than 25 case reports of unintended pregnancies have been attributed to concomitant use of ampicillin and oral contraceptives. Concomitant administration of ampicillin, as well as other antibiotics, may decrease the effectiveness of combined oral contraceptives, resulting in pregnancy. The American Medical Association recommends that women be counseled about the potential risk of antibiotics decreasing efficacy of oral contraceptives. If the patient desires, the pharmacist should recommend a backup method of contraception until menses occurs.

10. B. Ortho-Novum 10/11 is a biphasic oral contraceptive.

11. C. Nor-QD is a progestin-only oral contraceptive.

12. D. Too little progestin may result in breakthrough bleeding late in the menstrual cycle. She should be changed to a product with a higher progestin content.

13. E. The highest dose of estrogen (ethinyl estradiol) offered in an oral contraceptive is 50 mcg.

14. B. Fibrocystic breast changes are not a contraindication to using combined oral contraceptives.

15. B. Unopposed estrogen is not recommended in women with an intact uterus because of an increased risk of endometrial hyperplasia and endometrial cancer. Women with an intact uterus should receive a product containing estrogen plus progestin.

16. C. Thromboembolic disease is a definite contraindication to the use of hormone replacement therapy in postmenopausal women.

17. E. Breast tenderness and nausea are the most common side effects associated with estrogen replacement.

18. D. The WHI study was not terminated because of an increased risk of uterine cancer.

19. B. Vagifem dosage is 1 tablet vaginally once daily for 2 weeks; then 1 tablet vaginally twice weekly.

20. E. Macrolide antibiotics, itraconazole, and ketoconazole may result in increased pharmacologic effect of estrogen by inhibiting CYP450 3A4.

15-7. References

Postmenopausal Hormone Replacement Therapy

Kalantaridou SN, Davis SR, Calis KA. Hormone replacement therapy in women. In: Dipiro JT, Talbert RL, Yee GC, et al., eds. *Pharmacotherapy: A Pathophysiologic Approach*. 7th ed. New York: McGraw-Hill; 2008:1351–68.

Klasco RK, ed. DRUGDEX® System (electronic version). Greenwood Village, Colo.: Thomson Micromedex.

Loose DS, Stancel GM. Estrogens and progestins. In: Brunton LL, ed. *Goodman and Gilman's the Pharmacological Basis of Therapeutics*. 11th ed. New York: McGraw-Hill; 2006:1541–71.

North American Menopause Society. Estrogen and progestogen use in postmenopausal women: July 2008 position statement of the North American Menopause Society. *Menopause*. 2008;15:584–602. Available at: www.menopause.org.

O'Mara NB, Tom WC. Estrogen-containing hormone replacement products for postmenopausal women. *Pharmacist's Letter*. 2008;24(12):240407.

O'Neil CK. Health issues in older women. In: Dunsworth T, Richadrson M, Chant C, et al., eds. *Pharmacotherapy Self-Assessment Program*. 6th ed. Book 7: *Women's and Men's Health*. Lenexa, Kans.: American College of Clinical Pharmacy, 2008;143–57.

Parent-Stevens L, Sagraves R. Gynecologic and other disorders of women. In: Koda-Kimble MA, Young LY, eds. *Applied Therapeutics: The Clinical Use of Drugs*. 7th ed. Philadelphia: Lippincott Williams & Wilkins; 2005:48-28 to 48-44.

Warren MP. A comparative review of the risks and benefits of hormone replacement therapy regimens. *Am J Obstet Gynecol*. 2004;190:1141–67.

Contraception

Allen J, Cupp M. Hormonal contraception. *Pharmacist's Letter*. 2007;23(12):231207.

American College of Obstetricians and Gynecologists. The use of hormonal contraception in women with coexisting medical conditions. *Obstet Gynecol*. 2006;107(6):1453–72.

Dickerson LM, Shrader SP, Diaz VA. Contraception. In: Dipiro JT, Talbert RL, Yee GC, et al., eds. *Pharmacotherapy: A Pathophysiologic Approach*. 7th ed. New York: McGraw-Hill; 2008:1313–27.

Hardman JL. Contraception. In: Koda-Kimble MA, Young LY, eds. *Applied Therapeutics: The Clinical Use of Drugs*. 8th ed. Philadelphia: Lippincott Williams & Wilkins; 2005:45-1 to 45-26.

Klasco RK, ed. DRUGDEX® System (electronic version). Greenwood Village, Colo.: Thomson Micromedex.

Osteoporosis

Klasco RK, ed. DRUGDEX® System (electronic version). Greenwood Village, Colo.: Thomson Micromedex.

MacLaughlin EJ, Raehl CL. ASHP therapeutic position statement on the prevention and treatment of osteoporosis in adults. *Am J Health-Syst Pharm.* 2008;65:343–57.

National Osteoporosis Foundation. Clinician's Guide to Prevention and Treatment of Osteoporosis, 2008. Available at: www.nof.org/professionals/Clinicians_Guide.htm.

O'Connell MB, Vondracek SF. Osteoporosis and other metabolic bone diseases. In: Dipiro JT, Talbert RL, Yee GC, et al., eds. *Pharmacotherapy: A Pathophysiologic Approach.* 7th ed. New York: McGraw-Hill; 2008:1483–504.

Kidney Disease 16

Joanna Q. Hudson, PharmD, BCPS, FASN

16-1. Acute Kidney Injury

Acute renal failure, now increasingly referred to as acute kidney injury (AKI), is defined as rapid (hours to days) deterioration of kidney function resulting in azotemia (retention of nitrogenous waste products such as urea) and failure of the kidney to maintain fluid, electrolyte, and acid-base homeostasis.

A reduced urine output is frequently seen: oliguria (urine output < 400 mL/d), anuria (urine output < 50 mL/d), and nonoliguria (urine output > 400 mL/d).

The classification system proposed to distinguish between mild or severe and early or late cases of AKI is known as RIFLE: *R*isk of kidney dysfunction, *I*njury to the kidney, *F*ailure or *L*oss of kidney function, and *E*nd-stage renal disease (ESRD):

- *Risk:* A 1.5-fold increase in the serum creatinine or a decrease of the glomerular filtration rate (GFR) by 25 percent or urine output < 0.5 mL/kg/h for 6 hours
- *Injury:* A twofold increase in the serum creatinine or a decrease of GFR by 50% or urine output < 0.5 mL/kg/h for 12 hours
- *Failure:* A threefold increase in the serum creatinine, a decrease of GFR by 75% or urine output of < 0.5 mL/kg/h for 24 hours, or anuria for 12 hours
- *Loss:* Complete loss of kidney function (e.g., need for renal replacement therapy) for more than 4 weeks
- *ESRD:* Complete loss of kidney function (e.g., need for renal replacement therapy) for more than 3 months

A modification of RIFLE that includes slightly adapted diagnostic criteria and a staging system was proposed by the Acute Kidney Injury Network. The classification or staging system corresponds to risk (stage 1), injury (stage 2), and failure (stage 3) of the RIFLE criteria. Loss and ESRD were removed from the staging system and defined as outcomes.

Epidemiology

Incidence and prevalence

- Community-acquired AKI accounts for 1% of hospital admissions.
- Hospital-acquired AKI occurs in 5–7% of hospitalized patients.

Mortality

- The best prognosis is when renal replacement therapy is not required.
- The mortality rate is 40–50% for patients who require renal replacement therapy.
- The mortality rate is > 50% for patients with multiple organ failure.

Types and Classifications

AKI is classified according to the area of the kidney affected:

- *Prerenal AKI* is characterized by a decrease in perfusion to the kidney with or without systemic arterial hypotension. It is the most common type of AKI and is usually reversible.
- *Intrinsic or intra renal AKI* is the result of structural damage to the parenchymal tissue of the

kidney. It is divided into vascular, glomerular, interstitial, and tubular disorders (most common).

■ *Postrenal AKI* is an obstruction of urine flow occurring at any level of the urinary outflow tracts.

Clinical Presentation

■ Decreased urine output
■ Signs of hypovolemia (prerenal causes), such as tachycardia, decreased venous and arterial pressure, and orthostasis
■ Unique color and composition of urine: cola-colored urine (suggesting bleeding) and foaming (indicating proteinuria)
■ Symptoms of uremia (a clinical syndrome resulting from azotemia), including weakness, shortness of breath, fatigue, mental status changes, nausea and vomiting, bleeding, loss of appetite, and edema
■ Flank pain
■ Increased weight (suggesting fluid accumulation)
■ Increased blood pressure (suggesting fluid accumulation)
■ Signs and symptoms of electrolyte abnormalities (hyperkalemia) and metabolic acidosis (see Chapter 17 on fluids and electrolytes)
■ Bladder distention or prostate enlargement (postrenal causes)
■ Other findings specific to the cause of AKI (see section on pathophysiology)

Pathophysiology and Etiologies

Prerenal AKI

Prerenal AKI is caused by conditions that decrease glomerular hydrostatic pressure, leading to a decrease in GFR (see discussion on etiologies). Hypoperfusion leads to increased sodium and water reabsorption by the kidney and stimulates compensatory mechanisms.

The following compensatory mechanisms increase glomerular hydrostatic pressure and GFR:

■ Vasodilation of the afferent arteriole (mediated primarily by prostaglandins)
■ Vasoconstriction of the efferent arteriole (mediated primarily by angiotensin II)

Alterations in afferent and efferent arteriolar tone can affect compensatory mechanisms. Nonsteroidal anti-inflammatory drugs (NSAIDs) and cyclooxygenase-2 (COX–2) inhibitors can prevent compensatory vasodilation of the afferent arteriole. Angiotensin-converting enzyme inhibitors (ACEIs), angiotensin receptor blockers (ARBs), and renin inhibitors can prevent compensatory vasoconstriction of the efferent arteriole.

Etiologies of prerenal AKI are as follows:

■ Intravascular volume depletion related to excessive diuresis, vomiting, excessive gastrointestinal (GI) fluid loss, and bleeding
■ Severe hypotension
■ Decreased effective blood volume (volume sensed by arterial baroreceptors) as occurs with congestive heart failure, cirrhosis, nephrotic syndrome, and hepatorenal syndrome
■ Systemic vasodilatation as occurs with sepsis, liver failure, and anaphylaxis
■ Large-vessel renal vascular disease, including renal artery thrombosis or embolism and renal artery stenosis
■ Medications (see Table 16-1).

Intrinsic acute renal failure

The primary anatomic sites of the kidney are prone to structural damage from prolonged ischemia and direct toxicity because of the high metabolic activity and concentrating ability of the kidney.

Etiologies by anatomic site are as follows:

■ *Vascular:* Inflammation and emboli
■ *Glomerular (glomerulonephritis):* Systemic lupus erythematosus and medications (see Table 16-1)
■ *Interstitial:* Ischemia, allergic interstitial nephritis, infections, and medications (see Table 16-1)
■ *Tubular—accounts for 90% of intrinsic cases:* Intrarenal vasoconstriction, direct tubular toxicity, and intratubular obstruction; prolonged ischemia from prerenal causes; and toxins
■ *Endogenous:* Myoglobin, hemoglobin, and uric acid
■ *Exogenous:* Medications (see Table 16-1; aminoglycosides are common nephrotoxins leading to nonoliguric AKI after 5–7 days of therapy); radiocontrast-induced AKI; other causes such as ethylene glycol and pesticides

Postrenal acute kidney disease

This disease is an obstruction of urinary flow at any level from the urinary collecting system to the urethra. It must involve both kidneys (or one kidney in a patient with a single functioning kidney).

Etiologies by anatomic site are as follows:

■ *Renal pelves or tubules:* Crystal deposition
■ *Ureteral:* Tumor, stricture, and stones
■ *Bladder neck obstruction:* Prostatic hypertrophy and bladder carcinoma
■ *Medications:* See Table 16-1.

Table 16-1. Drug-Induced Causes of Kidney Disease

Clinical syndrome	Causative drugs[a]
Prerenal kidney disease	ACEIs, ARBs, COX-2 inhibitors, cyclosporine, diuretics, NSAIDs, radiocontrast dye, renin inhibitors, and tacrolimus
Intrinsic kidney disease	
Vascular	Amphetamines, cisplatin, cyclosporine, and mitomycin C
Glomerular	Gold, heroin, lithium, NSAIDs, and phenytoin
Interstitial nephritis	Analgesic combinations, aristolochic acid (Chinese herbs), cyclosporine, lithium, NSAIDs, penicillins, sulfonamides, and tacrolimus
Acute tubular necrosis	Aminoglycosides, amphotericin B, chemotherapeutic agents, cidofovir, cocaine, foscarnet, ifosfamide, radiocontrast dye, and tacrolimus
Postrenal kidney disease	
Obstructive	Acyclovir, methotrexate, oxalate, sulfonamides, and uric acid
Nephrolithiasis	Allopurinol, indinavir, sulfadiazine, and triamterene

a. This list does not include all potential nephrotoxins.

Diagnostic Criteria

Table 16-2 shows the diagnostic tests and the findings associated with AKI. A diagnosis requires the following steps:

- *Evaluate physical findings:* Assess for signs and symptoms listed in clinical presentation.
- *Take medication history (including OTC medication and herbals):* Identify potentially nephrotoxic agents (Table 16-1).
- *Estimate GFR:* Normal is 100–125 mL/min/1.73 m².
  - Consider limitations in using serum creatinine as a marker of kidney function (e.g., conditions of poor muscle mass) and in using equations to estimate GFR in patients with unstable kidney function.

- Other assessment equations and methods (e.g., Jelliffe equation) are available to estimate GFR in patients with unstable kidney function.

Creatinine clearance

Creatinine clearance (CrCl) is measured using urine collection methods:

$$CrCl = \frac{U_{Cr} \times V}{S_{Cr} \times t}$$

where U_{Cr} = urinary creatinine concentration (mg/dL)
V = volume of urine (mL)
S_{Cr} = serum creatinine concentration (mg/dL)
t = time period of urine collection (minutes)

Table 16-2. Laboratory Findings to Differentiate Prerenal and Intrinsic Kidney Disease

Diagnostic test	Prerenal kidney disease	Intrinsic kidney disease
BUN:Cr ratio	> 20:1	< 15:1
Urinalysis	Normal with few cells or casts (hyaline casts normal)	Granular casts with tubular epithelial cells
Urine osmolality	> 500 mOsm/kg	≤ 300–350 mOsm/kg
Urinary Cr:Plasma Cr ratio	> 40:1	< 20:1
Specific gravity	> 1.020	< 1.015
Urine sodium	< 20 mEq/L	> 40 mEq/L
FE_Na	< 1%	> 2%

Note: BUN, blood urea nitrogen; CR, creatinine; FE_Na, fractional excretion of sodium.

CrCl is estimated using the Cockcroft–Gault equation (assumes stable kidney function):

$$CrCl = \frac{(140 - age)(BW \text{ in kg})}{72 \times S_{Cr}(\text{mg/dL})}$$

where BW = body weight in kg. Ideal body weight is recommended if patient's body weight is more than 30% above the ideal body weight. Multiply the result of the Cockcroft–Gault equation by 0.85 for females.

Blood tests

- *Elevated:* Blood urea nitrogen (BUN), serum creatinine, and electrolytes (potassium and phosphorus)
- *Decreased:* Calcium (consider albumin concentration) and bicarbonate

Urinalysis

- An elevated specific gravity and osmolality are indicative of prerenal causes and stimulation of sodium and water retention.
- Proteinuria includes microalbuminuria (> 30 mg/d), overt proteinuria (> 300 mg/d), and nephrotic range proteinuria (> 3 g/d).
- Hematuria is indicated by red blood cells.
- Glucose and ketones may be present.
- Urine sediment consisting of granular casts and cellular debris suggests structural damage.
- White blood cells suggest inflammation.
- Eosinophils are associated with acute allergic interstitial nephritis.
- Consider whether fluids or diuretics were previously administered when interpreting urinalysis.

Urine chemistries

Evaluate urine sodium, potassium, chloride, creatinine, and urinary anion gap.

Fractional excretion of sodium (FE_{Na}) is useful to differentiate prerenal AKI from acute intrinsic kidney injury. A low value (< 1%) suggests retention of sodium and water (prerenal etiology) versus intrinsic cause.

$$FE_{Na} = \frac{U_{Na} \times P_{Cr} \times 100}{U_{Cr} \times P_{Na}}$$

where U_{Na} = urine sodium
U_{Cr} = urine creatinine

P_{Cr} = plasma creatinine
P_{Na} = plasma sodium

Other tests

Radiographic procedures include ultrasound, plain film radiograph, radioisotope scan, and computed tomography.

Renal biopsy is indicated for patients without cause of AKI identified by other diagnostic tests.

Treatment Principles and Goals

Prevention

Risk factors must be identified:

- Volume depletion
- Exposure to nephrotoxic medications
- Preexisting kidney or hepatic disease

Surgical procedures can be a risk factor. Consider baseline kidney function, age, cardiovascular status, and volume status.

Diagnostic tests requiring radiocontrast media can put patients at risk. Risk factors for contrast nephropathy are diabetes, heart failure, age > 75, and an estimated GFR < 60 mL/min/1.73 m². In addition to being given hydration, high-risk patients should receive oral acetylcysteine (Mucomyst) 600 mg twice daily for 2 days beginning the day before exposure to radiocontrast dye. Bicarbonate may also be added to the hydration fluid.

Treatment Goals

- Correct underlying causes of AKI (e.g., discontinue nephrotoxic agents, correct fluid status, treat underlying infection, and address cause of urinary tract obstructions).
- Return to baseline kidney function or highest kidney function possible.
- Prevent development of chronic kidney disease and the need for chronic renal replacement therapies (dialysis or transplantation).
- Avoid nephrotoxic agents or take measures to reduce exposure if possible.
- Adjust doses of medications on the basis of kidney function.
- Avoid agents contraindicated in patients with kidney disease, such as metformin (Glucophage).
- Address complications of AKI, such as electrolyte abnormalities (hyperkalemia), fluid overload, metabolic acidosis (see Chapter 17 on fluids and electrolytes), hyperphosphatemia (see Section 16-2 on chronic kidney disease).

Strategies for treatment

- Address underlying cause of AKI.
- Provide supportive care with diuretic therapy (loop diuretics) and replacement fluids as needed to maintain hemodynamic stability.

Drug Therapy

Diuretics

Select diuretics are shown in Table 16-3.

Mechanism of action

Loop diuretics are delivered to the tubular lumen of the kidney by proximal tubular cells and cause inhibition of sodium and chloride reabsorption in the thick ascending limb of the loop of Henle to promote water excretion.

Osmotic diuretics are freely filtered into the tubular lumen in the proximal tubule and increase the osmolarity of the glomerular filtrate, which inhibits tubular reabsorption of water and electrolytes and increases urinary output.

Thiazide and thiazide-like diuretics inhibit the Na^+-Cl^- cotransport in the early distal convoluted tubules. They are generally used in combination with loop diuretics for resistant edema and fluid overload, particularly metolazone, which is effective at GFRs < 30 mL/min. Other thiazide diuretics are generally not effective when GFR is < 30 mL/min.

Adverse drug events

Loop diuretics

Adverse drug events are as follows:

- Hypokalemia, hypomagnesemia, hyponatremia, hypovolemia, hyperuricemia, and hyperglycemia
- Hypercalciuria
- Orthostatic hypotension and dehydration
- Metabolic alkalosis (partly attributable to extracellular fluid volume contraction)
- Ototoxicity
- Diarrhea and nausea

Furosemide, bumetanide, and torsemide have a sulfonamide substituent (potential for hypersensitivity reactions). Ethacrynic acid is generally reserved for patients allergic to sulfa compounds.

Table 16-3. Diuretics as Drug Therapy for AKI by Drug Classification

Generic name	Trade name	Daily dosage range	Dosage forms	Frequency of administration
Loop diuretics[a]				
Furosemide	Lasix	20–400 mg	po	q 6–12 hours
		20–200 mg (up to 1–3 g/d in AKI)	IV	
Bumetanide	Bumex	0.5–10 mg	po, IV	q 12–24 hours
Torsemide	Demadex	10–200 mg	po, IV	q 24 hours
Ethacrynic acid	Edecrin	50–400 mg	po	q 8–12 hours
		50–100 mg	IV	
Osmotic diuretics				
Mannitol	Osmitrol, Resectisol	Initial test dose: 12.5–25 g over 3–5 minutes; maintenance dose: 0.25–0.5 g/kg (20–200 g/d)	IV	q 4–6 hours
Thiazide				
Hydrochlorothiazide	Microzide	25–200 mg	po	qd, bid
Chlorothiazide	Diuril	500 mg–2 g	po	qd, bid
		250–1,000 mg	IV	
Thiazide-like diuretics				
Metolazone	Zaroxolyn	5–20 mg	po	qd

a. Loop diuretics are also administered as a continuous infusion. Higher dose ranges for intermittent dosing are reserved for patients who are unresponsive to initial smaller doses.

Osmotic diuretics

The following adverse drug events may occur:

- Acute expansion of extracellular fluid volume and increased risk of pulmonary edema
- Acute rise in serum K^+, nausea and vomiting, headache, blurred vision, and rash

Thiazide and thiazide-like diuretics

Adverse drug events include the following:

- Hypokalemia, hyponatremia, and hypercalcemia
- Hypovolemia and orthostatic hypotension
- Hyperglycemia, hypochloremic alkalosis, and hyperlipidemia
- Hypersensitivity reactions from sulfonamide substituents
- Chest pain (metolazone; more common with Mykrox, which is more rapidly and extensively absorbed than Zaroxolyn)

Drug–drug and drug–disease interactions

- Loop diuretics and aminoglycosides have an increased potential for ototoxicity.
- Diuretics and other nephrotoxins have an increased risk of nephrotoxicity if hypovolemia occurs.
- Diuretics and lithium used concomitantly may result in decreased renal clearance of lithium. Monitor lithium concentrations more closely.
- For diuretics and digoxin, hypokalemia from diuretic use may increase risk of toxicity with digoxin. Monitor potassium and digoxin.
- Loop and thiazide diuretics may increase gout attacks because of hyperuricemia.
- For thiazide diuretics and diabetes, hyperglycemia may result from thiazides. Increase glucose monitoring.
- The following conditions decrease secretion of the diuretic to its site of action in the renal tubule:
  - Proteinuria (diuretic binds to protein and is not available at its site of action)
  - Decreased renal blood flow
  - Competitive inhibition of transport system (NSAIDs, probenecid, and cephalosporins)

Parameters to monitor

- Blood pressure (sitting and standing), pulse, urine output, fluid intake, serum creatinine, serum electrolytes, blood urea nitrogen, bicarbonate, calcium, glucose, and uric acid
- In the case of osmotic diuretics, serum osmolality (310–320 mOsm/kg); assess urine output after initial test dose (goal urine flow is at least 30–50 mL/h)

Pharmacokinetics

Loop diuretics

- **Oral bioavailability:** Furosemide (60%), bumetanide (85%), and torsemide (85%)
- **Oral:intravenous dose ratios:** Furosemide (1.5), bumetanide (1), and torsemide (1)
- **Equivalent doses:** 1 mg bumetanide = 20 mg torsemide = 40 mg furosemide
- **Elimination route:** Furosemide (primarily renal), bumetanide (hepatic and renal), torsemide (primarily hepatic), and ethacrynic acid (hepatic and renal)

Thiazide and thiazide-like diuretics

Metolazone absorption differs between brands. Mykrox (available outside the United States) is more rapidly and extensively absorbed than Zaroxolyn.

Other factors

Patients with kidney disease generally require larger doses of diuretics to achieve adequate concentrations of the drug at the site of action in the kidney.

The brands of metolazone (Zaroxolyn and Mykrox) are not bioequivalent and should not be interchanged.

Dopamine

The use of dopamine in AKI is controversial because benefits have not consistently been demonstrated.

Nondrug Therapy

Fluid management

Fluid intake and output should be evaluated and adjustments made to maintain hemodynamic stability (consider sensible and insensible losses).

Fluid selection (e.g., crystalloids, colloids, or normal saline) and rate of correction depend on the clinical condition of the patient.

Nutritional therapy

A high-calorie diet is generally required (patient-specific).

Restriction of sodium, potassium, and phosphorus should be considered.

Renal replacement therapies

Renal replacement therapies are procedures by which the blood is artificially cleared of waste and some essential metabolic products to augment the function of failed or failing kidneys. They include hemodialysis and hemofiltration, in which the semipermeable membrane is a dialyzer, and peritoneal dialysis, in which the peritoneal cavity serves as this membrane. Procedures may be intermittent or continuous. Hemodialysis and hemofiltration are the most common modalities for patients with AKI. Kidney transplantation is also considered a form of renal replacement therapy.

The potential for drug removal by dialysis must be considered.

Indications for renal replacement therapy

Any of the following refractory to more conservative measures are indications for renal replacement therapy:

- Acidosis
- Electrolyte abnormalities (hyperkalemia)
- Intoxication (drug-induced kidney failure), if drug can be removed by dialysis
- Volume overload
- Uremia (BUN >100 mg/dL) or uremic symptoms (pericarditis, encephalopathy, bleeding, dyscrasia, nausea, vomiting, and pruritus)

16-2. Chronic Kidney Disease

Chronic kidney disease (CKD) is kidney damage with or without a decrease in GFR or a GFR < 60 mL/min/1.73 m^2 for ≥ 3 months. *Kidney damage* is defined as pathologic abnormalities or markers of damage, including abnormalities in blood or urine tests or in imaging studies.

CKD is classified into five stages on the basis of kidney damage and GFR (Table 16-4). End-stage renal disease occurs when patients require renal replacement therapy (either dialysis or transplantation) to sustain life.

Epidemiology of Chronic Kidney Disease

Incidence and prevalence

Approximately 26 million American adults have CKD. The number of patients with CKD continues to increase, with a 50% increase in the number of patients with ESRD expected by 2020. The incidence of CKD is approximately four times higher in the African American population. The incidence is greatest in individuals age 45–64.

Approximately 500,000 patients are being treated for ESRD (including patients receiving hemodialysis, peritoneal dialysis, and transplantation).

Mortality

Life expectancy is four to five times shorter in dialysis patients than in the general population. The primary causes of death in the ESRD population are cardiovascular diseases and infection. Comorbidities, estimated GFR, and albumin at initiation of dialysis are strong predictors of mortality in the dialysis population.

Clinical Presentation

- Changes in urine output (may not occur in earlier stages of CKD)
- Foaming of urine, which indicates proteinuria (Table 16-5):
  - *Microalbuminuria:* Albumin in the urine in amounts of 30–300 mg/d

Table 16-4. Stages of Chronic Kidney Disease

Stage	Description	GFR (mL/min/1.73 m^2)	Action
—	Increased risk	≥ 90 (with CKD risk factors)	Screening and CKD risk reduction
1	Kidney damage with normal or increased GFR	≥ 90	Diagnosis and treatment, treatment of comorbid conditions, slowing of progression, and cardiovascular disease risk reduction
2	Kidney damage with mildly decreased GFR	60–89	Estimation of progression
3	Moderately decreased GFR	30–59	Evaluation and treatment of complications
4	Severely decreased GFR	15–29	Preparation for kidney replacement therapy
5	Kidney failure (defined as ESRD if renal replacement therapy is needed)	< 15 (or need for renal replacement therapy)	Renal replacement therapy (if uremia is present)

Table 16-5. Definitions of Proteinuria and Albuminuria

Condition	Total protein			Albumin		
	24-hour collection (mg/d)	Spot urine dipstick (mg/dL)	Spot urine protein: Cr ratio (mg/g)	24-hour collection (mg/d)	Spot urine dipstick (mg/dL)	Spot urine albumin: Cr ratio (mg/g)
Normal	< 300	< 30	< 200	< 30	< 3	< 17 (men); < 25 (women)
Microalbuminuria	n.a.	n.a.	n.a.	30–300	> 3	17–250 (men); 25–355 (women)
Albuminuria or clinical proteinuria	> 300	> 30	> 200	> 300	n.a.	> 250 (men); > 355 (women)

Note: n.a., not applicable.

- *Albuminuria:* Albumin in the urine in amounts > 300 mg/d
  - *Clinical proteinuria: Total* protein (in addition to albumin) in the urine in amounts > 300 mg/d
- Increased blood pressure (hypertension is a common etiology and result of CKD)
- Signs and symptoms of hyperglycemia and glucosuria (diabetes is a common etiology)
- Signs and symptoms associated with fluid and electrolyte abnormalities (e.g., hyperkalemia and fluid overload; see Chapter 17 on fluids and electrolytes)
- Development of secondary complications of CKD:
  - *Anemia:* Decreased hemoglobin and hematocrit, iron deficiency common
  - *CKD mineral and bone disorder:* Increased serum phosphorus, decreased serum calcium (at risk for hypercalcemia as kidney disease progresses), increased intact parathyroid hormone (iPTH), and vitamin D deficiency
  - *Metabolic acidosis:* Decreased serum bicarbonate and increased anion gap
  - *Malnutrition:* Decreased albumin and prealbumin (see Chapter 19 on nutrition)
- Signs of uremia (see Section 16-1) in later stages of CKD (stages 4 and 5 CKD)

Pathophysiology of Progressive Kidney Disease and Selected Secondary Complications

Progressive kidney disease

Progressive loss of nephron function results in adaptive changes in remaining nephrons to increase single nephron glomerular filtration pressure. Over time, the compensatory increase in single nephron GFR leads to hypertrophy from sustained increases in pressure and loss of individual nephron function.

Proteinuria, one of the initial diagnostic signs, may also contribute to the progressive decline in kidney function. Loss of kidney function is usually irreversible.

Etiology of progressive kidney disease
Each of the following may result in damage to the kidney that leads, over time, to a decrease in functioning nephrons and in total GFR:

- Diabetes (accounts for primary cause in 44% of patients with ESRD)
- Hypertension (accounts for primary cause in 26% of patients with ESRD)
- Glomerulonephritis
- Cystic kidney disease
- HIV (human immunodeficiency virus) nephropathy
- Other contributing factors (smoking, obesity, genetic factors, and gender differences)

Anemia of chronic kidney disease

The primary etiology is a decrease in production of the hormone erythropoietin by the kidney as kidney disease progresses. More than 90% of erythropoietin production occurs in the kidney and approximately 10% in the liver.

CKD results in a normochromic, normocytic anemia. Red blood cell lifespan is also decreased from 120 days to approximately 60 days in patients with kidney failure. Other contributors include iron deficiency and blood loss (e.g., from uremic bleeding, dialysis).

CKD Mineral and Bone Disorder

As kidney function declines, phosphorus elimination decreases. Hyperphosphatemia causes a reciprocal decrease in serum calcium concentrations (hypocalcemia). Hypocalcemia stimulates the release of iPTH by the parathyroid glands.

Conversion of the vitamin D precursor to the active form (1,25-dihydroxyvitamin D_3) occurs in the kidney. As kidney disease progresses, there is a decline in the 1α-hydroxylase enzyme that promotes the final hydroxylation step in the kidney, resulting in a deficiency in active vitamin D. Deficiencies in the precursor form of vitamin D have also been observed in stages 3 and 4 CKD. Active vitamin D (1,25-dihydroxyvitamin D_3) promotes increased intestinal absorption of calcium and suppresses production of parathyroid hormone by the parathyroid gland; therefore, vitamin D deficiency leads to worsening secondary hyperparathyroidism.

Increased iPTH promotes the following:

- Decreased phosphorus reabsorption within the kidney
- Increased calcium reabsorption by the kidney
- Increased calcium mobilization from bone

As kidney disease progresses, the following occur:

- Hyperphosphatemia and subsequent hypocalcemia progressively worsen, and secondary hyperparathyroidism becomes more severe.
- The renal effects of PTH on phosphorus and calcium are no longer maintained, and PTH predominantly stimulates calcium resorption from bone.
- Decreased production of active vitamin D worsens hypocalcemia and secondary hyperparathyroidism.
  - In more severe CKD (stages 4 and 5), patients are prone to develop hypercalcemia, in part because of the use of calcium-containing phosphate binders.
  - Patients with stage 5 CKD are at risk for calcifications and calciphylaxis.
- Uncontrolled secondary hyperparathyroidism leads to hyperplasia of the parathyroid gland and renal osteodystrophy (from sustained effects of iPTH on bone).

Metabolic acidosis

- Decreased excretion of acid by the kidney
- Accumulation of endogenous acids attributable to impaired kidney function (e.g., phosphates and sulfates)

Diagnostic Criteria

Progressive kidney disease

There is a progressive increase in serum creatinine: > 1.1–1.2 mg/dL for females and > 1.2–1.3 mg/dL for males. Consider factors that may alter serum creatinine, such as decreased muscle mass and nutritional status.

There is a decreased GFR (see Table 16-4 for CKD classifications). Consider the assessment method used:

- Measured creatinine clearance (see discussion of diagnostic criteria for acute kidney injury in Section 16-1)
- Cockcroft–Gault equation (see discussion of diagnostic criteria for acute kidney injury in Section 16-1)
- Modification of diet in renal disease abbreviated equation

$$GFR = 186 \times (\text{serum creatinine})^{-1.154}$$
$$\times (\text{age in years})^{-0.203}$$
$$\times 1.210 (\text{if patient is black})$$
$$\times 0.742 (\text{if patient is female})$$

- Schwartz equation (children)

$$CrCl(mL/min) = \frac{k \times \text{length} (\text{in centimeters})}{\text{serum creatinine}}$$

where $k = 0.55$ for children aged 1–13 years

- Microalbuminuria, albuminuria, or clinical proteinuria (Table 16-5)
- Abnormal serum chemistries:
  - Increased serum creatinine and BUN
  - Increased potassium, decreased serum bicarbonate, increased phosphorus, and decreased calcium (indicative of secondary complications)
- Development of secondary complications (e.g., anemia, CKD mineral and bone disorder, and fluid and electrolyte abnormalities)

Anemia of chronic kidney disease

Testing for anemia is recommended in all patients with CKD. Guidelines for anemia management in patients with CKD recommend further evaluation for anemia when hemoglobin is < 12 g/dL in females and < 13.5 g/dL in males.

For iron deficiency, evaluate red blood cell indices and iron indices to identify iron deficiency as a contributing factor; iron deficiency manifests as a microcytic anemia.

- Red blood cell count: < 4.2×10^6 cells per mm^2
- Mean corpuscular volume: < 80 femoliters

- Serum iron: < 50 mg/dL
- Total iron binding capacity: < 250 mg/dL
- Transferrin saturation (TSat): < 16%
- Serum ferritin: < 12 ng/mL

Transferrin saturation and serum ferritin should be maintained at higher values for CKD patients receiving erythropoietin therapy (TSat > 20% and serum ferritin >100 ng/mL for CKD patients not on dialysis and for peritoneal dialysis patients; and TSat > 20% and serum ferritin >200 ng/mL for hemodialysis patients).

Evaluate for folate and vitamin B_{12} deficiencies (manifests as a macrocytic anemia), sources of blood loss (e.g., GI bleeding), and confounding disease states (e.g., cancer and HIV).

CKD Mineral and Bone Disorder

- Serum phosphorus: > 4.6 mg/dL (> 5.5 mg/dL in stage 5 CKD)
- Calcium abnormalities:
  - Hypocalcemia: Corrected serum calcium < 8.5 mg/dL
  - Hypercalcemia (a concern in stages 4 and 5 CKD): Corrected calcium = measured serum calcium + 0.8 × (normal serum albumin – measured serum albumin); normal serum albumin = 4.0 g/dL
- Elevated calcium × phosphorus product: > 55 mg^2/dL^2 (elevated product increases risk for metastatic calcifications)
- Intact parathyroid hormone: > 70 pg/mL (stage 3 CKD), > 110 pg/mL (stage 4 CKD), and > 300 pg/mL (stage 5 CKD)
- Radiographic evidence of bone abnormalities (e.g., osteitis fibrosa cystica)

Metabolic acidosis

Serum bicarbonate (HCO_3^-) is < 20 mEq/L.

Typically have an increased anion gap: anion gap = $[Na^+] - ([Cl^-] + [HCO_3^-])$.

Signs and symptoms of chronic metabolic acidosis that develop as CKD progresses are generally not of the same magnitude as those of acute metabolic acidosis (e.g., hyperventilation, cardiovascular and central nervous system manifestations).

Treatment Principles and Goals

Progressive kidney disease

Treatment principles

- Control underlying cause of progressive CKD (e.g., diabetes and hypertension; see Chapters 8 and 13, respectively).

- Meet blood pressure goal: < 130/80 mm Hg for patients with evidence of kidney disease and/or diabetes.
- Prevent or minimize microalbuminuria or proteinuria.
- Slow the rate of progression of CKD (by achieving diabetes and hypertension goals and minimizing proteinuria).
- Prevent drug-induced causes of kidney disease:
  - Avoid chronic use of combinations of analgesics.
  - Minimize use of agents known to cause AKI (patients can develop an acute-on-chronic kidney disease).
- Manage secondary complications of CKD (anemia, mineral and bone disorders, and electrolyte abnormalities).
- Control hyperlipidemia.
- Address cardiovascular risk factors (cardiovascular disease is the leading cause of death in the CKD population).
- Adjust drug doses on the basis of kidney function.
- Avoid medications contraindicated in patients with reduced kidney function. For example, metformin (Glucophage) is contraindicated in patients with elevated serum creatinine (> 1.5 mg/dL for men and > 1.4 mg/dL for women) because of the increased risk of lactic acidosis.
- Prepare patient for renal replacement therapy (i.e., dialysis and transplantation) as needed.
- Start dialysis if stable GFR < 15 mL/min/1.73 m^2 and based on other indications (see Section 16-2 on indications for renal replacement therapy).
- Recommend smoking cessation.

Treatment strategies

- Diuretics for fluid balance and management of hypertension (diuretic selection based on kidney function)
- Antihypertensives with diet and lifestyle modifications for control of blood pressure (see Chapter 8 on hypertension)
- Antidiabetic agents with diet and lifestyle modifications for control of blood glucose (see Chapter 13 on diabetes)
- ACEIs and ARBs to delay progression of kidney disease (recommended for patients with diabetes and individuals with hypertension and proteinuria; see Table 16-5)
- Protein restriction to 0.6–0.8 g/kg/d:
  - Consider for patients with > 1 g/d proteinuria despite optimal blood pressure control with a regimen that includes an ACEI or ARB.
  - Be cautious about maintaining adequate caloric intake and avoid malnutrition.

- Do not implement for patients < 80% of their ideal body weight or with > 10 g/d proteinuria.
- Renal replacement therapy:
  - Consider plans for dialysis therapy (hemodialysis or peritoneal dialysis) during stage 4 CKD (when GFR < 30 mL/min) (see Section 16-2 for general description of dialysis).
  - Evaluate candidacy for kidney transplantation.

Anemia of chronic kidney disease

Target hemoglobin is 11–12 g/dL, and target hematocrit is 33–36% (based on the Kidney Disease Outcome Quality Initiative Guidelines). *Note:* The FDA labeling for all erythropoietic stimulating agents states the goal hemoglobin as 10–12 g/dL.

Iron indices are transferrin saturation > 20% and serum ferritin > 100 ng/mL for CKD patients not on dialysis and for peritoneal dialysis patients. The goal for serum ferritin in hemodialysis patients is > 200 ng/mL). *Note:* Ferritin is an acute phase reactant and may be elevated during conditions of infection or inflammation.

Treatment strategies
Erythropoietic stimulating agents
Erythropoietic stimulating agents (ESAs) stimulate red blood cell production in the bone marrow.

ESAs may be administered subcutaneously (SC) or intravenously (IV). SC is generally preferred for patients not on hemodialysis (i.e., peritoneal dialysis and early stage CKD patients who do not have IV access).

Epoetin alfa (Epogen and Procrit): Initial doses are 50–100 units/kg IV or SC three times per week.

Darbepoetin alfa (Aranesp): Initial dose is 0.45 mcg/kg IV or SC administered once weekly. Alternatively, for patients not on dialysis, an initial dose of 0.75 mcg/kg may be administered SC every two weeks.

Dose conversion is from epoetin alfa (units/week) to darbepoetin alfa (mcg/week)(Table 16-6).

The darbepoetin package insert states that for patients receiving epoetin alfa 2–3 times per week, darbepoetin alfa should be administered weekly. For patients receiving epoetin alfa once per week, darbepoetin alfa should be administered once every two weeks. In this situation, the weekly epoetin dose should be multiplied by 2 and that dose should be used in Table 16-6 to determine the appropriate darbepoetin dose.

For dose titration, allow at least 2–4 weeks before making a change in the dose of epoetin alfa or darbepoetin alfa based on the change in hemoglobin or hematocrit. If a change in hemoglobin is < 1 g/dL in a 4-week period and iron stores are adequate, increase the ESA dose by 25%. If a change in hemoglobin is > 1 g/dL in a 2-week period, or the hemoglobin is approaching 12 g/dL, reduce the ESA dose by 25%.

Table 16-6. Estimated Starting Doses of Darbepoetin Alfa Based on Previous Epoetin Alfa Dose

Epoetin alfa dose (units/wk)	Darbepoetin alfa dose (mcg/wk)	
	Adult	Pediatric
< 1,500	6.25	—a
1,500–2,499	6.25	6.25
2,500–4,999	12.5	10.0
5,000–10,999	25.0	20.0
11,000–17,999	40.0	40.0
18,000–33,999	60.0	60.0
34,000–89,999	100.0	100.0
≥ 90,000	200.0	200.0

a. Insufficient data.

Iron supplementation
Iron supplementation prevents iron deficiency as a cause of resistance to therapy with erythropoietic stimulating agents. Iron deficiency should be corrected prior to making changes in the dose of the erythropoietic stimulating agent.

Oral iron supplementation is limited by poor absorption and is often inadequate to achieve goal iron indices. It may be reasonable for stages 3 and 4 CKD patients and the peritoneal dialysis population (patients without IV access). The recommended dose is 200 mg elemental iron per day.

Intravenous iron supplementation is preferred for treatment of absolute iron deficiency and in hemodialysis patients with regular intravenous access. One may administer a full course of iron, typically a total dose of 1 g divided over 8–10 hemodialysis sessions (100 mg per dose for iron sucrose [Venofer] and iron dextran [InFeD and Dexferrum] or 125 mg per dose for sodium ferric gluconate [Ferrlecit]). Weekly doses of 25–125 mg may be administered as maintenance doses of iron in hemodialysis patients.

- ***Iron sucrose:*** The 100 mg dose may be diluted in 100 mL of 0.9% NaCl (sodium chloride) administered IV over at least 15 minutes or administered undiluted over 2–5 minutes.

■ *Iron dextran:* The 100 mg dose may be administered over 2 minutes IV push. One must administer a 25 mg test dose because of the risk of anaphylactic reactions.

■ *Sodium ferric gluconate:* The 125-mg dose may be diluted in 100 mL of 0.9% NaCl and administered IV over 1 hour or administered undiluted as an IV injection at a rate up to 12.5 mg/min. Dosing in pediatric patients is 1.5 mg/kg in 25 mL of 0.9% NaCl over 60 minutes (maximum dose 125 mg).

IV iron regimens differ in peritoneal dialysis patients and patients with CKD not requiring dialysis. A total dose of 1 g is recommended for iron-deficient patients, administered in divided doses. Iron sucrose has an approved regimen in these populations.

The approved dosing regimen for iron sucrose in nondialysis CKD patients is 200 mg over 2–5 minutes on five different occasions within a 14-day period. Peritoneal dialysis patients should receive 300 mg in 0.9% NaCl administered IV over 1.5 hours, followed by a second infusion of 300 mg 14 days later and then by a 400 mg dose administered over 2.5 hours 14 days later.

Ferumoxytol (Feraheme) is an IV form of iron approved in 2009 for treatment of iron deficiency anemia in adults with chronic kidney disease. The approved dose is 510 mg (17 mL) as a single dose, followed by a second 510 mg dose 3–8 days after the initial dose.

Blood transfusions may be required for more severe anemia or when blood loss is a major contributing factor.

CKD Mineral and Bone Disorder

■ Goal serum phosphorus is 2.7–4.6 mg/dL for stages 3 and 4 CKD and 3.5–5.5 mg/dL for stage 5 CKD.
■ Goal serum corrected calcium is approximately 8.5–10 mg/dL (normal range) for stages 3 and 4 CKD and 8.4–9.5 mg/dL for stage 5 CKD (recommend a lower range in stage 5 CKD because of risk of hypercalcemia and calcifications).
■ Calcium × phosphorus product is < 55 mg^2/dL^2.
■ Goal iPTH is as follows:
  • *Stage 3 CKD:* iPTH 35–70 pg/mL
  • *Stage 4 CKD:* iPTH 70–110 pg/mL
  • *Stage 5 CKD:* iPTH 150–300 pg/mL

Treatment strategies
■ Follow a dietary phosphorus restriction of 800–1,000 mg/d phosphorus (consult with dietitian).

■ Use phosphate binding agents—elemental (calcium, lanthanum, aluminum, and magnesium) and nonelemental (sevelemer):
  • Titrate doses on the basis of phosphorus and calcium × phosphorus product.
  • Limit use of calcium-containing phosphate binders if hypercalcemia occurs.
  • Aluminum is not a first-line agent; prescribe it only if needed for short-term use (< 30 days) to minimize the risk of accumulation.
■ Remove phosphorus by dialysis for ESRD patients. Continue phosphorus restriction and use of phosphate binding agents with dialysis.
■ Maintain goal calcium and phosphorus concentrations.
■ Provide vitamin D supplementation depending on the stage of CKD. Supplementation with the active form (calcitriol) or a vitamin D analog (doxercalciferol or paricalcitol) may be necessary in more severe stages of CKD (stages 4 and 5). Supplementation with a vitamin D precursor (e.g., ergocalciferol) may be sufficient in earlier stages.
■ Use a calcimimetic agent (cinacalcet [Sensipar]) to help control iPTH in ESRD patients. Initial dose is 30 mg po daily. The dose of cinacalcet should be titrated no more frequently than every 2–4 weeks through sequential doses of 60, 90, 120, and 180 mg once daily to target iPTH (150–300 pg/mL).
■ Control metabolic acidosis (which causes bone demineralization if not controlled).

Metabolic acidosis

■ *Serum bicarbonate:* 22–26 mEq/L
■ *pH:* 7.35–7.45

Treatment strategies
■ *Administration of sodium bicarbonate or other alkali preparation:* Gradual correction (over days to weeks) is usually appropriate for asymptomatic patients with mild to moderate acidosis (serum bicarbonate 12–20 mEq/L and pH 7.2–7.4).
■ *Dialysis:* Bicarbonate or lactate contained within the dialysate solution diffuses from dialysate to plasma and effectively treats metabolic acidosis.

Monitoring
Progressive kidney disease

■ Patients at high risk for CKD (e.g., patients with diabetes or hypertension) or patients diagnosed with CKD should have the following monitored regularly:

- *Serum creatinine:* Consider limitations.
- *Estimated GFR:* Assess rate of progression (mL/min per year).
- *Proteinuria:* Monitor annually in patients with type 1 diabetes with diabetes duration of ≥ 5 years and at diagnosis for patients with type 2 diabetes.
- *Serum electrolytes:* Assess levels.
- *Blood pressure:* Assess in individuals with hypertension.
- *Blood glucose:* Assess in individuals with diabetes.
- *Drug regimens:* Evaluate and adjust on the basis of kidney function.

Anemia of chronic kidney disease

- Monitor hemoglobin and hematocrit every 1–2 weeks after initiation of erythropoietic therapy or following a dose change and every 2–4 weeks once stable target hemoglobin and hematocrit are achieved.
- Monitor iron indices (transferrin saturation and serum ferritin).
- Evaluate patient for signs and symptoms of anemia.

CKD Mineral and Bone Disorder

- Phosphorus
- Calcium
- Parathyroid hormone
- Vitamin D (measure precursor levels, 25 hydroxy-vitamin D, in patients with stages 3 and 4 CKD)

Metabolic acidosis

- Serum bicarbonate
- Potassium

Drug Therapy

Progressive kidney disease

- ACEIs and ARBs (see Chapter 8 on hypertension and Chapter 13 on diabetes)
- Antihypertensive agents (see Chapter 8 on hypertension)
- Antidiabetic agents (see Chapter 13 on diabetes)

Anemia

Anemia is treated with erythropoietic stimulating agents (Table 16-7).

Mechanism of action
These agents stimulate the division and differentiation of erythroid progenitor cells and induce the release of reticulocytes from the bone marrow into the bloodstream, where they mature into erythrocytes.

Adverse drug events
Adverse drug events include the following:

- Hypertension
- Red blood cell aplasia
- Seizures (rare)
- Polycythemia
- Thrombocytosis

Drug–drug and drug–disease interactions
Causes of resistance to erythropoietic therapy are as follows:

- Iron deficiency
- Secondary hyperparathyroidism
- Inflammatory conditions
- Aluminum accumulation
- Other disease states causing anemia (e.g., cancer and HIV)

Parameters to monitor
The following should be monitored:

- Hemoglobin and hematocrit
- Iron indices
- Blood pressure

Table 16-7. Erythropoietic Stimulating Agents

Generic name	Trade name	Starting dose	Route of administration	Frequency of administration
Epoetin alfa	Epogen, Procrit	50–100 units/kg	IV or SC	1–3 doses per week
Darbepoetin alfa	Aranesp	0.45 mcg/kg	IV or SC	Once weekly or once every other week (may prolong interval to every 3–4 weeks)

Pharmacokinetics

Erythropoietic stimulating agents have the following half-lives:

- *Epoetin alfa:* Approximately 8.5 hours IV and 24 hours SC
- *Darbepoetin alfa:* Approximately 25 hours IV and 48 hours SC

The effect on hematologic parameters is observed over approximately 7 days to 6 weeks.

Steady-state conditions depend on the lifespan of red blood cells and the rate of red blood cell production.

Strengths and dosage forms

Epoetin alfa is supplied as single-dose, preservative-free solution (in vials of 2,000, 3,000, 4,000, 10,000, and 40,000 units/mL) and as a multidose, preserved solution (in vials of 10,000- and 20,000 units/mL).

Darbepoetin alfa is available in two solutions. A polysorbate solution and an albumin solution are supplied as single-dose vials (of 25, 40, 60, 100, 200, 300, and 500 mg/mL and of 150 mg/0.75 mL); as single-dose prefilled syringes; and as prefilled autoinjectors (syringes and autoinjectors available in doses of 25, 40, 60, 100, 150, 200, 300, and 500mcg). They contain no preservatives.

Iron supplementation

Iron supplements are described in Table 16-8.

Mechanism of action

Supplies a source of elemental iron necessary for the function of hemoglobin, myoglobin, and specific enzyme systems, and allows transport of oxygen via hemoglobin.

Patient instructions and counseling

- Oral iron may cause stools to be dark in color.
- Take between meals to increase absorption.
- Oral iron may be taken with food if GI upset occurs.
- Do not take with dairy products or antacids.

Adverse drug events

- Oral iron may cause stomach cramping, constipation, nausea, vomiting, and dark stools.
- In the case of intravenous iron, anaphylactic reactions have occurred with iron dextran (InFed and Dexferrum); administer a 25 mg test dose prior to administration of the full dose. A reduced incidence of hypersensitivity reactions exists with sodium ferric gluconate (Ferrlecit), iron sucrose (Venofer), and ferumoxytol (Feraheme). For all preparations, observe patients for diaphoresis,

---

Table 16-8. Iron Supplements

Generic name	Trade name	Dose	Dosage forms	Frequency of administration[a]
Ferrous sulfate	Fer-In-Sol, Feosol, Slow FE	200 mg elemental iron per day	po	bid–tid
Ferrous fumarate	Femiron, Vitron-C	200 mg elemental iron per day	po	bid–tid
Ferrous gluconate	Fergon	200 mg elemental iron per day	po	bid–tid
Polysaccharide iron	Hytinic, Niferec	200 mg elemental iron per day	po	qd–bid
Heme iron polypeptide	Proferrin	200 mg elemental iron per day	po	tid–qid
Sodium ferric gluconate	Ferrlecit	62.5–125.0 mg	IV	Weekly, three times per week, or monthly[b]
Iron sucrose	Venofer	20–200 mg	IV	Weekly, three times per week, or monthly[b]
Iron dextran	InFeD, Dexferrum	25–1,000 mg	IV	Weekly, three times per week, or monthly[b]
Ferumoxytol	Feraheme	510 mg × 1 followed by 2nd 510 mg dose 3–8 days after 1st dose	IV	As needed to treat iron deficiency in CKD.

a. For oral formulations, frequency of administration depends on the amount of elemental iron per unit; 200 mg elemental iron per day is necessary.
b. Three times per week is common in iron-deficient hemodialysis patients.

nausea, vomiting, lower back pain, dyspnea, and hypotension.

■ Iron overload may be treated with deferoxamine (Desferal).

Drug–drug and drug–disease interactions

GI absorption of oral iron is decreased when given with antacids, quinolones, and tetracycline and increased when administered with vitamin C.

Intravenous iron has a potential to increase risk of infection. Administration to patients with severe systemic infections is controversial.

Parameters to monitor

■ Ferritin and transferrin saturation.
■ Hemoglobin and hematocrit.
■ Monitor for anaphylactic or hypersensitivity reactions after IV administration.

Strengths and dosage forms

■ Ferumoxytol (Feraheme) is supplied in 17 mL single-dose vials containing 30 mg of elemental iron per milliliter.
■ Iron dextran (InFeD and Dexferrum) is supplied in 2 mL single-dose vials containing 50 mg of elemental iron per milliliter.
■ Iron sucrose (Venofer) is supplied in 5 mL single-dose vials containing 100 mg elemental iron (20 mg/mL).
■ Sodium ferric gluconate (Ferrlecit) is supplied as colorless glass ampules containing 62.5 mg elemental iron in 5 mL (12.5 mg/mL).

CKD Mineral and Bone Disorder

Phosphate binding agents are used to treat this disorder (Table 16-9).

Mechanism of action

These agents combine with dietary phosphate in the GI tract to form an insoluble complex that is excreted in the feces.

Patient instructions and counseling

■ Take with meals and snacks.
■ Do not take with oral iron salts or certain antibiotics (quinolones, tetracyclines).
■ Aluminum and magnesium products are generally for short-term use because of concern of accumulation in patients with kidney disease.
■ Use in conjunction with dietary phosphorus restriction.

Adverse drug events

■ Calcium products can result in hypercalcemia, nausea, vomiting, abdominal pain, and constipation.
■ Sevelamer hydrochloride (Renagel) and sevelamer carbonate (Renvela) can result in decreased LDL (low-density lipoprotein) cholesterol, increased HDL (high-density lipoprotein) cholesterol (may be a beneficial effect), nausea, and vomiting. *Note:* Sevelamer carbonate (Renvela) has less risk of lowering serum bicarbonate levels than does sevelamer hydrochloride (Renagel). The new formulation will eventually replace Renagel.

Table 16-9. Phosphate Binding Agents

Generic name	Trade name	Starting dosage range[a]
Calcium carbonate (40% elemental calcium)	Tums, Os-Cal-500, Nephro-Calci, Caltrate 600, CalCarb HD, CaCO$_3$ (multiple preparations)	0.8–2.0 g elemental calcium
Calcium acetate (25% elemental calcium)	Phos-Lo	1,334–2,001 mg
Sevelamer carbonate	Renvela	800–1,600 mg
Sevelamer hydrochloride	Renagel	800–1,600 mg
Lanthanum carbonate	Fosrenol	250–500 mg
Aluminum hydroxide	AlternaGel, Alu-Cap, Alu-tab, Amphojel, Basaljel	300–600 mg
Magnesium carbonate	Mag-Carb	70 mg
Magnesium hydroxide (milk of magnesia)	Various	300–400 mg

Note: All agents are taken orally and should be taken with meals.
a. Dose per meal.

- Lanthanum carbonate (Fosrenol) may cause nausea, vomiting, diarrhea, abdominal pain, and constipation.
- Aluminum may cause constipation, aluminum toxicity, chalky taste, cramps, nausea, and vomiting.
- Magnesium products may cause diarrhea, hypermagnesemia, cramps, and muscle weakness.
- All products may cause hypophosphatemia.

Drug–drug and drug–disease interactions

Calcium, lanthanum, aluminum, and magnesium are elemental compounds that may bind with antibiotics (quinolones and tetracyclines) in the GI tract, thus decreasing their absorption.

Sevelamer hydrochloride (Renagel) may contribute to metabolic acidosis and decreased LDL cholesterol. There is less risk of metabolic acidosis with sevelamer carbonate (Renvela).

Parameters to monitor

- Phosphorus, calcium, and iPTH
- Aluminum and magnesium (if receiving aluminum- or magnesium-containing products)
- For sevelamer (Renvela and Renagel), serum bicarbonate and LDL cholesterol

Vitamin D therapy

Vitamin D therapy is described in Table 16-10.

Mechanism of action (active vitamin D)

This therapy increases intestinal absorption of calcium, increases tubular reabsorption of calcium by the kidney (in patients with sufficient kidney function), suppresses synthesis of parathyroid hormone, and increases intestinal phosphorus absorption.

Patient instructions and counseling

- Use in conjunction with dietary phosphorus restriction and phosphate binding agents; therapy may need to be temporarily discontinued if calcium and phosphorus are elevated.
- Notify health care provider of any of the following signs of hypercalcemia: weakness, headache, decreased appetite, and lethargy.

Adverse drug events

- *Hypercalcemia:* Decreased incidence with vitamin D analogs (paricalcitol, doxercalciferol)
- *Hyperphosphatemia:* Decreased incidence with vitamin D analogs
- *Adynamic bone disease:* Caused by oversuppression of PTH

Drug–drug and drug–disease interactions

- Cholestyramine may decrease intestinal absorption of oral products.
- Magnesium absorption may be increased with concomitant administration.

Table 16-10. Vitamin D Therapy

Generic name	Trade name	Dosage range	Dosage forms	Frequency of administration
Vitamin D precursor				
Ergocalciferol	Drisdol	400–50,000 IU	po	Daily, weekly, or monthly
Ergocalciferol	Calciferol	400–50,000 IU	po or IV	Daily, weekly, or monthly
Active vitamin D				
Calcitriol	Calcijex	0.5–5 mcg	IV	Three times per week
Calcitriol	Rocaltrol	0.25–5 mcg	po	Daily, every other day, or three times per week
Vitamin D analogs				
Paricalcitol	Zemplar	1–4 mcg	po	Daily or three times per week
		2.5–15 mcg	IV	Three times per week
Doxercalciferol	Hectorol	5–20 mcg	po	Daily or three times per week
		2–8 mcg	IV	Three times per week

IU, international units.

Parameters to monitor
- iPTH
- Calcium
- Phosphorus
- Calcium × phosphorus product (vitamin D therapy may need to be temporarily discontinued or the dose decreased if the calcium × phosphorus product is elevated)
- Alkaline phosphatase
- Signs of vitamin D intoxication and hypercalcemia (e.g., weakness, headache, somnolence, nausea, vomiting, bone pain, and polyuria)

Pharmacokinetics
- Calcitriol (Calcijex):
  - Half-life 3–8 hours; protein binding 99.9%
- Paricalcitol (Zemplar):
  - Half-life: Healthy subjects 4–6 hours (oral); Stage 3 and 4 CKD 17–20 hours (oral); Stage 5 CKD 14–15 hours (IV)
  - Protein binding: > 99%
- Doxercalciferol (Hectorol):
  - Half-life of active metabolite: 32–37 hours

Ergocalciferol requires hydroxylation within the liver to form calcifediol and a second hydroxylation within the kidney to form active vitamin D.

Doxercalciferol requires conversion to its active form 1α, 25-dihydroxyvitamin D_2 in the liver.

Strengths and dosage forms
- Calcitriol (Calcijex): 1 mcg/mL ampules
- Calcitriol (Rocaltrol): 0.25 and 0.5 mcg capsules and 1 mcg/mL oral solution
- Paricalcitol (Zemplar): IV—2 and 5 mcg/mL vials; po—1, 2, and 4 mcg capsules
- Doxercalciferol: IV—2 mcg/mL ampules; po—0.5 and 2.5 mcg capsules

Calcimimetics: Cinacalcet (Sensipar)

Cinacalcet is approved for patients with stage 5 CKD who are on dialysis. It is used in conjunction with phosphate binder therapy and vitamin D. The dose range is 30–180 mg/d; initial dose is 30 mg titrated every 2–4 weeks on the basis of iPTH levels. Do not start therapy if corrected serum calcium is < 8.4 mg/dL.

Mechanism of action
Cinacalcet binds with the calcium-sensing receptor on the parathyroid gland and increases sensitivity of the receptor to extracellular calcium, thereby decreasing the stimulus for PTH secretion.

Patient instructions and counseling
- Cinacalcet should be taken with food or shortly after a meal.
- Tablets should be taken whole and should not be divided.

Adverse drug events
- Hypocalcemia (use with caution in patients with seizure disorder)
- Nausea and vomiting
- Diarrhea
- Myalgias

Drug–drug and drug–disease interactions
Cinacalcet is metabolized by multiple cytochrome P450 (CYP) enzymes, primarily CYP3A4, CYP2D6, and CYP1A2. Adjustments in dose may be required for patients taking agents that inhibit metabolism of cinacalcet (e.g., ketoconazole). Dose reductions of drugs with a narrow therapeutic range and with a metabolism dependent on these enzymes may also be required (e.g., tricyclic antidepressants, flecainide, and thioridazine).

Parameters to monitor
Serum calcium and serum phosphorus should be measured within 1 week and iPTH should be measured 1–4 weeks after initiation or dose adjustment of cinacalcet. The dose of cinacalcet should be titrated no more frequently than every 2–4 weeks through sequential doses of 60, 90, 120, and 180 mg once daily to target iPTH (150–300 pg/mL).

Pharmacokinetics
- The maximum concentration is achieved in approximately 2–6 hours following administration and is increased with food.
- Half-life is 30–40 hours.
- Volume of distribution is approximately 1,000 L.
- Cinacalcet is approximately 93–97% bound to plasma proteins.
- Cinacalcet is metabolized primarily by CYP3A4, CYP2D6, and CYP1A2.

Strengths and dosage forms
Cinacalcet is available in 30-, 60-, and 90-mg tablets.

Metabolic acidosis

See Chapter 17 on critical care.

Vitamin supplementation (specific to the dialysis population)

Water-soluble vitamins for dialysis patients are described in Table 16-11.

Mechanism of action

Vitamin supplementation replaces water-soluble vitamins lost during dialysis without providing supratherapeutic amounts of fat-soluble vitamins.

Patient instructions and counseling

- Take daily to replace water-soluble vitamins.
- Hemodialysis patients should take after dialysis.

Adverse drug events

- *General:* Nausea, headache, pruritus, and flushing (depending on specific vitamin)
- *Vitamin B$_6$ (pyridoxine):* Neuropathy and increased aspartate transaminase
- *Vitamin C (ascorbic acid):* Hyperoxaluria, dizziness, diarrhea, fatigue, and nausea
- *Folic acid:* Headache, rash, and pruritus

Drug–drug and drug–disease interactions

Folic acid may decrease phenytoin concentrations by increasing the metabolism.

Nondrug Therapy

- Preparation for renal replacement therapy when patients reach stage 4 CKD:
  - Choice of chronic dialysis (hemodialysis or peritoneal dialysis) if patient is a candidate for both modalities and discussion of transplantation
  - Placement of dialysis access (fistula or graft for hemodialysis, catheter for peritoneal dialysis)

Table 16-11. Water-Soluble Vitamin Supplements for Dialysis Patients

Generic name	Trade name
Vitamin B complex, vitamin C, and folic acid	Nephrocaps, Nephrovite, Nephrovite Rx, Renavite, Biotin Forte
Vitamin B complex, vitamin C, folic acid, and iron	Nephrovite Rx + Iron, NephrPlex Rx
Vitamin B complex	Allbee with C

Note: All these supplements are taken orally, 1 capsule or tablet once per day.

- Patient education regarding choice of renal replacement therapy and complications of CKD

Diet

- Risks and benefits of protein restriction (0.6–0.8 g/kg/d) should be considered in patients with stage 4 CKD.
- Increased protein requirements should be considered for patients on dialysis (approximately 1.2 g/kg/d) and even greater requirements for peritoneal dialysis patients because of increased protein loss with the dialysis procedure.
- Nutritional supplementation should be taken as needed.
- Counseling by a renal dietitian may be beneficial to tailor a diet based on the stage of CKD.

Renal replacement therapies

Hemodialysis

The intermittent hemodialysis procedure is generally performed three times per week for 3–5 hours for patients with stage 5 kidney disease (end-stage renal disease). It requires a viable permanent access site (graft or fistula) or a temporary site for patients requiring immediate dialysis or experiencing failed permanent access sites. Fistulas are the preferred access for chronic hemodialysis.

Complications include infection, hypotension during dialysis, clotting, and dialyzer reactions. Drug removal by hemodialysis is most likely to occur for drugs with small molecular weight, low protein binding, and small volume of distribution.

Peritoneal dialysis

Peritoneal dialysis requires insertion of a catheter into the peritoneum. Types include continuous ambulatory peritoneal dialysis and automated peritoneal dialysis (which includes continuous cycling, nocturnal tidal, and nightly intermittent peritoneal dialysis).

Several complications are possible:

- Peritonitis
  - Most common gram-positive organisms are *Staphylococcus epidermidis* and *Staphylococcus aureus*.
  - Most common gram-negative organisms are *Enterobacteriacae* and *Pseudomonas aeruginosa*.
  - Empiric therapy should include gram-positive coverage (first-generation cephalosporin or vancomycin if MRSA [methicillin-resistant *Staphylococcus aureus*] is prevalent) and gram-negative coverage (e.g., ceftazidime and aminoglycoside).

- Intraperitoneal administration of antibiotics is recommended.
- Hyperglycemia from glucose content of dialysate solution
- Malnutrition from increased protein loss

Transplantation
See Chapter 20 for information on transplantation.

16-3. Key Points

Acute Kidney Injury

- Prevention of kidney dysfunction in high-risk patients is the most effective strategy to address AKI.
- Conditions that put patients at increased risk of AKI include decreased perfusion of the kidney (attributable to dehydration or poor effective circulating volume such as with congestive heart failure) and administration of potentially nephrotoxic agents, particularly under conditions of decreased perfusion.
- Nephrotoxic agents should be avoided when possible in patients at risk for AKI.
- Immediate recognition and treatment of AKI may prevent irreversible kidney damage.
- Goals of treatment for patients with AKI are achievement of baseline kidney function and prevention of both chronic kidney disease and the need for chronic renal replacement therapy.
- Diuretics are often used in patients with AKI to maintain fluid balance and hemodynamic stability.
- A review of medications is frequently necessary to ensure appropriate dose adjustments based on kidney function (see Appendix B for drugs in renal failure).

Chronic Kidney Disease

- Chronic kidney disease is classified in stages 1 through 5 on the basis of estimated glomerular filtration rate and evidence of pathological abnormalities or markers of kidney damage, including abnormalities in blood or urine tests or in imaging studies.
- Screening for microalbuminuria and proteinuria is important for identifying patients with kidney disease and monitoring progression of the disease.
- Therapy to delay progression of kidney disease includes control of diabetes and hypertension,

initiation of therapy with angiotensin-converting enzyme inhibitors or angiotensin receptor blockers, and protein restriction if indicated.

- Common secondary complications of CKD include anemia, fluid and electrolyte abnormalities, hyperphosphatemia, secondary hyperparathyroidism, and malnutrition.
- Management of anemia includes administration of erythropoietic stimulating agents (epoetin alfa [Epogen and Procrit] and darbepoetin alfa [Aranesp]) and iron supplementation with oral iron (multiple preparations) or intravenous iron (sodium ferric gluconate [Ferrlecit], iron sucrose [Venofer], ferumoxytol [Feraheme], or iron dextran [InFeD and Dexferrum]) to achieve target hemoglobin (11–12 g/dL), while preventing iron deficiency.
- Hyperphosphatemia is managed by dietary phosphorus restriction; use of phosphate binding agents (calcium-containing products, lanthanum carbonate [Fosrenol], or sevelemer carbonate [Renvela]); and dialysis.
- Management of secondary hyperparathyroidism includes control of serum calcium and phosphorus and administration of vitamin D therapy—including vitamin D precursors in early CKD based on kidney function (ergocalciferol [Drisdol and Calciferol])—and active vitamin D therapy for more severe kidney disease (calcitriol [Calcijex and Rocaltrol], paricalcitol [Zemplar], or doxercalciferol [Hectorol]). The calcimimetic agent cinacalcet (Sensipar) is indicated for management of secondary hyperparathyroidism in patients with stage 5 CKD who are on dialysis and is used in conjunction with phosphate binders and vitamin D.
- Nutritional requirements must be reevaluated on the basis of severity of kidney disease (e.g., protein restriction to delay progression of CKD versus increased protein requirements for patients on dialysis).

16-4. Questions

1. R. T. is a 45-year-old female admitted to the hospital after fainting at work. Her past medical history includes type 2 diabetes and rheumatoid arthritis. Her only complaint is that she has had difficulty over the past 5 days keeping down anything she eats or drinks. She has also noticed a decrease in urination over

the past 24 hours. Regular medications include aspirin 325 mg qd, ibuprofen 600 mg qd for arthritis, metformin 500 mg qd, glyburide 5 mg qd, and Tylenol prn for headache. Laboratory values in the emergency department showed a serum creatinine of 2.0 mg/dL and BUN of 56 mg/dL, consistent with acute kidney injury. Her lab tests from 1 month ago at a regular checkup were normal. The most likely etiology of R. T.'s acute kidney injury is

A. dehydration from poor oral intake.
B. trauma from fainting.
C. age-related decreases in kidney function.
D. kidney failure caused by diabetes.
E. obstruction of urine outflow.

2. Which of the following medications may have contributed to R. T.'s acute kidney injury?

A. Aspirin
B. Ibuprofen
C. Metformin
D. Glyburide
E. Tylenol

3. Which of the following diuretics may retain its effectiveness at a glomerular filtration rate < 30 mL/min?

A. Hydrochlorothiazide
B. Chlorothiazide
C. Metolazone
D. Spironolactone
E. Aldactone

4. Which of the following fluid and electrolyte abnormalities typically occur in patients with severe kidney dysfunction (i.e., creatinine clearance <15 mL/min)?

I.   Metabolic alkalosis --
II. Hyperkalemia
III. Hyperphosphatemia

A. I only
B. III only
C. I and II only
D. II and III only
E. I, II, and III

5. Which set of laboratory values is most consistent with a patient in acute intrinsic kidney disease?

A. Urinary granular casts absent, FE_{Na} < 1, urinary osmolality 600 mOsm/kg

B. Urinary granular casts absent, FE_{Na} > 1, urinary osmolality 600 mOsm/kg
C. Urinary granular casts present, FE_{Na} < 1, urinary osmolality 300 mOsm/kg
D. Urinary granular casts present, FE_{Na} > 1, urinary osmolality 300 mOsm/kg
E. Acute intrinsic kidney failure can only be diagnosed by biopsy.

6. Which of the following diuretics would be most appropriate for the initial treatment of a patient with acute kidney injury?

I.   Metolazone
II. Spironolactone
III. Furosemide

A. I only
B. III only
C. I and II only
D. II and III only
E. I, II, and III

7. A patient with nephrotoxicity caused by tobramycin would likely present with an increase in serum creatinine

A. immediately after starting therapy and with nonoliguria.
B. immediately after starting therapy and with oliguria.
C. 5–7 days after starting therapy and with oliguria.
D. 5–7 days after starting therapy and with nonoliguria.
E. within 24 hours with excessive diuresis.

8. Lisinopril may cause hemodynamically mediated kidney disease by preventing which of the following compensatory mechanisms by the kidney?

A. Vasodilation of the afferent arteriole
B. Vasoconstriction of the afferent arteriole
C. Vasodilation of the efferent arteriole
D. Vasoconstriction of the efferent arteriole
E. Vasodilation of both the afferent and the efferent arterioles

9. The estimated creatinine clearance for a 47-year-old male patient with an ideal body weight of 176 pounds (slightly less than actual body weight) and a serum creatinine of 2.2 mg/dL is

A. 32 mL/min.
B. 40 mL/min.

C. 47 mL/min.

D. 93 mL/min.

E. 120 mL/min.

10. D. K. is a 53-year-old black female (body weight = 65 kg) with hypertension and hyper-cholesterolemia who is seen in the outpatient nephrology clinic for evaluation of kidney disease progression. Her current blood pressure is 156/82 mm Hg, SCr is 2.6 mg/dL (stable for the past 4 months), BUN is 44 mg/dL, and urinary protein is 800 mg/d. Her medications are enalapril 20 mg/d × 1 year and simvastatin 20 mg qd × 2 years. On the basis of D. K.'s estimated creatinine clearance, she would be classified in which of the following stages of chronic kidney disease?

   A. Stage 1
   B. Stage 2
   C. Stage 3
   D. Stage 4
   E. Stage 5

11. The recommended target blood pressure for D. K. is

   A. < 110/70 mm Hg.
   B. < 130/90 mm Hg.
   C. < 130/80 mm Hg.
   D. < 140/95 mm Hg.
   E. < 140/90 mm Hg.

12. Which of the following would be most beneficial in a patient with type 1 diabetes and micro-albuminuria to delay progression of CKD?

   I. Angiotensin-converting enzyme inhibitor
   II. Angiotensin receptor blocker
   III. Loop diuretic

   A. I only
   B. III only
   C. I and II only
   D. II and III only
   E. I, II, and III

13. Epoetin alfa and darbepoetin alfa stimulate erythropoiesis by which of the following?

   A. Prevention of excessive red blood cell destruction
   B. Prevention of degradation of bone marrow stem cells
   C. Differentiation of peritubular interstitial cells of the kidney

D. Increase in size of red blood cells produced in the bone marrow

E. Differentiation of erythroid progenitor stem cells in the bone marrow

14. When administered intravenously, darbepoetin alfa has a terminal half-life approximately _____ that of epoetin alfa.

   A. equal to
   B. twofold longer than
   C. twofold shorter than
   D. threefold longer than
   E. threefold shorter than

15. One of the most commonly reported adverse reactions with epoetin alfa and darbepoetin alfa is

   A. nausea.
   B. hypertension.
   C. constipation.
   D. anemia.
   E. anaphylaxis.

16. At least _____ should be allowed to lapse before a change in dose of epoetin alfa or darbepoetin alfa is made on the basis of a change in hemoglobin and hematocrit.

   A. 1 week
   B. 2–4 weeks
   C. 6–8 weeks
   D. 2 months
   E. 4 months

17. R. A. is a 42-year-old 70-kg male on hemodialysis tiw who receives epoetin alfa for treatment of anemia. He has been stable on an epoetin dose of 4,000 units intravenously tiw with an average hemoglobin of 11 g/dL (hematocrit of 33%). Over the past 3 months, his hematocrit has dropped to 28%. Iron indices reveal the following: serum ferritin 78 ng/mL and transferrin saturation 12%. The best initial treatment for R. A. is to

   A. increase the dose of epoetin alfa to maintain a hemoglobin of 11–12 g/dL (hematocrit of 33–36%).
   B. withhold epoetin alfa therapy until hemoglobin increases to 12 g/dL.
   C. administer intravenous iron (sodium ferric gluconate) at a maintenance dose of 125 mg per week.

D. administer a 1 g total dose of intravenous iron in divided doses.

E. begin oral ferrous sulfate 325 mg tid.

18. In the gastrointestinal tract, calcitriol

A. promotes absorption of calcium and inhibits absorption of phosphorus.

B. promotes absorption of phosphorus and inhibits absorption of calcium.

C. promotes absorption of both calcium and phosphorus.

D. promotes decreased binding of calcium and phosphorus.

E. promotes increased elimination of calcium and phosphorus.

19. J. T. is a 63-year-old female with stage 5 CKD (end-stage kidney disease) receiving peritoneal dialysis. Her most recent laboratory analysis reveals the following: BUN 58 mg/dL, SCr 5.2 mg/dL, phosphorus 7.4 mg/dL, calcium 9.0 mg/dL, albumin 2.5 g/dL, and iPTH 542 pg/mL. In addition to dietary restriction of phosphorus, which of the following agents is best for initial management of J. T.'s hyperphosphatemia?

I. Sevelamer carbonate
II. Lanthanum carbonate
III. Calcium carbonate

A. I only
B. III only
C. I and II only
D. II and III only
E. I, II, and III

20. J. T. should be instructed to take her phosphate binder

A. with meals to enhance systemic absorption of phosphorus.

B. with meals to minimize systemic absorption of phosphorus.

C. between meals to avoid food–drug interactions.

D. between meals to minimize GI side effects.

E. There are no specific instructions to follow with regard to meals.

21. Which of the following agents is appropriate for a patient with stage 5 CKD and secondary hyperparathyroidism requiring treatment to reduce iPTH?

I. Calcitriol
II. Paricalcitol
III. Ergocalciferol

A. I only
B. III only
C. I and II only
D. II and III only
E. I, II, and III

22. Cinacalcet is a calcimimetic that works by which of the following mechanisms?

A. It decreases the sensitivity of the calcium-sensing receptors on the parathyroid gland to calcium, which prevents secretion of PTH.

B. It increases the sensitivity of the calcium-sensing receptors on the parathyroid gland to calcium, which prevents secretion of PTH.

C. It stimulates the breakdown of iPTH and prevents the effects of PTH on bone turnover.

D. It inhibits the breakdown of iPTH to provide a negative feedback system and suppress PTH synthesis.

E. It increases calcium concentrations, which suppresses secretion of PTH from the parathyroid gland.

23. A drug with which of the following characteristics is most likely to be removed by hemodialysis (Vd = volume of distribution)?

A. f_u 0.05, Vd 0.2 L/kg
B. f_u 0.05, Vd 0.6 L/kg
C. f_u 0.30, Vd 0.6 L/kg
D. f_u 0.95, Vd 0.2 L/kg
E. f_u 0.95, Vd 6 L/kg

24. The best antibiotic selection for empiric treatment of peritonitis in a peritoneal dialysis patient is

A. cefazolin + vancomycin.
B. cefazolin + ceftazidime.
C. vancomycin alone.
D. cefazolin alone.
E. gentamicin alone.

25. Which of the following supplements should be recommended daily in a patient with stage 5 CKD requiring chronic hemodialysis?

A. Multivitamin
B. Nephrocaps
C. Vitamin A
D. Nephrocaps + vitamin A
E. Folic acid only

16-5. Answers

1. **A.** Dehydration is the most likely cause of AKI in R. T. because she has had a decrease in oral intake over the past 5 days. Dehydration would be classified as a prerenal cause of AKI. Fainting was likely a result of dehydration and not the cause of her decline in kidney function. A serum creatinine of 2.0 mg/dL would not be considered normal in a 45 year old, eliminating age as a rationale for kidney disease. Diabetes would be more likely to cause a chronic decrease in her kidney function as opposed to an acute change (lab tests from 1 month ago were normal, ruling out evidence of chronic kidney disease). She has had some urine output in the past 24 hours, which rules out obstruction.

2. **B.** NSAIDs are associated with hemodynamic changes (in particular, they prevent the compensatory vasodilation of the afferent arteriole that occurs in conditions of prerenal acute kidney disease). Metformin is not a cause of AKI in this case but would need to be discontinued at this time because of the risk of lactic acidosis in a patient with decreased kidney function (serum creatinine > 1.4 mg/dL in females and > 1.5 mg/dL in males).

3. **C.** There is some evidence that metolazone is beneficial in patients with kidney disease and a GFR < 30 mL/min. This is not the case with other thiazide or thiazide-like diuretics or with potassium-sparing diuretics. Metolazone is frequently used in combination with loop diuretics for this reason.

4. **D.** Hyperkalemia and hyperphosphatemia are common electrolyte abnormalities observed as kidney function decreases. Metabolic acidosis is also common, but not metabolic alkalosis.

5. **D.** Acute intrinsic kidney disease is generally characterized by the presence of granular casts (indicating structural damage), a fractional excretion of sodium > 1, and a urine osmolality similar to that of plasma osmolality (indicating changes in concentrating ability of the kidney).

6. **B.** A patient with acute kidney disease generally requires aggressive diuresis (while avoiding dehydration). Furosemide is a loop diuretic that is more potent than a thiazide-like diuretic (metolazone) or a potassium-sparing diuretic (spironolactone) and would be a rational choice for initial therapy of AKI. Spironolactone may also cause hyperkalemia in a patient with AKI.

7. **D.** Aminoglycoside-induced nephrotoxicity is characterized by a delay in changes in serum creatinine (approximately 5–7 days) and relatively normal urine output (nonoliguria).

8. **D.** Angiotensin-converting enzyme inhibitors may contribute to development of AKI in patients with conditions resulting in prerenal kidney disease (e.g., conditions resulting in decreased perfusion of the kidney, hypovolemia, heart failure, liver disease, and so forth). ACEIs (and angiotensin receptor blockers) prevent the compensatory vasoconstriction of the efferent arteriole mediated by angiotensin II that occurs in an attempt to increase GFR.

9. **C.** Using the Cockcroft–Gault equation to estimate creatinine clearance, one finds that this patient has an estimated creatinine clearance of 47 mL/min. For females, multiply the calculated value by 0.85.

$$CrCl = \frac{(140 - age)(BW\ in\ kg)}{72 \times SCr\ (mg/dL)}$$

$$BW\ (kg) = 176\ lbs/2.2 = 80\ kg$$

$$SCr = 2.2\ mg/dL$$

10. **D.** D. K.'s estimated creatinine clearance determined using the Cockcroft–Gault equation is 26 mL/min, classified as stage 4 CKD (GFR 15–29 mL/min/1.73 m^2).

$$CrCl = \frac{(140 - age)(BW\ in\ kg)}{72 \times SCr\ (mg/dL)}$$

with the result multiplied by 0.85 for a female. *Note:* The estimated GFR determined using the Modification of Diet in Renal Disease equation is 25 mL/min/1.73m^2.

11. **C.** The recommended blood pressure for D. K. is < 130/80 mm Hg because she has stage 4 CKD.

12. **C.** ACEIs and ARBs are advocated for patients with diabetes and microalbuminuria. The decreases in glomerular pressure caused by these agents that are detrimental in patients with AKI are beneficial in a chronic condition such as diabetes, in which sustained elevations in glomerular pressure result in worsening kidney disease over time.

13. **E.** Erythropoietic agents including epoetin alfa and darbepoetin alfa work in the bone marrow to stimulate differentiation of erythroid progenitor stem cells and result in an increase in red blood cell production (increase erythrocytes).

14. **D.** The half-life of darbepoetin alfa is three times longer than that of epoetin alfa, giving this agent the added benefit of reduced frequency of administration.

15. **B.** Hypertension is the most common adverse effect in patients receiving erythropoietic agents.

16. **B.** Stimulation of erythropoiesis by epoetin alfa and darbepoetin alfa occurs immediately; however, it will take at least 2–4 weeks before substantial changes in hemoglobin and hematocrit are observed as a result of any change in dose of erythropoietic therapy.

17. **D.** R. A. is iron deficient, as indicated by his low serum ferritin (< 100 ng/mL) and transferrin saturation (< 20%). No change in epoetin alfa should be made until the iron deficiency is corrected (this is the leading cause of resistance to epoetin alfa and darbepoetin alfa therapy). R. A. will require a full course of iron (1 g administered intravenously in divided doses with each dialysis session) as opposed to a maintenance dose, which should be administered once R. A. is iron replete. Sodium ferric gluconate may be administered in doses of 125 mg per dialysis session for eight sessions to give the total 1 g dose (iron sucrose would be administered in 100 mg increments over 10 hemodialysis sessions). Ferumoxytol would be administered as two 510 mg doses given 3–8 days apart. Absorption of oral iron is poor, making intravenous iron preferred in this hemodialysis patient.

18. **C.** Active vitamin D (calcitriol) promotes absorption of both calcium and phosphorus in the GI tract. This is one reason that therapy with calcitriol or a vitamin D analog may need to be withheld if the calcium × phosphorus product is elevated.

19. **C.** Sevelamer carbonate (Renvela) or lanthanum carbonate would be better options than a calcium-containing binder for initial management because J. T. has a corrected calcium of 10.2 mg/dL [corrected calcium = measured serum calcium + 0.8 × (normal serum albumin – measured serum albumin)] and a calcium × phosphorus product of 75 mg^2/dL^2. This elevated product increases the risk of metastatic calcifications. She requires a phosphorus binding agent without calcium to minimize calcium absorbed in the GI tract.

20. **B.** Phosphate binders should be taken with meals to minimize systemic absorption of phosphorus from the GI tract.

21. **C.** Calcitriol and paricalcitol are active forms of vitamin D that do not require conversion in the liver or kidney. Ergocalciferol is a vitamin D precursor that does require activation and would not be recommended for a patient with stage 5 CKD without the necessary activity of the enzyme in the kidney (1α-hydroxylase) responsible for final conversion to the active form.

22. **B.** The calcimimetic agent cinacalcet (Sensipar) works by binding with the calcium-sensing receptor on the parathyroid gland and increases the sensitivity of this receptor to calcium, thereby suppressing secretion of PTH.

23. **D.** Drug characteristics that make an agent more likely to be removed by dialysis include low protein binding, small volume of distribution, and low molecular weight. Among the choices given, the agent that best meets these criteria is choice D, which has a high fraction unbound in the plasma and a low volume of distribution.

24. **B.** Empiric therapy should include antibiotics with gram-positive and gram-negative coverage. Choice B is most appropriate.

25. **B.** Nephrocaps include water-soluble vitamins (vitamin B complex + vitamin C + folic acid) recommended for a patient with kidney failure. Supplementation with fat-soluble vitamins is not recommended in patients with kidney failure because of toxicities associated with accumulation.

16-6. References

Acute Kidney Injury and Drug-Induced Kidney Disease

Lameire N, Van Viesen W, Vanholder R. Acute renal failure. *Lancet*. 2005;365(9457):417–30.

Nolin TD, Himmelfarb J. Drug-induced kidney disease. In: DiPiro J, Talbert RL, eds. *Pharmacotherapy: A Pathophysiologic Approach*. 7th ed. New York: McGraw-Hill; 2008:795–810.

Ricci Z, Cruz D, Ronco C. The RIFLE criteria and mortality in acute kidney injury: A systematic review. *Kidney International*. 2008;73:538–46.

Wood AJJ. Diuretic therapy. *N Engl J Med*. 1998; 339:387–95.

Chronic Kidney Disease and Progression

Abosaif NY, Arije A, Atray NK, et al. K/DOQI clinical practice guidelines on hypertension and antihypertensive agents in chronic kidney disease. *Am J Kidney Dis*. 2004;43(suppl 1):S1–290.

Chobanian AV, Bakris GL, Black HR, et al. and the National High Blood Pressure Education Program Coordinating Committee. The seventh report of the Joint National Committee on Prevention, Detection, Evaluation, and Treatment of High Blood

Pressure: The JNC 7 report. *JAMA*. 2003;289: 2560–72.

Levey AS, Beto JA, Coronado BE, et al. Controlling the epidemic of cardiovascular disease in chronic renal disease: What do we know? What do we need to learn? Where do we go from here? *Am J Kidney Dis*. 1998;32:853–906.

National Kidney Foundation. NKF-K/DOQI clinical practice guidelines for chronic kidney disease: Evaluation, classification, and stratification. *Am J Kidney Dis*. 2002;39(suppl 1):S1–266.

U.S. Renal Data System. *USRDS 2008 Annual Data Report: Atlas of End-Stage Renal Disease in the United States*. Bethesda, Md.: National Institutes of Health, National Institute of Diabetes and Digestive and Kidney Diseases; 2008.

Anemia

American Reagent Laboratories. Venofer (iron sucrose injection) package insert. Shirley, N.Y.: American Reagent Laboratories; 2007.

Amgen. Aranesp (darbepoetin alfa) package insert. Thousand Oaks, Calif.: Amgen; 2008.

Macdougall IC, Gray SJ, Elston O, et al. Pharmacokinetics of novel erythropoiesis stimulating protein compared with epoetin alfa in dialysis patients. *J Am Soc Nephrol*. 1999;10:2392–95.

National Kidney Foundation. K/DOQI clinical practice guidelines and clinical practice recommendations for anemia in chronic kidney disease. *Am J Kidney Dis*. 2006 May;47(5 suppl 3):S1–145.

Watson Pharmaceuticals. Ferrlecit (sodium ferric gluconate complex in sucrose injection) package insert. Corona, Calif.: Watson Pharmaceuticals; 2006.

Hyperphosphatemia and Secondary Hyperparathyroidism

Amgen. Sensipar (cinacalcet HCl) tablets package insert. Thousand Oaks, Calif: Amgen; 2007.

Eknoyan G, Levin A, Levin NW. Bone metabolism and disease in chronic kidney disease. *Am J Kidney Dis*. 2003;42(4 suppl 3):S1–201.

Nutrition

National Kidney Foundation. K/DOQI clinical practice guidelines for nutrition in chronic renal failure. *Am J Kidney Dis*. 2000;35(suppl 2):S1–140.

Other

Aronoff GR, Bennett WM, Berns JS, et al. *Drug Prescribing in Renal Failure: Dosing Guidelines for Adults and Children*. 5th ed. Philadelphia: American College of Physicians; 2007.

Ifudu O. Care of patients undergoing hemodialysis. *N Engl J Med*. 1998;339:1054–62.

National Kidney Foundation Kidney Disease Outcomes Quality Initiative. *Clinical Practice Guidelines for Peritoneal Dialysis Adequacy: Update 2006*. New York: National Kidney Foundation. Available at: http://www.kidney.org/professionals/kdoqi/index.cfm.

Critical Care, Fluids, and Electrolytes

G. Christopher Wood, PharmD, FCCP, BCPS with Added Qualifications in Infectious Diseases

17-1. Sedation, Analgesia, and Neuromuscular Blockade

Definition and Classifications

- *Pain:* Critically ill patients may experience acute pain, chronic pain, or both.
- *Anxiety or agitation:* Patients may experience psychophysiological response to real or imagined danger. The term *agitation* is used in this chapter.
- *ICU delirium:* Delirium presented in the intensive care unit (ICU). See discussion of clinical presentation. The term *delirium* is used in this chapter.

Clinical Presentation

- Pain, agitation, or both in patients with impaired consciousness: pulling of tubes or lines, writhing, kicking, restlessness, hypertension, tachycardia, tachypnea, diaphoresis, moaning
- Delirium: fluctuating, disorganized thinking or inattentiveness not caused by an obviously reversible cause; with or without agitation

Pathophysiology

- Injuries
- Medical procedures and equipment (e.g., mechanical ventilation equipment or catheters)
- Mental status changes (e.g., fear, infection, hypoxia, sleep deprivation, or adverse drug effects or withdrawal)
- Preexisting medical conditions (e.g., chronic pain)

Diagnostic Criteria

- *Pain:* Use a verbal or visual scale to assess severity. For unconscious patients, use physical signs and symptoms.
- *Agitation:* Use a validated scale to assess (e.g., Riker Sedation-Agitation Scale).
- *Delirium:* Use Confusion Assessment Method for the ICU (CAM-ICU) scale.

Treatment Goals

- Find and remove the cause of pain, agitation, and delirium.
- Achieve a balance between patient comfort, adverse effects, and ability to provide care.
- Reserve neuromuscular blocking (NMB) agents for patients who are not controlled with maximum doses of sedation and analgesia.

Drug Therapy

Selected drug therapy is described in Table 17-1.

Mechanism of action

- *Opiates, nonsteroidal anti-inflammatory drugs (NSAIDs):* See Chapter 23 on pain management.
- *Benzodiazepines, haloperidol:* See Chapter 25 on psychiatric disease.
- *Propofol:* Mechanism of action is unknown—possibly γ-aminobutyric acid (GABA)-related activity.
- *NMB agents:* These are postsynaptic cholinergic receptor antagonists; they do not provide analgesia or sedation.

Table 17-1. Selected Drug Therapy Based on Guidelines for Use in ICU Patients

Generic name	Trade name	Dosage range	Forms[a]	Schedule[b]	Notes on usage
Morphine sulfate		0.5–10.0 mg	IV, IM, po	Continuous; q6h	General opiate of choice
Hydromorphone	Dilaudid	0.3–1.5 mg	IV	Continuous; q6h	Used in morphine intolerance, hemodynamic instability, or renal dysfunction
Fentanyl	Sublimaze	50–200 mcg/h	IV	Continuous	Used in morphine intolerance, hemodynamic instability, or renal dysfunction
Acetaminophen	Tylenol	Up to 4 g/d	po, PR	q4–6h	NSAIDs may be added to opiates
Ketorolac	Toradol	10–30 mg	IV, IM, po	q6h	Maximum use 5 days
Lorazepam	Ativan	0.5–4.0 mg	IV, po	Continuous; q6h	Long-term sedation (> 24–72 hours)
Midazolam	Versed	1–5 mg	IV	Continuous; q2h	Acute and short term (< 24–72 hours)
Propofol	Diprivan	1–5 mg/kg/h	IV	Continuous	Used when rapid awakening needed
Haloperidol	Haldol	2–5 mg	IV, po	q1–4h	Drug of choice for delirium
Pancuronium	Pavulon	0.05–0.1 mg/kg	IV	Continuous; q2h	General NMB agent of choice (low cost); causes tachycardia
Vecuronium	Norcuron	0.05–0.1 mg/kg	IV	Continuous; q1h	Used in hemodynamic instability, renal dysfunction, cardiac disease
Cisatracurium	Nimbex	0.05–0.10 mg/kg	IV	Continuous; q1h	Used in renal and hepatic dysfunction

a. Long-acting drugs and dosage forms generally not used in ICU (e.g., fentanyl patch, controlled-release morphine, doxacurium).
b. Continuous analgesia and sedation with frequent titration (patient-controlled analgesia pump, IV infusion, or scheduled) preferred to prn therapy alone. NMB agents used prn are preferred.

Patient instructions

When patient-controlled analgesia pumps are used, make sure the patient understands how to activate the device.

Adverse drug events

- *Opiates, NSAIDs:* See Chapter 23 on pain management.
- *Benzodiazepines, haloperidol:* See Chapter 25 on psychiatric disease.
- *Propofol:* Adverse events include respiratory depression, hypotension, and hypertriglyceridemia. The maximum dose is 5 mg/kg/h.
- *NMB agents:* Adverse events include respiratory depression, prolonged weakness or paralysis after discontinuation, and tachycardia with pancuronium.

Drug interactions

- *Opiates, NSAIDs:* See Chapter 23 on pain management.

- *Benzodiazepines, haloperidol:* See Chapter 25 on psychiatric disease.
- *Propofol:* Actions are potentiated by other sedatives.
- *NMB agents:* Actions are potentiated by corticosteroids, aminoglycosides, clindamycin, calcium channel blockers, anesthetics; actions are inhibited by anticholinesterase inhibitors (e.g., neostigmine).

Parameters to monitor

- *Opiates, NSAIDs:* Use a visual or verbal scale to assess efficacy. Also monitor heart rate (HR), blood pressure (BP), and respiratory rate (RR). See also Chapter 23 on pain management.
- *Benzodiazepines, haloperidol:* Use a validated scale. Also monitor HR, BP, and RR. See also Chapter 25 on psychiatric disease.
- *Propofol:* Use a validated scale. Also monitor BP, HR, RR, intracranial pressure (ICP), and serum triglycerides at baseline and 1–2 times a week during long-term use.
- *NMB agents:* Monitor movement and spontaneous breathing. Also monitor BP, HR, and ICP (acute

increases may indicate suboptimal sedation or analgesia). Peripheral nerve stimulation monitoring ("train of four") is highly recommended.

■ *Note:* In patients with continuous sedation, a daily wakening and assessment period results in decreased sedative use and a shorter length of stay in ICU.

Kinetics

■ *Opiates, NSAIDs:* See Chapter 23 on pain management.

■ *Benzodiazepines, haloperidol:* See Chapter 25 on psychiatric disease.

■ *Propofol:* Medication is highly lipophilic (may accumulate long term), has a rapid onset (1 minute), and has a short duration (about 10 minutes).

■ *NMB agents:* Onset for all NMB agents is < 5 minutes. Duration is 60–90 minutes for pancuronium and 30–60 minutes for vecuronium and cisatracurium. Excretion of pancuronium is mostly renal; for vecuronium, it is about 50:50, hepatic:renal. Excretion of cisatracurium is not organ dependent.

Other aspects

Propofol

Propofol is in a lipid vehicle (provides 1 kcal/mL). It should be used with caution in patients with egg allergy. It is a potential growth medium for bacteria; the maximum hang time for a bottle is 12 hours.

Dexmedetomidine

A newer agent (not discussed in depth in current guidelines), dexmedetomidine (Precedex), is available. It is a central alpha-2 agonist administered as a continuous IV infusion for up to 24 hours.

The potential advantage of dexmedetomidine is less respiratory depression than found with other agents. Adverse events include hypotension and bradycardia.

Newer data suggest the agent is safe for use longer than 24 hours and results in less delirium and shorter ICU stay than midazolam.

17-2. Traumatic Brain Injury

Definition

Traumatic brain injury is defined as neurologic deficit secondary to brain trauma.

Classifications

■ Severe
■ Mild or moderate

Clinical Presentation

■ Use the Glasgow Coma Scale (GCS) for assessment: sum of eye, motor, and verbal scores (range 3–15).

■ Traumatic brain injury has a wide range of presentation from mild confusion to totally nonresponsive coma.

Pathophysiology

■ Traumatic brain injury results from motor vehicle accidents (most common), falls and accidents, assaults, and gunshot wounds.

■ It is most common in 15- to 24-year age group.

■ Every year 375,000 cases and 75,000 deaths occur.

■ Traumatic brain injury consists of direct neuronal damage ± edema ± secondary ischemia-related neuronal death.

Diagnostic Criteria

■ Computed tomography (CT) scan
■ GCS
■ ICP monitoring in severe patients (GCS score 3–8)

Treatment Goals

■ Keep ICP < 20 mm Hg and cerebral perfusion pressure (CPP) > 50 mm Hg (CPP = mean arterial pressure − ICP).

■ Prevent seizures.

Strategies to decrease ICP

■ Osmotic agents and diuretics
  • Mannitol 0.25–1.0 g/kg intravenous (IV) q4h
  • Loop diuretics IV (e.g., furosemide)
  • Hypertonic NaCl IV (e.g., 3.0%, 7.5%)

■ Sedation
  • Short-acting agents are preferred to allow frequent patient assessment (e.g., propofol, fentanyl).
  • Pentobarbital (1–3 mg/kg/h IV) is a long-acting agent for refractory intracranial hypertension.

■ NMB agents:
  • A short-acting agent is preferred (vecuronium).

- Such agents are used for refractory intracranial hypertension.

Nondrug interventions

- Raising of the head of the bed (30 degrees)
- Ventricular drainage of cerebrospinal fluid via ventriculostomy
- Mild or moderate hyperventilation (pCO_2 30–35 mm Hg)
- Surgery

Strategies to increase mean arterial pressure

- Maximize fluid status. The overall goal is euvolemia.
- Vasopressors and inotropes may be used in shock after fluid status is optimized.

Seizure prevention

- Seizure prevention may be started on the basis of severity and type of injury.
- Phenytoin (Dilantin, generic) can be used: 20 mg/kg IV loading dose plus 4–8 mg/kg/d for 7 days.
  - Continue beyond 7 days if the patient has a seizure.
  - An alternative agent is carbamazepine.
- See Chapter 24 on seizure control for the mechanism of action, adverse drug events, drug interactions, and kinetics.

Parameters to monitor

The overall goal is CPP > 50 mm Hg and ICP < 20 mm Hg. Drug classes are covered elsewhere.

Other Aspects

Nimodipine (Nimotop) is a calcium channel blocker given for 21 days. It is indicated for treating aneurysmal subarachnoid hemorrhage. It may also provide some benefit in traumatic subarachnoid hemorrhage.

17-3. Acute Spinal Cord Injury

Definition

Acute spinal cord injury is traumatic spinal cord injury with neurologic impairment.

Classifications

- *Complete:* Total loss of motor and sensory function occurs in affected areas.
- *Incomplete:* Some motor or sensory function is retained in affected areas.
- *Paraplegia:* Neurologic deficit occurs in the lower extremities.
- *Quadriplegia:* Neurologic deficit occurs in the upper and lower extremities.
- *Central cord syndrome:* Symptoms are atypical.

Clinical Presentation

- Loss of motor function, loss of sensory function, or both, from nerves distal to level of vertebral injury
- Usually bilaterally symmetrical symptoms

Pathophysiology

See discussion of traumatic brain injury in Section 17-2.

Diagnostic Criteria

- Physical examination consistent with spinal cord injury
- CT or radiographic evidence of injury

Treatment Goals

Treatment goals are the reservation or restoration of motor and sensory function.

Drug Therapy

Drug therapy is considered optional in current treatment guidelines:

- A loading dose of methylprednisolone 30 mg/kg IV is given.
- If the loading dose is given within 3 hours of the injury, a 5.4 mg/kg/h IV infusion is continued for a total of 24 hours.
- If the loading dose is given within 3 hours of the injury, a 5.4 mg/kg/h IV infusion is continued for a total of 48 hours.
- No methylprednisolone is if > 8 hours have passed from the injury or in the case of penetrating injuries.

Mechanism of action

The mechanism of action is unknown. The medication is thought to protect neurons by inhibiting lipid peroxidation.

Adverse drug effects

- Increased infections (48 hours worse than 24 hours)
- Hyperglycemia

Parameters to monitor

- Neurologic status
- Serum glucose

17-4. Venous Thromboembolism Prophylaxis

Definition

Venous thromboembolism (VTE) is pathogenic blood clot formation.

Classifications

- *Deep venous thrombosis (DVT):* VTE in a large vein, generally in a lower extremity
- *Pulmonary embolism (PE):* DVT that has embolized to the pulmonary vasculature (much less common)

Clinical Presentations

- DVT is often asymptomatic:
  - Unilateral leg symptoms such as swelling, pain, tenderness, erythema, warmth, ± palpable cord
  - Pain behind the knee upon dorsiflexion (Homans' sign)
- PE is often asymptomatic:
  - Pulmonary symptoms such as chest pain, cough, dyspnea, tachypnea, hemoptysis
  - May proceed rapidly to life-threatening shock and hypoxia

Pathophysiology

Three general risk factors can be identified:

- Hypercoagulable states:
  - Clotting factor deficiencies or abnormalities (e.g., protein C or S deficiency)
  - Malignancy, pregnancy, estrogen use
- Direct vessel trauma
- Venous stasis (i.e., poor blood flow allows clot formation)

Specific Risk Factors

- Risk increases with age (see Table 17-2).
- Immobility, previous VTE, cancer, obesity, congestive heart failure, pregnancy, estrogen therapy, and smoking are risk factors.
- Major surgery or trauma are risk factors, particularly in the case of lower extremities or the pelvis, genito-urinary injury, and neurologic injury.

Epidemiology

- About 600,000 hospitalizations take place in the United States yearly with about 60,000 deaths (10% mortality).
- Incidence of DVT ranges from 2% to 80% depending on risk factors.

Diagnostic Criteria

- *Radiocontrast dye studies:* Such studies (venography for DVT, pulmonary angiography for PE) are invasive, are expensive, and require expertise, and adverse events common (e.g., nephropathy). A ventilation/perfusion scan (for PE) is less invasive, but inconclusive results are common.
- *Ultrasonography:* Used for DVT, ultrasonography is noninvasive, is inexpensive, is performed at the bedside, but is less sensitive.
- *Serum D-dimer concentrations:* Normal levels may rule out VTE.

Treatment Goals

- Goals are to decrease morbidity (VTE recurrence, progression to PE); mortality; and costs of VTE.
- VTE prophylaxis is underused: only 35% to 50% of at-risk patients receive it.

Drug Therapy to Treat VTE

Heparin

Therapy consists of full-dose IV heparin (80 units/kg load + 18 units/kg/h) or full-dose low molecular weight heparin (LMWH) subcutaneous (SC) (e.g., enoxaparin 1 mg/kg q12h or 1.5 mg/kg qd). LMWH may be used on an outpatient basis in stable DVT patients. Full-dose heparin may be given SC bid, but this is rarely done.

Warfarin

Begin warfarin concurrently. Discontinue heparin or LMWH when the international normalized ratio (INR) is therapeutic (usually 2–3) and stable. Duration is as follows:

- Reversible, 3 months
- Idiopathic, 6–12 months (consider longer)
- High risk, 12 months to indefinite

Direct thrombin inhibitors

Use direct thrombin inhibitors in place of heparin for heparin-induced thrombocytopenia.

Thrombolytic therapy

Reserve thrombolytic therapy for very severe cases. Therapy is highly individualized.

Inferior vena cava filter

Reserve this treatment for selected patients with contraindication to anticoagulation.

Drug Therapy to Prevent VTE

Drug therapy for prevention of VTE is described in Table 17-2.

Mechanism of action

- Heparin binds to antithrombin and potentiates its anticoagulation (anti-IIa activity > anti-Xa activity).

Table 17-2. Drug and Nondrug Therapy for Prevention of Venous Thromboembolism

Patient group	Recommended therapy[a]
Medical conditions	
General medical patient with risk factor	LDUH or LMWH; alternatives: IPC, ES
Acute myocardial infarction	LDUH or full-dose IV heparin
Ischemic stroke	LDUH or LMWH; alternatives: IPC, ES
General surgery (begin preoperatively; generally continue until patient is ambulatory or discharged)	
Low risk	
Minor procedure without risk factors	Early ambulation
Moderate risk	
Minor procedure + risk factor or > 40 years old; major procedure	LDUH, LMWH, or fondaparinux; alternatives: IPC, ES
High risk	
Major procedure + multiple risk factors or > 40 years old; minor procedure + multiple risk factors or > 60 years old	LDUH, LMWH, or fondaparinux plus IPC, ES (combine drug + mechanical), or both
Orthopedic surgery or trauma (recommended duration if available)	
Hip replacement (28–35 days)	LMWH or fondaparinux or warfarin (INR 2–3) ± IPC or ES
Knee replacement (minimum 10 days); hip fracture (28–35 days)	LMWH or fondaparinux or warfarin (INR 2–3); alternative: IPC
Neurosurgery	IPC ± ES; add LDUH or LMWH when bleeding is stopped
Major trauma (until discharge)	LMWH; alternative: IPC ± ES if bleeding risk; may use warfarin (INR 2–3) during rehabilitation if major impairment
Acute spinal cord injury (throughout rehabilitation)	LMWH ± IPC, ES; convert to warfarin (INR 2–3) in rehabilitation

a. ES (elastic compression stockings) may add to efficacy of drugs. IPC (intermittent pneumatic compression) may add to efficacy of drugs but noncompliance is high. LDUH (low-dose unfractionated heparin [generic]) dosing is 5,000 units SC q8–12h. Fondaparinux (Arixtra) dosing is 2.5 mg SC qd. LWMH (low molecular weight heparin) dosing is as follows: for dalteparin (Fragmin), 2,500–5,000 units SC qd; for enoxaparin (Lovenox), 30 mg SC q12h or 30–40 mg SC qd. In case of major trauma, start therapy within 36 hours of injury; routine vena cava filter placement is not recommended.

- LMWHs are the same as heparin but anti-Xa activity is > anti-IIa activity. Some controversy exists over the interchangeability of these drugs because of differences in Xa:IIa activity ratios.
- Fondaparinux is a factor Xa inhibitor.
- For warfarin, see Chapter 10 on cardiac arrhythmias.
- Direct thrombin inhibitors (lepirudin [Refludan], bivalirudin [Angiomax], argatroban) directly inhibit thrombin.

Patient instructions and counseling

- For heparin, fondaparinux, thrombin inhibitors, and thrombolytics, patient instructions and counseling are not necessary.
- For LMWHs and fondaparinux, patients can be taught to self-inject after hospital discharge:
  - Monitor for signs and symptoms of bleeding or VTE recurrence.
  - Avoid NSAIDs.
- For warfarin, see Chapter 10 on cardiac arrhythmias.

Adverse drug events

- *Bleeding:* Occurs with all agents:
  - Low-dose unfractionated heparin (LDUH) and low-dose LMWH have similar bleeding risks.
  - Protamine sulfate reverses heparin and LMWH.
- *Heparin-induced thrombocytopenia (HIT):* Occurs with heparin, LMWH:
  - Early onset occurs around the first week of therapy. It is transient, and no therapy is needed.
  - Late onset (> 50% decrease from baseline) is immune mediated. If the event is severe, heparin or LMWH must be discontinued:
    - Switch to direct thrombin inhibitor until platelets > 150,000/mcL, then possibly short-term warfarin (4 weeks).
    - Adverse events are less frequent with LMWH.
    - HIT may result in severe thrombosis or limb amputation.
    - HIT may happen immediately upon rechallenge with heparin or LMWH.
    - Spinal hematoma can occur with epidural catheters. LMWH or full anticoagulation is worse than LDUH; do not use LMWH.
    - Osteoporosis can occur with long-term therapy. Heparin is worse than LMWH.
- *Hypersensitivity (reexposure):* Occurs with lepirudin.

Drug interactions

- NSAIDs may increase bleeding risk with all agents.
- For warfarin, see Chapter 10 on cardiac arrhythmias.

Parameters to monitor

- Heparin (full-dose IV) and thrombin inhibitors:
  - Goal is partial thromboplastin time (PTT) that corresponds to an anti-Xa level of 0.3–0.7 units/mL (check with each lab for therapeutic range).
  - Monitor q6h until therapeutic; then once or twice daily.
  - LDUH does not affect PTT.
- LMWHs:
  - Goal is an anti-Xa level of 0.6–1 units/mL.
  - No routine monitoring is needed, but monitoring may be necessary in cases of renal impairment, obesity, prolonged use, and pregnancy.
- Fondaparinux:
  - No monitoring is necessary.
  - Fondaparinux affects anti-Xa levels.
- Direct thrombin inhibitors:
  - *Argatroban:* Goal is PTT that is 1.5–3.0 times control. Argatroban falsely elevates INR.
  - *Bivalirudin:* There are no recommendations in HIT. Bivalirudin elevates PTT and INR.
  - *Lepirudin:* Goal PTT is 1.5–2.5 times control.
- Warfarin (see Chapter 10 on cardiac arrhythmias).

Kinetics

- *Heparin:* Cleared by endothelial cell enzymes (half-life about 90 minutes); higher doses also renally cleared.
- *LMWHs:* Renally cleared; half-life 2–4 times longer than heparin.
- *Fondaparinux:* Renally cleared; longer half-life (about 24 hours).
- *Direct thrombin inhibitors:* Half-life 30–90 minutes; lepirudin renally cleared; others hepatically cleared.

17-5. Stress Ulcer Prophylaxis

Definition

Stress ulcer prophylaxis refers to gastrointestinal (GI) mucosal damage related to metabolic stress in the ICU.

Clinical Presentation

Presentation is similar to that of peptic ulcer disease (see Chapter 21 on gastrointestinal disorders).

Pathophysiology

Shunting of blood from the GI tract to vital organs during critical illness results in breakdown of gastric mucosal defenses (e.g., bicarbonate production, epithelial cell turnover).

Risk Factors

- Mechanical ventilation > 48 hours
- Coagulopathy
- Other disease states or organ dysfunction where GI perfusion may be compromised (e.g., sepsis, burns, traumatic brain injury)

Diagnostic Criteria

Diagnosis is based on signs and symptoms and can be confirmed with endoscopy.

Treatment Goals

The goal is to prevent stress ulcers.

Drug Therapy

- See Chapter 21 on GI disorders for full drug information.
- Histamine-2 (H2) antagonists or sucralfate are traditional standards of therapy; H2 antagonists may be more effective. Sucralfate administration can be difficult in ICU patients.
- Proton pump inhibitors are equivalent to H2 antagonists.
- Optimal duration of therapy is unknown (usually until risk factors have resolved or transfer from ICU).
- Antacids are less effective and are not recommended. They have higher aspiration risk and require frequent dosing.

17-6. Severe Sepsis and Septic Shock

Definition and Classifications

Severe sepsis is sepsis (see Chapter 29 on infectious disease) plus dysfunction of one or more major organs (e.g., hypotension responsive to fluids, oliguria, acute mental status change, lactic acidosis, respiratory insufficiency, coagulopathy).

Septic shock is severe sepsis plus hypotension that is not fully responsive to fluids (i.e., requires vasopressor therapy).

Clinical Presentation

See sepsis criteria (in Chapter 29) and the definitions of severe sepsis and septic shock.

Pathophysiology

Progression is seen in the systemic manifestations of sepsis. Imbalances in the inflammatory, immune, and coagulation systems lead to organ hypoperfusion and organ dysfunction with or without refractory hypotension.

Causative organisms vary by institution, but broad patterns are known:

- Common community-acquired organisms include *Streptococcus pneumoniae, Staphylococcus aureus, Haemophilus influenzae, Escherichia coli,* and "atypicals" (*Mycoplasma pneumoniae, Chlamydia pneumoniae, Legionella* spp.).
- Common nosocomial or health care–associated organisms include *Pseudomonas aeruginosa, S. aureus* (methicillin resistance more common), *Enterobacter* spp., *Klebsiella* spp., *Proteus* spp., *Citrobacter* spp., *Serratia* spp., and *Candida* spp.

Diagnostic Criteria

See sepsis criteria (in Chapter 29) and the definitions of severe sepsis and septic shock.

Treatment Goals

- Rapidly stabilize hemodynamic parameters and organ dysfunction within 6 hours.
- Identify causative organism or organisms, start appropriate antimicrobial therapy within 1 hour, and eliminate the source of infection, if applicable (e.g., vascular or urinary catheter, abscess). Duration of antimicrobial therapy is typically 7–14 days.
- Modulate inflammatory, coagulating, and hormonal derangements, if applicable.

Drug and Nondrug Therapy

See Chapter 29 on infectious disease for antimicrobial information (mechanism of action, dosing, adverse effects, etc.). Empiric antimicrobial selection is also covered in Chapter 29. Definitive therapy should be streamlined to a narrower spectrum agent, if possible, on the basis of the final culture and sensitivity reports.

See Section 17-7 for details on fluid therapy. Fluid therapy for severe sepsis and septic shock can be colloids, isotonic crystalloids, or both. Vasopressors should be used only after appropriate fluid therapy fails to adequately normalize BP (Table 17-3).

Mechanism of action

- Vasopressors and inotropes are adrenergic-receptor agonists.
- Drotrecogin alfa is recombinant human-activated protein C (an endogenous anticoagulant). The exact method of action is unknown, but it modulates coagulation and inflammatory cascades.

Adverse drug events

- *Vasopressors and inotropes:* Tachycardia, arrhythmias, organ and extremity ischemia, hypertension

- *Drotrecogin alfa:* Bleeding (contraindicated in active internal bleeding, recent trauma, stroke, or other clinical condition at high bleeding risk or presence of epidural catheter)

Drug–drug interactions

- *Vasopressors and inotropes:* None
- *Drotrecogin alfa:* Increased bleeding risk with concomitant anticoagulation or antiplatelet therapy

Parameters to monitor

- *Vasopressors and inotropes:* Monitor BP, HR, cardiac output, urine output, and extremity perfusion on physical exam.
- *Drotrecogin alfa:* Note signs and symptoms of bleeding on physical exam and monitor BP and HR. Monitor improvement in signs and symptoms of infection, temperature, white blood count (WBC), and organ dysfunction. Drotecogin alfa may prolong activated PTT.

Table 17-3. Vasopressors and Inotropes Used in Severe Sepsis and Septic Shock

Name	Dosage range	Adrenergic-receptor activity	Comments
Dopamine	< 5 mcg/kg/min	Increased renal perfusion (dopaminergic receptors)	Preferred agent; use of low-dose "renal tonic" dopamine is not recommended.
	5–10 mcg/kg/min	Increased cardiac output/HR (β_1) > increased BP (α_1)	
	10–20 mcg/kg/min	Increased cardiac output/HR and BP	
Norepinephrine	0.01–3 mcg/kg/min	Increased BP (α_1) > increased cardiac output/HR (β_1)	Preferred agent.
Epinephrine	0.01–0.5 mcg/kg/min	Increased cardiac output/HR and BP (all receptors)	Second-line agent (because of tachycardia, gut ischemia).
Phenylephrine	0.01–5 mcg/kg/min	Increased BP only (α_1)	
Dobutamine	5–20 mcg/kg/min	Increased cardiac output/HR (β_1)	
Vasopressin	0.01–0.04 units/min (0.03 most studied)	None; acts on vasopressin receptors	Add to catecholamine vasopressor in nonresponsive patients. Do not exceed maximum dose.

Immunomodulator used in severe sepsis and septic shock

Drotrecogin alfa (Xigris)	Dosing regimen: 24 mcg/kg/h × 96 h IV infusion		Add to antimicrobial therapy within 48 hours of onset of severe sepsis; decreases mortality. Limit use to highly severe illness (i.e., APACHE II score > 25); monitor for bleeding; very expensive but likely cost-effective.

Note: All catecholamine vasopressors are given as continuous IV infusions and are titrated to effect. APACHE = Acute Physiology, Age, and Chronic Health Evaluation.

Kinetics

For drotrecogin alfa, dose adjustment is not required in renal or hepatic dysfunction.

Other aspects

Low-dose hydrocortisone (200–300 mg × 7 days ± fludrocortisone 50 mcg/d) is recommended for patients with septic shock who are not responsive to fluids and vasopressors. Patients with a poor response to cosyntropin stimulation testing (serum cortisol increase of < 9 mcg/dL) may respond better to corticosteroid supplementation.

Vasopressin infusion (0.03 units/min) may be used to increase BP in patients refractory to high doses of traditional pressors. Doses > 0.04 units/min are associated with severe adverse events (e.g., cardiac arrest). New data suggest that patients receiving lower doses of catecholamine vasopressors (i.e., < 15 mcg/min of norepinephrine) benefit more from vasopressin than do patients on higher doses of norepinephrine.

17-7. Fluid and Electrolyte Abnormalities in Critically Ill Patients

See also Chapter 16 on kidney disorders (for hyperphosphatemia), Chapter 18 on nutrition, and chapter 19 on oncology (for hypercalcemia).

Definition

Fluid and electrolyte abnormalities are pathologic alterations in fluid and electrolyte homeostasis.

Classifications

Fluid and electrolyte abnormalities are classified by electrolyte (see the discussion on clinical presentation).

Clinical Presentation

In all cases, mild to moderate abnormalities are usually asymptomatic.

Sodium (normal range: 135–145 mEq/L)

In cases of hyponatremia or hypernatremia, lethargy, nausea, headache, dry mucous membranes, poor skin turgor (depends on hydration status), and confusion may occur.

Coma, seizures, or central pontine myelinolysis may occur in severe hyponatremia or if sodium increases or decreases rapidly (> 12 mEq/L/d).

Chloride (normal range: 96–106 mEq/L)

Symptoms are related to acid-base or fluid abnormalities, not chloride itself.

Water (moves osmotically with sodium)

In cases of dehydration, dry mucous membranes, poor skin turgor, lethargy, nausea, headache, hypotension, and tachycardia occur. Seizures, coma, or death can occur if dehydration is severe. Decreased urine output, metabolic acidosis, and hypotension are also found.

For edema or fluid overload, see Chapter 9 on heart failure.

Potassium (normal range: 3.5–5.0 mEq/L)

In cases of hypokalemia, confusion, muscle cramps, weakness, and cardiac arrhythmias occur.

In cases of hyperkalemia, muscle cramps, weakness, and cardiac arrhythmias occur.

Magnesium (normal range: 1.5–2.2 mEq/L)

With hypomagnesemia, presentation is similar to that of hypocalcemia.

In cases of hypermagnesemia, lethargy, weakness, and cardiac arrhythmias occur. Coma is possible in severe cases.

Phosphorus (normal range: 2.6–4.5 mg/dL)

In cases of hypophosphatemia, confusion, anxiety, weakness, respiratory depression, paresthesias, and lethargy occur. Seizures and coma are possible if hypophosphatemia is severe.

For hyperphosphatemia, see Chapter 16 on kidney disorders.

Calcium (normal range: 8.5–10.5 mg/dL)

In cases of hypocalcemia, confusion, anxiety, paresthesias, muscle cramps, and tetany occur. Coma and cardiac arrhythmias may occur in severe cases.

For hypercalcemia, see Chapter 19 on oncology.

Pathophysiology

Normal distribution of fluids and electrolytes

- Electrolytes with high serum concentrations are primarily extracellular (Na, Cl); those with low serum concentrations are mostly intracellular or in bone (K, P, Mg, Ca).
- Total body water is approximately 60–70% of total body weight (differs by age, gender, disease states).
  - Of all water, intracellular is approximately two-thirds; extracellular is approximately one-third.
  - Of extracellular water, approximately three-fourths is interstitial; approximately one-fourth is intravascular (plasma).
- Typical fluid requirements for adults are approximately 35 mL/kg/d; they can be much higher in critical illness because of extrarenal losses (GI tract, wounds) and fluid shifts (trauma, sepsis).
- Primary hormonal controls are aldosterone (sodium retention) and antidiuretic hormone (water retention).

Hyponatremia

The first three forms of hyponatremia listed below are hypotonic:

- *Hypovolemic (sodium and water loss):* This condition is characterized by high urine osmolality. It is related to extrarenal fluid losses (GI, wounds); diuretics; and adrenal insufficiency.
- *Euvolemic (moderate water retention):* This condition occurs with syndrome of inappropriate antidiuretic hormone (SIADH) release, renal failure, carbamazepine, NSAIDs, chlorpropamide.
- *Hypervolemic (sodium and water retention):* This condition occurs with congestive heart failure, cirrhosis, nephrotic syndrome, and glucocorticoids.
- *Hypertonic:* This condition is the dilutional effect of abnormal osmotic agents in the vasculature (severe hyperglycemia).

Hypernatremia

Hypernatremia occurs in cases of water loss or excessive sodium intake (e.g., from IV fluids). It is related to extrarenal fluid losses (GI, wounds) and diabetes insipidus.

Hypochloremia

Hypochloremia occurs with GI losses.

Hypokalemia

Hypokalemia is related to diuretics, β_2-agonists, amphotericin B, glucocorticoids, cisplatin, and GI losses.

Hyperkalemia

Hyperkalemia is related to renal dysfunction, acidosis, angiotensin-converting enzyme (ACE) inhibitors, potassium-sparing diuretics, trimethoprim, orally taken salt substitutes, and adrenal insufficiency.

Hypomagnesemia

Hypomagnesemia occurs with GI losses, diuretics, amphotericin B, alcohol, and cisplatin. It should be treated prior to treating hypokalemia; Na/K-ATPase pumps require magnesium to work.

Hypermagnesemia

Hypermagnesemia is related to renal dysfunction, magnesium-containing antacids, adrenal insufficiency, and hyperparathyroidism.

Hypophosphatemia

Hypophosphatemia is related to refeeding syndrome, phosphate binders, diuretics, hypercalcemia, vitamin D deficiency, and glucocorticoids.

Hypocalcemia

Hypocalcemia occurs with hypoparathyroidism, hypomagnesemia, vitamin D deficiency, and loop diuretics. Total calcium is artificially low in hypoalbuminemia (calcium is highly albumin bound).

Diagnostic Criteria

- Criteria include serum concentration, signs, and symptoms.
- Sodium analysis may use urine sodium and urine osmolality.

Treatment Goals

- Find and treat the underlying cause of abnormality.
- Treat abnormality to avoid sequelae.

Drug and Nondrug Therapy

Fluid replacement

Administer fluids as follows:

- *Crystalloids:* Salt solutions—½ or ¼ normal saline (NS) ± dextrose 5% ± KCl 20 mEq/L (approximates urine electrolytes), NS (154 mEq/L of Na), lactated Ringer's (LR), ¼ NS, or dextrose 5%—are chosen on the basis of sodium and fluid needs. NS or LR are typically used for fluid resuscitation (sodium is the major osmotic cation in plasma).
- *Colloids:* Osmotic agents—albumin 5–25% or hetastarch—are used for fluid resuscitation or to raise oncotic pressure (e.g., cirrhosis).
- *Vasopressors ± isotropic activity:* After fluids are optimized, vasopressors ± isotropic activity may be used (see Chapter 9 on heart failure).

Edema

Fluid restriction ± diuretics may be used. See Chapter 9 on heart failure and and Chapter 16 on kidney disorders.

Hyponatremia

If the case is severe, titrate 3% NaCl to maximum serum sodium increase of 12 mEq/d. Treat specific forms as follows:

- *Hypovolemic:* Replace fluid losses with IV NS (0.9% NaCl, 154 mEq/L).
- *Euvolemic (SIADH):* Use fluid restriction ± demeclocycline.
- *Hypervolemic:* Use fluid restriction ± diuretics.
- *Hypertonic:* Correct hyperglycemia.

Hypernatremia

Titrate low-sodium fluids (e.g., dextrose 5%, ¼NS) to a normal serum sodium. In cases of diabetes insipidus, use DDAVP (desmopressin).

Hyperchloremia

Give sodium acetate or LR instead of NS, especially if acidemic (acetate is converted to bicarbonate by the liver).

Hypokalemia

Administer IV (KCl) or po (KCl, K phosphate, or K acetate). Each 10 mEq dose increases serum potassium by about 0.1 mEq/L. IV administration faster than 10 mEq/h requires electrocardiogram (ECG) monitoring for arrhythmias.

Hyperkalemia

Treat hyperkalemia as follows:

- *Potassium removal (slower onset of action):* Use Na polystyrene sulfonate (Kayexalate) po or PR (per rectum), loop diuretics, or hemodialysis (if severe).
- *Intracellular potassium shifting (rapid onset of action):* Administer regular insulin + dextrose IV, albuterol, or Na bicarbonate.
- *Potassium antagonism of cardiac effects (rapid onset of action):* Administer IV calcium.

Hypomagnesemia

Dosages are described below. A large percentage of the dose is renally wasted. Repletion requires 3–days of treatment.

- *IV:* 0.5–1 mEq/kg/d (8 mEq = 1 g); administration rate = 8 mEq/h
- *IM:* Can give IM but painful
- *po:* Magnesium-containing antacid or laxative tid–qid as tolerated or magnesium oxide 300–600 mg bid–qid

Hypermagnesemia

Treat with diuretics, IV calcium, or hemodialysis (similar to hyperkalemia).

Hypophosphatemia

If the case is severe, use IV sodium or potassium phosphate 0.16–0.64 mmol/kg at 7.5 mmol/h to avoid potassium overdose (if potassium phosphate is used), calcium precipitation, or both.

Administer po 1–2 g/d (5–60 mmol/d), for example, Neutra-Phos, Neutra-Phos-K, or Fleet Phospho-soda.

Hyperphosphatemia

See Chapter 16 on kidney disorders for information about hyperphosphatemia.

Hypocalcemia

If patient is symptomatic, administer IV calcium gluconate (2–3 g) or IV calcium chloride (1 g) over 10 minutes. In addition, the following may be administered:

- IV infusion of 0.5–2.0 mg/kg/h of elemental calcium

■ Calcium salts such as calcium carbonate (po 1–3 g elemental calcium/d ± vitamin D)

Patient counseling

In cases of po administration, advise patient about potential adverse events.

Adverse drug events

■ *Sodium:* Edema or central pontine myelinolysis can occur if serum Na changes rapidly (> 12 mEq/d).
■ *Crystalloids:* Vein irritation is possible with hypotonic (¼ NS, ½ NS) or hypertonic fluids (3% NaCl). Dextrose 5% is approximately isotonic and is often added to low-sodium fluids.
■ *Potassium:* Events include cardiac arrhythmias (> 10 mEq/h), vein irritation (IV), GI upset (po; worse with wax matrix controlled-release tablets), and bad taste (po liquid). With sodium polystyrene sulfonate, constipation may occur (medication is usually mixed with sorbitol).
■ *Magnesium:* Events include diarrhea (po), flushing, sweating (IV), and vein irritation (IV).
■ *Phosphorus:* Events include diarrhea (po) and calcium phosphate precipitation (IV).
■ *Calcium:* IV calcium gluconate is less irritating than calcium chloride. Cardiac dysfunction can occur if medication is administered > 60 mg/min (elemental calcium). Events also include calcium phosphate precipitation (IV) and constipation (po).

Drug interactions

■ Hypokalemia and hypomagnesemia can predispose the patient to digoxin toxicity.
■ Binding of drugs in the GI tract by calcium or magnesium is possible (see Chapter 18 on nutrition).

Parameters to monitor

■ Serum concentrations
■ Resolution of signs and symptoms
■ With fluid replacement, normalization of the following: BP, HR, urine output (goal > 0.5 mL/kg/h), skin turgor, mucous membrane hydration, edema, cardiac output, pulmonary artery wedge pressure (see Chapter 9 on heart failure), and serum lactate/base deficit

Other aspects

Glucose control in critically ill patients
Tight glucose control (80–110 mg/dL) with insulin infusion was originally shown to reduce mortality in one large trial; however, recent large trials have not seen such a benefit. Hypoglycemia is common with intensive glucose control.

Anemia of critical illness
This common complication is caused by blood loss, bone marrow dysfunction (e.g., erythropoietin resistance), and hemodilution. Red blood count (RBC) transfusion is not recommended until hemoglobin is < 7.0 g/dL (unless patient is symptomatic). No benefit is gained from transfusing sooner, and transfusions are associated with increased infections and higher mortality.

Recombinant erythropoietin (40,000 units SC per week) has been shown to decrease the need for RBC transfusions by about 20% in a large trial; however, this benefit was not seen in a large follow-up trial. Until further data are available, erythropoietin is not recommended for routine use in the ICU, but it may be used if the patient has another indication for it (e.g., renal failure).

17-8. Key Points

■ Appropriate sedation and analgesia are essential because pain and agitation are common in critically ill patients. Drug selection should be based on clinical guidelines and patient parameters.
■ Sedation and analgesia should be monitored using a validated assessment tool.
■ NMB agents should be used only after sedation and analgesia have been maximized.
■ Neuromuscular blockade should be monitored using peripheral nerve stimulation in addition to observation of clinical signs and symptoms.
■ Appropriate stress ulcer prophylaxis is recommended for patients at risk.
■ Appropriate VTE prophylaxis is recommended for patients at risk. Optimal therapy is determined by clinical guidelines and patient risk factors.
■ High-dose methylprednisolone therapy within 8 hours of injury may improve outcomes after acute spinal cord injury.
■ ICP and CPP should be optimized after severe traumatic brain injury using drug and nondrug therapies. Phenytoin is effective at preventing early post-traumatic seizures.
■ Severe sepsis and septic shock are progressions of sepsis. Therapy includes hemodynamic stabilization, appropriate antimicrobial agents, and removal of infectious foci, if possible.
■ Drotrecogin alfa may decrease mortality as an adjunctive agent in patients with severe sepsis and a high severity of illness.

- Maintaining adequate fluid status is vital to maintaining tissue perfusion and organ function. However, many clinical factors can affect fluid and electrolyte status in critically ill patients. Finding and treating underlying causes of fluid and electrolyte abnormalities are essential.
- Fluid and electrolyte abnormalities are generally asymptomatic unless severe.
- Fluid and electrolyte therapy should be monitored closely because of patient instability and the risk of iatrogenic abnormalities (e.g., cardiac arrhythmias, fluid overload).

17-9. Questions

1. In most critically ill patients, the opiate of choice for analgesia is

    A. morphine.
    B. hydromorphone.
    C. fentanyl.
    D. acetaminophen.
    E. ketorolac.

2. In which situations should hydromorphone or fentanyl be used for analgesia in critically ill patients?

    I.   Morphine allergy
    II. Renal dysfunction
    III. Hemodynamic instability

    A. I only
    B. III only
    C. I and II only
    D. II and III only
    E. I, II, and III

3. What is the maximum duration of therapy for ketorolac?

    A. 5 days
    B. 7 days
    C. 14 days
    D. 30 days
    E. There are no restrictions on length of use.

4. Which agent is recommended for general long-term sedation in the ICU (> 24–72 hours)?

    A. Diazepam
    B. Propofol
    C. Midazolam

    Versed

D. bentobarbital
E. Lorazepam

5. In most critically ill patients, which of the following is the NMB agent of choice?

    A. Propofol
    B. Vecuronium
    C. Cisatracurium
    D. Pancuronium
    E. Any agent may be used first line.

6. The primary advantage of cisatracurium over pancuronium and vecuronium is that

    A. elimination is not organ dependent.
    B. it has a shorter duration of action.
    C. it has a longer duration of action.
    D. it is more effective.
    E. it does not require monitoring.

7. Which of the following is preferred as a first-line sedative agent for ICP control in patients with traumatic brain injury?

    A. Pentobarbital
    B. Lorazepam
    C. Propofol
    D. Vecuronium
    E. Sedation is not recommended.

8. The regimen of choice for post-traumatic seizure prophylaxis is

    A. phenytoin indefinitely.
    B. phenytoin × 7 days.
    C. carbamazepine × 7 days.
    D. benzodiazepines prn if seizures occur.
    E. propofol × 7 days.

9. Which of the following best describes the use of high-dose methylprednisolone in acute spinal cord injury?

    A. Duration of therapy is 24 hours if started within 12 hours of injury.
    B. Duration of therapy is 48 hours if started within 8 hours of injury.
    C. Duration of therapy is 24 hours if started 0–3 hours from injury and 48 hours if started 3–8 hours from injury.
    D. High-dose methylprednisolone may be started at any time after injury.
    E. Both blunt and penetrating spinal cord injuries should be treated with high-dose methylprednisolone.

Use Patient Profile 1 to answer questions 10 and 11.

Patient Profile 1—City Hospital

Patient name: Dennis Green

Age: 24 years

Sex: M

Race: Caucasian

Diagnosis:

Injury from motor vehicle accident:

  Multiple rib fractures

  Moderate liver contusion

Lab/diagnostic tests: CT scan of liver shows no active bleeding

Address: 42 Spring Street

Height: 5′10″

Weight: 70 kg

Allergies: NKDA

Medication orders:

  Cimetidine 300 mg IV q8h

  Morphine 1-4 mg IV q1h prn pain

Dietary: N/A

Additional orders: Pharmacy consult for VTE prophylaxis

Pharmacist notes: N/A

---

10. Which of the following is the most appropriate VTE prophylaxis regimen for Mr. Green?

    A. Low-dose LMWH
    B. Heparin 5,000 units SC q12h
    C. Full-dose IV heparin infusion
    D. Warfarin to INR 2–3
    E. Intermittent pneumatic compression and elastic stocking

11. The following day, Mr. Green requires placement of an epidural catheter for pain control for his rib fractures. Which of the following is true regarding VTE prophylaxis in Mr. Green?

    A. LMWH should be started and monitored closely with anti-Xa levels.
    B. LMWH should be avoided because of the risk of perispinal hematoma.
    C. Full-dose IV heparin should be used for VTE prophylaxis.
    D. Warfarin should be started.
    E. A full-dose direct thrombin inhibitor should be started.

Use Patient Profile 2 to answer questions 12 and 13:

Patient Profile 2—Suburb Hospital

Patient name: Ann Collins

Age: 65 years

Sex: F

Race: Caucasian

Diagnosis:

  Severe community-acquired pneumonia

  Acute pain and swelling in left leg 7 days after admission

Lab/diagnostic tests: Bedside ultrasound shows acute DVT in left leg

Address: 34 Summer Street

Height: 5′4″

Weight: 60 kg

Allergies: Penicillin (rash)

Medication orders:

  Ranitidine 50 mg IV q8h

  Heparin 5,000 units SC q12h changed to IV heparin infusion 1,100 units/h after DVT is diagnosed

  Gatifloxacin 400 mg IV qd

Dietary: N/A

Additional orders: N/A

Pharmacist notes: N/A

A comparison of Mrs. Collins's complete blood count (CBC) on admission and day 7 follows:

	Admission	Day 7
WBC	18.0	4.0
% neutrophils/% bands	80/10	60/0
Hematocrit (%)	42	48
Platelets	175,000	8,000

12. Which of Mrs. Collins's hematologic changes over time is most likely due to heparin?

    A. Leukopenia
    B. Leukocytosis
    C. Increased hematocrit
    D. Bandemia (left shift)
    E. Thrombocytopenia

13. What should be done regarding heparin therapy in Mrs. Collins?

    A. Switch to a direct thrombin inhibitor.
    B. Continue heparin; monitor CBC closely.
    C. Switch to high-dose LMWH.
    D. Switch to aspirin.
    E. Discontinue heparin; do not anticoagulate.

14. In most patients with an acute DVT who are hemodynamically stable, what is the initial treatment of choice?

    A. Heparin 5,000 units SC q12h
    B. Full-dose IV heparin or full-dose LMWH
    C. Thrombolytic therapy (e.g., recombinant tissue plasminogen activator)
    D. Aspirin
    E. Low-dose LMWH

15. All of the following are risk factors for the development of stress ulcers *except*

    A. sepsis.
    B. coagulopathy.
    C. mechanical ventilation.
    D. age > 40 years.
    E. burns.

16. Which of the following is correct regarding stress ulcer prophylaxis?

    A. H2 antagonists or sucralfate are equally effective and considered drugs of choice.
    B. Proton pump inhibitors are more effective than H2 antagonists or sucralfate.

    C. Antacids have the most direct effect on gastric pH and are considered drugs of choice.
    D. Sucralfate is more effective and causes less pneumonia than do H2 antagonists.
    E. All agents (H2 antagonists, sucralfate, proton pump inhibitors, and antacids) are equally effective.

17. Which of the following is the most likely adverse event associated with drotrecogin alfa use in severe sepsis?

    A. Renal dysfunction
    B. Allergy and anaphylactic shock
    C. Tachycardia
    D. Bleeding
    E. Rash

18. Which of the following will *not* increase blood pressure via α_1-adrenergic activation?

    A. Phenylephrine
    B. Dopamine
    C. Epinephrine
    D. Norepinephrine
    E. Dobutamine

19. M. W. is a 25-year-old pregnant female who is admitted to the medical ICU following several days of severe nausea and vomiting. She is hypotensive, tachycardic, and confused, and her urine output is very low. Her serum sodium is 128 mEq/L. Which of the following should be given to treat her fluid and sodium abnormality?

    A. IV normal saline or lactated Ringer's
    B. IV 5% dextrose in water
    C. po water
    D. IV furosemide
    E. Desmopressin

20. Common fluid and electrolyte abnormalities associated with loop diuretics include all of the following *except*

    A. hypokalemia.
    B. hyperkalemia.
    C. hypomagnesemia.
    D. dehydration.
    E. hypocalcemia.

21. R. T. is a 40-year-old male admitted to the medical ICU following a severe asthma exacerbation. RT's serum phosphorus is 0.9 mEq/L and his body weight is 70 kg (100% of ideal). Which of the following acute phosphorus supplementation regimens is most appropriate?

    A. 45 mmol of sodium phosphate IV over 6 hours
    B. 45 mmol of sodium phosphate IV over 10 minutes
    C. 15 mmol of po phosphorus (e.g., Neutraphos) over the next 24 hours
    D. 15 mmol of IV sodium phosphate over 2 hours
    E. No acute phosphorus therapy is required.

22. The most common electrolyte abnormality associated with ACE inhibitors is

    A. hypomagnesemia.
    B. hypokalemia.
    C. hyperkalemia.
    D. hyperphosphatemia.
    E. hypernatremia.

23. All of the following are useful in the rapid treatment of severe hyperkalemia *except*

    A. potassium restriction.
    B. IV calcium.
    C. IV regular insulin and dextrose.
    D. IV sodium bicarbonate.
    E. Oral Kayexalate.

24. Which of the following electrolyte abnormalities are most commonly associated with amphotericin?

    I. Hypokalemia
    II. Hypomagnesemia
    III. Hypocalcemia

    A. I only
    B. III only
    C. I and II only

D. II and III only
E. I, II, and III

25. All of the following are side effects of potassium replacement therapy *except*

    A. constipation (po).
    B. GI upset (po).
    C. cardiac arrhythmias (IV).
    D. vein irritation (IV).
    E. poor taste (po liquid).

26. Which of the following best describes GI side effects of antacids containing magnesium and calcium salts?

    A. Mg causes constipation; Ca causes diarrhea.
    B. Mg causes diarrhea; Ca causes constipation.
    C. Both cause diarrhea.
    D. Both cause constipation.
    E. Neither has GI side effects.

17-10. Answers

1. **A.** Morphine is recommended by the current Society of Critical Care Medicine (SCCM) guidelines on sedation and analgesia as the opiate of choice for most critically ill patients. Morphine is inexpensive, relatively short acting, and well tolerated by many patients.

2. **E.** Under SCCM guidelines, hydromorphone or fentanyl is recommended for critically ill patients with any of the three conditions mentioned. Morphine may cause more hemodynamic instability than does hydromorphone or fentanyl because of more histamine release. In addition, morphine has a renally excreted, partially active metabolite that may accumulate in renal dysfunction. Hydromorphone and fentanyl do not have such a metabolite. The reason for using these agents in morphine allergy is self-explanatory.

3. **A.** According to the manufacturer, ketorolac should not be used longer than 5 days because of the high risk of GI bleeding with this drug.

4. **E.** According to SCCM guidelines, lorazepam is the sedative of choice in most critically ill patients requiring long-term sedation. Lorazepam is less expensive than propofol and has a longer duration of action than propofol or midazolam.

5. **D.** Under SCCM guidelines, pancuronium is the NMB agent of choice for most critically ill patients. Pancuronium is less expensive than the other agents.

6. **A.** Cisatracurium is metabolized by nonspecific plasma esterases, whereas pancuronium and vecuronium have varying degrees of hepatic and renal elimination. Thus, SCCM guidelines recommend cisatracurium for use in patients with renal and hepatic dysfunction.

7. **C.** According to SCCM guidelines, propofol is the sedative of choice for patients who require neurologic assessment often. Patients with traumatic brain injury may require multiple neurologic assessments daily. The short duration of action of propofol allows rapid wakening.

8. **B.** According to the Brain Trauma Foundation guidelines, phenytoin for 7 days postinjury is the regimen of choice for post-traumatic seizure prophylaxis in patients requiring such therapy.

9. **C.** This regimen is based on the results of the National Acute Spinal Cord Injury Study III trial. Some controversy exists regarding the study design of this trial and the actual efficacy of the drug for this indication; however, most clinicians treat acute spinal cord injury with high-dose methylprednisolone.

10. **A.** According to American College of Chest Physicians (ACCP) guidelines, low-dose LMWH is the drug of choice for VTE prophylaxis in a patient with multiple trauma. LMWH is acceptable in this patient because the organ injury is not actively bleeding. If the patient had active bleeding, then mechanical methods (intermittent pneumatic compression and elastic stocking) would be indicated instead of LMWH.

11. **B.** Manufacturers of LMWHs do not recommend using these agents in patients with epidural catheters because of case reports of clinically significant spinal hematomas. Full anticoagulation should also be avoided.

12. **E.** Thrombocytopenia is a common hematologic side effect of heparin. A severe drop in platelets during the first 7–14 days is a typical presentation.

13. **A.** According to ACCP guidelines, all forms of heparin must be discontinued. However, this patient requires acute, full anticoagulation for treatment of an active DVT. A direct thrombin inhibitor should be started. These agents do not cross react with heparin and potentiate thrombocytopenia.

14. **B.** According to ACCP guidelines, rapid, full anticoagulation with IV heparin or SC LMWH is recommended in most patients with uncomplicated DVT. Thrombolytic therapy is recommended only in selected patients with hemodynamic instability or a massive VTE.

15. **D.** Increased age is not an independent risk factor for stress ulcers.

16. **A.** According to American Society of Health-System Pharmacists guidelines, H2 antagonists and sucralfate are generally considered to be equally effective and are the drugs of choice. However, some controversy exists over the effect of H2 antagonists on pneumonia development. Therefore, some clinicians prefer sucralfate.

17. **D.** Drotrecogin alfa is a recombinant form of the endogenous anticoagulant activated protein C. The anticoagulant activity increases the risk of bleeding.

18. **E.** Dobutamine has no α_1-adrenergic (vasoconstriction) activity.

19. **A.** M. W. is hyponatremic, and her clinical signs and symptoms indicate severe dehydration from GI losses of water and sodium. She requires rapid fluid resuscitation with a fluid that has an approximately physiologic amount of sodium (either NS 154 mEq/L or LR 130 mEq/L). This amount of sodium will increase her serum sodium into the normal range over time, and the osmotic effect will hold water in the extracellular compartment (the vasculature and interstitium) to help restore organ perfusion.

20. **B.** Loop diuretics enhance renal excretion of water, potassium, magnesium, and calcium.

21. **A.** R. T. is severely hypophosphatemic and requires high-dose IV therapy (0.64 mmol/kg × 70 kg = 44.8 mmol). The dose should be infused at 7.5 mmol/h (total time: 6 hours) to avoid precipitation with calcium.

22. **C.** ACE inhibitors cause hyperkalemia because of aldosterone inhibition.

23. **E.** Oral Kayexalate (sodium polystyrene sulfonate) does not act very quickly. It requires transit time through the intestines to bind potassium and create a gradient that pulls more potassium into the lumen of the GI tract.

24. **C.** Amphotericin B causes renal wasting of potassium and magnesium.

25. **A.** Oral potassium replacement therapy does not normally cause constipation. Cardiac arrhythmias are a concern if IV potassium is given faster than 10 mEq/h.

26. **B.** Magnesium salts (e.g., milk of magnesia) are often used as osmotic laxatives and may cause diarrhea. Calcium salts may cause constipation.

17-11. References

Allen ME, Kopp BJ, Erstad BL. Stress ulcer prophylaxis in the postoperative period. *Am J Health Syst Pharm.* 2004;61:588–96.

American Association of Neurological Surgeons and Congress of Neurological Surgeons. Pharmacological therapy after acute cervical spinal cord injury. *Neurosurgery.* 2002;50(3 suppl):S63–72.

American Society of Health-System Pharmacists Commission on Therapeutics. ASHP therapeutic guidelines on stress ulcer prophylaxis. *Am J Health Syst Pharm.* 1999;56:347–79.

Boucher BA, Clifton GD, Hanes SD. Critical care therapy. In: Helms RA, Quan DJ, Herfindal ET, Gourley DR, eds. *Textbook of Therapeutics: Drug and Disease Management.* 8th ed. Philadelphia: Lippincott Williams & Wilkins; 2006:655–73.

Boucher BA, Timmons SD. Acute management of the brain injury patient. In: DiPiro JT, Talbert RL, Yee GC, et al., eds. *Pharmacotherapy: A Pathophysiologic Approach.* 7th ed. New York: McGraw-Hill; 2008:965–76.

Brain Trauma Foundation, American Association of Neurological Surgeons, Congress of Neurological Surgeons. *Guidelines for the Management of Severe Traumatic Brain Injury.* New York: Brain Trauma Foundation; 2003.

Brophy DF, Gehr TWB. Disorders of potassium and magnesium homeostasis. In: DiPiro JT, Talbert RL, Yee GC, et al., eds. *Pharmacotherapy: A Pathophysiologic Approach.* 7th ed. New York: McGraw-Hill; 2008:877–88.

Corwin HL, Gettinger A, Fabian TC, et al. Efficacy and safety of epoetin alfa in critically ill patients. *New Engl J Med.* 2007;357:965–76.

Coyle JD, Joy MS. Disorders of sodium, water homeostasis. In: DiPiro JT, Talbert RL, Yee GC, et al., eds. *Pharmacotherapy: A Pathophysiologic Approach.* 7th ed. New York: McGraw-Hill; 2008:845–60.

Dellinger RP, Levy MM, Carlet JM, et al. Surviving Sepsis Campaign: International guidelines for management of severe sepsis and septic shock: 2008. *Crit Care Med.* 2008;36:296–327.

Geerts WH, Bergqvist D, Pineo GF, et al. Prevention of venous thromboembolism: American College of Chest Physicians evidence-based clinical practice guidelines (8th edition). *Chest.* 2008;133(suppl):381S–453S.

Jacobi J, Fraser GL, Coursin DB, et al. Clinical practice guidelines for the sustained use of sedatives and analgesics in the critically ill adult. *Crit Care Med.* 2002;30:119–41.

Kang-Birken SL, DiPiro JT. Sepsis and septic shock. In: DiPiro JT, Talbert RL, Yee GC, et al., eds. *Pharmacotherapy: A Pathophysiologic Approach.* 7th ed. New York: McGraw-Hill; 2008:1943–56.

Lau A, Chan LN. Electrolytes, other minerals, and trace elements. In: Lee M, ed. *Basic Skills in Interpreting Laboratory Data.* 3rd ed. Bethesda, Md.: American Society of Health-System Pharmacists; 2004:183–232.

Murray MJ, Cowen J, DeBlock H, et al. Clinical practice guidelines for sustained neuromuscular blockade in the critically ill patient. *Crit Care Med.* 2002;30:142–56.

Pai AB, Rohrscheib, Joy MS. Disorders of calcium and phosphorus homeostasis. In: DiPiro JT, Talbert RL, Yee GC, et al., eds. *Pharmacotherapy: A Pathophysiologic Approach.* 7th ed. New York: McGraw-Hill; 2008:861–76.

Nutrition

Rex O. Brown, PharmD, BCNSP

18-1. Overview

General Nutrition

U.S. dietary guidelines (food pyramid)

- Maintain a healthy weight.
- Maintain a low-fat diet (< 30% of total calories).
- Eat plenty of fruits, vegetables, and grain products.
- Use salt, sugar, and alcohol in moderation.

Malnutrition

- Causes of undernutrition (protein-calorie malnutrition):
  - Depressed intake of nutrients (starvation, semistarvation)
  - Alteration in nutrient metabolism (trauma, major infection)
- Causes of obesity:
  - Excessive caloric intake (especially carbohydrate and fat)
  - Alteration in nutrient metabolism (genetic predisposition)
  - Sedentary lifestyle

Dietary reference intakes (DRIs) of selected nutrients

- *Fiber:* 20–35 g/d (many people find this goal unpalatable)
- *Calcium:* 1,200–1,500 mg/d in adolescents and young adults; 1,000 mg/d in men until age 65 and women until age 50; 1,200–1,500 mg/d for life thereafter (usually requires supplements)

- **Multivitamins:** Helpful to meet daily requirements of pregnant and lactating women, elderly persons, and those who eat vegetarian or low-calorie diets

Nutritional assessment components

History and physical examination
- Dietary intake (anorexia, bullemia, hyperphagia, taste alterations)
- Underlying pathology affecting nutrition (cancer, burns)
- End-organ effects (diarrhea, constipation)
- General appearance (edema, cachexia)
- Skin appearance (scaling skin, decubitus ulcers)
- Musculoskeletal effects (depressed muscle mass, growth retardation)
- Neurologic effects (depressed sensorium, encephalopathy)
- Hepatic effects (jaundice, hepatomegaly)

Anthropometrics
- Skinfold measurements for assessment of fat (triceps, calf)
- Arm muscle circumference for assessment of skeletal muscle
- Weight for height to determine undernutrition or obesity
- Head circumference in infants to document appropriate growth
- Percentage of ideal body weight (IBW) after calculation of IBW for patient:
  - IBW of males (kg) = 50 + (2.3 × height in inches over 5 feet)
  - IBW of females (kg) = 45.5 + (2.3 × height in inches over 5 feet)

- Body mass index (BMI) for assessment of under-nutrition or obesity calculated from body weight (kg) and height (m): BMI = weight (kg)/height^2 (m^2)

Biochemical assessment

Serum albumin concentration

- Good prognostic indicator and good for assessment of long-term nutritional status
- Poor for repletion marker because of long half-life (21 d) and large body pool

Serum prealbumin concentration

- Good for short-term assessment of nutrition support because of short half-life (2 d) and small body pool

Serum transferrin concentration

- Good for short-term assessment of nutrition support because of short half-life (7 d) and small body pool
- Elevated in iron-deficiency anemia

Creatinine height index

- Requires 24-hour urine collection to determine levels of creatinine

Other methods of nutritional assessment

- Muscle strength testing
- Bioelectrical impedance (i.e., a low-grade electrical current runs through the body to identify body protein stores and fat stores)

Types of malnutrition

- *Marasmus:* Features depleted fat and muscle stores, normal biochemical measurements, and intact immune status
- *Kwashiorkor:* Features normal or elevated fat and body weight with abnormally low biochemical measurements and depressed immune function
- *Kwashiorkor–marasmus mix:* All measurements depressed
- *Obesity:* Demonstrated as elevated body weight to at least 120% of IBW or BMI > 27.8 (male) or > 27.3 (female)
  - Class I obesity: BMI > 30 and < 35
  - Class II obesity: BMI > 35 and < 40
  - Class III obesity: BMI > 40

Selected definitions

- *Hypermetabolism:* An increase in energy expenditure above normal (usually > 10% above normal)

- *Hypercatabolism:* An increase in protein losses above normal (usually via urinary excretion of urea nitrogen)
- *Specialized nutrition support:* Parenteral nutrition (PN) or enteral nutrition (EN)
- *Basal energy expenditure (BEE):* A calculation of the normal energy needs of healthy adult men or women using sex, age, height, and weight
- *Harris–Benedict equations for BEE:*
  - Male (kcal/d) = 66 + 13.7 (weight in kg) + 5 (height in cm) – 6.8 (age in years)
  - Female (kcal/d) = 655 + 9.6 (weight in kg) + 1.8 (height in cm) – 4.7 (age in years)
- *Mifflin equations for energy expenditure:*
  - Male (kcal/d) = 10 (weight in kg) + 6.25 (height in cm) – 4.9 (age in years) + 5
  - Female (kcal/d) = 10 (weight in kg) + 6.25 (height in cm) – 4.9 (age in years) – 161
- *Resting energy expenditure (REE):* A measured value of energy expenditure (generally ~10% above BEE or Mifflin in health, but can be 100% above BEE in severe burns)
- *Respiratory quotient (RQ):* The value that results when carbon dioxide production (VCO$_2$) is divided by oxygen consumption (VO$_2$)
  - RQ for carbohydrate oxidation = 1.0
  - RQ for fat oxidation = 0.7
  - RQ for protein oxidation = 0.8
  - RQ for fat synthesis = 8.0
- *Body cell mass:* Lean, metabolically active tissue (skeletal muscle, body organs)
- *Lean body mass:* Body cell mass, extracelluar fluid, and extracellular solids (bone, serum proteins)
- *RDI:* Recommended daily intake

18-2. Nutritional Requirements

Calorie Requirements

- Most clinicians dose specialized nutrition support in total calories (i.e., using carbohydrate, fat, and protein-calorie contributions to obtain the desired dose).
  - 25 kcal/kg/d for adults with little stress (e.g., elective surgery)
  - 30 kcal/kg/d for patients with infections, skeletal trauma
  - 35 kcal/kg/d for patients with major trauma (head injury, long-bone fractures)
  - 40 kcal/kg/d for patients with major thermal injury (> 50% total body surface area burn)

- Multiply BEE by the stress factor to determine calorie requirements:
  - $1.0 \times$ BEE for patients with little stress
  - $1.3 \times$ BEE for patients with minor trauma, infections
  - $1.5 \times$ BEE for patients with major trauma
  - $2 \times$ BEE for patients with severe thermal injury
- Measure the REE via indirect calorimetry for calorie requirements.

Caloric Contribution of the Major Macronutrients

- *Glucose:* 3.4 kcal/g because hydrated glucose is used in PN (glucose powder would be 4 kcal/g)
- *Fat:* 9 kcal/g
- Protein: 4 kcal/g
  - Protein requirements are usually dosed in grams per kilogram per day.
  - 0.8 g/kg/d is the adult recommended daily allowance (RDA) for protein in the United States.
  - 1.0 g/kg/d is the adult RDA for patients with minor stress (elective operations).
  - 1.5 g/kg/d is the adult RDA for patients with major trauma or infection.
  - 2.0 g/kg/d is the adult RDA for patients with severe head injury, sepsis, or severe thermal injury.

Measurement of Nutritional Efficacy Using Nitrogen Balance (NB)

NB = nitrogen in − nitrogen out

- Nitrogen in (grams) is determined by dividing the grams of protein taken in on the day of balance by 6.25.
- Nitrogen out (grams) is determined by measuring the grams of urea nitrogen excreted during a 24-hour urine collection and then adding a factor of 2 or 4 g for insensible nitrogen loss or stool loss.
- Positive NB can be used to document adequacy of nutritional support:
  - In undernourished patients, +4 to +6 g/d is desired.
  - Nitrogen equilibrium (−2 to +2 g/d) is usually adequate in critically ill patients.

Other Requirements during Nutrition Support

Water

- Up to 35 mL/kg/d for average-sized adults
- 40 mL/kg/d for smaller adults and adolescents
- > 40 mL/kg/d for patients with extrarenal losses (e.g., gastrointestinal drains)

Electrolytes

- Sodium requirements:
  - 60–100 mEq/d in adults
  - 2–6 mEq/kg/d in children
- Chloride requirements:
  - 60–100 mEq/d in adults
  - 2–6 mEq/kg/d in children
- Potassium requirements:
  - 60–100 mEq/d in adults
  - 2–5 mEq/kg/d in children
- Calcium requirements:
  - 5–15 mEq/d in adults
  - 2–3 mEq/kg/d in children
- Phosphorus requirements:
  - 20–45 mmol/d in adults
  - 1–2 mmol/kg/d in children
- Magnesium requirements:
  - 10–20 mEq/d in adults
  - 0.25–1.00 mEq/kg/d in children

Vitamins

- Vitamins are provided daily in both PN (added) and EN (endogenous).
- Most enteral formulations provide the DRI for vitamins in a volume of 1,000–1,500 mL.
- For parenteral vitamin products:
  - Adult products contain 12 (MVI-12) or 13 vitamins (Infuvite Adult, MVI-Adult); vitamin K is added separately when the product with 12 vitamins is used.
  - Pediatric products (MVI-Pediatric, Infuvite Pediatric) contain all 13 vitamins.

Trace elements

- *Zinc:* 3–5 mg/d in adults with PN; 50–250 mcg/kg/d in children with PN
- *Copper:* 0.5–1.2 mg/d in adults with PN; 20 mcg/kg/d in children with PN (maximum of 300 mcg/d)
- *Chromium:* 10–15 mcg/d in adults with PN; monitored but not given to children
- *Manganese:* 50–100 mcg/d in adults with PN; monitored but not given to children
- *Selenium:* 40–80 mcg/d in adults with PN; 1.5–3.0 mcg/kg/d in children with PN

18-3. Specialized Nutrition Support

Parenteral Nutrition

Indications

PN is generally used for patients who cannot be fed via the gastrointestinal tract.

Severe acute pancreatitis
- Oral or tube feeding will usually exacerbate this condition unless given via the jejunum (e.g., nasojejunal feeding tube or jejunostomy).

Short bowel syndrome
- This condition requires PN from a few weeks to lifelong, as needed.

Ileus
- This condition is secondary to lack of bowel function (e.g., acute renal failure secondary to sepsis)

Other indications
- Crohn's disease exacerbation with fistula or obstruction
- Neonates who cannot eat in the first day of life
- Preoperatively for undernourished patients who are undergoing an elective operation and for whom there is no direct access to the gastrointestinal tract (e.g., partial small bowel obstruction from cancer)
- Pregnancy with severe hyperemesis gravidarum (i.e., there is an inability to tolerate oral or enteral nutrition)
- Gastrointestinal fistulae where oral or enteral nutrition should be restricted

Components of parenteral nutrition

Protein
- Protein should be included in all PN formulations.
- Standard amino acids from 10%, 15%, or 20% stock solutions can be used for most patients.
- Final concentrations in the PN formulation vary from 2% to 7%.
- Doses > 2 g/kg/d are rarely needed.

Fat
- Fat is provided as intravenous fat emulsion either as a separate infusion or admixed with the rest of the PN formulation, making a total nutrient admixture (TNA).
- Products are manufactured as 10%, 20%, and 30% fat emulsions. (In the United States, 30% can be used only for TNAs, not for direct infusion.)
- Fat provides essential fatty acids to the patient who is most likely not eating by mouth.
- Fat provides nonprotein calories other than glucose.
- Common doses used in adults are ~1 g/kg/d (9–10 kcal/kg/d).
- Intravenous fat emulsions contain phospholipid to emulsify the product and glycerol to make the emulsion isotonic. (Both of these components provide modest calories.)

Dextrose
- Common doses of dextrose in critically ill patients are 3–4 mg/kg/min (~15–20 kcal/kg/d).
- Dextrose is in all PN formulations for obligate needs (central nervous system, renal medulla, white blood cells, red blood cells, and wound healing)
- PN formulations are usually made from 70% dextrose in water.
- Final concentrations in the PN formulation vary from D10W to D35W.
- Dextrose should never exceed a dose of 5 mg/kg/min (~25 kcal/kg/d).

Sodium
- Sodium can be provided as chloride, acetate, or phosphate salts in PN.
- After phosphate addition, the remaining anions are added on the basis of acid–base status. They are split between chloride and acetate with a normal pH, predominantly acetate with metabolic acidosis, and predominantly chloride with metabolic alkalosis.
- Requirements can be increased when the patient has extrarenal losses from nasogastric suction, abdominal drains, or ostomy losses.

Potassium
- Potassium can be provided as chloride, acetate, or phosphate salts in PN
- Requirements can be increased with administration of potassium-wasting drugs (diuretics, steroids) or in severe undernutrition.
- Like sodium, the remaining potassium can be added as acetate or chloride on the basis of acid–base status after the proper dose of phosphate is determined.

Calcium
- Most practitioners add calcium as the gluconate salt.
- Higher doses of calcium (~20–25 mEq/d) are needed in patients receiving long-term PN to help prevent metabolic bone disease.
- Addition of calcium is limited in PN formulations because of the potential to precipitate with phosphate salts, which ultimately results in insoluble calcium phosphate.

Phosphate
- Phosphate is added as the sodium or potassium salt.
- Higher doses of phosphorus (e.g., 30 mmol/L) are needed to prevent refeeding syndrome in severely undernourished patients.
- Phosphorus should be decreased or removed in patients with renal failure.
- Most practitioners prefer sodium phosphate over potassium phosphate because of the higher concentration of aluminum in the latter product, especially in chronic use of PN.
- Addition of phosphorus is limited in PN formulations because of the potential to precipitate with calcium or magnesium salts to form an insoluble compound.

Magnesium
- Most practitioners add magnesium as the sulfate salt.
- Higher doses should be used in patients with alcoholism or large bowel losses or in patients receiving drugs causing renal wasting of magnesium (cisplatin, amphotericin B, aminoglycosides, loop diuretics).
- Magnesium should be restricted or deleted in patients with renal failure.

Multivitamins
- Multivitamins are given daily as part of PN.
- Parenteral multivitamin preparations contain 12 or 13 vitamins. (Vitamin K should be administered separately if the 12-vitamin preparation is used.)
- Additional thiamine and folic acid are often given to alcoholic patients who are receiving PN.
- Additional folic acid (at least 600 mcg/d) should be given to pregnant patients receiving PN.

Trace elements
- Trace elements are given daily as a cocktail of four or five trace metals.
- Extra zinc should be given in patients with ostomy or diarrhea losses.
- Copper and manganese should be reduced or eliminated in patients with cholestasis.
- Extra selenium is usually needed in homebound PN patients.

Total nutrient admixtures versus two-in-one admixtures
Advantages of TNAs
- Decreased nursing time for administration
- Potentially decreased touch contamination
- Decreased pharmacy preparation time (assuming a 24-hour hang time)
- Financial savings (use of only one pump and one intravenous administration set)

Disadvantages of TNAs
- TNAs are better media for bacterial growth than are two-in-one admixtures.
- It is impossible to visualize particulate matter.
- Filter formulation with a 0.22-micron filter is not possible.
- Some additives like calcium and phosphorus are less compatible in TNAs.

Central vein PN versus peripheral vein PN
Advantages of central vein PN
- Central vein PN can maximize caloric intake.
- Volume restriction of patients is possible.
- Long-term catheter can be maintained.

Disadvantages of central vein PN
- Mechanical complications during catheter placement (e.g., pneumothorax)
- Potential hyperosmolar complications (e.g., from using hypertonic dextrose)
- Potential septic catheter complications

Advantages of peripheral vein PN
- It is easier to place the catheter (i.e., peripheral vein stick).
- Hyperosmolar complications are avoided because dilute formulations must be used.

Disadvantages of peripheral vein PN
- Incidence of thrombophlebitis is high.
- Frequent vein rotation is necessary.
- Energy intake is limited.
- Volume restriction is not possible (using dilute formulations).

- Cost is higher because more lipid calories are generally used. (Lipids are isotonic.)

Parenteral nutrition calculations

D20W (final concentration of PN formulation)
- D20W = 20% dextrose = 20 g/100 mL = 200 g/L × 3.4 kcal/g = 680 dextrose kcal/L
- 2 L/d of $D_{20}W$ (final concentration of PN formulation) = 1,360 dextrose kcal/d

Amino acids 5% (final concentration of PN formulation)
- 5% amino acids = 5 g/100 mL = 50 g/L × 4 kcal/g = 200 protein kcal/L
- 2 L/d of 5% amino acids = 100 g/d = 400 protein kcal/d

Lipid 2% (final concentration of TNA formulation)
- 2% lipid will deliver 200 kcal/L (includes calories from glycerol/phospholipid)
- 2 L/d of lipid 2% = 400 fat kcal/d

Lipid 20% infused at 20 m L/h × 24 h (separate infusion given with two-in-one PN formulations)
- 20% lipid = 2 kcal/mL
- 20 mL/h × 24 h = 480 mL/d
- 480 mL/d × 2 kcal/mL = 960 fat kcal/d

Example: $D_{30}W$; amino acids 4%; lipid 3%, at 60 mL/h
- 60 mL/h × 24 h/d = 1,440 mL/d (1.44 L/d)
- D30W = 30% dextrose = 300 g/L × 3.4 kcal/g = 1,020 kcal/L × 1.44 L = 1,469 dextrose kcal
- 4% amino acids = 40 g/L = 160 kcal/L × 1.44 L = 230 protein kcal
- 3% lipid = 300 kcal/L × 1.44 L = 432 fat kcal
- 1,469 kcal + 230 kcal + 432 kcal = 2,131 total kcal/d from the above PN formulation

Example: dextrose 400 g; amino acids 100 g; lipids 40 g; at 85 mL/h
- Dextrose 400 g × 3.4 kcal/g = 1360 kcal/d
- Amino acids 100 g × 4 kcal/g = 400 kcal/d
- Lipids 40 g × 10 kcal/g (includes phospholipid and glycerol) = 400 kcal/d

General principles of compounding parenteral nutrition

- Each component of the PN prescription should be reviewed to ensure a balanced PN formulation is provided.
- Each component should be assessed for dose and potential compatibility programs.

- All compounded PN formulations should be visually inspected to ensure no gross contamination or precipitation is present.
- Manufacturers of automated compounders should provide the additive sequence to ensure safety in PN preparation.

General principles of stability and compatibility of parenteral nutrition

- Parenteral multivitamins should be added shortly before dispensing and administering the PN formulation because vitamins A and C degrade fairly quickly.
- Preparation of TNAs using dual-chambered bags (lipid is kept in a separate compartment until administration) can enhance the shelf life of a PN formulation.
- Dibasic calcium phosphate ($CaHPO4$) can precipitate in PN formulations if the amounts of calcium gluconate and sodium or potassium phosphate are excessive.
- Generally, phosphate should be added first to the PN formulation.
- Generally, calcium should be added last to the PN formulation.
- Calcium chloride should not be used in PN because it is highly reactive with phosphate.
- Iron dextran can be added to two-in-one PN formulations but should not be added to TNAs.

Parenteral nutrition filtration

- Filters are used to prevent administration of particulate matter, microorganisms, and air.
- Use a new 0.22-micron filter each day with two-in-one PN formulations (0.22-micron filters with positive charged nylon can be used for up to 96 hours in two-in-one PN formulations).
- Use a new 1.2-micron filter each day with TNAs.

Complications of parenteral nutrition

Metabolic
Hyperglycemia
- Patients with stress of trauma or infection or those with diabetes often need regular human insulin added to the PN formulation to control hyperglycemia.
- Regular insulin continuous infusions are often needed to control hyperglycemia.

Electrolyte disorders

Hypokalemia

- Patients often require extra potassium in PN (e.g., 60 mEq/L).

Hypophosphatemia

- Patients often require extra phosphorus in PN (e.g., 30 mmol/L).

Hypomagnesemia

- Patients often require extra magnesium in PN (e.g., 16 mEq/L).

Hyponatremia

- Diagnosis of sodium disorders must include an assessment of extracellular fluid status (i.e., volume status).
  - *Volume depleted:* Add sodium and water to PN, or increase intravenous fluid administration.
  - *Volume overloaded:* Remove sodium from PN and concentrate the formulation.
  - *Euvolemic:* Generally, water restriction is first-line therapy (concentrate the PN formula).

Acid–base disorders

- Increase acetate and decrease chloride anions if the patient has metabolic acidosis.
- Increase chloride and decrease acetate anions if the patient has metabolic alkalosis.

Essential fatty acid deficiency

- During PN, at least 4% of total calories need to be provided as intravenous lipid (easily attained when lipid is used daily as a calorie source).

Trace element disorders

- Patients with increased ostomy output or chronic diarrhea need extra zinc.
- Hold copper and manganese in patients with cholestasis.

Hepatic steatosis

- Fatty infiltration of the liver has been reported with long-term PN.
- Hepatic steatosis is thought to be primarily caused by administration of excessive dextrose calories.
- The key to prevention is through administration of an appropriate dose of dextrose (e.g., < 5 mg/kg/min).

Mechanical complications

- Pneumothorax (punctured lung) can occur during central vein canulation.
- Subclavian artery injury can occur when the artery is cannulated instead of the vein.
- Subclavian vein thrombosis can occur with long-term central vein access. (Heparin is used in some PN patients to prevent this condition.)

Infectious complications

- Such complications are usually due to catheter-related breakdown in sterile technique.
- They are rarely solution related.

Monitoring of parenteral nutrition

Frequency and intensity of monitoring is based on the patient's condition, as assessed by

- Electrolyte balance and glucose control
- Acid–base status via arterial blood gases
- Intake and output for assessment of fluid balance
- Serum prealbumin concentrations, nitrogen balance, or both to document efficacy

Enteral Nutrition

Indications

- EN is generally used in patients who cannot or will not eat but have a functional and accessible gastrointestinal tract.
- Neonates should begin EN as early as possible, even if receiving PN.
- EN is used in elderly patients who lack the ability to ingest food orally.

Cardiac

- Cardiac patients may need fluid-restricted EN with fluid overload.

Pulmonary failure

- EN is used frequently in patients receiving mechanical ventilation.

Hepatic failure

- EN is used frequently in this population.
- In severe hepatic encephalopathy, use a formulation with high branched-chain amino acids and low aromatic amino acids.
- In the absence of encephalopathy or mild encephalopathy, use EN with standard protein.

Gastrointestinal failure
- In short bowel syndrome, EN is used to enhance small bowel hypertrophy after major bowel resection.
- In inflammatory bowel syndrome, EN is the preferred method of nutrition support.

Neurologic impairment
- EN is preferred because the patient may not be able to eat, but the gastrointestinal tract is functional and accessible.

Cancer or HIV infection
- Use EN (if possible) in these patients to prevent or treat undernutrition.

Types of enteral access

- Feeding enterostomy
  - Feeding enterostomy is used for long-term EN.
  - Gastrostomy requires a G-tube or PEG (percutaneous endoscopic gastrostomy).
  - Jejunostomy requires an exploratory laparotomy to place.
- Oral route (by drinking supplements)
- Nasal tube feeding
  - Nasal tube feeding is usual for short-term EN.
  - Nasogastric, nasoduodenal, or nasojejunal tubes are used.

Products for enteral nutrition

- Polymeric, nutritionally complete tube feeding is used for patients with normal digestive processes (e.g., 1 kcal/mL).
- Concentrated, nutritionally complete tube feeding is used for patients who need severe fluid restriction (e.g., 2 kcal/mL).
- Polymeric, nutritionally complete, oral supplements are used to supplement an oral diet (e.g., 1.0 or 1.5 kcal/mL).
- Chemically defined, nutritionally complete tube feeding is used for patients with impaired digestive processes such as short bowel syndrome or pancreatic insufficiency (e.g., 1 kcal/mL).
- Fiber-containing, nutritionally complete tube feeding is beneficial in patients who receive long-term tube feeding (can prevent diarrhea and constipation; e.g., 1.0 or 1.2 kcal/mL).
- Concentrated, low-protein, low-electrolyte tube feeding is generally used for patients with renal failure.

- A high branched-chain amino acid, low aromatic amino acid EN formula is used for patients with liver failure and severe hepatic encephalopathy (e.g., 1.0 or 1.5 kcal/mL).
- High-fat, low-carbohydrate, nutritionally complete tube feeding is helpful in management of diabetic or other glucose-intolerant patients (e.g., 1.0 or 1.2 kcal/mL).
- Immune-enhancing formulas that contain arginine, glutamine, and omega-3 fatty acids are marketed and used in patients with high metabolic stress (e.g., severe trauma or infection; 1.0 or 1.3 kcal/mL).

Complications of enteral nutrition

Pulmonary (e.g., aspiration pneumonia)
- The most severe complications of EN are pulmonary.
- Pulmonary complications are caused by regurgitation of gastric contents into the lung (with or without tube feeding).
- Prevention is important.
  - Elevate the head of the bed to 30° if possible.
  - Frequently assess the patient's abdomen to ensure tolerance.
  - Frequently assess the placement of the feeding tube (especially nasally placed tubes).

Gastrointestinal
- Diarrhea is often associated with the administration of EN, but EN is not necessarily the cause of the diarrhea.

Increased frequency or volume of stools
- Pharmacotherapy is often the cause, because of sorbitol in liquid vehicles.
- Lack of fiber and excessive infusion rate advancements can also be causes.
- Decreasing (or at least not advancing) the infusion rate is appropriate.
- Change to a fiber-containing formulation if the patient is not receiving one.
- Pseudomembranous enterocolitis can occur from antibiotic therapy.
- Use pharmacotherapeutic treatment if the above factors are ruled out (bismuth subsalicylate, loperamide, diphenoxylate).

Constipation (decrease in stool frequency)
- Lack of fiber can be a cause.
- Lack of water can be a cause.
- Poor mobility and drugs with anticholinergic activity can contribute.

- Keep patient well hydrated and use a fiber-containing EN formulation.

Mechanical

- In the event of nasal necrosis, use a small-bore feeding tube and do not tape it too firmly to the nose.
- To prevent esophageal injury, use a small-bore feeding tube.
- To prevent it from clogging, frequently flush the feeding tube with warm water.
- In the event of tube displacement, discourage removing the tube; the tube may have to be anchored with a bridle.

Metabolic

Hyperglycemia

- Use regular human insulin.
- Consider a high-fat, low-carbohydrate EN formulation.
- Regular insulin continuous infusions are sometimes necessary

Hypokalemia

- Provide additional potassium as an intravenous (IV) or per tube supplement.
- Some institutions allow the addition of potassium salts to the EN formulation.

Hypophosphatemia

- Provide additional phosphorus as an IV supplement (e.g., potassium phosphate).
- Some institutions allow the addition of phosphorus salts to the EN formulation (e.g., injectable sodium or potassium phosphate).

Monitoring of enteral nutrition

The intensity of monitoring will be dictated by the condition of the patient:

- Electrolyte balance and glucose control
- Acid–base status via arterial blood gases (critical care only)
- Intake and output for assessment of fluid balance
- Assessment of the patient's abdomen is required:
  - Positive bowel sounds usually should be present.
  - The abdomen should be soft, nontender, and nondistended in most cases.
  - A profoundly distended abdomen usually requires the EN to be decreased or discontinued temporarily.

- Serum prealbumin concentrations, nitrogen balance, or both should be assessed to document efficacy.

Home Nutrition Support

Parenteral nutrition

- PN can be given from weeks to a lifetime (e.g., severe short bowel syndrome).
- PN is usually cycled at night over 10–16 hours.
- Patient must be monitored closely for iron deficiency because iron supplementation is not routinely added to PN.
- Regular assessment of hemoglobin, hematocrit, and mean corpuscular volume is required.
- Serum iron, total iron-binding capacity, and ferritin are commonly used in the diagnosis of iron deficiency.
- Metabolic bone disease is another long-term complication of home PN.
  - Supplemental calcium in the PN formulation is usually required (15–25 mEq/d).
  - Adequate vitamin K for osteocalcin is important on a long-term basis.

Enteral nutrition

- EN can be given indefinitely as full nutrition support or as a supplement to an oral diet.
- Permanent feeding ostomies are used almost exclusively in home EN.
- Patients in nursing homes and extended care facilities usually receive EN as a continuous (24 hours) or intermittent (e.g., 12 hours) infusion.
- Patients who receive home EN via gastrostomy usually receive bolus feeding (e.g., two 240-mL cans tid via PEG).
- Patients who receive home EN as a supplement to oral intake are often cycled at night (e.g., 1,000 mL at 85 mL/h from 7:00 pm to 7:00 am each night).

18-4. Major Drug–Nutrient Interactions

Phenytoin and Enteral Tube Feeding

- It has been demonstrated that enteral feeding will bind to phenytoin, thus impairing the absorption dramatically, possibly because of the protein component of EN (caseinates).

Management of Phenytoin–Enteral Nutrition Interaction

- Hold the EN 2 hours before and after the daily dose of phenytoin capsules.
- Hold the EN 1 hour before and after each dose of phenytoin suspension (usually given bid or tid).
- Increase the EN infusion rate to allow the desired nutritional dose of EN to be given (i.e., to make up for the lost time while the EN is being held for drug administration).

Warfarin and Enteral Tube Feeding

- It has been reported that adequate anticoagulation with warfarin is very difficult to achieve with concurrent EN (low international normalized ratios).

Management of Warfarin–Enteral Nutrition Interaction

- Hold EN 1 hour before and after the daily warfarin dose. If this is done, the EN rate should be increased to attain the desired nutritional dose.

Management of Grapefruit Juice–Drug Interaction

- Grapefruit juice interacts with many drugs (e.g., amlodipine, carbamazepine, cyclosporine)
- Grapefruit juice from frozen concentrate has been reported to inhibit gastrointestinal cytochrome P450-3A4, resulting in enhancement of oral absorption of some drugs (toxicity).
- When taking drugs that are known to interact with grapefruit juice, patients should be advised to avoid these grapefruit products (i.e., substitute another fruit juice such as apple or orange juice).

18-5. Key Points

- Malnutrition can present as either undernutrition or obesity.
- The components of a nutritional assessment include a history and physical exam, anthropometric measurements, and biochemical tests.
- An increase in energy expenditure (energy needs) is defined as *hypermetabolism,* and an increase in nitrogen excretion (protein needs) is defined as *hypercatabolism.*

- Most patients receiving specialized nutrition support (parenteral or enteral nutrition) require 25–30 kcal/kg/d and 1–2 g protein/kg/d.
- The water requirement for most adult patients without substantial extrarenal losses is 30–40 mL/kg/d.
- PN should be reserved for patients whose gastrointestinal tracts are not functional or accessible (e.g., severe acute pancreatitis, severe short bowel syndrome).
- TNAs contain dextrose, amino acids, lipid emulsion, electrolytes, vitamins, and trace elements in one container.
- The advantages of TNAs include decreased nursing administration time, decreased potential for touch contamination, and reduced expense (the patient needs only one pump and one intravenous administration set).
- The advantages of central vein PN over peripheral vein PN include the ability to concentrate the formulation, administer adequate calories and protein, and use the catheter for long-term administration.
- For PN calculations: 1 g hydrated dextrose = 3.4 kcal, 1 g amino acids = 4 kcal, and 1 g lipid = 9 kcal. (Intravenous fat emulsion actually provides 10 kcal/g because it includes calories provided as glycerol and phospholipid.)
- All PN formulations should be filtered during administration (0.22-micron filter for two-in-one PN formulations and 1.2-micron filter for TNAs).
- Enteral nutrition support is generally used in patients who cannot or will not eat but have a functional and accessible gastrointestinal tract.
- Enteral tube feeding can be provided by one of the following methods: nasogastric, nasoduodenal, nasojejunal, gastrostomy, or jejunostomy.
- Diarrhea associated with enteral tube feeding is often caused by pharmacotherapy (e.g., sorbitol in liquid drug preparations as a vehicle).
- Patients receiving phenytoin or warfarin concurrently with enteral tube feeding should have the tube feeding held at least 1 hour before and after each dose.

18-6. Questions

1. What is the most appropriate calcium intake (mg/d) for adults over 65 years of age?

    A. 600–800 mg
    B. 800–1,000 mg
    C. 1,000–1,200 mg
    D. 1,200–1,500 mg
    E. 1,500–1,800 mg

Case Study for Questions 2 and 3

A patient presents for a comprehensive nutritional assessment. She is 35 years old, is 5 feet 8 inches, and weighs 52 kg. She has a history of Crohn's disease involving both the small bowel and colon. She has had no surgeries but has intermittent diarrhea.

Medications

- Prednisone 5 mg qod
- Mesalamine 1 g tid
- Loperamide 2 mg q6h prn diarrhea

Measurements

- Triceps skinfold = 3 mm (normal, 10–14 mm)
- Calf skinfold = 4 mm (normal, 10–15 mm)
- Serum albumin concentration = 2.5 g/dL
- Serum prealbumin concentration = 13 mg/dL (normal, 15–45 mg/dL)

2. The triceps skinfold measurement for this patient is an anthropometric measurement for assessment of

   A. somatic protein stores.
   B. fat stores.
   C. visceral protein stores.
   D. immune competence.
   E. body cell mass.

3. What type of malnutrition does this patient have?

   A. Kwashiorkor
   B. Marasmus
   C. Obesity
   D. Kwashiorkor–marasmus mix
   E. Fat overload syndrome

4. A patient with a bone fracture and gram-negative pneumonia excretes 15 g (normal, 6–8 g/d) of urea nitrogen during a 24-hour urine collection. On the basis of these data, the patient is

   A. hypercatabolic.
   B. hypermetabolic.
   C. hypocatabolic.
   D. hypometabolic.
   E. euvolemic.

5. During nutritional assessment, the measurement of body cell mass includes

   A. bone.
   B. interstitial fluid.
   C. skeletal muscle.
   D. intravascular fluid.
   E. extracellular fluid solids.

Case Study for Questions 6–9

Following major gastrointestinal resection, a patient with severe short bowel syndrome is started on parenteral nutrition (PN). It is anticipated that this patient may need this therapy for 6 months to 1 year. The PN prescription for this patient includes

- D20W amino acids 5% (final concentrations) at 105 mL/h (2,500 mL/d)
- Intravenous fat emulsion 20% at 10 mL/h × 24 h (240 mL/d)
- 0.45% sodium chloride injection at 50 mL/h × 24 h (1,200 mL/d)

6. How many calories from dextrose will this patient receive each day?

   A. 1,100
   B. 1,300
   C. 1,500
   D. 1,700
   E. 1,900

7. How many grams of protein will this patient receive each day?

   A. 25
   B. 50
   C. 75
   D. 100
   E. 125

8. How many calories from intravenous lipid will this patient receive each day?

   A. 240
   B. 360
   C. 480
   D. 600
   E. 720

9. Calculate the daily nitrogen balance (grams per day) in this patient if she excretes 12 g of urea nitrogen during the urine collection and 4 g are used as insensible and stool loss each day.

   A. –4
   B. –2
   C. 0
   D. 2
   E. 4

10. What would be an appropriate water or fluid requirement for a 60-kg patient with no extrarenal fluid losses?

    A. 800 mL
    B. 1,200 mL
    C. 2,400 mL
    D. 3,600 mL
    E. 4,800 mL

11. Which of the following disease states or clinical conditions would usually require the administration of parenteral nutrition?

    A. Severe acute pancreatitis
    B. Motor vehicle crash resulting in femur fracture and head injury
    C. 20% body surface area burn from a house fire
    D. Laparoscopic cholecystectomy
    E. Acute exacerbation of hepatic encephalopathy

12. What is the maximum dose (in kilocalories per kilogram per day) of dextrose in parenteral nutrition for adult patients?

    A. 5
    B. 10
    C. 15
    D. 20
    E. 25

13. In a patient with metabolic acidosis, what anion salt would you use to add the majority of sodium and potassium to a PN formulation?

    A. Chloride
    B. Gluconate
    C. Phosphate
    D. Acetate
    E. Sulfate

14. If excessive amounts of calcium are added to a standard parenteral nutrition formulation, it will likely precipitate with

    A. phosphate.
    B. gluconate.
    C. magnesium.
    D. chloride.
    E. sodium.

15. Which vitamin should be supplemented above standard amounts during nutrition support of a pregnant patient?

    A. Cyanocobalamin
    B. Folic acid
    C. Biotin
    D. Chromium
    E. Pantothenic acid

16. Which of the following is an advantage of central vein parenteral nutrition over peripheral vein parenteral nutrition?

    A. Allows easier catheter placement
    B. Does not require a pump for administration
    C. Allows for fluid restriction
    D. Does not have to be filtered
    E. Uses dilute formulations in most cases

17. Which component of a total nutrient admixture should be added last before storing it in a refrigerator?

    A. Phosphorus
    B. Magnesium
    C. Trace elements
    D. Calcium
    E. Intravenous fat emulsion

18. Which of the following are advantages of using a 0.22-micron filter when administering a two-in-one parenteral nutrition formulation?

    I. Traps particulate matter
    II. Prevents precipitates from entering the patient
    III. Filters most bacteria

    A. I only
    B. III only
    C. I and II only
    D. II and III only
    E. I, II, and III

19. Which trace element should be reduced or removed in patients with cholestasis who are receiving parenteral nutrition?

    A. Zinc
    B. Chromium
    C. Selenium
    D. Copper
    E. Iodine

20. A 70-year-old female who has mild congestive heart failure, gastroesophageal reflux disease (GERD), type II diabetes mellitus, and rheuma-

toid arthritis had a recent cerebral vascular accident. She will not regain her premorbid degree of mental status, so a decision is made to give her long-term nutritional support. Which method would be most appropriate for this patient?

A. Central parenteral nutrition
B. Nasogastric tube feeding
C. Peripheral parenteral nutrition
D. Jejunostomy tube feeding
E. Nasoduodenal tube feeding

21. A common cause of diarrhea in patients receiving enteral nutrition is from the

A. osmotic load of the enteral nutrition formulation.
B. sorbitol in drug vehicles.
C. addition of fiber to the enteral nutrition formulation.
D. solute load from the protein component of the enteral nutrition formulation.
E. improper placement of a nasogastric feeding tube.

22. What is the drug of choice for enhancing gastric emptying in a patient receiving enteral nutrition support?

A. Bismuth subsalicylate
B. Azithromycin
C. Metoclopramide
D. Loperamide
E. Acyclovir

23. A patient is receiving phenytoin capsules 300 mg each day for seizure control. She requires tube feeding with a 1 kcal/mL formulation at 85 mL/h (2,000 mL/d). What would be the most appropriate intervention to maintain a therapeutic drug concentration and maintain the required nutrition support?

I. Increase the dose of phenytoin to 600 mg/d.
II. Hold the enteral nutrition 2 hours before and after the dose.
III. Increase the enteral nutrition to 100 mL/h × 20 hours.

A. I only
B. III only
C. I and II only
D. II and III only
E. I, II, and III

24. What is the mechanism for grapefruit juice to inhibit the metabolism of some drugs that can result in drug toxicity?

A. Decreased renal excretion of drug
B. Inhibition of gastrointestinal cytochrome P450-3A4
C. Decreased systemic clearance of drug
D. Inhibition of hepatic cytochrome P450-3A4
E. Expanded apparent volume of distribution

18-7. Answers

1. D. Calcium requirements are 1,000 mg/d for male adults until age 65, when they increase to 1,200–1,500 mg/d. Calcium requirements are 1,000 mg/d for female adults until age 50, when they increase to 1,200–1,500 mg/d.

2. B. Skinfold measurements measure body fat stores, which assess the lipid component of the body. Visceral protein stores are serum proteins. Body cell mass and somatic protein stores assess skeletal muscle and visceral organs. Immune competence assessment requires a skin test with a common antigen.

3. D. All measurements of nutritional assessment are depressed (i.e., weight for height, anthropometric measurements, and biochemical serum markers of protein status).

4. A. Catabolism is related to loss of body protein. Because it is increased, the patient would be considered hypercatabolic in this case.

5. C. Lean body mass includes bone, skeletal muscle, visceral organs, and extracellular solids. Body cell mass includes only the lean, metabolically active tissue such as skeletal muscle and visceral organs (e.g., liver).

6. D. $D_{20}W$ = 20 g/100 mL = 200 g/L × 2.5 L/d = 500 g/d × 3.4 kcal/g = 1,700 kcal/d.

7. E. 5% amino acids = 5 g/100 mL = 50 g/L × 2.5 L/d = 125 g/d.

8. C. Intravenous lipid emulsion 20% = 2 kcal/mL × 240 mL/d = 480 kcal/d.

9. E. The nitrogen intake is calculated by dividing the protein intake (125 g) by 6.25, which results in 20 g. The nitrogen output would be the sum of the urinary urea nitrogen and insensible losses (12 g + 4 g = 16 g/d). Therefore, the nitrogen balance would be 20 g − 16 g = 4 g. A nitrogen balance of +4 would be suggestive of nutritional adequacy with this PN formulation.

10. **C.** Water requirements are 30–40 mL/kg/d for patients without extrarenal fluid losses: 60 kg × 40 mL/kg/d = 2,400 mL/d.

11. **A.** It is difficult to feed patients with severe pancreatitis enterally unless there is access to the small bowel (e.g., jejunostomy). The other clinical conditions, such as trauma and burns, would occur in patients in whom the gastrointestinal tract could and should be used for nutrition support. A patient receiving laparoscopic cholecystectomy would not need nutrition support. Most patients with hepatic encephalopathy can be fed enterally if they require nutrition support.

12. **E.** The dose of dextrose in PN should never exceed 5 mg/kg/min in adult patients. This dose can be converted to 25 kcal/kg/d.

13. **D.** Acetate is converted to bicarbonate in the liver and would thus help or at least not exacerbate the metabolic acidosis.

14. **A.** Calcium phosphate is a relatively insoluble compound, so manufacturer guidelines for the concentrations of these two elements must be followed closely to prevent precipitation. The order of mixing these components in the PN formulation is also important.

15. **B.** Folic acid should be given at a dose of at least 600 mcg/d during pregnancy. Many practitioners administer 1 mg/d above what the patient is eating or receiving via nutrition support. This practice has been shown to prevent neural tube defects in the newborn.

16. **C.** Hyperosmolar nutrients (dextrose, amino acids) can be used to concentrate the PN formulation, but the PN would have to be administered via a central vein.

17. **D.** If calcium is added last, the PN formulation will contain the final volume, including all other nutrients. The chance of calcium causing a precipitate will be decreased because all other components (e.g., phosphorus) are diluted in the entire volume of the PN.

18. **E.** A 0.22-micron filter will do all three. In contrast, a 1.2-micron filter (used with TNAs) will not filter most bacteria.

19. **D.** Copper is excreted via the biliary tract. Patients with severe cholestasis should have copper removed during short-term parenteral nutrition. In long-term PN, copper may be required in reduced doses to prevent anemia. Serum copper concentrations should be monitored regularly in long-term patients who have cholestasis.

20. **D.** She is not a candidate for long-term PN because her gastrointestinal tract would be accessible and functional. Nasogastric and nasoduodenal methods are used only for short-term enteral nutrition. A jejunostomy would be ideal because she also has GERD and perhaps gastroparesis from her diabetes.

21. **B.** Several liquid preparations for drugs contain sorbitol as a pharmaceutical vehicle. These liquid preparations are commonly used in patients with tubes because the drugs can be given easily this way, especially if the patient cannot swallow. Most enteral nutrition formulations are close to being isotonic (i.e., the osmotic load or solute load is not a major factor causing diarrhea). Fiber will prevent or improve diarrhea in most cases.

22. **C.** Metoclopramide enhances gastric emptying and is commonly used in patients with gastrointestinal intolerance. This is true in both diabetics and nondiabetics.

23. **D.** Phenytoin absorption is markedly impaired when it is given concurrently with enteral tube feeding. The enteral tube feeding should be held 2 hours before and after the daily dose of phenytoin capsules. To maintain the current dose of enteral nutrition, the rate of feeding should be increased to 100 mL/h × 20 h (2,000 mL/d).

24. **B.** Drugs such as amlodipine, carbamazepine, and cyclosporine are profoundly metabolized in the gastrointestinal tract before absorption. Grapefruit juice from frozen concentrate has been shown to inhibit gastrointestinal cytochrome P 450-3A4 and thus allows more of the drug to be absorbed, thereby causing drug toxicity for drugs with a narrow therapeutic index.

18-8. References

American Society for Parenteral and Enteral Nutrition Board of Directors and Clinical Guidelines Task Force. Guidelines for the use of parenteral and enteral nutrition in adult and pediatric patients. *J Parenter Enteral Nutr.* 2002;26(suppl 1):1SA–138SA.

Brown RO. Parenteral and enteral nutrition in adult patients. In: Helms RA, Quan DJ, Herfindal ET, Gourley DR, eds. *Textbook of Therapeutics: Drug and Disease Management.* 8th ed. Philadelphia: Lippincott, Williams & Wilkins; 2006:749–66.

Brown RO, Dickerson RN. Drug-nutrient interactions. *Am J Managed Care.* 1999;5:345–51.

Chessman KH, Kumpf VJ. Assessment of nutrition status and nutrition requirements. In: Dipiro JT, Talbert RL, eds. *Pharmacotherapy: A Pathophysiologic Approach.* 7th ed. New York: McGraw-Hill; 2008:2349–66.

Hodges BM, Delegge M. Nutritional considerations in major organ failure. In: Dipiro JT, Talbert RL, eds. *Pharmacotherapy: A Pathophysiologic Approach.* 7th ed. New York: McGraw-Hill; 2008: 2417–36.

Kumpf VJ, Chessman KH. Enteral nutrition. In: Dipiro JT, Talbert RL, eds. *Pharmacotherapy: A Pathophysiologic Approach.* 7th ed. New York: McGraw-Hill; 2008:2399–415.

Mattox TW, Reiter PD. Parenteral nutrition. In: Dipiro JT, Talbert RL, eds. *Pharmacotherapy: A Pathophysiologic Approach.* 7th ed. New York: McGraw-Hill; 2008:2379–97.

McCarter DN, Marshall LL. General nutrition and vitamins/minerals. In: Helms RA, Quan DJ, Herfindal ET, Gourley DR, eds. *Textbook of Therapeutics: Drug and Disease Management.* 8th ed. Philadelphia: Lippincott, Williams & Wilkins; 2006:721–48.

Sacks G, Crill CM. Prevalence and significance of malnutrition. In: Dipiro JT, Talbert RL, eds. *Pharmacotherapy: A Pathophysiologic Approach.* 7th ed. New York: McGraw-Hill; 2008:2367–77.

Task Force for the Revision of Safe Practices for Parenteral Nutrition. Safe practices for parenteral nutrition. *J Parenter Enteral Nutr.* 2004;28 (suppl):S39–70.

Van den Berghe G, Wouters P, Weekers F, et al. Intensive insulin therapy in critically ill patients. *N Engl J Med.* 2001;345:1359–67.

Oncology 19

J. Aubrey Waddell, PharmD, FAPhA, BCOP
Jaclyn S. King, PharmD

19-1. Overview

Definition

Oncology can be defined as the science dealing with the etiology, pathogenesis, and treatment of cancers (synonymous with malignant neoplasms). It encompasses more than 100 different diseases that share characteristics of uncontrollable cell proliferation, invasion of local tissues, and metastases (e.g., spread from original site).

In the United States, men have roughly a one-in-two cumulative lifetime risk of developing cancer and women have a one-in-three risk. In 2009, approximately 1,479,350 new cases of cancer will be diagnosed, and about 562,340 cancer deaths will occur. The most common types of cancer are prostate, lung, and colorectal in men and breast, lung, and colorectal in women.

Classifications

Neoplastic malignancies arise from four tissue types (epithelial, connective, lymphoid, and nerve) and are classified on the basis of this origin. Table 19-1 lists the tissue origin of each type of malignancy and the corresponding medical terminology.

Clinical Presentation

The first signs and symptoms of cancer (solid tumors) develop when the tumor has grown to approximately 10^9 cells (1 cm in diameter or 1 g mass). The type of cancer determines the presentation of signs and symptoms, which vary widely across tumor types.

Positive screening tests (see Section 19-3) or generalized signs of anorexia, fatigue, fever, weight loss, and anemia must also be evaluated. Boxes 19-1 and 19-2 show the American Cancer Society's seven warning signs of cancer for adults and the warning signs for children.

Pathophysiology and Etiology

The following factors promote cancer:

- **External factors:** Tobacco, chemicals, radiation, infectious organisms, and diet
- **Internal factors:** Genetics, hormones, and immune conditions

Development of cancer is genetically regulated and is a multistage process:

- **Initiation:** Normal cells are exposed to chemical, physical, or biological carcinogens. Such exposure results in irreversible damage, genetic mutations, and selective growth advantages.
- **Promotion:** Reversible environmental changes favor the growth of the mutated cells.
- **Transformation:** The cells become cancerous.
- **Progression:** Additional genetic changes occur, resulting in increased cancerous proliferation. Tumors invade local tissues, and metastasis occurs.

Genetic alterations are necessary for the development and growth of cancer. Some of the most common are the following:

- Oncogenes promote growth advantages in mutated cells and cause excessive proliferation (e.g., ras, c-myc).
- Inactivation of tumor suppressor genes (TSGs) results in inappropriate cell growth, because TSGs normally regulate the cell cycle (e.g., p53).

Table 19-1. Tissue Origin of Malignant Tumor Types

Origin	Tissue type	Malignant tumor
Epithelial	Surface epithelium	Carcinoma
	Glandular tissue	Adenocarcinoma
Connective	Fibrous	Fibrosarcoma
	Bone	Osteosarcoma
	Smooth or striated muscle	Leiomyosarcoma or rhabdomyosarcoma
	Fat	Liposarcoma
Lymphoid	Bone marrow	Leukemia
	Lymphoid	Hodgkin and non-Hodgkin lymphoma
	Plasma cell	Multiple myeloma
Neural	Glial	Glioblastoma and astrocytoma
	Nerve sheath	Neurofibrosarcoma
	Melanocytes	Malignant melanoma
Mixed	Gonadal tissue	Teratocarcinoma

Source: Adapted from Balmer et al., 2002.

- Anti-apoptotic genes are activated (e.g., bcl-2).
- DNA (deoxyribonucleic acid) repair genes experience reduced activity.

Malignant tumor cells do not resemble their tissue of origin (in contrast to benign tumors). They are unstable and are incapable of performing normal cell functions.

Diagnostic Criteria

A sample of suspected malignant tissues or cells is needed for a definitive diagnosis. Sampling can be done with a biopsy, fine-needle aspiration, or exfoliative cytology. This tissue sample is examined by a pathologist, who assigns a stage to the cancer. This process is called *pathological staging*.

Radiation or chemotherapy should not begin without proper clinical and pathological staging. Clinical staging can be accomplished by imaging studies, which may include the following:

- A chest x-ray evaluates the spread of cancer to bones or lungs.
- Computed tomography (CT) assesses the size, shape, and position of tumor and detects masses in lymph nodes, brain, or adrenal glands through a three-dimensional view.
- Magnetic resonance imaging (MRI) evaluates the spread of cancer to the brain or spinal cord.
- Positron emission tomography (PET) evaluates lymph and other metastatic involvement.
- A bone scan assesses for the presence of bone metastasis.

Laboratory work may include complete blood counts (CBCs), blood chemistries, and tumor markers (see Section 19.3).

Box 19-1. Warning Signs of Cancer in Adults

*C*hange in bowel or bladder habits
A sore that does not heal
*U*nusual bleeding or discharge
*T*hickening of lump in breast or elsewhere
*I*ndigestion or difficulty swallowing
*O*bvious change in wart or mole
*N*agging cough or hoarseness

Source: American Cancer Society, 2009

Box 19-2. Warning Signs of Cancer in Children

*C*ontinued, unexplained weight loss
*H*eadaches with vomiting in the morning
*I*ncreased swelling or persistent pain in bones or joints
*L*ump or mass in abdomen, neck, or elsewhere
*D*evelopment of a whitish appearance in the pupil of the eye
*R*ecurrent fevers not caused by infection
*E*xcessive bruising or bleeding
*N*oticeable paleness or prolonged tiredness

Source: American Cancer Society, 2009.

If a diagnosis of cancer is made, the malignancy will need to be staged or categorized on the basis of severity of the disease and the results of the pathological staging tests. Staging guides the oncology practitioner in determining the prognosis and the treatment regimen for the patient.

The tumor, node, metastasis (TNM) staging system is the most commonly used tool for solid tumors. Tumors are scored numerically on the basis of the size of the tumor, the extent of lymph node involvement, and presence or absence of metastases. This score allows classification of tumors by stage, from 0 to IV, with stage IV denoting the presence of metastasis (e.g., most severe disease). A stage 0 tumor is called a carcinoma in situ, where the malignancy has not yet invaded the basement membrane of the epithelial surface.

Lymphoid tumors are staged differently and are beyond the scope of this review. Refer to Adams et al. (2002) for more information.

Treatment Principles and Goals

Treatment regimens are based on the type of cancer, stage, the age of the patient, and other prognostic factors (e.g., presence of a tumor marker, poor performance status, and ethnicity, among others).

Primary therapy is the initial and mainstay approach to treat cancer. It usually consists of removal of the tumor or debulking through surgery.

Neoadjuvant therapy is given prior to the primary therapy. The goal is to reduce the size of the tumor, thereby increasing the efficacy of the primary treatment. Examples include chemotherapy or radiation.

Adjuvant therapy is additional therapy given after the main treatment. The goal is to ensure that all residual disease has been eradicated.

The four main cancer treatments are surgery, radiation, chemotherapy, and biologic therapy. Most regimens are a combination of these modalities:

- *Surgery* alone is reserved for solid localized tumors, where the entire cancer can be resected. It may also be combined with other modalities in later stages of disease. It is not an option for patients with lymphoid-based disease (e.g., Hodgkin lymphoma).
- *Radiation* alone is also reserved for curing localized tumors because it treats a very focused area. It also can be combined with other treatments as neoadjuvant or adjuvant therapy to reduce disease-related symptoms or to reduce the incidence of disease recurrence.

- *Chemotherapy* is a means of systemic treatment, in contrast to the two types of local treatment just described. It can be used to treat the primary tumor as well as metastases. Chemotherapy is generally not administered to patients with local disease that can be fully resected.
- *Biologic therapy* is another systemic treatment and includes agents such as monoclonal antibodies, interferons, interleukins, and tumor vaccines. It is a relatively new type of treatment and acts by stimulating the host immune system.

The goals of cancer therapy are based on the type and stage of cancer, as well as on patient characteristics (e.g., an older patient with a short life expectancy may not be offered intense treatment that may impair quality of life). Goals may be as follows:

- *Localized or regional disease* (i.e., stages 0, I, II, and early III): Provide curative intent and inhibit recurrence of disease. Stage 0 diseases are often not treated, but monitored until clinically apparent.
- *Advanced or metastasized disease* (i.e., advanced stage III and all stage IV): Palliate symptoms, reduce tumor load, prolong survival, and increase quality of life.

Survival and response to treatment

In 2009, more than 1,500 people per day will die of a cancer-related cause, which accounts for one in four deaths. Survival depends on patient characteristics, type of disease, stage of disease, and treatment regimen. Older patients with more severe disease, a poor performance status, and faster-growing tumors have a poor prognosis.

Response to treatment modalities for solid tumors are classified as follows:

- *Cure:* 5 years of cancer-free survival for most tumor types
- *Complete response:* Absence of all neoplastic disease for a minimum of 1 month after cessation of treatment
- *Partial response:* ≥ 50% decrease in tumor size or other disease markers for a minimum of 1 month
- *Stable disease:* No change or no meeting of criteria for partial response or progression
- *Progression:* ≥ 25% increase in tumor size or new lesion

Response to treatment for hematologic cancers is measured by the elimination of abnormal cells, a decrease in tumor markers to normal, and the improved function of affected cells.

19-2. Drug Therapy

Chemotherapy

Chemotherapeutic agents have a very narrow therapeutic index and a toxic side-effect profile. They are generally more effective in combination because of synergism through biochemical interactions. It is important to choose drugs with different mechanisms of action, resistance, and toxicity profiles to get the full benefit of combination therapy.

Chemotherapy has the greatest effect on rapidly dividing cells, because most of the potent chemotherapy drugs act by damaging DNA. These agents are more active in different phases of the cell cycle. A therapeutic effect is seen on cancer cells, but adverse effects are also seen on human cells that rapidly divide (e.g., hair follicles, gastrointestinal (GI) tract, and blood cells). Agents can be phase specific or phase nonspecific. Nonspecific agents are effective in all phases.

Cell Cycle Phases

- G_0 = *resting phase:* No cell division occurs, and cancer cells are generally not susceptible to chemotherapy. This lack of susceptibility is problematic for slow-growing tumors that exist primarily in this phase.
- G_1 = *postmitotic phase:* Enzymes for DNA synthesis are manufactured, lasting 10–24 hours.
- S = *DNA synthesis phase:* DNA separation and replication occurs, lasting 10–20 hours.
- G_2 = *premitotic phase:* Specialized proteins and RNA (ribonucleic acid) are made, lasting 2–10 hours.
- M = *mitosis:* Actual cell division occurs, lasting 30–60 minutes.

Drug Classes

There are numerous chemotherapy agents. Drugs are grouped by class. Refer to the corresponding table for each class of drugs.

Alkylating agents

Table 19-2 provides summary information about alkylating agents.

Mechanism of action
Alkylating agents cause covalent bond formation of drugs to nucleic acids and proteins, which results in the cross-linking of one or two DNA strands and inhibition of DNA replication. These agents are not phase specific. The most commonly used agents include cyclophosphamide, ifosfamide, carmustine, dacarbazine, and temozolomide.

Patient instructions and counseling
- All drugs are carcinogenic, teratogenic, and mutagenic.
- Medications may cause sterility.
- Let your dentist know you are on chemotherapy because of an increased risk of bleeding and infections.
- Hydration and mesna therapy are recommended for cyclophosphamide and ifosfamide.
- Let your doctor know if you have burning on urination.

Adverse drug events
The following adverse events may occur: myelosuppression, primarily leukopenia; mucosal ulceration; pulmonary fibrosis (carmustine) and interstitial pneumonitis; pyrexia and fatigue (bendamustine); alopecia; nausea and vomiting; amenorrhea and azoospermia; hemorrhagic cystitis with cyclophosphamide and ifosfamide; encephalopathy with ifosfamide; and seizures (polifeprosan and carmustine).

Drug interactions
Drugs with specific interactions of moderate to major severity include the following:

- *Altretamine:* Tricyclic antidepressants and monoamine oxidase inhibitors
- *Bendamustine:* Strong cytochrome P450 (CYP450) 1A2 inhibitors
- *Busulfan:* Itraconazole, phenytoin, and acetaminophen
- *Carmustine:* Cimetidine, ethyl alcohol, phenytoin, and amphotericin B
- *Cyclophosphamide:* Allopurinol, barbiturates, digoxin, phenytoin, and warfarin
- *Ifosfamide:* Allopurinol, phenytoin, and warfarin
- *Streptozocin:* Nephrotoxic agents

Monitoring parameters
Monitor pulmonary function tests, renal and hepatic tests, chest x-rays; CBC with differential (baseline and expected nadir prior to next cycle) and electrolytes, urinalysis for red blood count detection from hemorrhagic cystitis, signs of bleeding (bruising and melena), infection (sore throat and fever), and nausea or vomiting.

Table 19-2. Alkylating Agents

Generic name	Trade name	Dosage range	Dosage form	Frequency	Diseases[a]
Nitrogen mustard					
Mechlorethamine	Mustargen	6–10 mg/m²	IV	Days 1, 8 q 4 wk	HL, NHL
Cyclophosphamide	Cytoxan, Neosar	500–2,000 mg/m², 40–100 mg/m²	IV, po	q 3 wk, qd 2–14 days	ALL, CLL, HL, NHL, myeloma, testis, neuroblastoma, breast, ovary, lung, cervix
Ifosfamide	Ifex	1.2 g/m²	IV	qd × 5 d q 3 wk	HL, NHL, lung, bladder, sarcoma
Melphalan	Alkeran	16 mg/m², 6 mg/m²	IV, po	q 4 wk, qd 4 days q 4 wk	Myeloma, breast, ovary
Chlorambucil	Leukeran	0.1–0.2 mg/kg	po	qd × 3–6 wk	CLL, HL, NHL
Bendamustine	Treanda	100–120 mg/m²	IV	qd × 2 d, q 21–28 d	CLL, NHL
Ethylenimines and methylmelamines					Ovarian
Altretamine	Hexalen	260 mg/m²	po	qd × 14–21 d	
Thiotepa	Thioplex	10–20 mg/m²	IV	q 3–4 wk	Bladder, breast, ovarian, HL, NHL
Alkyl sulfonates					CML, BMT
Busulfan	Myleran, Busulfex	4–8 mg/kg	IV, po	qd	
Nitrosureas					HL, NHL, brain, myeloma
Carmustine	BiCNU	150–200 mg/m²	IV	q 6 wk	Islet cell carcinoma
Streptozocin	Zanosar	500 mg/m²	IV	qd 5 d q 6 wk	Glioblastoma multiforme
Polifeprosan 20 with carmustine implant	Gliadel	7.7 mg	Implant	n.a.	

ALL, acute lymphocytic leukemia; BMT, bone marrow transplant; CLL, chronic lymphocytic leukemia; CML, chronic myelogenous leukemia; HL, Hodgkin lymphoma; n.a., not applicable; NHL, non-Hodgkin lymphoma.

a. Appearance of disease in list does not indicate U.S. Food and Drug Administration approval for drug's use in treatment of that disease, but does indicate use of that drug in that disease in clinical practice.

Antimetabolites: S-phase specific

See Table 19-3 for general information about antimetabolites.

Mechanism of action

These agents are structural analogues of natural metabolites and act by falsely inserting themselves in place of a pyrimidine or purine ring, causing interference in nucleic acid synthesis. Phase-specific agents are most active in the S phase and in tumors with a high growth fraction. They are subdivided into three groups: folate, purine, and pyrimidine antagonists.

Patient instructions and counseling

- Avoid crowds and sick people.
- You may be asked to chew ice if receiving fluorouracil (5-FU) to reduce damage to the mucosal lining in your mouth.
- Contact your doctor if you have uncontrollable nausea or vomiting; excessive diarrhea; or pain, swelling, or tingling in palms of hands and soles of feet (hand-foot syndrome).
- Call your doctor if you feel dizzy or lightheaded or have trouble urinating (clofarabine).
- You should be receiving folic acid and vitamin B$_{12}$ injections if you are receiving pemetrexed.
- Nelarabine may cause sleepiness and dizziness.

Adverse drug events

Adverse events include hand-foot syndrome, stomatitis (5-FU and capecitabine); severe diarrhea, GI mucosal damage, nausea, vomiting, fatigue, myelosuppression, alopecia, neurotoxicity (nelarabine, cytarabine, fludarabine, and methotrexate); rash, fever, and flu-like symptoms (gemcitabine); renal toxicity and mucositis (5-FU and methotrexate); conjunctivitis

Table 19-3. Antimetabolites

Generic name	Trade name	Dosage range	Dosage form	Frequency	Disease[a]
Folic acid antagonists					
Pemetrexed	Alimta	500–600 mg/m²	IV	q 21 d	Malignant mesothelioma, NSCLC, breast, NHL, sarcoma, ALL
Methotrexate	Rheumatrex	10–12 mg, 1–10 g/m², 25 mg/m², 10 mg/m²	Intrathecal, IV, IM, po	q wk, q 3 wk, q wk, q wk	
Pyrimidine analogs					
Azacitidine	Vidaza	75–100 mg/m²	SC, IV	qd × 7 d q 4 wk	Myelodysplastic syndrome
Fluorouracil, 5-FU	Adrucil	450 mg/m²	IV	qd × 5 d	Colorectal, breast, head, neck
Cytarabine	Cytosar-U, DepoCyt	3 gm/m², 100–200 mg/m², 50 mg	IV, Continuous IV, intrathecal	q 12 hr days 1, 3, 5 q 6 w, qd × 7 d, q 14 d	ALL, AML, CML
Capecitabine	Xeloda	2,500 mg/m²	po	qd × 14 d, q 3 wk	Breast, colorectal
Gemcitabine	Gemzar	1,000–1,250 mg/m²	IV	q wk	Pancreatic, NSCLC, bladder
Decitabine	Dacogen	15 mg/m²	IV	q8h × 3 d, q 6 wk	Myelodysplastic syndrome
Purine analogs					
Clofarabine	Clolar	52 mg/m²	IV	qd × 5 d q 4 wk	ALL (pediatric)
Mercaptopurine	Purinethol	1.5–2.5 mg/kg	po	Qd	ALL
Thioguanine	Tabloid	2–3 mg/kg	po	Qd	ALL, AML
Pentostatin	Nipent	4 mg/m²	IV	q 2 wk	CLL, hairy cell leukemia, ALL
Cladribine	Leustatin	0.09–0.10 mg/kg	IV	qd × 7 d	NHL, hairy cell leukemia, CLL
Fludarabine	Fludara	25 mg/m²	IV	qd × 5 d q 4 wk	CLL, NHL
Guanosine analogs					
Nelarabine	Arranon	Children: 650 mg/m²/d Adults: 1,500 mg/m²/d	IV IV	qd × d, q 21 d d 1, 3, 5, q 21 d	T-cell ALL or NHL

ALL, acute lymphocytic leukemia; AML, acute myelogenous leukemia; CLL, chronic lymphocytic leukemia; CML, chronic myelogenous leukemia; NHL, non-Hodgkin lymphoma; NSCLC, non–small cell lung cancer.

a. Appearance of disease in list does not indicate U.S. Food and Drug Administration approval for drug's use in treatment of that disease, but does indicate use of that drug in that disease in clinical practice.

(cytarabine, especially in high doses); hemolytic uremic syndrome (gemcitabine); opportunistic infections (cladribine and fludarabine); and tumor lysis syndrome, systemic inflammatory response syndrome, or capillary leak (clofarabine).

Interactions
Drugs with specific interactions include the following:

- ***Capecitabine:*** Warfarin and phenytoin
- ***Cytarabine:*** Digoxin
- ***Fluorouracil:*** Warfarin
- ***Mercaptopurine:*** Warfarin and allopurinol
- ***Methotrexate:*** Nonsteroidal anti-inflammatory drugs (NSAIDs), amiodarone, amoxicillin, sulfasalazine, doxycycline, erythromycin, hydrochlorothiazide, mercaptopurine, omeprazole, phenytoin, and folic acid
- ***Pentostatin:*** Cyclophosphamide and fludarabine

Monitoring parameters
Note any complaints of mucositis or mouth soreness; monitor for neurotoxicity (e.g., ask the patient to write his or her name), CBC with differential prior to each dose of drug, and hepatic and renal function; and monitor for tingling or swelling of palms of hands and soles of feet, bruising or bleeding, and international normalized ratio (capecitabine). Monitor weight and question patient about diarrhea, jaundice, and hepatomegaly (mercaptopurine). Continuous intravenous (IV) fluids and allopurinol for prevention of tumor lysis syndrome should be administered

to patients taking clofarabine, and those patients should also receive prophylactic corticosteroids for systemic inflammatory response syndrome and capillary leak. Pemetrexed toxicities are reduced by lowering plasma homocysteine levels with concomitant folic acid and vitamin B12. Dexamethasone should be given to prevent cutaneous reactions caused by pemetrexed.

Antitumor antibiotics

For additional information about antitumor antibiotics, consult Table 19-4.

Mechanism of action
Anthracyclines block DNA and RNA transcription through the intercalation (insertion) of adjoining nucleic acid pairs in DNA, which results in DNA strand breakage. They also inhibit the topoisomerase II enzyme. Mitomycin is an alkylating-like agent that cross-links DNA. Dactinomycin blocks RNA synthesis. Bleomycin inhibits DNA synthesis in mitosis and

G_2 stages of growth. Bleomycin is the only cell cycle–specific agent.

Patient instructions and counseling
- Contact your doctor if you have fast, slow, or irregular heartbeats or breathing difficulties.
- Anthracyclines may cause a change of urine color or change the whites of eyes to a blue-green or orange-red.
- Bleomycin may cause a change in skin color or nail growth.

Adverse drug events
Events include severe nausea and vomiting, alopecia, and stomatitis. Anthracyclines may cause cardiac toxicity, acute or chronic (doxorubicin = daunorubicin > idarubicin > epirubicin > mitoxantrone). All anthracyclines have limits on cumulative lifetime dosing, are vesicants, and are associated with secondary acute myelogenous leukemia (AML); avoid in patients with a cardiac history. Myelosuppression risk exists with all agents, although mitomycin demonstrates a delayed

Table 19-4. Antitumor Antibiotics

Generic name	Trade name	Dosage range	Dosage form	Frequency	Disease[a]
Anthracyclines					
Doxorubicin	Adriamycin, Doxil (liposomal)	60–75 mg/m², 20–50 mg/m² (liposomal)	IV	q 3 wk	ALL, AML, NHL, HL, solid tumors of every major organ
Daunorubicin	Cerubidine, Daunoxome (liposomal)	45 mg/m², 40 mg/m² (liposomal)	IV	qd × 3 d, q 2 wk	ALL, AML, NHL
Epirubicin	Ellence, Pharmarubicin	60–120 mg/m²	IV	q 3 wk	Breast, bladder, lung, ovarian, gastric
Idarubicin	Idamycin	12–13 mg/m²	IV	qd × 3 d	AML, ALL, breast
Mitoxantrone	Novantrone	12–14 mg/m²	IV	q 3 wk	Prostate, NHL, AML, breast
Valrubicin	Valstar	800 mg	Intravesical	q wk × 6 wk	Bladder
Alkylating-like					
Mitomycin	Mutamycin	10–20 mg/m²	IV, intravesical	q 6–8 wk	Bladder, breast, NSCLC, cervix, pancreatic, colon
Chromomycin					
Dactinomycin	Cosmegen	12–15 mcg/kg	IV	qd × 5 d	Wilms' tumor, testis, sarcoma
Miscellaneous					
Bleomycin	Blenoxane	10–20 USP units/m²/wk	IM, IV, and SC	q wk	HL, NHL, testis, head, neck, lung, skin

ALL, acute lymphocytic leukemia; AML, acute myelogenous leukemia; HL, Hodgkin lymphoma; NHL, non-Hodgkin lymphoma; NSCLC, non–small cell lung cancer.
a. Appearance of disease in list does not indicate U.S. Food and Drug Administration approval for drug's use in treatment of that disease, but does indicate use of that drug in that disease in clinical practice.

effect. Dactinomycin may cause renal toxicity, leukopenia, and increased pigmentation of previously radiated skin. Bleomycin may cause pulmonary fibrosis and interstitial pneumonitis. Mitomycin may cause hemolytic uremic syndrome.

Drug interactions
Drugs with specific interactions include the following:

- Bleomycin: Phenytoin and digoxin
- Doxorubicin: Cisplatin, digoxin, paclitaxel, phenytoin, phenobarbital, trastuzumab, and zidovudine
- Epirubicin: Cimetidine and trastuzumab
- Idarubicin: Probenecid and trastuzumab

Monitoring parameters
Monitor hepatic and renal function, CBC with differential, and pulmonary function tests before and after treatment with bleomycin. Provide cardiac monitoring through left ventricular ejection fraction measurements for anthracyclines as well as monitoring of the cumulative lifetime dose, and be alert for extravasation and necrosis with anthracyclines. Adjust anthracycline dosing on the basis of elevated total bilirubin.

Pharmacokinetics
Anthracyclines are extensively bound in the tissue, have large volumes of distribution and long half-lives, and are excreted in the bile. Dosing adjustments are necessary in patients with hepatic impairment. Bleomycin is renally excreted and requires dosing adjustments in impaired patients.

Other factors
Lifetime doses of doxorubicin should not exceed 450–550 mg/m², taking into account other anthracycline agents received. The lifetime maximum for epirubicin is 900 mg/m²; for idarubicin, it is 150 mg/m².

Hormones and antagonists

Table 19-5 provides information about hormones and antagonists.

Mechanism of action
This diverse group of compounds acts on hormone-dependent tumors by inhibiting or decreasing the production of the disease-causing hormone.

Patient instructions and counseling
- Avoid use in pregnant women; several agents may cause weight gain and menstrual irregularities in women.

- Be aware of leg swelling or tenderness (e.g., signs of a deep vein thrombosis), breathing problems, and sweating.
- Transient muscle or bone pain, problems urinating, and spinal cord compression may occur initially in patients receiving luteinizing hormone-releasing hormone (LHRH) agonists.
- Take exemestane after meals.

Adverse drug events
Events include edema, menstrual disorders, hot flashes, transient muscle or bone pain, tumor flare, and transient increase in serum testosterone (LHRH agonists); thromboembolic events, gynecomastia, elevated liver enzymes, nausea and vomiting, diarrhea, erectile impotence, decreased libido, endometrial cancers with tamoxifen, bone loss (LHRH and aromatase inhibitors); and risk of ventricular arrhythmias and QT prolongation.

Interactions
Drugs with specific interactions include the following:

- *Aminoglutethimide:* Dexamethasone, warfarin, tamoxifen, and theophylline
- *Bicalutamide:* Warfarin
- *Degarelix:* Amiodarone, procainamide, quinidine, and sotalol
- *Fluoxymesterone:* Cyclosporine, anticoagulants, and valerian
- *Flutamide:* Warfarin
- *Medroxyprogesterone acetate:* Aminoglutethimide and rifampin
- *Megestrol:* Dofetilide contraindication
- *Nilutamide:* Alcohol
- *Tamoxifen:* Anticoagulants and cyclophosphamide
- *Toremifene:* CYP450 3A4 inducers (carbamazepine and phenytoin)

Monitoring parameters
Check white blood counts (WBCs) with differential, platelets, liver function tests, thyroid function, and serum creatinine regularly. Note any weight changes, abnormal vaginal bleeding, body or bone pain, galactorrhea, or decreased libido. Monitor for embolic disorders and uterine cancer (in females). Check prostate-specific antigen (PSA) and testosterone levels in males. Monitor bone mineral density for LHRH agonist and aromatase inhibitors.

Pharmacokinetics
The majority of agents are available orally with longer half-lives, allowing once-daily dosing.

Table 19-5. Hormones and Antagonists

Generic name	Trade name	Dosage range	Dosage form	Frequency	Disease[a]
Adrenocorticoids					
Aminoglutethimide	Cytadren	250 mg	po	qd	Adrenal, breast, prostate
Progestins					
Megestrol acetate	Megace	40 mg, 40–320 mg	po	qid, qd divided	Breast, endometrial
Medroxyprogesterone acetate	Provera, Depo-Provera	400–1,000 mg	IM	q wk	Endometrial
Estrogens					
Ethinyl estradiol	Estinyl	150 mcg–3 mg, 100 mcg to 1 mg	po	qd	Prostate, breast
Antiestrogen					
Tamoxifen	Nolvadex	20–40 mg	po	qd	Breast
Fulvestrant	Faslodex	250 mg	IM	q mo	Breast
Toremifene	Fareston	60 mg	po	qd	Breast
Third Generation					
Aromatase inhibitors					
Exemestane	Aromasin	25 mg	po	qd	Breast
Anastrozole	Arimidex	1 mg	po	qd	Breast
Letrozole	Femara	2.5 mg	po	qd	Breast
Androgens					
Testosterone propionate	Delatestryl	200–400 mg	IM	qd	Breast
Fluoxymesterone	Halotestin	10–40 mg	po	q 2–4 wk	Breast
Antiandrogens					
Flutamide	Eulexin	250 mg	po	tid	Prostate
Bicalutamide	Casodex	50 mg	po	qd	Prostate
Nilutamide	Nilandron	300 mg, 150 mg	po	qd × 30 days, qd	Prostate
LHRH agonists					
Triptorelin	Trelstar	3.75, 11.25 mg	IM	q 28 d, q 84 d	Prostate
Leuprolide	Lupron, Eligard	7.5, 22.5, 30.0, 45, 65 mg	IM and SC	q mo, q 3 mo, q 4 mo, q 6 mo, q 12 mo	Prostate, breast
Goserelin	Zoladex	3.6, 10.8 mg	SC	q mo, q 3 mo	Prostate, breast
GNRH antagonist					
Degarelix		240 mg, 80 mg	SC	First month, then q 28 d	Prostate

GNRH, gonadotropin-releasing hormone; LHRH, luteinizing hormone–releasing hormone.

a. Appearance of disease in list does not indicate U.S. Food and Drug Administration approval for drug's use in treatment of that disease, but does indicate use of that drug in that disease in clinical practice.

Other factors

Agents are often contraindicated if the patient has more than one hormone-dependent tumor. With the exception of tamoxifen, third generation aromatase inhibitors, and LHRH agonists, the majority of agents are not indicated for first-line therapy.

Plant alkaloids

See Table 19-6 for information about plant alkaloids.

Mechanism of action

These agents inhibit the replication of cancerous cells. Taxanes and vincas interfere with microtubule assembly in the M phase. Camptothecins and epipodophyllotoxins inhibit topoisomerase I and II enzymes, respectively, causing DNA strand breaks. Topoisomerase I and II affect G_2 and S phases, respectively.

Patient instructions and counseling

■ Contact doctor for uncontrollable diarrhea (irinotecan), nausea or vomiting, or signs and symptoms of an infection.

■ Patients should receive prophylaxis for emesis and pretreatment for anaphylaxis or peripheral edema (taxanes).

■ Patients should receive a prescription for loperamide for delayed diarrhea with irinotecan therapy.

Adverse drug events

Adverse events include myelosuppression, mucositis, nausea and vomiting, alopecia, edema, hand-foot syndrome (docetaxel); hypotension or hypersensitivity on administration (paclitaxel); neurotoxicity (vincristine); peripheral neuropathy and myalgia or arthralgia (ixabepilone and paclitaxel); diarrhea, headache, and secondary malignancies (topoisomerase II inhibitors); and syndrome of inappropriate antidiuretic hormone secretion (SIADH) (vinca alkaloids)

Interactions

Drugs with specific interactions include the following:

■ ***Docetaxel:*** CYP450 3A4 inducers and inhibitors
■ ***Etoposide:*** Cyclosporine, St. John's wort, and warfarin

Table 19-6. Plant Alkaloids

Generic name	Trade name	Dosage range	Dosage form	Frequency	Disease[a]
Taxanes					
Docetaxel (gastric)	Taxotere	60–100 mg/m²	IV	q 3 wk	NSCLC, breast, ovarian, head, neck, gastric
Paclitaxel	Taxol	135–175 mg/m²	IV	q 3 wk	NSCLC, breast, ovarian, head
Paclitaxel	Abraxane	260 mg/m²	IV	q 3 wk	Breast
Epothilones					
Ixabepilone	Ixempra	40 mg/m² (maximum 88 mg)	IV	q 3 wk	Breast
Epipodophyllotoxins					
Etoposide	VePesid	100 mg/m², 50 mg/m²	IV, po	qd × 3–5 d q 3 wk, qd × 21 d q 4 wk	SCLC, testis, NSCLC
Teniposide	Vumon	165 mg/m²	IV	q wk × 4 doses	ALL, SCLC
Camptothecins					
Irinotecan	Camptosar	100–125 mg/m²	IV	q wk	Colorectal, NSCLC, SCLC
Topotecan	Hycamtin	1.5 mg/m²	IV	qd × 5 d q 21 d	Ovarian, lung, AML, cervical
Vinca alkaloids					
Vincristine	Oncovin	1.4 mg/m²	IV	q wk	ALL, HL, NHL, CLL
Vinblastine	Velban	6 mg/m²	IV	q 2–3 wk	HL, NHL, testis
Vinorelbine	Navelbine	25–30 mg/m²	IV	q wk	NSCLC, breast, ovarian

ALL, acute lymphocytic leukemia; AML, acute myelogenous leukemia; CLL, chronic lymphocytic leukemia; HL, Hodgkin lymphoma; NHL, non-Hodgkin lymphoma; NSCLC, non–small cell lung cancer; SCLC, small cell lung cancer.
a. Appearance of disease in list does not indicate U.S. Food and Drug Administration approval for drug's use in treatment of that disease, but does indicate use of that drug in that disease in clinical practice.

- *Irinotecan:* St. John's wort
- *Ixabepilone:* CYP450 3A4 inducers and inhibitors
- *Paclitaxel:* CYP450 3A4 inducers and inhibitors
- *Teniposide:* CYP450 3A4 inducers and inhibitors
- *Vinblastine:* Phenytoin, erythromycin, mitomycin, and zidovudine
- *Vinca alkaloids:* CYP450 3A4 inhibitors; itraconazole, and voriconazole
- *Vincristine:* Phenytoin, l-asparaginase, carbamazepine, digoxin, filgrastim, nifedipine, and zidovudine

Monitoring parameters

Monitor WBCs with differential for all agents; peripheral neuropathy, liver and renal function, painful mouth sores, and blood pressure (taxanes and epipodophyllotoxins); acute and late-onset diarrhea or dyspnea on exertion (irinotecan); bilirubin elevations (taxanes and camptothecins); fluid retention (docetaxel); and neuropathy, shortness of breath, bronchospasm, and SIADH (vincas).

Pharmacokinetics

Taxanes and epipodophyllotoxins are extensively bound to plasma and tissues.

Other factors

Drug resistance may occur through p-glycoprotein pumps for all agents. Topotecan needs dose adjustments for patients with a creatinine clearance < 40 mL/min. Vincas are vesicants and need close monitoring for extravasation. Vincristine should not be administered intrathecally. In adult patients, vincristine doses are often capped at 2 mg.

Dose adjustments may be needed for patients with liver impairment.

Biologic response modifiers and monoclonal antibodies

Table 19-7 provides information about biologic response modifiers and monoclonal antibodies.

Table 19-7. Biologic Response Modifiers and Monoclonal Antibodies

Generic name	Trade name	Dosage range	Dosage form	Frequency	Disease[a]
Immune therapies					
Aldesleukin	Proleukin	600,000 units/kg	IV	q 8 h × 14 doses	Metastatic renal cell, metastatic melanoma
Interferon alfa-2b	Intron A	20×10^6 units/m², 10×10^6 units/m², 2×10^6 units	IV, SC, SC	qd × 5 d per wk × 4 wk,[b] 3 × wk × 11 mo, 3 × wk × 6 mo	Malignant melanoma and hairy cell leukemia
Thalidomide	Thalomid	200 mg	po	qd	Multiple myeloma, erythema nodosum leprosum
Lenalidomide	Revlimid	10 mg	po	qd	Myelodysplastic syndrome
		25 mg	po	qd d 1–21, q 28 d	Multiple myeloma
Monoclonal antibodies					
Rituximab	(Rituxan)	375 mg/m²	IV	q wk × 4–8 doses, q 3 wk	NHL, CLL
Trastuzumab	(Herceptin)	2–6 mg/kg	IV, SC	q wk	Metastatic breast
Gemtuzumab	(Mylotarg)	9 mg/m²	IV	q 2 wk	AML
Alemtuzumab	(Campath)	3–10 mg	IV	qd, then 30 mg 3 × wk	B-cell CLL
Bevacizumab	(Avastin)	5–15 mg/kg	IV	q 2 wk *or* q 3 wk	Colorectal, NSCLC, breast, glioblastoma, renal cell carcinoma
Cetuximab	(Erbitux)	250–500 mg/m²	IV	q 1–2 wk	Colorectal, head and neck
Denileukin diftitox	(Ontak)	9 or 18 mcg/kg	IV	qd × 5 d q 21 d	T-cell lymphoma
Ibritumomab tiuxetan	(Zevalin)[c]				NHL
Tositumomab	(Bexxar)[c]				NHL

AML, acute myelogenous leukemia; CLL, chronic lymphocytic leukemia; NHL, non-Hodgkin lymphoma; NSCLC, non–small cell lung cancer.
a. Appearance of disease in list does not indicate U.S. Food and Drug Administration approval for drug's use in treatment of that disease, but does indicate use of that drug in that disease in clinical practice.
b. Induction dose.
c. See package insert for range, form, and frequency of dosing.

Mechanism of action

Biologic response modifiers activate the body's immune-mediated host defense mechanisms to malignant cells. In contrast to immunotherapy, these agents have direct biological effects on malignancies. Monoclonal antibodies bind to specific antigens and kill malignant cells through the activation of apoptosis, an antibody-mediated toxicity, or complement-mediated lysis.

Patient instructions and counseling

- Let your doctor know if you have severe fatigue, trouble breathing, or irregular heart rhythms.
- Chills, fever, depression, and flu-like symptoms are common.
- Monoclonal antibodies can cause infusion-related reactions such as fever and chills.
- If you receive bevacizumab, you should have your blood pressure checked regularly and have tests that check for protein in your urine.
- You should wear sunscreen and avoid excessive sunlight if you are receiving cetuximab.
- You should receive medication for your thyroid if you are going to receive tositumomab.
- For both men and women, do not try to conceive until 12 months after finishing therapy.
- With thalidomide and lenalidomide, do not get pregnant. Two forms of birth control must be used, both by women and by men on the drug who have sexual contact with women of childbearing age.

Adverse drug events

Events include hypotension and hypersensitivity on infusion; cardiac, pulmonary, and renal impairment; and mental status changes (e.g., depression), fever, chills, nausea, and musculoskeletal pain with all agents. Other events include tumor lysis syndrome (rituximab); bleeding, hemorrhage, hypertension, proteinuria, and skin rash (bevacizumab); cutaneous and severe infusion reactions and interstitial lung disease (cetuximab); and hypothyroidism (tositumomab). Avoid use in patients with autoimmune disorders.

Additional events include neurotoxicity (thalidomide), neutropenia (thalidomide and lenalidomide), and deep-vein thrombosis and pulmonary embolism (thalidomide and lenalidomide).

Interactions

Drugs with specific drug interactions include the following:

- **Aldesleukin:** Glucocorticoids, NSAIDs, and antihypertensives

- **Ibritumomab:** Antiplatelets and anticoagulants
- **Interferon-alfa 2b:** Zidovudine, theophylline, phenytoin, and phenobarbital
- **Tositumomab:** Antiplatelets and anticoagulants
- **Trastuzumab:** Anthracyclines, cyclophosphamide, and warfarin

Monitoring parameters

Monitor baseline and follow-up pulmonary, cardiac, and renal function tests. Check CBCs with differential, liver function tests, thyroid-stimulating hormone, electrolytes, and glucose regularly. Premedicate with acetaminophen and diphenhydramine for monoclonal antibodies. Observe blood pressure during infusion (hypotension concerns) for all agents. Perform blood pressure monitoring (hypertensive concerns) and urine dipstick analysis (bevacizumab). Monitor for vital signs, itching, and swelling. Check for trouble breathing (cetuximab and ibritumomab).

Other factors

Ensure that the correct form of interferon alfa is being used (four forms). Do not administer gemtuzumab and alemtuzumab as an IV push or bolus.

Miscellaneous Agents

Miscellaneous agents are described in Table 19-8.

Platinum compounds

These compounds are alklyating-like agents that cause the inhibition of DNA synthesis. They include cisplatin, carboplatin, and oxaliplatin. Adverse effects include nephrotoxicity, peripheral neurotoxicity, myelosuppression, ototoxicity, nausea, and vomiting.

Cisplatin needs hydration therapy and premedications. It interacts with doxorubicin, rituximab, tacrolimus, topotecan, and aminoglycosides.

Carboplatin needs monitoring for thrombocytopenia. It interacts with aminoglycosides.

Oxaliplatin has unique neurotoxicities (e.g., bronchial spasms).

Sorafenib

Sorafenib inhibits multiple tyrosine kinases and is used for treatment of advanced renal cell cancer. Take tablets on an empty stomach. Sorafenib causes diarrhea, fatigue, rash, hand-foot syndrome, hypertension, nausea and vomiting, neutropenia, and alopecia. It can decrease doxorubicin and irinotecan levels.

Sunitinib

Sunitinib inhibits multiple tyrosine kinases and is used for treatment of advanced renal cell cancer and GI

Table 19-8. Miscellaneous Agents

Generic name	Trade name	Dosage range	Dosage form	Frequency	Disease[a]
Platinum compounds					
Cisplatin	Platinol-AQ	50–100 mg/m^2	IV	q 3–4 wk	NSCLC, ovarian, testis, bladder, head, neck, lung
Carboplatin	Paraplatin	300–400 mg/m^2, AUC 6	IV	q 3–4 wk	Ovarian, testis, NSCLC, head, neck, lung
Oxaliplatin	Eloxatin	85–130 mg/m^2	IV	q 2 wk	Colorectal
Enzymes					
Asparaginase	Elspar	6,000 IU/m^2	IM	3 × wk	ALL
	Oncaspar	2,500 IU/m^2	IM	Q 14 d	ALL
Cell-specific					
Hydroxyurea	Hydrea	20–30 mg/kg	po	qd	CML, AML, head, neck
MTOR inhibitors					
Temsirolimus	Torisel	25 mg	IV	q wk	Renal cell carcinoma
Tyrosine kinase inhibitor					
Imatinib mesylate	Gleevec	400–600 mg	po	qd	CML, gastrointestinal stromal tumors
Erlotinib	Tarceva	150 mg	po	qd	NSCLC
Gefitinib	Iressa	250–500 mg	po	qd	NSCLC
Sunitinib	Sutent	50 mg	po	qd × 28 d, 14 d off	Kidney, gastrointestinal stromal tumors
Dasatinib	Sprycel	70 mg	po	bid	CML or AML resistant to or intolerant to imatinib
Sorafenib	Nexavar	400 mg	po	bid	renal cell, hepatocellular carcinoma
Lapatinib	Tykerb	1,250 mg	po	qd × 21 d	Breast
Nilotinib	Tasigna	400 mg	po	q12h	CML
26S Proteasome inhibitor					
Bortezomib	Velcade	1.3 mg/m^2	IV	Days 1, 4, 8, 11	Multiple myeloma, mantle cell lymphoma

AML, acute myelogenous leukemia; CML, chronic myelogenous leukemia; MTOR, mammalian target of rapamycin; NSCLC, non–small cell lung cancer.
a. Appearance of disease in list does not indicate U.S. Food and Drug Administration approval for drug's use in treatment of that disease, but does indicate use of that drug in that disease in clinical practice.

stromal tumors. Take it with or without food. It causes neutropenia, rash changes in skin color, fatigue, myalgia, headaches, hypertension, nausea and vomiting, diarrhea, and increased liver enzymes. It is extensively metabolized by CYP3A4; CYP3A4 inhibitors may increase levels, and CYP3A4 inducers may decrease levels. Ketoconazole increases levels, and rifampin reduces levels.

Dasatinib

Dasatinib specifically targets BCR-ABL mutations (including those resistant to imatinib), thereby inhibiting leukemic cell growth. It is used for treatment of chronic myelogenous leukemia (CML) and pH+ acute lymphocytic leukemia (ALL). It causes rash neutropenia, thrombocytopenia, edema, diarrhea, nausea and vomiting, weight changes, arthralgia, myalgia, cough, shortness of breath, infection, electrolyte changes, and arrhythmias. Significant drug interactions occur with CYP3A4 inhibitors; avoid concurrent use or reduce dose. Avoid acid reduction therapies because they will reduce absorption. Avoid medications that prolong QT interval.

Lapatinib

Lapatinib inhibits multiple tyrosine kinases and is used in combination with capecitabine to treat human epidermal growth factor receptor–2 (HER2) positive breast cancer. Common adverse effects include fatigue, diarrhea, nausea, vomiting, myelosuppression, increased liver enzymes, and palmar-plantar erythrodysesthesia. Significant drug interactions occur with strong CYP450 3A4 inhibitors and inducers; avoid concurrent use or reduce dose. These agents should be taken by mouth, on an empty stomach, 1 hour prior to or 2 hours after a meal.

Nilotinib

Nilotinib selectively inhibits BCR-ABL kinase and is used for the treatment of pH+ CML. Adverse effects include headache, fatigue, rash, pruritus, constipation, nausea, vomiting, and diarrhea. Significant drug interactions occur with strong CYP450 3A4 inhibitors and inducers; avoid concurrent use or reduce dose. Capsules should be taken by mouth, on an empty stomach, and swallowed whole; do not crush or open.

Asparaginase

Asparaginase removes exogenous asparagines from leukemic cells that are required for their survival. Intradermal skin testing is needed because of severe anaphylactic reactions. Adverse effects include myelosuppression, hyperuricemia, hyperglycemia, and renal problems. Drug interactions occur with methotrexate, prednisolone, prednisone, and vincristine.

Hydroxyurea

Hydroxyurea inhibits DNA synthesis without interfering with RNA and protein synthesis. Adverse effects include myelosuppression (leukopenia), development of secondary leukemias, nausea, vomiting, diarrhea, constipation, mucositis, and rare but fatal hepatotoxicity and pancreatitis. Drug interactions occur with didanosine and stavudine.

Imatinib mesylate

Imatinib mesylate is a selective inhibitor of the Philadelphia chromosome (biomarker in CML). It causes hepatotoxicity, fluid retention (pleural effusions and weight gain), neutropenia, GI effects, muscle cramps, nausea, and vomiting. Drug interactions occur with CYP450 3A4 substrates (cyclosporine, simvastatin, erythromycin, and itraconazole) and CYP450 2C9 substrates (warfarin).

Erlotinib

Erlotinib is an HER1 and epidermal growth factor receptor (EGFR) tyrosine kinase inhibitor. For oral therapy, take 1 hour before or 2 hours after meals. Erlotinib causes rash, diarrhea, anorexia, stomatitis,

and interstitial lung disease. Drug interactions occur with CYP450 3A4 inducers and inhibitors. Monitor hepatic function.

Gefitinib

Gefitinib is an EGFR tyrosine kinase inhibitor and a third-line agent for non–small cell lung cancer (NSCLC). It causes diarrhea, rash, acne, and dry skin. Drug interactions occur with CYP450 3A4 inducers and inhibitors and with warfarin.

Bortezomib

Bortezomib inhibits the 26S proteasome and stabilizes regulatory proteins causing apoptosis and disrupting cell proliferation. It causes nausea, vomiting, thrombocytopenia, neuropathy, hypotension, and diarrhea.

Temsirolimus

Temsirolimus inhibits the mammalian target of rapamycin (MTOR) and is used for the treatment of renal cell carcinoma. Adverse effects include myelosuppression, anorexia, rash, mucositis, edema, hyperglycemia, dyslipidemia, and nausea. Drug interactions occur with angiotensin-converting enzyme inhibitors and strong CYP450 3A4 inhibitors and inducers.

Common Toxicities and Treatments

Common toxicities of chemotherapeutic agents are outlined in Table 19-9. They can be classified as acute, subacute, chronic, cumulative, or chronic and cumulative. Rapidly dividing cells, including mucous membranes, hair, skin, GI tract, and bone marrow, are the most common acute toxicities. Examples of delayed or cumulative toxicities include nephrotoxicity, neurotoxicity, cardiomyopathy, pulmonary fibrosis, and secondary malignancies.

The prevention and treatment of chemotherapy-induced nausea and vomiting (CINV) constitute an important area in which pharmacists may play a role in drug selection in oncology patients. The selection of antiemetic agents should be based primarily on the emetogenic potential of the drug regimen. Other factors that increase the risk of CINV include sex (female), young age, prior chemotherapy exposure, lack of chronic alcohol use, combination chemotherapy, high dosage and numerous cycles, and short infusion times. It is important that patients also receive prescriptions to prevent delayed CINV.

Table 19-10 summarizes the pertinent antiemetic drugs used in the prophylactic setting.

Table 19-9. Common Toxicities of Chemotherapeutic Agents

Toxicity	Causative drugs[a]	Recommended therapy
Alopecia	Cyclophosphamide, doxorubicin, paclitaxel, mechlorethamine	n.a.
Cardiac toxicity	Anthracyclines, trastuzumab	Limit cumulative doses
Diarrhea	Irinotecan, fluorouracil	Premedicate with atropine (irinotecan); treat with loperamide
Edema	Docetaxel	Administer prophylactic dexamethasone
Extravasation	Anthracyclines, mitomycin, vinca alkaloids, paclitaxel, mechlorethamine	Treat with heat packs for vincas and with cold compresses for all other drugs
Hemorrhagic cystitis	Cyclophosphamide, ifosfamide	Premedicate with hydration therapy, mesna
Hepatotoxicity	Asparaginase, cytarabine, mercaptopurine, methotrexate, imatinib, erlotinib	n.a.
Hypersensitivity	Paclitaxel, asparaginase, cisplatin, carboplatin, etoposide, teniposide	Premedicate with ranitidine or cimetidine, diphenhydramine, dexamethasone, or test dose; treat with emergency resuscitation
Infertility	Cyclophosphamide, chlorambucil, melphalan, mechlorethamine	n.a.
Myelosuppression	Alkylating agents, fluorouracil, methotrexate, lomustine, cyclophosphamide, methotrexate	Treat with G-CSF, platelet transfusions, red blood cell transfusions, erythropoietin-stimulating agents (unless cancer is curable)
Nausea and vomiting	Cisplatin, cyclophosphamide, cytarabine, dacarbazine, ifosfamide, melphalan, mitomycin, mechlorethamine	Premedicate with dexamethasone, phenothiazines (e.g., Compazine), 5-HT$_3$-receptor antagonists (e.g., granisetron), and neurokinin-1 antagonists
Neurotoxicity	Paclitaxel, cisplatin, cytarabine, methotrexate, vincristine, asparaginase	Dose reductions
Pulmonary toxicity	Bleomycin, busulfan, carmustine, mitomycin, trastuzumab	Treat with corticosteroids
Renal toxicity	Cisplatin, ifosfamide, methotrexate, streptozocin	Premedicate with hydration therapy
Stomatitis	Fluorouracil, methotrexate	Hold ice chips in mouth; administer palifermin[b]

n.a., not applicable.
a. Adverse effects are not limited to the listed drugs.
b. Use for hematologic malignancies that need myelotoxic therapy requiring hematopoietic agents only.

For highly to moderately emetogenic drug regimens, dexamethasone and 5-HT$_3$ receptor antagonists are recommended—at a minimum—for the prevention of acute CINV. Aprepitant should also be considered, especially for highly emetogenic regimens.

For low to minimally emetogenic drug regimens, dexamethasone and a phenothiazine are recommended.

For prevention of delayed CINV (> 24 hours after administration of highly emetogenic and some moderately emetogenic chemotherapy), aprepitant and dexamethasone are recommended.

All patients receiving agents with emetogenic potential should receive prophylactic therapy for CINV, with rescue medication readily available.

Miscellaneous Commonalities across Chemotherapy Agents

- Patients should not receive live and rotavirus vaccines during chemotherapy because of immune suppression.
- The majority of agents are teratogenic and mutagenic.

Table 19-10. Pharmacologic Management for the Prevention of Acute Chemotherapy-Induced Nausea and Vomiting

Generic name	Trade name	Dosage range	Dosage form[a]	Frequency	Side effects
5-HT₃ receptor antagonists					
Dolasetron	Anzemet	100–200 mg	IV, po	30 min before treatment	Headache, dizziness, constipation, blurred vision, elevated liver enzymes
Granisetron	Kytril	1–2 mg	IV, po	30 min before treatment	Headache, dizziness, constipation, blurred vision, elevated liver enzymes
Ondansetron	Zofran	8–16 mg / 16–24 mg	IV / po	30 min before treatment	Headache, dizziness, constipation, blurred vision, elevated liver enzymes
Palonosetron	Aloxi	0.25, 0.5 mg	IV, po	Day 1 (not to be repeated within 7 d)	Diarrhea, headache, fatigue, insomnia, arrhythmias
Phenothiazines					
Prochlorperazine	Compazine	10–25 mg	IV, po, PR	q4h prn	Sedation, hypotension, extra-pyramidal effects, lethargy
Chlorpromazine	Thorazine	25–50 mg	po	q4–6h prn	Sedation, hypotension, extra-pyramidal effects, lethargy
Promethazine	Phenergan	12.5–25 mg	IV, po, PR	q4–6h prn	Sedation, hypotension, extra-pyramidal effects, lethargy
Butyrophenones					
Droperidol	Inapsine	1.25–2.5 mg	IM, slow IV	q4h prn	Sedation, tachycardia, hypotension
Haloperidol	Haldol	2 mg	IV, IM, po	q4–6h prn	Sedation, tachycardia, hypotension
Corticosteroids					
Dexamethasone	Decadron	4 mg, 10–20 mg	IV, po	Varies	Anxiety, insomnia, GI upset, psychosis
Cannabinoids					
Dronabinol	Marinol	10–20 mg	po	q3–6h	Drowsiness, euphoria, dry mouth
Nabilone	Cesamet	1–2 mg	po	bid	Drowsiness, euphoria, dry mouth
Benzodiazepines					
Lorazepam	Ativan	2 mg	po	q6h	Sedation, amnesia
Benzamides					
Metoclopramide	Reglan	20 mg	po	tid–qid	Diarrhea, sedation, agitation
Neurokinin-1 antagonist					
Aprepitant	Emend	80–125 mg	po	Day 1 (125 mg); days 2–3 (80 mg daily)	Somnolence, fatigue, diarrhea

a. Most agents are available in more than one dosage form. Because of space limitations, oral dosing has been given preference.

- Patients should avoid becoming pregnant or breast-feeding during and immediately after chemotherapy.
- Patients should have laboratory studies done on a regular basis to check for common toxicities, such as myelosuppression, renal and hepatic impairment, and electrolyte disturbances.

19-3. Nondrug Therapy

As mentioned previously, cancer treatment is generally a combination of modalities. Chemotherapy is an important component, because most patients present with advanced disease on diagnosis. Surgery plays a role in resecting primary tumors or metastases. It can

Table 19-11. American Cancer Society Screening Recommendations

Disease[a]	Sex	Age (years)	Procedure	Frequency
Colorectal	M and F	50+	Fecal occult blood test	Every year
	M and F	50+[b]	Flexible sigmoidoscopy, colonoscopy, double contrast barium enema, CT colonography	Every 5 years (flexible sigmoidoscopy, CT colonography, and double contrast barium enema, followed by colonoscopy if positive result), every 10 years (colonoscopy)
Breast	F	20+	Breast self-exam	Every month
	F	20–39 or 40+	Clinical breast exam	Every 3 years or every year
	F	40+	Mammography	Every year
Cervical	F	21+[c]	Pap smear and pelvic exam	Every year
Prostate	M	50+	Digital rectal exam	Every year
	M	50+	Prostate-specific antigen test	Every year

Adapted from the American Cancer Society, 2009.
a. No specific screening recommendations have been made for lung, skin, and testicular cancer in patients with average risk. However, after age 40, it is recommended that all men and women receive health counseling and a physical exam every year.
b. Screening should be done earlier if there is a strong family history of prostate cancer.
c. Screening should be done earlier if patient is sexually active.

also be used for diagnostic purposes to biopsy tumors or for other exploratory purposes. Radiation is used to shrink primary tumors in local disease or metastases. It can be used both in neoadjuvant therapy to downsize tumors and in adjuvant therapy to eradicate residual disease.

Screening is also an important part of cancer therapy, because it can allow the detection of disease in very early stages, when the survival rates are much higher. Table 19-11 refers to American Cancer Society screening recommendations for patients at average risk of developing cancer.

Tests can also be performed to screen and monitor tumor markers. They are found in the plasma, serum, or other body fluids and may be used to identify neoplastic growth. These markers are often not sensitive enough to diagnose cancer and may produce false positive results (i.e., falsely identify people with a disease that they do not have). However, they are helpful in identifying the recurrence of advanced disease in patients who had elevated levels on diagnosis. Table 19-12 lists some commonly used tumor markers.

19-4. Key Points

■ Oncology includes more than 100 diverse diseases that share properties of abnormal and detrimental cell growth.

Table 19-12. Common Tumor Markers and Associated Cancers

Tumor marker	Abnormal level	Cancer
Alpha-fetoprotein (AFP)	> 20 ng/mL	Hepatocellular, ovarian
β-2 microglobulin (β2M)	> 3 ng/mL	Multiple myeloma, lymphoma
CA 15-3	> 25 U/mL	Breast
CA 125	> 30 U/mL	Ovarian
CA 19-9	> 37 U/mL	Pancreatic, colorectal
Calcitonin[a]	> 70 pg/mL	Thyroid
Carcinoembryonic antigen (CEA)	> 5 U/mL	Colorectal, breast, non–small cell lung
Chromogranin A	> 76 ng/mL (males); > 51 (females)	Neuroendocrine, lung, prostate
Gamma globulin	> 2–3 g/100 mL	Multiple myeloma
HER2/neu	> 450 fmol/mL	Breast
Human chorionic gonadotropin (HCG)	> 5 mIU/mL	Testicular
Prostate-specific antigen (PSA)[a]	> 4–10 ng/mL	Prostate
Thyroglobulin	> 10 ng/mL	Thyroid

a. PSA can be used to diagnose early disease.

- Diseases are classified on the basis of the tissue in which they originate (e.g., breast cancer metastasized to the brain is classified as breast cancer).
- Signs and symptoms of cancer do not follow a specific pattern. A health care provider should evaluate any unusual or persistent change in body appearance or function.
- Before a diagnosis of cancer can be made and systemic treatment can begin, a positive biopsy or blood examination must confirm the presence of the disease.
- Further imaging and laboratory work-up should be done to evaluate the extent of the disease (i.e., determine the stage of disease).
- Cancer therapy must be individualized to each patient on the basis of the type and severity of disease, patient characteristics, and patient and family preferences.
- Surgery, radiation, chemotherapy, and biologic therapy are all cancer treatment modalities. They are often used in combination.
- Pharmacists can affect patients' chemotherapy and biologic therapy by counseling the patients and educating health care providers on details of the individual drug regimens.
- Chemotherapy is often used in combinations to take advantage of different mechanisms of action, prevent resistance, and minimize toxicities.
- Most chemotherapy is aimed at rapidly proliferating cancerous cells. However, many chemotherapy-related side effects occur in normal highly proliferative cells of the body, such as hair follicles, the gastrointestinal tract lining, and blood cells.
- Patients should be aware of expected toxicities of chemotherapy, which include alopecia, diarrhea, nausea and vomiting, infertility, myelosuppression, neurotoxicity, nephrotoxicity, hepatotoxicity, stomatitis, and pulmonary toxicity.
- The importance of laboratory studies and follow-up appointments to treatment should be stressed to the patient.
- All prophylactic and post-treatment medications for chemotherapy-related complications should be made available to the patient. Counsel the patient to keep a diary of events that occur prior to and after treatments. Use this record to make interventions and monitor the patient's quality of life.
- All pharmacists should be aware of the accepted cancer screening recommendations and should discuss these with patients. Many diseases can be cured if they are caught early enough.
- It is the pharmacist's responsibility to ensure that the patient and family are adequately educated to participate in making decisions about their care.

19-5. Questions

Use Patient Profile 1 to answer questions 1–5.

Patient Profile 1—Medication Profile: Community

Patient name: Tina Tiny

Age: 33

Sex: Female

Diagnosis:
1. Diagnosis on 12/03 of metastatic breast cancer
2. Mastectomy to right breast on 12/15/03
3. Weight loss of 20 lbs
4. Allergies

Address: 234 Small Street

Height: 5'8"

Weight: 150 lbs

Allergies: Sulfa, penicillin

Pharmacist notes:

Date	Note
01/04	Patient complained of soreness after mastectomy and swelling of right arm.
03/04	Patient did not pick up birth control last month (2/04).
03/04	Patient is receiving Zoladex 3.6 mg SC q28d at oncology clinic. Received dose today.

Medication record:

Date	Rx no.	Physician	Drug and strength	Quantity	Sig	Refills
12/03	12345	Buford	Percocet 5/325	30	1–2 q4h prn	0
03/04	12347	Buford	Tamoxifen 20 mg	30	1 po qd	2
03/04	12349	Buford	Megace 40 mg/mL	80 mg/d	—	2
03/04	12350	Charles	Celebrex 10 mg	30	1 po qd	2

1. Which of the following agents that Ms. Tiny is taking can be used to treat breast and prostate cancer?

   I.   Zoladex
   II. Tamoxifen
   III. Celebrex

   A. I only
   B. III only
   C. I and II only
   D. II and III only
   E. I, II, and III

2. When Ms. Tiny presents the tamoxifen prescription, you notice that the directions are missing. You call the doctor to clarify what the instructions are for this patient. Which of the following is a correct choice?

   A. 10 mL po qd
   B. 20 mL po qd
   C. 40 mg po bid
   D. 20 mg po qd
   E. 5 mg po bid

3. Ms. Tiny presents to your pharmacy with complaints of lower leg calf pain that is tender to the touch and red. You suspect a deep-vein thrombosis. Which of the following agents is most likely to be associated with this condition?

   I.   Megace
   II. Goserelin
   III. Tamoxifen

   A. I only
   B. III only
   C. I and II only
   D. II and III only
   E. I, II, and III

4. Ms. Tiny calls you 2 days after her 03/04 visit to your pharmacy. She has been feeling a lot of bone pain and describes an "achy, creaky feeling all over." She is worried that her cancer has spread to her bones. What advice can you give her?

   I.   She should call her oncology caretaker and be formally evaluated.
   II. This could be a side effect of her Zoladex therapy, and the pain should subside.
   III. This could be a side effect of her Celebrex therapy, and the pain should subside.

   A. I only
   B. III only
   C. I and II only
   D. II and III only
   E. I, II, and III

5. Ms. Tiny's mother (age 59) is worried that she will develop breast cancer like her daughter. Which of the following is *not* an appropriate initial screening test for breast cancer?

   A. Monthly breast self-examination
   B. Clinical breast examination
   C. Mammography
   D. Biopsy
   E. Mammography and clinical breast examination

6. Which of the following classes of agents is best known for causing infusion-related reactions, such as fever and chills?

   I.   Monoclonal antibodies
   II. Alkylating agents
   III. Vinca alkaloids

   A. I only
   B. III only
   C. I and II only
   D. II and III only
   E. I, II, and III

7. Your patient has just received 5-FU and irinotecan for the treatment of colorectal cancer. Before he leaves the clinic, you ensure that he has a prescription to prevent or treat which of the following side effects from irinotecan?

   A. Nausea with Aloxi
   B. Diarrhea with loperamide
   C. Headache with aspirin
   D. Delayed allergic reaction with epinephrine
   E. Change in urine color: no treatment available

8. Which of the following drugs is an oral prodrug of 5-FU?

   A. Fluorouracil
   B. Xeloda
   C. Fludara
   D. Cytoxan
   E. Alkeran

9. An elderly male patient comes to your pharmacy and is worried that he might have prostate cancer. He just had some laboratory studies done, and his doctor told him that some level was abnormal, indicating potential prostate cancer. Which lab test might he be talking about?

    I.   PSA
    II. Cortisol
    III. ESR

    A. I only
    B. III only
    C. I and II only
    D. II and III only
    E. I, II, and III

10. *Stomatitis* is the clinical term for which of the following chemotherapy-related adverse effects?

    I.   Nausea and projectile vomiting
    II. Obstruction of the lower esophageal sphincter
    III. Inflammation of the mucosal lining of the mouth

    A. I only
    B. III only
    C. I and II only
    D. II and III only
    E. I, II, and III

11. Which of the following does *not* describe characteristics of most chemotherapy agents?

    A. They have a wide therapeutic index.
    B. They interfere with DNA synthesis and replication.
    C. They are more effective in combination.
    D. Acute adverse effects occur primarily in rapidly dividing normal cells.
    E. They have both phase-specific and non-phase-specific actions

Use Patient Profile 2 to answer questions 12–17.

Patient Profile 2—Medication Profile: Institution

Patient name:	Cassimer Migash
Age:	60
Sex:	Male
Diagnosis:	1. Diagnosis on 02/04 of metastatic non–small cell lung cancer
	2. Chronic obstructive pulmonary disease
	3. Asthma
Address:	579 Hunter's Ridge
Height:	180 cm
Weight:	200 lbs
Allergies:	NKDA

Lab and diagnostic tests:

Date	Test
05/04	WBC: 2,500/mcL
05/04	RBC: 2.8×10^6/mm³
05/04	PLT: 100×10^3/mcL
05/04	Theophylline: 10 mcg/mL
05/04	Hgb: 9 g/dL
05/04	Hct: 30%

Medication record:

Date	Route	Drug	Sig
04/04	IV	Paclitaxel 175 mg/m²	175 mg/m² over 3 h q 3 wk
04/04	IV	Carboplatin AUC 6	AUC 6 over 2 h q 3 wk
04/04	po	Theophylline SR 400 mg	1 tab po bid
04/04	INH	Albuterol inhaler	2 puffs prn
04/04	INH	Cromolyn inhaler	1 puff qid
04/04	INH	Beclomethasone inhaler	2 puffs qid
04/04	po	Dexamethasone 20 mg	1 tab 12 h and 6 h prior to chemo
04/03	IV	Diphenhydramine 50 mg	Infuse 30 min and 60 min prior to chemo
04/03	IV	Cimetidine 300 mg	Infuse 30 min and 60 min prior to chemo

12. A nurse would like to know if she can administer the diphenhydramine and the cimetidine to Mr. Migash in the same IV line simultaneously. Which of the following resources will provide you with this information?

    I.   Wolters Kluwer Health's Facts & Comparisons
    II. Trissel's *Handbook on Injectable Drugs*
    III. Micromedex

    A. I only
    B. III only
    C. I and II only
    D. II and III only
    E. I, II, and III

13. Which of the following agents being taken by Mr. Migash requires the premedication regimen of dexamethasone, diphenhydramine, and ranitidine or cimetidine to prevent an anaphylactic reaction?

    I.   Taxotere
    II. Paraplatin
    III. Taxol

    A. I only
    B. III only
    C. I and II only
    D. II and III only
    E. I, II, and III

14. On the basis of the patient's weight and height, you calculate Mr. Migash's body surface area to be 2.1 m². Paclitaxel is supplied as 6 mg/mL in 5 mL, 16.7 mL, and 50 mL vials. Your pharmacy has all quantities available. What is the best way to correctly dose this patient?

    A. One 50 mL vial and one 16.7 mL vial
    B. One 50 mL vial and one 5 mL vial
    C. Two 16.7 mL vials
    D. Two 16.7 mL vials and one 5 mL vial
    E. Four 16.7 mL vials

15. You are concerned that Mr. Migash will develop nausea and vomiting from his chemotherapy regimen. Which of the following regimens would be suitable to prevent acute CINV?

    A. Dexamethasone, granisetron, and aprepitant
    B. Granisetron and prochlorperazine
    C. Metoclopramide, dexamethasone, and aprepitant
    D. Palonosetron and granisetron
    E. Lorazepam and droperidol

16. On the basis of the patient's laboratory values, which of the following adverse reactions appear to have occurred as a likely result of the chemotherapy?

    I.   Thrombocytopenia
    II. Leukopenia
    III. Anemia

    A. I only
    B. III only
    C. I and II only
    D. II and III only
    E. I, II, and III

17. The goal of Mr. Migash's treatment regimen is

    I.   to cure his disease.
    II. to palliate his disease-related symptoms.
    III. to increase his quality of life.

    A. I only
    B. III only
    C. I and II only
    D. II and III only
    E. I, II, and III

18. Doxorubicin is an antineoplastic agent that

    A. is not related to epirubicin and daunorubicin.
    B. interacts with the microtubules of cells during mitosis.
    C. has an oral dosage form commercially available.
    D. causes cumulative cardiac toxicity.
    E. can also be used to treat tuberculosis.

19. Which of the following agents is used in cancer regimens but is not considered an antineoplastic agent?

    A. Methotrexate
    B. Leucovorin
    C. Doxorubicin
    D. Cyclophosphamide
    E. Gemcitabine

20. Methotrexate (Rheumatrex) is *not* available as which of the following dosage forms?

    A. An intravenous injection
    B. An oral tablet or capsule
    C. An intrathecal injection
    D. An ointment
    E. An intramuscular injection

19-6. Answers

1. **A.** Zoladex (goserelin) is an LHRH agonist that can be used to treat both breast and prostate cancer. LHRH agonists are approved by the U.S. Food and Drug Administration (FDA) for premenopausal women because they inhibit estrogen production from the ovaries.

2. **D.** The FDA-approved dose for breast cancer therapy is 20 mg po qd. The drug is not available in a liquid form.

3. **E.** All three agents are hormonal products and are associated with thromboembolic side effects. It is important that patients on these products are aware of the signs and symptoms of deep-vein thrombosis.

4. **C.** Although the bone pain is most likely a side effect of her Zoladex therapy, Ms. Tiny should notify her oncology practitioner so he or she can document this side effect. If other factors point to metastatic disease, she may need additional evaluation.

5. **D.** Biopsies should never be performed as initial screening tests. However, if results from the mammography and other tests point to disease, a biopsy is needed to make a diagnosis. There is some debate about the usefulness of clinical breast examinations for women who are reluctant to perform breast self-examinations; however, clinical breast examinations should be offered.

6. **A.** Monoclonal antibodies are commonly associated with infusion-related reactions. Patients should receive premedication, such as acetaminophen, to prevent this.

7. **B.** Diarrhea is a dose-limiting toxicity of irinotecan. Late-onset diarrhea can be life threatening. All patients should receive a prescription for loperamide to treat delayed-onset diarrhea. Patients should be instructed to take 2 mg po q2h while awake and 4 mg po q4h during the night until the diarrhea has stopped for at least 12 hours. Acute-onset diarrhea can be treated with atropine.

8. **B.** Xeloda (generic name capecitabine) is an oral prodrug of 5-FU. Fluorouracil is another name for 5-FU. Fludara is the brand name for fludarabine and is used to treat chronic lymphocytic leukemia and non-Hodgkin lymphoma intravenously. Cytoxan is the brand name for cyclophosphamide and is available in IV and po dosage forms. Alkeran is the brand name for melphalan and is also available in IV and po dosage forms.

9. **A.** PSA (prostate-specific antigen) is a lab test that is commonly done in men over age 40. It should be performed annually in men over age 50 to check for prostate cancer.

10. **B.** *Stomatitis* is used to describe an irritation or ulceration of the mucosal lining. This side effect is common with fluorouracil and methotrexate. Having the patient hold ice chips in his or her mouth during treatment can prevent it. The cold is thought to cause vasoconstriction of the lining and prevent damage.

11. **A.** Chemotherapy agents have a very narrow therapeutic index. This is one of the main reasons these drugs have so many toxic effects. They can be phase specific or non-phase-specific drugs and can cause many adverse reactions to normal cells that undergo rapid proliferation.

12. **D.** Both Trissel's *Handbook on Injectable Drugs* and the Micromedex IV compatibility tool can be used to assess whether diphenhydramine and cimetidine are compatible.

13. **B.** Taxol is the brand name of paclitaxel. This agent has been shown to cause hypersensitivity reactions in patients. It is unclear if these reactions are due to the drug itself or the drug's vehicle (Cremophor). All patients receiving paclitaxel should receive a premedication regimen of dexamethasone, diphenhydramine, and ranitidine or cimetidine. Taxotere is the brand name of docetaxel. This agent also requires premedications with a minimum of a corticosteroid. However, this regimen is given to prevent peripheral edema, not an anaphylactic reaction.

14. **A.** The patient requires 367.5 mg of drug. Both choice A and choice E will provide 400 mg of drug; however, using one large vial and one medium vial is more economical than using four medium vials.

15. **A.** This patient's regimen contains carboplatin and paclitaxel. Together these agents have a high likelihood of causing acute (and delayed) CINV. The patient should receive a corticosteroid, a 5-HT$_3$ antagonist, and a neurokinin-1 inhibitor, which makes choice B incorrect because it contains a 5-HT3 antagonist and a dopamine antagonist. Aprepitant is approved in combination with a corticosteroid and a 5-HT$_3$ antagonist, which makes choice C incorrect because it adds a corticosteroid and a dopamine antagonist to the aprepitant. Choice D contains two 5-HT$_3$ antagonists. Therapy should include more than

one class of agent. Choice E agents are not efficacious in moderate to severe CINV.

16. **E.** Myelosuppression is a common adverse reaction to most chemotherapy agents. Both paclitaxel and carboplatin can cause anemia, thrombocytopenia, and leukopenia. It is very important to monitor blood levels in these patients. If myelosuppression is too severe, the length of time between chemotherapy cycles may be increased so that all or some of the blood cells can return to normal levels.

17. **D.** Mr. Migash has metastatic disease. When a solid tumor is diagnosed as stage IV, this finding is representative of the fact that the disease is incurable. The treatment goals for these patients include relieving any disease-related symptoms, minimizing toxicity from treatments, and increasing the patient's quality of life through treatment or supportive care measures.

18. **D.** Doxorubicin is an antitumor antibiotic related to epirubicin and daunorubicin. These agents act by binding tightly to DNA through intercalation and by inhibiting the topoisomerase II enzyme. Doxorubicin does have a liposomal IV product, but it is not available orally. All anthracyclines are associated with cardiac toxicity and have cumulative dosing limits to prevent this.

19. **B.** Leucovorin is a reduced folate agent that is used in combination with 5-FU to potentiate the therapeutic effects of 5-FU and as a rescue treatment for high-dose methotrexate.

20. **D.** Methotrexate is not commercially available for topical use. It is available in all of the other dosage forms.

19-7. References

Adams VR, Yee GC. Lymphomas. In: Dipiro JT, Talbert RL, Yee GC, et al, eds. *Pharmacotherapy: A Pathophysiologic Approach.* 5th ed. New York: McGraw-Hill; 2002:2331–56.

American Cancer Society. Cancer facts & figures 2009. Available at: www.cancer.org.

Balmer CM, Valley AW. Cancer treatment and chemotherapy. In: Dipiro JT, Talbert RL, Yee GC, et al., eds. *Pharmacotherapy: A Pathophysiologic Approach.* 5th ed. New York: McGraw-Hill; 2002: 2175–222.

Chabner BA, Amrain PC, Druker B, et al. Antineoplastic agents. In: Brunton LL, Lazo JS, Parker KL, eds. *Goodman & Gilman's: The Pharmacological Basis of Therapeutics.* 11th ed. New York: McGraw-Hill; 2006:1315–404.

DeVita VT, Hellman S, Rosenberg SA, eds. *Cancer: Principles & Practices of Oncology.* 8th ed. Philadelphia: Lippincott Williams & Wilkins; 2008.

Dorr RT, Fritz WL. *Cancer Chemotherapy Handbook.* New York: Elsevier; 1980.

Medina PJ, Fausel C. Cancer treatment and chemotherapy. In: Dipiro JT, Talbert RL, Yee GC, et al., eds. *Pharmacotherapy: A Pathophysiologic Approach,* 7th ed. New York: McGraw-Hill; 2008:2085–120.

Mueller BA, Schumock GT, Bertch KE, et al., eds. *Pharmacotherapy Self-Assessment Program.* 4th ed. Book 10, Hematology/oncology. Lenexa, Kans.: American College of Clinical Pharmacy; 2002.

National Comprehensive Cancer Network. NCCN clinical practice guidelines—Antiemesis. Ver. 3. 2009. Available at: www.nccn.org.

Solid Organ Transplantation

Benjamin Duhart, Jr, MS, PharmD

20

20-1. Organ Transplantation

Principles of Transplantation

Types of allografts

- *Heart:* First successful transplant occurred in 1968. In 2007, 2,141 heart transplants were performed in the United States.
- *Intestines:* First successful transplant occurred in 1987. In 2007, 57 intestinal transplants were performed in the United States.
- *Kidney:* First successful cadaveric transplant occurred in 1954. In 2007, 16,119 kidney transplants were performed in the United States.
- *Liver:* First successful cadaveric transplant occurred in 1967. In 2007, 5,890 liver transplants were performed in the United States.
- *Lung:* First successful cadaveric single-lung transplant occurred in 1983. In 2007, 1,461 lung transplants were performed in the United States.
- *Pancreas:* First successful solitary pancreas transplant occurred in 1968. In 2007, 1,304 pancreas transplants were performed in the United States.

Goal

The goal is to improve patients' quality of life and survival by stabilizing and improving end-organ failure–related complications.

Patient and Graft Outcomes

Table 20-1 shows the patient and graft survival rates for transplant recipients.

Definitions

- *Acute rejection:* A systemic immunologic response to donor antigens primarily mediated by T-lymphocytes
- *Adaptive immunity:* Involves the stimulation of cells and soluble mediators in response to specific antigens with a markedly enhanced response on repeat exposure
- *Complement:* An enzyme system that is a crucial part of the basic immune response on primary exposure to an antigen and that also provides augmented signaling during memory immunity
- *Human leukocyte antigen (HLA):* Antigen-binding proteins that rescue protein fragments from intracellular catabolism (class I or II) or select antigens from the extracellular milieu that are then presented to lymphocytes (class II)
- *Induction:* Administration of short-term antibody therapy prior to and during the initial transplant as prophylaxis for acute rejection
- *Innate immunity:* Involves the stimulation of cells and soluble mediators that nonspecifically recognize antigens and have no ability to alter response with repeat exposure
- *Major histocompatibility complex (MHC):* A group of genes that encode for HLAs class I and II
- *Opsonization:* Occurs when antigens or immune complexes become coated with a molecule that facilitates binding with a phagocyte
- *Panel reactive antibody (PRA):* A test that quantifies a patient's immunologic reactivity to a given pool of antigens
- *Phagocytosis:* A process by which recognized antigens are engulfed and subsequently undergo intracellular catabolism

Table 20-1. Kaplan–Meier Patient and Graft Survival Rates for Transplant Recipients

Organ	Patient survival (%)	Graft survival (%)
Heart		
1 year	87.8	87.3
3 years	80.2	79.3
Intestinal		
1 year	81.0	73.4
3 years	67.4	54.3
Kidney: cadaveric		
1 year	94.8	90.0
3 years	88.4	78.9
Kidney: living		
1 year	98.0	95.1
3 years	94.7	88.5
Liver: cadaveric		
1 year	86.9	82.3
3 years	78.9	73.7
Liver: living		
1 year	90.6	84.1
3 years	83.8	77.1
Lung:		
1 year	84.0	82.3
3 years	68.0	65.4
Pancreas		
1 year	96.7	80.1
3 years	91.9	55.9

Based on data from U.S. Organ Procurement and Transplantation Network and the Scientific Registry of Transplant Recipients as of May 1, 2007.

Basic Immunology and Acute Rejection

Fundamental types of immunity

Innate immunity
Cellular components

- **Macrophages:** Phagocytic cells found throughout the body, which may function as antigen-presenting cells
- **Neutrophils:** Highly motile cells whose major physiologic role is the destruction of invading microorganisms through phagocytosis or opsonization
- **Natural killer cells:** A subset of non-B- and non-T-lymphocytes that survey for the normal biosynthesis and expression of HLA class I, making them important in immunity against viral infection and malignancy

Humoral components

- **Complement:** Activation leads to formation of lipophilic complexes, called *membrane-attack complexes,* in the cell membrane of the target cell and results in osmotic leakage.
- **Physiologic function:** Humoral component provides a defense against pyogenic bacterial infections.
  - Bridges innate and adaptive immunity
  - Mediates disposal of immune complexes
  - Consists of acute phase proteins

Adaptive immunity
Cellular components

- **Thymus-derived lymphocytes (T-cells):** Mature T-cells become activated when they encounter an antigen-presenting cell (APC). T-cells do not recognize antigens directly.
  - CD4+ T-cells (*helper T-cells*) recognize antigen presented via HLA class II.
  - CD8+ T-cells (*cytotoxic T-cells*) recognize antigen presented via HLA class I.
- **Bone marrow–derived lymphocytes (B-cells):** B-cells encounter the antigen to which their surface immunoglobulin has specificity, through either its APC function or by interaction with an activated CD4+ T-cell. B-cell–CD4+ T-cell interaction is required for translocation into a follicle within secondary lymphoid tissue, where a germinal center forms and where high-affinity memory B-cells and plasma cells are produced and selected (somatic hypermutation).

Humoral components

- **Complement:** See the previous section on innate immunity.
- **Immunoglobulin (Ig):** This complex protein of various isotypes is formed as a consequence of B-cell activation for the purpose of binding and elimination of the activating antigen.

Acute rejection

Pathophysiology
During transplantation, the recipient is exposed to donor antigens to which he or she has no previous exposure. Although undesirable, acute rejection is the normal physiologic response of the immune system to these donor antigens. This response can be divided into five basic phases:

1. *Recognition:* Foreign antigen is recognized via self- or nonself-recognition mediated through MHC.
2. *Presentation:* On recognition, APC present antigens in association with native HLA class II to inactive CD4+ T-cells.
3. *Activation and proliferation:* Activation depends on antigen–HLA binding to the T-cell receptor (TCR) complex and the subsequent binding of a second signal or "co-stimulatory pathway." Subsequently, the active CD4+ T-cell produces and releases various lymphokines, particularly interleukin-2 (IL-2), which is important for activation and proliferation of numerous lymphocyte lineages.
4. *Recruitment:* Recruitment is mediated through several lymphokines produced as a consequence of lymphocyte activation.
5. *Antigen and tissue destruction:* Tissue injury is mediated through induction of polyclonal immune response.

Incidence
The incidence is organ specific and depends on many pre- and post-transplant factors. Several known factors increase risk:

- Increased HLA mismatch
- Factors affecting previous sensitization (e.g., history of pregnancy, previous transplantation, previous rejection, or panel reactive antibody > 20%)
- Ethnicity (i.e., African American recipients)
- Age (i.e., pediatric recipients)
- Donor source (i.e., cadaveric donor)
- Prolonged preservation time
- Noncompliance

Immunosuppressive Strategies

Balance of immunosuppression

Selection of an immunosuppression regimen for the prevention of acute rejection should be individualized on the basis of known risk and potential for toxicity. Subsequent adjustment must focus on the balance of the triad: rejection, infection, and toxicity.

Phases of preventive immunosuppression

Induction
The early phase is intended to provide highly potent, multifocal suppression of the immune system for several days to a few weeks. Commonly used agents include the following:

- Corticosteroids
- Monoclonal antibody (muromonab, basiliximab, daclizumab)
- Polyclonal antibody (antithymocyte globulin— equine or rabbit)

Maintenance
The immunosuppression regimen is designed to provide chronic, balanced immunodeficiency. Some commonly used regimens include the following:

- Double therapy:
  - Calcineurin inhibitor + steroids
  - Calcineurin inhibitor + antimetabolite
  - Calcineurin inhibitor + mTOR (mammalian target of rapamycin) inhibitor
  - mTOR inhibitor + steroids
  - mTOR inhibitor + antimetabolite
  - Antimetabolite + steroids
- Triple therapy:
  - Calcineurin inhibitor + antimetabolite + steroids
  - mTOR inhibitor + calcineurin inhibitor + steroids
  - mTOR inhibitor + antimetabolite + steroids

Phases of immunosuppression during treatment

Treatment
Selection of the agents is organ specific and depends on the severity of acute rejection. Commonly used agents include the following:

- Corticosteroids
- Calcineurin inhibitor
  - Tacrolimus may be used as the primary treatment of acute rejection in liver recipients.
  - Tacrolimus may also have a role as adjuvant therapy in refractory acute rejection in various other solid organ recipients.
- Monoclonal antibody (muromonab)
- Polyclonal antibody (antithymocyte globulin— equine or rabbit)

Maintenance reevaluation
The decision to heighten maintenance immunosuppression depends on the cause for rejection (i.e., failure of regimen versus noncompliance).

Immunosuppressive Complications

Infectious

Infectious complications are an important cause of early morbidity and mortality. The incidence is organ specific and is closely linked to the net degree of immunodeficiency. Prevention is a key management strategy following transplantation. A list of infectious complications follows:

- Bacterial
  - Tuberculosis: *Mycobacterium tuberculosis*
  - Nocardiosis: Various species of *Nocardia*
- Fungal
  - Aspergillosis: Various species of *Aspergillus*
  - Blastomycosis: *Blastomyces dermatitidis*
  - Candidiasis: Various species of *Candida*
  - Coccidioidomycosis: *Coccidioides immitis*
  - Cryptococcosis: *Cryptococcus neoformans*
  - Histoplasmosis: *Histoplasma capsulatum*
  - Mucormycosis: Various species of *Mucor*
  - *Pneumocystis* pneumonia: *Pneumocystis carinii (Pneumocystis jiroveci)*
- Parasitic
  - Toxoplasmosis: *Toxoplasma gondii*
- Viral
  - Cytomegalovirus
  - Epstein-Barr virus: including post-transplant lymphoproliferative disease
  - Herpes simplex virus
  - Varicella-zoster virus
  - Human herpes viruses (i.e., HHV-6, HHV-8)
  - Parvovirus
  - Polyomavirus

Noninfectious

The noninfectious complications are specific to the agents included in the immunosuppressive regimen.

20-2. Immunosuppressants

Immunosuppressant drugs are described in Table 20-2.

Calcineurin Inhibitors

Cyclosporine

Mechanism of action

Cyclosporine inhibits calcineurin-dependent translocation of the cytosolic subunit of NFAT (nuclear factor of activated T-cells), the promoter gene for IL-2, into the nucleus, thereby inhibiting transcription and synthesis of IL-2; thus, it inhibits IL-2-mediated monoclonal T-cell proliferation and polyclonal T-cell activation.

Administration

- Intravenous
  - Administer 5–6 mg/kg per day divided every 12 hours or as a continuous infusion. Each milliliter of IV concentrate should be diluted in 20–100 mL of normal saline (NS) or 5% dextrose in water (D_5W) in a glass container. For bolus dosing, the dose should be infused over 2–6 hours.
- Oral
  - *Capsules:* Administer the daily dose as two equally divided doses every 12 hours with meals.
  - *Oral solution:* Administer the daily dose as two equally divided doses every 12 hours with meals. The solution may be diluted with chocolate milk or orange juice in a glass container. Additional diluent should be used to rinse the container to ensure administration of the total dose.

Drug–drug interactions

The drug is metabolized primarily via cytochrome P450 (CYP450) 3A isoenzymes. Substances known to alter functionality of these enzymes will alter bioavailability and elimination of this drug (Table 20-3).

Drug interactions lead to altered exposure of other drugs by cyclosporine (Table 20-4).

Drug–disease interactions

- *Altered biliary flow:* Diversion of biliary flow can significantly reduce adsorption. This more profoundly affects cyclosporine USP (United States Pharmacopeia) than it does cyclosporine USP (modified).
- *Diabetes mellitus:* Administration worsens glycemic control in patients with preexisting diabetes.
- *Vaccination:* In general, immunosuppressants may affect efficacy of vaccinations. The use of live vaccines should be avoided.

Adverse drug reactions

- *Central nervous system (CNS):* Seizure, hallucinations, insomnia, tremor, paresthesias
- *Head, ears, eyes, nose, and throat (HEENT):* Gingival hyperplasia
- *Cardiovascular (CV):* Hypertension
- *Gastrointestinal (GI):* Hepatotoxicity
- *Renal:* Nephrotoxicity
- *Endocrine and metabolic:* Diabetes mellitus, hyperlipidemia, hyperuricemia, hyperkalemia, hypomagnesemia
- *Dermatologic:* Hirsutism, hypertrichosis, acne

Table 20-2. Immunosuppressant Drugs

Generic name	Trade name	Dosage forms	Dose	Generic products
Calcineurin inhibitors				
Cyclosporine USP	Sandimmune	Injection: 50 mg/mL; oral solution: 100 mg/mL; capsules: 25, 50, 100 mg	Intravenous: 5–6 mg/kg/d; oral: 8–14 mg/kg/d divided q12h; adjusted to desired trough concentration	Injection: 50 mg/mL; capsules: 25, 100 mg
Cyclosporine USP (modified)	Neoral	Oral solution 100 mg/mL; capsules: 25 and 100 mg	Oral: 5–10 mg/kg/d divided q12h; adjusted to desired trough concentration	Oral solution: 100 mg/mL; capsules: 25, 100 mg
Tacrolimus	Prograf	Injection: 5 mg ampoules; capsules: 0.5, 1.0, and 5.0 mg	Intravenous: 0.03–0.05 mg/kg/d as continuous infusion; oral: 0.1–0.2 mg/kg/d divided q12h; adjusted to desired trough concentration	Not available
MTOR inhibitor				
Sirolimus	Rapamune	Oral solution: 1 mg/mL; tablets: 1, 2 mg	Initial: 6–15 mg po; maintenance: 2–5 mg po qd; adjusted to desired trough concentration	Not available
Antiproliferative agents				
Azathioprine	Imuran	Injection: 100 mg vial; tablets: 50 mg	Initial: 3–5 mg/kg IV or po; maintenance: 1–2 mg/kg IV or po qd	Injection: 100 mg vial; tablets: 50 mg
Mycophenolate mofetil	CellCept	Injection: 500 mg vial; oral suspension: 200 mg/mL; capsules: 250 mg; tablets: 500 mg	Maintenance: adults: 2–3 g/d divided q8–12h IV or po; children: 1,200 mg/m² divided q8–12h IV or po	Capsules: 250 mg; tablets: 500 mg
Mycophenolate sodium	Myfortic	Tablets: 180, 360 mg	Maintenance: adults: 720 mg po q12h; children: 400 mg/m² po q12h (maximum dose of 720 mg po q12h)	Not available
Monoclonal antibodies				
Muromonab-CD3	Orthoclone OKT 3	Injection: 5 mg ampoules	Induction:[a] 2.5–5.0 mg IV qd × 7–10 d; acute rejection: 2.5–5.0 mg IV qd × 10–14 d	Not available
Basiliximab	Simulect	Injection: 10 and 20 mg vials	Induction: adults and children > 35 kg: 20 mg IV on day 0 and day 4; children < 35 kg: 10 mg IV on day 0 and day 4	Not available
Daclizumab	Zenapax	Injection: 25 mg vials	Induction: 1 mg/kg IV q 2 wk for a total of 5 doses	Not available
Polyclonal antibodies				
Antithymocyte globulin (equine)	Atgam	Injection: 50 mg vials	Induction:[a] 15 mg/kg IV qd × 7–14 d; acute rejection: 10–15 mg/kg IV qd × 14 d	Not available
Antithymocyte globulin (rabbit)	Thymoglobulin	Injection: 25 mg vials	Induction:[a] 1.5 mg/kg IV qd × 3–7 d; acute rejection: 1.5 mg/kg IV qd × 7–14 d	Not available

a. Medication is not FDA-approved for induction.

Table 20-3. Drug Interactions Leading to Altered Exposure of CYP450 3A Isoenzyme Substrates

CYP450 3A4 enzyme inducers[a]	CYP450 3A4 enzyme inhibitors[b]
Anticonvulsants: phenytoin, phenobarbital, carbamazepine	Antidepressants: nefazodone
Antimicrobial agents: rifampin, rifabutin	Antiviral agents: delavirdine, indinavir, nelfinavir, ritonavir, saquinavir
Antiviral agents: nevirapine, efavirenz	Azole antifungal agents: voriconazole, posaconazole, ketoconazole, fluconazole, itraconazole, clotrimazole
Herbal products: St. John's wort	
	Calcium channel blockers: diltiazem, nicardipine, verapamil
	Macrolide antimicrobial agents: erythromycin, clarithromycin
	Food–drug interaction: grapefruit juice

Note: The table shows examples only. Numerous other interactions are associated with CYP450 3A4 substrates. See current journals or drug interaction texts for a more detailed list.
a. Inducers result in increased metabolism and decreased bioavailability of substrates of the same system.
b. Inhibitors result in decreased metabolism and increased bioavailability of substrates of the same system.

Patient instructions
- Keep cyclosporine stored in its original container.
- Take the prescribed dose twice daily with meals.
- Keep timing of dosing consistent.
- Make sure you take or do not take your medication at the appropriate time prior to therapeutic drug monitoring.
- Many medications interact with this medication. Do not take anything prescribed by another physician until you verify that there are no drug interactions.

Monitoring
- C_0 *(trough):* Goals depend on multifactorial risk assessment and assay type.
- C_2 *(concentration 2 hours after dose):* Goals depend on multifactorial risk assessment and assay type.

Pharmacokinetics
- ***Cyclosporine USP:*** Highly lipoprotein bound
  - Bioavailability: significant intra- and inter-patient variability

Table 20-4. Drug Interactions Leading to Altered Exposure of Other Drugs by Cyclosporine

Mechanism	Drug	Comment
CYP450 3A4 enzyme substrates	HMG-CoA reductase inhibitors: lovastatin, simvastatin, atorvastatin	Coadministration of these agents with CsA results in significant increases in HMG-CoA reductase inhibitor exposure and may place patients at increased risk of rhabdomyolysis.
CYP450 3A4 enzyme substrates	Sirolimus	Simultaneous administration increased C_{max} and area under the curve of sirolimus by 120–500% and 140–230%, respectively; administration 4 hours apart increased C_{max} and area under the curve of sirolimus by 30–40% and 35–80%, respectively.
Alteration in enterohepatic recycling	Mycophenolate mofetil	CsA coadministration inhibits MPAG excretion via hepatocytes, thus interfering with MPA enterohepatic recycling and leading to reduced exposure of the active metabolite, MPA.

Note: The table shows examples only. Numerous other interactions are associated with CYP450 3A4 substrates. See current journals or drug interaction texts for a more detailed list. CsA, cyclosporine A; HMG-CoA, 3-hydroxy-3-methyglutaryl coenzyme A; MPA, mycophenolic acid; MPAG, phenolic glucuronide of MPA.

- Mean F = 30%, range 5% to 92%
- Elimination: half-life = 19 hours; range 10–28 hours (increased with hepatic dysfunction)
- *Cyclosporine USP (modified):* Highly lipoprotein bound
  - Bioavailability: improved and more consistent absorption (60–70% increased C_{max})
  - Elimination: half-life = 8 hours; range 5–18 hours (increased with hepatic dysfunction)

Tacrolimus

Mechanism of action

Tacrolimus inhibits translocation of the cytosolic sub-unit of NFAT, the promoter gene for IL-2, into the nucleus via its binding with FKBP-12 and a calcium-calmodulin-calcineurin complex, thereby inhibiting transcription and synthesis of IL-2. Thus, it inhibits IL-2-mediated monoclonal T-cell proliferation and polyclonal T-cell activation.

Administration

- *Intravenous:* Dilute in NS or D_5W to a concentration between 0.004 and 0.02 mg/mL, and administer as a continuous infusion via a PVC (polyvinylchloride)–free container and tubing.
- *Oral:* Administer two equally divided doses po every 12 hours consistently, with or without food.

Drug–drug interactions

Because tacrolimus is metabolized primarily via CYP450 3A isoenzymes, substances known to alter functionality of these enzymes will alter bioavailability and elimination of this drug (Table 20-3).

Drug–disease interactions

- *Diabetes mellitus:* Administration worsens glycemic control in patients with preexisting diabetes.
- *Vaccinations:* In general, immunosuppressants may affect efficacy of vaccinations. The use of live vaccines should be avoided.

Adverse drug reactions

- *CNS:* Seizure, hallucinations, insomnia, tremor, depression, psychosis, anorexia
- *HEENT:* Alopecia
- *CV:* Hypertension
- *GI:* Hepatotoxicity
- *Renal:* Nephrotoxicity

- *Endocrine and metabolic:* Diabetes mellitus, hyperlipidemia, hyperkalemia, hypercalcemia, hypomagnesemia, hypophosphatemia
- *Hematologic:* Anemia

Patient instructions

- Take the prescribed dose at a consistent time twice daily, with or without food, but always in the same way to maintain consistency.
- Make sure you do not take your medication prior to therapeutic drug monitoring.
- Many medications interact with this medication. Do not take anything prescribed by another physician until you verify that there are no drug interactions.

Monitoring

Monitor C_0 (trough). Goals depend on multifactorial risk assessment (in general, 5–20 ng/mL).

Pharmacokinetics

- Highly protein bound
- Bioavailability: F = 14–32%
- Elimination: half-life = 8 hours; range 6–11 hours (increased with hepatic dysfunction)

mTOR Inhibitor

Sirolimus

Mechanism of action

Sirolimus binds to FKBP-12 to form a complex that binds and inhibits activation of its target protein, mTOR (mammalian target of rapamycin), a kinase that is critical in IL-2-mediated cell-cycle progression.

Administration

- To limit variability, administer consistently with or without food.
- With tablets, administer daily dose po once a day.
- With oral solution, dilute the dose in 2 oz of water or orange juice, stir vigorously, and drink at once. Then refill container with 4 oz of the chosen fluid, stir vigorously, and drink.

Drug–drug interactions

Because sirolimus is metabolized primarily via CYP450 3A isoenzymes, substances known to alter functionality of these enzymes will alter bioavailability and elimination of this drug (Table 20-3).

Additionally, the pharmacokinetic profile of sirolimus is significantly altered by concomitant cyclosporine (Table 20-4).

Drug–disease interactions

- *Liver transplantation:* Sirolimus is associated with increased incidence of mortality, graft loss, and hepatic artery thrombosis in de novo liver transplant recipients.
- *Lung transplantation:* There have been cases of fatal bronchial anastomotic dehiscence in de novo lung transplant recipients.
- *Vaccinations:* In general, immunosuppressants may affect efficacy of vaccinations. The use of live vaccines should be avoided.

Adverse drug reactions

- *CNS:* Anorexia
- *HEENT:* Oral ulcers
- *GI:* Diarrhea, esophagitis, gastritis, gastroenteritis, hepatotoxicity, hepatic artery thrombosis in de novo liver transplant recipients
- *Renal:* Synergistic nephrotoxicity with calcineurin inhibitors
- *Endocrine and metabolic:* Hyperlipidemia, hypertension, hyperkalemia
- *Dermatologic:* Rash, acne
- *Hematologic:* Leukopenia, thrombocytopenia, pancytopenia, thrombosis
- *Other:* Lymphocele, pneumonitis, bronchial anastomotic dehiscence in de novo lung transplant recipients

Patient instructions

- Take the prescribed dose at a consistent time once daily, with or without food, but in the same way to maintain consistency.
- Make sure you do not take your medication prior to therapeutic drug monitoring.
- Many medications interact with this medication. Do not take anything prescribed by another physician until you verify that there are no drug interactions.

Monitoring

Monitor C_0 (trough). Goal depends on multifactorial risk assessment and assay type (in general, 5–20 ng/mL).

Pharmacokinetics

- Bioavailability: tablet: F = 27%; oral solution: F = 15%
- Elimination: half-life = 57–63 hours (increased with hepatic dysfunction)

Antiproliferative Agents

Azathioprine

Mechanism of action

Azathioprine is a purine analogue prodrug, which is cleaved to 6-mercaptopurine; 6-mercaptopurine is activated intracellularly to several active metabolites, which can be incorporated directly into DNA (deoxyribonucleic acid) as thiopurine as well as interfere with the RNA (ribonucleic acid) and DNA biosynthesis directly and via feedback inhibition.

Administration

- *Intravenous:* Dilute dose in NS or D_5W and administer IV infusion over 5–60 minutes.
- *Oral:* Administer daily dose po once a day.

Drug–drug interactions

Xanthine oxidase is responsible for the elimination of the active metabolites of azathioprine. Concomitant use of allopurinol with azathioprine results in significantly increased azathioprine-induced toxicity. Reduce dose of azathioprine by 65–75%.

Drug–disease interactions

- *Renal insufficiency:* Bioavailability is significantly reduced in uremic patients.
- *Vaccinations:* In general, immunosuppressants may affect efficacy of vaccinations. The use of live vaccines should be avoided.

Adverse drug reactions

- *HEENT:* Retinopathy
- *GI:* Nausea, vomiting, diarrhea, anorexia, pancreatitis, hepatotoxicity
- *Dermatologic:* Rash, skin cancer
- *Hematologic:* Leukopenia, thrombocytopenia, pancytopenia

Patient instructions

- Take the prescribed dose at a consistent time once daily, with or without food, but take in the same way to maintain consistency.
- Do not take anything prescribed by another physician until you verify that there are no drug interactions.

Monitoring

No clinically important pharmacokinetic or pharmacodynamic monitoring exists.

Pharmacokinetics
- Bioavailability: F = 41–47%
- Bioavailability in uremic patients: F = 17%

Mycophenolate mofetil

Mechanism of action
Mycophenolate mofetil is metabolized to mycophenolic acid (MPA), which causes noncompetitive, reversible inhibition of inosine monophosphate dehydrogenase, a critical enzyme in the de novo pathway of purine synthesis, which is crucial during lymphocyte activation and proliferation.

Administration
- **Intravenous:** Dilute in D_5W to a concentration of 6 mg/mL and infuse over at least 2 hours.
- **Oral:** Administer as equally divided doses po every 8–12 h consistently with or without food.

Drug–drug interactions
- **Cyclosporine:** See Table 20-4.
- **Cholestyramine:** Because of the interruption of enterohepatic recirculation, administration can decrease MPA exposure.
- **Colestipol and colesevelam:** Simultaneous administration can decrease MPA exposure.
- **Antacids:** Simultaneous administration with magnesium- or aluminum-containing antacids reduces absorption and decreases MPA exposure.
- **Note:** Efficacy of oral contraceptives may decrease with therapy. Additional birth control methods are recommended.

Drug–disease interactions
- **Severe renal impairment:** Mycophenolate mofetil reduces protein binding of MPA.
- **Vaccinations:** In general, immunosuppressants may affect efficacy of vaccinations. The use of live vaccines should be avoided.

Adverse drug reactions
- **GI:** Nausea, vomiting, diarrhea, abdominal pain
- **Hematologic:** Leukopenia, thrombocytopenia, anemia, pancytopenia

Patient instructions
- Take the prescribed dose at consistent times during the day, with or without food, but in the same way to maintain consistency.

- Make sure you do not take your medication prior to therapeutic drug monitoring.

Monitoring
No clinically important pharmacokinetic or pharmacodynamic monitoring exists.

Pharmacokinetics
- MPA is highly protein bound.
- Bioavailability: F = 94%
- Elimination: half-life = 16–18 hours

Mycophenolate sodium

Mechanism of action
Delayed-release tablets deliver MPA, which causes noncompetitive, reversible inhibition of inosine monophosphate dehydrogenase, a critical enzyme in the de novo pathway of purine synthesis, which is crucial during lymphocyte activation and proliferation.

Administration
Administer as equally divided doses po every 12 hours consistently without food.

Drug–drug interactions
- **Cholestyramine:** Administration interrupts enterohepatic recirculation and decreases MPA exposure.
- **Antacids:** Simultaneous administration with magnesium- or aluminum-containing antacids reduces absorption and decreases MPA exposure.
- **Note:** Efficacy of oral contraceptives may decrease with therapy. Additional birth control methods are recommended.

Drug–disease interactions
- **Severe renal impairment:** Mycophenolate sodium reduces protein binding of MPA.
- **Vaccinations:** In general, immunosuppressants may affect efficacy of vaccinations. The use of live vaccines should be avoided.

Adverse drug reactions
- **GI:** Nausea, vomiting, diarrhea, abdominal pain
- **Hematologic:** Leukopenia, thrombocytopenia, anemia, pancytopenia

Patient instructions
- Take the prescribed dose at consistent times during the day, either 30 minutes before or 2 hours

after meals, but take the same way each day to maintain consistency.

■ Make sure you do not take your medication prior to therapeutic drug monitoring.

Monitoring

No clinically important pharmacokinetic or pharmacodynamic monitoring exists.

Pharmacokinetics

■ MPA is highly protein bound.
■ Bioavailability: F = 72% to 92%
■ Elimination: half-life = 8–16 hours

Corticosteroids

Selection of agent

Selection of the corticosteroid used is based on the ratio of glucocorticoid to mineralocorticoid potency.

Intravenous agents are methylprednisolone and dexamethasone. Oral agents are prednisone, prednisolone, and dexamethasone.

Mechanism of action

Corticosteroids bind to cytosolic glucocorticoid receptors, which translocate to the nucleus, where the complexes bind to regulatory DNA sequences, glucocorticoid-responsive elements (GREs) within the promoter section of various genes. Activation of these GREs modifies activities of promoter genes such as NFAT, AP-1, and NF-κB, which results in down-regulation of expression of HLA and numerous cell adhesion molecules, as well as decreased synthesis of numerous lymphokines responsible for activation, proliferation, and migration (i.e., IL-1, IL-2, IL-6, IL-8, IFN-γ, TNF-α).

Administration

Administration depends on the individual agent.

Drug–drug interactions

Because corticosteroids are metabolized primarily via CYP450 3A isoenzymes, substances known to alter functionality of these enzymes will alter bioavailability and elimination of these drugs (Table 20-3).

Drug–disease interactions

■ *Diabetes mellitus:* Administration worsens glycemic control in patients with preexisting diabetes.
■ *Osteopenia and osteoporosis:* Administration alters calcium and phosphate absorption and excretion, as well as osteoblast activity, resulting

in progression of bone loss that is common in metabolic diseases such as end-stage renal disease and liver failure.

■ *Vaccinations:* In general, immunosuppressants may affect efficacy of vaccinations. The use of live vaccines should be avoided.

Adverse drug reactions

The incidence and extent of most adverse drug reactions with corticosteroids depend on the ratio of glucocorticoid to mineralocorticoid potency. Adverse drug events include the following:

■ *CNS:* Seizure, psychosis, delirium, hallucinations, mood swings, insomnia, pseudotumor cerebri
■ *HEENT:* Cataracts, glaucoma
■ *CV:* Hypertension, cardiomyopathy
■ *GI:* Increased appetite, gastroesophageal reflux disease, peptic ulcer disease, pancreatitis
■ *Renal:* Edema, alkalosis, hyperkalemia
■ *Endocrine and metabolic:* Diabetes mellitus, hyperlipidemia, hypothalamic-pituitary-adrenal axis suppression, growth suppression
■ *Dermatologic:* Hirsutism, acne, skin atrophy, impaired wound healing
■ *Hematologic:* Transient leukocytosis
■ *Musculoskeletal:* Arthralgia, myopathy, osteoporosis, avascular necrosis

Patient instructions

■ When taking orally, take daily dose in the morning with food.
■ Many drugs interact with these agents. Do not take anything prescribed by another physician until you verify that there are no drug interactions.

Monitoring

No clinically important pharmacokinetic or pharmacodynamic monitoring exists.

Pharmacokinetics

Pharmacokinetics depend on the individual agent.

Monoclonal Antibodies

Orthoclone OKT3

Mechanism of action

Murine monoclonal IgG binds to and facilitates removal of cell lines expressing CD3. CD3, part of the T-cell receptor complex, is an important molecule that distinguishes T-cells. CD3 is important in antigen recognition and antigen-specific signal transduction.

Administration
- Premedication:
  - *Dose 1:* Intravenous steroids, acetaminophen, and antihistamines taken 1 hour prior to the dose are strongly recommended to modify first-dose reactions.
  - *Subsequent doses:* Take acetaminophen and antihistamines 1 hour prior to the dose with steroids as needed for infusion-related reactions.
- Dosing:
  - Prior to administration, volume status must be carefully assessed.
  - Patients with evidence of volume overload or uncompensated congestive heart failure on chest x-ray should not receive this drug.
  - The dose should be administered via IV bolus over less than a minute.

Drug–drug interactions
No clinically significant interactions occur.

Drug–disease interactions
- Uncompensated congestive heart failure or volume overload presents risk of fatal pulmonary edema.
- In general, immunosuppressants may affect efficacy of vaccinations. The use of live vaccines should be avoided.

Adverse drug reactions
- **CNS:** Dizziness, headache
- **HEENT:** Photophobia
- **CV:** Tachycardia
- **Hematologic:** Transient lymphopenia, pancytopenia
- **Musculoskeletal:** Rigor, tremor
- **Other:** Fever, chills, dyspnea, pulmonary edema

Patient instructions
Report any shortness of breath, palpitations, lightheadedness, tremor, fever, or itching to your medical care provider immediately.

Monitoring
Monitor CD3 (suppression of CD3 lineage < 25 cells/mm^3).

Pharmacokinetics
Elimination: half-life = 18 hours

Basiliximab

Mechanism of action
Chimeric (murine and human), monoclonal IgG specifically binds to the subunit, CD25, of the human high-affinity IL-2 receptor, which is expressed only on activated lymphocytes. In this way, basiliximab competitively inhibits IL-2 and facilitates preferential elimination of activated lymphocytes.

Administration
Dilute to a concentration of 0.4 mg/mL in NS or D$_5$W. Administer peripherally or centrally as a bolus or continuous infusion over 20–30 minutes.

Drug–drug interactions
No clinically significant drug interactions occur.

Drug–disease interactions
In general, immunosuppressants may affect efficacy of vaccinations. The use of live vaccines should be avoided.

Adverse drug reactions
Severe acute hypersensitivity reactions, including anaphylaxis, may occur within the 24 hours following administration of the initial dose or on repeat exposure.

Patient instructions
Report any shortness of breath, palpitations, lightheadedness, or itching to your medical care provider immediately.

Monitoring
No clinically important pharmacokinetic or pharmacodynamic monitoring exists.

Pharmacokinetics
- **Adults** (following a 20 mg IV infusion over 20 minutes):
  - Mean C_{max} = 7.1 ± 5.1 mg/L
  - Mean half-life = 7.2 ± 3.2 days
- **Children:** Mean half-life = 11.5 ± 6.3 days

Pharmacodynamics
- **Adults:** CD25 saturation is at or above serum concentration of 0.2 mcg/mL. Mean duration of saturation depends on concomitant immunosuppressive regimen.
- **Children:** CD25 saturation is similar to that seen in adults.

Daclizumab

Mechanism of action

Humanized monoclonal IgG specifically binds to the subunit, CD25, of the human high-affinity IL-2 receptor, which is expressed only on activated lymphocytes. In this way, daclizumab competitively inhibits IL-2 and facilitates preferential elimination of activated lymphocytes.

Administration

Dilute in 50 mL of NS and administer peripherally or centrally as a continuous infusion over 15 minutes.

Drug–drug interactions

No clinically significant drug interactions occur.

Drug–disease interactions

In general, immunosuppressants may affect efficacy of vaccination. The use of live vaccines should be avoided.

Adverse drug reactions

Severe acute hypersensitivity reactions, including anaphylaxis, have rarely occurred within the 24 hours following administration of the initial dose or on repeat exposure.

Patient instructions

Report any shortness of breath, palpitations, lightheadedness, or itching to your medical care provider immediately.

Monitoring

No clinically important pharmacokinetic or pharmacodynamic monitoring exists.

Pharmacokinetics

- **Adults** (at recommended dosing):
  - Mean C_{max}: dose 1 = 21 ± 14 mg/mL; dose 5 = 32 ± 22 mg/mL
  - Mean C_{min}: dose 5 = 7.6 ± 4.0 mg/mL
  - Half-life = 20 days
- **Children** (at recommended dosing):
  - Mean C_{max}: dose 1 = 16 ± 12 mg/mL; dose 5 = 21 ± 14 mg/mL
  - Mean C_{min}: dose 5 = 5.0 ± 2.7 mg/mL
  - Half-life = 13 days

Pharmacodynamics

- **Adults:** CD25 saturation is at serum concentrations of 5–10 mg/mL. At recommended dosing, saturation occurs for approximately 120 days.
- **Children:** CD25 saturation is at serum concentrations of 5–10 mg/mL. At recommended dosing, saturation occurs for approximately 90 days.

Polyclonal Antibodies

Antithymocyte globulin (equine)

Mechanism of action

This antithymocyte globulin is purified, sterile, polyclonal IgG harvested from horses immunized with human thymocytes. The preparation includes IgG directed against cell surface markers such as CD2, CD3, CD4, CD8, CD11a, and CD 18. In this way, horse antithymocyte globulin targets multiple phases of immunity, including T-cell activation, homing, and cytotoxic activities.

Administration

- Premedication:
  - **Dose 1:** Giving intravenous steroids, acetaminophen, and antihistamines 1 hour prior to the dose is strongly recommended to modify first-dose reactions.
  - **Subsequent doses:** Give acetaminophen and antihistamines 1 hour prior to the dose with steroids as needed for infusion reactions.
- Dosing:
  - Dilute the dose to a concentration not to exceed 4 mg/mL in ½NS or D_5W.
  - Administer centrally over 4–6 hours.

Drug–drug interactions

No clinically significant drug interactions occur.

Drug–disease interactions

In general, immunosuppressants may affect the efficacy of vaccinations. The use of live vaccines should be avoided.

Adverse drug reactions

Most adverse drug reactions with antithymocyte globulin (equine) are infusion-related reactions (i.e., fever, chills, and dyspnea); leukopenia; thrombocytopenia; or rash.

Patient instructions

Report any shortness of breath, palpitations, lightheadedness, tremor, fever, or itching to your medical care provider immediately.

Monitoring

The goal for treatment of acute rejection is suppression of CD3 lineage to <50 cells/mm^3.

Pharmacokinetics

Elimination: half-life = 36 hours–12 days

Antithymocyte globulin (rabbit)

Mechanism of action

This antithymocyte globulin is purified, pasteurized, polyclonal IgG harvested from pathogen-free rabbits immunized with human thymocytes. This preparation includes IgG directed against cell surface markers, such as TCRab, CD2, CD3, CD4, CD5, CD6, CD7, CD8, CD11a, CD18, CD28, CD45, CD49, CD54, CD58, CD80, CD86, HLA class I, and β_2 microglobulin. In this way, rabbit antithymocyte globulin targets multiple phases of immunity, including T-cell activation, homing, and cytotoxic activities.

Administration

- Premedication:
  - *Dose 1:* Giving intravenous steroids, acetaminophen, and antihistamines 1 hour prior to the dose is strongly recommended to modify first-dose reactions.
  - *Subsequent doses:* Give acetaminophen and antihistamines 1 hour prior to the dose with steroids as needed for infusion reactions.
- Dose:
  - Dilute dose to a concentration of 0.5 mg/mL in NS or D_5W.
  - Administer centrally over 4–6 hours.

Drug–drug interactions

In the case of immunoglobulin, administration may decrease the degree of lymphocyte depletion achieved.

Drug–disease interactions

In general, immunosuppressants may affect efficacy of vaccinations. The use of live vaccines should be avoided.

Adverse drug reactions

Most adverse drug reactions with antithymocyte globulin (rabbit) are infusion-related reactions (i.e., fever, chills, and dyspnea); leukopenia; thrombocytopenia; or rash.

Patient instructions

Report any shortness of breath, palpitations, lightheadedness, tremor, fever, or itching to your medical care provider immediately.

Monitoring

The goal for treatment of acute rejection is suppression of CD3 lineage to < 50 cells/mm^3.

Pharmacokinetics

A two-compartment model is used. For terminal elimination, half-life = 2–3 days for first dose; range = 14–45 days with multiple doses.

20-3. Key Points

- The goal of solid organ transplantation is to improve patients' quality of life and survival by stabilizing or improving complications related to end-organ failure.
- The immune system is a highly intricate system with mechanisms for antigen recognition in a highly specific manner, as well as in a nonspecific manner.
- Acute rejection is a normal physiologic immune response to transplantation of donor antigens.
- The incidence of acute rejection is organ specific and depends on multiple pre- and post-transplant factors.
- Selection of the post-transplant immunosuppression regimen for prevention of acute rejection should be individualized on the basis of known risk and potential toxicity.
- Adjustment in the post-transplant immunosuppression regimen should focus on the balance between acute rejection, infection, and toxicity.
- Selection of the agent to be used to treat acute rejection is organ dependent and depends on the severity of acute rejection.
- Immunosuppressive complications, both infectious and noninfectious, are an important cause of early morbidity and mortality and require close management following transplantation.
- Many agents commonly included in immunosuppression regimens require a clinician with expertise in immunosuppressive therapeutic drug monitoring to optimize efficacy and reduce toxicity.
- Many agents commonly included in immunosuppression regimens have the potential for numerous pharmacokinetic and pharmacodynamic drug interactions.

Patient Profile 1—City Hospital

Patient name: Doe, John
Age: 52
Gender: Male
Ethnicity: African American
Diagnoses:

    h/o ESRD s/p cadaveric renal transplant 3 mo ago
    DM × 20 yrs
    HTN × 30 yrs
    Drug-induced hyperkalemia
    Current laboratory results:
    SCr = 1.2
    K = 5.3
    WBC 3.8
    Plt 120

Address: 101 South First Street
Height: 5′11″
Weight: 240 lb
Allergies: Sulfa
Medications prior to hospital admission:

    Prograf 4 mg po bid
    Amaryl 4 mg po bid
    Cellcept 750 mg po bid
    Metoprolol 100 mg po bid
    Diflucan 200 mg po qd
    Dapsone 100 mg po qd
    Valcyte 450 mg po qd
    EC ASA 81 mg po qd
    Prednisone 5 mg po qd

Additional medications prescribed during hospital course:

    Lasix 40 mg po bid
    Imuran 100 mg po qd

20-4. Questions

Use Patient Profile 1 to answer questions 1–4.

1. Which medication(s) should be given with caution because of the patient's sulfonamide allergy?

    I.   Lasix
    II. Dapsone
    III. Amaryl

    A. I only
    B. II only
    C. I and III only
    D. II and III only
    E. I, II, and III

2. Which of the following combinations of drugs represent therapeutic duplication?

    A. Prograf and Imuran
    B. Azathioprine and CellCept
    C. Dapsone and Valcyte
    D. Amaryl and Tacrolimus
    E. Prednisone and CellCept

3. Which of the following combinations of drugs interact?

    I.   Diflucan and tacrolimus
    II. Diflucan and Valcyte
    III. Dapsone and Lasix

    A. I only
    B. II only
    C. I and II only
    D. II and III only
    E. I, II, and III

4. Mr. Doe was diagnosed with drug-induced hyperkalemia. Which medication on his profile could be responsible for this?

    A. CellCept
    B. Lasix
    C. Prednisone
    D. Prograf
    E. EC ASA

5. Which medication(s) is (are) classified as a calcineurin inhibitor?

    I.   Rapamune
    II. Cyclosporine
    III. Tacrolimus

A. I only
B. II only
C. III only
D. II and III
E. I and III

6. Which medication(s) cause myelosuppression?

   I. Sirolimus
   II. Mycophenolate mofetil
   III. Valcyte

   A. I only
   B. II only
   C. III only
   D. I, II, and III
   E. II and III

7. Which medication(s) require bile for emulsification and absorption?

   A. Imuran
   B. Cyclosporine
   C. Prograf
   D. Prednisone
   E. All of the above

8. All of the following are known adverse effects of cyclosporine *except*

   A. hirsutism.
   B. nephrotoxicity.
   C. oral ulceration.
   D. gingival hyperplasia.
   E. hyperlipidemia.

9. All of the following are contraindications or precautions associated with Rapamune *except*

   A. de novo lung transplant recipient.
   B. hyperlipidemia.
   C. diabetes mellitus.
   D. de novo liver transplant recipient.
   E. allergy to sirolimus.

10. What is the generic name for Imuran?

    A. Mycophenolate mofetil
    B. Azathioprine
    C. Cyclosporine
    D. Tacrolimus
    E. Prednisone

11. Which of the immunosuppressive medication(s) listed may cause diabetes mellitus?

    I. Prednisone
    II. Azathioprine
    III. Tacrolimus

A. I only
B. II only
C. III only
D. I and III
E. I, II, and III

12. Which medication(s) require(s) therapeutic drug monitoring via trough concentrations?

    A. Mycophenolate mofetil
    B. Prograf
    C. Daclizumab
    D. Basiliximab
    E. Mycophenolate mofetil and Prograf

13. Which medication(s) select(s) for destruction of activated lymphocytes by binding to the CD25 subunit of the high affinity IL-2 receptor?

    I. Antithymocyte globulin (rabbit)
    II. Antithymocyte globulin (equine)
    III. Daclizumab

    A. I only
    B. II only
    C. III only
    D. I and II
    E. I, II, and III

14. All of the following increase the risk of acute rejection *except*

    A. pediatric recipient.
    B. HLA mismatch.
    C. living donor.
    D. noncompliance.
    E. history of previous transplantation.

15. Which of the following produces a significant pharmacokinetic interaction when administered with azathioprine?

    A. Allopurinol
    B. Diflucan
    C. Sirolimus
    D. Probenecid
    E. Allopurinol and probenecid

16. Which of these conditions alter(s) the pharmacokinetic profile of cyclosporine?

    I. Biliary obstruction
    II. Malnutrition
    III. Hyperglycemia

A. I only
B. II only
C. III only
D. I and II
E. I, II, and III

17. Which of the following medication(s) interact(s) with sirolimus?

  I.   Erythromycin
  II. Prevalite
  III. Diltiazem

  A. I only
  B. II only
  C. III only
  D. I and III
  E. II and III

18. Which of the following immunosuppressants should *not* be administered at the same time secondary to an interaction related to timing of doses?

  I.   Prograf and mycophenolate mofetil
  II. Rapamune and cyclosporine
  III. Neoral and azathioprine

  A. I only
  B. II only
  C. III only
  D. None of these interact.
  E. II and III

19. Which type of immunity involves stimulation of cells and soluble mediators that nonspecifically recognize alloantigens with no altered response on repeat exposure?

  A. Autoimmunity
  B. Innate immunity
  C. Adaptive immunity
  D. Acute rejection
  E. Hyperacute rejection

20. Which group of genes encodes for antigens that are responsible for self- or nonself-recognition?

  I.   Class I human leukocyte antigen (HLA)
  II. Class II human leukocyte antigen (HLA)
  III. Major histocompatibility complex (MHC)

  A. I only
  B. II only
  C. III only
  D. I and II
  E. I, II, and III

21. On binding of antigen displayed by the antigen-presenting cell to the T-cell receptor complex, what additional step is required for T-helper-cell activation?

  I.   Binding of the co-stimulatory pathway (i.e., CD58/CD2)
  II. Activation of the promoter gene NFAT
  III. Transcription of the IL-2 gene

  A. I only
  B. II only
  C. III only
  D. No additional step is required.
  E. I and II

22. Which cytokine released by activated CD4$^+$ lymphocytes plays a major role in the subsequent activation of numerous lymphocyte lineages?

  A. Interleukin-1 (IL-1)
  B. Tumor necrosis factor-α (TNF-α)
  C. Interleukin-2 (IL-2)
  D. Interferon-γ (IFN-γ)
  E. Complement

23. Which solid organ was the first to be successfully transplanted?

  A. Heart
  B. Liver
  C. Kidney
  D. Lung
  E. Pancreas

24. What is the 1-year patient survival rate for renal transplant recipients?

  A. > 90%
  B. 60–70%
  C. 25–50%
  D. < 25%
  E. Limited data available; currently an experimental procedure

20-5. Answers

1. **C.** Lasix and Amaryl are structurally similar to sulfonamides and would be expected to elicit a similar allergic response. Dapsone is a sulfone and would not be expected to elicit an allergic response.

2. **B.** Both azathioprine and CellCept are classified as antiproliferative agents. Both agents

inhibit purine biosynthesis and would not act synergistically.

3. **A.** Diflucan is an inhibitor of cytochrome P450 3A isoenzymes, which is the enzyme system that is responsible for metabolism of tacrolimus.

4. **D.** Hyperkalemia (incidence 20–40%) is a well-documented adverse drug reaction with Prograf.

5. **D.** Both cyclosporine and tacrolimus are calcineurin inhibitors.

6. **D.** All of the listed agents have myelosuppressive properties when administered individually. When they are administered concurrently, the myelosuppression is synergistic.

7. **B.** Cyclosporine is highly lipophilic and requires bile for emulsification and absorption.

8. **C.** Hirsutism, nephrotoxicity, gingival hyperplasia, and hyperlipidemia are known adverse effects of cyclosporine. Oral ulceration is not an adverse effect of cyclosporine.

9. **C.** The use of Rapamune (sirolimus) in de novo lung and liver transplant recipients is contraindicated because of an increased incidence of fatal adverse drug reactions. Additionally, use of Rapamune in patients with uncontrolled hyperlipidemia is strongly discouraged because of its profound effects on lipid biosynthesis and catabolism.

10. **B.** Azathioprine is the generic name for Imuran.

11. **D.** Prednisone and tacrolimus may cause diabetes mellitus. Azathioprine does not produce a diabetogenic effect.

12. **B.** Prograf requires therapeutic drug monitoring via trough concentrations to obtain desired therapeutic effects.

13. **C.** Daclizumab selects for destruction of activated lymphocytes by binding to the CD25 subunit of the high-affinity IL-2 receptor.

14. **C.** Of the listed parameters, all are considered to increase the risk of acute rejection except a living donor as the donor source.

15. **A.** Xanthine oxidase is responsible for the elimination of the active metabolites of azathioprine. Concomitant use of allopurinol with azathioprine results in significantly increased azathioprine-induced toxicity. Reduce the dose of azathioprine by 65–75%.

16. **D.** Both biliary obstruction and severe malnutrition would change the pharmacokinetic profile of cyclosporine. Cyclosporine requires bile for emulsification and absorption. If bile flow is obstructed, then the bioavailability is significantly decreased. Additionally, cyclosporine is a highly lipoprotein-bound drug. In severe malnutrition, total protein stores are depleted, thereby increasing the total free drug.

17. **D.** Both erythromycin and diltiazem are inhibitors of P450 3A isoenzymes, which is the enzyme system that is responsible for sirolimus metabolism.

18. **B.** Simultaneous administration of Rapamune (sirolimus) and cyclosporine increases C_{max} and area under the curve of sirolimus by 120–500% and 140–230%, respectively. Administration 4 hours apart increases C_{max} and area under the curve of sirolimus by 30–40% and 35–80%, respectively.

19. **B.** Innate immunity is the fundamental type of immunity in which antigens are recognized in a nonspecific manner. This type of immunity is not augmented on repeat exposure.

20. **C.** Class I and II HLA are the actual antigens important for self- and nonself-recognition. The group of genes that encode for these antigens is the major histocompatibility complex.

21. **A.** Activation is dependent on antigen–HLA binding to the T-cell receptor complex and the subsequent binding of a second signal or "costimulatory pathway."

22. **C.** Active CD4+ T-cells produce and release various lymphokines, particularly IL-2, which is important for activation and proliferation of numerous lymphocyte lineages.

23. **C.** The kidney was the first organ to be successfully transplanted, in 1954.

24. **A.** According to Table 20-1, the 1-year patient survival rates for both cadaveric and living donor renal transplant recipients are 94.8% and 98.0%, respectively.

20-6. References

Budde K, Curtis J, Knoll G, et al. Enteric-coated mycophenolate sodium can be safely administered in maintenance renal transplant patients: Results of a 1-year study. *Am J Transplant*. 2003;4:237–43.

Christians U, Jacobsen W, Benet LZ, Lampen A. Mechanisms of clinically relevant drug interactions associated with tacrolimus. *Clin Pharmacokinet*. 2002;41:813–51.

Cotts WG, Johnson MR. The challenge of rejection and cardiac allograft vasculopathy. *Heart Fail Rev*. 2001;6:227–40.

Delves PJ, Roitt IM. The immune system: First of two parts. *N Engl J Med*. 2000;343:37–49.

Delves PJ, Roitt IM. The immune system: Second of two parts. *N Engl J Med*. 2000;343:108–17.

Dunn CJ, Wagstaff AJ, Perry CM, et al. Cyclosporin: An updated review of the pharmacokinetic properties, clinical efficacy, and tolerability of a microemulsion-based formulation (Neoral) in organ transplantation. *Drugs*. 2001;61:1957–2016.

Galley BJ, Perez RV, Ramsamooj R. Acute renal transplant injury and interaction between antithymocyte globulin and pooled human immunoglobulin. *Clin Transplant*. 2004;18:327–31.

Kelly P, Kahan BD. Review: Metabolism of immunosuppressant drugs. *Curr Drug Metab*. 2002;3:275–87.

Klupp J, Holt DW, van Gelder T. How pharmacokinetic and pharmacodynamic drug monitoring can improve outcome in solid organ transplant recipients. *Transpl Immunol*. 2002;9:211–14.

Neuberger J. Incidence, timing, and risk factors for acute and chronic rejection. *Liver Transpl Surg*. 1999;5(suppl 1):S30–36.

Salvadori M, Holzer H, de Mattos A, et al. Enteric-coated mycophenolate sodium is therapeutically equivalent to mycophenolate mofetil in de novo renal transplant patients. *Am J Transplant*. 2003; 4:231–6.

Gastrointestinal Diseases

21

Christa M. George, PharmD, BCPS, CDE

21-1. Peptic Ulcer Disease

Definition and Incidence

Peptic ulcer disease (PUD) is a group of disorders of the upper gastrointestinal (GI) tract characterized by ulcerative lesions that depend on acid and pepsin for their formation.

Approximately 1.5 million to 2 million Americans have an active ulcer at any given time. Annually in the United States, 500,000 new cases are diagnosed.

The U.S. lifetime prevalence of PUD ranges from 11% to 20% for men and from 8% to 11% for women. PUD has been estimated to cost $10 billion per year in the United States.

Classification

Ulcers are either duodenal or gastric in nature. Duodenal ulcers are more common.

Duodenal and gastric ulcers are classified as *Helicobacter pylori* related, nonsteroidal anti-inflammatory drug (NSAID) related, non–*H. pylori* related, non-NSAID related, or stress related.

Clinical Presentation

Epigastric pain occurring 1–3 hours after meals that is relieved by ingestion of food or antacids is the classic presentation of PUD. Pain typically occurs in episodes lasting weeks to months and may be followed by variable periods of spontaneous remission and recurrence.

Ten percent of patients with PUD present with complications and have no prior history of pain.

Pathophysiology

Duodenal ulcers result from the imbalance between duodenal acid load and the acid-buffering capacity of the duodenum. Duodenal ulcers are more frequently associated with an antrum-predominant gastritis.

H. pylori is a gram-negative microaerophilic bacterium that inhabits the area between the stomach's mucosal layer and epithelial cells. The bacteria can be found anywhere gastric epithelium is present.

Over 50% of the world's population is colonized by *H. pylori*, but only 15% of colonized individuals develop clinical symptoms of PUD. The prevalence of *H. pylori* is decreasing in developed countries. It has been estimated that 30–40% of the U.S. population is infected with *H. pylori*.

H. pylori causes duodenal inflammation, increases duodenal acid load, and impairs duodenal bicarbonate secretion, which leads to duodenal ulcers. It causes inflammation of gastric epithelium, particularly in the antrum-corpus area. The inflammation disrupts mucosal defense, which also leads to gastric ulcers.

NSAIDs are the leading cause of PUD in patients negative for *H. pylori* infection. They are directly toxic to gastric epithelium and inhibit the synthesis of prostaglandins.

Inhibition of prostaglandin synthesis leads to decreased secretion of bicarbonate and mucus, decreased mucosal perfusion, decreased epithelial proliferation, and decreased mucosal resistance to injury.

NSAIDs may cause gastric or duodenal ulcers (more frequently gastric). Gastric ulcers are associated with a corpus-predominant (i.e., diffuse-predominant) gastritis. This pattern of gastritis is associated with low acid output, gastric atrophy, and adenocarcinoma.

Diagnostic Criteria

Upper GI endoscopy is used to diagnose PUD. The procedure is usually reserved for patients with symptoms of PUD who are over 55 years of age or who have alarm symptoms (bleeding, anemia, early satiety, unexplained weight loss, progressive dysphagia, odynophagia, recurrent vomiting, family history of GI cancer, previous esophagogastric cancer).

Patients with symptoms of PUD who are under 55 years of age and have no alarm symptoms may be tested for the presence of *H. pylori* and treated with eradication therapy if results are positive.

Available tests for *H. pylori* are divided into two groups: those that require endoscopy and those that do not.

- Histology and rapid urease testing may be performed on biopsy samples taken during endoscopy.
  - Rapid urease testing may be performed in patients who have *not* taken a proton pump inhibitor (PPI) within 1–2 weeks or an antibiotic or bismuth within 4 weeks of the endoscopy. Histology should be performed on patients who have recently taken PPIs, antibiotics, or bismuth.
  - Culture and polymerase chain reaction testing are not yet widely available for clinical use and are thus not routinely recommended.
- Antibody testing, urea breath tests, and fecal antigen tests do not require endoscopy.
  - Antibody testing should be avoided in populations with a low prevalence of *H. pylori* because of the low positive predictive value in these populations.
  - Urea breath tests and fecal antigen tests may be used to confirm eradication of *H. pylori* no sooner than 4 weeks after completion of the treatment regimen.

Treatment Principles and Goals

The goals of PUD therapy include healing the ulcer and eliminating its cause. Additional considerations include preventing complications and relieving symptoms.

Use of PPIs is associated with faster healing rates and symptom relief than treatment with histamine 2–receptor antagonists (H2RAs). (Note: H2RAs are less expensive.)

Choice of PUD therapy is based on the etiology of the case. For *H. pylori*–related PUD, antibacterial therapy is used with antisecretory therapy.

- Eradication of *H. pylori* reduces the recurrence of PUD and is of prime importance.

- The American College of Gastroenterology treatment guidelines for *H. pylori* eradication in PUD recommend initial triple therapy with a PPI, clarithromycin, and either amoxicillin or metronidazole for 14 days or quadruple therapy with bismuth, metronidazole, tetracycline, and either an H2RA or a PPI for 10–14 days.
- Sequential therapy starting with a PPI and amoxicillin for 5 days followed by a PPI and clarithromycin for an additional 5 days requires further study.
- The eradication of *H. pylori* should be confirmed with urea breath testing or fecal antigen testing no sooner than 4 weeks after completing eradication therapy.
- If a patient has persistent *H. pylori* infection after the initial eradication therapy regimen, salvage therapy with bismuth quadruple therapy for 7–14 days should be administered.

For NSAID-related PUD, discontinuation of the offending agent is imperative.

- Antisecretory therapy with a PPI or an H2RA should be administered for 4 weeks to promote healing and to relieve symptoms.
- If *H. pylori* is also present, antibacterial therapy should be initiated. Eradication of *H. pylori* does not prevent NSAID-related complications or recurrence.
- PPIs, H2RAs, or misoprostol should be used to prevent PUD in patients who require chronic NSAIDs and who are at risk of developing PUD (e.g., patients who are elderly or who have concomitant cardiovascular disease, patients with a history of PUD, patients using high-dose NSAID therapy, and patients who concomitantly use corticosteroids or anticoagulants).

Sucralfate may also be used to aid in ulcer healing, but it requires multiple daily dosing and is associated with many significant drug interactions.

Non–*H. pylori*, non-NSAID-related PUD should be treated with antisecretory therapy.

Drug Therapy

Mechanism of action

PPIs suppress gastric acid secretion specifically by inhibiting the H^+-K^+-ATPase enzyme system of the secretory surface of the gastric parietal cell.

H2RAs suppress gastric acid secretion by reversibly blocking histamine-2 receptors on the surface of the gastric parietal cell.

Clarithromycin, amoxicillin, metronidazole, tetracycline, bismuth subsalicylate, and furazolidone exhibit antibacterial effects against *H. pylori*.

When exposed to gastric acid, sucralfate forms a viscous adhesive that binds positively charged protein molecules in the ulcer crater, thus forming a protective barrier that protects against back-diffusion of hydrogen ions.

See Table 21-1 for selected medications.

Patient counseling

Educate patients about the importance of completing the entire course of therapy to ensure the eradication of *H. pylori* and to avoid bacterial resistance.

PPIs are best taken before eating. Lansoprazole and dexlansoprazole granules may be sprinkled onto applesauce for patients who have trouble swallowing pills. Lansoprazole orally disintegrating tablets should not be crushed or chewed. Omeprazole capsules should be swallowed whole. Omeprazole over-the-counter (OTC) tablets should not be crushed or chewed. Omeprazole–sodium bicarbonate capsules should be swallowed whole.

If antacids are being used to control breakthrough symptoms, the dose should be taken no less than 1–2 hours before or after an H2RA is taken. H2RAs may be taken without regard to meals.

Amoxicillin, clarithromycin, and metronidazole may be taken without regard to meals; however, taking clarithromycin and metronidazole with meals often reduces the incidence of stomach upset.

Tetracycline is best taken on an empty stomach. Antacids, dairy products, or iron-containing products should be taken 2 hours before or after tetracycline.

Sucralfate should be taken 1 hour before meals and at bedtime.

Adverse drug effects

- Side effects occur in 15–20% of patients, but they are usually minor.
- PPIs and H2RAs are generally well tolerated, but headache, diarrhea, and nausea have been reported.

Table 21-1. Selected Medications Used in Peptic Ulcer Disease

Generic name	Trade name	Classification	Dosage range and frequency	Dosage forms
Omeprazole	Prilosec	Proton pump inhibitor	20–40 mg qd	C, G
Omeprazole	Prilosec OTC	Proton pump inhibitor	20 mg qd × 14 days	T
Omeprazole + sodium bicarbonate	Zegerid	Proton pump inhibitor and antacid	20–40 mg qd	C, P
Esomeprazole	Nexium	Proton pump inhibitor	20–40 mg qd	C, IV, G
Lansoprazole	Prevacid, Prevacid SoluTab	Proton pump inhibitor	15 mg qd–30 mg bid	C, ODT, L, ST
Dexlansoprazole	Kapidex	Proton pump inhibitor	30–60 mg qd	C
Rabeprazole	Aciphex	Proton pump inhibitor	10–20 mg qd	T
Pantoprazole	Protonix	Proton pump inhibitor	40–80 mg qd	T, G, IV
Cimetidine	Tagamet	H2-receptor blocker	300 mg qid–800 mg hs	T, L, IV
Ranitidine	Zantac	H2-receptor blocker	150 mg bid–300 mg hs	T, L, IV, C, EfT
Nizatidine	Axid	H2-receptor blocker	150 mg bid–300 mg hs	C, L, T
Famotidine	Pepcid	H2-receptor blocker	20 mg bid–40 mg hs	T, C, P, IV
Clarithromycin	Biaxin	Antibacterial	500 mg bid × 10–14 d	T, G
Amoxicillin	Amoxil	Antibacterial	1 g bid × 10–14 d	C, P, CT
Metronidazole	Flagyl	Antibacterial	500 mg tid × 10–14 d	T, C, IV,
Tetracycline	Various trade names	Antibacterial	500 mg qid × 10–14 d	C
Sucralfate	Carafate	Cytoprotective	1 g qid	T, L

C, capsule; CT, chewable tablet; EfT, effervescent tablet; G, granules for oral suspension; IV, intravenous; L, liquid; ODT, orally disintegrating tablet; P, powder for oral suspension; ST, SoluTab; T, tablet.

- Antibiotics may cause diarrhea, nausea, dysgeusia, rash, and monilial vaginitis.
- Bismuth subsalicylate may cause black, tarry stools.
- Constipation is the most common side effect of sucralfate.

Drug interactions

- Omeprazole inhibits the cytochrome P450 (CYP450) enzyme system, which decreases the elimination of warfarin, phenytoin, diazepam, and cyclosporine. Lansoprazole has been reported to increase theophylline clearance by approximately 10%.
- PPIs and H2RAs may alter the bioavailability of drugs that require an acidic environment for absorption (e.g., ketoconazole, digoxin, and iron).
- Cimetidine is a potent inhibitor of the CYP450 enzyme system, which decreases the elimination of numerous drugs (e.g., warfarin, theophylline, and phenytoin).
- Amoxicillin and tetracycline may decrease the effectiveness of oral contraceptives.
- Clarithromycin is a potent inhibitor of the CYP450 enzyme system, which decreases the elimination of warfarin, digoxin, cyclosporine, carbamazepine, theophylline, and cisapride (no longer on the market).
- Tetracycline may decrease the effectiveness of oral contraceptives. Antacids, iron products, and dairy products bind to tetracycline, decreasing its effectiveness. Tetracycline can also increase the therapeutic effect of warfarin. Tetracycline can increase or decrease lithium levels.
- Metronidazole produces a disulfiram-like reaction when ingested with alcohol and increases the therapeutic effect of warfarin and lithium.
- Sucralfate leads to the absorption of small amounts of aluminum, which may accumulate if given to patients with renal insufficiency (especially when combined with aluminum-containing antacids).
- Sucralfate alters the absorption of numerous drugs, including warfarin, digoxin, phenytoin, ketoconazole, quinidine, and quinolones.
- Disulfiram-like reactions have been reported with the concurrent ingestion of alcohol and furazolidone.

Monitoring parameters

Patients should monitor for the return of PUD symptoms and for the side effects of medications, as discussed in the earlier sections.

Pharmacokinetics

Several medications are substrates for or have effects on the CYP450 enzyme system in the liver, as discussed in the drug interactions section.

Nondrug Therapy and Complications

Patients should be counseled to decrease psychological stress and to discontinue smoking and drinking alcohol, taking NSAIDs, and ingesting food or beverages that may exacerbate PUD symptoms.

Major complications occur in approximately 25% of patients with PUD (hemorrhage, perforation, penetration, and obstruction):

- Patients with active bleeding who are hemodynamically stable should receive intravenous PPI therapy and undergo endoscopy to evaluate the risk of bleeding recurrence.
- Patients with active bleeding who are hemodynamically unstable should receive intravenous fluids and blood transfusions. They should undergo emergency endoscopy for coagulation of bleeding sites. Various modalities may be used to achieve bleeding-site coagulation.
- As soon as patients tolerate oral intake, intravenous PPI therapy should be changed to oral therapy.
- Surgery is reserved for those patients who have refractory ulcers, recurrent bleeding, or a perforated ulcer.

21-2. Gastroesophageal Reflux Disease

Definition and Incidence

Gastroesophageal reflux disease (GERD) is a condition that develops when the reflux of stomach contents causes troublesome symptoms or complications.

The prevalence of GERD is highest in Western countries. It occurs equally in men and women, except that its incidence is higher in pregnant women. The incidence of GERD is higher and more frequently severe in Caucasians than in African Americans. Obesity has been strongly correlated to the incidence of GERD. GERD may also occur in children. The risk of experiencing complications from GERD increases with age.

Approximately 20% of the U.S. population experiences heartburn or regurgitation of gastric acid weekly.

Approximately 30–50% of pregnant women have symptomatic esophageal reflux; 50% experience heartburn daily.

Classification

The manifestations of GERD are divided into esophageal and extraesophageal syndromes.

Esophageal syndromes

Esophageal syndromes comprise those that are only symptomatic in nature and those that are symptomatic with esophageal injury on endoscopy. Symptomatic syndromes include the typical reflux syndrome and the reflux chest pain syndrome:

- The *typical reflux syndrome* is defined by the presence of troublesome heartburn, regurgitation, or both. Patients may have other symptoms, such as epigastric pain or sleep disturbance.
- The *reflux chest pain syndrome* occurs when GERD causes chest pain that is similar to ischemic cardiac pain. This pain can occur without concurrent heartburn or regurgitation.

Symptomatic syndromes with esophageal injury include GERD complications such as reflux esophagitis, reflux stricture, Barrett's esophagus, and esophageal adenocarcinoma.

- *Reflux esophagitis* is characterized by visible breaks in the distal esophageal mucosa.
- A *reflux stricture* is defined as a persistent luminal narrowing of the esophagus caused by GERD.
- *Barrett's esophagus* occurs when esophageal squamous epithelium from the gastroesophageal junction is replaced with metaplastic columnar epithelium. It is a risk factor for the development of *esophageal adenocarcinoma*.

Extraesophageal syndromes

Extraesophageal syndromes include those syndromes that have established associations with GERD and those with proposed associations with GERD.

Esophageal syndromes that have established associations with GERD include reflux cough syndrome, reflux laryngitis syndrome, reflux asthma syndrome, and reflux dental erosion syndrome.

Esophageal syndromes that have proposed associations with GERD include pharyngitis, sinusitis, idiopathic pulmonary fibrosis, and recurrent otitis media.

Clinical Presentation

Heartburn and regurgitation are the common characteristic symptoms of the typical reflux syndrome.

Heartburn is defined as a burning sensation in the retrosternal area. *Regurgitation* is defined as the perception of flow of refluxed gastric content into the mouth or hypopharynx.

Symptoms usually occur shortly after having a meal, when reclining after a meal, or on lying down at bedtime. Symptoms often awaken patients from sleep.

Symptoms are exacerbated by eating a large meal (especially a high-fat meal), by bending over, and occasionally by exercising.

Symptoms suggestive of complications from GERD include continuous pain, dysphagia, odynophagia, bleeding, unexplained weight loss, and choking.

Symptom severity does not correlate with the degree of esophagitis present on endoscopy, but severity usually does correlate with the duration of reflux.

Pathophysiology

The effortless movement of gastric contents into the esophagus is a physiologic process that occurs numerous times daily throughout life and does not produce symptoms. It occurs more frequently in patients with GERD.

The pathophysiology of GERD involves the prolonged contact of esophageal epithelium with refluxed gastric contents containing acid and pepsin. Prolonged contact between esophageal epithelium and gastric contents can overwhelm esophageal defense mechanisms and produce symptoms.

Higher-potency gastric refluxate may produce symptoms during times of esophageal contact of normal duration. The presence of refluxate in an esophagus with impaired defense mechanisms may also produce symptoms.

Esophageal defenses consist of the antireflux barrier, luminal clearance mechanisms, and tissue resistance.

- Components of the antireflux barrier are the lower esophageal sphincter (LES) and the diaphragm. The LES is a thickened ring of circular smooth muscle localized to the distal 2–3 cm of the esophagus. It is contracted at rest, thereby serving as a barrier to refluxate. The diaphragm encircles the LES and acts as a mechanical support, especially during physical exertion.
- Luminal clearance factors include gravity, esophageal peristalsis, and salivary and esophageal gland secretions (which contain acid-neutralizing bicarbonate).
- The three areas of tissue resistance are pre-epithelial, epithelial, and postepithelial defense. Preepithelial and epithelial tissues limit the rate

of diffusion of H+ between cell membranes. Postepithelial defense is provided by the blood supply, which removes HCl and supplies oxygen, nutrients, and bicarbonate.

Diagnostic Criteria

For patients who present with troublesome symptoms of GERD, a trial of empiric therapy is appropriate. A diagnosis of GERD may be assumed for patients who respond to empiric treatment.

Diagnostic testing with endoscopy should be performed in patients who present with troublesome GERD symptoms and dysphagia, weight loss, or epigastric mass on physical examination. It should also be performed on patients who do not respond to empiric treatment.

- Endoscopy is the preferred method for evaluating the esophageal mucosa for esophagitis and for evaluating for the presence of complications. It is a highly specific test, but it is not extremely sensitive. Patients with symptoms may have normal esophageal mucosa.
- Esophageal manometry may be performed in patients with persistent symptoms despite an empiric trial of twice-daily PPI therapy with normal esophageal mucosa on endoscopy. It consists of passing a tube into the stomach and subsequently measuring pressures as the tube is pulled back across the LES, esophagus, and pharynx. Esophageal manometry is often performed to facilitate placement of ambulatory pH probes. It is always performed to aid in determining the best procedure in antireflux surgery candidates.
- Ambulatory pH monitoring may be used to confirm the diagnosis of GERD in patients with persistent GERD symptoms despite an empiric trial of PPI therapy, with normal esophageal mucosa on endoscopy, and no abnormalities on esophageal manometry testing. It is performed by passing a small electrode to measure pH intranasally to the level of 5 cm above the LES. This test allows patient symptoms to be correlated with the timing of episodes of decreased pH levels in the esophagus. It may not be available at all institutions.

Treatment Principles and Goals

Goals of therapy are to alleviate or eliminate symptoms, decrease frequency and duration of reflux, promote healing of the injured mucosa, and prevent the development of complications.

Therapy is directed at increasing lower esophageal pressure, improving esophageal acid clearance and gastric emptying, protecting esophageal mucosa, decreasing the acidity of refluxate, and decreasing the amount of gastric contents being refluxed.

Acid suppression is the mainstay of therapy for patients with esophageal GERD syndromes. GERD is considered a chronic condition, and most patients will require chronic therapy. Chronic therapy should be titrated down to the lowest effective dose.

PPIs provide faster symptomatic relief and heal esophagitis more effectively than H2RAs. H2RAs are more effective than placebo.

Antacids are appropriate self-treatment for patients with symptoms of GERD that are not troublesome to the patient.

An empiric trial of once-daily PPI therapy is appropriate for patients with troublesome GERD symptoms. If patients do not respond to once-daily therapy, twice-daily therapy may be used.

Patients with esophageal GERD syndromes and troublesome dysphagia should undergo endoscopy to evaluate for the presence of reflux esophagitis, reflux stricture, Barrett's esophagus, or esophageal adenocarcinoma.

An empirical trial of twice-daily PPI therapy may be used for patients with suspected reflux chest pain syndrome after cardiac causes have been thoroughly considered.

Acute or maintenance therapy with once- or twice-daily PPIs may be used in patients with a suspected extraesophageal GERD syndrome who also have esophageal GERD syndrome.

Antireflux surgery may be performed when a patient is responsive to, but intolerant of, acid suppressive therapy or has persistent troublesome symptoms of GERD.

Drug Therapy

Mechanism of action

For information on H2RAs and PPIs, see the section on PUD.

Antacids neutralize gastric acid (which increases LES tone) and inhibit the conversion of pepsinogen to pepsin, thus raising the pH of gastric contents.

Alginic acid reacts with sodium bicarbonate in saliva to form sodium alginate viscous solution, which floats on the surface of gastric contents. The solution acts as a barrier to protect the esophagus from the corrosive effects of gastric reflux.

See Table 21-2 for selected medications.

Table 21-2. Selected Antacids and Absorbents

Generic name	Trade name	Classification	Dosage range and frequency	Dosage forms
Magnesium hydroxide	Milk of magnesia	Antacid	15–30 mL prn	T, L
Aluminum hydroxide	Amphojel, ALternaGEL	Antacid	15–30 mL prn	T, L
Aluminum carbonate	Basaljel	Antacid	15–30 mL prn	T, L
Magnesium hydroxide + aluminum hydroxide	Maalox	Antacid	15–30 mL prn	T, L
Magaldrate	Riopan	Antacid	15–30 mL prn	T, L
Calcium carbonate	Tums, Titralac	Antacid	15–30 mL prn	T, L
Sodium bicarbonate	Various trade names	Antacid	15–30 mL prn	T, L
Alginic acid + aluminum hydroxide + magnesium hydroxide	Gaviscon	Absorbent + antacid	15–30 mL prn; 2 after meals	T, L

L, liquid; T, tablet.

Patient counseling

For information on H2RAs and PPIs, see the section on PUD.

Antacids and alginic acid are appropriate for the initial management of symptoms of GERD that are not troublesome to the patient. Symptoms persisting longer than 2 weeks require further evaluation and treatment with prescription medications.

Refrigeration of liquid antacids may aid in palatability. Chewable tablets may be more effective than liquids because of increased adherence of antacid and saliva to the distal esophagus. Antacids must be taken at least 2 hours apart from tetracyclines, iron, and digoxin. Antacids and quinolones should be taken 4–6 hours apart.

Alginic acid is effective for the relief of GERD symptoms, but no data indicate esophageal healing on endoscopy. Alginic acid is ineffective if the patient is in the supine position and must not be taken at bedtime.

Adverse drug effects

For information on H2RAs and PPIs, see the section on PUD.

Magnesium-containing antacids frequently cause diarrhea. Aluminum-containing antacids frequently cause constipation and bind to phosphate in the gut, which can lead to bone demineralization. Antacids may also cause acid–base disturbances.

Magnesium and aluminum toxicity may occur when used chronically in patients with renal insufficiency. Sodium bicarbonate may cause sodium overload, particularly in patients with hypertension, congestive heart failure, and chronic renal failure. It may also lead to systemic alkalosis. It should be used on a short-term basis, if at all.

Drug interactions

For information on H2RAs and PPIs, see the section on PUD.

When taken with antacids, the absorption and effectiveness of tetracycline, ferrous sulfate, and quinolones are reduced because the antacids form chelates with them. Antacids decrease the absorption of azoles and sucralfate by increasing gastric pH. Antacids increase urine pH, which decreases the renal clearance of quinidine. Antacids decrease the systemic absorption of digoxin and H2RAs when taken concomitantly with them. Large doses of antacid may decrease the absorption of phenytoin.

Digoxin and phenytoin levels should be monitored frequently when antacids are used concomitantly. Suspected adverse effects of antacids should be reported to a health care provider.

Monitoring parameters

Patients should monitor for the return of GERD symptoms and for the side effects of medications as discussed in the previous section.

Pharmacokinetics

Several medications are substrates for or have effects on the CYP450 enzyme system in the liver. See the discussion under drug interactions in Section 21-1.

Nondrug Therapy

- Lifestyle modifications alone are unlikely to control GERD symptoms. Lifestyle modifications should be tailored to the circumstances of the individual patient.
- Weight loss should be recommended for overweight or obese patients with esophageal GERD syndromes.
- Patients who experience GERD symptoms when recumbent should be advised to elevate the head of the bed.
- Patients should be advised to avoid foods that exacerbate GERD symptoms (alcohol, coffee, chocolate, high-fat foods, spicy foods, acidic foods, and carbonated drinks).
- Patients should be advised to adopt behaviors that reduce esophageal acid exposure, such as to stop smoking, to avoid lying down for 2–3 hours after meals, and to eat smaller meals.
- Calcium channel blockers, β-blockers, nitrates, barbiturates, anticholinergics, and theophylline decrease LES pressure. Tetracyclines, NSAIDs, aspirin, bisphosphonates, iron, quinidine, and potassium chloride have direct irritant effects on the esophageal mucosa.

21-3. Inflammatory Bowel Disease

Definition and Incidence

Idiopathic inflammatory bowel disease (IBD) is divided into two major types:

- *Ulcerative colitis* (UC) is defined as a chronic mucosal inflammatory condition confined to the rectum and colon.
- *Crohn's disease* (CD) is defined as a transmural inflammation of the GI tract that can affect any part of the GI tract from mouth to anus.

The prevalence of UC is approximately 37.5–229.0 cases per 100,000 persons. The prevalence of CD is approximately 50 cases per 100,000 persons.

Approximately 500,000 persons have CD and 500,000 persons have UC in the United States. UC is slightly predominant in men; CD is predominant in women. The overall incidence of IBD is similar between men and women.

North America, Scandinavia, and Great Britain have the highest incidence rates for IBD.

UC typically occurs in persons between 30 and 40 years of age. CD typically occurs between ages 20 and 30. Both may be diagnosed at any stage in life, but of all cases of IBD, 10–15% are diagnosed before adulthood.

The incidence of IBD is low for Hispanics and Asian Americans. Its incidence in African Americans has increased and is equal to that of Caucasians. In addition, its incidence rate is high among the Jewish population in North America, Europe, and Israel.

Classification

The two major types of IBD are ulcerative colitis and Crohn's disease. Clinical presentation and diagnostic tests help distinguish one form from the other.

Clinical Presentation

IBD is characterized by acute exacerbations of symptoms followed by periods of remission that are spontaneous or secondary to changes in medical therapy.

Ulcerative colitis

The hallmark clinical symptom of UC is bloody diarrhea, which is often accompanied by rectal urgency and tenesmus.

The extent and severity of UC are characterized by clinical and endoscopic findings. Clinical symptoms are categorized as mild, moderate, severe, and fulminant. Endoscopic findings are categorized as distal (limited to below the splenic flexure) or extensive (extending proximal to the splenic flexure).

- *Mild UC* is characterized by fewer than four stools per day with or without blood, without systemic disturbance and with a normal erythrocyte sedimentation rate (ESR).
- *Moderate UC* is characterized by more than four stools per day with minimal signs of toxicity.
- *Severe UC* is characterized by more than six stools per day with blood; systemic disturbance (e.g., fever, tachycardia, anemia); and ESR greater than 30.
- *Fulminant UC* is characterized by more than 10 bowel movements per day, continuous bleeding, toxicity, abdominal tenderness and distension, blood transfusion requirement, and colonic dilation on abdominal plain films.

Crohn's disease

The presentation of CD is variable and its onset is often insidious. Typical symptoms include chronic or nocturnal diarrhea and abdominal pain. Additional typical symptoms include weight loss, fever, and rectal bleeding.

Clinical signs may include pallor, abdominal mass or tenderness, cachexia, perianal fissure, fistula, or abscess.

Extraintestinal symptoms include inflammation of the skin, joints, and eyes.

Symptoms differ depending on the site and severity of inflammation:

- *Mild to moderate:* Patients are ambulatory and tolerate oral alimentation without dehydration; toxicity (fever, rigors, or prostration); abdominal tenderness; painful mass or obstruction; or weight loss > 10%.
- *Moderate to severe:* Patients fail to respond to treatment for mild to moderate disease or have fever, weight loss, abdominal pain, nausea, vomiting (without obstruction), or anemia.
- *Severe to fulminant:* Patients have persistent symptoms despite the use of steroids or biologic agents as outpatients, or individuals present with high fever, persistent vomiting, evidence of obstruction, rebound tenderness, cachexia, or abscess.

Symptomatic remission occurs when a patient is asymptomatic or without any symptomatic inflammatory sequelae.

The ileum and colon are the most commonly affected sites. Ileitis may mimic appendicitis. Intestinal obstruction and inflammatory masses or abscesses may also develop. Patients with colonic CD commonly have rectal bleeding, perianal lesions, and extraintestinal manifestations (e.g., spondylarthritis, peripheral arthritis, erythema nodosum, pyoderma gangrenosum, uveitis, fatty liver, chronic active hepatitis, cirrhosis, primary sclerosing cholangitis, gallstones, cholangiocarcinoma, and hypercoagulability).

Oral CD is characterized by lesions ranging from a few aphthous ulcers to deep linear ulcers with edema and induration. Gastroduodenal involvement may mimic PUD.

Pathophysiology

The etiology of UC and CD is unclear, but similar factors may contribute to both diseases. These factors include infectious agents, genetics, environmental factors, immune deficits, and psychological factors. Major etiologic theories involve a combination of infectious and immunologic factors.

UC is confined to the rectum and colon and affects only the mucosa and submucosa. The primary lesion of UC is a crypt abscess, which forms in the crypts of the mucosa. CD most commonly affects the terminal ileum and involves extensive damage to the bowel wall.

UC and CD complications can be local or systemic. Local complications of UC include hemorrhoids, anal fissures, and perirectal abscesses. Toxic megacolon can lead to perforation and is a major complication that affects 1–3% of patients with UC or CD. Colonic strictures and hemorrhage may also occur. Small bowel strictures, obstruction, and fistulae are common in CD. Systemic complications (extraintestinal) can occur with UC and CD.

Diagnostic Criteria

UC is diagnosed on the basis of clinical symptoms, proctosigmoidoscopy or colonoscopy, tissue biopsy, and bacteria-negative stool studies. CD is diagnosed on the basis of clinical symptoms, contrast radiography or endoscopy, tissue biopsy, and bacteria-negative stool studies. Abdominal ultrasonography, computed tomography, and magnetic resonance imaging aid in the identification of masses, abscesses, and perianal complications in UC and CD.

Treatment Principles and Goals

Treatment of IBD involves medications that target inflammatory mediators and alter immunoinflammatory processes. These medications include anti-inflammatory, immunosuppressive, and biologic agents.

Nutritional considerations are also important because many patients with IBD may be malnourished.

Goals of therapy for UC and CD include induction and maintenance of remission of symptoms, induction and maintenance of mucosal healing, improved quality of life, resolution of complications and systemic symptoms, and prevention of future complications. For patients with CD, remission means that patients are asymptomatic or without inflammatory sequelae, including patients who have responded to medical intervention. Patients who require steroids to maintain their condition are considered steroid dependent, not in remission.

In UC patients, remission is likely to last at least 1 year with medical therapy. Without medical therapy, up to two-thirds of patients will relapse within 9 months. For mild CD, up to 40% of patients improve in 3–4 months with observation alone. Most will remain in remission for prolonged periods without medical therapy.

The treatment of choice for distal UC that involves only the rectum (proctitis) is topical therapy with aminosalicylates:

- Treatment is initiated with a nightly suppository or enema. Improvement usually occurs within 2–3 weeks. Most patients will require maintenance therapy with topical aminosalicylates to remain in remission.
- Rectally administered steroids may be used in combination with aminosalicylates when patients do not respond to aminosalicylates alone.
- For patients who do not respond to or who cannot tolerate topical therapy, oral therapy with steroids or aminosalicylates is necessary.

Mild to moderate distal colitis may be treated with oral aminosalicylates, topical mesalamine, or topical steroids; however, topical aminosalicylates are more effective than topical steroids or oral aminosalicylates.

- Combining oral and topical aminosalicylates is more effective than using them individually.
- Patients who are refractory to maximum doses of these agents may require oral steroid treatment.
- For the maintenance of remission, mesalamine enemas may be used every 1–2 days. Oral aminosalicylates are also effective for maintaining remission. Combining oral and topical aminosalicylates is more effective at maintaining remission than using them individually. Topical steroids are not effective at maintaining remission.

For moderate to severe distal colitis, twice-daily enemas are required. Combining oral and topical aminosalicylates may also be required.

For severe distal colitis, combining oral and topical aminosalicylates is required.

- Oral corticosteroids are reserved for patients who fail initial aminosalicylate therapy.
- Corticosteroids are tapered after remission is achieved, and topical and oral aminosalicylates are continued as maintenance therapy.

Extensive UC (pancolitis) requires oral therapy; however, topical therapy is still a useful adjunct in controlling rectal disease.

For mild to moderate extensive UC, oral aminosalicylates are first-line therapy.

- Patients who fail to respond require the addition of high-dose oral corticosteroid therapy.
- Azathioprine and 6-mercaptopurine may be used in patients who do not respond to, or cannot be

weaned from, corticosteroids. These drugs may also be used to maintain remission.

- Corticosteroid tapering should begin only when complete remission is achieved.
- Corticosteroids do not have a role in maintenance therapy; aminosalicylates are usually effective at maintaining remission.
- For patients who fail oral therapy, hospitalization and intravenous steroid therapy is necessary.

For moderate to severe UC refractory to conventional therapy, infliximab may be used to avoid or reduce corticosteroid use and to induce remission.

For severe or fulminant colitis, hospitalization and complete bowel rest are required.

- Intravenous (IV) steroids are the mainstays of therapy.
- Topical therapy may be added for patients with significant rectal symptoms.
- In patients who do not respond to 7 days of IV steroids, surgery or IV cyclosporine should be considered. Patients who respond to IV cyclosporine are converted to oral cyclosporine and a steroid taper.
- Azathioprine may be added to maintain remission.

Abdominal x-ray should be performed to exclude toxic megacolon. Surgery is often required for patients with toxic megacolon, and preoperative antibiotics are recommended to reduce the chance of septic complications.

For CD, clinical improvement should be evident within 2–4 weeks. Maximal clinical improvement should occur within 12–16 weeks. Treatment for acute disease should be continued until remission is achieved or the patient's symptoms fail to improve.

For mild to moderate CD localized to the ileum or right colon, controlled-release oral budesonide is appropriate initial therapy.

- Controlled-release oral budesonide is more effective than oral mesalamine and placebo. It has similar efficacy to conventional oral corticosteroids.
- Oral mesalamine has been used as first-line therapy; however, new evidence indicates that it is only minimally more effective than placebo and less effective than corticosteroids.
- Oral sulfasalazine is more effective than placebo but less effective than corticosteroids for ileocolonic and colonic CD.
- Rectal aminosalicylates are often used to treat distal colonic CD; however, controlled studies showing efficacy are lacking.
- Although metronidazole and ciprofloxacin are widely used in the treatment of CD, clinical trials have not consistently demonstrated efficacy.

- No controlled data exist regarding the treatment of mild to moderate oral CD. Lidocaine lozenges may provide symptomatic relief. Lesions will respond to systemic steroids or azathioprine in 50% of patients.
- For CD of the stomach, esophagus, duodenum, and jejunum, PPIs, oral corticosteroids, mercaptopurine, azathioprine, methotrexate, infliximab, adalimumab, and certolizumab pegol have improved symptoms in uncontrolled trials.
- When remission is achieved, maintenance therapy should be initiated. For patients who do not respond, treatment with alternative agents for mild to moderate disease may be initiated or the treatment may be advanced to agents used for moderate to severe disease.

For patients with moderate to severe disease, oral corticosteroids are the mainstay of therapy.

- Prednisone 40–60 mg daily should be given until symptoms resolve and weight gain resumes. Steroids are not appropriate maintenance therapy.
- Infections or abscesses should be treated with appropriate antibiotics or surgical drainage.
- Azathioprine and 6-mercaptopurine may be added to oral corticosteroids to maintain a steroid-induced remission. They are also effective for steroid-dependent or steroid-refractory patients.
- Parenteral methotrexate is effective for inducing remission and allowing steroid dose reduction in patients with steroid-dependent and steroid-refractory CD.
- Infliximab, adalimumab, and certolizumab pegol may be used in patients who do not respond to oral corticosteroids or immunosuppressive agents. They may also be used as an alternative to oral corticosteroids when the side effects of oral corticosteroids need to be avoided.
- Natalizumab may be used when patients are intolerant or unresponsive to oral corticosteroids, immunosuppressants, and biologic therapies.
- Enteral nutrition should be used to support the patient's overall nutrition status, not to induce remission of CD.
- When remission is achieved, maintenance therapy should be initiated.

For severe to fulminant CD, hospitalization for intravenous steroids and hydration is required.

- Intravenous steroids equivalent to 40–60 mg/day of prednisone should be administered.
- Parenteral fluid and electrolyte therapy should be administered to restore hydration.

- Parenteral or enteral nutrition support should be administered after 5–7 days if the patient cannot meet adequate nutritional requirements.
- Anemic patients may require blood transfusions.
- Intestinal obstructions related to adhesions should be managed with bowel rest and nasogastric tube suctioning. Obstructions related to inflammatory strictures require antibiotic therapy and IV steroids. Surgery should be considered if obstructive symptoms do not respond to therapy.
- Abscesses should be drained and appropriate antibiotic therapy instituted.
- High-dose metronidazole or ciprofloxacin may be used in the management of fistulas. Chronic therapy may be required to prevent recurrent drainage.
- Azathioprine, 6-mercaptopurine, and infliximab may also be used in the management of fistulas.
- If patients do not respond to IV steroids after 5–7 days of therapy, cyclosporine or tacrolimus therapy may be instituted.
- When symptoms respond to initial treatment, the patient should be converted to an equivalent oral corticosteroid regimen.
- Patients who do not respond to therapy require surgical intervention.

Maintenance therapy should be initiated when remission is achieved.

- Corticosteroids should not be used as long-term maintenance therapy.
- Sulfasalazine and mesalamine have not shown consistent benefit as maintenance therapy.
- Azathioprine, 6-mercaptopurine, and methotrexate have shown benefit as maintenance therapy.
- Azathioprine may be used as maintenance therapy in steroid-naive patients who achieved remission with infliximab.
- Infliximab, adalimumab, and certolizumab pegol are effective maintenance therapies.
- Natalizumab may be used for maintenance therapy after it has been successfully used to induce remission.

Drug Therapy

See Table 21-3 for selected medications used in IBD.

Mechanism of action

Sulfasalazine is cleaved to sulfapyridine (excreted in the urine) by bacteria in the gut and mesalamine (the

Table 21-3. Selected Medications Used in Inflammatory Bowel Disease

Generic name	Trade name	Classification	Dosage range and frequency	Dosage forms
Sulfasalazine	Azulfidine	Aminosalicylate	4–6 g/d	T
Mesalamine	Asacol	Aminosalicylate	2.4–4.8 g/d	DT
Mesalamine	Pentasa, Rowasa	Aminosalicylate	2–4 g/d	DC
Mesalamine	Salofalk, Claversal	Aminosalicylate	1–4 g/d	EN, SU
Mesalamine	Lialda	Aminosalicylate	2.4–4.8 g/d	DT
Mesalamine	Canasa	Aminosalicylate	500–1,000 mg	SU
Balsalazide	Colazal	Aminosalicylate	6.75 g/d	DC
Metronidazole	Flagyl	Antibacterial	10–20 g/d (Crohn's disease)	T, IV
Ciprofloxacin	Cipro	Antibacterial	500 mg bid (Crohn's disease)	T, IV
Prednisone	Various trade names	Corticosteroid	40–60 mg/d	T
Methylprednisolone	Solu-Medrol	Corticosteroid	16 mg q8h	IV
Budesonide	Entocort EC	Corticosteroid	9 mg qd	C
Azathioprine	Imuran	Immunosuppressive	1.0–2.5 mg/kg/d	T, IV
6-mercaptopurine	Purinethol	Immunosuppressive	1.5 mg/kg/d	T
Methotrexate	Abitrexate	Antimetabolite	25 mg/wk	IM, SC
Infliximab	Remicade	Immunomodulator	Induction: 5 mg/kg at 0, 2, and 6 wks; maintenance: 5 mg/kg q 8 wks	IV
Adalimumab	Humira	Immunomodulator	Induction: 160 mg as 4 injections over 1–2 days then 80 mg 2 wks later; maintenance: 40 mg q other wk starting on day 29	SC
Certolizumab pegol	Cimzia	Immunomodulator	Induction: 400 mg (given as 2 separate doses of 200 mg each) at 0, 2, and 4 wks; maintenance: 400 mg q 4 wks	SC
Natalizumab	Tysabri	Immunomodulator	300 mg over 1 h every 4 wks	IV
Cyclosporine	Neoral, Sandimmune	Immunosuppressive	4 mg/kg/d	IV, C, L

C, capsule; DT, delayed-release tablet; DC, delayed-release capsule; EN, enema; IV, intravenous; IM, intramuscular; L, liquid; SC, subcutaneous; SU, suppository; T, tablet.

active component). The sulfapyridine molecule is responsible for the many side effects associated with sulfasalazine.

Mesalamine's mechanism of action is poorly understood. Mesalamine inhibits cyclooxygenase and may also inhibit production of cyclooxygenase, thromboxane synthetase, platelet-activating factor synthetase, and interleukin-1 in macrophages. It may also act as a superoxide free-radical scavenger.

Corticosteroids have immunomodulatory effects and inhibit the production of cytokines and other inflammatory mediators.

Corticosteroids, azathioprine, 6-mercaptopurine, cyclosporine, and tacrolimus are immunosuppressive agents. For full discussion of their mechanism of action, patient counseling, side effects, drug interactions, and pharmacokinetics, see Chapter 20 on transplantation.

The exact mechanism of action of metronidazole and ciprofloxacin in IBD is not known. One theory suggests that antibacterials interrupt the role of bacteria in the inflammatory process.

Methotrexate inhibits dihydrofolate reductase and purine synthesis, reduces the production of leukotriene-B_4 and interleukin-1 and -2, and may induce T-cell apoptosis.

Infliximab is a chimeric monoclonal antibody that inhibits human tumor necrosis factor, which inhibits subsequent cytokine-triggered inflammatory processes.

Adalimumab is a recombinant monoclonal antibody that inhibits human tumor necrosis factor, which inhibits subsequent cytokine-triggered inflammatory processes.

Certolizumab pegol is a pegylated humanized antibody Fab fragment of tumor necrosis factor monoclonal antibody. It inhibits human tumor necrosis factor activity, which inhibits subsequent cytokine-triggered inflammatory processes. Pegylation delays elimination and prolongs the half-life of the drug.

Natalizumab is a monoclonal antibody against the alpha-4 subunit of integrin molecules. It blocks the association of integrin with vascular receptors, which limits adhesion and transmigration of leukocytes.

Patient counseling

Sulfasalazine should be taken after meals. Patients should avoid sun exposure while taking it. Folic acid supplementation should be given during sulfasalazine treatment to avoid anemia. Sulfasalazine may cause orange discoloration of urine and skin.

Mesalamine tablets should be swallowed whole. Suppositories should not be handled excessively and foil wrappers should be removed before insertion. Suspension enemas should be shaken well before use.

Antacids and ciprofloxacin should be taken 4–6 hours apart. Iron- or zinc-containing products should be taken 4 hours before or 2 hours after taking ciprofloxacin. Patients should avoid excessive exposure to sunlight.

Patients taking methotrexate should avoid alcohol, salicylates, and prolonged exposure to sunlight. Female patients of childbearing age should be counseled on appropriate contraceptive measures during methotrexate therapy.

Patients receiving therapy with infliximab should be counseled on the possibility of infusion reactions, delayed hypersensitivity reactions, and increased risk of infections. Live vaccines should not be administered to patients taking infliximab.

Patients taking adalimumab should be counseled on the increased risk of infections and to report any symptoms of infection to their physician immediately. They should also be counseled on the potential for injection site reactions and be taught proper injection technique and proper sharps disposal. Live vaccines should not be administered to patients taking adalimumab.

Patients taking certolizumab pegol should be counseled on the increased risk of infections and to report any symptoms of infection to their physician immediately. They should also be counseled on the potential for injection-site reactions and be taught proper injection technique and sharps disposal. Live vaccines should not be administered to patients taking certolizumab pegol.

Patients taking natalizumab should be counseled on the risk of acute hypersensitivity infusion reactions. They should also be counseled on the increased risk of infections, particularly progressive multifocal leukoencephalopathy. Patients should report symptoms of infection to their physician immediately.

Adverse drug effects

Sulfasalazine may cause nausea, vomiting, anorexia, and headaches. The sulfapyridine moiety leads to hypersensitivity reactions (e.g., rash, fever, agranulocytosis, pancreatitis, nephritis, and hepatitis) and altered spermatogenesis in males.

Mesalamine is better tolerated than sulfasalazine. Olsalazine may cause self-limited watery diarrhea. Balsalazide causes abdominal pain in 10% of patients.

Ciprofloxacin may cause nausea, diarrhea, headache, and vaginal candidiasis.

Methotrexate frequently causes nausea and leukopenia. Asymptomatic elevations in liver function tests may occur.

Infliximab may cause infusion-related reactions, upper respiratory infections, headache, rash, cough, and stomach pain. Allergic reactions have been reported. Infliximab increases the risk of serious infections (bacterial, viral, and fungal infections; tuberculosis) and certain types of cancer. New onset or exacerbation of preexisting heart failure, hepatotoxicity, neuropathy, anemia, and lupus-like syndrome have also been reported.

Adalimumab may cause injection-site reactions, upper respiratory infections, headaches, rash, and nausea. Allergic reactions have been reported. Adalimumab increases the risk of serious infections (bacterial, viral, and fungal infections; tuberculosis) and certain types of cancer. New onset or exacerbation of preexisting heart failure, neuropathy, anemia, and lupus-like syndrome have also been reported.

Certolizumab pegol may cause injection-site reactions, upper respiratory tract infections, rash, and urinary tract infections. Allergic reactions have been reported. Certolizumab increases the risk of serious infections (bacterial, viral, and fungal infections; tuberculosis) and certain types of cancer. New onset or exacerbation of preexisting heart failure, neuropathy, anemia, and lupus-like syndrome have also been reported.

Natalizumab increases the risk of developing progressive multifocal leukoencephalopathy. Serious allergic reactions (usually within 2 hours of infusion) and hepatotoxicity have been reported. Natalizumab increases the risk of serious infections (bacterial, viral, and fungal infections; tuberculosis).

Drug interactions

Sulfasalazine may decrease the bioavailability of digoxin by inhibiting its absorption.

Azathioprine is converted into 6-mercaptopurine in vivo; 6-mercaptopurine then undergoes hepatic first-pass metabolism, which is catalyzed by xanthene oxidase. By inhibiting xanthene oxidase, allopurinol increases the bioavailability of azathioprine. The azathioprine dose should be lowered by 25–50% when the two agents are used concurrently.

Ciprofloxacin binds with antacids, zinc, and iron products. It also increases the therapeutic effects of warfarin, cyclosporine, and theophylline.

Corticosteroids should not be administered with natalizumab because of the increased risk of serious infections.

The use of methotrexate and concurrent NSAIDs has caused fatal interactions. Methotrexate may increase levels of 6-mercaptopurine.

Infliximab should not be administered with etanercept or anakinra because of the increased risk of serious infections. Live vaccines should not be administered to patients taking infliximab. The herbal supplement echinacea may decrease the effectiveness of infliximab.

Adalimumab should not be administered with anakinra because of the increased risk of serious infections. Live vaccines should not be administered to patients taking adalimumab. The herbal supplement echinacea may decrease the effectiveness of adalimumab. Methotrexate may decrease the clearance of adalimumab; however, this effect has not been shown to be clinically significant.

Certolizumab pegol should not be administered with anakinra, abatacept, rituximab, or natalizumab because of the increased risk of serious infections. Live vaccines should not be administered to patients taking certolizumab. The herbal supplement echinacea may decrease the effectiveness of certolizumab. Certolizumab may falsely elevate the activated partial thromboplastin time and the lupus anticoagulant assays.

Natalizumab should not be administered with other immunosuppressants, such as 6-mercaptopurine, azathioprine, cyclosporine, and methotrexate, or with tumor necrosis factor inhibitors because of the increased risk of progressive multifocal leukoencephalopathy. The herbal supplement echinacea may decrease the effectiveness of natalizumab.

Monitoring parameters

Serum chemistries, complete blood counts, liver function tests, blood glucose concentrations, ESR, response to therapy, and the presence of adverse effects should be monitored. Tuberculosis skin testing should be performed before administering biologic agents.

Pharmacokinetics

- Sulfasalazine is metabolized by intestinal flora to sulfapyridine and 5-aminosalicylic acid. Unchanged drug and metabolites are excreted in the urine.
- Mesalamine is metabolized in the liver and gut to 5-aminosalicylic acid. The metabolite is eliminated via the urine and feces.
- Azathioprine is thought to be hepatically metabolized to 6-mercaptopurine by glutathione S-transferase; 6-mercaptopurine is further metabolized by hypoxanthine guanine phosphoribosyltransferase, xanthene oxidase, and thiopurine methyltransferase. Metabolites are excreted in the urine.
- Ciprofloxacin is partially metabolized in the liver. Unchanged drug and metabolites are excreted in the urine and feces.
- Metronidazole is metabolized in the liver and is excreted in the urine and feces.
- Prednisone is metabolized in the liver and excreted in the urine.
- Methotrexate is primarily eliminated by the kidneys.

Nondrug Therapy

Patients with UC and CD are often malnourished because of malabsorption or maldigestion caused by chronic bowel inflammation, "short gut" syndrome from multiple bowel surgeries, or bile salt deficiency in the gut. The catabolic effects of the disease process can also lead to malnutrition.

Individuals should eliminate foods that exacerbate symptoms. Patients with lactase deficiency should avoid dairy products or take lactase supplements to avoid symptoms.

Enteral or parenteral supplementation may be used in patients with severe UC or CD to maintain adequate nutritional status.

Surgery may be necessary for patients with severe UC or CD. Surgery involves removing diseased segments of bowel, repairing fistulas, and draining abscesses.

- In UC, surgery is indicated for patients who fail maximum medical therapy to correct complications (perforation, strictures, obstruction, hemorrhage, toxic megacolon). It is also used as prophylaxis against the development of cancer (in patients with long-standing UC) and in patients with premalignant changes found on bowel biopsies.
- In CD, surgery is indicated for neoplastic or pre-neoplastic lesions, obstructing stenoses, suppurative complications, or CD that does not respond to pharmacotherapy. Smoking cessation should be encouraged to reduce the risk of recurrence of CD after surgery (as well as for overall health benefits).

21-4. Irritable Bowel Syndrome

Definition and Incidence

Irritable bowel syndrome (IBS) is defined as abdominal pain or discomfort that occurs in association with altered bowel habits over a period of 3 months.

IBS is a prevalent and expensive condition. It significantly impairs health-related quality of life and leads to reduced work productivity.

IBS patients visit physicians more frequently, have more diagnostic tests performed, take more medications, miss more workdays, show lower work productivity, are hospitalized more frequently, and consume more direct health care costs than patients without IBS.

The worldwide prevalence of IBS is 7–10%. Most cases of IBS are diagnosed before age 50. IBS is 1.5 times more common in women than in men. It is also more common in patients from lower socioeconomic groups.

Classifications

No symptom-based diagnostic criteria have ideal accuracy for diagnosing IBS. Traditional criteria (Kruis, Manning) are at least as accurate as the more recent Rome I criteria. Rome II and III criteria have been proposed, but their accuracy has not been evaluated.

Because of the lack of ideal accuracy of symptom-based diagnostic criteria, the American College of Gastroenterology proposed a new definition of IBS (see previous section).

Once the diagnosis is made, IBS may be classified according to its predominant symptom: diarrhea predominant, constipation predominant, or mixed (symptoms may alternate). Symptoms may also be further categorized as mild, moderate, or severe.

Clinical Presentation

IBS is a heterogeneous disorder with various clinical presentations:

- Abdominal pain is generally described as crampy or achy, and the intensity and location are highly variable. Pain may be exacerbated by meals and may last from 1 to 3 hours. Stress and emotional turmoil can also exacerbate pain.
- Patients typically present with diarrhea, constipation, or alternating periods of both.
- Upper GI symptoms occur more frequently in patients with constipation (heartburn, dyspepsia, early satiety, and nausea). Women experience abdominal distention, bloating, and nausea more often than men.
- Extraintestinal symptoms are common. They include genitourinary symptoms (e.g., pelvic pain, dysmenorrhea, dyspareunia, urinary frequency, nocturia, and sensation of incomplete bladder evacuation); impaired sexual function (e.g., decreased libido); and musculoskeletal complaints (e.g., lower back pain, headaches, and chronic fatigue).
- Alarm features include rectal bleeding, weight loss, iron deficiency anemia, nocturnal symptoms, family history of colorectal cancer, IBD, or celiac sprue. These symptoms may indicate the presence of an organic disease.

Pathophysiology

The pathogenesis is multifactorial and includes abnormal gut sensorimotor activity, central nervous system (CNS) dysfunction, psychological disturbances, genetic predisposition, enteric infection, and other luminal factors:

- Colonic motor abnormalities commonly occur in IBS. Patients with IBS may exhibit an exaggerated gastrocolonic response lasting up to 3 hours.
- Small intestinal motor patterns are frequently disturbed in patients with IBS. Small intestinal transit

is delayed in constipation-predominant IBS and is accelerated in diarrhea-predominant IBS.

- Bloating may be the result of abnormal retrograde reflux of intestinal gas, enhanced perception of the presence of intestinal gas, or obstructive intestinal motor patterns.
- Motor dysfunction of other smooth muscles may occur in IBS. The following abnormalities may also be found: lowered LES sphincter pressures, abnormal esophageal body peristalsis, gastric slow-wave dysrhythmias, delayed gastric and gallbladder emptying, and dysfunction of the sphincter of Oddi.
- It is theorized that IBS results from sensitization of visceral afferent fibers, which causes normal physiologic events to be perceived as painful. It is unknown if sensorineural dysfunction is generalized or localized to the gut afferent fibers.
- It is unknown whether IBS is primarily a CNS disorder with centrally directed changes in gut sensorimotor function or primarily a gut disorder with inappropriate CNS input. Further investigation is needed in this area.
- Eighty percent of patients with IBS exhibit psychiatric disturbances. The onset of psychiatric disturbances usually predates or occurs concurrently with the onset of IBS. Psychological stress triggers symptoms in many patients. IBS is also associated with a history of sexual abuse.
- Other factors that may contribute to IBS are alterations in gut flora (controversial), antecedent GI infection, carbohydrate malabsorption, food allergies, neurohumoral disturbances, genetic factors, and abnormal stool characteristics (low concentrations of bile or short-chain fatty acids).

Relief of pain with defecation, looser stool with pain onset, more frequent stools with pain onset, and abdominal distention are significantly more common in IBS than in organic disease.

Diagnostic Criteria

- Physical examination is usually normal.
- Routine diagnostic testing with complete blood count, serum chemistries, thyroid function tests, stool for ova and parasites, and abdominal imaging are not recommended in patients with typical IBS symptoms and no alarm symptoms because of the low probability of diagnosing organic disease.
- Serologic screening for celiac sprue should be pursued in patients with diarrhea-predominant or mixed-symptom IBS.

- Lactose breath testing may be considered when lactose intolerance is suspected after dietary modification.
- Colonoscopy should be performed in patients with IBS with alarm symptoms to rule out CD, ulcerative colitis, and colorectal cancer.
- Colonoscopy should be performed in patients with IBS over the age of 50 to rule out colon cancer.

Treatment Principles and Goals

Treatment should be offered to patients seeking medical care if the patient and physician believe that the IBS symptoms decrease the patient's quality of life. Goals of therapy include improving IBS symptoms and improving patient quality of life.

Evidence from small clinical trials is inconsistent regarding the effectiveness of anticholinergic and antimuscarinic agents (dicyclomine and hyoscyamine) in the management of IBS; however, they are often used as first-line therapy in patients with mild symptoms. They may provide short-term relief of abdominal pain and discomfort. They should be used with caution in patients with constipation.

Psyllium has been shown to be moderately effective for IBS, although the evidence is weak.

Calcium polycarbophil was shown to improve symptoms in one small study. Polyethylene glycol was shown to improve stool frequency, but not abdominal pain, in a small study of adolescents with constipation-predominant IBS. It may be used as adjunctive therapy in patients with constipation-predominant IBS.

Loperamide significantly improves stool consistency and decreases stool frequency in patients with diarrhea-predominant IBS. It has no effect on abdominal pain or global IBS symptoms.

Tegaserod improves global IBS symptoms, bloating, abdominal pain, and altered bowel habits in patients with constipation-predominant IBS. It was withdrawn from the U.S. market in March 2007 because of an increased incidence (0.11%) of cardiovascular events in patients taking the drug. It is available only through the U.S. Food and Drug Administration (FDA) under an emergency investigational drug protocol.

Tricyclic antidepressants (TCAs) improve abdominal pain in patients with IBS. They also improve global IBS symptoms in patients with diarrhea-predominant IBS but not constipation-predominant IBS.

Selective serotonin reuptake inhibitors (SSRIs) improve abdominal pain in patients with IBS and are also effective in the treatment of comorbid psychiatric disorders in patients with IBS. SSRIs are recommended for patients with moderate to severe abdominal pain or those with psychiatric comorbidities. Several types of psychological counseling and therapy are effective in some patients with IBS.

Alosetron improves global IBS symptoms, abdominal discomfort, stool consistency, and stool frequency in women with diarrhea-predominant IBS. Because of the incidence of colon ischemia and complicated constipation, alosetron is available only through a prescribing program regulated by the FDA and administered by the drug's manufacturer. It is approved only for use in women with chronic, severe, diarrhea-predominant IBS who do not respond to other therapies.

Lubiprostone has been shown to relieve global IBS symptoms in women with constipation-predominant IBS.

Drug Therapy

Table 21-4 shows selected medications used to treat IBS.

Mechanism of action

The antispasmodic agent dicyclomine decreases GI motility by relaxing smooth muscle in the gut.

Hyoscyamine is an anticholinergic agent that decreases GI motility by decreasing smooth muscle tone through antimuscarinic activity in the gut.

Tricyclic antidepressants, such as amitriptyline, delay intestinal transit and may blunt perception of visceral distention. The effect of TCAs on the cerebral processing of visceral pain is unknown.

Tegaserod maleate, a partial 5-HT$_4$ agonist that stimulates the peristaltic reflex and intestinal secretion, inhibits visceral sensitivity by binding to 5-HT$_4$ receptors in the gut.

Lactulose, milk of magnesia, and polyethylene glycol solutions are osmotic laxatives that aid in the treatment of IBS patients with constipation.

Fiber supplements (bulk laxatives) increase stool bulk and water content.

Loperamide inhibits peristalsis by directly affecting the circular and longitudinal muscles of the intestinal wall.

Diphenoxylate is a meperidine congener that directly affects the circular smooth muscle in the gut, which slows GI transit time.

Alosetron is a selective 5-HT$_3$ receptor antagonist that inhibits activation of nonselective cation channels in the gut, thereby modulating the enteric nervous system.

Table 21-4. Selected Medications Used in Irritable Bowel Syndrome

Generic name	Trade name	Classification	Dosage range and frequency	Dosage forms
Dicyclomine	Bentyl	Antispasmodic, anticholinergic	10–20 mg qid prn	T, C, L
Hyoscyamine	Various trade names	Anticholinergic	0.25–0.5 mg bid–qid	T, L
Amitriptyline	Elavil	Tricyclic antidepressant	10–50 mg qhs	T
Paroxetine	Paxil	SSRI	10–60 mg/d	T, L, DT
Tegaserod	Zelnorm	Serotonin (5-HT$_4$) receptor antagonist	6 mg bid	T
Lactulose	Various trade names	Osmotic laxative	30–45 mL bid–qid prn	L
Polycarbophil	Fibercon	Bulking agent	1 g qd–qid prn	T
Polyethylene glycol	Various trade names	Osmotic laxative	250 mL q 10 min up to 4 L	L
Alosetron	Lotronex	Serotonin (5-HT$_3$) receptor antagonist	1 mg qd–bid	T
Lubiprostone	Amitiza	C-2 chloride channel activator	8 mcg bid	C
Loperamide	Imodium	Antidiarrheal	2 mg after each loose stool; maximum 16 mg/d	T, C, L
Diphenoxylate/atropine	Lomotil	Antidiarrheal	15–20 mg/d of diphenoxylate in 3–4 divided doses	T, L

C, capsule; DT, delayed-release tablet; L, liquid; T, tablet.

SSRIs inhibit the neuronal uptake of serotonin in the CNS. Citalopram has peripheral effects on colonic tone and sensitivity. Paroxetine has potent anticholinergic effects.

Lubiprostone is the only C-2 chloride channel activator available. By activating C-2 chloride channels in the gut, lubiprostone increases secretion of saltwater into the intestinal lumen. It is approved only for women with constipation-dependent IBS.

Patient counseling

Antispasmodics and anticholinergic agents are best used on an as-needed basis up to three times per day during acute attacks or before meals when postprandial symptoms are present.

Patients taking a TCA should avoid prolonged exposure to sunlight and avoid concurrent use of CNS depressants.

Tegaserod should be taken 30 minutes before meals and should not be initiated during an acute exacerbation of IBS. It is available only through an emergency investigational drug protocol from the FDA.

Osmotic laxatives should be used on an as-needed basis. Lactulose may be mixed with water or juice to increase palatability. Patients should drink plenty of water.

Patients must be enrolled in the manufacturer's prescribing program to receive alosetron. Patients should not initiate therapy with alosetron if they are currently constipated. Alosetron should be discontinued if no improvement in symptoms is seen after 4 weeks of therapy.

See Chapter 25 on psychiatric disease for a full discussion of SSRIs.

Lubiprostone should be taken with food and water. Softgel capsules should be swallowed whole.

Adverse drug effects

Dicyclomine, hyoscyamine, and TCAs may cause anticholinergic side effects (CNS depression, dry mouth, urinary retention, constipation, and decreased sweating).

Tegaserod may cause diarrhea, nausea, headache, and abdominal pain. It was associated with an increased risk of cardiovascular events in clinical trials.

Osmotic laxatives may cause abdominal pain and cramping.

Alosetron may cause constipation, abdominal pain, and nausea. Intestinal obstruction, perforation, toxic megacolon, ischemic colitis, and death have occurred.

See Chapter 25 on psychiatric disease for a full discussion of SSRIs.

Lubiprostone's most common side effects are nausea, diarrhea, and headache. Allergic reactions and dyspnea within 1 hour of the first dose have also been reported. Though dyspnea may recur with repeated doses, it usually resolves within 3 hours.

Drug interactions

Anticholinergics and antispasmodics may decrease the effectiveness of antipsychotic medications. Side effects from anticholinergics are increased when they are given concurrently with a TCA.

TCA concentrations may be increased or decreased by medications that induce or inhibit the activity of the CYP450 enzyme system in the liver. TCAs should not be given concurrently with monoamine oxidase inhibitors or sympathomimetic agents.

No significant drug interactions with tegaserod have been reported.

Other medications should not be taken within 1 hour of the start of therapy with osmotic laxatives.

The levels of alosetron may be decreased by concurrent administration of rifamycin derivatives.

There are no known drug interactions with lubiprostone.

Monitoring parameters

Patients should monitor for the presence of IBS symptoms and for the side effects of medications, as discussed in the section on adverse drug effects.

Pharmacokinetics

Dicyclomine, hyoscyamine, amitriptyline, paroxetine, tegaserod, alosetron, loperamide, and diphenoxylate/atropine undergo hepatic metabolism.

Lubiprostone is metabolized in the stomach and small intestine.

Nondrug Therapy

An effective physician–patient relationship is necessary for successful treatment. Education should be provided regarding disease pathophysiology and treatment and reassurance that the symptoms are real.

Although evidence supporting exclusion diets is lacking, patients may be counseled to avoid foods that exacerbate IBS symptoms. Foods commonly implicated are fatty foods, beans, gas-producing foods, alcohol, caffeine, lactose (in lactase-deficient individuals), and occasionally excess fiber.

Cognitive behavioral therapy, dynamic psychotherapy, and hypnotherapy are more effective than usual care in relieving global symptoms of IBS. Although the quality of the evidence regarding such therapy is low, the potential benefit outweighs the potential risks.

21-5. Key Points

Peptic Ulcer Disease

- PUD is a group of disorders of the upper GI tract characterized by ulcerative lesions that require acid and pepsin for their formation.
- Duodenal and gastric ulcers are classified as *Helicobacter pylori* related, NSAID related, non–*H. pylori* related, non-NSAID related, or stress related.
- Epigastric pain occurring 1–3 hours after meals that is relieved by ingestion of food or antacids is the classic symptom of PUD.
- *H. pylori* is a gram-negative microaerophilic bacterium inhabiting the area between the mucous layer and epithelial cells in the stomach. It can be found anywhere gastric epithelium is present.
- NSAIDs are the leading cause of PUD in patients who are negative for *H. pylori* infection.
- NSAIDs are directly toxic to gastric epithelium and inhibit the synthesis of prostaglandins.
- The goals of PUD therapy are ulcer healing and eliminating the cause. Additional considerations are prevention of complications and relief of symptoms.
- Upper GI endoscopy is used to diagnose PUD. The procedure is usually reserved for patients with symptoms of PUD who are over 55 years of age or who have alarm symptoms (bleeding, anemia, early satiety, unexplained weight loss, progressive dysphagia, odynophagia, recurrent vomiting, family history of gastrointestinal cancer, or previous esophagogastric cancer).
- Patients with symptoms of PUD who are less than 55 years of age and have no alarm symptoms may be tested for the presence of *H. pylori* and treated with eradication therapy if results are positive.
- Histology and rapid urease testing may be performed on biopsy samples obtained during endoscopy to test for *H. pylori*.
- Serum antibody tests, urea breath tests, and fecal antibody testing do not require endoscopy to test for *H. pylori*.
- The American College of Gastroenterology treatment guidelines for *H. pylori* eradication in PUD recommend initial triple therapy with a PPI, clarithromycin, and either amoxicillin *or* metronidazole for 14 days or quadruple therapy with bismuth, metronidazole, tetracycline, and either an H2RA or a PPI for 10–14 days.
- NSAID-related PUD treatment consists of discontinuing the offending agent and issuing antisecretory therapy for symptom relief.
- Antisecretory therapy with a PPI or an H2RA should be administered for 4 weeks to promote healing and to relieve symptoms.
- Patients with active bleeding who are hemodynamically stable should receive intravenous PPI therapy and undergo endoscopy to evaluate the risk of bleeding recurrence.
- Patients with active bleeding who are hemodynamically unstable should receive intravenous fluids and blood transfusions. They should undergo emergency endoscopy for coagulation of bleeding sites. Various modalities may be used to achieve bleeding-site coagulation.
- Surgery is reserved for patients who have refractory ulcers, recurrent bleeding, or a perforated ulcer.
- Patients should be counseled on the importance of adherence to treatment regimens, proper dosing, and the side effects of medications.
- Patients should be counseled to decrease psychological stress, to discontinue smoking and drinking alcohol, to stop using NSAIDs, and to avoid food or beverages that exacerbate PUD symptoms.

Gastroesophageal Reflux Disease

- GERD is a condition that develops when the reflux of stomach contents causes troublesome symptoms or complications.
- Approximately 20% of the U.S. population experiences heartburn or regurgitation of gastric acid weekly.
- The manifestations of GERD are divided into esophageal and extraesophageal syndromes.
- Esophageal syndromes consist of those that are only symptomatic in nature and those that are symptomatic with esophageal injury on endoscopy. Symptomatic syndromes include the typical reflux syndrome and the reflux chest pain syndrome.
- The typical reflux syndrome is defined by the presence of troublesome heartburn or regurgitation. Patients may also have other symptoms, such as epigastric pain or sleep disturbance.
- The pathophysiology of GERD involves the prolonged contact of esophageal epithelium with

refluxed gastric contents that contain acid and pepsin.

- Esophageal defenses consist of the antireflux barrier, luminal clearance mechanisms, and tissue resistance. Increased contact time of refluxate and esophageal mucosa or impaired defense mechanisms can lead to the symptoms of GERD.

- For patients who present with troublesome symptoms of GERD, a trial of empiric therapy is appropriate. A diagnosis of GERD may be assumed for patients who respond to empiric treatment.

- Diagnostic testing with endoscopy should be performed in patients who present with troublesome GERD symptoms and dysphagia, weight loss, or epigastric mass on physical examination. It should also be performed on patients who do not respond to empiric treatment.

- Goals of therapy are to alleviate or eliminate symptoms, decrease frequency and duration of reflux, promote healing of the injured mucosa, and prevent the development of complications.

- An empiric trial of once-daily PPI therapy is appropriate for patients with troublesome GERD symptoms. If patients do not respond to once-daily therapy, twice-daily therapy may be used.

- Antireflux surgery may be performed when a patient is responsive to, but intolerant of, acid suppressive therapy or has persistent troublesome symptoms of GERD.

- Patients should be counseled on medication dosing and administration, side effects, drug interactions, monitoring of GERD symptoms, and lifestyle modifications.

- Lifestyle modifications alone are unlikely to control GERD symptoms. Lifestyle modifications should be tailored to the circumstances of the individual patient.

- GERD is considered a chronic condition, and most patients will require chronic therapy with antisecretory agents. Antisecretory therapy should be titrated to the lowest effective dose.

Inflammatory Bowel Disease

- Idiopathic IBD is divided into two major types: (1) ulcerative colitis and (2) Crohn's disease.
- UC is a mucosal inflammatory condition confined to the rectum and colon.
- CD is a transmural inflammation of the GI tract that can affect any part (mouth to anus).
- The hallmark clinical symptom of UC is bloody diarrhea, often with rectal urgency and tenesmus.

- Clinical symptoms are categorized as mild, moderate, or severe. Endoscopic findings are categorized as distal (limited to below the splenic flexure) or extensive (extending proximal to the splenic flexure).

- Typical symptoms of CD include chronic or nocturnal diarrhea and abdominal pain. Additional typical symptoms include weight loss, fever, and rectal bleeding.

- Symptoms differ depending on the site of inflammation and are categorized as mild, moderate, or severe.

- The etiology of IBD is unclear, but similar factors may contribute to both UC and CD. The diagnosis of IBD is made on the basis of negative stool evaluation for infectious causes.

- Treatment of IBD involves medications that target inflammatory mediators and alter immunoinflammatory processes. These medications include anti-inflammatory agents, immunosuppressive agents, and biologic agents.

- Goals of therapy for UC and CD include inducing and maintaining remission of symptoms, improving quality of life, resolving complications and systemic symptoms, and preventing future complications.

- Patients should be counseled on medication dosing and administration, side effects, drug interactions, monitoring of IBD symptoms, and proper nutrition.

- Patients with IBD are often malnourished because of malabsorption or maldigestion caused by chronic bowel inflammation, "short gut" syndrome from multiple bowel surgeries, or bile salt deficiency in the gut.

- Surgery may be necessary for patients with severe UC or CD. Surgery (proctocolectomy) is curative for UC but not for CD.

Irritable Bowel Syndrome

- IBS is abdominal pain or discomfort that occurs in association with altered bowel habits over a period of 3 months.
- IBS is a prevalent and expensive condition. It significantly impairs health-related quality of life and leads to reduced work productivity.
- IBS is a heterogeneous disorder with various clinical presentations. Common symptoms include abdominal pain, diarrhea, and constipation.
- The pathogenesis is multifactorial, including abnormal gut sensorimotor activity, CNS dysfunction, psychological disturbances, genetic

predisposition, enteric infection, and other luminal factors.

- No symptom-based diagnostic criteria have ideal accuracy for diagnosing IBS. Traditional criteria (Kruis, Manning) are at least as accurate as the more recent Rome I criteria. Rome II and III criteria have been proposed, but their accuracy has not been evaluated.

- Alarm features include rectal bleeding, weight loss, iron-deficiency anemia, nocturnal symptoms, family history of colorectal cancer, IBD, or celiac sprue. These symptoms may indicate the presence of an organic disease.

- Treatment should be offered to patients seeking medical care if the patient and physician believe that the IBS symptoms decrease the patient's quality of life.

- Goals of therapy include improving IBS symptoms and patient quality of life.

- Anticholinergic and antimuscarinic agents provide short-term relief of abdominal pain and discomfort. Psyllium has been shown to be moderately effective for IBS. Calcium polycarbophil was shown to improve symptoms in one small study. Polyethylene glycol was shown to improve stool frequency. Loperamide decreases stool frequency in patients with diarrhea-predominant IBS. TCAs improve abdominal pain in IBS patients. SSRIs are recommended for patients with moderate to severe abdominal pain or psychiatric comorbidities. Tegaserod improves global IBS symptoms, bloating, abdominal pain, and altered bowel habits in patients with constipation-predominant IBS. Alosetron improves global IBS symptoms, abdominal discomfort, stool consistency, and stool frequency in women with diarrhea-predominant IBS. Lubiprostone has been shown to relieve global IBS symptoms in women with constipation-predominant IBS.

- Patients should be counseled on medication dosing and administration, side effects, drug interactions, and monitoring of IBS symptoms.

- An effective physician–patient relationship is necessary for successful treatment.

- Education regarding disease pathophysiology and treatment, and reassurance that the symptoms are real should be provided.

- Patients should be counseled to avoid foods that exacerbate symptoms.

- Cognitive behavioral therapy, dynamic psychotherapy, and hypnotherapy are more effective than usual care in relieving global symptoms of IBS.

21-6. Questions

1. H. B. is a 59-year-old black male recently diagnosed with PUD on endoscopy. Tissue biopsy is positive for *H. pylori*. H. B. has no known drug allergies. Which of the following is the ideal therapeutic regimen for *H. pylori*–related PUD in H. B.?

   A. PPI, clarithromycin, amoxicillin
   B. PPI, bismuth, metronidazole, tetracycline
   C. Omeprazole, amoxicillin
   D. Omeprazole, bismuth, clarithromycin, furazolidone
   E. Omeprazole, sucralfate, clarithromycin, furazolidone

2. If H. B. were allergic to penicillin, which treatment recommendation would you choose?

   A. PPI, clarithromycin, amoxicillin
   B. PPI, bismuth, metronidazole, tetracycline
   C. Omeprazole, metronidazole
   D. Clarithromycin, metronidazole, tetracycline
   E. Clarithromycin, metronidazole, furazolidone

3. Which one of the following is the leading cause of PUD in *H. pylori*–negative patients?

   A. Mineralocorticoids
   B. NSAIDs
   C. DMARDs
   D. Antibiotics
   E. Corticosteroids

4. Which of the following are true of NSAIDs?

   I. They inhibit production of prostaglandins.
   II. They are directly toxic to gastroduodenal epithelium.
   III. They require dose adjustments in renal insufficiency.
   IV. They cause only gastric ulcers.
   V. They allow healing of PUD during continued therapy.

   A. I, II, and III only
   B. I and III only
   C. II and IV only
   D. V only
   E. All are correct.

5. Which of the following are goals of therapy for PUD?

    I.   Reduce episodes of diarrhea.
    II. Eliminate symptoms.
    III. Reduce risk of gastric cancer.
    IV. Heal ulcerations.
    V.   Avoid spreading *H. pylori*.

    A. I, II, and III only
    B. I and III only
    C. II and IV only
    D. V only
    E. All are correct.

6. Which of the following tests do *not* require endoscopy to test for *H. pylori* infection?

    I.   Serum antibody test
    II. Fecal antigen test
    III. Urea breath test
    IV. Histology test
    V.   Rapid urease test

    A. I, II, and III only
    B. I and III only
    C. II and IV only
    D. V only
    E. All are correct.

7. A. B. is a 45-year-old white female with a past medical history significant only for seizure disorder. She has experienced heartburn after meals intermittently for the past 2 weeks. It becomes worse when she is reclining at bed-time. Her medications include phenytoin 300 mg hs. A. B. says her symptoms are not troublesome and she is going to self-treat with over-the-counter medications. Which one of the following should *not* be recom-mended to A. B.?

    A. Aluminum hydroxide
    B. Cimetidine
    C. Famotidine
    D. Ranitidine
    E. Magnesium hydroxide

8. A. B.'s symptoms are not relieved after 2 weeks of OTC treatment with famotidine and lifestyle modifications. A. B. states her symptoms are becoming "troublesome." Which of the fol-lowing is the best choice?

    A. Add the prokinetic agent metoclopramide to famotidine.

    B. Endoscopy should be performed because A. B. has symptoms suggestive of compli-cations from GERD.
    C. Add alginic acid 2 tablets qhs to famotidine.
    D. Discontinue current therapy and initiate therapy with omeprazole 20 mg daily.
    E. Continue famotidine for 1 more week to achieve maximum effectiveness.

9. Which of the following are the most common symptoms of esophageal GERD syndromes?

    I.   Heartburn
    II. Belching
    III. Regurgitation
    IV. Hypersalivation
    V.   Hoarseness

    A. I, II, and III only
    B. I and III only
    C. II and IV only
    D. V only
    E. All are correct.

10. Which of the following diagnoses carries an increased risk for developing esophageal adenocarcinoma?

    I.   Typical reflux syndrome
    II. Reflux cough syndrome
    III. Reflux laryngitis
    IV. Nontroublesome symptoms of GERD
    V.   Barrett's esophagus

    A. I, II, and III only
    B. I and III only
    C. II and IV only
    D. V only
    E. All are correct.

11. Which of the following may exacerbate GERD symptoms by lowering the LES pressure?

    A. Quinidine
    B. Iron
    C. Potassium chloride
    D. Diltiazem
    E. Tetracycline

12. Which of the following is the best choice for the initial treatment of troublesome symptoms of the typical reflux syndrome?

    A. Nizatidine 75 mg qd
    B. Pantoprazole 40 mg qd
    C. Metoclopramide 10 mg qid

D. A 3-month trial of lifestyle modifications

E. Pantoprazole 40 mg qd with metoclopramide 10 mg qid

13. A. Y. is a 32-year-old white male who presents with bloody diarrhea (less than four stools per day) for 2 days. Complete blood counts and ESR are normal. Physical exam is normal. Colonoscopy reveals distal colitis. Which of the following is the best choice for initial therapy for A. Y.?

A. Prednisone 40 mg po qd

B. Sulfasalazine 4–6 g po qd

C. Mesalamine 1–4 g PR qhs

D. Mesalamine 4–6 g po qd

E. Methylprednisolone 16 mg IV q8h

14. A. Y. continues to have bloody diarrhea (without systemic disturbances). Which one of the following is the best choice?

A. Add prednisone 40 mg po qd and discontinue enema.

B. Add mesalamine 2–4 g po qd and continue enema.

C. Add methylprednisolone 16 mg IV q8h until remission is achieved.

D. Add mesalamine 2–4 g po qd and discontinue enema.

E. Add azathioprine 1.0–2.5 mg/kg per day and discontinue enema.

15. Which of the following are true for UC?

I. Aminosalicylates are the drugs of choice for maintenance therapy.

II. Oral corticosteroids are the drugs of choice for maintenance therapy.

III. Azathioprine often allows reduction in corticosteroid dose.

IV. Topical aminosalicylates are the drugs of choice for severe or fulminant disease.

V. Ciprofloxacin is alternative first-line therapy for mild to moderate disease.

A. I, II, and III only

B. I and III only

C. II and IV only

D. V only

E. All are correct.

16. Which of the following is true for CD?

I. Infliximab is the drug of choice for mild to moderate disease.

II. Oral corticosteroids are the drugs of choice for maintenance therapy.

III. Topical aminosalicylates are the drugs of choice for mild to moderate disease.

IV. Oral cyclosporine is the drug of choice for maintenance therapy.

V. Budesonide should be used as initial therapy for CD of the ileum and right colon.

A. I, II, and III only

B. I and III only

C. II and IV only

D. V only

E. All are correct.

17. Which of the following is true for moderate to severe CD?

A. Azathioprine is the drug of choice for initial therapy.

B. Budesonide is appropriate maintenance therapy.

C. Oral corticosteroids are the drugs of choice for initial therapy.

D. Methotrexate has no role in CD therapy.

E. Topical aminosalicylates are appropriate maintenance therapy.

18. Which of the following is associated with the development of progressive multifocal leukoencephalopathy?

A. Prednisone

B. Sulfasalazine

C. Mesalamine

D. Methotrexate

E. Natalizumab

19. J. J. is a 39-year-old female who presents with mild abdominal pain and diarrhea for 12 weeks. J. J. has no significant past medical history and occasionally misses days from her full-time job. Her symptoms are worse after meals. Which of the following is the best choice for initial therapy?

I. Paroxetine 10 mg qd

II. Amitriptyline 10 mg hs

III. Tegaserod 6 mg bid

IV. Alosetron 1 mg qd

V. Dicyclomine 10 mg qid after meals

A. I, II, and III only

B. I and III only

C. II and IV only

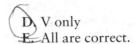

D. V only
E. All are correct.

20. J. J.'s symptoms are controlled for several months until she loses her job. Her abdominal pain then returns. She has five episodes of diarrhea per day and complains of fatigue and insomnia. Which of the following are the most appropriate for J. J.?

    I.   Initiate psychological counseling.
    II. Prescribe amitriptyline 10–50 mg hs.
    III. Add loperamide 2 mg after each loose stool (16 mg/d maximum).
    IV. Add alosetron 1 mg qd.
    V.   Start tegaserod 6 mg bid.

    A. I, II, and III only
    B. I and II only
    C. II and IV only
    D. V only
    E. All are correct.

21. Which of the following is indicated for constipation-predominant IBS?

    A. Tegaserod 6 mg bid
    B. Alosetron 1 mg bid
    C. Loperamide 2–16 mg/d
    D. Paroxetine 10–40 mg qd
    E. Diphenoxylate + atropine 2 tabs qid

22. Which of the following is affected by medications that induce or inhibit the cytochrome P450 enzyme system?

    A. Tegaserod
    B. Alosetron
    C. Fibercon
    D. Polyethylene glycol
    E. Amitriptyline

23. Which life-threatening complication caused the restriction of alosetron?

    A. Stevens–Johnson syndrome
    B. Toxic epidermal necrolysis
    C. Aplastic anemia
    D. Ischemic colitis
    E. Chronic diarrhea

24. Alosetron is indicated for which group of IBS patients?

    A. Women with diarrhea-predominant IBS
    B. Men with diarrhea-predominant IBS
    C. Women with constipation-predominant IBS
    D. Men with constipation-predominant IBS
    E. Children with diarrhea-predominant IBS

21-7. Answers

1. **A.** Triple-drug therapy with a PPI, clarithromycin, and amoxicillin is recommended by the American Gastroenterological Association as initial therapy for *H. pylori*. Quadruple therapy with a bismuth-based regimen is less convenient but may be used first line in patients who are penicillin allergic. Two-drug regimens are less effective and are not recommended. Furazolidone is unavailable in the United States.

2. **B.** The patient is allergic to penicillin; therefore, amoxicillin cannot be used. Two-drug regimens are less effective and not recommended. Antisecretory therapy is an integral part of *H. pylori* regimens to promote ulcer healing. Furazolidone is unavailable in the United States.

3. **B.** NSAIDs are the leading cause of PUD in patients who are negative for *H. pylori* infection.

4. **A.** NSAIDs inhibit production of prostaglandins and are directly toxic to gastroduodenal epithelium. NSAIDs require dose adjustments in renal insufficiency. NSAIDs may cause gastric or duodenal ulcers and must be discontinued to allow for ulcer healing.

5. **C.** Elimination of symptoms and healing of ulcerations are goals of therapy for PUD.

6. **A.** The serum antibody test, fecal antigen test, and urea breath test do not require endoscopy.

7. **B.** Cimetidine is a potent inhibitor of the cytochrome P450 enzyme system and will increase serum concentrations of phenytoin in A. B.

8. **D.** Prokinetic agents are useful mainly in patients with concurrent gastric motility disorders and are not routinely recommended. A. B. does not currently exhibit symptoms of GERD complications. Alginic acid is ineffective when the patient is lying in the supine position and should not be given at bedtime. Nonprescription medications for GERD should be discontinued if symptoms are not relieved after a 2-week trial.

9. **B.** Heartburn and regurgitation are the most common symptoms of the typical reflux syndrome.

10. **D.** Patients with Barrett's esophagus have an increased risk of developing esophageal adenocarcinoma.

11. **D.** Calcium channel blockers decrease LES pressure. Quinidine, iron, potassium chloride, and tetracycline have direct irritant effects on the esophageal mucosa.

12. **B.** The correct dose of nizatidine (prescription strength) would be 150 mg bid. Metoclopramide is not routinely recommended for the treatment of the typical reflux syndrome. When patients find their symptoms "troublesome," pharmacologic therapy should be initiated.

13. **C.** Topical aminosalicylates (answer C) are more effective than oral aminosalicylates (answer B) and topical steroids for mild distal UC (although oral aminosalicylates or topical steroids may be used first line if the patient prefers). Oral and IV steroids (answers A and E) are reserved for more severe cases of UC or cases that do not respond to oral and topical aminosalicylates. The oral dose of mesalamine in answer D is incorrect.

14. **B.** Oral aminosalicylates should be added if no response is achieved with topical aminosalicylates. Oral and IV steroids are reserved for moderate to severe UC or for patients with systemic disturbances. Azathioprine may be added if UC is refractory to aminosalicylates and to allow corticosteroid dose reduction.

15. **B.** Aminosalicylates are the drugs of choice for maintenance therapy of UC, not corticosteroids. Azathioprine often allows a reduction in dose of corticosteroids in the management of active UC. Severe or fulminant UC requires oral, not topical, therapy. Ciprofloxacin may be used as an alternative first-line therapy in the treatment of mild to moderate CD, not UC.

16. **D.** Budesonide is the treatment of choice for mild to moderate CD of the ileum and right colon. Infliximab is reserved for moderate to severe disease in patients who do not respond to oral corticosteroids or immunosuppressive agents. It may also be used in patients in whom side effects from oral corticosteroids must be avoided. Oral corticosteroids should not be used for long-term maintenance therapy. Oral budesonide is the drug of choice for mild to moderate CD, not topical corticosteroids. Oral cyclosporine has no role in CD; IV cyclosporine may be used in severe or fulminant CD that does not respond to 5–7 days of IV corticosteroids.

17. **C.** Moderate to severe disease initially requires oral corticosteroid therapy. Corticosteroids have no role in maintenance therapy. Topical aminosalicylates may be used as adjuncts in colonic CD. Methotrexate is used as maintenance therapy for moderate to severe CD.

18. **E.** Natalizumab has been associated with the development of progressive multifocal leukoencephalopathy.

19. **D.** J. J. has mild, diarrhea-predominant IBS. Symptomatic treatment with dicyclomine is appropriate initial therapy, especially since her symptoms are meal related. A TCA may be added to dicyclomine if needed. Tegaserod is indicated for constipation-predominant IBS. Alosetron is reserved for patients with severe, diarrhea-predominant disease who have failed other therapies. Paroxetine may be added if initial therapies are ineffective or if J. J. develops severe abdominal pain or psychiatric comorbidities.

20. **A.** Alosetron is reserved for patients with severe, diarrhea-predominant disease who have failed other therapies. Several types of psychotherapy have been shown to be more effective than usual care in IBS. TCAs improve abdominal pain in IBS and may also help with insomnia. Loperamide may be used on an as-needed basis for diarrhea. Tegaserod is indicated for constipation-predominant IBS.

21. **A.** Alosetron is approved for restricted use in diarrhea-predominant IBS. Loperamide and diphenoxylate + atropine are antidiarrheal medications that will exacerbate constipation. Paroxetine is an SSRI with potent anticholinergic effects, which could worsen constipation. Another drug should be chosen if an SSRI is needed for depression.

22. **E.** TCA serum concentrations are affected by drugs that alter cytochrome P450 activity.

23. **D.** Severe constipation, ischemic colitis, and death have been reported with alosetron.

24. **A.** Alosetron is approved for women with diarrhea-predominant IBS. It was not found to be effective in men and is not approved for use in children.

21-8. References

Peptic Ulcer Disease

Berardi RR, Welage LS. Peptic ulcer disease. In: Dipiro JT, Talbert RL, Yee GC, et al., eds. *Pharmacotherapy: A Pathophysiologic Approach.* 7th ed. New York: McGraw-Hill; 2008:569–87.

Chey WD, Wong BC. American College of Gastroenterology guideline on the management of

Helicobacter pylori infection. *Am J Gastroenterol.* 2007; 102:1808–25.

Del Valle, J. Peptic ulcer disease and related disorders. In: Fauci AS, Braunwald E, Kasper DL, et al., eds. *Harrison's Principles of Internal Medicine.* 17th ed. New York: McGraw-Hill; 2008.

Malfertheiner P, Megraud F, O'Morain C, et al. Current concepts in the management of *Helicobacter pylori* infection: The Maastricht III Consensus Report. *Gut.* 2007;56:772–81.

NIH Consensus Conference. *Helicobacter pylori* in peptic ulcer diseases: NIH Consensus Development Panel on Helicobacter Pylori in Peptic Ulcer Disease. *JAMA.* 1994;272:65–69.

Ramakrishnan K, Salinas RC. Peptic ulcer disease. *Am Fam Physician.* 2007;76:1005–12.

Rokkas T, Sechopoulos P, Robotis I, et al. Cumulative *H. pylori* eradication rates in clinical practice by adopting first- and second-line regimens proposed by the Maastrict III consensus and a third-line empirical regimen. *Am J Gastroenterol.* 2009;104: 21–25.

Shiotani A, Graham DY. Pathogenesis and therapy of gastric and duodenal ulcer disease. *Med Clin North Am.* 2002;86:1447–66.

Singh G, Triadafilopoulos G. Epidemiology of NSAID-induced GI complications. *J Rheumatol.* 1999; 26(suppl 26):18–24.

Vakil, N. *H. pylori* treatment: New wine in old bottles? *Am J Gastroenterol.* 2009;104:26–30.

Wolfe MM, Lichtenstein DR, Singh G. Gastrointestinal toxicity of nonsteroidal anti-inflammatory drugs. *N Engl J Med.* 1999;340:1888–89.

Gastroesophageal Reflux Disease

Cappell MS. Clinical presentation, diagnosis, and management of gastroesophageal reflux disease. *Med Clin North Am.* 2005;89:243–91.

DeVault KR, Castell DO. Updated guidelines for the diagnosis and treatment of gastroesophageal reflux disease. *Am J Gastroenterol.* 2005;100:190–200.

Goyal RK. Diseases of the esophagus. In: Fauci AS, Braunwald E, Kasper DL, et al., eds. *Harrison's Principles of Internal Medicine.* 17th ed. New York: McGraw-Hill; 2008.

Kahrilas PJ, Shaheen NJ, Vaezi MF. American Gastroenterological Association institute technical review on the management of gastroesophageal reflux disease. *Gastroenterol.* 2008;135:1392–413.

Kahrilas PJ, Shaheen NJ, Vaezi MF, et al. American Gastroenterological Association medical position statement on the management of gastroesophageal reflux disease. *Gastroenterol.* 2008;135:1383–91.

Locke GR, Talley NH, Fett SL, et al. Prevalence and clinical spectrum of gastroesophageal reflux: A population-based study in Olmstead county. *Gastroenterol.* 1997;112:1448–56.

Vakil N, van Zanten SV, Kahrilas P, et al. The Montreal definition and classification of gastroesophageal reflux disease: A global, evidence-based consensus. *Am J Gastroenterol.* 2006;101:1900–20.

Williams DB, Schade RR. Gastroesophageal reflux disease. In: Dipiro JT, Talbert RL, Yee GC, et al., eds. *Pharmacotherapy: A Pathophysiologic Approach.* 7th ed. New York: McGraw-Hill; 2008:555–67.

Inflammatory Bowel Disease

Ardizzone S, Porro GB. Inflammatory bowel disease: New insights into pathogenesis and treatment. *J Intern Med.* 2002;252:475–96.

Banerjee S, Peppercorn MA. Inflammatory bowel disease: Medical therapy for specific clinical presentations. *Gastroenterol Clin North Am.* 2002; 31:185–202.

Drug therapy for ulcerative colitis. *Pharmacist's/ Prescriber's Letter.* 2007;23:230308.

Friedman S, Blumberg RS. Inflammatory bowel disease. In: Fauci AS, Braunwald E, Kasper DL, et al., eds. *Harrison's Principles of Internal Medicine.* 17th ed. New York: McGraw-Hill; 2008.

Hemstreet BA, DiPiro JT. Inflammatory bowel disease. In: Dipiro JT, Talbert RL, Yee GC, et al., eds. *Pharmacotherapy: A Pathophysiologic Approach.* 7th ed. New York: McGraw-Hill; 2008:589–605.

Kornbluth A, Sachar DB. Ulcerative colitis practice guidelines in adults (update): American College of Gastroenterology, Practice Parameters Committee. *Am J Gastroenterol.* 2004;99:1371–85.

Lichtenstein GR, Hanauer SB, Sandborn WJ, et al. Management of Crohn's disease in adults: American College of Gastroenterology Practice guidelines. *Am J Gastroenterol.* 2009;104:465–83.

Rutgeerts P, Vermeire S, Van Assche, G. Biological therapies for inflammatory bowel diseases. *Gastroenterol.* 2009;136:1182–97.

Irritable Bowel Syndrome

Brandt LJ, Chey WD, Foxx-Orenstein AE, et al. An evidence-based position statement on the management of irritable bowel syndrome. *Am J Gastroenterol.* 2009;104(suppl 1): S1–7.

Brandt LJ, Chey WD, Foxx-Orenstein AE, et al. An evidence-based systematic review on the management of irritable bowel syndrome. *Am J Gastroenterol.* 2009;104(suppl 1):S8–S35.

Drossman DA, Camilleri M, Mayer EA, Whitehead WE. AGA technical review on irritable bowel syndrome. *Gastroenterol.* 2002;123:2108–31.

Owyang C. Irritable bowel syndrome. In: Fauci AS, Braunwald E, Kasper DL, et al., eds. *Harrison's Principles of Internal Medicine.* 17th ed. New York: McGraw-Hill; 2008.

Palsson OS, Drossman DA. Psychiatric and psychological dysfunction in irritable bowel syndrome and the role of psychological treatments. *Gastroenterol Clin North Am.* 2005;34:281–303.

Spruill WJ, Wade WE. Diarrhea, constipation, and irritable bowel syndrome. In: Dipiro JT, Talbert RL, Yee GC, et al., eds. *Pharmacotherapy: A Pathophysiologic Approach.* 7th ed. New York: McGraw-Hill; 2008:617–32.

Rheumatoid Arthritis, Osteoarthritis, Gout, and Lupus

Kevin L. Freeman, PharmD, BCNSP

22-1. Rheumatoid Arthritis

Rheumatoid arthritis (RA) is a highly variable, chronic autoimmune disorder of unknown etiology characterized by symmetric, erosive synovitis. Manifestations may extend to extra-articular sites.

Incidence

RA affects 1% of the population and is two to three times more common in women than in men. It has a peak incidence in women between 30 and 60 years of age. Certain families, monozygotic twins, and people with specific HLA (human leukocyte antigen) genetic markers have a greater incidence of RA, which suggests a genetic predisposition.

Clinical Presentation

The onset of RA is unpredictable and varies from rapid to insidious progression. The course of the disease is likewise variable: 10–20% of patients have a short course with remission, 70–80% have mild to moderate disease with cyclic exacerbations, and 10–20% develop progressively destructive disease.

RA usually affects diarthrodial joints such as the proximal interphalangeal (PIP) joints, metacarpophalangeal (MCP) joints, metatarsophalangeal (MTP) joints, wrists, and ankles. Also commonly involved are the elbows, shoulders, sternoclavicular joints, temporomandibular joints, hips, and knees.

The initial complaints may include generalized fatigue and multiple joint pain.

Morning stiffness is a hallmark of RA. Patients describe it as a gel-like sensation in the joints that occurs after attempting to move upon awakening.

Ulnar deviation, swan-neck deformities, boutonnière deformities, hammertoe formation, and ankylosis are common irreversible joint abnormalities that occur in RA.

The extra-articular features that occur in RA include rheumatoid nodules, vasculitis, anemia, thrombocytopenia, Felty's syndrome, and Sjögren's syndrome.

Etiology

The cause of RA remains a mystery. Factors that may be responsible are of environmental, genetic, endocrinologic, gastrointestinal, atmospheric, and infectious origin.

RA is widely held to have a strong genetic component. This assertion is supported by the fact that a greater prevalence of RA is found in patients with the major histocompatibility complex antigen HLA-DR4. This class II antigen is expressed on the surface of helper T-lymphocytes and macrophages. In combination with environmental factors, an inappropriate immune response may occur, resulting in chronic inflammation.

Patients with RA have been demonstrated to have increased antibody titers to *Mycobacterium tuberculosis, Proteus mirabilis, Escherichia coli, Klebsiella pneumoniae,* normal human gut flora antigen, Epstein–Barr virus, and the superantigen staphylococcal enterotoxin B.

Female patients are at greater risk of RA after breast-feeding, which supports the theory that endocrinologic risk factors are involved.

Gastrointestinal (GI) factors may be responsible for hyperactivity of the immune system—that is, antibodies to enteric organisms and gluten develop in the GI tract.

Atmospheric changes are associated with symptomatic changes in the disease course.

Pathophysiology

Because of causes still unknown, the body's immune system (starting with macrophages) attacks the cells within the joint capsule, thereby causing synovitis (as indicated by the warmth, swelling, redness, and pain associated with RA). Specifically, helper T-lymphocytes stimulate B-cells to attack antigen (in this case, the body's own collagen). In addition, helper T-lymphocytes release cytokines (interleukins and tumor necrosis factor, or TNF), which cause further inflammation and injury in the joints. During the inflammatory process, the cells of the synovium grow and divide abnormally, causing a normally thin synovium to become thick (pannus). These abnormal synovial cells begin to invade and destroy the cartilage and bone within the joint. These effects are responsible for the pain and deformities seen in patients with RA.

Diagnostic Criteria

Patients meeting four of the following criteria are classified as having RA:

- Morning stiffness of or near joints lasting 1 hour before maximum improvement. This condition must be present for at least 6 weeks.
- Three or more joint areas, including the right or left PIP joint, MCP joint, wrist, elbow, MTP joint, ankle, or knee, must have arthritis, as demonstrated by soft tissue swelling or fluid. This condition must be present for at least 6 weeks and observed by a physician.
- Arthritis, as demonstrated by soft tissue swelling or fluid in the hand joints (MCP, PIP, or wrist), must be present for at least 6 weeks and observed by a physician.
- Symmetric arthritis must occur in the areas noted in the second criterion. This condition must be present for at least 6 weeks and observed by a physician.
- Subcutaneous nodules (rheumatoid nodules) over bony prominences, extensor surfaces, or in juxta-articular regions must be present.
- Positive rheumatoid factor (antibodies that collect in the synovium of the joint) must be present, as demonstrated by a positive test in less than 5% of normal subjects.
- Radiologic changes of the hands or wrists (e.g., erosions or bone decalcification in or next to involved joints) must be present.

Treatment Goals

According to the American College of Rheumatology (ACR), the goals in managing RA are to prevent or control joint damage, prevent loss of function, and decrease pain.

Monitoring

At each visit, the patient should be evaluated for subjective evidence of active disease on the basis of the following criteria:

- Degree of joint pain
- Duration of morning stiffness
- Duration of fatigue
- Presence of actively inflamed joints on examination
- Limitation of function

Periodically, the patient should be evaluated for disease activity or progression:

- Evidence of disease progression on physical examination (loss of motion, instability, malalignment, deformity)
- Erythrocyte sedimentation rate or C-reactive protein elevation
- Progression of radiographic damage of involved joints

Other parameters for assessing response to treatment (outcomes):

- Physician's global assessment of disease activity
- Patient's global assessment of disease activity
- Functional status or quality-of-life assessment using standardized questionnaires

The majority of clinical studies use a benchmark of 20% improvement in the preceding criteria, also known as ACR 20.

Drug Therapy

Aggressive use of disease-modifying antirheumatic drugs (DMARDs) is suggested (Table 22-1).

The ACR recommendations focus on the use of biologic and nonbiologic therapies for the treatment of RA. The use of nonmedical therapies and anti-inflammatory drugs as well as other analgesics is still a part of the optimal treatment regimen; however, it was not evaluated as part of the 2008 recommendations (Figures 22-1 and 22-2).

The 2008 ACR recommendations for the initiation or reinstitution of biologic and nonbiologic therapies depend on three factors:

Table 22-1. Disease-Modifying Antirheumatic Drugs

Generic name	Trade name	Dosage range	Administration schedule	Dosage forms
Nonbiologic				
Hydroxychloroquine	Plaquenil	200–400 mg	1–2 doses per day	po
Sulfasalazine	Azulfidine	2,000–4,000 mg	2–3 doses per day	po
Methotrexate	Rheumatrex	7.5–25.0 mg	Once weekly	po, IM, SC, IV
Gold sodium thiomalate	Myochrysine	25–50 mg	Every 2–4 weeks	IM
Auranofin	Ridaura	3–6 mg	1–2 doses per day	po
Azathioprine	Imuran	50–150 mg	1–2 doses per day	po, IV
Penicillamine	Cuprimine	250–750 mg	2–3 doses per day	po
Minocycline	Minocin	100–200 mg	2 doses per day	po
Leflunomide	Arava	10–20 mg	1–2 doses per day	po
Biologic				
Etanercept	Enbrel	25 mg	Twice weekly or 50 mg once weekly	SC
Infliximab	Remicade	3 mg/kg	Weeks 0, 2, and 6, then every 8 weeks	IV
Anakinra	Kineret	100 mg	1 dose per day	SC
Adalimumab	Humira	40 mg	Every other week	SC
Abatacept	Orencia	< 60 kg = 500 mg; 60–100 kg = 750 mg; > 100 kg = 1,000 mg	Weeks 0, 2, and 4, then every 4 weeks	IV
Rituximab		1,000 mg IV	Every 2 weeks for two doses	IV

- Disease duration:
  - Early (< 6 months)
  - Intermediate (6–24 months)
  - Long or longer (> 24 months)
- Disease activity:
  - Available indices:
    - Disease Activity Score in 28 Joints
    - Simplified Disease Activity Index
    - Clinical Disease Activity Index
  - Mild disease: typically fewer than six inflamed joints, no extra-articular disease, and no radiographic evidence of erosions
  - Severe disease: typically more than 20 inflamed joints, elevation in C-reactive protein, and positive rheumatoid factor, extra-articular disease, or both
- Prognostic factors:
  - Physical examination, health questionnaire, and laboratory analysis
  - Poor prognosis: functional limitation, extra-articular disease, elevated rheumatoid factor or anti-cyclic citrullinated peptide (CCP) antibodies (anti-CCP may be more specific than rheumatoid factor)

Nonsteroidal anti-inflammatory drugs

Salicylates, nonsteroidal anti-inflammatory drugs (NSAIDs), and selective cyclooxygenase-2 (COX-2) inhibitors are agents with analgesic and anti-inflammatory properties useful in the management of RA. These agents reduce joint pain and swelling; however, they do not inhibit joint destruction or otherwise alter the course of the disease. For this reason, they should not be considered as a sole treatment option. These agents act by inhibiting prostaglandin synthesis and release. Cyclooxygenase is present in many cells, including platelets, endothelial cells, and cells of the gastric and intestinal mucosa. The initial choice of agent is based on the efficacy, safety, cost, and convenience for any given patient. A wide range of interpatient variability exists with regard to clinical effect; several NSAIDs may need to be tried before achieving patient satisfaction. See Table 22-2.

Aspirin

Mechanism of action

Aspirin prevents prostaglandin formation by inhibiting the action of the enzyme cyclooxygenase. The

Figure 22-1. Nonbiologic DMARD Use

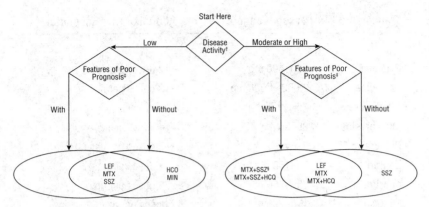

A = disease duration < 6 months

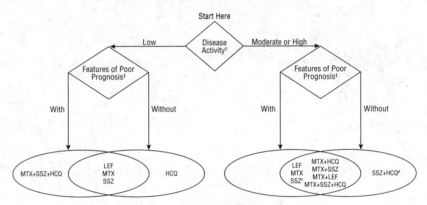

B = disease duration 6–24 months

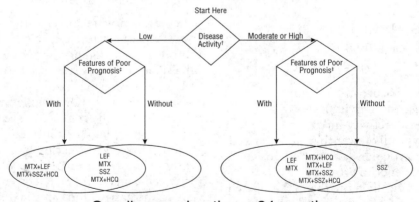

C = disease duration > 24 months

Note: DMARD, disease-modifying antirheumatic drug; HCQ, hydroxychloroquine; LEF, leflunomide; MTX, methotrexate; SSZ, sulfasalazine; MIN, minocycline; †, see text; ‡, includes functional limitation (defined using standard measurement scales such as Health Assessment Questionnaire score or variations of this scale), extra-articular disease (presence of rheumatoid nodules, secondary Sjögren's syndrome, RA vasculitis, Felty's syndrome, and RA lung disease), rheumatoid factor positivity, positive anticyclic citrullinated peptide antibodies, or bony erosions by radiography; §, patients with high disease activity and poor prognosis; ǁ, patients with moderate disease activity and high disease activity without features of poor prognosis; #, patients with high disease activity without features of poor prognosis.

Source: Reprinted with permission from American College of Rheumatology. Recommendations for the use of nonbiologic and biologic disease-modifying antirheumatic drugs in rheumatoid arthritis. *Arthritis Rheum.* 2008;59:762–84.

Figure 22-2. Biological DMARD Use

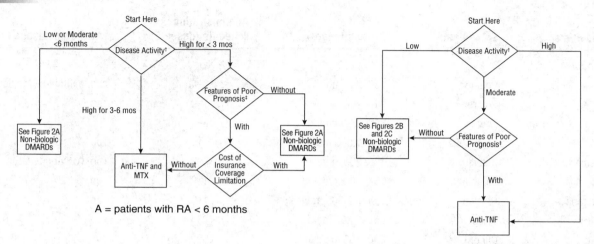

A = patients with RA < 6 months

B = patients with RA > 6 months who failed prior methotrexate therapy

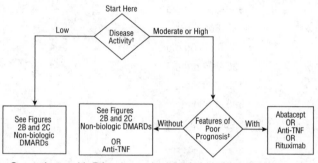

C = patients with RA > 6 months who failed prior methotrexate combination therapy or after administration of alternative DMARDs

Note: DMARD, disease-modifying antirheumatic drug; MTX, methotrexate; SSZ, sulfasalazine; TNF, tumor necrosis factor; †, see text; ‡, includes functional limitation (defined using standard measurement scales such as Health Assessment Questionnaire score or variations of this scale), extra-articular disease (presence of rheumatoid nodules, secondary Sjögren's syndrome, RA vasculitis, Felty's syndrome, and RA lung disease), rheumatoid factor positivity, positive anticyclic citrullinated peptide antibodies, or bony erosions by radiography; §, patients with high disease activity and poor prognosis; ‖, patients with moderate disease activity and high disease activity without features of poor prognosis; #, patients with high disease activity without features of poor prognosis.

Source: Reprinted with permission from American College of Rheumatology. Recommendations for the Use of Nonbiologic and Biologic Disease-Modifying Antirheumatic Drugs in Rheumatoid Arthritis. *Arthritis Rheum.* 2008;59:762–84.

antithrombotic effect of aspirin occurs by an irreversible inhibition of platelet cyclooxygenase. This irreversible inhibition is unique to aspirin, because the remaining NSAIDs do so in a reversible manner.

Dosage
The usual daily dosage needed to achieve anti-inflammatory effects is 3–5 g per day.

Patient instructions
Aspirin should be taken with food or milk to decrease gastrointestinal intolerance. Patients should report any dark or black stools, abdominal pain, or swelling to their physician immediately.

Adverse drug events
Aspirin irreversibly inhibits platelet activity, and serious bleeding may result. Dyspepsia, GI bleeding, tinnitus, hepatitis, and renal damage have been reported.

Drug–drug and drug–disease interactions
■ *Warfarin:* Aspirin may enhance the hypoprothrombinemic effects of warfarin.

Table 22-2. Drug Therapy with Nonsteroidal Anti-Inflammatory Drugs

Generic name	Trade name	Dosage range	Administration schedule (doses/d)	Available dosage forms
Acetic acids				
Diclofenac	Voltaren	150–200 mg/d	3–4	po, ophthalmic, topical gel
	Votaren XR	100–200 mg/d	1–2	po
Etodolac	Lodine	600–1,200 mg/d	2–4	po
	Lodine XL	400–1,000 mg/d	1	po
Indomethacin	Indocin	100–200 mg/d	2–3	po, IV, suppository
	Indocin SR	75–150 mg/d	1–2	po
Nabumetone	Relafen	1,000–2,000 mg/d	1–2	po
Tolmetin	Tolectin	600–1,800 mg/d	3	po
Sulindac	Clinoril	300–400 mg/d	2	po
Propionic acids				
Fenoprofen	Nalfon	900–3,200 mg/d	3–4	po
Flurbiprofen	Ansaid	200–300 mg/d	2–4	po
Ibuprofen	Motrin	1,200–3,200 mg/d	3–4	po
Ketoprofen	Orudis	150–300 mg/d	3–4	po
Ketoprofen SR	Oruvail	100–200 mg/d	1	po
Naproxen	Naprosyn	500–1,500 mg/d	2–3	po
Oxaprozin	Daypro	1,200–1,800 mg/d	1	po
Fenamates				
Meclofenamate	Meclomen	200–400 mg/d	3–4	po
Oxicams				
Piroxicam	Feldene	10–20 mg/d	1–2	po
COX-2 selective				
Celecoxib	Celebrex	200–400 mg/d	1–2	po

- *Uricosuric agents:* The uricosuric effects of agents such as probenecid are antagonized by aspirin.
- *Methotrexate:* Aspirin may displace methotrexate from its protein binding sites, thereby increasing serum methotrexate concentrations.

Parameters to monitor
Complete blood count (CBC) as well as creatinine should be monitored at least yearly.

Other NSAIDs

Mechanism of action
The mechanism of action is the same as described for aspirin.

Patient instructions
Patient instructions are the same as described for aspirin. Studies indicate that the optimal times for taking an NSAID might be after the evening meal and immediately on awakening. Patients with a hypersensitivity to aspirin should not take NSAIDs.

Adverse drug events
Compared with patients with osteoarthritis, patients with RA on NSAID therapy are at increased risk for a serious complication.

As with aspirin, NSAIDs cause platelet dysfunction. Unlike aspirin, however, this effect is readily reversible with discontinuation of the medication.

All NSAIDs are capable of causing GI intolerance and peptic ulceration. Risk factors for the development of peptic ulcer disease include advanced age, history of previous ulcer, concomitant use of corticosteroids or anticoagulants, higher dosage of NSAID, use of multiple NSAIDs, or serious underlying disease. Options to decrease the risk of developing GI ulceration include adding a high-dose histamine blocker such as ranitidine or a proton pump inhibitor such as lansoprazole to the patient's regimen. Lansoprazole and esomeprazole both have U.S. Food and Drug Administration (FDA) approval for reducing the risk of NSAID-induced gastric ulcers in those patients who had a previous risk of ulceration and who continue to require NSAID treatment. Misoprostol, an oral prostaglandin analogue, may be added at a dose of 100–200 mcg four times daily to prevent ulceration. Misoprostol is available in combination with diclofenac and sold under the trade name Arthrotec. Some evidence exists that, compared with other NSAIDs, ibuprofen, nabumetone, and naproxen carry lower risks of ulceration and GI symptoms. Piroxicam, in contrast, appears to carry a higher risk of serious GI consequences. A 2008 joint consensus statement by the American College of Cardiology Foundation, the American Heart Association, and the American College of Gastroenterology recommends that patients with a history of ulcer disease or with risk factors for ulceration be treated with a proton pump inhibitor while on NSAID therapy.

Hepatic failure has been reported with NSAID use.

Renal blood flow can be decreased by NSAIDs, which may lead to permanent renal damage. Prostaglandins are responsible for maintaining the patency of the afferent renal tubule. Inhibition by NSAIDs decreases glomerular filtration pressure, resulting in decreased blood flow. Because of this mechanism, patients with hypertension, severe vascular disease, and kidney or liver problems and those taking diuretics must be monitored closely.

Central nervous system (CNS) side effects such as dizziness, drowsiness, and confusion may occur with all NSAIDs.

Within the class, some drug-specific adverse reactions occur. Meclofenamate, for example, has a high incidence (> 10%) of abdominal cramping and diarrhea. Paradoxically, indomethacin tends to have more severe CNS adverse effects, such as headache.

Concern exists about NSAIDs and their risk of cardiovascular events. The FDA now requires that manufacturers include a black box warning regarding the potentially serious cardiovascular and GI adverse events associated with these drugs.

Drug–drug interactions

Interactions are the same as those described for aspirin. Ibuprofen may diminish the antiplatelet mech-

anism of aspirin if it is taken before aspirin or taken daily on a scheduled basis. It is recommended that aspirin be taken 2 hours before taking ibuprofen.

COX-2 inhibitors

COX-1 is the isoenzyme constitutively found in most tissues that produce the prostaglandins PGI_2 and PGE_2, which protect the gastric barrier, and thromboxane A_2, which is responsible for platelet function. COX-2 is the inducible isoenzyme present at sites of inflammation. COX-2 is also found in the brain, kidneys, and reproductive organs. Celecoxib (Celebrex) has been shown to have lower incidence of endoscopically demonstrated gastroduodenal lesions than do ibuprofen, naproxen, and diclofenac. The lower risk for GI complications is apparently eliminated when patients take low-dose aspirin concomitantly.

Celecoxib

Mechanism of action

Celecoxib selectively inhibits prostaglandin synthesis by specifically targeting the COX-2 isoenzyme.

Patient instructions

Patients with a history of allergic reaction to sulfonamides should avoid the use of celecoxib.

Adverse drug events

Although the rates of GI ulceration have been demonstrated to be lower with COX-2 inhibitors than with traditional NSAIDs, the risk is not completely eliminated. In addition, the risk of dyspepsia, abdominal pain, and nausea is not significantly less with COX-2 inhibitors than with traditional NSAIDs. Celecoxib now contains a black box warning regarding cardiovascular and GI risk associated with its use (as described later).

Drug–drug interactions

Interactions are the same as those associated with aspirin.

Parameters to monitor

CBC as well as creatinine should be monitored at least yearly.

Other aspects

The FDA recommended the voluntary removal of valdecoxib (Bextra) from the market in 2005 because of the lack of adequate data on the cardiovascular safety of its long-term use and the recent data demonstrating increased cardiovascular risk in short-term coronary artery bypass graft (CABG) patients. This risk is in addition to that of potentially life-threatening skin reactions. Merck removed rofecoxib (Vioxx) from the market in September 2004 because its use was shown to be associated with an increased cardiovascular risk in the VIGOR (Vioxx Gastrointestinal Outcomes Research), APPROVE (Adenomatous Polyp Prevention on Vioxx), and VICTOR (Vioxx in Colorectal Therapy, Definition of Optimal Regimen) trials. The FDA has concluded that the benefits of celecoxib outweigh the risks in properly selected and informed patients. Celecoxib contains a black box warning about cardiovascular and GI risk. Patients with a high risk of cardiovascular events should not use celecoxib, including CABG patients. Low doses of celecoxib (200 mg per day) do not seem to be associated with increased risk.

Disease-modifying antirheumatic drugs

Unlike the NSAIDs, DMARDs have the ability to reduce or prevent joint damage and preserve joint integrity and function. The ACR recommends that patients with an established diagnosis of RA be offered treatment with DMARDs. Biologic DMARDs are reserved for use after failure of nonbiologic agents, unless the patient has early disease with high activity and poor prognosis risk factors. Methotrexate is typically selected for initial therapy because of its track record to induce long-term response. Methotrexate or leflunomide may be used as monotherapy in patients with all disease durations and activity regardless of poor prognostic features. Unfortunately, all DMARDs tend to lose effectiveness over time. It is rare for a patient to use one medication for longer than 2 years.

Nonbiologic DMARDs

Hydroxychloroquine
Mechanism of action
Hydroxychloroquine (Plaquenil) may inhibit interleukin-1 release by monocytes, thereby decreasing macrophage chemotaxis and phagocytosis.

Patient instructions
Beneficial effect may not be seen until 1–6 months of use. Patients should report any changes in vision to their physician immediately.

Adverse drug events
The most serious potential adverse effect associated with hydroxychloroquine is retinal damage that can lead to vision loss. This damage is caused by the deposition of the drug in the melanin layer of the cones. A cumulative dose of 800 g and age > 70 years increase

the risk. Hydroxychloroquine may also cause rash, abdominal cramping, diarrhea, myopathy, skin pigment changes, and peripheral neuropathy.

Parameters to monitor
Ophthalmic evaluations should be performed at baseline. If the patient has no risk factors (liver disease, retinal disease, age > 60) and the baseline exam is normal, the American College of Ophthalmology recommends no further testing for 5 years. High-risk patients should have annual exams.

Dose
The dose is 6.0–7.5 mg/kg of lean body weight daily or 200 mg bid (maximum dose).

Sulfasalazine
Mechanism of action
The intestinal flora breaks sulfasalazine (Azulfidine) down to 5-aminosalicylic acid and sulfapyridine, the active moiety in RA. Sulfapyridine likely inhibits endothelial cell proliferation, reactive oxygen species, and cytokines. In addition, it has been shown to slow radiographic progression of RA.

Patient instructions
Sulfasalazine may produce effects more quickly (within 1 month) than hydroxychloroquine. A coated tablet form may help reduce adverse GI effects.

Adverse drug events
The most common adverse reactions associated with sulfasalazine include headache, GI intolerance, dysgeusia, rash, leukopenia, and thrombocytopenia.

Drug–drug interactions
Sulfasalazine may inhibit the absorption of folic acid.

Parameters to monitor
Patient tests should include baseline CBC, liver function tests (LFTs), and glucose-6-phosphate dehydrogenase (G6PD) levels. Patients should then have a CBC every 2–4 weeks for the first 3 months and then once every 3 months thereafter. Patients should receive a pneumococcal vaccination prior to initiation.

Dose
Begin with 500 mg daily, titrated up to 1–3 g per day divided tid or qid.

Methotrexate
Mechanism of action
Methotrexate (Rheumatrex) inhibits dihydrofolate reductase. It reduces dihydrofolate to tetrahydrofolate, which can be used as a carrier of single carbon

units for the synthesis of nucleotides and thymidylate. Therefore, methotrexate interferes with DNA synthesis, repair, and cellular replication.

Patient instructions
Patients should be instructed not to change the amount of methotrexate taken without first consulting their physician.

Adverse drug events
- *Liver:* Methotrexate may cause liver damage. People with diabetes, liver problems, obesity, and psoriasis and those who are elderly or alcoholic are at higher risk. If LFTs are more than three times the upper limit of normal, methotrexate should be discontinued.
- *Bone marrow:* Leukopenia, thrombocytopenia, and pancytopenia are rare but serious adverse events associated with methotrexate therapy.
- *Lung:* Pulmonary toxicity occurs in up to 5% of people who take methotrexate. Risk factors for the development of pulmonary toxicity include age, diabetes, rheumatoid involvement of the lungs, protein in the urine, and previous use of sulfasalazine, oral gold, or penicillamine.
- *GI:* Nausea, vomiting, and stomatitis occur with an incidence of 5–30%.

Drug–drug interactions
Aspirin and other NSAIDs may increase methotrexate concentrations by as much as 30–35%. Trimethoprim-sulfamethoxazole may cause additive hematologic abnormalities because of its similar affinity for dihydrofolate reductase.

Parameters to monitor
CBC, LFTs, albumin, and creatinine should be monitored every 2–4 weeks for the first 3 months and every 8–12 weeks thereafter. Patients at risk for hepatitis B and C should be screened prior to initiation.

Other aspects
Taking folate supplements may help minimize adverse effects such as liver toxicity. Folic acid in doses up to 3 mg per day has proven effective and does not diminish methotrexate activity. Patients should receive a pneumococcal vaccination prior to initiation.

Dose
The dose is 7.5–25.0 mg once weekly.

Leflunomide
Mechanism of action
Leflunomide (Arava) inhibits dihydroorotate dehydrogenase (an enzyme involved in de novo pyrimidine synthesis) and has antiproliferative activity. Several in vivo and in vitro experimental models have demonstrated its anti-inflammatory effect.

Patient instructions
Leflunomide is under pregnancy category X. Women taking leflunomide who wish to become pregnant should follow the drug elimination procedure outlined under "Other aspects."

Adverse drug events
Diarrhea, elevated LFTs, alopecia, hypertension, and rash have been reported with leflunomide therapy.

Drug–drug interactions
An increased risk of liver toxicity exists when leflunomide is used in conjunction with methotrexate. Rifampin causes a 40% increase in levels of leflunomide's active metabolite, M1.

Parameters to monitor
CBC, LFTs, albumin, and creatinine should be monitored every 2–4 weeks for the first 3 months and every 8–12 weeks thereafter. If alanine aminotransferase exceeds two times the upper limit of normal, reduce the dose of leflunomide to 10 mg per day. Patients at risk for hepatitis B and C should be screened prior to initiation.

Kinetics
After absorption, 80% of the parent compound is converted to the active metabolite, M1, which is responsible for all of leflunomide's activity. Because the half-life is 2 weeks, a loading dose is necessary. In addition, M1 undergoes extensive enterohepatic recirculation.

Other aspects
Begin the following drug elimination procedure if a patient decides to become pregnant: 8 g of cholestyramine three times daily for 11 days; plasma levels of M1 < 0.02 mg/L must be verified on two separate occasions at least 14 days apart.

Many randomized controlled trials have established leflunomide as an alternative to methotrexate as monotherapy.

Patients should receive a pneumococcal vaccination prior to initiation.

Dose
100 mg daily for 3 days (loading dose), then 20 mg daily

D-penicillamine
Mechanism of action
How penicillamine (Cuprimine) induces therapeutic effects in RA is currently unknown. It is known,

however, that penicillamine significantly reduces immunoglobulin M rheumatoid factor and appears to suppress disease activity.

Patient instructions

Penicillamine should be taken on an empty stomach and at least 2 hours from any dose of antacids or iron supplements.

Adverse drug events

- *Bone marrow:* Penicillamine may cause thrombocytopenia and leukopenia approximately 6 months into therapy. Rarely, aplastic anemia develops and is associated with its use.
- *Renal:* Proteinuria may occur in up to 32% of patients on penicillamine therapy.
- *Dermatologic:* Skin rash may occur 6–9 months after therapy commences.
- *Other:* Penicillamine causes stomatitis, dysgeusia, and polymyositis.

Drug–drug interactions

Absorption decreases approximately 70% with concomitant administration of antacids, iron, and zinc. Penicillamine may increase digoxin levels. In addition, penicillamine's chelating effects in combination with oral gold compounds may cause gold from deep tissue compartments to mobilize, which can increase toxicity.

Parameters to monitor

Patients should have CBC, platelet count, creatinine, and urine dipstick for protein lab testing done before initiating therapy. Afterward, the patient should have a CBC and urine dipstick for protein every 2 weeks until the dosage is stable and then every 1–3 months.

Other aspects

Penicillamine may take up to 1 year to be effective. Note that more than half the patients who take it withdraw because of side effects.

Dose

Begin with 125–250 mg/d, and increase by 125–250 mg/d every 8–10 weeks, not to exceed a maximum dose of 750 mg/d.

Gold compounds

The intramuscular (IM) gold compounds are gold sodium thiomalate (Myochrysine) and aurothioglucose (Solganal). Auranofin (Ridaura) is given orally.

Mechanism of action

The mechanism of action of gold compounds is currently unknown; they appear to suppress the synovi-tis seen in RA. Current research indicates that they may stimulate specific protective factors, such as interleukin-6 and interleukin-10.

Patient instructions

Patients receiving gold therapy should avoid prolonged sun exposure, which may increase the risk of serious rash.

Adverse drug events
IM gold

Patients may experience an immediate "nitroid reaction" (i.e., flushing, weakness, dizziness, sweating, syncope, and hypotension). Rash is the single-largest adverse effect associated with gold therapy. The rash may range from simple erythema to exfoliative dermatitis. Gold therapy may also cause proteinuria or microscopic hematuria. Rarely, immunologic glomerulonephritis may occur, in which case gold therapy should be permanently discontinued. Leukopenia and thrombocytopenia occur with a 1–3% incidence.

Oral gold

Adverse reactions are similar to those associated with the IM formulation. However, GI complaints of nausea, diarrhea, emesis, and dysgeusia are higher.

Drug–drug interactions

Patients receiving concomitant penicillamine therapy may be subject to an increased risk of toxicity associated with gold therapy. The risk of rash is higher when gold therapy is used with hydroxychloroquine.

Parameters to monitor

At baseline, all patients should have a CBC, platelet count, creatinine, and urine dipstick for protein. For patients receiving IM therapy, a CBC, platelet count, and urine dipstick are recommended every 1–2 weeks for the first 20 weeks and then again at the time of each (or every other) injection. Those on oral therapy should have a CBC, platelet count, and urine dipstick for protein every 4–12 weeks.

Other aspects

Aurothioglucose may have a lower rate of injection reactions; its sesame seed formulation slows absorption.

Dosing
IM gold

A 10 mg test dose IM is followed by a 25 mg test dose on week 2 and then weekly 50 mg doses until a cumulative dose of 1 g is achieved. The maintenance regimen is 50 mg every 2 weeks for 3 months or until 1.5 g is given; then every 3 weeks; and then monthly.

Oral gold
The dose is 3 mg bid up to 3 mg tid.

Biologic DMARDs

Antitumor necrosis factor therapy

The drugs used in antitumor necrosis factor (anti-TNF) therapy are infliximab (Remicade), etanercept (Enbrel), and adalimumab (Humira).

Mechanism of action

Composed of human constant and murine variable regions, infliximab binds specifically to human tumor necrosis factor (TNF).

Similarly, by binding specifically to TNF, etanercept binds and blocks its interaction with the cell surface's TNF receptors. It is produced by recombinant technology in Chinese hamster ovaries.

Adalimumab is a recombinant human immunoglobulin G_1 monoclonal antibody that binds to TNF with high affinity.

Patient instructions

Patients should not receive live vaccines during treatment. Therapy should be temporarily discontinued in the event of an acute infection.

Adverse drug events

Therapy has been associated with serious mycobacterial, fungal, and opportunistic infectious complications such as sepsis and tuberculosis, leading to requirement of an FDA black box warning to that effect in 2008. Other adverse reactions include rash, headache, nausea, and cough. Although rare, both etanercept and infliximab have been associated with nerve damage that resembles the disease process in multiple sclerosis. Lymphoma has been reported with all three TNF antagonists.

Drug–drug interactions

Live vaccines may interact with these drugs.

Parameters to monitor

Be clinically alert for tuberculosis, histoplasmosis, and other opportunistic infections.

Other aspects

Patients should be tested for tuberculosis (skin testing, chest radiograph, or both) and hepatitis B (if risk factors are present) before initiating therapy with any biologic agent. Currently, infliximab is approved for therapy only in combination with methotrexate. Increased mortality in heart failure patients taking infliximab has been shown. The ACR recommends against the use of anti-TNF agents in patients with class III–IV heart failure.

Dose

The dosage for infliximab is 3 mg/kg intravenous (IV) initially, at weeks 2 and 6, and then every 8 weeks in combination with methotrexate.

The dosage for etanercept is 25 mg subcutaneous (SC) twice weekly or 50 mg SC once weekly.

The dosage for adalimumab is 40 mg SC every second week.

Anakinra

Mechanism of action

Anakinra (Kineret) blocks the biologic activity of interleukin-1 by competitively inhibiting interleukin-1 binding to the interleukin-1 type I receptor.

Patient instructions

Kineret is supplied in a single-use, prefilled syringe that should be stored in the refrigerator. Any syringe left unrefrigerated for more than 24 hours should be discarded.

Adverse drug events

Like the anti-TNF agents, anakinra increases the risk of serious infections. Injection-site reactions are extremely common. Headache, nausea, diarrhea, sinusitis, flu-like symptoms, and abdominal pain have also been reported.

Drug–drug interactions

Live vaccines can interact with anakinra.

Parameters to monitor

Patients should have a CBC checked at baseline, then monthly for 3 months, and then once every 3 months for the first year of therapy.

Dose

The dose is 100 mg daily SC.

Abatacept

Mechanism of action

Abatacept (Orencia) selectively modulates T-cell activation causing downregulation and an anti-inflammatory effect.

Adverse drug events

Like the other biologic DMARDs, abatacept increases the risk of infections, especially upper respiratory infections. Nausea and headache are also frequently reported. In addition, patients with chronic obstructive pulmonary disease developed adverse effects more frequently than with placebo. More cases of lung cancer were observed in patients treated with abatacept than with placebo. The lymphoma rate was higher as well.

Drug–drug interactions

Use of abatacept is contraindicated with other biologic DMARDs because of increased risk of infection. Live vaccines are contraindicated as well.

Other aspects

Abatacept contains maltose and may falsely elevate blood glucose readings. Monitors that do not react to maltose, such as those based on glucose dehydrogenase nicotine adenine dinucleotide, glucose oxidase, or glucose hexokinase test methods, are recommended.

Dose

Dose is based on weight (< 60 kg = 500 mg; 60–100 kg = 750 mg; > 100 kg = 1,000 mg). Infusions are given over 30 minutes. After the initial dose, give at 2 and 4 weeks, followed by every 4 weeks.

Rituximab
Mechanism of action

Rituximab (Rituxan) causes a transient depletion of B-lymphocytes by binding to the CD20 surface antigens.

Other aspects

Rituximab should be used only in patients with moderate to severe RA who have had an inadequate response or a contraindication to anti-TNF products.

Dose

Give 1,000 mg every 2 weeks for two doses; patients may be premedicated with a glucocorticoid to decrease infusion-related reactions.

Other agents

Azathioprine

Azathioprine (Imuran) is a purine analogue immunosuppressive agent that is generally reserved for refractory RA. It is associated with dose-related bone marrow suppression, stomatitis, diarrhea, rash, and liver failure. Patients must have a baseline CBC, creatinine, and liver profile. Patients should then have a CBC and platelet count every 1–2 weeks after any change in dosage and every 1–3 months thereafter. Azathioprine should not be administered with allopurinol because xanthine oxidase metabolizes 6-mercaptopurine.

Cyclosporine A

By blocking T-cell activation, cyclosporine A (Sandimmune) produces powerful immunosuppressive effects and is beneficial as monotherapy in the treatment of RA. Serious adverse effects such as hypertension, nephrotoxicity, glucose intolerance, and hepatotoxicity have limited its use.

Corticosteroids

Low-dose oral corticosteroids (< 10 mg per day of prednisone or the equivalent) and local injections of glucocorticoids are highly effective. Studies indicate that corticosteroids decrease the progression of RA. They may be useful for acute flare-ups and in patients with significant systemic manifestations of RA. RA is associated with an increased risk of osteoporosis (independent of steroid therapy), and the addition of steroidal anti-inflammatory agents increases the risk. Patients on glucocorticoids should receive 1,500 mg of elemental calcium per day and 400–800 international units (IU) of vitamin D per day.

Nondrug Therapy
Surgery

Prosorba column

A device called the *Prosorba column* removes inflammatory antibodies from the patient's blood.

Joint surgery

Patients may have arthroscopy performed to clean out the bone and cartilage fragments that cause pain within the joint capsule. Patients may eventually require complete joint replacement surgery.

Lifestyle modifications

A mild exercise regimen can be an effective therapy.

Some evidence suggests a moderate increase in daily protein intake may be beneficial in RA.

Patients with RA benefit from a formal support group.

22-2. Osteoarthritis

Osteoarthritis (OA), a disease that affects the weight-bearing joints of the peripheral and axial skeleton, is the most common form of arthritis in the United States. OA is also known as *degenerative joint disease*.

Incidence

According to radiologic evidence, approximately 60–80% of people over the age of 65 have OA. Before the age of 50, men have a higher incidence; however, after the age of 50, women have a higher incidence.

Clinical Presentation

Pain is a common initial finding in patients with OA. This pain typically worsens with weight-bearing activity and improves with rest of the affected joint. Changes in weather and barometric pressure tend to influence the severity of pain.

Joint stiffness, including morning stiffness, is another common complaint. This stiffness differs from that of RA. It is relatively short in duration, is related to periods of inactivity, and resolves with movement.

Crepitus is common, especially when the knee joint is involved.

Joint deformities also occur in OA. Heberden's nodes, Bouchard's nodes, and osteophytes on the distal interphalangeal and proximal interphalangeal joints are commonly seen.

Pathophysiology

Although the causes of OA are not completely understood, biomechanical stresses affecting the articular cartilage and subchondral bone are thought to be the primary factors in the development of OA. In addition, inflammatory, biochemical, and immunologic components play a role. The function of the normal cartilage—that is, to dissipate the force and stress caused by normal weight-bearing activity—is impaired in OA.

- Collagen fibers are destroyed and subsequently release proteoglycans. The hydration of the cartilage increases, and the cartilage becomes thick.
- Metalloproteinases, which degrade the proteoglycans, are released to initiate the reparation process. This degradation causes an increase in chondrocyte activity.
- The resulting cartilage is thin because the chondrocyte activity cannot match the rate at which proteoglycan degradation occurs.
- With this ever-thinning layer of cartilage now exposing bone, the grinding motion stimulates osteoclast and osteoblast activity, thereby causing bone resorption and vascular changes. Ultimately, these changes lead to the formation of osteophytes.

Diagnostic Criteria

Osteoarthritis of the hip

According to the ACR classification criteria, osteoarthritis of the hip exists if the patient has hip pain and at least two of the following:

- Erythrocyte sedimentation rate < 20 mm/h
- Radiographic femoral or acetabular osteophytes
- Radiographic joint space narrowing

Other criteria include one of the following:

- Hip pain and radiographic femoral or acetabular osteophytes
- Hip pain and radiographic joint space narrowing and erythrocyte sedimentation rate < 20 mm/h

Osteoarthritis of the knee

According to ACR classification criteria, osteoarthritis of the knee exists if the patient has knee pain, radiographic osteophytes, and at least one of the following:

- Age > 50 years
- Morning stiffness ≤ 30 minutes in duration
- Crepitus on motion

Other criteria include one of the following:

- Knee pain and radiographic osteophytes
- Knee pain and age ≥ 40 years, morning stiffness ≤ 30 minutes in duration, and crepitus on motion

Treatment Principles

Treatment of patients with OA focuses on symptom control. Currently, no therapeutic options are known to change the course of the disease.

Drug Therapy

Pain relief is the primary treatment goal for patients with OA. The recommended initial drug of choice is acetaminophen. For those patients who do not respond fully, the addition of an NSAID (see discussion of this class in Section 22-1) is made. Box 22-1 outlines pharmacologic therapy for patients with osteoarthritis.

Acetaminophen

Mechanism of action
Acetaminophen centrally inhibits prostaglandin synthesis.

Patient instructions
Patients with hepatic disease or viral hepatitis are at risk of toxicity from chronic acetaminophen use.

Adverse drug events
Hepatotoxicity is the most severe side effect associated with acetaminophen therapy. For this reason,

---

Box 22-1. Pharmacologic Therapy for Patients with Osteoarthritis

Oral
- Acetaminophen 4 g/d
- COX-2-specific inhibitor
- Nonselective NSAID plus misoprostol or a proton pump inhibitor
- Nonacetylated salicylate
- Other pure analgesics
  Tramadol (Ultram) 50 mg/dose (up to 400 mg/d)
  Ultracet 37.5 mg/dose (up to 300 mg/d)
- Alternative therapy: glucosamine 1,500 mg/d (alone or in combination with chondroitin)

Intra-articular
- Glucocorticoids
- Hyaluronan

Topical
- Capsaicin
- Methyl salicylate

---

patients should not ingest more than 4 g of acetaminophen per day. Long-term therapy has also been linked to renal failure.

Other aspects
Acetaminophen is generally considered the initial drug of choice; however, there have been no clinical trials comparing its side effects, potential toxicity, or pain-relieving properties with those of NSAIDs.

Tramadol

Tramadol is a central opioid agonist that binds to mu receptors and weakly inhibits norepinephrine and serotonin reuptake.

Adverse drug events
Nausea, vomiting, constipation, and seizures are associated with tramadol use. Withdrawal symptoms may occur with abrupt discontinuation.

Drug interactions
Tramadol is contraindicated in patients taking monoamine oxidase inhibitors because of the risk of serotonin syndrome.

Other aspects
Tramadol is available as an immediate-release product (Ultram), as an extended-release product (Ultram ER), and in combination with acetaminophen 325 mg (Ultracet).

Topical agents (capsaicin)

Mechanism of action
Derived from the pepper plant, capsaicin works by exciting the nociceptive C-afferent neurons, which, in turn, causes the release of substance P, which is responsible for transmitting pain from the peripheral to the central nervous system.

Patient instructions
Patients should avoid contact with eyes. It is important to wash hands thoroughly after use.

Adverse drug events
Patients will experience mild burning and stinging at the site of application.

Other aspects
Patients usually derive benefit after several weeks of application. Capsaicin is often used in conjunction with oral agents.

Glucosamine sulfate and chondroitin

Mechanism of action
Glucosamine is found naturally in articular cartilage and acts as a substrate in the synthesis of proteoglycans. Chondroitin, another constituent in the cartilage, attracts and retains water, which provides shock absorption. In addition, chondroitin prevents the breakdown of cartilage and stimulates RNA (ribonucleic acid) synthesis of chondrocytes.

Patient instructions
Patients taking anticoagulants concomitantly may be at increased risk of bleeding.

Adverse drug events
Adverse events tend to be mild but include dyspepsia and euphoria.

Other aspects
This combination is available over the counter and has some clinical literature to support its use. The Arthritis Foundation, however, does not currently recognize it as a treatment for OA.

Other agents

The FDA has approved hyaluronic acid derivatives for the treatment of pain associated with OA of the knee. These agents may be an option after all conventional therapies for OA have been exhausted. The injection of this product into the synovium appears to replenish the viscosity to the space, thus enabling normal tissue to regenerate.

Nondrug Therapy

Nondrug therapy for OA consists of the following:

- Patient education
- Self-management programs (e.g., Arthritis Foundation Self-Management Program)
- Personalized social support through telephone contact
- Weight loss (if overweight)
- Aerobic exercise programs
- Physical therapy (i.e., range-of-motion exercises)
- Muscle-strengthening exercises
- Assistive devices for ambulation
- Patellar taping
- Appropriate footwear
- Lateral-wedged insoles (for genu varum)
- Bracing
- Occupational therapy
- Joint protection and energy conservation
- Assistive devices for activities of daily living

22-3. Gout

Gout, a systemic disease caused by the buildup of uric acid in the joints, causes inflammation, swelling, and pain. *Hyperuricemia* is defined as a urate level > 8 mg/dL in men and 7 mg/dL in women.

Incidence

Gout has been known as "the disease of kings and the king of diseases" and can be traced to the time of Hippocrates. Gout occurs in approximately 1% of the population. The vast majority of gout patients are men.

Clinical Presentation

Pain in one joint of the lower extremity is the most common first symptom of gout. The initial period of pain, usually monarticular and self-limiting, is followed by a period in which the patient is completely asymptomatic.

Termed *intercritical periods,* the time between acute gouty arthritis attacks may be 3 months to 2 years. The length of time shortens as the disease progresses.

The first attack is typically at night or in the early morning.

Gout commonly affects the ankle, heel, knee, wrist, finger, elbow, and instep. The most common site of the initial attack is the first MTP joint and is known as *podagra.*

The patient may experience fever, chills, and malaise during an acute gouty arthritis attack. Left untreated, the attack may last 1–2 weeks.

The skin over the affected joint becomes red, hot, swollen, and tender. As the patient recovers from the attack, local desquamation may occur.

Pathophysiology

Uric acid is the end product of purine metabolism (Figure 22-3). Xanthine oxidase is the rate-limiting step in the formation of uric acid. Uric acid, which serves no known biological function, has a body content of 1.0–1.2 g.

Approximately 70% of uric acid is excreted via the kidneys. At physiologic pH, uric acid primarily exists as monosodium urate (MSU) salt.

Approximately 95% of serum uric acid is filtered across the glomerulus. Of this filtered amount, almost 100% is reabsorbed in the early part of the proximal tubule, only to be secreted back into the lumen in the more distal part of the tubule.

Primary gout is a result of an innate defect in purine metabolism or uric acid excretion. In this case,

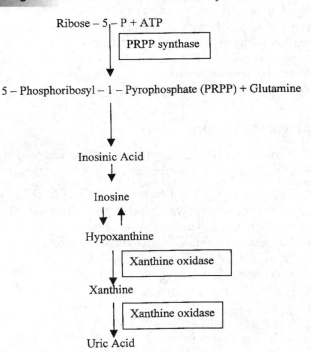

Figure 22-3. Ribose–Uric Acid Pathway

hyperuricemia may result from uric acid overproduction (in "overproducers"), impaired renal clearance of uric acid (in "underexcreters"), or a combination of both. In rare instances, enzyme defects of either hypoxanthine guanine phosphoribosyltransferase or 5-phosphoribosyl-1-pyrophosphate may cause primary gout (Figure 22-3).

Secondary gout is associated with increased nucleic acid turnover, decreased renal function, increased purine production, or drug-induced decreased elimination of uric acid. Hematologic disorders that are lymphoproliferative and myeloproliferative in nature are known causes of secondary hyperuricemia. Salicylates such as aspirin may inhibit tubular secretion of uric acid at low doses. All diuretics, with the exception of spironolactone, may cause hyperuricemia. Ethambutol, pyrazinamide, nicotinic acid, ethanol, niacin, and cyclosporine are known to cause an increase in serum uric acid.

Acute gout attacks are caused by the deposition of monosodium urate (MSU) in the synovium of the joint. This deposition results in the stimulation of the body's inflammatory cascade. The MSU crystals undergo phagocytosis by polymorphonuclear leukocytes. These leukocytes, damaged by the sharp crystals, burst and release their contents (interleukin-1, lysosomes, and prostaglandins) into the synovium, resulting in the inflammatory reaction—that is, pain, swelling, and erythema.

If left untreated, deposits of MSU crystals, also known as *tophi,* lead to joint deformity and disability. Ultimately, patients may develop one of two types of renal disease: urate nephropathy or uric acid nephropathy. Urate nephropathy results from the deposition of MSU crystals in the renal interstitium. Uric acid nephropathy results from the deposition of uric acid in the collecting tubules.

Diagnostic Criteria

The American Rheumatism Association lists the following criteria for the diagnosis of gout:

- **Definite:** Sodium urate crystals in the affected joint appear negatively birefringent when viewed through a polarized light source.
- **Suggestive:** A minimum of six of the following criteria should be met.
  - More than one attack of arthritis
  - Development of maximum inflammation within 1 day
  - Oligoarthritis attack
  - Redness over joint
  - Painful or swollen first MTP joint
  - Unilateral attack on first MTP joint
  - Unilateral attack on tarsal joint
  - Tophus
  - Hyperuricemia
  - Asymptomatic swelling within a joint

Ruling out pseudogout is also important. In pseudogout, crystals deposited into the joint synovium cause intense pain and inflammation, but the culprit is calcium pyrophosphate dihydrate, not monosodium urate.

Treatment Goals

- Relieve pain and inflammation.
- Reduce serum uric acid concentration.
- Prevent recurrent gout attacks.

Drug Therapy

Drugs for the treatment of gout are outlined in Table 22-3.

Acute gouty arthritis attack

Three treatments are available: colchicine, NSAIDs (indomethacin in particular), and corticosteroids. Avoiding treatments that affect serum uric acid concentrations is best during an acute attack.

Colchicine
Mechanism of action
Colchicine inhibits the phagocytosis of urate crystals by leukocytes. Colchicine also inhibits the release of chemotactic factor, thus reducing the adhesion of polymorphonuclear leukocytes. The net result makes colchicine an anti-inflammatory agent without analgesic activity.

Patient instructions
Patients should immediately stop taking colchicine if abdominal cramping or diarrhea occurs. Patients should never exceed a total of 8 mg during an acute gouty arthritis attack.

Adverse drug events
Nausea, bloating, emesis, and diarrhea occur in up to 80% of patients taking colchicine. Rarely, it may cause bone marrow suppression. This effect occurs with a higher incidence in those patients with underlying renal or hepatic dysfunction. When colchicine is given intravenously, possible extravasation may cause local skin necrosis. In addition, the intravenous route has been associated with bone marrow suppression,

Table 22-3. Drugs for the Treatment of Gout

Generic name	Trade name	Classification	Normal dose	Comments	Dosage forms
Colchicine		Anti-inflammatory	1.2 mg po followed by 0.6 mg 1 hour later. Maximum dose is 1.8 mg over 1 hour.	Drug may be used for chronic suppressive therapy; dose must be adjusted for renal insufficiency.	po, IV
Probenecid	Benemid	Uricosuric agent	250–500 mg bid	Avoid salicylates; take with plenty of water.	po
Sulfinpyrazone	Anturane	Uricosuric agent	50–200 mg bid	Avoid salicylates; take with plenty of water.	po
Allopurinol	Zyloprim	Xanthine oxidase inhibitor	100–300 mg qd or divided dose	Drug may cause rash; reduce dosage in renal failure.	po
Indomethacin	Indocin	NSAID	50 mg tid	Drug may cause fluid retention, GI bleeding.	po, IV, suppository

disseminated intravascular coagulation, seizures, and death.

Drug–drug and drug–disease interactions
Patients with active peptic ulcer disease should not take colchicine.

Parameters to monitor
With long-term therapy, patients should have a serum creatinine test, liver function test, and complete white blood cell count check periodically.

Dose
For the treatment of an acute gouty arthritis attack, patients should take 1.2 mg orally followed by 0.6 mg in 1 hour. Maximum dose is 1.8 mg.

Other aspects
Colchicine is most effective when initiated within 12–36 hours of the attack.

Indomethacin
Indomethacin is the most extensively studied NSAID in the treatment of an acute gouty arthritis attack. Unlike colchicine, indomethacin is effective at any point during the acute attack. For more information, see the review of NSAIDs in Section 22-1.

Corticosteroids
For the treatment of acute gout pain, corticosteroids are effective when given intra-articularly, intravenously, or orally. Their use is limited to treatment failures of colchicine and NSAIDs. Intramuscular corticotropin (adrenocorticotropic hormone) is also effective when given (40 units) to treat an acute gouty arthritis attack.

Gout prophylaxis (intercritical period)

Patients with asymptomatic hyperuricemia should not be routinely treated with pharmacologic agents. These patients should undergo a workup to determine the cause of hyperuricemia. The use of low-dose (0.6–1.2 mg/d) colchicine can prevent subsequent attacks of gout. Patients in the intercritical period (after an acute gouty arthritis attack) are candidates for long-term prophylactic therapy directed at affecting serum uric acid levels. Choice of therapy is based on the patient's pathophysiologic cause of hyperuricemia. Patients are generally classified as *overproducers* or *underexcreters*. Placing the patient on a purine-restricted diet and performing a 24-hour urine collection to measure uric acid concentration may identify overproducers of uric acid. Those patients who excrete more than 600 mg of uric acid are considered overproducers. Once this diagnosis is made, patients are treated with one of two classes of agents: xanthine oxidase inhibitors or uricosurics.

Probenecid
Mechanism of action
Probenecid (Benemid) is a uricosuric agent that promotes the excretion of uric acid by blocking its reuptake at the proximal convoluted tubule.

Patient instructions
Patients should drink at least 2 liters of water per day to decrease the risk of uric acid stone formation.

Patients should take probenecid with food if GI intolerance occurs.

Adverse drug events

Probenecid is generally well tolerated and is associated with very few adverse side effects. Up to 10% of patients receiving probenecid therapy develop uric acid stones. Probenecid may cause abdominal discomfort, but patients can often avoid it by taking probenecid with food.

Drug–drug interactions

Because probenecid prevents the tubular secretion of many weak organic acids, it has potential drug interactions—for example, with the penicillins, cephalosporins, nitrofurantoin, and rifampin. Although the interaction between probenecid, penicillins, and cephalosporins has been used therapeutically, the interaction with nitrofurantoin reduces nitrofurantoin's effectiveness. Using probenecid and aspirin together, even in low doses, is not advisable because aspirin blocks uric acid excretion. A crossover study in patients with gouty arthritis concluded that low-dose aspirin did not significantly interfere with the uricosuric effects of probenecid. Avoiding the combination would be reasonable, however. Additionally, the diuretic effects of furosemide and hydrochlorothiazide are magnified when probenecid is taken concomitantly. Finally, patients receiving sulfonylureas should be monitored closely for hypoglycemia when started on probenecid.

Other aspects

Patients should never begin uricosuric therapy during an acute gouty arthritis attack because of the risk of exacerbating the attack. Probenecid should not be used in patients with a creatinine clearance less than 50 mL/min.

Sulfinpyrazone
Mechanism of action

Sulfinpyrazone (Anturane) is a uricosuric agent that promotes the excretion of uric acid by blocking its reuptake at the proximal convoluted tubule.

Patient instructions

Patients should drink at least 2 liters of water per day to decrease the risk of uric acid stone formation. Patients should take sulfinpyrazone with food if GI intolerance occurs. Patients who are sensitive to aspirin should not take this agent because of the risk of bronchoconstriction.

Adverse drug events

Like probenecid, sulfinpyrazone is generally well tolerated. The most common reported adverse effects are GI discomfort and uric acid stone formation. In addition, rarely, sulfinpyrazone has been associated with bone marrow suppression and immunoallergic interstitial nephritis.

Drug–drug interactions

Sulfinpyrazone decreases the effectiveness of nitrofurantoin. When sulfinpyrazone is taken with aspirin, the effect of sulfinpyrazone is lessened.

Parameters to monitor

Patients should have complete blood work periodically because of the rare risk of bone marrow suppression associated with sulfinpyrazone therapy.

Other aspects

Patients should never start uricosuric therapy during an acute gouty arthritis attack; uricosuric therapy may exacerbate the attack. When increasing the dose of sulfinpyrazone, titrate upward slowly to minimize the risk of uric acid stone formation. Because uricosuric therapy may precipitate an acute gouty arthritis attack, patients should take an NSAID or colchicine for the first 6–12 months of therapy. Patients with a creatinine clearance of less than 50 mL/min should not use sulfinpyrazone.

Allopurinol
Mechanism of action

Allopurinol (Zyloprim) and its metabolite, oxypurinol, inhibit xanthine oxidase formation (the rate-limiting step in uric acid synthesis), thereby facilitating the clearance of the more water-soluble precursors of uric acid, oxypurines.

Patient instructions

Patients should immediately report any signs of rash to their health care providers. Allopurinol should be taken with food to minimize GI discomfort.

Adverse drug events

Allopurinol is generally well tolerated; the overall occurrence of adverse effects is less than 1%. Patients should be advised that rash, the most common adverse effect, might occur at any time during therapy. The rash may be as simple as a maculopapular eruption or as serious as the life-threatening Stevens–Johnson syndrome (which is exfoliative and erythematous). Rarely, allopurinol may cause alopecia, neutropenia, and hepatitis.

Drug–drug interactions

The chemotherapeutic agents azathioprine and 6-mercaptopurine are metabolized via the xanthine oxidase pathway; therefore, allopurinol and its metabolite oxypurinol may increase serum levels of these agents. The concomitant administration of ampicillin or amoxicillin with allopurinol increases the risk of rash to approximately 20%.

Parameters to monitor

Patients should be encouraged to report the first signs of rash to their physicians immediately. Patients should have serum creatinine as well as liver function tests drawn periodically.

Kinetics

With a half-life of 30 hours, allopurinol is rapidly converted to its active metabolite (oxypurinol). This speed allows for once-daily dosing.

Other aspects

To reduce the risk of precipitating an acute gouty arthritis attack, allopurinol should be initiated at a dose of 100 mg per day and increased at 100 mg intervals weekly to an average dose of 300 mg per day. Patients with renal insufficiency require a dose adjustment. Assuming the target dose is 300 mg per day, patients with a creatinine clearance of 10–20 mL/min should receive 200 mg per day. Those with a clearance of less than 10 mL/min should receive 100 mg per day.

Febuxostat (Uloric) was approved in February 2009 for the chronic management of hyperuricemia in patients with gout. It is also a xanthine oxidase inhibitor; however, unlike allopurinol, it is not a purine-based analogue.

Secondary hyperuricemia

As discussed earlier, hyperuricemia may be caused by lymphoproliferative and myeloproliferative disorders, as well as their chemotherapeutic treatments (e.g., tumor lysis syndrome). Allopurinol is commonly added to the prescribed chemotherapeutic regimen to prevent complications of hyperuricemia, for example, an acute gouty arthritis attack. Rasburicase (Elitek) is an approved therapeutic agent that is used to prevent hyperuricemia in children with leukemia, lymphoma, and solid-tumor malignancies. Rasburicase is a recombinant urate oxidase enzyme that converts uric acid to allantoin, thereby allowing it to be eliminated. Patients with G6PD deficiency should not use rasburicase.

22-4. Systemic Lupus Erythematosus

Systemic lupus erythematosus (SLE) is a chronic autoimmune inflammatory disorder that can affect any system in the body, including the skin, joints, and internal organs.

Classification

The workup of SLE must include the consideration of an alternative diagnosis. Because other autoimmune diseases have similar characteristics and because the features of SLE, RA, and scleroderma overlap, a thorough assessment is warranted. Drug-induced lupus must be ruled out as well.

Clinical Presentation

Signs and symptoms consistent with SLE include the following:

- Malar rash (a butterfly-shaped rash over the cheeks and across the bridge of the nose)
- Discoid rash (scaly, disk-shaped sores on the face, neck, or chest)
- Photosensitivity
- Oral ulcers
- Arthritis
- Serositis (inflammation of the lining around the heart, lungs, or abdomen that causes pain and shortness of breath)
- Proteinuria
- Central nervous system problems
- Antinuclear antibodies (autoantibodies that react against the body's own cells)
- Anemia
- Fatigue
- Fever
- Skin rash
- Muscle aches
- Nausea
- Vomiting and diarrhea
- Anorexia
- Raynaud's phenomenon
- Weight loss

Patients typically present with chronic fatigue and depression. Dermatitis and arthritis (in multiple joints) are the most common clinical manifestations. The arthritic pain patients describe is generally out of proportion to the amount of synovitis present. Although it is rare, serious renal abnormalities can occur in patients with SLE. CNS involvement, also rare, can be serious. Lupus-related encephalopathy may occur from scarring of arterioles in the subcortical white matter. In addition, patients with SLE are at risk of stroke because of the thromboembolic nature of the antiphospholipid antibody.

Pathophysiology

The exact pathophysiology of SLE remains unknown. It is an autoimmune disease (type III hypersensitivity) in which patients have an overactivity of B cells. The result is hypergammaglobulinemia that ultimately precipitates immune complexes on the vascular membranes, thereby causing activation of complement. Drugs, procainamide being the most predominant, may also cause SLE. Other such medications include phenytoin, chlorpromazine, hydralazine, quinidine, methyldopa, and isoniazid.

Diagnostic Criteria

Criteria for diagnosing SLE are as follows:

- Characteristic rash across the cheeks
- Discoid lesion rash
- Photosensitivity
- Oral ulcers
- Arthritis
- Inflammation of membranes in lungs, heart, or abdomen
- Evidence of kidney disease
- Evidence of severe neurologic disease
- Blood disorders, including low red blood cell, white blood cell, and platelet counts
- Immunologic abnormalities
- Positive antinuclear antibody

A patient must experience four of the criteria before a classification of SLE can be made. These criteria, proposed by the ACR, should not be the sole characteristics for diagnosis, however.

Therapy

Therapy for each case of SLE is based on the particular symptoms of any given patient. Arthritis is commonly treated with NSAIDs or glucocorticoids. Dermatologic complications can be treated with hydroxychloroquine (see Section 22-1). Hydroxychloroquine may also be used for musculoskeletal manifestations that do not respond to NSAIDs. Thrombocytopenia generally responds to glucocorticoid therapy. Immunosuppressive agents are used

in patients with lupus nephritis. Most commonly, cyclophosphamide is used, sometimes in combination with glucocorticoids.

22-5. Key Points

Rheumatoid Arthritis

- RA, a highly variable autoimmune disease characterized by symmetric, erosive synovitis, often affects extra-articular sites.
- RA usually affects diarthrodial joints (e.g., PIP joints, MCP joints, MTP joints, wrists, and ankles). Also commonly involved are the elbows, shoulders, sternoclavicular joints, temporomandibular joints, hips, and knees.
- Morning stiffness is the hallmark of RA.
- According to the ACR, the goals in managing RA are to prevent or control joint damage, prevent loss of function, and decrease pain.
- The ACR recommends the aggressive use of DMARDs.
- Unlike the NSAIDs, DMARDs can reduce or prevent joint damage and preserve joint integrity and function. DMARDs carry the risk of various toxicities, and they must be monitored on a regular basis.

Osteoarthritis

- OA is the most common form of arthritis in the United States.
- Joint stiffness, a common complaint in osteoarthritis, differs from that in RA because it is relatively short in duration and resolves with movement.
- Unlike RA, pain relief is the primary treatment goal in OA. The initial drug of choice is acetaminophen.

Gout

- Gout, a systemic disease caused by the buildup of uric acid in the joints, causes inflammation, swelling, and pain.
- Primary gout is a result of an innate defect in purine metabolism or uric acid excretion.
- Patients with gout are classified as *overproducers* or *underexcreters* on the basis of 24-hour uric acid concentration levels.
- Treatment of an acute gouty arthritis attack involves the use of colchicine, NSAIDs, or glucocorticoids.

■ Uricosuric agents, xanthine oxidase inhibitors, or both are used to prevent further gout attacks. These agents should not be used during an acute gouty arthritis attack.

Systemic Lupus Erythematosus

■ SLE is a chronic autoimmune inflammatory disorder that can affect any system in the body.
■ Therapy for SLE is primarily driven by the clinical manifestations of the disease.

22-6. Questions

1. A 45-year-old man presents to his local physician with a complaint of extreme stiffness in the morning that lasts until noon on most days for the past 2 months. He also states that he feels "drained" all the time and that both of his knees are swollen and painful. On examining the patient, the physician documents the presence of rheumatoid nodules. The patient's laboratory workup is significant for thrombocytopenia and a positive rheumatoid factor. He states that he has been taking over-the-counter ibuprofen at a dose of 200 mg two or three times daily without relief. Which of the following represents the best drug therapy option for this patient?

   A. Increase the dose of ibuprofen to 800 mg three times daily.
   B. Increase the dose of ibuprofen and add methotrexate 25 mg twice daily.
   C. Increase the dose of ibuprofen and add celecoxib 100 mg twice daily.
   D. Increase the dose of ibuprofen and add leflunomide at a dose of 100 mg daily for 3 days, followed by 20 mg daily.

2. Which of the following represents the best way to decrease potential liver toxicity with methotrexate while achieving optimal therapeutic benefit?

   A. Add 1–3 mg of folic acid per day to the patient's regimen.
   B. Decrease the dose of methotrexate to 25 mg once monthly.
   C. Add monthly injections of leucovorin to the patient's regimen.
   D. Add leflunomide to the patient's regimen.

3. Because combination DMARD therapy may be more efficacious in the refractory RA population, which of the following represents the *best* choice for combination therapy?

   A. Arava 20 mg once daily + Rheumatrex 25 mg once weekly
   B. Remicade 3 mg/kg IM + Rheumatrex 25 mg once weekly
   C. Myochrysine IM + Plaquenil 200 mg twice daily
   D. Remicade 3 mg/kg IV + Rheumatrex 25 mg once weekly

4. A physician inquires about the recommended monitoring parameters for patients started on Ridaura. Which of the following represents the most appropriate response?

   A. Baseline ophthalmologic exam, CBC, and serum creatinine, followed by a yearly CBC, serum creatinine, and ophthalmologic exam
   B. Baseline liver function tests, CBC, and albumin, followed by monthly liver function tests
   C. Baseline CBC, serum creatinine, and urine dipstick for protein, followed by a CBC and urine dipstick for protein every 1–2 months
   D. No recommended monitoring parameters at this time

5. All of the following represent methods used to decrease the GI toxicity associated with NSAIDs *except*

   A. changing patients from a nonselective cyclooxygenase inhibitor to a type II–specific inhibitor such as Celebrex.
   B. adding a proton pump inhibitor such as Prevacid to the patient's NSAID.
   C. adding Cytotec to the patient's NSAID.
   D. instructing the patient to take his or her NSAID at night, when acid secretion is limited.

6. Which of the following is (are) true concerning diclofenac?

   I. It is available as an extended-release product, Voltaren XR.
   II. It is available as an injectable product, Voltaren IM.
   III. It is available in combination with misoprostol, Arthrotec.

A. I only
B. I and II only
C. I, II, and III
D. I and III only

7. Which of the following would be a contra-indication for the use of Enbrel?

   A. Renal insufficiency
   B. Active infection
   C. Patient over the age of 65
   D. Patient with class I or II congestive heart failure

8. Regarding the biologic DMARDs, the following statements are correct *except*

   A. Kineret is packaged as a single-use prefilled syringe that should be kept in the refrigerator.
   B. patients should have a tuberculin skin test completed before initiation.
   C. it is acceptable to use FluMist for influenza prevention.
   D. patients receiving therapy are at increased risk for opportunistic infections.

9. The use of glucocorticoids is associated with numerous adverse effects and long-term consequences. All of the following are initiatives to treat, prevent, or minimize these adverse effects *except*

   A. instructing patients to take the glucocorticoid once daily instead of dividing the total daily dose into two to four doses.
   B. instructing patients on long-term therapy to add 1,500 mg of elemental calcium and 400–800 IU of ergocalciferol to their regimen.
   C. suggesting adding a bisphosphonate to their therapy.
   D. informing patients that stopping glucocorticoid abruptly is contraindicated.

10. A young lady enters your pharmacy and informs you that she plans on becoming pregnant and would like you to review her medication profile to see if any would be potentially harmful. On reviewing her profile, you notice that she is taking Arava for RA. Which is the most appropriate response?

    A. Arava is a category C drug and could potentially harm the fetus. She should

    discuss the risks and benefits of becoming pregnant with her physician first.
    B. Arava is a category X drug, and she should undergo the drug elimination procedure with cholestyramine before trying to become pregnant.
    C. Arava is a category X drug with no active metabolites and a short half-life; therefore, she should discontinue the drug and wait 1–2 weeks before trying to become pregnant.
    D. Arava is a category B drug, and the risk of toxicity to the fetus is extremely low.

11. R. Y. is a 67-year-old man with chief complaints of a swollen big left toe and extreme pain. The area is erythematous and tender. Laboratory analysis reveals a uric acid level of 10 mg/dL. Review of R. Y.'s past medical history reveals hypertension and congestive heart failure. A diagnosis of gout is made. Which is the best choice for the treatment of R. Y.'s acute gouty arthritis attack?

    A. Probenecid 500 mg now, followed by 500 mg twice daily
    B. Indomethacin 50 mg now, followed by 50 mg three to four times daily
    C. Allopurinol 100 mg once daily
    D. Colchicine 1.2 mg followed by 0.6 mg in 1 hour if symptoms persist

12. The following symptoms are consistent with the diagnosis of gout *except*

    A. the presence of negatively birefringent crystals in the affected synovial joint fluid.
    B. the presence of calcium pyrophosphate in the affected synovial joint fluid.
    C. the presence of tophi.
    D. the presence of hyperuricemia.

13. Which of the following best describes Benemid?

    A. Like allopurinol, it decreases the body's production of uric acid.
    B. Like Anturane, it is a uricosuric agent that aids in the tubular reabsorption of uric acid.
    C. It blocks the excretion of uric acid in the urine.
    D. Like Anturane, it is a uricosuric agent that blocks reuptake of uric acid at the proximal convoluted tubule.

14. Which of the following represents a therapeutically ineffective combination that should be avoided?

    A. Benemid + penicillin G
    B. Benemid + cephalexin
    C. Anturane + Macrobid
    D. Benemid + colchicine

15. All of the following statements are true regarding Zyloprim *except*

    A. it works to decrease the formation of uric acid by inhibiting xanthine oxidase.
    B. it does not require dosage adjustment in patients with renal insufficiency.
    C. skin reactions, including Stevens–Johnson syndrome, have been reported with its use.
    D. it should not be used for the treatment of an acute gouty arthritis attack.

16. Which of the following represent potentially dangerous drug interactions with Zyloprim?

    I. Amoxicillin
    II. Imuran
    III. Essidrex

    A. I only
    B. I and II only
    C. I, II, and III
    D. III only

17. All of the following are consistent with the diagnosis of osteoarthritis *except*

    A. the presence of morning stiffness that is not associated with immobility and may last for several hours.
    B. a common initial finding of pain that typically worsens with weight-bearing activity and subsides with rest.
    C. it commonly occurs in the knees or the hips.
    D. crepitus is common.

18. Which of the following medication combinations is (are) contraindicated?

    I. Tylenol + Ultram
    II. Glucosamine sulfate and chondroitin
    III. Ultram + Parnate

    A. All of the above
    B. II only
    C. III only
    D. I and II only

19. Concerning treatment of osteoarthritis, which of the following statements is *incorrect*?

    A. Tylenol is generally considered the initial drug of choice.
    B. Tylenol is considered safe and effective, and it has minimal adverse effects, especially in doses greater than 4 g per day.
    C. Muscle-strengthening exercises may be helpful.
    D. Hyaluronic acid derivatives have been approved by the FDA for the treatment of pain associated with osteoarthritis.

20. The following medications are considered to be DMARDs *except*

    A. Plaquenil.
    B. Cuprimine.
    C. Myochrysine.
    D. Nalfon.

22-7. Answers

1. **D.** Although the patient currently has room to increase his dose of the NSAID, he would benefit from the addition of a DMARD. This patient has a disease duration of less than 6 months with moderate disease and poor prognostic factors. Methotrexate represents a viable option; however, the dose of 25 mg twice daily is excessive (it should be dosed once weekly). The addition of leflunomide is the best choice.

2. **A.** The addition of folic acid to the methotrexate regimen has been demonstrated to reduce the risk of liver toxicity. Lowering the dose of methotrexate is likely to decrease risk but is also likely to decrease its effectiveness. Leucovorin, an injectable formulation of folate, is used only to reverse methotrexate toxicity.

3. **D.** Arava plus methotrexate (Rheumatrex) may be a very efficacious combination, but it increases the risk of liver toxicity significantly. Gold therapy in combination with Plaquenil increases the risk of rash. Remicade, approved only for use in combination with Rheumatrex, is given IV and not IM; this combination represents the best choice.

4. **C.** Gold therapy is associated with glomerulonephritis, thrombocytopenia, and leukopenia; therefore, a baseline renal evaluation and periodic testing should occur during the entire course of therapy.

5. **D.** Adding a proton pump inhibitor, adding Cytotec, or changing to a selective COX-II inhibitor has been demonstrated to lower the risk of significant GI adverse effects. Timing of the dose of an NSAID has never been demonstrated to affect the risk of GI toxicity.

6. **D.** Diclofenac is available as an immediate-release product, an extended-release product, and in combination with misoprostol. It is not available in an injectable formulation.

7. **B.** Because of its effects on tumor necrosis factor, Enbrel may decrease a patient's ability to fight infection. Enbrel is contraindicated in patients with an active infection. Its use should be temporarily discontinued until the acute process has resolved.

8. **C.** FluMist is a live weakened flu vaccine. Live vaccines are contraindicated in patients receiving biologic DMARDs.

9. **A.** Patients taking glucocorticoids are at risk of developing osteoporosis. Efforts to minimize this adverse effect include the addition of calcium and vitamin D to the patient's regimen as well as adding a bisphosphonate (e.g., Fosamax) to suppress bone resorption. Because of adrenal suppression that occurs with long-term glucocorticoid therapy, patients should taper off the agent.

10. **B.** Because Arava is a teratogenic agent with an active metabolite with a long half-life, a drug elimination procedure should be performed before becoming pregnant.

11. **D.** Both probenecid and allopurinol may exacerbate an acute gouty arthritis attack and should be reserved for the prevention of further attacks only. Indomethacin is an option for the treatment of an acute gouty arthritis attack; however, because of NSAIDs' tendency to cause fluid retention in the renal tubules, it would not be the ideal agent in a patient with congestive heart failure. Colchicine represents the best option from this list.

12. **B.** The presence of calcium pyrophosphate is consistent with the diagnosis of pseudogout, not gout.

13. **D.** Benemid is a uricosuric agent that blocks reuptake of uric acid at the proximal convoluted tubule. It does not affect the body's ability to produce uric acid. Answer B is incorrect because Benemid does not promote the reabsorption of uric acid.

14. **C.** Benemid does prevent the tubular secretion of penicillin and cephalexin. However, these interactions are used therapeutically to increase the duration of action of a single dose. The combination of Benemid and colchicine (marketed under the trade name Colbenemid) has been used therapeutically to prevent the manifestation of an acute gouty arthritis attack. Finally, a combination of Anturane and Macrobid will inhibit Macrobid from reaching its site of action, thus diminishing its therapeutic efficacy.

15. **B.** Zyloprim must be adjusted in patients with renal insufficiency. Its use has been associated with serious skin reactions that may occur at any point during therapy. Zyloprim should never be used in the treatment of an acute gouty arthritis attack.

16. **B.** The coadministration of amoxicillin and allopurinol increases the risk of rash up to 20%. Imuran is metabolized via xanthine oxidase, whose activity is inhibited by allopurinol, thus increasing the risk of toxicity associated with Imuran. Although Essidrex may increase uric acid levels, there is no direct drug–drug interaction associated with allopurinol.

17. **A.** The morning stiffness associated with osteoarthritis is usually of short duration, is associated with periods of inactivity, and resolves with movement.

18. **C.** Tylenol + Ultram is marketed therapeutically as Ultracet. Glucosamine sulfate with or without chondroitin is recommended as an alternative therapy in the treatment of osteoarthritis. The combination of Ultram and Parnate, a monoamine oxidase inhibitor, is contraindicated because of the risk of serotonin syndrome.

19. **B.** Tylenol is generally considered to be safe and effective; however, its use is associated with hepatic failure and the rare incidence of renal failure. Patients should be advised to take *less* than 4 g per day to limit the risk of hepatic failure.

20. **D.** Nalfon, also known as *fenoprofen*, is an NSAID, not a DMARD.

22-8. References

Rheumatoid Arthritis

American College of Rheumatology. Recommendations for the use of nonbiologic and biologic disease-modifying antirheumatic drugs in rheumatoid arthritis. *Arthritis Rheum.* 2008;59:762–84.

Bhatt DL, Scheiman J, Abraham NS, et al. ACCF/ACG/AHA 2008 expert consensus document on reducing the gastrointestinal risks of antiplatelet therapy and NSAID use. *Am J Gastroenterol.* 2008; 103:2890–907.

Boyce EG. Rheumatoid arthritis. In: Helms RA, Quan DJ, Herfindal ET, et al., eds. *Textbook of Therapeutics: Drugs and Disease Management.* 8th ed. Baltimore: Lippincott Williams & Wilkins; 2006:1705–36.

Goekoop YP, Allaart CF, Breedveld FC, et al. Combination therapy in rheumatoid arthritis. *Curr Opin Rheumatol.* 2001;30:249–54.

Kremer JM. Rational use of new and existing disease-modifying agents in rheumatoid arthritis. *Ann Intern Med.* 2001;134:695–706.

Kwoh CK, Anderson LG, Greene JM, et al. Guidelines for the management of rheumatoid arthritis. *Arthritis Rheum.* 2002;46:328–46.

Olsen NJ, Stein CM. New drugs for rheumatoid arthritis. *N Engl J Med.* 2004;21:2167–79.

Saag KG, Teng GG, Patkar NM, et al. American College of Rheumatology 2008 recommendations for the use of nonbiologic and biologic disease-modifying antirheumatic drugs in rheumatoid arthritis. *Arthritis Rheum.* 2008;59:762–84.

Sims RW, Kwoh CK, Anderson LG, et al. Guidelines for monitoring drug therapy in rheumatoid arthritis. *Arthritis Rheum.* 1996;39:723–31.

Wolfe F, Rehman W, Lane NE, et al. Starting a disease-modifying antirheumatic drug or a biologic agent in rheumatoid arthritis: Standards of practice for RA treatment. *J Rheumatol.* 2001;28:1704–11.

Osteoarthritis

Altman RD, Hochberg MC, Moskowitz RW, et al. Recommendations for the medical management of osteoarthritis of the hip and knee. *Arthritis Rheum.* 2000;43:1905–15.

Boh LE. Osteoarthritis. In: Dipiro JT, Talbert RL, Yee GC, et al., eds. *Pharmacotherapy: A Pathophysiologic Approach.* 4th ed. New York: McGraw-Hill; 1997:1441–59.

Roberts LJ, Morrow JD. Analgesic-antipyretic and antiinflammatory agents and drugs employed in the treatment of gout. In: Hardman JG, Limbird LE, Gilman AG, eds. *Goodman and Gilman's The Pharmacological Basis of Therapeutics.* 10th ed. New York: McGraw-Hill; 2001:687–732.

Small RE. Osteoarthritis. In: Helms RA, Quan DJ, Herfindal ET, et al., eds. *Textbook of Therapeutics: Drugs and Disease Management.* 8th ed. Baltimore: Lippincott Williams & Wilkins; 2006:1737–52.

Gout

American College of Rheumatology. 2008. Gout. www.rheumatology.org/public/factsheets/diseases_and_conditions/gout.asp.

Becker MA, Schumacher HR, Wortmann RL, et al. Febuxostat compared with allopurinol in patients with hyperuricemia and gout. *N Engl J Med.* 2005; 353:2450–61.

Emmerson BT. The management of gout. *N Engl J Med.* 1996;334:445–51.

Harris M, Bryant LR, Danaher, et al. Effect of low-dose aspirin on serum urate levels and urinary excretion in patients receiving probenecid for gouty arthritis. *J Rheumatol.* 2000;27:2873–6.

Hawkins DW, Rahn DW. Gout and hyperuricemia. In: Dipiro JT, Talbert RL, Yee GC, et al., eds. *Pharmacotherapy: A Pathophysiologic Approach.* 4th ed. New York: McGraw-Hill; 1997:1460–5.

McCloskey WW, Kostka-Rokosz MD. Gout and hyperuricemia. In: Helms RA, Quan DJ, Herfindal ET, et al., eds. *Textbook of Therapeutics: Drugs and Disease Management.* 8th ed. Baltimore: Lippincott Williams & Wilkins; 2006:1753–66.

Terkeltaub RA, Edwards NL, Pratt PW, et al. Gout. In: Klippel JH, Weyand CM, Wortmann RL, eds. *Primer on the Rheumatic Diseases.* 11th ed. Atlanta: Arthritis Foundation; 1998:230–43.

Systemic Lupus Erythematosus

Burlingame MB, Delafuente JC. Systemic lupus erythematosus. In: Dipiro JT, Talbert RL, Yee GC, et al., eds. *Pharmacotherapy: A Pathophysiologic Approach.* 4th ed. New York: McGraw-Hill; 1997:1378–92.

Krikoria S. Systemic lupus erythematosus. In: Helms RA, Quan DJ, Herfindal ET, et al., eds. *Textbook of Therapeutics: Drugs and Disease Management.* 8th ed. Baltimore: Lippincott Williams & Wilkins; 2006:1767–87.

Lupus Foundation of America. Lupus. www.lupus.org/.

Pain Management and Migraines

23

Elizabeth S. Miller, PharmD

23-1. Pain

Pain is any unpleasant sensory and emotional experience associated with actual or potential tissue damage, or defined in terms of such damage, or both. Chronic pain is a largely unrecognized problem in American society.

Currently, about 75 million individuals suffer from some form of chronic benign pain. Between one-third and one-half of chronic pain sufferers have pain severe enough to require daily medication.

Types and Clinical Presentation

Pain can be classified as acute, chronic benign, or malignant.

Acute pain is caused by an injury, illness, or surgery. It responds to medications and usually resolves when the underlying cause has been treated or healed. It is often associated with physiologic symptoms such as tachycardia, hypertension, diaphoresis, and mydriasis.

Chronic benign pain exists beyond an expected time for healing, typically 3–6 months or more. It is often associated with psychological effects, including social isolation, depression, and anxiety. Chronic pain syndromes are often not responsive to traditional analgesics and require the use of adjuvant medications.

Malignant pain may be acute, chronic, or intermittent and is often related to cancer progression or chemotherapy.

Pain is also defined by source. Such a classification divides pain into somatic, visceral, and neuropathic pain.

Somatic pain originates from the skin, muscles, tendons, ligaments, and bones. It is localized and described as sharp, stabbing, throbbing, or aching in nature. Although somatic pain can be severe, it tends to respond well to treatment with opioids.

The body's internal organs such as the liver, intestines, or stomach generate *visceral pain*. Visceral pain tends to be poorly localized and more likely to generate referred pain felt some distance away from the actual problem. Opioids are not as effective for visceral pain as they are for somatic pain.

Neuropathic pain results when the nerves themselves are damaged. It is typically burning in nature, although it may also be numb, be aching, or cause a sensation like an electric shock. Opioid medications are often ineffective for treating neuropathic pain, and adjuvant analgesics play a significant role in treatment.

Pathophysiology

Nociception, the pain sensation, begins when a sensory nerve ending is stimulated and sends repetitive signals to the spinal cord along ascending nerve fibers. An individual nerve does not transmit directly to the brain but instead connects to secondary nerves in the dorsal horn of the spinal cord. The secondary nerves eventually connect to nerve cells in the brain stem.

A descending antinociceptive pathway also exists. Neurotransmitters from the descending fibers inhibit the transmission of the pain signal. Opioids chemically resemble these neurotransmitters.

Chronic pain is not a prolonged version of acute pain. As pain signals are repeatedly generated, neural pathways undergo changes that make them hypersensitive to pain signals and resistant to antinociceptive input.

Diagnostic Criteria

The individual's self-report of pain is the primary source of information in acute pain.

Chronic pain assessment should include a detailed history of the pain's intensity and characteristics, a physical examination emphasizing the neurological exam, and a psychosocial assessment (Figure 23-1).

The purpose of diagnostic tests, such as x-rays, computed tomography, or magnetic resonance imag-ing scans, or laboratory tests differs depending on the type of pain. In cancer patients, the major purpose of diagnostic testing is to visualize the disease progression. In chronic benign pain, the major purpose of diagnostic testing is to rule out the presence of any diseases for which there is a curative treatment.

Goals of Pain Management

Acute pain

The goal in acute pain management is to provide patients with pain relief that allows them to rest comfortably and allows rehabilitation postsurgery or postinjury. This goal can be accomplished with short-acting medications administered as needed.

Malignant pain

A major goal of cancer pain management is to relieve the patient's pain without inducing disabling side effects.

The World Health Organization (WHO) has developed a three-step hierarchy for analgesic pain management in cancer pain patients (Figure 23-2). In general, this program includes using nonopioid analgesics as a baseline, supplementing with opioid anal-

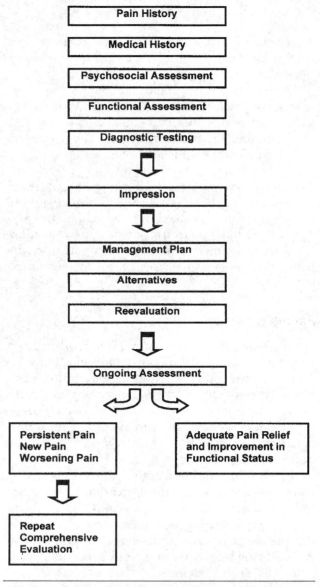

Figure 23-1. Algorithm for Comprehensive Evaluation and Management of Chronic Pain

Reproduced with permission from the Pain Management Center of Paducah.

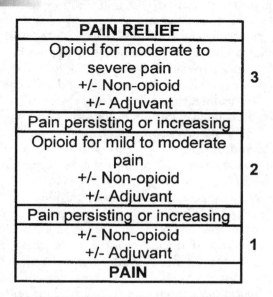

Figure 23-2. The WHO's Three-Step Hierarchy for Analgesic Pain Management in Cancer Patients

Reproduced with permission from WHO 1996.

gesics as needed, and adding adjunctive medications when appropriate.

Cancer patients may suffer from constant pain that continues for months or years. For this reason, treatment with long-acting agents is more appropriate than treatment with short-acting medications. However, short-acting agents, referred to as "breakthrough" or "rescue" doses, are often available in addition to the long-acting medications.

Chronic benign pain

The goal of chronic benign pain treatment is to restore the patient to the highest degree of function possible.

Multimodal therapy, the use of several different types of treatment, is usually required. Multimodal therapies include nerve blocks, rehabilitation, physical therapy, pharmacotherapy, acupuncture, and psychotherapy. Basic pharmacotherapy follows the WHO guidelines for treating cancer pain (Figure 23-2).

Analgesics are categorized into nonopioid analgesics, opioid analgesics, and adjuvant analgesics. Nonopioid analgesics such as acetaminophen and nonsteroidal anti-inflammatory drugs (NSAIDs) relieve all types of mild to moderate pain. Unless contraindicated, all pain patients should first be given a trial of nonopioid analgesics. Nonopioids and opioids relieve pain via different mechanisms. Thus, combination therapy offers the potential for improved relief with fewer side effects. Nonopioids do not produce tolerance, physical dependence, or addiction.

Adjuvant analgesics are drugs with a primary indication other than pain. Commonly used analgesic adjuvants include antiepileptic drugs, tricyclic antidepressants, and local anesthetics.

Principles of opioid use

Opioids have no ceiling effect of analgesia.

Oral medications should be used whenever possible. Intramuscular injections are painful and should be avoided.

When patients have constant or near-constant pain, analgesics should be given around the clock. Long-acting opioid analgesics are often used for this purpose.

The use of short-acting opioids as rescue medication is controversial in chronic benign pain. If allowed, doses of rescue medications should range from 10% to 15% of the total daily long-acting opioid dose.

Mixed agonist–antagonist opioids are not used in chronic pain. They may induce a withdrawal syndrome in patients tolerant to opioids.

Drug Therapy
Mechanism of action

Morphine and other opioid agonists are thought to produce analgesia by mimicking the action of endogenous opioid peptides that bind at opioid receptors in the antinociceptive pathway.

Opioid receptors are located in the central nervous system (CNS), pituitary gland, and gastrointestinal (GI) tract. They are abundant in the periaqueductal gray matter of the brain and the dorsal horn of the spinal cord, two areas that are very active in pain reduction.

When a drug binds to one of these receptors as an agonist, it produces analgesia. When a drug binds to one of these receptors as an antagonist, analgesia and other effects are blocked.

The three major types of opioid receptor sites involved in analgesia are mu (μ), delta (δ), and kappa (κ):

- Binding to the μ receptor produces analgesia, sedation, euphoria, respiratory depression, physical dependence, constipation, and other effects.
- Activation of the κ receptor produces analgesia and respiratory depression. In addition, psychotomimetic effects such as anxiety, strange thoughts, nightmares, and hallucinations are more common.
- Activation of δ receptors produces analgesia without many adverse events. However, there is no available δ-receptor agonist.

Opioid analgesics

Opioids are classified by activity at the receptor site; that is, they are classified as pure opioid agonists, agonist–antagonists, or pure opioid antagonists.

Pure opioid agonists primarily activate μ receptors, although they may produce some κ-receptor activation (Table 23-1). Pure opioid agonists are the most clinically useful opioid analgesics.

Morphine is the prototypical pure opioid agonist. Methadone is an opioid agonist with additional antagonist activity at the NMDA (N-methyl-D-aspartate) receptor. The NMDA receptor is believed to be active primarily in chronic pain.

Mixed agonist–antagonists bind as agonists at the κ receptor, producing weak analgesia. They bind as weak antagonists at the μ receptor (Table 23-2). The result is more dysphoria and psychotomimetic effects with a lower risk of respiratory depression.

Pentazocine is the prototypical agonist–antagonist opioid. Buprenorphine is actually a partial agonist at

Table 23-1. Starting Doses for Strong Opioids for Severe Pain in Adults: Mu Agonists

Generic name	Common product name and strength	Dosing interval	Equianalgesic dose IV	Equianalgesic dose po	Oral starting dose
Fentanyl (synthetic)					
Injection	Sublimaze 50 mcg/mL	0.5–2 hours IM or IV	0.1 mg	Not applicable	
Transdermal	Duragesic 12, 25, 50, 75, 100 mcg/h	q 2–3 days			
Transmucosal lozenge	Actiq 200, 400, 600, 800, 1,200, 1,600 mcg	prn			100 to 200 mcg
Disintegrating tablet	Fentora 100, 200, 400, 600, 800 mcg	prn			100 mcg
Hydromorphone (semisynthetic)					
Tablet	Dilaudid 2, 4, 8 mg	4–6 hours po; 6–8 hours IM, SC, or IV	1.5 mg	7.5 mg	4–8 mg
Liquid	Dilaudid 1 mg/mL; HP 10 mg/mL				
Injection	Dilaudid 1, 2, 4 mg/mL				
Levorphanol (semisynthetic)					
Tablet	Levo-Dromoran 2 mg	6–8 hours po; 3–4 hours IV; 6–8 hours IM or SC	2 mg	4 mg	2–4 mg
Injection	Levo-Dromoran 2 mg/mL				
Meperidine (synthetic)					
Tablet	Demerol 50, 100 mg	3–4 hours po; 3–4 hours IM or SC	75 mg	300 mg	50–150 mg (not recommended)
Liquid	Demerol 10 mg/mL				
Injection	Demerol 25, 50, 75, 100 mg/mL				
Methadone (synthetic)					
Tablet	Dolophine 5, 10 mg; Methadose 5, 10 mg; 40 mg dispersible	3–8 hours po; 4–12 hours IM, SC, or IV	Acute: 10 mg acute; chronic: 2–4 mg	Acute: 20 mg; chronic: 2–4 mg	2.5–10.0 mg
Liquid	Methadose 10 mg/mL; methadone hydrochloride (HCl) 1, 2, 10 mg/mL				
Injection	Methadone HCl 10 mg/mL				
Morphine (natural)					
Immediate-release tablet	MSIR 15, 30 mg	2–4 hours po; 4 hours IM, SC, or IV; 4 hours per rectum	10 mg	30 mg	5–30 mg
Liquid	MSIR 2, 4, 20 mg/mL; morphine sulfate 2, 5 mg/mL; Roxanol 20 mg/mL				
Injection	Duramorph, Astramorph PF 0.5, 1 mg/mL				
Suppository	RMS 5, 10, 20, 30 mg				
Controlled-release tablet	Avinza 30, 45, 60, 75, 90, 120 mg	24 hours po			
	Kadian 10, 20, 30, 50, 60, 80, 100, 200 mg	12–24 hours po			
	MsContin 15, 30, 60, 100, 200 mg	8–12 hours po			
	Oramorph SR 15, 30, 60, 100 mg	8–12 hours po			

Table 23-1. Starting Doses for Strong Opioids for Severe Pain in Adults: Mu Agonists *(Continued)*

Generic name	Common product name and strength	Dosing interval	Equianalgesic dose IV	Equianalgesic dose po	Oral starting dose
Oxycodone (semisynthetic)					
Tablet	Roxicodone 5, 15, 30 mg	4–6 hours po	Not applicable	20 mg	5–30 mg
Capsule	OxyIR 5 mg				
Liquid	Roxicodone 1, 20 mg/mL; OxyFast 20 mg/mL				
Tablet (oxycodone/ acetaminophen)	Magnacet 2.5/400, 5/400, 7.5/400, 10/400 mg				
Tablet (oxycodone/ acetaminophen)	Roxicet 5/325, 5/500 mg; Percocet 2.5/325, 5/325, 7.5/325, 10/325 mg				
Capsule (oxycodone/ acetaminophen)	Tylox 5/500 mg				
Liquid (oxycodone/ acetaminophen)	Roxicet 5/325 per 5 ml				
Controlled-release tablet	Oxycontin 10, 15, 20, 40, 80 mg	12 hours po			
Oxymorphone (semisynthetic)					
Injection	Oxymorphone HCl 1, 1.5 mg/ml; Opana 1 mg/ml	4–6 hours po; 4 hours IM, SC, or IV	1 mg	10 mg	5–20 mg
Immediate-release tablet	Opana 5, 10 mg	12 hours po			
Controlled-release tablet	Opana ER 5, 7.5, 10, 15, 20, 30, 40 mg				

μ and κ receptors. This opioid has limited efficacy in pain management and is primarily used in detoxification programs.

Opioid antagonists block the μ and κ receptors (Table 23-3). These drugs do not produce analgesia. They are used to reverse respiratory and CNS depression caused by overdose with opioid agonists. Naloxone and naltrexone are opioid antagonists.

Opioid analgesic adverse effects

Central nervous system

Opioids produce a number of CNS effects, including sedation, euphoria, dysphoria, changes in mood, and mental clouding. Confusion, disorientation, and cognitive impairment are also possible.

Chronic sedation can be treated with CNS stimulants such as methylphenidate or dextroamphetamine. Modafinil also promotes daytime wakefulness.

Mild to moderate muscle jerks are common in patients on high doses of opioids. Myoclonus can be treated by changing the opioid dose, changing the opioid, or giving low doses of a benzodiazepine.

Neuroendocrine

Morphine acts in the hypothalamus to inhibit the release of gonadotropin-releasing hormone and corticotropin-releasing factor, thus decreasing levels of luteinizing hormone, follicle-stimulating hormone, adrenocorticotropic hormone, and β-endorphins.

Changes in hormone levels may cause decreased levels of testosterone and cortisol, disturbances in menstruation, and sexual dysfunction.

High doses of morphine and related opioids produce convulsions. Most convulsions occur at doses far in excess of those required to produce analgesia.

Table 23-2. Opioid Dosing for Mild to Moderate Pain in Adults

Generic name	Common product name and strength	Dosing interval	IV starting dose	Oral starting dose
Moderate-mild opioids				
Codeine (natural)				
Tablet	Codeine sulfate 15, 30, 60 mg (CII)	4–6 hours	15–30 mg	15–60 mg
Injection	Codeine phosphate 15, 30 mg/mL			
Tablet (codeine/ acetaminophen)	Tylenol with Codeine #1 (300/7.5 mg), #2 (300/15 mg), #3 (300/30 mg), #4 (300/60 mg)			
Liquid (codeine/ acetaminophen)	Tylenol with Codeine Elixir 8/160 mg per 5 mL			
Hydrocodone (semisynthetic)				
Tablet (hydrocodone/ acetaminophen)	Vicodin 5/500 mg; Vicodin ES 7.5/750 mg; Vicodin HD 10/660 mg; Norco 5/325, 7.5/325, 10/325 mg; Lortab 2.5/500, 5/500, 7.5/500, 10/500 mg; Lorcet 10/650 mg	4–6 hours	Not applicable	5–10 mg
Liquid (hydrocodone/ acetaminophen)	Hycet 7.5/325 mg per 15 mL; Lortab Elixir 7.5/500 mg per 15 mL			
Tablet (hydrocodone/ ibuprofen)	Zydone 5/400, 7.5/400, 10/400 mg; Vicoprofen 7.5/200 mg; Reprexain 2.5/200, 5/200, 10/200 mg			
Propoxyphene (synthetic)				
Tablet (propoxyphene/ acetaminophen)	Darvocet N 50 (50/325 mg); Darvocet N 100 (100/650 mg)	4–6 hours	Not applicable	65–130 mg; maximum 600 mg/d
Capsule (propoxyphene/ acetaminophen)	Darvon 65 mg			
Agonists-antagonists				
Pentazocine				
Tablet (pentazocine/ naloxone)	Talwin NX 50/0.5 mg	4 hours		50–100 mg; maximum 600 mg/d
Tablet (pentazocine/ aspirin)	Talwin Compound 12.5/325 mg	6–8 hours	30 mg IM, SC, or IV; maximum 360 mg/d	12.5–25 mg
Injection	Talwin 30 mg/mL	3–4 hours		
Butorphanol				
Injection	Stadol 1, 2 mg/mL	3–4 hours	0.5–2 mg	
Nasal spray	Butorphanol tartrate 1 mg/spray			1 spray in 1 nostril
Nalbuphine injection	Nalbuphine HCl 10, 20 mg/mL	3–6 hours	10 mg	
Buprenorphine injection	Buprenex 0.3 mg/mL	6–8 hours	0.3–0.6 mg	
Miscellaneous				
Tablet	Ultram 50 mg	4–6 hours		50–100 mg; maximum 400 mg/d
Controlled-release tablet	Ultram ER, Ryzolt 100, 200, 300 mg	24 hours		100 mg; maximum 300 mg/d
Tablet (tramadol/ acetaminophen)	Ultracet 325/37.5 mg			

Table 23-3. Opioid Antagonists

Generic name	Common product name and strength	Dosing interval	IV starting dose	Oral starting dose
Naloxone injection	Naloxone HCl 0.4 mg/mL	Every 2–3 min	Opioid overdose: 0.4–2 mg; postoperative narcotic depression: 0.1–0.2 mg	
Naltrexone				
Tablet	Revia 50 mg; naltrexone HCl 25, 50, 100 mg	qd, qod, q3d		Alcoholism: 50 mg qd; narcotic addiction: 50 mg qd, 100 mg qod, or 150 mg q3d
Injection	Vivitrol 380 mg/vial	Monthly	Alcoholism: 380 mg monthly	

Respiratory

Respiratory depression is the most serious opioid-induced adverse effect. Opioids depress respiration by a direct effect on the brain-stem respiratory centers, making the brain stem less responsive to carbon dioxide.

The μ receptor is the primary receptor involved in respiratory depression, although activation of the κ receptor also contributes.

At equianalgesic doses, all of the pure opioid agonists depress respiration to the same degree. The agonist–antagonists have a ceiling effect (i.e., a dose beyond which no further respiratory depression or analgesia is produced), but this level is usually above recommended doses.

Opioids depress cough by inducing a direct effect on the cough reflex in the medulla.

Cardiovascular

Therapeutic doses of many opioids produce peripheral vasodilation, reduced peripheral resistance, and inhibition of the baroreceptor reflexes.

Peripheral vasodilation results primarily from opioid-induced release of histamine. Orthostatic hypotension and fainting can result. The naturally occurring and semisynthetic products are potent histamine releasers. Fentanyl has little propensity to release histamine.

Methadone has been associated with torsades de pointes, an atypical rapid ventricular tachycardia, at an average daily dose of 400 mg. Methadone should be used cautiously in patients on other QTc-prolonging medications.

Gastrointestinal

All clinically significant μ agonists produce some degree of nausea and vomiting by direct stimulation of the chemoreceptor trigger zone in the medulla, sensitization of the vestibular system, and slowing of GI motility.

Nausea and vomiting commonly occur in ambulatory patients (15–40% of patients with nausea and vomiting are ambulatory). Both can be pretreated with an antiemetic such as promethazine or prochlorperazine.

Opioids promote constipation by delaying gastric emptying, slowing bowel motility, and decreasing peristalsis. Opioids may also reduce secretions from the colonic mucosa. At its worst, gastrointestinal dysfunction results in ileus, fecal impaction, and obstruction.

Because transdermal delivery bypasses absorption from the GI tract, constipation has been reported to be less frequent with this delivery method than with other methods.

Patients on opiates do not develop tolerance to constipation. All patients taking around-the-clock opioid analgesics should be placed on prophylactic bowel regimens. Bowel regimens include increased fluid and fiber intake, daily stool softeners, and mild laxatives.

Severe constipation is managed with osmotic laxatives such as magnesium citrate and milk of magnesia.

Genitourinary

Opioids increase smooth muscle tone in the bladder and ureters and may cause bladder spasm and urgency.

An opioid-induced increase in sphincter tone can make urination difficult. Urinary retention is most common in elderly men.

Biliary

Opioids increase smooth muscle tone in the biliary tract, especially in the sphincter of Oddi, which regulates the flow of bile and pancreatic fluids. This effect can result in a decrease in biliary and pancreatic secretions and a rise in the bile duct pressure. Patients may experience epigastric distress and occasionally biliary spasm.

All opioids are capable of causing constriction of the sphincter of Oddi and the biliary tract. Although morphine may cause more biliary constriction in animals than do other opioids, this finding has never been shown to be clinically useful in humans.

Skin and eye

Therapeutic doses of morphine dilate cutaneous blood vessels, which causes flushing on the face, neck, and upper thorax. Sweating and pruritus may also occur. These changes may be caused in part by release of histamine. Histamine release may induce or worsen asthmatic attacks in predisposed patients and can lead to wheezing, bronchoconstriction, and status asthmaticus.

Skin rash around the transdermal fentanyl patch is a common side effect caused by the patch adhesive.

Following a toxic dose of μ agonists, miosis is marked and pinpoint pupils are pathognomonic; however, mydriasis occurs when asphyxia intervenes.

Overdose

Acute overdose with opioids is manifested by respiratory depression; somnolence progressing to stupor or coma; skeletal muscle flaccidity; cold, clammy skin; constricted pupils; and sometimes pulmonary edema, bradycardia, hypotension, and death.

An opioid antagonist may be given to block opioid receptors and reverse the effects of overdose.

Antagonist administration may cause a complete reversal of opioid effects and precipitate an acute withdrawal syndrome in persons physically dependent on opioids.

Antagonists are dosed to patient response every few minutes. If no response is observed after 10 mg, the diagnosis of opioid-induced toxicity should be questioned.

Infusion may be useful in cases of overdose with long-acting drugs such as methadone. The infusion rate for adults is approximately 100 mL/h (0.4 mg/h).

Tolerance and physical dependence

The use of opioids is often limited by concerns regarding tolerance, physical dependence, and addiction.

Tolerance can be defined as a state in which a larger dose is required to produce the same response that could formerly be elicited by a smaller dose. Tolerance to analgesia is demonstrated by the need for an increased dosage of a drug to produce the same level of analgesia. Tolerance to analgesia develops more slowly than tolerance to other opioid effects.

Tolerance to adverse effects of opioids occurs after 2–3 weeks of continuous administration. Tolerance to the constipating and neuroendocrine effects of opioids does not occur.

Physical dependence is the occurrence of a withdrawal syndrome after an opioid is stopped or quickly decreased without titration. Warn patients to avoid abrupt discontinuation of such drugs.

Addiction is the psychological dependence on the use of a substance. It is characterized by impaired control over drug use, compulsive use, craving, and continued use despite harm.

Pharmacokinetics of Selected Opioids

Morphine

Compared with other opioids, morphine is relatively insoluble in lipids (i.e., in adults, only small amounts of the drug cross the blood–brain barrier).

Morphine does not accumulate in tissues when given in normal dose and therefore does not cause increasing toxicity with frequent dosing.

Morphine is primarily metabolized by glucuronidation during the first pass through the liver. Approximately 50% of morphine is converted by the liver to morphine-3-glucuronide and 15% to morphine-6-glucuronide (M6G). The pharmacologic effects of morphine (both analgesia and side effects) are in part caused by M6G.

Much of an oral dose is inactivated during this first pass through the liver; consequently, oral doses need to be much larger than parenteral doses to produce the same analgesic effects.

Fentanyl

Fentanyl is highly soluble in lipids. It accumulates in skeletal muscle and fat and is released slowly into the blood. Plasma half-life is 3–4 hours after parenteral administration.

Fentanyl is rapidly metabolized, primarily by dealkylation, to inactive metabolites in the liver. This process is mediated through the cytochrome P450 (CYP450) 3A4 hepatic enzyme system. The presence of inactive metabolites makes fentanyl a preferred drug in patients with liver dysfunction.

Fentanyl is not used orally because of low oral bioavailability.

Transdermal fentanyl

The uptake of fentanyl through the skin is relatively slow and constant. The skin does not metabolize the drug, and 92% of the dose is delivered into the bloodstream as intact fentanyl.

Because of temperature-dependent increases in fentanyl release from the patch system as well as increased skin permeability, an increase in body temperature to 40°C (104°F) theoretically may increase serum fentanyl concentrations by approximately one-third.

Fentanyl is absorbed into the upper layers of the skin, forming a depot. Fentanyl then becomes available to systemic circulation. Serum fentanyl concentrations are measurable within 2 hours after application of the first patch, and analgesic effects can be observed 8–16 hours after application. Steady state is reached after several sequential patch applications.

Transmucosal fentanyl citrate lozenge

The absorption pharmacokinetics of fentanyl from the oral transmucosal dosage form is a combination of initial rapid absorption from buccal mucosa and delayed absorption of fentanyl from the GI tract. Normally 25% of the total dose is available by buccal absorption, and 25% is available from the GI tract, making the total bioavailability 50%.

Analgesia begins in 10–15 minutes, peaks in 20 minutes, and persists for 1–2 hours.

Transmucosal fentanyl is indicated only for those already receiving and who are tolerant to around-the-clock opioid therapy.

Fentanyl citrate buccal tablet

Following buccal administration, fentanyl is readily absorbed with an absolute bioavailability of 65%. Approximately 50% of the total dose administered is absorbed transmucosally and becomes systemically available. The remaining half of the total dose is swallowed and undergoes more prolonged absorption from the GI tract.

Buccal tablets are indicated only for those already receiving around-the-clock opioid therapy.

Methadone

After therapeutic doses, about 90% of methadone is bound to plasma protein and is widely distributed in tissues. Methadone is found in low concentrations in the blood and the brain, with higher concentrations in the kidney, spleen, liver, and lung. Terminal half-life is extremely variable (15–55 hours); therefore, accumulation is possible, and dosing intervals need to be carefully monitored.

Methadone is extensively metabolized in the liver, mainly by N-demethylation. This process appears to be mediated primarily by CYP450 3A4 and to a lesser extent by CYP450 2D6. The major metabolites are excreted in the bile and urine.

Analgesic efficacy does not correspond to the half-life of the drug. Methadone may be dosed every 3 hours for pain control.

Oxycodone

Oxycodone is metabolized to noroxycodone, oxymorphone, and their glucuronides via the CYP450 enzyme system. The major circulating metabolite is noroxycodone. Noroxycodone is reported to be a weaker analgesic than oxycodone. Oxymorphone, although possessing good analgesic activity, is present in the plasma only in low concentrations. Its metabolism is mediated by CYP450 2D6.

Hydromorphone

Hydromorphone is metabolized to three major metabolites: hydromorphone 3-glucuronide, hydromorphone 3-glucoside, and dihydroisomorphine 6-glucoside. Whether hydromorphone is metabolized by the CYP450 system is not known. Hydromorphone is a poor inhibitor of CYP450 isoenzymes and is not expected to inhibit the metabolism of other drugs.

Meperidine

Normeperidine, a metabolite of meperidine, produces anxiety, tremors, myoclonus, and generalized seizures when it accumulates with repetitive dosing. Patients with compromised renal function are particularly at risk. Naloxone does not reverse this hyperexcitability. For these reasons, meperidine should not be used for more than 48 hours in patients with renal or CNS disease or at doses greater than 600 mg every 24 hours.

Propoxyphene

Propoxyphene is appropriate for short-term mild to intermittent pain. It produces a toxic metabolite, norpropoxyphene, with effects similar to normeperidine.

Drug Interactions and Drug–Disease Interactions

Drug interactions

All drugs with CNS depressant actions (barbiturates, benzodiazepines, alcohol) can intensify sedation and respiratory depression caused by morphine and other opioids.

Antihistamines, tricyclic antidepressants, and atropine-like drugs can exacerbate morphine-induced constipation and urinary retention.

Antihypertensive drugs and others that lower blood pressure can exacerbate opioid-induced hypotension.

The combination of meperidine and a monoamine oxidase (MAO) inhibitor has produced a syndrome characterized by excitation, delirium, hyperpyrexia, convulsions, and severe respiratory depression. Death has also occurred. Although this syndrome has not been reported with other opioids, combinations containing opioids and MAO inhibitors should be avoided.

Agonist–antagonists can precipitate a withdrawal syndrome if administered to an individual who is physically dependent on a pure opioid agonist.

CYP450 enzymes metabolize codeine, hydrocodone, fentanyl, methadone, and oxycodone. Although not well documented, drug interactions through this system may exist. In particular, transdermal fentanyl should be used with caution in a patient on a CYP450 3A4 inhibitor. The patient should be monitored over an extended period and dose adjustments made as appropriate.

Codeine, hydrocodone, and oxycodone require metabolism through CYP450 2D6 to active drug (Table 23-4). Approximately 7% of Caucasians, 3% of African Americans, and 1% of Asians are poor metabolizers of CYP450 2D6; they produce no CYP450 2D6 or produce undetectable levels of it. Poor metabolizers may experience little or no analgesia from drugs requiring 2D6 for conversion to active metabolites.

About 5% of the patients have multiple copies of the CYP450 2D6 gene, making them ultrafast metab-

Table 23-4. CYP450 2D6 Enzyme Activity

Substrates	Inhibitors	Inducers
Codeine	Celecoxib	Carbamazepine
Hydrocodone	Cimetidine	Ethanol
Meperidine	Citalopram	Phenobarbital
Methadone	Fluoxetine	Phenytoin
Oxycodone	Methadone	Rifampin
Propoxyphene	Paroxetine	
Tramadol	Propoxyphene	
	Sertraline	

olizers. The clearance of some opioids may be increased, making more frequent dosing of the medications necessary.

Drug–disease interactions

In view of the extensive hepatic metabolism of opioids, their effects may be increased in patients with liver disease, particularly those with severe liver failure. Most opioids require dose reduction in severe liver disease.

Fentanyl, morphine, and methadone require dosing adjustment in renal impairment. Doses of fentanyl and morphine should be reduced 25% when creatinine clearance (CrCl) is 10–50 mL/min and by 50% when CrCl is < 10 mL/min. The dosing interval of methadone should be increased to at least every 6 hours when CrCl is 10–50 mL/min and to every 8 hours when CrCl is < 10 mL/min.

Renal impairment slows the clearance of morphine conjugates, resulting in accumulation of the active metabolite M6G. For this reason, dosage reduction may be advisable in the presence of clinically significant renal impairment.

Methadone appears to be firmly bound to protein in various tissues, including the brain. After repeated administrations, methadone gradually accumulates in tissues. The risk of accumulation is greater in patients with impaired renal or hepatic function because both organs are involved in the metabolism of methadone.

Patient Counseling

Respiratory depression is increased by concurrent use of other drugs with CNS-depressant activity (e.g., alcohol, barbiturates, and benzodiazepines). Outpatients should be warned against the use of alcohol with all other CNS depressants.

Inform patients about symptoms of hypotension (lightheadedness, dizziness). Patients should minimize hypotension by moving slowly when changing from a supine to an upright position.

Fentanyl transdermal patch

The fentanyl transdermal patch must be applied to a clean, nonhairy site on the upper torso. Only water should be used to clean the area. Soap or alcohol can increase the effects of the medication and should not be used. The patch should not be applied to oily, broken, burned, cut, or irritated skin. It must be held in place for a minimum of 30 seconds to ensure adhesion.

Each new patch should be applied to a different area of skin to avoid irritation. If a patch comes off or causes irritation, it should be removed and a new patch applied to a different site.

To dispose of the patch, fold it in half and flush down the toilet.

Do not cut or damage the patch.

Temperature-dependent increases in fentanyl release from the patch could result in an overdose. Advise patients to avoid exposing the patch to direct external heat sources such as heating pads, electric blankets, heat lamps, saunas, hot tubs, and heated waterbeds. In addition, patients who develop a high fever while wearing the patch should contact their physician immediately.

Long-acting opioid formulations

The long-acting formulations should be swallowed whole (i.e., not broken, chewed, or crushed).

Avinza, a long-acting morphine capsule formulation, contains fumaric acid. Doses above 1,600 mg per day contain a quantity of fumaric acid that has not been demonstrated to be safe and may result in serious renal toxicity.

Kadian and Avinza (long-acting morphine sulfate) may be opened and the beads ingested with a small amount of applesauce (sprinkle administration). In addition, Kadian is approved for sprinkle administration through a gastrostomy tube.

Patients must not consume alcoholic beverages or any medications containing alcohol while on Opana ER therapy. The co-ingestion of alcohol with Opana ER may result in increased plasma levels and a potentially fatal overdose of oxymorphone. In addition, food increases the Opana ER maximum concentration by approximately 50%. Opana ER should be ingested 1 hour before and 2 hours after a meal.

Transmucosal fentanyl citrate lozenge

The lozenge is used by placing it in the mouth between the cheek and the gum. Consumption of the lozenge should take 15 minutes. Another lozenge may be used 30 minutes after the start of the first one. Tell the patient not to bite or chew the lozenge.

To dispose of a finished lozenge, discard the handle in a place that is out of reach of children and pets. If medicine remains on the handle, place the handle under hot running tap water until the medicine is dissolved. Never leave unused or partly used lozenges where children or pets can get to them.

Fentanyl citrate buccal tablet

Once removed from the blister pack, the lozenge must be used right away. It is placed in the mouth above the back molars and between the upper cheek and gum. It is left in place until it dissolves, which may take between 14 and 25 minutes. After 30 minutes, any remaining tablet is swallowed with a glass of water.

Parameters to monitor

Evaluate for pain control 1 hour after opioid administration. If analgesia is insufficient, consider a dosage increase. Patients taking opioids chronically should be evaluated regularly for adequate doses.

Monitor the patient for respiratory depression. Higher risk for respiratory depression exists in patients who are not tolerant to opioid analgesics. Consider treatment when the respiratory rate is less than 8–12 respirations per minute for 30 minutes or longer despite stimulation or if oxygen saturation is less than 90%.

If a patient is easily arousable, he or she is unlikely to have respiratory depression.

Tramadol

Tramadol is an analogue of codeine, whose mechanism of action is not completely understood. Analgesia is apparently mediated by binding of the parent molecule and the O-desmethyltramadol (M1) active metabolite to μ opioid receptors, as well as by weak inhibition of neuronal uptake of norepinephrine and serotonin. Tramadol is not a federally controlled substance.

The liver extensively metabolizes tramadol. The formation of the M1 active metabolite is dependent on CYP450 2D6. M1 appears to be up to 6 times more potent than tramadol in producing analgesia and 200 times more potent in binding to μ opioid receptors. CYP450 3A4 and CYP450 2B6 also play a role in tramadol metabolism. Caution should be exercised when administering tramadol to patients on CYP450 2D6 and CYP450 3A4 inhibitors.

The most common adverse effects are sedation, dizziness, headache, dry mouth, and constipation. Respiratory depression is minimal. Seizures have been reported; avoid use of tramadol in patients with seizure disorders or recognized risk for seizure (such as head trauma, metabolic disorders, alcohol and drug withdrawal, and CNS infections).

23-2. Nonpharmacologic Treatment of Pain

General Principles of Nonpharmacologic Treatment

Nonpharmacologic strategies used in combination with appropriate drug regimens may improve pain relief by enhancing the therapeutic effects of medications and permitting use of lower doses.

Nonpharmacologic interventions should not be a substitute for analgesic use.

Physical Interventions

Physical therapy

Physical therapy is most commonly used to help restore physical strength and functioning after injury or surgery.

Physical therapy can provide pain relief for patients with musculoskeletal pain, some types of neuropathic pain, and sympathetically mediated pain.

Acupuncture

The National Institutes of Health recognize the benefit of acupuncture as an adjunct treatment of painful conditions.

Transcutaneous electrical nerve stimulation

In transcutaneous electrical nerve stimulation (TENS), a controlled, low-voltage electrical current is applied through electrodes placed on the skin. Theoretically, the current will interfere with the ability of nerves to transmit pain signals to the spinal cord and brain. After several decades of research, it still is not clear if TENS provides any better pain relief than placebo.

Neurostimulation

Neurostimulation involves implanting a computerized generator and electrodes near the spinal cord, near the peripheral nerves, or within the brain. Stimulators are most effective for patients with neuropathic pain and are not very beneficial in other types of pain.

Behavioral Techniques

Biofeedback

In biofeedback, electrodes connected to amplifiers are placed on the body or scalp. During biofeedback sessions, a therapist helps the patient learn to mentally control and change the signals from the electrodes, which helps the patient gain conscious control over normally unconscious functions. Biofeedback is most commonly used to relax muscles and reduce stress. Its advantages are that it is noninvasive, inexpensive, and safe; however, usually between 5 and 15 sessions are required before effective control is achieved.

Distraction and relaxation

Distraction and relaxation assist the patient in refocusing attention on nonpainful stimuli. Both are believed to improve mental health, which translates into improved pain control.

23-3. Migraine

Migraine is a chronic neurovascular disorder characterized by recurrent attacks of severe headache and autonomic nervous system dysfunction. Some patients also experience aura with neurologic symptoms. An estimated 18% of women and 6% of men experience migraine.

Clinical Presentation and Diagnostic Criteria

Migraine classification is based on whether an aura of visual or sensory symptoms is present. Migraine with aura is less common than migraine without aura.

Migraine headache manifests as moderate or severe throbbing pain that is localized in the temple or around the eye. It is accompanied by nausea in 90% of patients and vomiting in about half of patients.

Photophobia (increased sensitivity to light) and phonophobia (increased sensitivity to sound) also are frequent complaints. A prodrome of mood changes, stiff neck, fatigue, or other symptoms may occur hours or days before the onset of the headache.

Criteria for diagnosing migraine without aura

- The patient has at least five headaches lasting 4–72 hours each.
- The headaches have at least two of the following four characteristics:
  - Unilateral location
  - Pulsating quality
  - Moderate or severe intensity (inhibits or prohibits daily activities)
  - Aggravation with walking stairs or similar routine physical activity

■ During the headache, at least one of the following symptoms occurs:
  • Nausea or vomiting
  • Photophobia
  • Phonophobia
■ Symptoms cannot be consistent with other headache types.

Criteria for diagnosis of migraine with aura

■ The patient has at least two attacks with three of the following four criteria:
  • One or more completely reversible aura symptoms occur, indicating focal cerebral cortical or brain stem dysfunction (or both).
  • At least one aura symptom develops gradually (> 4 minutes) or two or more symptoms occur in succession.
  • No aura symptom lasts > 60 minutes.
  • Headache follows aura in < 1 hour.
■ There is no evidence of related organic disease.

Pathophysiology

Migraine and the brain

The pathogenesis of migraine is unclear and is thought to be multifactorial. The current thinking is that a primary neuronal dysfunction originates in the CNS, leading to a sequence of changes that account for the different stages of migraine.

The Cortical Spreading Depression theory explains that a wave of depolarization spreads across the cerebral cortex from occipital to frontal regions, resulting in brain ion dysfunction and secondary vasoconstrictor vascular events. These changes account for the progression and variety of symptoms that occur in patients with prodromal or aura phase.

The headache phase is probably related to trigeminovascular activation with the release of inflammatory neuropeptides, such as substance P, neurokinin A, and calcitonin gene-related peptide, in the trigeminal vascular system. This process, in turn, causes vasodilation.

It is suggested that the pain of headache is due to vasodilation as well as direct stimulation via the thalamus of the cortical pain areas situated in higher centers of the CNS. Not all migraine patients experience aura, so both direct effects and the secondary vasoactive responses account for the headache in patients who have migraine attacks without the aura.

The pathophysiology of the postdrome is unknown, but it may be caused by a gradual recovery from the extreme neurologic disruption that occurs during migraine.

Individuals prone to migraine may have a genetic migraine threshold that renders them susceptible to a migraine attack on exposure to some or any of a range of patient-specific triggers. Hormonal influences, environmental and physiologic stressors, low blood sugar, and fatigue are all thought to affect this threshold. Once the threshold is exceeded, trigeminovascular activation is thought to be responsible for inducing a migraine.

Treatment Principles

Abortive therapy

The U.S. Headache Consortium identifies the following goals for successful treatment of acute attacks of migraine:

■ Treat attacks rapidly and consistently and prevent recurrence.
■ Restore the patient's ability to function.
■ Minimize the use of rescue medication.
■ Optimize self-care and reduce subsequent use of resources.
■ Promote cost-effective therapies with minimal adverse effects.

Successful treatment of migraine depends on early intervention in relation to onset of headache and adequate dosing.

Preventive therapy

Preventive therapy should be considered in the following situations:

■ Attacks unresponsive to abortive medication
■ Attacks causing substantial disability
■ Attacks occurring twice or more monthly
■ Patient at risk for rebound headache
■ Trend in increasing frequency of attacks

Two-thirds of patients taking preventive medication will have a 50% decrease in the frequency of attacks.

The minimum duration of trial for a daily preventive medication is 2–3 months. No consensus exists on the duration of the prophylaxis trial period; however, prophylaxis efficacy may continue to improve when a medication is taken continuously for months to years.

The goals of migraine preventive therapy are as follows:

■ Reduce attack frequency, severity, and duration.
■ Improve responsiveness to treatment of acute attacks.
■ Improve function and reduce disability.

Rebound headaches

Persons who take abortive medications daily can develop drug rebound headaches, or headaches that begin upon discontinuation of a medication. Essentially all of the medications, with the possible exception of the triptans, cause rebound headache.

Drug Therapy

Abortive therapy: Nonprescription medications

Aspirin, acetaminophen, ibuprofen, and other aspirin-like analgesics provide adequate relief of mild to moderate migraines. Advil Migraine (ibuprofen 200 mg liquid-filled caps) and Motrin Migraine Relief (ibuprofen 200 mg) are examples of nonprescription medications indicated for migraine relief.

Combination products containing aspirin, acetaminophen, or both with caffeine are also available without a prescription. Caffeine has analgesic and possibly anti-inflammatory properties. It may also increase gastric acidity and perfusion, enhancing the absorption of aspirin. Excedrin Migraine (acetaminophen 250 mg, aspirin 250 mg, and caffeine 65 mg) is an example of an available combination nonprescription product.

Abortive therapy: Nonspecific prescription medications

Combination products containing an analgesic, caffeine, and butalbital or codeine are available. The butalbital may be useful for its sedative properties. Excessive use of these products can cause physical dependence and rebound headaches.

A combination of the vasoconstrictor isometheptene, the sedative dichloralphenazone, and acetaminophen (Midrin) may be useful for mild to moderate migraines. Isometheptene is also available in combination with acetaminophen and caffeine (Migraten). Both combinations are generally well tolerated.

Opioids are well recognized as good analgesics, but strong evidence exists only for the efficacy of butorphanol nasal spray for migraine. Although opioids are commonly used, surprisingly few studies of opioid use in headache pain document whether overuse and the development of dependence are as frequent as clinically perceived.

Given intravenously, the antiemetic metoclopramide may be appropriate as monotherapy for acute attacks, particularly in patients with significant nausea. Chlorpromazine and prochlorperazine may also be considered. Serotonin-receptor antagonists ($5\text{-}HT_3$) have not been shown to be useful migraine treatments.

Abortive therapy: Ergotamine

Mechanism of action

In cranial arteries, ergotamine acts directly to promote constriction and reduce the amplitude of pulsations. In addition, the drug can affect blood flow by depressing the vasomotor center. Antimigraine effects are possibly due to agonist activity at serotonin receptor subtypes $5\text{-}HT_{1B}$ and $5\text{-}HT_{1D}$.

Because of the risk of dependence, ergotamine should not be taken daily on a long-term basis.

Caffeine may be added to ergotamine to enhance vasoconstriction and ergotamine absorption (Table 23-5).

Pharmacokinetics

Oral ergotamine has poor bioavailability because of extensive first-pass metabolism. Sublingual administration may not provide therapeutic blood levels.

Although the half-life of ergotamine is only 2 hours, pharmacologic effects can be seen for 24 hours after administration.

The drug is eliminated primarily by hepatic metabolism. Metabolites are excreted in the bile.

Adverse effects

Ergotamine is well tolerated at usual therapeutic doses.

The drug can stimulate the chemoreceptor trigger zone to cause nausea and vomiting in about 10% of patients. Concurrent treatment with metoclopramide or a phenothiazine antiemetic can help suppress this response.

Other common side effects include weakness in the legs, myalgia, numbness and tingling in the periphery, angina-like pain, tachycardia, and bradycardia.

Overdose

Acute or chronic overdose can cause serious toxicity (ergotism). Symptoms include ischemia, myalgias, and paresthesias. Ischemia can progress to gangrene.

The risk of ergotism is highest in patients with sepsis, peripheral vascular disease, and renal or hepatic impairment.

Drug–drug and drug–disease interactions

Ergotamine should not be combined with selective serotonin-receptor agonists because of the risk of a prolonged vasospastic reaction.

Table 23-5. Agents Used in Migraine Treatment

Drug	Common brand names and strengths	Maximum daily dose (weekly maximum)	Dosing instructions
Ergot alkaloids			
Ergotamine sublingual tablet	Ergomar 2 mg	6 mg (10 mg) po	1 tablet at onset; then 1 every 30 min prn
Ergotamine/caffeine tablet	Cafergot 1/100 mg	Ergotamine 6 mg (10 mg)	2 tablets at onset; then 1 every 30 min prn
Ergotamine/caffeine suppository	Migergot 2/100 mg; Cafergot 2/100 mg	Ergotamine 4 mg (10 mg)	Insert 1 at onset; repeat in 1 hour prn
Dihydroergotamine	Injection: 1 mg/mL DHE 45 Nasal spray: Migranal 4 mg/mL	DHE 2 mg (6 mg IV or 3 mg IM)	0.5–1.0 mg IV or IM every hour as needed
		DHE 2 mg (6 mg)	Administer 1 spray (0.5 mg) in each nostril, followed in 15 min by an additional spray in each nostril
Miscellaneous agents			
Isometheptene/ dichloralphenazone/ acetaminophen capsule	Midrin 65/100/325 mg	5 capsules within a 12-hour period	2 capsules at once, followed by 1 capsule every hour until headache is relieved
Isometheptene/ acetaminophen/caffeine capsule	Migraten 65/325/100 mg	5 capsules within a 12-hour period	2 capsules at once, followed by 1 capsule every hour until headache is relieved

Separate doses of ergotamine and serotonin agonists by at least 24 hours.

Ergotamine is contraindicated for patients with hepatic or renal impairment, sepsis, coronary artery disease (CAD), and peripheral vascular disease.

Patient counseling
Monitor patients to avoid overuse of the medication.

Ergotamine and its derivatives are U.S. Food and Drug Administration (FDA) pregnancy category X. They should not be taken during pregnancy because of their ability to promote uterine contractions and cause fetal harm or abortion.

Teach patients to recognize signs of ergotism. Muscle pain, paresthesias, and cold or pale extremities should be reported immediately.

Abortive therapy: Dihydroergotamine

Mechanism of action
The action of dihydroergotamine (DHE) is similar to that of ergotamine. Like ergotamine, DHE alters transmission at serotonergic, dopaminergic, and α-adrenergic junctions.

In contrast to ergotamine, DHE causes minimal peripheral vasoconstriction, little nausea and vomiting, and no physical dependence. However, diarrhea is prominent.

Contraindications are the same as for ergotamine: CAD, peripheral vascular disease, sepsis, pregnancy, and hepatic or renal impairment.

As with ergotamine, do not administer DHE within 24 hours of a serotonin agonist.

Pharmacokinetics
DHE is not active orally because of extensive first-pass metabolism.

An active metabolite, 8′-hydroxydihydroergotamine, contributes to its therapeutic effects. The half-life of DHE plus its active metabolite is about 21 hours.

Concomitant administration of DHE with potent CYP450 3A4 inhibitors, including protease inhibitors and macrolide antibiotics, is contraindicated. Because CYP450 3A4 inhibition elevates the serum levels of DHE, the risk for vasospasm leading to cerebral ischemia or ischemia of the extremities is increased.

Abortive therapy: Selective serotonin-receptor agonists

The selective serotonin-receptor agonists, also known as *triptans,* are first-line drugs for terminating a migraine attack (Table 23-6). The triptans all activate 5-HT_{1B}/5-HT_{1D} and to a lesser extent 5-HT_{1A} or 5-HT_{1F} receptors. Triptans have no known affinity for 5-HT_2 or 5-HT_3 and other 5-HT receptor subclasses,

Table 23-6. Selective Serotonin Receptor Agonists (Triptans)

Drug	Brand name	Available strengths	Dosage (maximum daily dose)	Half-life	Onset	Metabolism
Almotriptan	Axert	Tablet: 6.25, 12.5 mg	12.5 mg; repeat in 2 hours (25 mg)	3.5 hours	60 min	CYP450: MAO
Sumatriptan	Imitrex	Tablet: 25, 50, 100 mg	50–100 mg; repeat in 2 hours (200 mg)	2.5 hours	60–120 min	MAO
		Nasal: 5, 20 mg	5 or 20 mg; repeat in 2 hours (40 mg)		15–20 min	
		Injection: 6 mg/mL; Statdose injection: 4, 6 mg/mL	4 or 6 mg; repeat in 1 hour (12 mg)		10–15 min	
Eletriptan	Relpax	Tablet: 20, 40 mg	20 mg; repeat in 2 hours (80 mg)	5 hours	60 min	CYP450 3A4
Frovatriptan	Frova	Tablet: 2.5 mg	2.5 mg; repeat in 2 hours (7.5 mg)	25 hours	60–120 min	Renal 50%
Rizatriptan	Maxalt	Tablet or wafer: 5, 10 mg	5 or 10 mg; repeat in 2 hours (30 mg)	2–3 hours	30 min	MAO
Zolmitriptan	Zomig	Tablet or wafer: 2.5, 5 mg	2.5 or 5 mg; repeat in 2 hours (10 mg)	2.5–4 hours	45 min	CYP450: MAO
		Nasal: 5 mg	5 mg; repeat in 2 hours (10 mg)	3 hours	10–15 min	CYP450: MAO
Naratriptan	Amerge	Tablet: 1, 2.5 mg	1 or 2.5 mg; repeat in 4 hours (5 mg)	6 hours	60 min	Renal 70%; CYP450
Miscellaneous agents						
Sumatriptan/naproxen	Treximet	Tablet: 85/500 mg	1 tablet; may repeat in 2 hours (2 tablets) The safety of treating more than 5 migraines in a 30-day period has not been established.	Sumatriptan 2 hours/ naproxen 19 hours	60–120 min	Sumatriptan: MAO; naproxen: no significant CYP450 induction

nor do they bind to adrenergic, dopaminergic, muscarinergic, or histaminergic receptors.

Pharmacokinetics

The pharmacokinetics of the different triptans vary somewhat. However, all are generally well tolerated and efficacious at appropriate doses.

Subcutaneous sumatriptan injection has the fastest onset of action when compared with other triptans. Sumatriptan nasal spray has a slightly slower onset than the injection.

The onset of the majority of oral triptans, including the dissolving wafers, is similar among the available agents. Rizatriptan may have a slightly faster onset of action at 1.0–1.5 hours.

Migraine recurrence rates may be lower with long-half-life triptans such as naratriptan and frovatriptan. However, triptans with longer half-lives tend to have a slower onset of action.

Adverse effects

Triptans are generally well tolerated. Most side effects are mild and transient.

The triptans differ slightly from one another in terms of tolerability but not in terms of safety.

The most frequent side effects are (1) tingling and paresthesias and (2) sensations of warmth in the head, neck, chest, and limbs. Less frequent effects are dizziness, flushing, and neck pain or stiffness.

Chest symptoms

About 50% of patients on sumatriptan experience unpleasant chest symptoms usually described as "heavy arms" or "chest pressure" rather than pain. These symptoms are transient and not related to ischemic heart disease. Possible causes are pulmonary vasoconstriction, esophageal spasm, intercostal muscle spasm, and bronchoconstriction.

Coronary vasospasm

Rarely, sumatriptan causes angina secondary to coronary vasospasm. Electrocardiographic changes have been observed in patients with CAD or Prinzmetal's (vasospastic) angina.

To reduce the risk of angina, do not give sumatriptan to patients who have risk factors for CAD. These patients include postmenopausal women, men over 40, smokers, and patients with hypertension, hypercholesterolemia, obesity, diabetes, or a family history of CAD.

Other adverse effects

Mild reactions include vertigo, malaise, fatigue, and tingling sensations.

Transient pain and redness may occur at sites of subcutaneous injection.

Intranasal administration may cause irritation in the nose and throat as well as an offensive or unusual taste.

Drug–drug and drug–disease interactions

All triptans and ergot alkaloids cause vasoconstriction. Accordingly, if one triptan is combined with another or with an ergot alkaloid, excessive and prolonged vasospasm could result.

Do not use triptans within 24 hours of an ergot derivative or another triptan.

MAO inhibitors can suppress degradation of triptans, which causes plasma levels to rise and results in toxicity. Furthermore, triptans should not be administered within 2 weeks of stopping an MAO inhibitor.

Triptans are contraindicated for patients with a history of ischemic heart disease, myocardial infarction, uncontrolled hypertension, or other heart disease. Do not use triptans during pregnancy.

Patient counseling

Patients should be counseled to contact a physician if pain or tightness in the chest occurs.

Patients should not exceed daily maximum doses. If migraines occur more than three times a month, prophylactic treatment should be considered.

Pain at the sumatriptan injection site should last less than 1 hour.

Migraine Prophylactic Therapy

Table 23-7 summarizes selected migraine preventive treatments.

β-adrenergic blocking agents

Propranolol is one of the drugs of choice for migraine prophylaxis. This agent can reduce the number and intensity of attacks in about 70% of patients.

Not all β-blockers are active against migraines. Recommended first-line agents include propranolol and timolol. Additional agents with demonstrated efficacy include atenolol and metoprolol.

Because not all β-blockers are effective, a mechanism other than β-blockade is apparently responsible for the beneficial effects.

Anticonvulsants

Good evidence supports the efficacy of divalproex sodium and sodium valproate. Adverse events with these therapies include weight gain, hair loss, tremor,

Table 23-7. Selected Migraine Preventive Treatments

Drug	Recommended dose/day	Selected side effects
β-adrenergic receptor antagonists		
Propranolol	80–240 mg	Reduced energy, tiredness, postural symptoms
Metoprolol	100–200 mg	
Timolol	20–30 mg	
Atenolol	100 mg	
Antidepressants		
Amitriptyline	25–150 mg	Drowsiness
Fluoxetine	10–20 mg	Headache, nausea, nervousness, insomnia, drowsiness
Serotonin antagonists		
Methysergide	1–6 mg (treatment must be discontinued for 1 month every 6 months)	Drowsiness, leg cramps, hair loss, retroperitoneal fibrosis
Calcium channel blockers		
Diltiazem	90–180 mg	Headache
Verapamil	160–320 mg	Constipation, peripheral edema, cardiac conduction disturbances
Anticonvulsants		
Divalproex	400–600 mg	Drowsiness, weight gain, tremor, hair loss, hematologic and liver abnormalities, teratogenicity
Valproate	500–1500 mg	
Gabapentin	900–2400 mg	Somnolence, dizziness
Topiramate	100 mg	Confusion, paresthesias, weight loss

Adapted from Goadsby P, Lipton R, Ferrari M 2002; D'Amico D, Tepper J 2008.

and teratogenic potential, such as neural tube defects. Both are considered first line for prevention.

Topiramate has good scientific evidence for clinical efficacy. It is FDA approved for migraine prevention. Side effects associated with use include paresthesia, fatigue, nausea, dizziness, and difficulty concentrating. Anorexia and weight loss may also occur.

Limited evidence indicates moderate efficacy of gabapentin. Gabapentin has no documented drug interactions and is excreted unchanged in the urine. Drowsiness and dizziness are common adverse events.

Antidepressants

Amitriptyline has been more frequently studied than the other antidepressants and is the only one with consistent support for efficacy in migraine prevention. It is considered a first-line treatment. There is limited evidence for the use of other tricyclic antidepressants (TCAs) such as nortriptyline, protriptyline, doxepin, clomipramine, or imipramine.

Drowsiness, weight gain, and anticholinergic symptoms are frequently reported with the TCAs.

Limited evidence exists that supports using fluoxetine at dosages ranging from 20 mg every other day to 40 mg per day. Although benefit may be seen in clinical practice, controlled trials offer no evidence for the use of fluvoxamine, paroxetine, sertraline, bupropion, mirtazapine, trazodone, or venlafaxine in this manner.

Calcium channel blockers

Several calcium channel blockers are moderately effective at reducing migraine attacks. They include verapamil and diltiazem. Beneficial effects develop slowly, reaching a maximum in 1–2 months.

Calcium channel blockers cause side effects in 20–60% of patients. Constipation and orthostatic hypotension are most common. Peripheral edema may occur as well.

Cardiovascular effects, including bradycardia, arrhythmias, QT prolongation, may necessitate appropriate monitoring.

Methysergide

Methysergide is an ergot alkaloid used in migraine prophylaxis. It is not effective for aborting an ongoing attack.

It is more efficacious than propranolol but has significantly more side effects.

The drug seems to activate serotonin receptors in the CNS. Suppression of pain pathways by this mechanism may explain its usefulness.

Methysergide causes a number of adverse effects. With long-term therapy, methysergide can cause retroperitoneal, pleuropulmonary, and cardiac fibrosis. Fibrotic changes, although rare, are most serious.

Other adverse effects include vascular insufficiency, insomnia, altered mood, depersonalization, hallucinations, nightmares, and GI disturbances such as nausea, vomiting, and diarrhea.

Ergot alkaloids, serotonin-receptor agonists, β-adrenergic blockers, dopamine, and drugs that inhibit the CYP450 3A4 subclass of hepatic metabolizing enzymes increase the risk of arterial spasm.

23-4. Nonpharmacologic Treatment of Migraines

General Principles of Nonpharmacologic Therapies

Nonpharmacologic approaches may be well suited to patients who have exhibited a poor tolerance or poor response to drug therapy; who have a contraindication to drug therapy; or who have a history of long-term, frequent, or excessive use of analgesics or other acute medications. Nonpharmacologic interventions may also be useful in patients who are pregnant, are planning to become pregnant, or are nursing.

Treatment Recommendations

Patients with migraine pain may experience relief by resting or sleeping in a cool, quiet, dark environment.

Half of migraine patients experience considerable relief by applying a cold compress to the head.

Relaxation training, thermal biofeedback combined with relaxation training, electromyographic biofeedback, and cognitive-behavioral therapies are somewhat effective in preventing migraine.

Evidence pertaining to the treatment of migraine with acupuncture is limited, and the results are mixed. Similarly, limited evaluation has been conducted with hypnosis, TENS, cervical manipulation, and hyperbaric oxygen.

Trigger Management

Trigger management is important in preventing migraine attacks. Triggering factors can cause migraine and if, recognized and avoided, may impede an impending attack.

Triggers vary from person to person. Examples of triggers include changes in weather or air pressure; bright sunlight, glare, or fluorescent lights; chemical fumes; menstrual cycles; and certain foods such as processed meats, red wine, beer, dried fish, broad beans, fermented cheeses, aspartame, and monosodium glutamate.

23-5. Key Points

Pain Management

- Opioids relieve pain by mimicking the actions of endogenous opioid peptides at μ, δ, and κ receptors.
- Opioids fall into three categories: pure μ agonists, agonist–antagonists, and pure antagonists. Pure μ agonists are the most pharmacologically useful.
- *Addiction* is a behavior pattern involving the continued use of a substance for nonmedical reasons despite harm. *Physical dependence* refers to the occurrence of an abstinence syndrome if the opioid is abruptly discontinued.
- With prolonged use, tolerance develops to analgesia, euphoria, sedation, respiratory depression, and other adverse effects—but not to constipation.
- Opioid overdose induces coma, respiratory depression, and pinpoint pupils. Naloxone and other pure opioid antagonists are used in cases of overdose to reverse most effects of opioids.
- Alcohol and other CNS depressants can intensify opioid-induced sedation and respiratory depression. TCAs and antihistamines may

worsen opioid-induced constipation and urinary retention.

■ Hydrocodone, codeine, fentanyl, methadone, and oxycodone are metabolized by the CYP450 system. Thus, drug interactions through the CYP450 enzymes may exist.

■ The liver extensively metabolizes opioids; dose adjustments may be required in liver dysfunction. Fentanyl, morphine, and methadone require dosing adjustments in renal dysfunction.

Migraine

■ The pathogenesis of migraine is unclear and is thought to be multifactorial. The current thinking is that a primary neuronal dysfunction originates in the CNS, leading to a sequence of changes that account for the different stages of migraine.

■ The goal of abortive therapy is to eliminate headache pain and associated nausea and vomiting. The goal of preventive therapy is to reduce the incidence of migraine attacks.

■ Nonopioid analgesics are effective for abortive therapy of mild to moderate pain.

■ Opioid analgesics are reserved for severe migraine that has not responded to other drugs.

■ Ergotamine is used for abortive therapy but should not be used daily. Overdose with ergotamine can cause ergotism, a serious condition in which generalized constriction of peripheral arteries and arterioles causes severe tissue ischemia.

■ Triptans are drugs of choice for abortive therapy of migraines. They activate $5-HT_{1B}/5-HT_{1D}$ receptors, thereby causing constriction of cranial blood vessels and suppression of inflammatory neuropeptides.

■ Triptans can cause coronary vasospasm and are contraindicated in patients with ischemic heart disease, prior myocardial infarction, and uncontrolled hypertension. If a triptan is combined with another triptan or with an ergot alkaloid, excessive prolonged vasospasms could result. Because of increased triptan toxicity, triptans should not be administered concurrently with MAO inhibitors and should not be given within 2 weeks of stopping an MAO inhibitor.

■ The most recently published clinical practice guidelines consider propranolol, amitriptyline, divalproex sodium, and timolol first line for prevention of migraines. Since the publication of the guidelines, topiramate has gained an FDA indication for migraine prevention.

23-6. Questions

1. Approximately how many people in the United States experience severe chronic pain?

   A. 10 million
   B. 23 million
   C. 40 million
   D. 50 million
   E. 75 million

2. Addiction is currently understood to be

   I. characterized by compulsive use of drugs.
   II. synonymous with physical dependence on a medication.
   III. the use of a substance for psychic effects.

   A. I only
   B. III only
   C. I and III only
   D. II and III only
   E. I, II, and III

3. The World Health Organization analgesic hierarchy emphasizes

   A. concurrent use of nonopioids, opioids, and adjuvant medications.
   B. avoiding opioid use.
   C. reserving opioid use only for severe pain.
   D. using single agents rather than a combination of medications.
   E. using nonopioids only for treatment of mild pain.

4. All of the following adverse effects are manifestations of μ opioid agonists *except*

   A. constipation.
   B. respiratory depression.
   C. atrial flutter.
   D. nausea.
   E. miosis.

5. The preferred route of opioid administration is

   A. oral.
   B. intravenous.
   C. subcutaneous.
   D. rectal.
   E. intramuscular.

6. Which of the following opioids has the longest duration of analgesic effect?

   A. Methadone
   B. Controlled-release morphine
   C. Hydromorphone
   D. Transdermal fentanyl
   E. Controlled-release oxycodone

7. All of the following opioids are metabolized through the cytochrome P450 hepatic enzyme system *except*

   A. hydrocodone.
   B. oxycodone.
   C. morphine.
   D. methadone.
   E. fentanyl.

8. The clearance of which opioid may be increased in patients with multiple copies of the CYP450 2D6 gene?

   A. Methadone
   B. Oxycodone
   C. Fentanyl
   D. Morphine
   E. Hydromorphone

9. Which of the following statements regarding methadone pharmacokinetics is true?

   A. The half-life corresponds to analgesic efficacy.
   B. It is highly plasma protein bound and widely distributed in tissue.
   C. The clearance of methadone is rapid, resulting in frequent dosing.
   D. Methadone has low bioavailability from the GI tract and therefore is not useful when given orally.
   E. Methadone is metabolized by hepatic glucuronidation.

10. Which agent can be used to reverse respiratory effects caused by opioid overdose?

    A. Naloxone
    B. Pentazocine
    C. Buprenorphine
    D. Naltrexone
    E. Tramadol

11. Which of the following opioids is not appropriate for use as an around-the-clock medication in chronic pain?

    A. Morphine
    B. Oxycodone
    C. Fentanyl
    D. Hydromorphone
    E. Methadone

12. Which of the following opioids has a toxic metabolite that can accumulate in renal dysfunction?

    A. Oxycodone
    B. Fentanyl
    C. Meperidine
    D. Hydromorphone
    E. Methadone

Use Case Study 1 to answer questions 13 and 14.

Case Study 1

Patient name: Mary Martin   **Address:** 815 Elm Street

Age: 65   **Sex:** Female

Allergies: NKDA

Diagnosis:

Chronic low back pain

Hypertension

Hypercholesterolemia

Chronic constipation

Date	Medication
3/3	Paxil 20 mg qd
3/3	Zocor 40 mg qd
3/3	Lotensin 20 mg qd
3/3	Premarin 0.625 mg
3/3	Morphine sulfate extended-release 60 mg bid
3/3	Senokot S
3/28	Elavil 50 mg qhs
4/1	Milk of magnesia

13. Which of Mrs. Martin's medications is most likely to worsen opioid-induced constipation?

    A. Paxil
    B. Zocor
    C. Lotensin
    D. Premarin
    E. Elavil

14. The physician recommends changing Mrs. Martin's opioid to one that is less constipating. Which of the following medications is least likely to cause constipation?

    A. Morphine extended release
    B. Methadone
    C. Oxycodone extended release
    D. Transdermal fentanyl patch
    E. Hydromorphone

15. The rationale of adding caffeine to a simple analgesic for migraine treatment is to

    I.   decrease the required dose of acetaminophen and aspirin.
    II. cause cerebral arterial vasoconstriction.
    III. increase gastric acidity and perfusion, enhancing aspirin absorption.

    A. I only
    B. III only
    C. I and III only
    D. II and III only
    E. I, II, and III

16. Which of the following agents is a selective serotonin agonist?

    A. Sumatriptan
    B. Ketorolac
    C. Dihydroergotamine
    D. Metoclopramide
    E. Caffeine

17. Which is true regarding the adverse effects of ergotamine?

    A. Ergotamine inhibits the chemoreceptor trigger zone to minimize nausea and vomiting.
    B. Ergotamine has minimal risk of dependence.
    C. Muscle weakness is an uncommon side effect of ergotamine.

    D. Angina-like pain reported with the triptans is not seen with ergotamine use.
    E. Overuse of ergotamine can result in ischemia.

18. Which statement about triptans is correct?

    A. Few contraindications exist to the use of triptans.
    B. Triptans are contraindicated in ischemic cardiovascular disease.
    C. Triptans are preferred for migraine treatment during pregnancy.
    D. Patients taking ergot alkaloids can use triptans concomitantly.
    E. Triptans are strictly contraindicated in patients with hypertension.

19. Which of the following statements is true regarding the use of opioids for migraines?

    A. Opioid use is not associated with rebound headaches.
    B. Butorphanol nasal spray is efficacious in migraine abortive therapy.
    C. Opioids in combination with butalbital and caffeine do not produce physical dependence.
    D. Opioids scheduled around the clock are useful for migraine prophylaxis.
    E. Opioids are not commonly prescribed for migraine treatment.

20. Which of the following agents is most likely to cause pulmonary fibrosis?

    A. Methysergide
    B. Amitriptyline
    C. Carbamazepine
    D. Propranolol
    E. Valproic acid

21. Which statement about Midrin is correct?

    I.   Midrin can be used concomitantly with over-the-counter products containing acetaminophen.
    II. Midrin dose is limited to 5 capsules per 12 hours.
    III. Midrin may cause sedation.

    A. I only
    B. III only
    C. I and III only

Use Case Study 2 to answer questions 23 and 24.

Case Study 2

Patient name: James Hunt   **Address:** 817 Elm Street
Age: 45   **Sex:** Male
Allergies: NKDA   **Diagnosis:** Migraine with aura, controlled hypertension
Medications:

Date	Drug	Sig	Quantity
1/1	Sumatriptan 100 mg tablet	Oral, use as directed	#9 tabs
1/1	Lisinopril 10 mg tablet	Oral, qd	#30 tabs
2/1	Sumatriptan 100 mg tablet	Oral, use as directed	#9 tabs
2/1	Lisinopril 10 mg tablet	Oral, qd	#30 tabs
3/1	Sumatriptan 100 mg tablet	Oral, use as directed	#9 tabs
3/1	Lisinopril 10 mg tablet	Oral, qd	#30 tabs
3/9	Sumatriptan 100 mg tablet	Oral, use as directed	#9 tabs
3/14	Sumatriptan 100 mg tablet	Oral, use as directed	#9 tabs

     D. II and III only
     E. I, II, and III

22. Dihydroergotamine differs from ergotamine in which of the following ways?

     A. DHE has higher incidence of nausea and vomiting.
     B. DHE has higher incidence of physical dependence.
     C. DHE has no contraindications for ischemic cardiovascular disease.
     D. DHE has a higher incidence of diarrhea.
     E. DHE can be administered concomitantly with a triptan.

23. Which of the following statements is true regarding initiation of prophylactic migraine therapy in Mr. Hunt?

     A. Mr. Hunt is at high risk for rebound headaches caused by excessive sumatriptan use.
     B. Mr. Hunt is limiting his sumatriptan use to 3 days per week and is not a candidate for prophylactic treatment.
     C. Mr. Hunt is a candidate for prophylactic therapy because of the increasing frequency of attacks.

     D. Mr. Hunt requires prophylactic therapy because his hypertension is a contraindication to using abortive therapies.
     E. Prophylactic treatment is contraindicated in migraines with aura.

24. Which medication is appropriate to give Mr. Hunt for migraine prophylaxis?

     A. Butorphanol
     B. Propranolol
     C. Dihydroergotamine
     D. Acetaminophen
     E. Hydrocodone

23-7. Answers

1. E. Currently, about 75 million individuals suffer from some form of chronic benign pain.
2. C. Physical dependence is the occurrence of a withdrawal syndrome after an opioid is stopped or quickly decreased without titration. Addiction is the psychological dependence on the use of substances for psychic effects and is characterized by compulsive use.
3. A. The WHO analgesic hierarchy involves choosing among three stepped levels of treatment. Mild pain may respond to nonopioid drugs

alone. Combining a low-dose opioid with a nonopioid can relieve pain of moderate severity. More severe pain requires the addition of a higher-dose opioid preparation to the nonopioid. At any step, analgesic adjuvants may be useful.

4. **C.** Atrial flutter is not a documented adverse effect of opioids. However, therapeutic doses of many opioids produce peripheral vasodilation, reduced peripheral resistance, and inhibition of the baroreceptor reflexes. Recently, methadone has been associated with torsades de pointes, an atypical rapid ventricular tachycardia.

5. **A.** Oral medications should be used whenever possible because of convenience, flexibility, and steady serum levels.

6. **D.** Transdermal fentanyl provides analgesia for up to 72 hours. The analgesic effects of methadone do not correlate with its long half-life.

7. **C.** Morphine is metabolized by hepatic glucuronidation.

8. **B.** Oxycodone is metabolized through CYP450 2D6 to active metabolites. Fast metabolizers—those with multiple copies of the CYP450 2D6 gene—would clear oxycodone and its metabolites quickly.

9. **B.** About 90% of methadone is bound to plasma protein and is widely distributed in tissues. Methadone has a long terminal half-life, resulting in slow clearance. This half-life does not correspond to analgesic dosing. It is metabolized via the CYP450 enzyme system.

10. **A.** Naloxone is a μ antagonist useful in opioid overdose. Naltrexone is also a μ antagonist, but it is reserved for use in alcoholism and opioid addiction.

11. **D.** Hydromorphone is an opioid with a short half-life with no available long-acting formulation. Thus, it is not useful as an around-the-clock medication.

12. **C.** Normeperidine, a metabolite of meperidine, can accumulate with chronic use, with renal impairment, and when the dose exceeds 600 mg every 24 hours.

13. **E.** The anticholinergic effects of tricyclic antidepressants such as Elavil can exacerbate opioid-induced constipation and urinary retention.

14. **D.** Because transdermal delivery bypasses absorption from the GI tract, constipation has been reported to be less frequent than with other opioids.

15. **C.** Caffeine has analgesic and possibly anti-inflammatory properties. Therefore, reduced doses of acetaminophen and aspirin may be required. Caffeine may also increase gastric acidity and perfusion, enhancing the absorption of aspirin.

16. **A.** Sumatriptan is a selective serotonin agonist.

17. **E.** Adverse effects of ergotamine include nausea and vomiting, physical dependence, muscle weakness, and angina-like pain. Overuse of ergotamine can result in ischemia that may progress to gangrene.

18. **B.** Triptans are contraindicated in pregnancy and ischemic cardiovascular disease. They cannot be used within 24 hours of another triptan or ergot alkaloid.

19. **B.** Good evidence exists for the efficacy of butorphanol nasal spray in migraine abortive therapy. Although opioids are commonly used for abortive therapy, they may be associated with rebound headaches and physical dependence.

20. **A.** With long-term therapy, methysergide can cause retroperitoneal, pleuropulmonary, and cardiac fibrosis. Fibrotic changes, although rare, are serious.

21. **D.** Midrin may be useful for mild to moderate migraines. It is generally well tolerated but may cause sedation. Because of Midrin's acetaminophen content, use of other acetaminophen products should be limited.

22. **D.** In contrast to ergotamine, DHE causes minimal peripheral vasoconstriction, little nausea and vomiting, and no physical dependence. However, diarrhea is prominent.

23. **C.** Prophylactic therapy should be considered because his migraines occur more than twice monthly and there is a trend toward increasing frequency of attacks.

24. **B.** Propranolol has been shown to be effective for migraine prophylaxis. This agent can reduce the number and intensity of attacks in about 70% of patients. Butorphanol, acetaminophen, dihydroergotamine, and hydrocodone are not approved for migraine prophylaxis.

23-8. References

Pain

American Pain Society. Acupuncture. In: *Principles of Analgesic Use in the Treatment of Acute Pain and Cancer Pain.* 4th ed. Glenview, Ill.: American Pain Society; 1999.

American Pain Society. *Principles of Analgesic Use in the Treatment of Acute Pain and Cancer Pain.*

6th ed. Glenview, Ill.: American Pain Society; 2008.

American Society of Anesthesiologists Task Force on Pain Management. Practice guidelines for chronic pain management. *Anesthesiology*. 1997; 86:995–1004.

Baumann TJ. Pain management. In: DiPiro JT, Talbert PE, Hayes PE, et al., eds. *Pharmacotherapy: A Pathophysiologic Approach*. 4th ed. New York: Elsevier; 1999:1014–25.

Bonica JJ, ed. *The Management of Pain*. 2nd ed. Philadelphia: Lea & Febiger; 1990.

Brookoff D. Chronic pain: 1. A new disease. *Hosp Pract (Off Ed)*. 2000;35:45–52, 59.

Chou R, Fanciullo GJ, Fine PG, et al. Clinical guidelines for the use of chronic opioid therapy in chronic noncancer pain. *J Pain*. 2009;10:113–30.

Duragesic [package insert]. Titusville, N.J.: Janssen Pharmaceutical Products; February 2005.

Fentora [package insert]. Frazer, Pa.: Cephalon; 2007.

Holdsworth M, Forman W, Killilea T, et al. Transdermal fentanyl disposition in elderly subjects. *Gerontology*. 1994;40:32–37.

Hutchison TA, Shahan DR, eds. DRUGDEX® System. MICROMEDEX, Greenwood Village, Colo. (vol. expired March 2003).

Jacox A, Carr DB. *Management of Cancer Pain: Clinical Practice Guideline No. 9*. AHCPR Publication No. 94-0492. Rockville, Md.: Agency for Health Care Policy and Research, U.S. Department of Health and Human Services, Public Health Service; 1994.

Joint Commission on Accreditation of Healthcare Organizations. *Pain Assessment and Management: An Organizational Approach*. Oakbrook Terrace, Ill.: Joint Commission on Accreditation of Healthcare Organizations; 2000.

Merskey H, Bogduk N, eds. *Classification of Chronic Pain: Descriptions of Chronic Pain Syndromes and Definitions of Pain Terms*. 2nd ed. Seattle: IASP Press; 1994.

National Institutes of Health. Acupuncture. NIH Consensus Statement Online, November 3–5, 1997; 15:1–34. Available at: http://consensus.nih.gov/ 1997/1997Acupuncture107html.htm.

Opana [package insert]. Chadds Ford, Pa.: Endo Pharmaceuticals; 2008.

Opana ER [package insert]. Chadds Ford, Pa.: Endo Pharmaceuticals; 2008.

Portenoy RK. Opioid therapy for chronic nonmalignant pain: A review of the critical issues. *J Pain Symptom Manage*. 1996;11:203–17.

Ryzolt [package insert]. Stamford, Conn.: Purdue Pharma; 2008.

Seddon S, Covington EC, Heit HA, et al. Definitions related to the use of opioids in treatment of pain: Consensus statement of the American Academy of Pain Medicine, the American Pain Society and the American Society of Addiction Medicine. 2001.

Turk DC, Melzack R, eds. *Handbook of Pain Assessment*. 2nd ed. New York: Guilford Press; 2001.

Ultram ER [package insert]. Raritan, N.J.: PriCara; January 2006.

Wolters Kluwer Health. Facts and comparisons online. Wolters Kluwer Health, St. Louis, Mo.

World Health Organization. *Cancer Pain Relief: With a Guide to Opioid Availability*. 2nd ed. Geneva: World Health Organization; 1996.

Migraines

Anthony M, Rasmussen BK. Migraine without aura. In: Olesen J, Tfelt-Hansen P, Welch KMA, eds. *The Headaches*. New York: Raven Press; 1993:255–61.

Barbanti P, Fabbrini G, Pesare M, Cerbo R. Unilateral cranial autonomic symptoms in migraine. *Cephalalgia*. 2002;22:256–9.

Brandes JL, Saper JR, Diamond M, et al. Topiramate for migraine prevention: A randomized controlled trial. *JAMA*. 2004;291:965–73.

Cady RK, Schreiber CP. Sinus headache or migraine? Considerations in making a differential diagnosis. *Neurology*. 2002;58(suppl 6):S10–14.

Campbell JK, Penzien DB, Wall EM. Evidence-based guidelines for migraine headache: Behavioural and physical treatments. American Academy of Neurology; 2000. Available at: http://www.aan. com/professionals/practice/pdfs/gl0089.pdf.

Center for Clinical Health Policy Research. *Drug Treatments for the Prevention of Migraine Headache*. Technical Review 2.3. Durham, N.C.: Duke University; 1999.

Couch JR. Sinus headache: A neurologist's viewpoint. *Semin Neurol*. 1988;8:298–302.

D'Amico D, Tepper J. Prophylaxis of migraines: General principles and patient acceptance. *Neuropsychiatr Dis Treat*. 2008;4:1155–67.

Diamond M. The role of concomitant headache types and non-headache comorbidities in the underdiagnosis of migraine. *Neurology*. 2002;58 (suppl 6):S3–9.

Goadsby P, Lipton R, Ferrari M. Migraine: Current understanding and treatment. *N Engl J Med*. 2002;346:257–70.

Hargreaves RJ, Shepheard SL. Pathophysiology of migraine: New insights. *Can J Neurol Sci*. 1999; 26(suppl 3):S12–19.

Headache Classification Subcommittee of the International Headache Society. The international classification of headache disorders: 2nd edition. *Cephalalgia.* 2004;24(suppl 7):1–160.

Hutchison TA, Shahan DR, eds. DRUGDEX® System. MICROMEDEX, Greenwood Village, Colo. (vol. expired March 2003).

International Headache Society. Revised classification proposal. Accessed at: http://ihs-classification.org.

Kaniecki RG, Totten J. Cervicalgia in migraine: Prevalence, clinical characteristics, and response to treatment. Poster presented at 10th Congress of the International Headache Society, New York; 2002.

Lipton RB, Diamond S, Reed M, et al. Migraine diagnosis and treatment: Results from the American Migraine Study II. *Headache.* 2001;41:638–45.

Lipton RB, Stewart WF, Diamond S, et al. Prevalence and burden of migraine in the United States: Data from the American Migraine Study II. *Headache.* 2001;41:646–57.

Matchar DB, Young WB, Rosenberg JH, et al. Evidence-based guidelines for migraine headache in the primary care setting: Pharmacological management of acute attacks. American Academy of Neurology; 2000. Available at: www.aan.com/professionals/practice/pdfs/gl0087.pdf.

Pietrobon D, Striessnig J. Neurobiology of migraine. *Nat Rev Neurosci.* 2003;4:386–98.

Ramadan NM, Silberstein SD, Freitag FG, et al. Evidence-based guidelines for migraine headache in the primary care setting: Pharmacological management for prevention of migraine. American Academy of Neurology; 2000. Available at: www.aan.com/professionals/practice/pdfs/gl0090.pdf.

Rasmussen BK, Jensen R, Schroll M, Olesen J. Interrelations between migraine and tension-type headache in the general population. *Arch Neurol.* 1992;49:914–8.

Silberstein SD. Practice parameter: Evidence-based guidelines for migraine headache (an evidence-based review)—Report of the Quality Standards Subcommittee of the American Academy of Neurology. *Neurology.* 2000;55:754–62.

Silberstein SD. Topiramate in migraine prevention: Evidence-based medicine from clinical trials. *Arch Neurol.* 2004;61:490–95.

Smith TR. Pitfalls in migraine diagnosis and management. *Clin Cornerstone.* 2001;4:26–35.

Snow V, Weiss K, Wall EM, Mottur-Pilson C. Pharmacological management of acute attacks of migraine and prevention of migraine headache. *Ann Intern Med.* 2002;137:840–49.

Spierings ELH, Ranke AH, Honkoop PC. Precipitating and aggravating factors of migraine versus tension-type headache. *Headache.* 2001;41:554–58.

Tepper S, Newman L, Dowson A, et al. The prevalence and diagnosis of migraine in a primary care setting in the United States: Insights from the Landmark Study. Poster presented at the Annual Scientific Meeting of the American Headache Society, June 21–23, Seattle; 2002.

Topamax [package insert]. Titusville, N.J.: Ortho-McNeil Neurologics; June 2005.

Wolters Kluwer Health. Facts and comparisons online. Wolters Kluwer Health, St. Louis, Mo.

Seizure Disorders

24

Stephanie J. Phelps, PharmD, BCPS

24-1. Epilepsy

Epilepsy occurs when neurons become depolarized and repetitively fire action potentials. It is involuntary and episodic. The term is applied after two unprovoked seizures. A seizure does not mean a person has epilepsy; however, epilepsy means a person has seizures. Anticonvulsants do not cure epilepsy.

Terminology

- *Aura:* A subjective sensation or motor phenomenon that marks a seizure onset and is generally associated with sensations that are localized in a particular region of the brain
- *Automatisms:* Purposeless movements seen with partial seizures
- *Postictal:* Symptoms and signs seen after a seizure

Types of Epilepsy

There are two main types of epilepsy: partial seizures and generalized seizures.

Partial seizures

Partial seizures begin in one hemisphere of the brain. They are unilateral, asymmetric movements, generally associated with an aura. Complex partial seizures are accompanied by altered consciousness.

Drugs for new-onset seizures
- *Monotherapy:* Carbamazepine (drug of choice), oxcarbazepine (> 4 years), phenobarbital, phenytoin, topiramate, valproic acid

- *Adjunctive therapy:* Gabapentin (> 12 years), lacosamide, lamotrigine (> 2 years), levetiracetam (> 4 years), oxcarbazepine (> 2 years), phenobarbital, phenytoin, tiagabine (> 4 years), topiramate (> 10 years), valproic acid, vigabatrin, zonisamide

Drugs for refractory seizures
- *Monotherapy:* Carbamazepine, felbamate, lamotrigine (conversion > 2 years), phenytoin, phenobarbital, topiramate, valproic acid
- *Adjunctive therapy:* Gabapentin, lamotrigine, lacosamide, levetiracetam, oxcarbazepine, phenobarbital, phenytoin, zonisamide

Generalized seizures

Generalized seizures begin simultaneously in both brain hemispheres. They are characterized by bilateral movements and have no aura.

Absence seizures

This type of generalized seizure has a sudden onset. It is brief (seconds) and characterized by a blank stare, upward rotation of the eyes, and lip smacking (confused with daydreaming). It has a three per second spike and wave on electroencephalography (EEG) and can be precipitated by hyperventilation.

Drugs
Historically, ethosuximide has been the drug of choice. If a patient has both absence and generalized tonic–clonic seizures and is older than 2 years of age, many consider valproic acid to be the drug of choice. Although not labeled, lamotrigine and topiramate have been used.

Primary generalized tonic–clonic seizure

This type of seizure has two phases:

- *Tonic phase:* Rigid, violent, sudden muscular contractions (stiff or rigid); crying or moaning; deviation of the eyes and head to one side; rotation of the whole body and distortion of features; suppression of respiration; falling to the ground; loss of consciousness; tongue biting; involuntary urination
- *Clonic phase:* Repetitive jerks; cyanosis continues; foaming at the mouth; small grunting respirations between seizures, but deep respirations as all muscles relax at the end of the seizure

Drugs of choice
- *Monotherapy:* Carbamazepine, phenobarbital, phenytoin, topiramate (> 10 years)
- *Adjunctive therapy:* Lamotrigine (> 2 years), levetiracetam (> 6 years), topiramate (> 2 years), valproic acid

Juvenile myoclonic epilepsy

Myoclonic seizures precede generalized tonic–clonic seizures; they generally occur on awakening. Sleep deprivation and alcohol commonly precipitate them.

Lifelong treatment is required with valproic acid, lamotrigine, levetiracetam, topiramate, or some combination.

Other less common seizure types

Catamenial epilepsy
Catamenial epilepsy is associated with hormonal changes during menstruation. It may be treated with acetazolamide.

Infantile spasms
Infantile spasms begin in the first 6 months of life. They occur in clusters, several times a day. Parents describe symptoms that sound like colic. Infantile spasms have high mortality and morbidity.

Treat this condition with adrenocorticotropic hormone (ACTH) or oral steroids, vigabatrin, or valproic acid (> 2 years). Although not labeled for this purpose, topiramate and zonisamide have been used.

Lennox–Gastaut Syndrome
This difficult-to-treat epilepsy most often appears between 2 and 6 years of age and is often accompanied by mental retardation and behavior problems.

It is characterized by frequent and different types of seizures.

Treat this condition with combination anticonvulsants that include felbamate (> 2 years), lamotrigine (> 2 years), rufinamide, and topiramate (> 2 years). Although not labeled by the Food and Drug Administration (FDA) for this purpose, zonisamide has been used.

Post-traumatic epilepsy
These seizures occur after head trauma. Patients may be started on phenytoin or fosphenytoin for a period of 7 days. If no seizures occur, phenytoin should be discontinued.

Etiologies for Epilepsy

- *Mechanical:* Birth injuries, head trauma, tumors, vascular abnormalities (stroke)
- *Metabolic:* Electrolyte disturbances (low sodium, elevated calcium); glucose abnormalities (low); inborn errors of metabolism
- *Genetic:* Benign familial neonatal seizures (chromosome 20), juvenile myoclonic epilepsy (chromosome 6), Baltic myoclonic (chromosome 21)
- *Other:* Fever; infection
- *Drugs:* These include the following:
  - Recreational drugs such as alcohol, cocaine and crack, ephedra, narcotics, methylphenidate
  - Carbapenems (imipenem), lindane, local anesthetics (lidocaine), metoclopramide, theophylline, tricyclic antidepressants
  - Meperidine (the metabolite normeperidine can cause seizures in patients with renal failure who receive normal doses)
  - Anticonvulsants that are used for treatment of a nonindicated seizure type (Table 24-1)

Criteria for Treating Epilepsy

Almost no child should be treated after one seizure.

Treat adults who have structural brain damage, a first seizure that was severe, or an occupation that places them at risk of injury should a second seizure occur.

Principles in the treatment of epilepsy

- *Monotherapy (one agent):* This form of treatment is always preferred.
- *Polytherapy (two agents):* Add an anticonvulsant with a different mechanism of action, provided serum concentrations (where appropriate)

	Seizure type		
Anticonvulsant	**Absence**	**Generalized tonic–clonic**	**Myoclonic**
Carbamazepine (Tegretol, Carbitrol)	Causes	Causes	Causes
Phenytoin (Dilantin, Phenytek)	Causes		
Phenobarbital	Causes		

Table 24-1. Seizures Caused by Anticonvulsants

and doses of the first anticonvulsant have been maximized. Begin to reduce the dose of the first drug slowly. This step is important if the patient has developed side effects or if the patient has not responded to the first anticonvulsant.

- *Polytherapy (three or more agents):* Although rarely needed, add a third anticonvulsant if (1) a combination of anticonvulsants is tolerated and significantly reduces seizure frequency or severity, but greater control might be achieved, or (2) the two anticonvulsants have been maximized. Reassess response, and discontinue unnecessary anticonvulsants as soon as possible.

Reasons for Treatment Failure

- Incorrect diagnosis
- Wrong anticonvulsant
- Inappropriate dose, route, or formulation
- Altered pharmacokinetics that require a dosage alteration
- Poor patient adherence
- Seizures that are refractory to therapy

Patient Counseling Information Applicable to All Anticonvulsants

- It is important that you keep a diary of your seizures and keep regular appointments with your doctor, so that he or she can determine whether your medication is working properly and whether you are experiencing unwanted side effects.
- The full effects of this medication may not be seen for several weeks. Continue to take the medication unless directed otherwise by your physician.
- Take with food or milk if upset stomach occurs.
- Do not drink alcohol or take central nervous system (CNS) depressants or illegal drugs with this medication.

- If this medication causes blurred vision or drowsiness, do not drive or operate heavy machinery while taking this medication until you have become accustomed to its effects
- Consult with your physician if you anticipate pregnancy, become pregnant, or plan to breast-feed while taking this medication.
- Some medications decrease the effectiveness of birth control pills. You should discuss this with your physician or pharmacist, who may recommend that you use a backup birth control method to prevent pregnancy.
- If you are a woman capable of having children, you should take 1 mg of folic acid a day.
- Do not stop taking this medication unless your doctor advises you to do so; some medicines have to be stopped slowly. Let your doctor or pharmacist know if you stop taking this medication.
- Check with your pharmacist or doctor before taking or starting any new medication (prescription, over-the-counter, or herbal product).
- If you miss a dose, take it as soon as you remember unless it is almost time for the next dose. If it is almost time for the next dose, skip the missed dose and resume your regular schedule. Do not take extra or double doses. If you miss two or more doses, contact your physician for further instructions.
- Contact your physician immediately if skin rash occurs.

Mechanisms of Action of Anticonvulsants

Anticonvulsants work through a variety of mechanisms including the following:

- Enhancing sodium channel inactivation
- Reducing current through T-type calcium channels
- Enhancing γ-aminobutyric acid (GABA) activity
- Enhancing antiglutamate activity

24-2. Medications Used to Treat Epilepsy

Carbamazepine

Carbamazepine is the most widely used anticonvulsant in adults and children. It is the drug of choice for complex partial seizures. It is effective in most generalized seizures but ineffective in absence seizures and febrile seizures.

Pharmacokinetics

- *Bioavailability:* Good (75–85%). Dispense in moisture-proof containers because studies show decreased bioavailability with high humidity (as may occur in medicine cabinets).
- *Protein binding:* 75–90% bound to alpha-1-acid glycoprotein; the 10,11-epoxide metabolite is 50% protein bound.
- *Metabolism:* Extensively hepatically metabolized to 10,11-epoxide, which is effective as an anticonvulsant and is capable of causing toxicity.
- *Renal elimination:* Low (1–3%).
- *Half-life:* About a day if used as monotherapy and about 12 hours if given with more than one anticonvulsant.
- *Reference range:* 4–12 mg/L (monotherapy, 8–12 mg/L; polytherapy, 4–8 mg/L).

Other aspects

Carbamazepine is one of a few drugs that can induce its own metabolism (i.e., autoinduction). Mean time to onset is 21 days (range: 17–31 days).

Side effects

Upon initiation, side effects are nausea, vomiting, drowsiness, dizziness, and neutropenia. A dose-related, transient, and reversible rash that rarely causes the drug to be discontinued may also occur.

With chronic therapy, the following side effects may occur:

- Syndrome of inappropriate antidiuretic hormone (SIADH) causing hyponatremia and water retention
- Osteomalacia (treat with vitamin D if alkaline phosphatase increase and 25-hydroxycholecalciferol decreases)
- Folate deficiency causing megaloblastic anemia

Some severe or life-threatening side effects are possible:

- *FDA black box warning:* Potentially fatal, severe dermatologic reactions (including Stevens–Johnson syndrome and toxic epidermal necrolysis) may occur. Over 90% of patients who experience these reactions do so within the first few months of treatment. Patients of Asian descent are at higher risk for toxic dermatologic reactions and should be screened for the variant HLA-B*1502 allele (genetic marker) prior to initiating therapy.
- *FDA black box warning:* Aplastic anemia may occur. In such cases, discontinuation of carbamazepine is recommended if white blood count < 2,000–3,000 or neutrophils < 1,000–1,500.
- *FDA warning:* Direct hepatotoxicity and multiorgan hypersensitivity reactions may occur. These side effects generally present within 1 month. Fever, rash, or fatalities may occur even if carbamazepine is discontinued. Stop carbamazepine if liver function tests increase more than three times above normal.
- *FDA warning:* Increased risk of suicidal behavior or ideation is possible. The FDA has analyzed suicidality reports from placebo-controlled studies involving 11 anticonvulsants (including carbamazepine) and found that patients receiving anticonvulsants had approximately twice the risk of suicidal behavior or ideation (0.43%) of patients receiving placebo (0.22%).
- *Teratogenic concerns:* Fetal carbamazepine syndrome is possible. Features include epicanthal folds, short nose, long philtrum, hypoplastic nails, microcephaly, and developmental delay. Carbamazepine is a pregnancy category D drug.

Drug–drug interactions

- Carbamazepine is a CYP3A4, CYP2C9, and CYP2C19 inducer.
- Erythromycin, cimetidine, lithium, and propoxyphene increase the serum concentration or effect of carbamazepine.
- Phenobarbital, primidone, and phenytoin decrease the anticonvulsant effect of carbamazepine.
- Carbamazepine may increase the serum concentration or effect of felbamate; felbamate will increase concentrations of the 10,11-epoxide metabolite carbamazepine and cause toxicity.

Commercially available formulations

Table 24-2 shows the commercially available formulations.

Table 24-2. Dosage Forms, Normal Maintenance Doses, and Dosing Interval for Older Anticonvulsants

Generic name	Trade name	Dosage form	Adult oral maintenance dose[a]	Interval[b]
Carbamazepine	Carbatrol, Equetro	Extended-release capsule: 100, 200, 300 mg	800–1,200 mg/d	bid
	Epitol	200 mg		
	Tegretol	Suspension: 100 mg/5 mL (5, 10, 450 mL) Chewable tablet: 100 mg Tablet: 200 mg		Suspension: qid Chewable tablet: tid–qid Tablet (200 mg): bid
	Tegretol XR	Extended-release tablet: 100, 200, 400 mg		Extended-release tablet: bid
Ethosuximide	Zarontin	Capsule: 250 mg	25–1,500 mg/d	bid
Fosphenytoin	Cerebyx	Injection:[c] 150 mg/2 mL; 750 mg/10 mL	NA	NA
Phenobarbital	Variety of generics	Elixir: 20 mg/5 mL (5, 7.5, 15, 480 mL) Tablet (15, 30, 60, 100 mg) Injection: 60, 65, 130 mg/mL (1 mL)	30–120 mg/d	bid–tid
Phenytoin	Dilantin	Suspension: 125 mg/5 mL (240 mL) Chewable tablet: 50 mg Prompt-release capsule: 30, 100 mg Extended-release capsule: 30, 100 mg Injection: 50 mg/mL	100–600 mg/d	bid–tid bid–tid bid–tid qd
	Phenytek	Extended-release capsule: 200 mg, 300 mg		
	Generic	Suspension: 100 mg/4 mL (4 mL); 125 mg/5 mL (240 mL) Prompt-release capsule: 100 mg Extended-release capsule: 100 mg Injection: 50 mg/mL		
Primidone	Mysoline	Suspension: 250 mg/5 mL Tablet: 50, 125, 250 mg Chewable tablet: 125 mg	250–750 mg/d	tid–qid
Valproic acid	Depacon	Injection: 100 mg/mL (5 mL)	NA	NA
	Depakene	Syrup: 250 mg/5 mL (5, 10, 480 mL) Gel capsule: 250 mg	250–4,000 mg/d	bid–qid
	Stavzor	Gel capsule: 125, 250, 500 mg		
Divalproex sodium	Depakote Sprinkles	Capsule: 125 mg		bid
	Depakote	Delayed-release tablet: 125, 250, 500 mg		bid
	Depakote ER	Extended-release tablet: 250, 500 mg		qd

NA, not applicable.

a. With the exception of the intravenous dosage forms, these anticonvulsants are begun at low doses and slowly titrated to a dose that will control the patient's seizures.

b. Interval may either decrease or increase in the presence of medications that induce or inhibit metabolism, respectively.

c. 150 mg of fosphenytoin = 100 mg phenytoin.

Patient counseling

See general counseling information. In addition, counsel the patient as follows:

- Shake suspension well.
- Do not store in areas of high humidity (e.g., medicine cabinets).
- Do not use with monoamine oxidase inhibitors.

Ethosuximide

Indications are absence and myoclonic seizures.

Pharmacokinetics

- *Bioavailability:* Good
- *Protein binding:* Very low (< 10%)
- *Metabolism:* 80% hepatically metabolized to three inactive metabolites
- *Renal elimination:* 50% as metabolites; 10% to 20% as unchanged drug
- *Half-life:* 30–60 hours
- *Reference range:* 40–100 mg/L

Side effects

Upon initiation, side effects are nausea, vomiting, dizziness, drowsiness, lethargy, headache, rashes (including Stevens–Johnson syndrome), and urticaria.
  With chronic therapy, anorexia and weight loss, as well as gum hypertrophy, could occur.

- *FDA warning:* Increased risk of suicidal behavior or ideation is possible. The FDA has analyzed suicidality reports from placebo-controlled studies involving 11 anticonvulsants (including ethosuximide) and found that patients receiving anticonvulsants had approximately twice the risk of suicidal behavior or ideation (0.43%) of patients receiving placebo (0.22%).

Drug–drug interactions

- CYP3A3/4 substrate
- Phenytoin, carbamazepine, primidone, and phenobarbital may increase the clearance of ethosuximide.
- Isoniazid may inhibit metabolism and increase ethosuximide serum concentrations.

Commercially available formulations

See Table 24-2 for commercially available formulations.

Felbamate

Felbamate should be used as adjunctive therapy only in severe refractory partial seizures, with or without secondary generalization, in patients older than 14 years of age and in partial or generalized seizures associated with Lennox–Gastaut syndrome.

Pharmacokinetics

- *Bioavailability:* Complete (> 90%)
- *Protein binding:* Low (20–25%)
- *Metabolism:* Hepatic via hydroxylation and conjugation
- *Renal elimination:* 40–50% excreted unchanged; 40% as inactive metabolites in urine
- *Half-life:* 20–30 hours; shorter (i.e., 14 hours) with concomitant enzyme-inducing drugs; prolonged (by 9–15 hours) in renal dysfunction
- *Reference range:* Not necessary to routinely monitor serum drug concentrations, but dose should be titrated to clinical response; therapeutic range not fully determined, but some have proposed 30–100 mg/L

Side effects

Upon initiation, nausea and vomiting, anorexia, headache, insomnia, and dizziness may occur.
  With chronic therapy, weight loss significant enough to warrant discontinuing the medication is possible.
  Severe or life-threatening side effects are possible:

- *FDA black box warning:* Direct hepatotoxicity may occur at any time; however, the earliest onset of severe liver dysfunction occurred 3 weeks after starting felbamate. It is not known if dose, duration, or use of concomitant medications affects the risk. Most cases require liver transplantation. Liver enzyme tests and bilirubin should be obtained before initiation and periodically, and felbamate should be immediately withdrawn if liver function tests become elevated.
- *FDA black box warning:* Aplastic anemia can develop at any point without warning. Risk may be 100-fold greater than the general population. Complete blood count with differential and platelet count should be taken before, during, and for a significant time after discontinuing felbamate therapy. Felbamate should be immediately withdrawn if bone marrow suppression occurs.
- *FDA warning:* Increased risk of suicidal behavior or ideation may occur. The FDA has analyzed

suicidality reports from placebo-controlled studies involving 11 anticonvulsants (including felbamate) and found that patients receiving anticonvulsants had approximately twice the risk of suicidal behavior or ideation (0.43%) of patients receiving placebo (0.22%).

Drug–drug interactions

- Felbamate induces CYP3A4.
- Felbamate inhibits CYP2C19, epoxide hydroxylase, and β-oxidation.
- Carbamazepine, phenobarbital, and phenytoin decrease the anticonvulsant effect of felbamate.
- Phenobarbital, phenytoin, and valproic acid increase the anticonvulsant effect of felbamate.
- Felbamate decreases carbamazepine concentrations but increases the concentration of carbamazepine epoxide (active metabolite), which may result in carbamazepine toxicity.
- Felbamate increases the serum concentrations of phenobarbital, phenytoin, and valproic acid. When felbamate is begun, a 20% reduction in phenytoin dose resulted in phenytoin concentrations comparable to those prior to initiation of felbamate.

Commercially available formulations

See Table 24-3 for commercially available formulations.

Patient counseling

See general counseling information. In addition, the patient or legal guardian should sign a consent form before taking this medication. A patient information consent form is included as part of the package insert and is available from the local representative or by calling 800-526-3840.

Fosphenytoin

Indications are for short-term parenteral administration for generalized convulsive status epilepticus.

Pharmacokinetics

- *Bioavailability:* Time for complete conversion to phenytoin is 15 minutes and 30 minutes after intravenous (IV) and intramuscular (IM) administration, respectively.
- *Protein binding:* Protein binding is high (95–99% primarily to albumin).
- *Metabolism:* Each millimole of fosphenytoin is metabolized to 1 millimole of phenytoin, phosphate, and formaldehyde. Formaldehyde is then converted to formate, which is metabolized by a folate-dependent mechanism. Conversion increases the dose and infusion rate, most likely because of a decrease in fosphenytoin protein binding.
- *Renal elimination:* None.
- *Half-life:* See the later discussion of phenytoin for the half-life of the active drug.
- *Reference range:* 10–20 mg/L (phenytoin).

Side effects

Upon initiation, side effects include hypotension (with rapid IV administration), vasodilation, tachycardia, and bradycardia; burning, pruritus, tingling, and paresthesia (predominately in the groin area); and rash and exfoliative dermatitis.

Chronic therapy does not result in additional side effects.

- *FDA warning:* Increased risk of suicidal behavior or ideation is possible. The FDA has analyzed suicidality reports from placebo-controlled studies involving 11 anticonvulsants (including fosphenytoin) and found that patients receiving anticonvulsants had approximately twice the risk of suicidal behavior or ideation (0.43%) of patients receiving placebo (0.22%).
- *FDA warning:* The FDA is investigating the possibility of an increased risk of serious skin reactions (e.g., Stevens–Johnson syndrome and toxic epidermal necrolysis) in patients given phenytoin who have the human leukocyte antigen allele HLA-B*1502. This allele occurs almost exclusively in individuals with ancestry across broad areas of Asia, including Han Chinese, Filipinos, Malaysians, South Asian Indians, and Thais. Until the FDA evaluation is finalized, fosphenytoin should be avoided as an alternative for carbamazepine in patients who test positive for HLA-B*1502.

Drug–drug interactions

See the later discussion of phenytoin for drug–drug interactions.

Commercially available formulations

See Table 24-2 for commercially available formulations.

Table 24-3. Dosage Forms, Normal Maintenance Doses, and Dosing Intervals for the Newer Anticonvulsants

Generic name	Trade name	Dosage form	Adult oral maintenance dose[a]	Interval[b]
Felbamate	Felbatol	Suspension: 600 mg/5 mL (240, 960 mL) Tablets: 400, 600 mg	1,200–3,600 mg/d	tid–qid
Gabapentin	Neurontin	Capsules:100, 300, 400 mg Oral solution: 250 mg/mL (480 mL) Tablets: 100, 300, 400, 600, 800 mg	900–3,600 mg/d[c]	tid
Lacosamide	Vimpat	Tablets: 50,100, 150, 200 mg Injection: 200 mg/20mL	200-400 mg/d	bid
Lamotrigine	Lamictal	Chewable tablets: 2, 5, 25 mg Tablets: 25, 100, 150, 200 mg	50–400/d	bid bid
	Lamictal ODT	Tablets: 25, 50, 100, 200 mg		bid
	Lamictal XR	Tablets: 25, 50, 100, 200 mg		qd
Levetiracetam	Keppra	Tablets: 250, 500, 750 mg Solution: 100 mg/mL	1,000–3,000 mg/d	bid
	Keppra XR	Extended release: 500 mg		Extended release: qd
Oxcarbazepine	Trileptal	Tablets: 150, 300, 600 mg Suspension: 300 mg/5mL (250 mL)	600–2,400 mg/d	bid
Pregabalin	Lyrica	Tablets: 100, 150, 200, 225, 300 mg	300–600 mg/d	bid–tid
Tiagabine	Gabitril	Tablets: 2, 4, 12, 16 mg	4–56 mg/d	bid–qid
Topiramate	Topamax	Sprinkle capsules:15, 25 mg Tablets: 25, 50, 100, 200 mg	200–400 mg/d[d]	bid
Rufinamide	Banzel	Tablets: 200, 400 mg	45 mg/kg/d	bid
Vigabatrin	Sabril	Tablets: 500 mg	400–600 mg/d	bid
Zonisamide	Zonegran	Capsules: 25, 50, 100 mg	100–600 mg/d	qd

a. With the exception of gabapentin, these anticonvulsants are begun at low doses and slowly titrated over weeks to a dose that will control the patient's seizures.
b. Interval may either decrease or increase in the presence of medications that induce or inhibit metabolism, respectively.
c. Much larger doses have been given.
d. The recommended maintenance doses for initial monotherapy and adjunctive therapy are 400 mg/d and 200–400 mg/d, respectively. Doses > 400 mg are no more effective than doses ≤ 400 mg.

Gabapentin

Indications are for adjunctive therapy for partial seizures.

Pharmacokinetics

- *Bioavailability:* Poor (60% with decreasing absorption as age decreases)
- *Protein binding:* Very low (< 3%)
- *Metabolism:* None
- *Renal elimination:* 100%
- *Half-life:* Short (< 12 hours); increases with decreased renal function (anuric patients: 132 hours; decreased during hemodialysis to about 4 hours)

- *Reference range:* Routine monitoring of serum concentrations not required; minimum effective concentration thought to be 2 mg/L

Side effects

Upon initiation, somnolence, dizziness, ataxia, fatigue, and nervousness may occur.

With chronic therapy, weight gain may occur. Neuropsychiatric events (i.e., emotional lability, hostility, hyperkinesias) are possible in children, especially those with mental retardation and attention deficit disorders. This problem generally resolves following a reduction in the dose.

- *FDA warning:* Increased risk of suicidal behavior or ideation is possible. The FDA has analyzed suicidality reports from placebo-controlled studies involving 11 anticonvulsants (including gabapentin) and found that patients receiving anticonvulsants had approximately twice the risk of suicidal behavior or ideation (0.43%) of patients receiving placebo (0.22%).

Drug–drug interactions

- No interactions affect metabolism; aluminum- and magnesium-containing antacids may decrease absorption.
- High protein intake can increase absorption.
- Although it is not a true drug interaction, combination with carbamazepine may cause dizziness. Reduce the dose of carbamazepine.

Commercially available formulations

See Table 24-3 for commercially available formulations.

Patient counseling

See general counseling information. In addition, the patient should be counseled as follows:

- Food may decrease the extent of absorption.
- If you take antacids, wait at least 2 hours before taking gabapentin.
- Refrigerate oral solution.

Lacosamide

Indications are for adjunctive therapy for partial seizures (> 17 years).

Pharmacokinetics

- *Bioavailability:* Complete
- *Protein binding:* Very low (< 15%)
- *Metabolism:* None
- *Renal:* 95% (40% as unchanged drug, 30% as inactive metabolite, 20% as uncharacterized metabolite)
- *Half-life:* About 13 hours

Side effects

Upon initiation, nausea and vomiting may occur, as well as dizziness, lack of coordination, and diplopia.

Severe or life-threatening include increased risk of suicidal behavior or ideation. An FDA warning has been issued: The FDA has analyzed suicidality reports from placebo-controlled studies involving 11 anticonvulsants (including lacosamide) and found that patients receiving anticonvulsants had approximately twice the risk of suicidal behavior or ideation (0.43%) of patients receiving placebo (0.22%).

Drug–drug interactions

Carbamazepine, phenobarbital, and phenytoin may decrease the serum concentration of lacosamide.

Commercially available formulations

See Table 24-3 for commercially available formulations.

Lamotrigine

Lamotrigine is indicated as adjunctive therapy for partial seizures (> 2 years), primary and secondary generalized tonic–clonic seizures (> 2 years), and seizures associated with Lennox–Gastaut syndrome. It is also approved for conversion to monotherapy. Although it is used for absence, atypical absence, atonic, and myoclonic seizures, it is not labeled for these indications.

Pharmacokinetics

- *Bioavailability:* Complete
- *Protein binding:* Low (55% to albumin)
- *Metabolism:* > 75% hepatically metabolized via glucuronidation; autoinduction possible
- *Renal:* 75–90% excreted as glucuronide metabolites and 10% as unchanged drug
- *Half-life:* Dependent on patient age and concomitant drug therapy
- *Reference range:* Proposed serum concentration of 1–5 mg/L, but clinical value of monitoring concentrations has not been established.

Side effects

Upon initiation, nausea and vomiting, dizziness, sedation, somnolence, and diplopia may occur.

No additional side effects are associated with chronic therapy.

Severe or life-threatening side effects are possible:

- *FDA black box warning:* Although rare, toxic epidermal necrolysis has been reported, and deaths have occurred. The risk of rash may be increased in those receiving valproic acid, large initial doses, or a rapid increase in dosage. The rash usually appears within 2–8 weeks of therapy initiation but has been reported after prolonged treatment (e.g., 6 months). Refer the patient to a physician if signs or symptoms of a rash develop. The physician may suggest holding a single dose until the rash is evaluated.

- *FDA warning:* Increased risk of suicidal behavior or ideation may occur. The FDA has analyzed suicidality reports from placebo-controlled studies involving 11 anticonvulsants (including lamotrigine) and found that patients receiving anticonvulsants had approximately twice the risk of suicidal behavior or ideation (0.43%) of patients receiving placebo (0.22%).

Drug–drug interactions

- Lamotrigine is a weak uridine diphosphate glucuronosyltransferase inducer.
- Valproic acid may increase the serum concentration or effect of lamotrigine.
- Carbamazepine, phenobarbital, phenytoin, and primidone decrease the serum concentration and effect of lamotrigine.
- Estrogen-containing oral contraceptives may decrease the serum concentration of lamotrigine.
- Lamotrigine may decrease the serum concentration or effect of valproic acid.
- Although not a true drug–drug interaction, the combination with carbamazepine may cause dizziness. Reduce the dose of carbamazepine.

Commercially available formulations

See Table 24-3 for commercially available formulations.

Patient counseling

See general counseling information. In addition, patients should be counseled to notify their physician immediately if a skin rash occurs.

Levetiracetam

Levetiracetam is indicated for adjunct for partial, primary generalized, and myoclonic seizures.

Pharmacokinetics

- *Bioavailability:* Complete
- *Protein binding:* Very low (< 10%)

- *Metabolism:* Not extensive; metabolites not active and renally eliminated
- *Renal:* Undergoes glomerular filtration and subsequent partial tubular reabsorption; 66% excreted unchanged and 27% as inactive metabolites
- *Half-life:* Short (4–8 hours)
- *Reference range:* Not established; clinical value of monitoring concentrations not established

Side effects

Upon initiation, dizziness, fatigue, and sedation may occur.

No additional side effects occur with chronic therapy.

Severe or life-threatening side effects include increased risk of suicidal behavior or ideation. The medication carries an FDA warning: The FDA has analyzed suicidality reports from placebo-controlled studies involving 11 anticonvulsants (including levetiracetam) and found that patients receiving anticonvulsants had approximately twice the risk of suicidal behavior or ideation (0.43%) of patients receiving placebo (0.22%).

Drug–drug interactions

No significant interactions have been identified.

Commercially available formulations

See Table 24-3 for commercially available formulations.

Oxcarbazepine

Oxcarbazepine is indicated for monotherapy (> 4 years) and adjunct therapy (> 2 years) for partial seizures.

Pharmacokinetics

- *Bioavailability:* Complete
- *Protein binding:* 67% (parent compound); 40%, monohydroxy metabolite (MHD) (primarily to albumin)
- *Metabolism:* Extensive to 10-MHD metabolite, which is active
- *Renal:* > 95%
- *Half-life:* 2 hours (oxcarbazepine); 9 hours (MHD)

Side effects

Upon initiation, nausea, vomiting, drowsiness, dizziness, and neutropenia (transient) may occur. On rare instances, a dose-related, transient, and reversible rash causes the drug to be discontinued. The frequency is less than that with carbamazepine, but cross-hypersensitivity reactions with carbamazepine may occur in 25% of patients.

With chronic therapy, the following side effects are possible:

- *SIADH:* This syndrome, causing hyponatremia and water retention, is more common than with carbamazepine.
- *Antiepileptic drug hypersensitivity syndrome:* A multiorgan involvement reaction occurs with rash, lymphadenopathy, fever, abnormal liver function tests, hepatitis, nephritis, oliguria, hepatorenal syndrome, hematological abnormalities, pruritus, asthenia, or arthralgia.
- *FDA warning:* Increased risk of suicidal behavior or ideation is possible. The FDA has analyzed suicidality reports from placebo-controlled studies involving 11 anticonvulsants (including oxcarbazepine) and found that patients receiving anticonvulsants had approximately twice the risk of suicidal behavior or ideation (0.43%) of patients receiving placebo (0.22%).

Drug–drug interactions

- Oxcarbazepine is an inhibitor of CYP2C19.
- Oxcarbazepine is an inducer of CYP3A4 and CYP3A5.
- Oxcarbazepine increases serum concentrations of phenobarbital and phenytoin.
- Oxcarbazepine may decrease serum concentrations of felodipine, lamotrigine, and oral contraceptives (i.e., ethinyl estradiol, levonorgestrel).
- Carbamazepine, phenobarbital, phenytoin, and valproic acid may decrease MHD concentrations.

Commercially available formulations

See Table 24-3 for commercially available formulations.

Patient counseling

This medication decreases the effectiveness of birth control pills. Use a supplemental birth control method to prevent pregnancy while taking oxcarbazepine or contact your physician about a high-estrogen oral contraceptive.

Phenobarbital

Phenobarbital is indicated for neonatal seizures and generalized seizures (except absence). Other anticonvulsants are more effective in complex partial seizures.

Pharmacokinetics

- *Bioavailability:* Good (70–90%)
- *Protein binding:* Low (30–50%)
- *Metabolism:* Hepatic via hydroxylation and glucuronide conjugation
- *Renal elimination:* 20–50% unchanged in urine; increases with alkalinization of the urine
- *Half-life:* Long (20–400 hours); increasing half-life with decreasing age
- *Reference range:* 15–40 mg/L

Side effects

Upon initiation, drowsiness, dizziness, light-headedness, lack of coordination, headaches, or nervousness may occur.

With chronic therapy, the following side effects are possible:

- Hyperactivity occurs, primarily in children; however, it rarely necessitates discontinuation of therapy.
- Lower memory and concentration abilities occur. The medication slightly lowers IQ.
- Folate deficiency may cause megaloblastic anemia.
- Vitamin K–deficient hemorrhagic disease is possible. Administer vitamin K to the mother before delivery and to the newborn.

Severe or life-threatening side effects are possible:

- *Hepatic failure:* Discontinue phenobarbital if liver function tests increase to more than three times above normal.
- *Stevens–Johnson syndrome:* Refer the patient to a physician if a rash develops. The physician may suggest holding a single dose until the rash is evaluated.
- *FDA warning:* Increased risk of suicidal behavior or ideation are possible. The FDA has analyzed suicidality reports from placebo-controlled studies involving 11 anticonvulsants (including phenobarbital) and found that patients receiving anticonvulsants had approximately twice the risk of suicidal behavior or ideation (0.43%) of patients receiving placebo (0.22%).
- *Teratogenic effects (phenobarbital syndrome):* Effects include developmental delay, short nose, low nasal bridge, low-set ears, wide mouth, protruding lips, and distal digital hypoplasia. The medication is pregnancy category D.

Drug–drug interactions

- Phenobarbital is an inducer of CYP1A2, CYP2B6, CYP2C8, CYP2C9, CYP2C19, CYP3A4, and uridine diphosphate glucuronosyltransferase.

- Chloramphenicol, felbamate, ketoconazole, methylphenidate, and valproic acid increase the serum concentration or effect of phenobarbital.
- Phenytoin decreases the anticonvulsant effect of phenobarbital.
- Phenobarbital may increase the serum concentration or effect of alcohol, caffeine, and monoamine oxidase inhibitors.
- Phenobarbital may decrease the serum concentration or effect of rifampin, birth control pills, corticosteroids, cyclophosphamide, cyclosporine, delavirdine, griseofulvin, haloperidol, lamotrigine, metronidazole, propranolol, quinidine, ritonavir, saquinavir, theophylline, and warfarin.

Other aspects

Phenobarbital is subject to control under the Federal Controlled Substances Act of 1970 as a schedule V (C–V) drug.

Commercially available formulations

See Table 24-2 for commercially available formulations.

Patient counseling

See general counseling information. In addition, this medication decreases the effectiveness of birth control pills. Counsel the patient to use a supplemental birth control method to prevent pregnancy while taking phenobarbital or contact a physician about a high-estrogen oral contraceptive.

Phenytoin

Phenytoin is indicated for all seizure types except absence and febrile seizures. It is also indicated for prevention of seizures following neurosurgery. It is frequently used to prevent post-traumatic epilepsy following head trauma, but is not approved for this indication.

Pharmacokinetics

- *Bioavailability:* Slow, variable, and formulation dependent; decreased in children
- *Protein binding:* Very high (90–95%); increased free fraction in neonates
- *Metabolism:* Hepatic
- *Renal elimination:* Low (< 5%)

- *Half-life:* Exhibits capacity-limited or saturable pharmacokinetics (i.e., Michaelis–Menten) and does not technically have a half-life
- *Reference range:* 10–20 mg/L

Side effects

Upon initiation, nausea, vomiting, drowsiness, and dizziness may occur.

With chronic therapy, the following side effects are possible:

- Peripheral neuropathy may occur.
- Hydantoin facies (thickening of subcutaneous tissues, enlargement of nose and lips) is possible.
- Acne, hirsutism, and gingival hyperplasia may occur. Suggest good oral hygiene.
- Osteomalacia may occur. Treat with vitamin D if alkaline phosphatase increases and 25-hydroxy-cholecalciferol decreases.
- Vitamin K–deficient hemorrhagic disease is possible. Administer vitamin K to the mother before delivery and to the newborn.
- Folate deficiency may cause megaloblastic anemia.

Severe or life-threatening side effects are as follows:

- *Hepatic failure:* Discontinue if liver function tests increase more than three times above normal.
- *Stevens–Johnson syndrome:* Refer the patient to a physician if signs or symptoms of a rash develop. The physician may suggest holding a single dose until the rash is evaluated.
- *FDA warning:* The FDA is investigating the possibility of an increased risk of serious skin reactions (e.g., Stevens–Johnson syndrome and toxic epidermal necrolysis) in patients given phenytoin who have the human leukocyte antigen allele HLA-B*1502. This allele occurs almost exclusively in individuals with ancestry across broad areas of Asia, including Han Chinese, Filipinos, Malaysians, South Asian Indians, and Thais. Until the FDA evaluation is finalized, phenytoin should be avoided as an alternative for carbamazepine in patients who test positive for HLA-B*1502.
- *FDA warning:* Increased risk of suicidal behavior or ideation may occur. The FDA has analyzed suicidality reports from placebo-controlled studies involving 11 anticonvulsants (including phenytoin) and found that patients receiving anticonvulsants had approximately twice the risk of suicidal behavior or ideation (0.43%) of patients receiving placebo (0.22%).

■ *Teratogenic effects (fetal hydantoin syndrome):* Features include craniofacial anomalies, broad nasal bridges, short upturned noses, low-set and prominent ears, distal digital hypoplasia, and intrauterine growth restriction. The medication is pregnancy category D.

Drug–drug interactions

■ Phenytoin induces CYP2C19, UTG.
■ Phenytoin inhibits CYP2C9.
■ Phenytoin displaces some drugs from albumin binding sites.
■ Acute alcohol use; amiodarone; chloramphenicol; chlordiazepoxide; diazepam; disulfiram; estrogens; felbamate; histamine antagonists (e.g., cimetidine); halothane; isoniazid; methylphenidate; phenothiazines; phenylbutazone; salicylates; succinimides; sulfonamides (sulfadiazine, sulfamethoxazole, and sulfisoxazole); tolbutamide; trazodone; warfarin; and zidovudine increase the serum concentration or effect of phenytoin.
■ Antacids, bleomycin, cisplatin, nevirapine, rifampin, ritonavir, vinblastine, zidovudine, and some herbals (i.e., shankhapushpi, kava kava, and valerian) decrease the effect of phenytoin.
■ Phenytoin may increase the serum concentration or effect of valproic acid.
■ Phenytoin may decrease the serum concentration or effect of phenobarbital.

Drug–nutrient interactions

Patients receiving tube feedings and oral phenytoin at the same time may have a significant decrease in absorption of phenytoin. If possible, discontinue feeding 2 hours before and after a dose of phenytoin.

Commercially available formulations

See Table 24-2 for commercially available formulations.

Patient counseling

See general counseling information. In addition, counsel the patient as follows:

■ Do not break, crush, or chew capsule before swallowing; swallow whole.
■ Shake suspension well.
■ This medication may alter your gums. Brush and floss daily, and have regular visits with your dentist.

Pregabalin

Pregabalin is indicated for adjunctive therapy in partial seizures.

Side effects

Upon initiation, nausea, vomiting, dizziness, drowsiness, and lethargy may occur.

With chronic therapy, increased appetite and weight gain are possible.

Severe or life-threatening side effects may occur:

■ *Angioedema:* There is some risk of angioedema (e.g., swelling of the face, tongue, lips, gums, and throat or larynx), with or without life-threatening respiratory compromise.
■ *FDA warning:* Increased risk of suicidal behavior or ideation may occur. The FDA has analyzed suicidality reports from placebo-controlled studies involving 11 anticonvulsants (including pregabalin) and found that patients receiving anticonvulsants had approximately twice the risk of suicidal behavior or ideation (0.43%) of patients receiving placebo (0.22%).

Drug–drug interactions

No known interactions.

Other aspects

Pregabalin is subject to control under the Federal Controlled Substances Act of 1970 as a schedule V (C–V) drug.

Commercially available formulations

See Table 24-3 for commercially available formulations.

Primidone

Primidone is indicated for generalized tonic–clonic, complex partial, and simple partial seizures.

Pharmacokinetics

■ *Bioavailability:* 60–80%
■ *Protein binding:* High (99%)
■ *Metabolism:* Hepatically metabolized to phenobarbital (active) and phenylethylmalonamide (PEMA)
■ *Renal elimination:* Urinary excretion of active metabolites and 15–25% unchanged primidone

- *Half-life:* Primidone, 10–12 hours for primidone; PEMA, 16 hours; phenobarbital, age dependent (20–400 hours)
- *Reference range:* 5–12 mg/L for primidone; 15–45 mg/L for phenobarbital

Side effects

Upon initiation, nausea, vomiting, dizziness, drowsiness, and lethargy may occur.

With chronic therapy, malignant lymphoma-like syndrome, megaloblastic anemia, and systemic lupus-like syndrome are possible.

- *FDA warning:* Increased risk of suicidal behavior or ideation is possible. The FDA has analyzed suicidality reports from placebo-controlled studies involving 11 anticonvulsants (including primidone and phenobarbital) and found that patients receiving anticonvulsants had approximately twice the risk of suicidal behavior or ideation (0.43%) of patients receiving placebo (0.22%).

Drug–drug interactions

- Primidone is an inducer of CYP1A2, CYP2B6, CYP2C, CYP2C8, CYP3A3/4, and CYP3A5-7.
- Primidone may decrease serum concentrations of ethosuximide, valproic acid, and griseofulvin.
- Methylphenidate may increase primidone serum concentrations.
- Phenytoin may decrease primidone serum concentrations.

Commercially available formulations

See Table 24-2 for commercially available formulations.

Tiagabine

Tiagabine is indicated for adjunctive therapy in the treatment of partial seizures.

Pharmacokinetics

- *Bioavailability:* Complete (> 95%)
- *Protein binding:* High (96%, mainly to albumin and alpha$_1$-acid glycoprotein)
- *Metabolism:* Hepatic via oxidation and glucuronidation; undergoes enterohepatic recirculation
- *Renal:* Low (about 2% excreted unchanged in urine)

- *Half-life:* 5–10 hours
- *Reference range:* Not established

Side effects

Upon initiation, nausea and vomiting, somnolence, impaired concentration, confusion, ataxia, and speech and language problems may occur.

No additional side effects have been associated with chronic therapy to date.

- *FDA warning:* Increased risk of suicidal behavior or ideation is possible. The FDA has analyzed suicidality reports from placebo-controlled studies involving 11 anticonvulsants (including tiagabine) and found that patients receiving anticonvulsants had approximately twice the risk of suicidal behavior or ideation (0.43%) of patients receiving placebo (0.22%).

Drug–drug interactions

- Tiagabine is a CYP3A substrate and may also be metabolized by CYP1A2, 2D6, or 2C19.
- Valproic acid may increase the serum concentration or effect of tiagabine.
- Carbamazepine, phenobarbital, primidone, and phenytoin may decrease the anticonvulsant effect of tiagabine.
- Tiagabine may decrease the serum concentration or effect of valproic acid.

Commercially available formulations

See Table 24-3 for commercially available formulations.

Topiramate

Topiramate is indicated for initial monotherapy (> 10 years of age) for partial onset seizures or primary generalized tonic–clonic seizures and for adjunctive therapy for patients (2–16 years) with partial onset seizures or primary generalized tonic–clonic seizures. It is also indicated for seizures associated with Lennox–Gastaut syndrome (> 2 years).

Pharmacokinetics

- *Bioavailability:* 80%
- *Protein binding:* 15–41%
- *Metabolism:* Minor hepatic (via hydroxylation, hydrolysis, and glucuronidation)
- *Elimination:* 70% excreted unchanged in urine; may undergo renal tubular reabsorption

- *Half-life:* About 20 hours
- *Reference range:* Not established; clinical value of monitoring concentrations not established

Side effects

Upon initiation, drowsiness, dizziness, difficulty with concentration, loss of appetite, mood changes, and paresthesias may occur.

With chronic therapy, the following side effects are possible:

- Hyperchloremic metabolic acidosis
- Acute myopia and secondary angle closure glaucoma
- Kidney stones (caution patient that adequate hydration may reduce stone formation)
- Paresthesia
- Word finding difficulties and decreased cognition (dose related)
- Significant weight loss

Severe or life-threatening side effects are as follows:

- *Oligohidrosis:* Children taking topiramate may not adequately sweat when overheated and could develop hyperthermia and heat stroke. Caution the parent to assess the child's ability to sweat, to be cautious about the child getting overheated, and to have the child drink plenty of water.
- *FDA warning:* Increased risk of suicidal behavior or ideation may occur. The FDA has analyzed suicidality reports from placebo-controlled studies involving 11 anticonvulsants (including topiramate) and found that patients receiving anticonvulsants had approximately twice the risk of suicidal behavior or ideation (0.43%) of patients receiving placebo (0.22%).

Drug–drug interactions

- Topiramate induces β-oxidation.
- Topiramate inhibits CYP2C19.
- CNS depressants (alcohol, morphine, codeine) and carbonic anhydrase inhibitors (acetazolamide) may increase the serum concentration or effect of topiramate.
- Phenobarbital, phenytoin, and valproic acid may decrease the anticonvulsant effect of topiramate.
- Topiramate may increase the serum concentration or effect of metformin.
- Topiramate may decrease the serum concentration or effect of oral contraceptives and valproic acid.

Commercially available formulations

See Table 24-3 for commercially available formulations.

Patient counseling

See general counseling information. In addition, counsel the patient as follows:

- If using the Topamax sprinkle capsule, sprinkle the contents on a small amount of cool, soft food (e.g., applesauce or yogurt) and swallow immediately without chewing.
- Drink plenty of fluids to avoid kidney stones.
- Confirm that children in hot climates can sweat.

Valproic Acid

Valproic acid is used for all types of generalized and partial seizures; along with ethosuximide, it is the drug of choice for absence seizures. It is rarely used in children < 2 years of age.

Pharmacokinetics

- *Bioavailability:* Complete
- *Protein binding:* High (80–90%; dose dependent)
- *Metabolism:* Extensive via hepatic glucuronide conjugation and oxidation
- *Renal:* Low (2–3% unchanged in urine)
- *Reference range:* 50–150 mg/L (curvilinear relationship between serum concentration and protein binding)

Side effects

Upon initiation, nausea and vomiting may occur.

With chronic therapy, the following side effects are possible:

- *Weight gain:* This side effect is at times significant enough to warrant discontinuing the medication.
- *Alopecia:* Effects may be partial or total. To prevent or treat alopecia, supplement with zinc and selenium.
- *Tremor:* This effect is dose dependent. Treat it by decreasing the dose, discontinuing the drug, or adding propranolol.
- *Thrombocytopenia:* A dose-dependent decrease in platelets may occur.
- *Elevation in liver enzymes:* This side effect may be transient and responds to discontinuation of valproic acid.

Severe or life-threatening side effects are possible:

- *FDA black box warning:* Fatal hepatotoxicity is possible. It is most common in children < 2 years of age who have severe epilepsy and are receiving multiple anticonvulsants.
- *FDA black box warning:* Fatal hemorrhagic pancreatitis may occur.
- *FDA black box warning:* Fetal valproate syndrome may occur. Features include craniofacial anomalies, small inverted noses, shallow philtrum, flat nasal bridge, long upper lip, congenital liver disease, and spina bifida. This medication is pregnancy category D.
- *FDA warning:* Increased risk of suicidal behavior or ideation may occur. The FDA has analyzed suicidality reports from placebo-controlled studies involving 11 anticonvulsants (including valproic acid) and found that patients receiving anticonvulsants had approximately twice the risk of suicidal behavior or ideation (0.43%) of patients receiving placebo (0.22%).

Drug–drug interactions

- Valproic acid inhibits CYP2C9, CYP 2C19, uridine diphosphate glucuronosyltransferase, epoxide hydroxylase, and β-oxidation.
- It displaces some drugs from albumin binding sites.
- Felbamate, phenytoin, and salicylates increase the serum concentration or effect of valproic acid.
- Carbamazepine, felbamate, lamotrigine, phenytoin, phenobarbital, and primidone decrease the anticonvulsant effect of valproic acid.
- Valproic acid may increase the serum concentration or effect of amitriptyline, carbamazepine, ethosuximide, felbamate, lamotrigine, phenobarbital, primidone, and zidovudine.
- Valproic acid may decrease the serum concentration or effect of phenytoin.

Commercially available formulations

See Table 24-2 for commercially available formulations.

Patient counseling

See general counseling information. Patients should also be counseled as follows:

- You may take this medication with food or milk to reduce stomach irritation. Do not take with carbonated drinks.

- Swallow valproic acid capsules whole with water only; do not break, chew, or crush.
- Swallow divalproex sodium delayed-released capsules whole or sprinkle the contents on a small amount of cool, soft food (e.g., applesauce or pudding) and swallow without chewing immediately after preparation.
- Swallow divalproex sodium delayed-release tablets whole; do not break, chew, or crush.
- You may mix valproic acid syrup with any liquid or add it to a small amount of food.
- Report any sore throat, fever, fatigue, bleeding, or bruising that is severe or persists to your physician.
- Your doctor may monitor your liver function with blood tests every 1–2 weeks initially and periodically thereafter.

Vigabatrin

Vigabatrin is indicated for infantile spasms; it is adjunctive therapy for complex partial seizures.

Pharmacokinetics

- *Bioavailability:* Complete
- *Protein binding:* Low
- *Metabolism:* Minimal
- *Renal:* 80% (unchanged)
- *Half-life:* 5–13 hours

Side effects

Upon initiation, fatigue, headache, drowsiness, dizziness, tremor, or agitation. Hyperactivity (e.g., hyperkinesia, agitation, excitation, or restlessness) has been reported in children.

With chronic therapy, permanent decrease in peripheral vision may occur. However, there is no effect on central vision or color.

- *FDA warning:* Increased risk of suicidal behavior or ideation is possible. The FDA has analyzed suicidality reports from placebo-controlled studies involving 11 anticonvulsants (including vigabitrin) and found that patients receiving anticonvulsants had approximately twice the risk of suicidal behavior or ideation (0.43%) of patients receiving placebo (0.22%).
- *FDA black box warning:* Medication may cause permanent vision loss in infants, children, and adults. Due to the risk of vision loss and because vigabatrin provides an observable symptomatic benefit when it is effective, the patient who fails

to show substantial benefit within a short period of time after initiation of treatment (2–4 weeks for infantile spasms; < 3 months in adults) should be withdrawn from therapy. If in the clinical judgment of the prescriber evidence of treatment failure becomes obvious earlier in treatment, vigabatrin should be discontinued at that time.

Commercially available formulations

See Table 24-3 for commercially available formulations.

Patient counseling

See general counseling information. In addition, counsel patients to notify their physician of any change in vision.

Zonisamide

Zonisamide is indicated for partial seizures.

Pharmacokinetics

- *Bioavailability:* Complete
- *Protein binding:* Low (40%)
- *Metabolism:* Undergoes acetylation and subsequent conjugation with glucuronide in the liver
- *Renal elimination:* 62% (35% as unchanged)
- *Half-life:* 50–70 hours
- *Reference range:* proposed therapeutic range, 10–20 mg/L; concentrations > 30 mg/L associated with adverse effects

Side effects

With chronic therapy, side effects are very similar to those of topiramate:

- Kidney stones (contraindicated in patients with a history of kidney stones; should be adequately hydrated)
- Weight loss
- Reversible or irreversible psychosis (rare)

Severe or life-threatening side effects may occur:

- *Oligohidrosis:* The medication carries an FDA warning. Children taking zonisamide may not sweat as needed and could develop hyperthermia. Warn parents of the need to be aware of children getting overheated and to have them drink plenty of water.

- *FDA warning:* Zonisamide may cause a dose-dependent metabolic acidosis, which has occurred at doses as small as 25 mg/d. Metabolic acidosis is usually asymptomatic; however, chronic untreated metabolic acidosis may result in decreased growth rates in children, as well as decreased fetal growth and fetal death following exposure during pregnancy. The FDA is now recommending a serum bicarbonate level prior to initiation and periodically during therapy. If metabolic acidosis develops, consider decreasing the dose or discontinuing use with appropriate dose tapering.
- *FDA warning:* Increased risk of suicidal behavior or ideation may occur. The FDA has analyzed suicidality reports from placebo-controlled studies involving 11 anticonvulsants (including zonisamide) and found that patients receiving anticonvulsants had approximately twice the risk of suicidal behavior or ideation (0.43%) of patients receiving placebo (0.22%).
- *Other:* Zonisamide is a sulfonamide. Life-threatening sulfonamide reactions may occur (e.g., Stevens–Johnson syndrome, toxic epidermal necrolysis, aplastic anemia, agranulocytosis, and fulminant hepatic necrosis).

Drug–drug interactions

- Zonisamide is a CYP3A4 substrate.
- Carbamazepine, phenobarbital, phenytoin, and valproic acid decrease the effect of zonisamide.
- Lamotrigine may inhibit the clearance of zonisamide and increase zonisamide serum concentrations.

Commercially available formulations

See Table 24-3 for commercially available formulations.

Patient counseling

See general counseling information. In addition, counsel the patient as follows:

- Notify your pharmacist or physician if you are allergic to sulfa medications.
- Drink plenty of fluids to help prevent kidney stones.
- Contact your doctor if your child is not sweating as usual.

24-3. Other Issues

Nondrug Treatment of Epilepsy

Nondrug treatments are as follows:

- Ketogenic diet
- Vagal nerve stimulator
- Surgical correction

Withdrawal of Anticonvulsants

Over half of patients who remain seizure free for 2 years can have their anticonvulsant successfully withdrawn. Most who are seizure free for 4 years can be successfully withdrawn from anticonvulsants.

Unless the patient is experiencing a severe or life-threatening adverse effect, *never* abruptly discontinue an anticonvulsant; taper slowly over 2–6 months.

Status Epilepticus

Status epilepticus is defined as a seizure that lasts longer than 5 minutes or two or more discrete seizures between which there is incomplete recovery of consciousness. It is a medical emergency. See Table 24-4 for suggested order of therapies.

Benzodiazepines

Benzodiazepines are first-line agents. Diazepam or lorazepam are preferred.

Hydantoin (phenytoin or fosphenytoin)

Phenytoin (intravenous)

Phenytoin can only be mixed with normal saline.

If an individual is not already receiving phenytoin, give a loading dose of 15–20 mg/kg. Because phenytoin contains propylene glycol and is in itself cardiotoxic, do not infuse faster than 50 mg/minute.

If the maintenance dose is to be given every 12 hours, give the first dose 12 hours after the end of the loading dose. If the maintenance dose is to be given every 24 hours, give the first dose 24 hours after the end of the loading dose.

The alkaline pH of phenytoin precludes IM administration.

Fosphenytoin

Fosphenytoin is a phenytoin prodrug that is converted to phenytoin within minutes after infusion. It can be admixed with any IV solution.

Fosphenytoin must be dosed in PE (phenytoin equivalents): 1 mg of phenytoin = 1.5 mg of fosphenytoin. It can be given at a rate of 150 mg/min (three times faster than phenytoin).

Phenobarbital

Phenobarbital may cause respiratory depression or arrest. The likelihood of such an effect may be increased if benzodiazepines have been given.

Phenobarbital-induced sedation may eliminate the ability to perform an accurate neurologic assessment.

Table 24-4. Treatment of Status Epilepticus

As soon as possible	■ Assess cardiorespiratory status; insert oral airway and administer oxygen as needed.
	■ Place secure IV and start infusion of normal saline.
	■ Obtain medical history; perform neurological examination.
	■ Obtain the following tests: if the patient has been on anticonvulsants as an outpatient, obtain blood for serum drug concentrations and a chemistry panel including electrolytes, glucose, blood urea nitrogen, and urine drug screen.
	■ Administer 25 g of glucose and 100 mg of thiamine IV.
If still seizing	■ Administer either diazepam or lorazepam up to maximum dosage until seizure stops.
If still seizing	■ Load with IV phenytoin (provided patient was not on phenytoin at home or has low serum concentrations) and begin maintenance doses.
	■ Monitor blood pressure and EEG.
If still seizing	■ Load with IV phenobarbital or begin a continuous infusion of midazolam.
If still seizing	■ Begin medically induced coma.
	■ Adjust EEG to burst suppression.
	■ Avoid hypotension during infusion of the barbiturate.

Because phenobarbital contains propylene glycol and is cardiotoxic, do not infuse faster than 60 mg/min in adults and 30 mg/min in children.

Midazolam

Because of midazolam's very short half-life, the loading dose should be followed by continuous infusion.

Medically induced coma

Medically induced coma is used for severe refractory status epilepticus. It is usually achieved with pentobarbital.

Give a loading dose (20–40 mg/kg) over 1–2 hours, followed by continuous infusion (1–4 mg/kg/hr).

If hypotension occurs, begin dopamine or slow the rate of infusion.

Titrate to burst suppression (isoelectric) on EEG.

Other therapies used for refractory status epilepticus

- Propofol
- Newer anticonvulsants (IV: levetiracetam; oral: topiramate)
- Magnesium
- Lidocaine
- IV immune globulin

Febrile Seizures

A febrile seizure is a benign seizure that occurs in the absence of CNS infection in a child with fever. It is the most common seizure disorder in childhood. The age of onset is 4 months to 5 years (peaks at 14–18 months).

A child is at risk if he or she has two of the following risk factors:

- A first- or second-degree relative with a history of a febrile seizure
- Developmental delay
- Delayed discharge (> 28 days) from a newborn center
- Day care attendance

Overall, the development of epilepsy in children who have experienced such seizures is rare (1–2%). However, about 15% of children who have complex febrile seizures (as defined below) will go on to develop epilepsy.

There are two types of febrile seizures:

- Simple febrile seizure:
  - Benign
  - A primary generalized seizure

- Less than 15 minutes in duration
- Does not recur within 24 hours
- Complex febrile seizure:
  - Focal (involves an arm, leg, or face on one side only or eye deviation toward one side)
  - Prolonged (> 15 minutes) or recurring within 24 hours of the initial seizure

Acute treatment of a simple or complex febrile seizure

Drugs of choice for prolonged febrile seizure are rectally administered benzodiazepines (rectal diazepam or lorazepam). Diastat is a commercially available gel of diazepam to be given rectally.

Prophylaxis for a simple or complex febrile seizure

If temperature is > 38C°, give the patient a nonaspirin antipyretic.

Daily anticonvulsants are not indicated for the prevention of recurrent febrile seizures.

Maintenance therapy

Maintenance therapy is not generally used. However, an anticonvulsant (i.e., phenobarbital) may be considered after a complex febrile seizure if epilepsy is suspected.

Carbamazepine and phenytoin are *not* effective in the prevention of recurrent febrile seizures.

24-4. Key Points

- Phenytoin can be mixed only with normal saline and should not be given faster than 50 mg/min.
- Gabapentin and levetiracetam are not associated with any significant drug interactions.
- As of September 2009, the following anticonvulsants carry a U.S. black box warning: carbamazepine (aplastic anemia, dermatologic reactions); valproic acid (liver failure, teratogenicity, pancreatitis); felbamate (aplastic anemia, hepatic failure); and lamotrigine (serious rash). FDA warnings have been given for Zonisamide and topiramate, which have been reported to cause oligohidrosis and hyperthermia. The FDA has found that 11 of the anticonvulsants are associated with an increased risk of suicidal behavior or ideation.
- Although absence seizures are frequently treated with ethosuximide or valproic acid (if ≥ 2 years of age), lamotrigine and topiramate are also used.

- Carbapenems (e.g., imipenem) and normeperidine (a metabolite of meperidine that accumulates in renal failure) may cause seizures.
- Carbamazepine undergoes autoinduction (i.e., it induces its own metabolism), and phenytoin has capacity-limited or saturable (i.e., Michaelis–Menten) pharmacokinetics.
- Because of the potential for severe life-threatening liver toxicity, valproic acid is generally not used in a patient < 2 years of age.
- There may be an association between folic acid deficiency and spina bifida; hence, all women with epilepsy who are of childbearing age should be on daily folic acid (1 mg).
- Unless a patient is experiencing a life-threatening adverse effect, an anticonvulsant should not be abruptly discontinued.
- Topiramate may cause significant weight loss, and valproic acid may cause significant weight gain.
- Topiramate and zonisamide may cause kidney stones.
- Patients with an allergy to sulfa medications should not be given zonisamide.

24-5. Questions

1. Which of the following is true regarding phenytoin?

    A. The maximum rate of intravenous administration is 50 mg/min.
    B. If intravenous access cannot be established, phenytoin can be given IM.
    C. Because phenytoin contains propylene glycol, it is soluble as any IV fluid.
    D. It is an inhibitor of the cytochrome P450 system.
    E. A major limitation to the use of the product in pediatric patients is the lack of a commercially available liquid formulation.

2. A 50 kg patient with no history of epilepsy presents in status epilepticus. The patient is given an adequate dose of lorazepam and is about to be given a loading dose of intravenous phenytoin. Assuming a phenytoin V_d of 0.6 L/kg, what dose of phenytoin should be given to achieve a serum phenytoin concentration of ~ 16–18 mg/L?

    A. 18 mg/kg
    B. 500 mg
    C. 30 mg/kg

    D. 50 mg
    E. 5 g

3. Which of the following is true regarding a patient with refractory status epilepticus who is placed in a medically induced coma with a barbiturate?

    A. If the patient is mechanically ventilated, the barbiturates will induce respiratory arrest.
    B. The goal of a coma that is medically induced with a barbiturate is to induce burst suppression (isoelectric) on EEG.
    C. If hypotension develops, the patient should be given nitroprusside.
    D. The barbiturates are not associated with drug interactions.
    E. A major problem with this type of therapy is kidney failure.

4. Which of the following is associated with autoinduction?

    A. Phenobarbital
    B. Phenytoin
    C. Carbamazepine
    D. Gabapentin
    E. Levetiracetam

5. Which of these agents reduces the likelihood of congenital malformations in epileptic women receiving valproate?

    A. Folic acid
    B. Vitamin B_{12}
    C. Ginkgo biloba
    D. Iron
    E. Selenium

6. A 33-year-old woman is being started on an anticonvulsant. She is already slightly overweight and is very concerned about the effects of the various medications on her weight. Which of the following is (are) true regarding anticonvulsants and their effect on weight?

    I.   Valproic acid increases weight.
    II. Topiramate decreases weight.
    III. Phenytoin increases weight.

    A. I
    B. I and II
    C. II
    D. III
    E. I, II, and III

7. A 24-year-old woman has complex partial seizures that are currently controlled with valproic acid, gabapentin, and topiramate. She calls your pharmacy to ask if any of her medications can cause nosebleeds since she has had one or two in the past week. You refer her to her local medical doctor, where her platelet count is reported to be 95,132/mm^3. Which of the following is true?

   A. None of her anticonvulsants cause thrombocytopenia.
   B. Valproate can cause a dose-related thrombocytopenia.
   C. Gabapentin has inhibited the metabolism of topiramate, and the elevated concentration of topiramate is responsible for the thrombocytopenia.
   D. Gabapentin can cause idiosyncratic thrombocytopenia.
   E. Topiramate can cause thrombocytopenia.

8. A patient has hypertension, diabetes mellitus, and chronic renal failure (serum Cr = 6.8), and has developed seizures. Which of the following anticonvulsants would require dosage adjustment in this patient?

   A. Gabapentin, topiramate
   B. Lamotrigine, felbamate
   C. Phenobarbital, gabapentin
   D. Phenytoin, valproic acid
   E. Phenobarbital, levetiracetam

9. Which of the following anticonvulsants is metabolized to phenobarbital?

   A. Ethosuximide
   B. Primidone
   C. Zonisamide
   D. Levetiracetam
   E. Carbamazepine

10. A 7-year-old boy on valproic acid for partial complex seizures with secondary generalization that are refractory to phenobarbital, phenytoin, carbamazepine, and gabapentin continued to have seizures and was started on lamotrigine 2 weeks ago. Today he presents with a diffuse maculopapular erythematous rash with lesions on the lips. Which of the following is correct?

    A. A rash associated with lamotrigine generally occurs within the first few days; hence, the rash is not associated with an anticonvulsant.
    B. The patient should be given diphenhydramine, and lamotrigine should be continued.
    C. Lamotrigine should be discontinued.
    D. The rash is secondary to a drug interaction between gabapentin and carbamazepine.
    E. All of the anticonvulsants are associated with life-threatening rash. To prevent status epilepticus associated with abrupt discontinuation of the anticonvulsants, the medications should be slowly discontinued.

11. A new anticonvulsant has just been approved by the FDA. Its bioavailability is > 95%, and it is highly protein bound to α_1-acid glycoprotein. It undergoes extensive hepatic metabolism by CYP450 2C9. Less than 5% is excreted unchanged in the urine. It is known to inhibit CYP450 3A4. A patient on this anticonvulsant has developed significant depression and is being started on an antidepressant that is 93% bound to albumin and is a potent inhibitor of CYP450 2C19. The antidepressant is metabolized by CYP450 3A4 to an active metabolite that is hepatically cleared by CYP450 2C9. The neurologist wants to know if any drug interactions may occur that would necessitate a reduction in drug dosage.

    A. No drug interactions should occur in this patient.
    B. The dose of the anticonvulsant should be reduced because of a potential protein binding interaction that would increase the serum concentration of the anticonvulsant.
    C. The dose of the anticonvulsant should be increased.
    D. The dose of the antidepressant should be reduced.
    E. Because of an interaction in the gut that decreases bioavailability, the dose should be increased.

12. Which of the following is (are) not associated with any drug–drug interactions?

    I. Gabapentin
    II. Carbamazepine
    III. Levetiracetam

    A. I
    B. II
    C. I and III
    D. II and III
    E. I and II
    F. III

13. A 42-year-old woman has been successfully treated with valproic acid for years, but she has experienced some undesirable side effects. She is slowly titrated onto a new anticonvulsant, and the valproic acid is slowly discontinued. She presents to the emergency department with severe flank pain and is diagnosed with a kidney stone. Which of the following may have precipitated her current situation?

    A. Gabapentin
    B. Lamotrigine
    C. Levetiracetam
    D. Topiramate
    E. Phenytoin

14. Which of the following drugs carries (carry) a black box warning?

    I.   Carbamazepine
    II. Felbamate
    III. Levetiracetam

    A. II
    B. III
    C. I
    D. I and II
    E. II and III

15. Which of the following carries a black box warning for pancreatitis?

    A. Carbamazepine
    B. Felbamate
    C. Zonisamide
    D. Valproic acid
    E. Phenytoin

16. What is the drug of choice for absence seizures in a child < 2 years of age?

    A. Phenytoin
    B. Phenobarbital
    C. Ethosuximide
    D. Valproic acid
    E. Primidone

17. Diastat is given by which of the following routes?

    A. Rectally
    B. Intramuscularly
    C. Intravenously
    D. Intranasally
    E. Subcutaneously

18. Which of the following is true?

    A. Febrile seizures must be accompanied by a CNS infection.
    B. Complex febrile seizures last > 15 minutes.
    C. Most children who have a febrile seizure go on to develop epilepsy.
    D. The drug of choice for a simple febrile seizure is carbamazepine.
    E. Simple febrile seizures should never be treated.

19. Which of the following anticonvulsants is (are) available in a liquid, chewable tablet, and intravenous formulation?

    I.   Carbamazepine
    II. Phenytoin
    III. Valproic acid

    A. II
    B. III
    C. I
    D. I and II
    E. I, II, and III

20. Patients should be told to drink plenty of fluid when taking which of the following?

    A. Carbamazepine
    B. Topiramate
    C. Levetiracetam
    D. Gabapentin
    E. Phenytoin

21. Which of the following medications may cause seizures in an adult patient with renal failure?

    A. Meperidine
    B. Phenobarbital
    C. Carbamazepine
    D. Lamotrigine
    E. Theophylline

22. Which of the following is associated with Michaelis–Menten pharmacokinetics?

    A. Carbamazepine
    B. Valproic acid
    C. Topiramate
    D. Phenytoin
    E. Phenobarbital

23. A patient on which of the following medications should be made aware of the importance of good oral hygiene?

 A. Felbamate
 B. Phenytoin
 C. Zonisamide
 D. Phenobarbital
 E. Levetiracetam

24-6. Answers

1. **A.** Because phenytoin contains propylene glycol and is itself cardiotoxic, the IV formulation should not be infused faster than 50 mg/min. Phenytoin is extremely alkaline (pH ~13). Not only is IM administration associated with tissue damage, it is erratically absorbed. Phenytoin can be admixed only with normal saline, is an inducer, and is also available as a suspension and a chewable tablet.

2. **B.** The equation for calculation of a loading dose is as follows: Dose = C_p (serum concentration) desired × V_d (volume of distribution). So C_p desired is ~ 17 × (0.6 L/kg × 50 kg) ≈ 510 mg.

3. **B.** The goal is to produce a "flat" EEG. If the patient is mechanically ventilated, the effect of a medication on respiration is not a factor in its administration. Although pentobarbital may cause hypotension if given too rapidly, nitroprusside is a vasodilator used to treat hypertension. The barbiturates are known inducers. Coma that is medically induced with a barbiturate does not cause kidney failure.

4. **C.** Carbamazepine induces its own metabolism, with peak effects seen about 21 days after beginning the medication or following an increase in dosage. Phenobarbital and phenytoin are inducers. Gabapentin and levetiracetam are not cleared hepatically.

5. **A.** Many of the anticonvulsants can cause folic acid deficiency. An association exists between folic acid deficiency and spina bifida; hence, all women with epilepsy who are of childbearing age should receive supplemental folic acid every day (1 mg).

6. **B.** Topiramate can cause significant weight loss, and valproate can cause significant weight gain. Phenytoin does not significantly affect weight.

7. **B.** Valproic acid can cause clinically significant thrombocytopenia. Gabapentin is not associated with any drug interaction that affects metabolism, and it does not cause a decrease in platelets. Topiramate does not cause thrombocytopenia.

8. **A.** Gabapentin and topiramate would require dosage adjustment because they are renally eliminated.

9. **B.** Primidone (Mysoline) is an active anticonvulsant, but it is also metabolized to phenobarbital.

10. **C.** Lamotrigine has a black box warning for severe rash. Because this patient has a diffuse rash and lesions on the lips, lamotrigine should be discontinued. Because the incidence of severe rash may be higher in children than in adults, current practice would be to discontinue lamotrigine and not "treat through" the rash with diphenhydramine. Gabapentin does not interact with lamotrigine. However, the combination of valproic acid and lamotrigine is associated with a higher incidence of rash. Although abrupt discontinuation of an anticonvulsant may induce status epilepticus, an anticonvulsant may be abruptly discontinued in the face of a life-threatening event.

11. **D** is correct because the new anticonvulsant inhibits CYP450 3A4 and the antidepressant is metabolized by this enzyme.

12. **C.** At this time, neither gabapentin nor levetiracetam is associated with significant drug–drug interactions. The absorption of gabapentin may be reduced by concurrent administration of aluminum- or magnesium-containing antacids; hence, antacids should be given 2 hours before or after a dose of gabapentin. Carbamazepine is an inducer that is associated with numerous drug–drug interactions.

13. **D.** Both topiramate and zonisamide may cause kidney stones. Although neither agent is contraindicated in an individual with a history of kidney stones, these drugs should be used cautiously in such patients. Patients should be counseled to remain adequately hydrated because doing so may decrease the risk of stone formation.

14. **D.** Both carbamazepine and felbamate are associated with aplastic anemia and hepatic failure. Levetiracetam has no black box warning.

15. **D.** Valproic acid may cause fatal hemorrhagic pancreatitis.

16. **C.** Although valproic acid is extremely effective and is frequently used as monotherapy for absence seizures, it should not be given to a patient < 2 years of age.

17. **A.** Diastat is a commercially available gel form of diazepam that is given rectally.

18. **B.** Unlike simple febrile seizures, which last a brief period, complex febrile seizures are prolonged (> 15 minutes) or recur within 24 hours of the initial seizure. Febrile seizures must occur in the absence of CNS infection in a child with fever. Most febrile seizures are benign, and children do not go on to develop epilepsy. Carbamazepine is ineffective in febrile seizures.

19. **A.** Only phenytoin is available as a liquid (125 mg/5 mL), as a chewable tablet (50 mg), and in an intravenous dosage form. Carbamazepine is not available in an IV dosage form, and valproic acid is not available as a chewable tablet.

20. **B.** Because topiramate may cause kidney stones, patients should be encouraged to drink plenty of fluids. This would also be true for zonisamide.

21. **A.** Normeperidine, a metabolite of meperidine, can accumulate in patients with renal failure who receive normal doses and cause seizures. The other agents listed are not eliminated renally in adults.

22. **D.** Phenytoin has capacity-limited or saturable (i.e., Michaelis–Menten) pharmacokinetics.

23. **B.** Phenytoin may cause gingival hyperplasia (i.e., overgrowth of the gums). Hence, patients should be instructed to brush and floss daily and to have regular visits with the dentist.

24-7. References

American Academy of Neurology, Quality Standards Subcommittee. Practice parameter: A guideline for discontinuing antiepileptic drugs in seizure-free patients—summary statement. *Neurology.* 1996;47:600–2.

Anderson GD. A mechanistic approach to antiepileptic drug interactions. *Ann Pharmacother.* 1998;32:554–63.

Baumann RJ, Duffner PK. Treatment of children with simple febrile seizures: The AAP practice parameter. *Pediatr Neurol.* 2000;23:11–17.

Brunbech L, Sabers A. Effect of antiepileptic drugs on cognitive function in individuals with epilepsy: A comparative review of newer versus older agents. *Drugs.* 2002;62:593–604.

Carroll MC, Yueng-Yue KA, Esterly NB, et al. Drug-induced hypersensitivity syndrome in pediatric patients. *Pediatrics.* 2001;108:485–92.

Commission on Antiepileptic Drugs, International League against Epilepsy. Guidelines for therapeutic monitoring on antiepileptic drugs. *Epilepsia.* 1993;34:585–87.

Deckers CL, Knoester PD, de Haan GJ, et al. Selection criteria for the clinical use of the newer antiepileptic drugs. *CNS Drugs.* 2003;17:405–21.

Johannessen SI, Battino D, Berry DJ, et al. Therapeutic drug monitoring of the newer antiepileptic drugs. *Ther Drug Monit.* 2003;25:347–463.

Perucca E. The clinical pharmacokinetics of the new antiepileptic drugs. *Epilepsia.* 1999;40(suppl 9):S7–13.

Working Group on Status Epilepticus. Treatment of convulsive status epilepticus: Recommendations of the Epilepsy Foundation of America's Working Group on Status Epilepticus. *JAMA.* 1993;270:854–59.

Psychiatric Disease

Jason Carter, PharmD

25-1. Axis Diagnosis

The fourth edition of the *Diagnostic and Statistical Manual of Mental Disorders* (DSM-IV) of the American Psychiatric Association organizes psychiatric diagnoses into five axes:

  I.   Clinical disorders
 II.   Personality disorders and mental retardation
III.   General medical conditions
 IV.   Psychosocial and environmental problems
  V.   Global assessment of functioning

25-2. Schizophrenia

Schizophrenia is a psychiatric disorder characterized by a profound disruption in perception, cognition, and emotion.

Epidemiology

Approximately 1% of the U.S. adult population has schizophrenia. There are 200,000 new cases reported yearly.

No gender or racial differences exist. Onset is earlier in males (average age, 18–24 years) than in females (average age, late 20s to early 40s).

Types and Classifications

Paranoid

Paranoid schizophrenia is characterized by prominent preoccupation with hallucinations (usually auditory) and one or more delusions.

Disorganized

Disorganized schizophrenia is characterized by disorganized speech and behavior, as well as blunted, flat, or inappropriate affect.

Catatonic

With catatonic schizophrenia, psychomotor disturbances are present that may involve catalepsy or stupor, excessive motor activity, rigid posture, mutism, peculiar or repetitive movements, and echolalia or echopraxia.

Undifferentiated

With undifferentiated schizophrenia, hallucinations or delusions are present but without prominent paranoid, disorganized, or catatonic symptoms.

Residual

With residual schizophrenia, hallucinations and delusions are not prominent, but there is continued evidence of an ongoing disturbance (flat affect, poverty of speech, or avolition).

Clinical Presentation

The onset of schizophrenia is typically characterized by deterioration in occupational and social situations over a period of 6 months or more.

Symptoms

Symptoms include the following:

- Hallucinations (auditory, visual, tactile, olfactory, or gustatory)

- Delusions (usually persecutory or grandiose)
- Disorganized thoughts or speech
- Impaired cognition, attention, concentration, judgment, and motivation

Symptoms are commonly referred to as *positive* (hallucinations or delusions); *negative* (flat affect, avolition, anhedonia, and poverty of thought); or *disorganized* (disorganized speech or behavior).

Most patients fluctuate between acute episodes and remission, but complete remission without any symptoms is uncommon.

Associated features

Morbidity
There are many comorbid disease states (mental and medical); for example, substance abuse is found in 60–70% of persons with schizophrenia.

Mortality
Shortened life expectancy is a feature of schizophrenia. Patients with schizophrenia are at increased risk of suicide (10% commit suicide). Risk factors for suicide are as follows:

- Male
- Socially isolated
- Comorbid psychiatric disorders
- Unemployed
- < 30 years of age

Etiology

The etiology is most likely multifactorial:

- Genetic
- Neurobiologic
- Developmental (season of birth, viral illness, traumatic injury)

DSM-IV Diagnostic Criteria

Two or more of the following symptoms prevail for at least 1 month:

- Hallucinations
- Delusions
- Disorganized speech
- Grossly disorganized or catatonic behavior
- Negative symptoms
- Anhedonia
- Flat affect
- Avolition

Significant social dysfunction exists:

- Signs of the disturbance are continuous and persist for 6 months.
- Schizoaffective disorders and mood disorders, mental retardation, substance abuse, and other causative medical disorders have been ruled out.

Treatment Principles and Goals

- All antipsychotics are equally effective if used properly.
- Clozapine is the only agent proven effective in treating refractory schizophrenia.
- The basis for choosing an antipsychotic medication is the following:
  - Past history of response (patient's response or a family member's response to a medication)
  - Side-effect profile of the antipsychotic
- Administer therapy with a trial of antipsychotics (at least 4–6 weeks at recommended doses).
- Do everything possible to simplify the drug regimen.
- Consider long-acting injectable preparations in situations of poor compliance.

Drug Therapy

Tables 25-1 and 25-2 provide an overview of drug therapy alternatives.

Mechanism of action

These drugs block postsynaptic dopamine-2 receptors. They share anticholinergic, antihistaminic, and α-blocking properties.

Other conventional agents

Though not commonly used, perphenazine (Trilafon), thiothixene (Navane), trifluoperazine (Stelazine), and loxapine (Loxitane) are conventional agents used to treat schizophrenia.

Management of adverse effects

Sedation
The level of sedation depends on the drug used. Low-potency drugs in this class are more sedating than high-potency drugs.

Sedation effects are worse initially, but become more tolerable over time.

Table 25-1. Typical (Conventional or Older) Antipsychotics

Drug and form	Trade name	Form	Potency	Dosage range	Equivalent oral dose	Clinical pearls
Chlorpromazine	Thorazine	10, 25, 50, 100, 200 mg tablets; 30, 75, 150, 200, 300 mg sustained release capsules; 10 mg/5 mL syrup; 30 mg/mL, 100 mg/mL concentrate; 25 mg, 100 mg rectal suppository; 25 mg/mL injection	Low	50–2000 mg/d	100 mg	First antipsychotic used clinically; contributed to deinstitutionalization of many patients in the 1950s; 100 mg of chlorpromazine is equivalent to 2 mg of haloperidol.
Thioridazine	Mellaril	10, 15, 25, 50, 100, 150, 200 mg tablets; 25 mg/5 mL, 100 mg/5 mL suspension; 30 mg/mL, 100 mg/mL concentrate	Low	50–800 mg/d	100 mg	Pigmentary retinopathy at daily doses > 800 mg/d; black box warning: QT prolongation
Perphenazine	Trilafon	2, 4, 8, 16 mg tablets; 5 mg/mL injection	Medium	4–64 mg/d in divided doses	10 mg	Moderate sedation, extrapyramidal symptoms; low anticholinergic effect, orthostasis
Fluphenazine	Prolixin	1.0, 2.5, 5.0, 10.0 mg tablets; 25 mg/mL decanoate injection; 2.5 mg/mL injection; 2.5 mg/5 mL elixir; 5 mg/mL concentrate	High	1–65 mg/d po; 12.5–75 mg IM (decanoate) every 2 weeks	2 mg	Decanoate injection every 2 weeks; immediate-release injection, 5–10 minutes onset
Haloperidol	Haldol	0.5, 1.0, 2.0, 5.0, 10.0, 20.0 mg tablets; 2 mg/mL concentrate; 50, 100 mg/mL decanoate injection; 5 mg/mL injection	High	1–100 mg/d po; 50–300 mg IM (decanoate) every 4 weeks	2 mg	Decanoate injection every 4 weeks; immediate-release injection, 5–10 min onset

Table 25-2. Adverse Effects of Typical Antipsychotic Medications

Drug	Extrapyramidal symptoms	Sedation	Orthostasis	Weight gain	Anticholinergic effect
Chlorpromazine	+++	++++	++++	++	+++
Thioridazine	+++	++++	++++	+	++++
Perphenazine	++++	++	+	+	++
Fluphenazine	++++	+	+	+	+
Haloperidol	++++	+	+	+	+

Orthostasis

Severity depends on the drug used. Low-potency formulations promote more orthostasis than do high potency formulations.

This condition is especially problematic in elderly patients.

Weight gain

Weight gain is very prominent in patients taking these medications. Low doses should be used. Appropriate diet and exercise should be encouraged to offset weight gain.

Anticholinergic effect

Severity depends on the drug used. Low-potency drugs of this type are more sedating than high-potency ones.

Dry mouth, blurred vision, constipation, and urinary hesitancy may occur. Use high-potency agents in patients bothered by anticholinergic side effects.

Extrapyramidal symptoms

Extrapyramidal symptoms (EPSs) are most likely attributed to an imbalance in dopamine and acetylcholine. Antipsychotics cause a hypodopaminergic state.

Dystonic reactions

Reactions usually occur within 24–96 hours of initiating or changing dose. They present as painful, involuntary muscle spasms in skeletal muscles (most commonly in the facial or neck muscles, but sometimes in the back, arm, and leg muscles).

Treatment is benztropine (Cogentin) 1–2 mg intramuscular (IM) or diphenhydramine (Benadryl) 25–50 mg IM every 30 minutes until the reaction is relieved. Prophylaxis with oral therapy is usually initiated.

Akathisia

Akathisia usually occurs within a few weeks of initiating antipsychotic therapy. It is described as a subjective feeling of discomfort, usually seen as motor restlessness of the legs (inability to stand still or sit still).

Akathisia is treated with lipophilic β-blockers (e.g., propranolol), benzodiazepines, clonidine, and anticholinergics.

Pseudoparkinsonism

Pseudoparkinsonism usually occurs after months or years of therapy. This condition resembles Parkinson's symptoms (e.g., cogwheel rigidity, bradykinesia, tremor, shuffling gait).

It is treated with amantadine (Symmetrel) 100 mg bid or anticholinergics.

Other adverse effects

Tardive dyskinesia

Tardive dyskinesia (TD) is an irreversible drug-induced movement disorder that occurs after years of antipsychotic therapy. It is caused by long-term suppression of dopamine.

A triad of symptoms characterize TD:

- Choreoathetosis (splayed, writhing fingers)
- Oral or buccal movements (grimacing, bruxism, lip-smacking)
- Protrusion of the tongue

The only treatment is prevention (i.e., use the lowest effective dose of antipsychotic). However, various therapies (vitamin E, lecithin, vitamin B_6) may help alleviate symptoms.

Monitor for TD by administering the Abnormal Involuntary Movement Scale (AIMS) to all patients taking antipsychotics.

Neuroleptic malignant syndrome

Neuroleptic malignant syndrome (NMS) has a low incidence and high mortality. It is thought to be due to dopamine blockade. Clinical presentation of NMS is as follows:

- Rapid progression (<24 hours)
- Body temperature > 104°F
- Lead-pipe rigidity
- Hypertension
- Diaphoresis
- Increased heart rate
- Incontinence
- Increased liver function test (LFT), creatinine phosphokinase (CPK), and white blood count (WBC)

Treatment is as follows:

- Transport patient to an emergency room immediately (STAT).
- Discontinue antipsychotic medication.
- Administer supportive therapy (cooling blankets, hydration); the dopamine agonist bromocriptine (Parlodel); and the smooth muscle relaxant dantrolene (Dantrium).

Endocrine and metabolic effects

Such effects include amenorrhea, galactorrhea, and gynecomastia caused by hyperprolactinemia.

Dopamine regulates prolactin release. When dopamine is blocked, prolactin is elevated.

Other effects include weight gain and decreased glucose tolerance.

Dermatologic effects (especially in long-term therapy)
Allergy to medication, photosensitivity, and pigmentation problems may occur.

Hypothalamic effects
Temperature dysregulation (i.e., sensitivity to extreme temperatures) is possible.

Cardiac effects
QT prolongation is possible. Effects are more common with thioridazine (black box warning).

The recommendation is to obtain an electrocardiogram (ECG) for all patients on antipsychotics.

Ophthalmologic effects
Pigmentary retinopathy is associated with daily thioridazine doses > 800 mg. Melanin deposits occur on the cornea and may lead to blindness.

Atypical (newer) antipsychotics
See Table 25-3 for an overview of these drugs.

No universally accepted definition of *atypical* exists, but these drugs generally have the following features.

- Side effects are less severe (little or no EPS, minimal to no prolactin increase, less risk of TD).
- More weight gain, more lipid abnormalities, and a greater risk of diabetes are seen with these drugs.
- A dose-dependent increased risk of ventricular arrhythmias and sudden cardiac death is seen, possibly because of prolongation of the QT interval similar to typical antipsychotics.

Table 25-3. Atypical Antipsychotics

Drug	Trade name	Form	Usual dose	Adverse effects	Clinical pearls
Clozapine	Clozaril, FazaClo (disintegrating clozapine tablets)	25, 100 mg tablets	12.5 mg titrated up to 300–900 mg/d	Sedation, weight gain, hypersalivation, black box: seizure risk (> 600 mg/d), agranulocytosis, orthostasis, myocarditis, respiratory and cardiac arrest; no EPS or TD	Indicated for refractory schizophrenia only. Weekly CBC with differential is required; if WBC < 3,500 or ANC < 1,500, patient *must* discontinue medication; if stable CBC with differential for 6 months, patient may go to biweekly dosage; if still stable for additional 6 months, patient may go to every-4-weeks dosage. Procyclidine [Kemadrin] 5 mg may help with hypersalivation.
Risperidone	Risperdal	0.25, 0.5, 1.0, 2.0, 3.0, 4.0 mg tablets; 1 mg/mL concentrate	1 mg bid up to 4–6 mg/d; maximum dose 16 mg/d	Dose-related EPS (> 8 mg/d), +/– weight gain, +/– sedation, prolactin elevation, orthostasis, Sedation, weight gain, possible dose-related EPS	Available in concentrate; do not mix with teas or colas; used commonly in dementia (0.25–1 mg); patient must overlap Consta with oral risperidone for at least 3 weeks.
	Risperdal-M (disintegrating risperidone tablets)	0.5, 1.0, 2.0 mg			
	Risperdal Consta (long-acting injection)	25.0, 37.5, 50.0 mg			

(continued)

Table 25-3. Atypical Antipsychotics *(Continued)*

Drug	Trade name	Form	Usual dose	Adverse effects	Clinical pearls
Olanzapine	Zyprexa	2.5, 5, 7.5, 10, 15, 20 mg tablets	10–20 mg/d; higher doses have been reported	Sedation, orthostasis, weight gain	Olanzapine is also indicated for acute manic episodes of bipolar disorder; Zyprexa Zydis is useful for patients who are unable to swallow or are "cheeking" medications.
	Zyprexa Zydis (disintegrating olanzapine tablets)	5, 10, 15, 20 mg tablets			
	Zyprexa IntraMuscular	10 mg/mL injection	10 mg IM × 1; may repeat in 2 and 4h; maximum IM daily dose 30 mg	Sedation, orthostasis	
Quetiapine	Seroquel	25, 100, 200, 300, 400 mg tablets	300–800 mg/d; higher doses have been reported	Sedation, dizziness, headache	Low EPS and prolactin elevation risk; cataract risk: do lens test at baseline and every 6 months.
	Seroquel XR (extended-release tablets)	200, 300, 400 mg			
Ziprasidone	Geodon	20, 40, 60, 80 mg capsules; 20 mg/mL injection	40–200 mg/d po; 20 mg IM × 1 dose (may repeat in 4 h; maximum IM daily dose 40 mg)	+/– sedation, +/– weight gain, QT prolongation warning in package insert	Use caution with other medications that prolong QT interval.
Aripiprazole	Abilify	2, 5, 10, 15, 20, 30 mg tablets; 1 mg/mL concentrate; 7.5-mg/mL injection	10–30 mg/d po; 5.25–15 mg/d IM; maximum IM daily dose 30 mg	Possible insomnia, +/– weight gain	Once-daily dosing benefit; partial dopamine agonist
	Abilify Discmelt (disintegrating tablets)	10, 15 mg			
Paliperidone	Invega	3, 6, 9 mg extended release tablets	6 mg/d; maximum dose 12 mg/d	Headache, tachycardia, somnolence, anxiety	Sustained release tablet: do not crush or chew; tablet shell may be seen in stool.

ANC, absolute neutrophil count; CBC, complete blood count.

- Decreased affinity for the dopamine receptor is present.
- Results from the CATIE (Clinical Antipsychotic Trials in Intervention Effectiveness) showed very high discontinuation rates for all antipsychotics secondary to inefficacy or intolerable side effects.

No difference was seen between perphenazine and atypicals (except olanzapine).
- There is a black box warning for increase in mortality with atypical antipsychotics in elderly patients with dementia, and atypical antipsychotics are not approved for the treat-

ment of patients with dementia-related psychosis.

Mechanism of action
These drugs are weak dopamine and dopamine-2 receptor blockers that block serotonin and α-adrenergic, histaminic, and muscarinic receptors in the central nervous system.

Treatment Strategies
Acute schizophrenia

- Decrease danger to self and others.
- Haloperidol or fluphenazine (immediate release) 5–10 mg IM and lorazepam 2 mg IM q4h prn may be used for psychosis or agitation. An anticholinergic may also be needed (e.g., benztropine or diphenhydramine for EPSs).
- Olanzapine 10 mg IM may be used and can be repeated in 2 hours and again 4 hours later, for a maximum of 30 mg/d for psychosis or agitation.
- Patients may use ziprasidone 10 mg IM administered every 2 hours or 20 mg IM administered every 4 hours, for a maximum of 40 mg/d for psychosis or agitation.

Maintenance

- Start an atypical antipsychotic at a recommended dose or continue a conventional agent (if it was effective for patient before hospital admission).
- Positive symptoms will respond first.
- Monitor for side effects and emphasize compliance.
- Lifelong therapy is usually needed.
- Use lowest effective dose to decrease risk of side effects (e.g., TD).

Recommended monitoring for patients on atypical antipsychotics

- Fasting glucose and lipids and blood pressure at baseline and at 12 weeks
- Weight (body mass index) at baseline, 4 weeks, 8 weeks, and 12 weeks, and then quarterly
- Waist circumference at baseline and then annually

Noncompliance and alternative dosing
Haloperidol decanoate (Haldol-D)
The dosage conversion from po to IM is as follows: po daily dose × 10 = IM dose every 4 weeks. For example, 20 mg daily dose × 10 = 200 mg every 4 weeks.

Steady state is reached in 8–12 weeks.

Fluphenazine decanoate (Prolixin-D)
The dosage conversion from po to IM is as follows: 1 mg po = 1.25 mg IM. For example, 20 mg daily dose × 1.25 mg = 25 mg IM every 2 weeks.

Steady state is reached in approximately 6 weeks.

Depot administration technique
Both medications are suspended in sesame seed oil. They are very viscous. Ensure that the patient has no allergy to sesame seed oil.

Administer in gluteal or deltoid muscle with a 16- or 18-gauge needle.

Risperidone long-acting injection (Risperdal Consta)
Overlap with po medication for 3 weeks.

The recommended dose is 25 mg every 2 weeks. The maximum dose is 50 mg every 2 weeks. Alternate IM administration between two buttocks.

Steady state is reached in approximately 8 weeks.

Use the diluent and needle supplied in the pack to reconstitute and administer injection.

25-3. Bipolar Disorder

Bipolar disorder (manic-depressive illness) is a recurrent mood disorder with a lifetime prevalence of 0.8%–1.6%. This disorder is associated with significant morbidity and mortality.

Incidence is equal in females and males. Onset is usually between ages 8 and 44. The first episode for females is usually marked by a depressive episode. For males, it is usually marked by a manic episode.

Types and Classifications

- *Bipolar I:* This type is characterized by the occurrence of manic episodes and major depressive episodes.
- *Bipolar II:* This type is characterized by the occurrence of hypomanic episodes and major depressive episodes.
- *Cyclothymia:* This type is defined as numerous episodes of hypomania and depressive episodes that cannot be classified as major depressive episodes. Diagnosis requires that cyclothymia occur for at least a 2-year period.

Clinical Presentation

See DSM-IV for complete diagnostic criteria.

Mania

Mania is characterized by heightened mood (euphoria), flight of ideas, rapid or pressured speech, grandiosity, increased energy, decreased need for sleep, irritability, and impulsivity. Judgment is significantly impaired (e.g., increased risk-taking behavior). Marked impairment also exists in social or occupational functioning.

Psychotic features are usually present. Hospitalization is needed.

Changes in sleeping patterns (especially insomnia) commonly initiate manic episodes.

Drug-induced causes include antidepressants (tricyclic antidepressants, selective serotonin reuptake inhibitors, monoamine oxidase inhibitors); bronchodilators (albuterol, salmeterol); stimulants; xanthines (caffeine, theophylline); dopamine agonists (bromocriptine, amantadine); and sympathomimetics.

Note: The STEP-BD (Systematic Treatment Enhancement Program for Bipolar Disorder) trial showed that antidepressants used in combination with mood stabilizers did not increase the risk of inducing mania in bipolar depression. However, this combination was not associated with increased efficacy.

Hypomania

Hypomania is a less severe form of mania. This disorder usually does not cause marked impairment in social or occupational functioning.

Many patients find this state highly desirable because they experience a great sense of well-being and feel productive, creative, and confident.

Dysphoric (mixed) mania

Dysphoric mania is characterized by manic and depressive features, mood variability, and mood lability. Symptoms usually include agitation, insomnia, suicidal ideation, psychosis, and appetite disturbances.

Major depression

See Section 25-4.

Rapid cycling

In rapid cycling, the patient experiences > 4 mood episodes in a year. Mood episodes may occur in any combination.

Rapid cycling primarily occurs in women (70–90%). The prognosis is usually poor.

Etiology

The etiology is unknown; however, the leading hypothesis supports genetic etiology. Other theories include neurotransmitter involvement, circadian rhythm, and kindling hypothesis.

Clinical Course

The mean age of onset is 21 years. The first episode for females is usually depression. For males, it is mania.

Untreated episodes may last from weeks to months. A high mortality rate exists because of suicide. Comorbid substance abuse is very common (60–70%).

Treatment Principles and Goals

Acute

In acute cases, the goal is to control the current episode (i.e., slow down the patient and reduce harm to self and others).

Maintenance

Maintenance goals are as follows:
- Prevent or minimize future episodes.
- Maintain drug therapy, and reduce adverse effects.
- Prevent drug interactions.
- Educate the patient and family about the disorder.
- Provide adequate follow-up services (including substance abuse treatment).
- Maximize the patient's functional status and quality of life.

Drug Therapy

Table 25-4 provides information about mood stabilizers.

Lithium

Indications
Lithium is indicated for acute treatment and prophylaxis of manic episodes associated with bipolar disorders. It is effective for both the manic and depressive components.

Mechanism of action
The mechanism of action is unknown. Various theories suggest that lithium facilitates γ-aminobutyric acid (GABA) function, alters cation transport across cell membranes in nerve and muscle cells, or influences reuptake of 5-hydroxytryptamine (5-HT) or norepinephrine (NE).

Table 25-4. Mood Stabilizers

Drug	Trade name	Form	Usual dose	Adverse effects	Clinical pearls
Lithium	Lithobid, Eskalith CR	150, 300, 600 mg caplets; 300 mg, 450 mg (CR) tablets; 300 mg (SR) tablets; syrup, as citrate 300 mg/5 mL (Cibalith-S)	Starting: 900–1,200 mg in divided doses; titrate to desired response or level	Tremor, polydipsia or polyuria, nausea or diarrhea, weight gain, hypothyroidism, mental dulling	Many drug interactions; toxicity is a concern (pregnancy category D); monitor blood levels—acute: 0.6–1.2 mEq/L, maintenance: 0.8–1.0 mEq/L
Divalproex sodium	Depakote	125, 250, 500 mg tablets; 250, 500 mg (ER) tablets	Starting: 500 mg bid–tid or 15 mg/kg; maximum dose 60 mg/kg/d; ER dosed daily	GI upset, sedation, tremor, weight gain, alopecia, transient elevation in LFTs	Black box warnings: hepatotoxicity, hemorrhagic pancreatitis, teratogenicity (pregnancy category D); monitor blood levels—50–125 mcg/mL
Carbamazepine	Tegretol	200 mg tablets; 100 mg chew tablets; 100, 200, 400 mg ER tablets; 100 mg/ 5 mL suspension	Starting: 200 mg bid; increase to 800–1,200 mg/d (tid–qid doses); usual range 400–1,600 mg/d	Ataxia, dizziness, sedation, slurred speech, aplastic anemia	See text for contraindications; many drug interactions (pregnancy category C); monitor blood levels—4–12 mcg/mL
Lamotrigine	Lamictal	25, 100, 150, 200 mg tablets; 2, 5, 25 mg chew tablets	Starting: 25 mg/d weeks 1 and 2; 50 mg/d week 5; 200 mg/d week 6; 200 mg/d usual dose	Dizziness, headache, ataxia, nausea, diplopia, rash	Black box warning: severe rashes such as Stevens–Johnson syndrome; start at 25 mg and titrate to 200 mg over 6 weeks to help prevent rash

CR, controlled release; ER, extended release; GI, gastrointestinal.

Contraindications

Contraindications include renal disease, severe cardiovascular disease, history of leukemia, first trimester of pregnancy, and hypersensitivity to lithium.

Precautions

Use with caution in patients who have thyroid disease, patients who have sodium depletion, patients who are receiving diuretics, or dehydrated patients.

Monitoring (baseline and follow-up)

- *Thyroid panel:* Lithium may cause hypothyroidism. Test baseline and thyroid-stimulating hormone (TSH) every 6–12 months or as clinically indicated.
- *Serum creatinine (SCr) and blood urea nitrogen (BUN):* Lithium is 100% renally eliminated. Test baseline and every 3 months for patients with renal dysfunction and every 12 months otherwise or as clinically indicated.
- *Complete blood count (CBC) with differential:* Lithium may cause leukocytosis and may

reactivate leukemia. Test baseline and every month for 3 months; then test as clinically indicated.

- *Electrolytes:* In the event of hyponatremia, lithium toxicity may occur.
- *ECG:* Lithium causes flattened or inverted T waves. This condition is reversible. Test baseline and every 6–12 months or as clinically indicated.
- *Urinalysis:* Lithium may decrease specific gravity.
- *Pregnancy test:* Lithium may cause cardiovascular defects (e.g., Ebstein's anomaly).
- *Lithium level:* Lithium reaches steady-state levels in 4–5 days (half-life = ~24 h). Obtain the level 2–8 hours after the dose (acute: 0.6–1.2 mEq/L; maintenance: 0.8–1.0 mEq/L). Draw the level weekly for 4 weeks and then monthly for 3 months or as clinically indicated.

Drug interactions

Table 25-5 summarizes the drug interactions associated with lithium.

Table 25-5. Drug Interactions with Lithium

Increase level of lithium	Decrease level of lithium
Nonsteroidal anti-inflammatory drugs	Theophylline
Angiotensin-converting enzyme inhibitors	Caffeine
Fluoxetine	Pregnancy
Metronidazole	Osmotic diuretics (mannitol and urea)
Diuretics (e.g., thiazides)	
Sodium depletion:	
Low sodium diet	
Excessive exercise or sweating	
Vomiting or diarrhea	
Salt deficiency	

In addition, several toxicity concerns are associated with the drug:

- *Mild toxicity (serum levels 1.5–2.0 mEq/L):* Gastrointestinal (GI) upset (nausea, vomiting, diarrhea); muscle weakness; fatigue; fine hand tremor; difficulty with concentration and memory
- *Moderate toxicity (serum levels 2.0–2.5 mEq/L):* Ataxia, lethargy, nystagmus, worsening confusion, severe GI upset, coarse tremors, increased deep tendon reflexes
- *Severe toxicity (serum levels > 3.0 mEq/L):* Severely impaired consciousness, coma, seizures, respiratory complications, death

Toxicity is treated as follows:

- Discontinue lithium and initiate gastric lavage.
- Correct electrolyte and fluid imbalances.
- Monitor neurologic changes.
- Give supportive care.
- Give dialysis if indicated.

Patient information
- Monitoring serum lithium levels routinely is important.
- Maintain a steady salt and fluid intake.
- Do not crush or chew extended- or slow-release dosage forms.

Divalproex sodium

Divalproex sodium is indicated for bipolar disorder. It is considered first-line treatment for acute manic episodes. It has unlabeled use for prophylaxis of manic episodes, is effective for rapid cyclers and patients with dysphoric mood, and is helpful in the management of agitation and aggression.

Mechanism of action
Its mechanism of action is unknown, but divalproex sodium is thought to increase GABA or mimic its action at the postsynaptic receptor site.

Contraindications
Contraindications include

- Hepatic dysfunction
- Hypersensitivity to divalproex sodium
- Patients < 2 years old
- Pregnancy

With respect to pregnancy, valproic acid (VPA) may cause neural tube defects. If the benefit outweighs the risk, supplement with 4–5 mg/d of folic acid to decrease risk of fetal damage.

Monitoring
VPA
- VPA level reaches steady state in 3–5 days (half-life = 9–16 h); 50–125 mcg/mL is optimal.
- Draw level weekly for 2–3 weeks, then every 3 months or as clinically indicated.

LFTs
- Test baseline and every month for 6 months, and then every 6 months or as clinically indicated.
- Divalproex sodium is hepatically eliminated; it carries a black box warning for hepatotoxicity.

CBC with differential
- Test baseline and every month for 6 months, and then every 6 months or as clinically indicated.
- VPA may cause thrombocytopenia.

Drug interactions
- Divalproex sodium is a cytochrome P450 (CYP450) 2C19 enzyme substrate, a CYP450 2C9 and 2D6 inhibitor, and a weak CYP450 3A3/4 inhibitor.
- Interactions occur with carbamazepine, lamotrigine, and phenytoin. Increased sedative effects occur with phenobarbital and benzodiazepines.

Patient information
- Take with food to avoid GI upset.
- Take a multivitamin with selenium and zinc if alopecia (hair loss) occurs.
- It is important to monitor VPA levels routinely.

Carbamazepine

Carbamazepine (CBZ) is considered second-line therapy for acute and prophylactic treatment of bipolar disorder.

Mechanism of action
The mechanism of action is unknown.

Monitoring
Monitor CBC with differential, electrolytes, LFTs, SCr or BUN, and ECG (if the patient is > 40 years old or has a preexisting heart disease).

CBZ is an autoinducer. Monitor levels routinely, especially during first few months of therapy. The optimal level is 4–12 mcg/mL.

Contraindications
Contraindications include history of previous bone marrow depression and hypersensitivity to CBZ.

Drug interactions
- CBZ is a CYP450 2C8 and 3A3/4 enzyme substrate.
- It is a CYP450 1A2, 2C, and 3A3/4 inducer.
- CBZ may induce the metabolism of benzodiazepines, clozapine, corticosteroids, oral contraceptives, VPA, warfarin, phenytoin, and tricyclic antidepressants (plus others).
- Cimetidine, clarithromycin, diltiazem, propoxyphene, verapamil, metronidazole, and lamotrigine (plus others) inhibit CBZ.

Lamotrigine (Lamictal)
Lamotrigine is approved for maintenance treatment of Bipolar I disorder. Titration of the dose is required to monitor for signs and symptoms of severe and potentially life-threatening skin rashes (Table 25-6). Coadministration with VPA increases the risk.

Drug interactions and effects
- CBZ, phenytoin, oral contraceptives, rifampin, and phenobarbital decrease lamotrigine concentrations.
- VPA increases lamotrigine concentrations.
- Adverse effects include nausea, headache, tremor or anxiety, and sedation.

Other therapies

Atypical antipsychotics
These agents are approved for treatment of bipolar disorder. Olanzapine or fluoxetine (Symbyax) is indicated for the treatment of depressive episodes associated with bipolar disorder.

Gabapentin (Neurontin)
This agent may be useful as adjunctive therapy for bipolar disorder. No significant drug interactions exist. No drug serum level monitoring is required.

Gabapentin is renally eliminated. It has mild sedative effects (sedation, ataxia, and fatigue).

Oxcarbazepine (Trileptal)
This agent is structurally similar to CBZ (keto-analogue of CBZ). It is sometimes used as a mood stabilizer in patients with bipolar disorder, but further studies are needed.

No autoinduction problems exist, and there are no drug serum levels to monitor. It appears to have fewer drug-drug interactions than CBZ.

Table 25-6. Lamotrigine Dose Titration

Timing	Patients not taking carbamazepine (or other enzyme-inducing drugs) or valproate (orange color)	Patients taking valproate (blue color)	Patients taking carbamazepine (or other enzyme-inducing drugs) and not taking valproate (green color)
Weeks 1 and 2	25 mg daily	25 mg every other day	50 mg daily
Weeks 3 and 4	50 mg daily	25 mg daily	100 mg daily, in divided doses
Week 5	100 mg daily	50 mg daily	200 mg daily, in divided doses
Week 6	200 mg daily	100 mg daily	300 mg daily, in divided doses
Week 7	200 mg daily	100 mg daily	Up to 400 mg daily, in divided doses

Topiramate (Topamax)

This agent may be useful for treatment of bipolar disorder, but further studies are needed. Doses are usually lower than those indicated for treating seizure disorders.

Topiramate may cause weight loss.

Calcium channel blockers

These agents are usually reserved as last-line therapy. Data in the literature are inconsistent about using verapamil for mania (other calcium channel blockers may be effective).

Although these agents are not routinely used, they could possibly be used in pregnancy.

25-4. Major Depression

Major depression is a prevalent and serious illness in the United States. It affects 10 million to 14 million people of all ages.

The condition is treatable but grossly undertreated. Most cases go unrecognized, which may be due to the social stigma surrounding depression. Several myths contribute to the problem of undertreatment (e.g., major depression is due to personal weakness or an inability to handle life's problems).

Epidemiology

The lifetime prevalence rate is 17%. One out of four females (10–24%) is affected. One out of 8 males (5%–12%) is affected.

Major depression is most common between the ages of 25 and 44.

Risk factors include the following:

- Family history
- Female
- Previous depressive episode
- Previous suicide attempt
- Comorbid medical or substance abuse disorder

Etiology

The etiology is unknown; however, there are many hypotheses, including the following:

- Dysregulation of neurotransmitters
- Decreased concentration of certain neurotransmitters
- Genetic basis for the disorder

Clinical Presentation

Physical findings

- Fatigue
- Pain (i.e., headaches, back pain, GI upset)
- Sleep disturbances (usually insomnia)
- Appetite disturbances (usually decreased appetite)
- Psychomotor retardation or agitation

Emotional symptoms

- Anhedonia
- Depressed mood for most of the day
- Hopelessness or helplessness
- Inappropriate feelings of guilt and worthlessness
- Anxiety or worry
- Suicidal ideation

Cognitive symptoms

- Decreased ability to concentrate
- Indecisiveness

Laboratory studies

There are no diagnostic laboratory tests for depression, but the following lab work should be conducted to rule out other medical illnesses that may manifest as depressive symptoms:

- CBC with differential
- Thyroid function tests
- Rapid plasma reagin (test for syphilis)
- Urine drug screen

Medical conditions that may contribute to the development or worsening of depression include the following:

- Myocardial infarction (MI)
- Cerebrovascular accident
- Parkinson's disease
- Multiple sclerosis
- Systemic lupus erythematosus
- Human immunodeficiency virus
- Rheumatoid arthritis
- Thyroid abnormalities
- Diabetes mellitus
- Cancer
- Vitamin deficiency

Possible drug-induced causes of depression should also be ruled out, including corticosteroids, oral contraceptives, propranolol, clonidine, and methyldopa.

Prognosis

Seventy percent of patients are responsive to antidepressant therapy. Following the first episode, 50–60% of patients will have another episode; following the second episode, 70–80% will have a third; and following the third, 90% will have another.

If untreated, an episode may resolve spontaneously within 6 to 24 months.

Approximately 15% of patients will commit suicide. Risk factors for suicide include being male, >50 years old, or unemployed; having recently lost a job or spouse; being socially isolated; having access to a weapon; and experiencing comorbid substance abuse.

Males are more likely to commit suicide, but females are more likely to attempt suicide. Males commonly use more violent means of suicide (e.g., firearms and hanging) than do females (e.g., slashing of wrists and drug overdoses).

DSM-IV Diagnostic Criteria

At least five symptoms (see previous discussion of clinical presentation) must be present mostly every day for a 2-week period and represent a change from previous functioning. At least one of the symptoms must be depressed mood or anhedonia.

Treatment Principles and Goals

Goals are as follows:

- Improve patient's ability to function and quality of life.
- Reduce or eliminate target symptoms with an antidepressant.
- Optimally, incorporate psychotherapy.
- Prevent relapse.

All antidepressants are equally effective in a given population:
Response varies from person to person.

- Each differs in side-effect and drug-interaction profiles.
- None are "speed" or "uppers."

Note: The U.S. Food and Drug Administration now requires all antidepressant drugs to include boxed warnings about increased risk of suicidal ideation and behavior in children and adolescents and in young adults (up to age 24), and a medication guide highlighting these risks is to be distributed with each new or refilled prescription for antidepressants in this population.

Basis for choosing an agent

- Past history of a patient's response or a family member's response to certain agents
- Side-effect profile and how it relates to any given patient's situation

Monitoring parameters

In the first week, the following should be noted:

- Decreased anxiety
- Trend toward normalization of appetite and sleep pattern

In the second to third week, the following should be noted:

- Increased energy
- Improved concentration and memory
- Improved somatic symptoms

Note: There is an increased risk for suicide at this time because the patient has the energy to carry out any ideations.

At 4–6 weeks, the following should be evident:

- Improved mood
- Decreased suicidal ideation
- Increased libido

Duration of therapy

Acute phase
The acute phase is usually 6–12 weeks or the length of time needed to stabilize depressive symptoms.

Maintenance phase
During this phase, maintain therapeutic doses of antidepressant. The duration is usually 1 year; you may taper antidepressant for a period of time and monitor for signs of relapse. The goal is to prevent relapse.

Prophylaxis

Chronic antidepressant therapy may be necessary for certain patients experiencing the following:

- A first-degree relative with bipolar disorder or recurrent depression
- Onset of depression before age 20 or after age 60

- Recurrence of depression within 1 year after medication discontinuation
- Severe, sudden, or life-threatening depression

Drug Therapy

Tricyclic antidepressants

Tricyclic antidepressants (TCAs) are described in Table 25-7.

Mechanism of action
TCAs increase the synaptic concentration of 5-HT or NE in the central nervous system (i.e., TCAs inhibit the presynaptic neuronal membrane's reuptake of 5-HT or NE).

Other information about TCAs
- Doses may be titrated to full dose range over 1–3 weeks.
- Many patients are dosed half-strength because of sedative effects; however, for patients with insomnia, the sedating effects may be helpful.

- These agents are deadly in overdose (blocks sinoatrial node in the heart).
- Drug serum levels are not commonly used in guiding therapy, but monitoring may be useful in patients taking amitriptyline, desipramine, imipramine, or nortriptyline.

Adverse effects
Effects include orthostatic hypotension, tachycardia, sedation, anticholinergic effects, arrhythmias (prolonged QT interval), weight gain, and sexual dysfunction.

Tertiary amines (e.g., amitriptyline, imipramine, doxepin, clomipramine) have more intense adverse effects compared to secondary amines (e.g., nortriptyline, desipramine).

Contraindications
Concomitant use of a monoamine oxidase inhibitor (MAOI) within the past 14 days, during pregnancy or lactation, and with narrow-angle glaucoma is contraindicated.

Table 25-7. Tricyclic Antidepressants

Drug	Trade name	Form	Indications	Initial dose	Dose range
Amitriptyline	Elavil	10, 25, 50, 75, 100, 150 mg tablets; 10 mg/mL injection (pregnancy category D)	Depression, chronic and neuropathic pain, migraine prophylaxis, peripheral neuropathy	50–75 mg/d	75–300 mg
Nortriptyline	Pamelor, Aventyl	10, 25, 50, 75 mg capsules; 10 mg/5 mL injection (pregnancy category D)	Depression, chronic pain	25–50 mg/d	40–200 mg
Imipramine	Tofranil	75, 100, 125, 150 mg pamoate capsule	Depression, childhood enuresis, chronic and neuropathic pain	50–75 mg/d	75–300 mg
	Tofranil-PM	10-, 25-, 50-mg tablets; 12.5-mg/mL injection (pregnancy category D)			
Doxepin	Sinequan	10, 25, 50, 75, 100, 150 mg capsules; 10 mg/mL concentrate; 5% cream (pregnancy category C)	Depression; anxiety; unlabeled: chronic and neuropathic pain	75 mg/d (in divided doses)	75–300 mg
Clomipramine	Anafranil	25, 50, 75 mg (pregnancy category C)	Obsessive-compulsive disorder; depression; panic attacks; chronic pain	25–100 mg qd, titrated up for 1–2 weeks	Usual effective dose 200–250 mg/d; maximum dose 250 mg because of dose-related increased risk of seizure
Desipramine	(Norpramin)	10, 25, 50, 75, 100, 150 mg tablets (pregnancy category C)	Depression; chronic pain; unlabeled: peripheral neuropathy	50–75 mg/d	75–300 mg

Precautions

Use with caution in patients with cardiac conduction disturbances, seizure disorders, hyperthyroidism, and renal or hepatic impairment. Avoid abrupt withdrawal in patients with prolonged use.

Drug interactions

- Increase in TCA level increases the levels of selective serotonin reuptake inhibitors (SSRIs), cimetidine, diltiazem, verapamil, labetalol, propoxyphene, quinidine, haloperidol, and methylphenidate.
- Decrease in TCA level affects CBZ, phenytoin, and barbiturate metabolism.
- Administration with MAOIs may cause serotonin syndrome.
- Monitoring blood pressure, pulse, ECG changes, and mental status changes is prudent; drug serum monitoring may be useful for amitriptyline, desipramine, imipramine, and nortriptyline.

Monoamine oxidase inhibitors

Table 25-8 summarizes information about MAOIs.

Mechanism of action

MAOIs increase the synaptic concentration of NE, 5-HT, and dopamine (DA) by inhibiting the breakdown enzyme—monoamine oxidase.

Note: MAOIs may be useful for patients who do not respond to other antidepressants or for treatment of atypical depression; however, they are rarely used because of the need for dietary restrictions, their side effect profile, and their potentially dangerous interactions with other medications.

Adverse effects

Effects include orthostatic hypotension, weight gain, sexual dysfunction, anticholinergic effects, and hypertensive crisis.

Contraindications

Be alert for renal or hepatic dysfunction, cardiovascular disease, and concomitant sympathomimetic therapy (e.g., pseudoephedrine, ephedra).

When a patient is switched from MAOIs to SSRIs, the MAOI must be discontinued 2 weeks prior to initiation of SSRI to prevent serotonin syndrome. When a patient is switched from SSRIs to MAOIs, the SSRI must be discontinued 2 weeks prior to initiation of MAOI, with the exception of fluoxetine, which requires 5 weeks because of its long half-life.

Precautions

Be aware of drug–food interaction with tyramine-containing foods (e.g., red wine, aged cheeses, and marmite).

Drug interactions

- TCAs
- SSRIs
- Sympathomimetics
- Meperidine

Selective serotonin reuptake inhibitors

See Table 25-9 for information about SSRIs.

Mechanism of action

These agents selectively inhibit the reuptake of 5-HT.

All SSRIs should be tapered upon discontinuation of treatment (over 2–4 weeks), except fluoxetine. Side effects with abrupt withdrawal include flu-like symptoms, dizziness, nausea, tremor, anxiety, and palpitations.

Adverse effects

Effects include GI complaints, nervousness, insomnia, headache, fatigue, and sexual dysfunction, but SSRIs are safer in overdose than TCAs.

Table 25-8. Monoamine Oxidase Inhibitors

Drug	Trade name	Form	Initial dose	Dose titration	Dose range
Phenelzine	Nardil	15 mg tablets	15 mg tid (>16 years old)	Increase by 15 mg/wk	60–90 mg/d
Tranylcypromine	Parnate	10 mg tablets	30 mg/d in divided doses	Increase by 10 mg/d every 1–3 weeks	30–60 mg/d

Table 25-9. Selective Serotonin Reuptake Inhibitors

Drug	Trade name	Form	Initial dose	Usual dose	Clinical pearls
Citalopram	Celexa	10, 20, 40 mg tablets; 10 mg/5 mL syrup	10 mg	20–40 mg/d; maximum dose 60 mg/d	Used in geriatric patients; fewer drug interactions
Escitalopram	Lexapro	5, 10, 20 mg tablets	10 mg	10–20 mg/d	S-isomer of citalopram; 40 mg Celexa = 10 mg Lexapro
Fluvoxamine	Luvox	50, 100 mg tablets	50 mg	100–300 mg/d	Available in generic; primarily used for obsessive-compulsive disorder drug interactions
Paroxetine	Paxil	10, 20, 30, 40 mg tablets; 10 mg/5 mL suspension	10–20 mg	10–40 mg; maximum dose 50 mg/d	Least-activating SSRI
Paroxetine	Paxil CR	12.5, 25.0, 37.5 mg tablets	12.5–25.0 mg	25.0–37.5 mg	Controlled-release formulation associated with fewer side effects; 10.0 mg Paxil = 12.5 mg Paxil CR
Fluoxetine	Prozac, Sarafem	10, 20, 40 mg capsules; 10, 20 mg tablets; 20 mg/5 mL syrup; 90 mg capsules	10–20 mg	20–80 mg/d	Longer half-life, so tapering unnecessary; 90 mg formulation given once weekly
Sertraline	Zoloft	25, 50, 100 mg tablets; 20 mg/mL concentrate	25–50 mg	50–100 mg/d; maximum dose 200 mg/d	Used in geriatric patients; fewer drug interactions

Drug interactions

Drug interactions exist with TCAs, MAOIs, and SSRIs. Interactions are variable depending on the SSRI. Reportedly there are fewer drug interactions with escitalopram and citalopram.

Serotonin–norepinephrine reuptake inhibitors

See Table 25-10 for information about serotonin–norepinephrine reuptake inhibitors (SNRIs).

Venlafaxine (Effexor, Effexor XR)
Mechanism of action
This agent inhibits the reuptake of 5-HT and NE (and also DA at higher doses). It is frequently referred to as an SNRI. Anticholinergic and antihistaminic effects are negligible. As the dose increases, NE and DA reuptake are more pronounced.

Adverse effects
Effects include GI upset, anxiety, insomnia, and headache. Elevation in blood pressure is possible; use with

Table 25-10. Serotonin–Norepinephrine Reuptake Inhibitors

Drug	Trade name	Form	Initial dose	Maximum dose	Clinical pearls
Venlafaxine	Effexor	25.0, 37.5, 50.0, 75.0, 100.0 mg capsules	37.5 mg bid	375 mg/d in divided doses	Take with food; monitor blood pressure
	Effexor XR	37.5, 75.0, 150.0, 225.0 mg capsules	75 mg/d	225 mg/d	Less GI upset than immediate release formulation; monitor blood pressure
Desvenlafaxine	Pristiq	50, 100 mg extended release tablets	50 mg daily	50 mg/d; CrCl < 30 mL/min every other day	Less drug interactions due to conjugation; monitor blood pressure
Duloxetine	Cymbalta	20, 30, 60 mg capsules	30 mg daily	120 mg/d	Also used for diabetic peripheral neuropathy; monitor blood pressure

CrCl, creatinine clearance

caution in patients with uncontrolled hypertension. An extended release formulation is available to minimize GI upset. Other side effects are similar to those of SSRIs. Withdrawal symptoms may occur if the medication is abruptly discontinued.

Drug interactions
Cimetidine inhibits venlafaxine metabolism. Cyproheptadine induces venlafaxine metabolism. Serotonin syndrome is seen in combination with sibutramine, sumatriptan, tramadol, and trazodone. PT/INR (prothrombin time per international ratio) elevations have been seen when venlafaxine is added to patients taking warfarin.

Other aspects
Venlafaxine is indicated for both generalized anxiety disorder and major depression. It is not recommended in patients with uncontrolled hypertension or recent MI or cerebrovascular disorders.

Desvenlafaxine (Pristiq)
Mechanism of action
The mechanism of action of desvenlafaxine is similar to that of venlafaxine.

Adverse effects
Common effects include GI upset, increased serum cholesterol and triglycerides, xerostomia, sleep disturbances, and erectile dysfunction. Serious effects include hypertension, hyponatremia, and abnormal bleeding.

Withdrawal symptoms may occur if the drug is abruptly discontinued.

Drug interactions
The primary metabolic pathway is conjugation; therefore, desvenlafaxine has fewer drug interactions than venlafaxine.

Serotonin syndrome is seen in combination with MAOIs, SSRIs, sibutramine, tramadol, triptans, and linezolid.

Use in combination with unfractionated heparin, glycoprotein IIb or IIIa receptor inhibitors, warfarin, and nonsteroidal anti-inflammatory drugs may increase the risk of bleeding.

Duloxetine (Cymbalta)
Mechanism of action
The mechanism of action of duloxetine is similar to that of venlafaxine. It is a potent inhibitor of 5-HT and NE, and it has no significant affinity for dopaminergic, adrenergic, cholinergic, or histaminergic receptors.

Adverse effects
Effects include GI upset, dry mouth, dizziness, decreased appetite, elevation in blood pressure, and other side effects similar to those of SSRIs. Urinary hesitation may occur. The patient may have withdrawal symptoms with abrupt discontinuation.

Drug interactions
CYP1A2 inhibitors (e.g., cimetidine, quinolone antibiotics) and CYP2D6 inhibitors (e.g., fluoxetine, quinidine) increase duloxetine levels. The combination of duloxetine with triptans and serotonergic drugs may cause serotonin syndrome.

Other aspects
Duloxetine is indicated for both major depression (20 or 30 mg bid or 60 mg qd) and diabetic peripheral neuropathic pain (60 mg qd). It is metabolized by CYP450 1A2 and 2D6; these inhibitors may increase plasma levels of duloxetine, causing increased side effects. Duloxetine is contraindicated in uncontrolled narrow-angle glaucoma.

Other classes of antidepressant medication

Bupropion (Wellbutrin, Wellbutrin SR, Wellbutrin XL, Zyban)
Mechanism of action
Bupropion, an inhibitor of NE and DA reuptake (effects on 5-HT reuptake are minimal), is referred to as a norepinephrine–dopamine reuptake inhibitor (NDRI).

Adverse effects
Effects include GI upset, insomnia, anxiety, headache, and psychosis (rare). Buproprion is less associated with sexual dysfunction than are SSRIs and other classes. It also decreases the seizure threshold.

Drug interactions
Cimetidine and ritonavir inhibit bupropion metabolism, and CBZ induces bupropion metabolism.

Other aspects
There is an increased risk of seizure with bupropion, especially in patients with a seizure disorder, eating disorder, or electrolyte imbalance. The maximum daily dose is 450 mg (400 mg SR). Titrate the dose slowly to minimize seizure risk. Bupropion is marketed as Zyban for smoking cessation.

Trazodone (Desyrel)
Mechanism of action
This agent inhibits 5-HT reuptake and blocks 5-HT$_{2A}$ receptors.

Adverse effects
Effects include extreme sedation, orthostatic hypotension, and priapism. There are no anticholinergic or cardiotoxic effects.

Drug interactions

Fluoxetine and ritonavir inhibit trazodone metabolism.

Other aspects

Because it causes excessive sedation, trazodone is not clinically used as an antidepressant; rather, it is commonly used to treat insomnia (usually dosed 25–150 mg qhs).

Nefazodone (Serzone)
Mechanism of action

This agent inhibits 5-HT and NE uptake and blocks 5-HT$_{2A}$ receptors.

Adverse effects

Effects include GI upset, sedation, dry mouth, constipation, and lightheadedness. Nefazodone is associated with minimal sexual dysfunction and orthostatic hypotension.

Drug interactions

Nefazodone is a potent inhibitor of CYP3A4 isoenzyme; use with caution with drugs metabolized through this enzyme (e.g., buspirone, 3-hydroxy-3-methyl-glutaryl-coenzyme A reductase inhibitors, alprazolam, triazolam, digoxin). Ritonavir inhibits nefazodone metabolism.

Other aspects

Nefazodone is usually dosed bid because of its short half-life. There is a black box warning for hepatotoxicity.

Mirtazapine (Remeron and Remeron Soltab)

Mirtazapine is available in 7.5, 15.0, 30.0, and 45.0 mg tablets.

Mechanism of action

This agent antagonizes presynaptic α_2 autoreceptors and heteroreceptors that prevent the release of 5-HT and NE (resulting in increased 5-HT and NE in the synapses). It antagonizes 5-HT$_{2A}$ and 5-HT$_3$ receptors, thereby resulting in less GI upset and less anxiety.

Adverse effects

Effects include sedation, increased appetite, weight gain, and constipation. Elevation in LFTs and increase in triglycerides may occur. There is also a small risk of agranulocytosis or neutropenia.

Other aspects

Mirtazapine may be useful in geriatric patients because it causes increased appetite, is sedating, and has no significant drug interactions.

Aripiprazole (Abilify)

Aripiprazole is approved for adjunct treatment of major depressive disorders. It is available in 2, 5, 10, 15, 20, and 30 mg tabs and in a 1 mg/mL concentrate. The maximum dose is 15 mg/d.

Mechanism of action

This agent's action is not fully understood; it partially antagonizes D2 and 5-HT$_{1A}$ receptors and antagonizes 5-HT$_{2A}$ receptors.

Adverse effects

See Section 25-2 on schizophrenia.

Selegiline (Emsam)

Selegiline is available in 6, 9, and 12 mg/24 hour patches.

Mechanism of action

This agent's mechanism of action is not fully understood; however, it is believed to be linked to selegiline's irreversible inhibition of monoamine oxidase.

Adverse effects

Effects include headache, insomnia, application-site reaction, diarrhea, and dry mouth.

Other aspects

There are no dietary restrictions for the 6 mg dose.

Psychostimulants

Methylphenidate has been used to treat depression (especially in the geriatric population) and has been shown to increase activity level as well as improve mood symptoms. It may cause GI upset, insomnia, and cardiovascular effects. It should be used with caution in anxious or psychotic patients. It inhibits TCA metabolism.

Nonpharmacologic Treatments
Psychotherapy

Psychotherapy is especially useful combined with drug therapy.

Electroconvulsive therapy

Electroconvulsive therapy (ECT) is very safe and effective for treating depression. It is believed to physically "reset" receptors in the brain. ECT is usually reserved for refractory or psychotic patients.

Procedure

The patient is anesthetized and paralyzed in an outpatient setting. The patient is monitored through an electroencephalogram (EEG) during the procedure, and a seizure is induced for 30–90 seconds.

Acute and maintenance treatment
The procedure is administered every other day for 6–9 treatments. Maintenance treatment is variable for each patient, but ECT is usually administered monthly after acute treatment.

Adverse effects
Effects include short-term memory loss and confusion on the day of treatment.

Relative contraindications
ECT increases intracranial pressure and, therefore, is not recommended in patients with recent MI, intracerebral hemorrhage, or cerebral lesions.

25-5. Anxiety Disorders

Anxiety disorders are serious, debilitating mental illnesses that include a group of conditions that share extreme anxiety as the primary mood disturbance.

Epidemiology

Anxiety disorders affect approximately 19 million adults in the United States. There are no racial or cultural differences, and gender differences depend on the specific anxiety disorder.

There is significant comorbidity with other psychiatric illnesses (e.g., substance abuse).

Types and Classifications

Generalized anxiety disorder

Generalized anxiety disorder (GAD) is characterized by unprovoked excessive worry and tension. Anxiety usually consumes the patient's day, thereby affecting social and occupational functioning. Physical complaints (e.g., GI upset, headache, muscle tension, tremors, insomnia, fatigue) are common. Incidence of GAD is higher in females than in males.

Panic disorder

Panic disorder (PD), with or without agoraphobia, is characterized by feelings of terror that suddenly strike without warning and usually last for approximately 10–15 minutes.

Physical symptoms include increased heart rate, sweating, tremors, shortness of breath, chest pain, and dizziness. The patient feels as if death is imminent.

Agoraphobia (fear of open or public places) usually develops later in the illness, especially if PD is not treated. Agoraphobic patients associate panic attacks with certain places and occasions, so they avoid going out and remain at home. Agoraphobia is more prevalent in females than in males.

Obsessive-compulsive disorder

Obsessive-compulsive disorder (OCD) is characterized by intrusive, recurrent, and repetitive thoughts that severely interfere with the patient's social and occupational functioning (e.g., preoccupation with contamination, order, counting, cleanliness, safety).

Compulsions (e.g., repetitive washing of hands and checking and rechecking) are acts that must be performed in an attempt to decrease the anxiety felt about the obsessions. Prevalence of OCD is equal in males and females.

Social anxiety disorder

Social anxiety disorder (SAD) is characterized by feelings of anxiety in social situations (e.g., speaking in front of others and attending social gatherings). Patients feel as though everyone is staring and judging them. People affected by SAD usually do not seek treatment and will, instead, self-medicate with alcohol. There is equal male and female prevalence.

Simple or specific phobias

Simple phobias are defined as specific fears (e.g., heights, dogs, mice, spiders, needles) that cause an extreme anxiety response. Affected persons usually do not seek treatment and will, instead, avoid situations that involve the phobia.

Exposure therapy to the perceived threat is common therapy. Incidence in females is greater than in males.

Post-traumatic stress disorder

Post-traumatic stress disorder (PTSD) is characterized by severe anxiety that is caused by an event outside of normal human experience (e.g., war, rape, natural disasters). Symptoms include vividly reliving the event to the extent that anxiety symptoms (i.e., flashbacks, nightmares or night terrors, extreme mood changes, feelings of fright) commonly occur. PTSD is often associated with strong guilt feelings, impaired relationships, social withdrawal, and personality changes. There is a greater prevalence in females than in males.

Anxiety due to a medical disorder

Anxiety is likely to be related to evidence of a medical condition (e.g., congestive heart failure, hyperthyroidism, chronic obstructive pulmonary disease [COPD]).

Substance-induced anxiety disorder

Anxiety symptoms are likely to be a direct result of use of an agent (e.g., amphetamines, toxin, medication). Symptoms may also occur with intoxication or withdrawal.

Associated features

High comorbidity exists with other psychiatric illnesses, especially depression. High comorbidity also exists with alcohol or substance abuse.

This disorder is associated with chronic medical illnesses (e.g., chronic pain syndromes, long-term illnesses, GI distress, headaches).

Etiology

This disorder's etiology is presently unknown. Most current evidence suggests the cause is primarily biologic (imbalance of GABA, 5-HT, and NE) with genetic predisposition.

Drug Therapy

Benzodiazepines

Benzodiazepines (BZDs), the most commonly used anxiolytics, are described in Table 25-11.

Mechanism of action

BZDs potentiate the actions of GABA by increasing the influx of chloride ions into neurons. It is hypothesized that, through their effects on neurons mediated by receptor complexes, BZDs reduce neuronal firing and, thus, the symptoms of anxiety.

Note: The rate of absorption varies with BZDs. The more lipophilic compounds (i.e., alprazolam, diazepam, clorazepate, flurazepam) are rapidly absorbed and result in quicker onset of action. The less lipophilic BZDs are chlordiazepoxide, clonazepam, and lorazepam.

Adverse effects

Effects include sedation, dizziness, confusion, blurred vision, diplopia, syncope, residual daytime sedation, and reduced psychomotor and cognitive dysfunction.

Metabolism

Lorazepam, oxazepam, and temazepam (LOT) are conjugated and are preferred in patients with hepatic dysfunction and elderly patients.

Table 25-11. Benzodiazepines

Drug	Trade name	Time to peak plasma concentration (h)	Half-life (h)	Usual daily dose (mg/d)	Metabolic pathway
Alprazolam	Xanax, Niravam	1–2	12–15	0.5–4.0	Oxidation
Chlordiazepoxide	Librium	2–4	5–30	5–200	Oxidation
Clonazepam	Klonopin	1–2	18–50	1–3	Nitro reduction
Clorazepate	Tranxene	1–2	Not significant	15–60	Oxidation
Diazepam	Valium	0.5–2	20–80	2–40	Oxidation
Estazolam	ProSom	2	10–24	0.5–2.0	Oxidation
Flurazepam	Dalmane	0.5–2	Not significant	15–30	Oxidation
Halazepam	Paxipam	1–3	7–14	80–160	Oxidation
Lorazepam	Ativan	1–6	10–20	2–6	Conjugation
Oxazepam	Serax	2–4	5–20	30–120	Conjugation
Prazepam	Centrax	6	1.2	20–60	Oxidation
Quazepam	Doral	2	25–41	7.5–30	Oxidation
Temazepam	Restoril	2–3	10–40	15–30	Conjugation
Triazolam	Halcion	1	1.5–5.0	0.125–0.5	Oxidation

Drug interactions

BZDs metabolized by CYP3A4 (e.g., alprazolam, diazepam, and triazolam) have decreased clearance if taken concomitantly with CYP3A4 inhibitors (e.g., ketoconazole, erythromycin, nefazodone). BZDs are deadly in overdose if taken concomitantly with alcohol.

Clinical pearls

■ BZDs may cause a paradoxical reaction in children, cognitively impaired elderly patients, mentally retarded patients, and post–head injury patients.
■ Never abruptly discontinue BZDs because doing so may precipitate status epilepticus. Always taper the dose to avoid seizure risk and withdrawal symptoms.
■ In elderly patients, the BZDs of choice are those that are conjugated (LOT). There is an increased risk of falls in this population.
■ It is best to avoid use of BZDs in pregnancy (especially first trimester) because of risk of cleft palate. BZDs are also present in breast milk and should be avoided in nursing females.
■ The abuse potential is great; BZDs are not recommended for patients with substance abuse issues.
■ Tolerance is common, and increasing doses are needed to control anxiety levels.
■ Alprazolam extended-release (Xanax XR) is dosed once daily; do not crush, chew, or break doses. It is also available as an orally disintegrating tablet (Niravam).

Buspirone (BuSpar)

Mechanism of action

The mechanism of action is poorly understood; 5-HT$_{1A}$ is a partial agonist, and buspirone reportedly stimulates presynaptic 5-HT$_{1A}$ receptors. In addition, the agent has a moderate affinity for D$_2$ receptors.

Buspirone does not interact with the BZD-GABA receptor complex.

Onset of anxiolytic effect is longer for buspirone than for BZD (2–3 weeks).

Adverse effects

Effects include GI upset, headache, and nervousness.

Benefits

Possible benefits over BZDs include the following:

■ Usually less sedating than BZDs
■ Little to no psychomotor or cognitive impairment
■ No association with withdrawal symptoms, abuse, or physical dependence
■ Not cross-tolerant with BZDs or alcohol

Antidepressants as treatment for anxiety disorders

TCAs are usually a third-line treatment because of side effects and the danger of overdose. Clomipramine is effective for OCD.

MAOIs are usually a third-line treatment because of side effects and drug–food interactions.

SSRIs and SNRIs are a first-line treatment for many anxiety disorders, especially in patients with comorbid depression and substance abuse problems.

Titrate doses of antidepressants slowly to decrease risk of initial anxiety symptoms. Ultimately, higher doses are commonly used for anxiety disorders.

Other classes of drugs used to treat anxiety disorders

β-blockers (e.g., propranolol and atenolol) ease peripheral symptoms of anxiety and may be useful for panic disorders and SAD.

Hydroxyzine reduces anxiety and is often used in patients with substance abuse issues.

Nonpharmacologic Treatment

■ Supportive psychotherapy (individual, group, family)
■ Cognitive behavioral therapy
■ Focus on coping with the fear of the symptoms of anxiety
■ Relaxation techniques
■ Exercise and lifestyle modifications (reduce caffeine and simple sugars)

25-6. Eating Disorders

Anorexia Nervosa

Characteristics

Patients suffering from anorexia nervosa refuse to maintain body weight at or above a minimal, normal weight for their age and height (85% or less of expected body weight). They experience intense fear of gaining weight or becoming fat, although they are underweight. There is a disturbance in self-perception of body weight, size, proportion, and attractiveness.

A female patient experiences amenorrhea for at least three consecutive cycles.

Types

- Restricting
- Binge eating and purging

Bulimia Nervosa

Characteristics

Recurrent episodes of binge eating occur (often followed by intense feelings of guilt). The patient may consume as much as 5,000–20,000 calories over 2–8 hours. Recurrent and inappropriate compensatory behavior occurs in order to prevent weight gain.

A person averages 2 binges per week for 3 months. Self-evaluation is primarily influenced by body shape and weight.

Types

- Purging (vomiting, abuse of laxatives or diuretics)
- Nonpurging (excessive exercise, fasting)

Binge Eating Disorder

Characteristics

Recurrent episodes of binge eating occur (patients are usually obese). The patient eats when not physically hungry, eats more rapidly than normal, and feels disgusted with himself or herself. Marked distress is present regarding binge eating.

Binge eating episodes occur, on average, at least 2 days per week for 6 months.

Etiology and Prevalence

The etiology of eating disorders is essentially unknown, but various theories have been proposed (genetic predisposition, environmental and societal issues, chemical imbalance in the brain). There is usually a defined event or situation that begins the disorder (e.g., a significant stressor such as starting college, divorce, or death of a loved one).

Eating disorders are most commonly seen in Caucasian, middle- to upper-class females.

The age of onset for anorexia nervosa is 13–20 years old. The male-to-female ratio is 1:10–20. For bulimia nervosa, the age of onset is 16–18 years old, and the male-to-female ratio is 1:10.

Medical Complications and Signs of Disease

- Eating disorders produce states of semistarvation and noticeable malnutrition, especially in anorexia.

- In bulimia, patients are more difficult to identify because they are commonly of normal body weight.
- Dehydration occurs.
- There is a high incidence of comorbid anxiety, depression, OCD, and substance abuse.
- Dental caries and enamel erosion occur because of stomach acid exposure.
- Calluses on the dorsum of the hand or fingers develop because of induction of vomiting.
- Mortality rate is about 10% from starvation (primarily because of electrolyte imbalances), arrhythmia, or suicide.
- Long-term complications include endocrine or metabolic, cardiovascular, renal, gastroenterologic, hematologic, pulmonary, musculoskeletal, immunologic, and dermatologic issues.

Treatment

Psychotherapy is the mainstay of treatment. Therapy can be individual, group, family, supportive, cognitive behavioral, or insight oriented. Primary objectives are to define and examine extent of problem. The patient learns to accept the condition, and treatment results in a reconstruction of self-identity and self-confidence.

Dietary intake is slowly normalized with the goal of restoring normal body weight. Nutritional counseling is used. Distorted ideas about caloric intake and body shape are corrected.

Relapse prevention focuses on developing and using coping mechanisms and avoiding high-risk situations.

Drug Therapy

SSRIs are primarily used and may be more effective for patients with bulimia. Antidepressants do not appear to be beneficial in helping severely malnourished anorexia nervosa patients gain weight, but they may help patients maintain weight after it has been gained.

Fluoxetine (Prozac) is indicated for the treatment of bulimia nervosa. Higher doses are used; titrate to 60 mg/d every morning.

Topiramate (Topamax) and zonisamide (Zonegran) may be beneficial in binge-eating disorder and bulimia nervosa.

Ideally, treatment of eating disorders includes both psychotherapy and pharmacotherapy.

25-7. Key Points

Schizophrenia

- Patients with schizophrenia have positive (hallucinations and delusions), negative (flat affect, avolition, anhedonia, poverty of thought), and disorganized speech and behavior symptoms. Positive symptoms usually respond to drug therapy first.

■ Antipsychotics (conventional or atypical) are essential treatment for schizophrenia; atypical medications (risperidone, olanzapine, quetiapine, ziprasidone, aripiprazole, and paliperidone) have been considered first-line medical treatment because they lower risk of EPSs and TD more than conventional medications and they appear to be more beneficial for negative symptoms.

■ Recent evidence has shown that schizophrenic patients discontinue medications frequently regardless of whether they are taking second-generation or first-generation antipsychotics. Such research questions whether the atypical antipsychotics are more effective at treating negative symptoms than are the typical medications.

■ Atypical antipsychotics (especially olanzapine) are associated with weight gain and with lipid and glucose abnormalities (ziprasidone and aripiprazole do not appear to have the weight gain and metabolic abnormalities).

■ Low-potency conventional agents (chlorpromazine, thioridazine) are used more often than high-potency agents (haloperidol, fluphenazine).

■ Low-potency agents have more sedation, orthostatic hypotension, and anticholinergic side effects and fewer EPS than high-potency agents. High-potency agents have more EPS and less sedation, orthostatic hypotension, and anticholinergic effects.

■ EPS consist of dystonic reactions (to be remedied by diphenhydramine 25–50 mg IM or benztropine 1–2 mg IM every 30 minutes until resolution); akathisia (to be treated with lorazepam, clonidine, or propranolol); and pseudoparkinsonism (ameliorated by amantadine or benztropine).

■ Clozapine is the only agent proven effective for refractory schizophrenia.

■ Consider long-acting injectable preparations in situations of poor compliance.

Bipolar Disorder

■ The acute treatment for bipolar disorder focuses on slowing down the patient and reducing harm to himself or herself and others

■ Maintenance treatment focuses on preventing or reducing the number of future episodes.

■ A mood stabilizer is an essential component in the treatment of bipolar disorder. First-line mood stabilizers include lithium and divalproex sodium (or valproic acid).

■ The risk of lithium side effects and toxicity can be prevented by monitoring the patient for signs and symptoms of problems and by obtaining regular blood-level readings.

■ Other drug therapies that may be used to treat the patient with bipolar disorder include atypical antipsychotics, gabapentin, carbamazepine, oxcarbazepine, topiramate, and lamotrigine (especially if the patient is depressed).

Major Depression

■ All antidepressants are equally effective in a given population.

■ Response varies from person to person. Antidepressants differ in side-effect and drug-interaction profiles, and none are "speed" or "uppers."

■ Choice of agent depends on the history of response of other family members to certain antidepressants (if available) and the particular side-effect profile (as it relates to any given patient).

■ First-line agents include SSRIs, bupropion, venlafaxine, and duloxetine; second-line agents may include mirtazapine and nefazodone; third-line agents may include TCAs and MAOIs.

■ The goal is to reduce or eliminate target symptoms with an antidepressant; incorporating psychotherapy is optimal.

■ The goal of treatment of depression is to improve the patient's ability to function and his or her quality of life.

Anxiety Disorders

■ Anxiety disorders are serious, debilitating mental illnesses that have extreme anxiety as the primary mood disturbance.

■ Various drug therapies include benzodiazepines, buspirone, antidepressants (especially SSRIs and venlafaxine), β-blockers, and hydroxyzine.

■ Nonpharmacologic therapy of anxiety disorders is an important aspect of care (e.g., supportive therapy, cognitive behavioral therapy, relaxation techniques, and exercise and lifestyle modifications).

Eating disorders

■ Anorexia nervosa is characterized by a refusal to maintain body weight (at or above a minimal normal weight for age and height), an intense fear of gaining weight, a disturbance in self-perception of body weight, and amenorrhea for at least three consecutive cycles.

- Bulimia nervosa is characterized by recurrent episodes of binge eating, recurrent and inappropriate compensatory behavior to prevent weight gain, an average of two binges per week for 3 months, and self-evaluation that is primarily influenced by body shape and weight.
- Eating disorders most commonly occur in young, Caucasian, middle- to upper-class females.
- Medical complications and comorbid psychiatric disorders (e.g., anxiety, depression, and substance abuse) are extremely common in this population.
- Medications such as antidepressants may be helpful in treating eating disorders (especially bulimia); optimal therapy should include psychotherapy in combination with drug therapy.

25-8. Questions

Select the single best response for questions 1–4.

1. S. J. is a 30-year-old white female with a 10-year history of schizophrenia. Her current therapy includes haloperidol 10 mg po bid. The psychiatrist wants to convert her to haloperidol decanoate. What would be the appropriate equivalent monthly dose of haloperidol decanoate?

   A. 100 mg
   B. 10 mg
   C. 500 mg
   D. 200 mg
   E. 12.5 mg

2. B. T. reports to the nursing station with his head pulled sharply to the side and rear. He complains of severe pain in his neck and back area. The most appropriate diagnosis and treatment would be which of the following?

   A. Akathisia; propranolol 20 mg IM until resolution
   B. Dystonic reaction; diphenhydramine 50 mg IM every 30 minutes until resolution
   C. Tardive dyskinesia; physical therapy
   D. Dystonic reaction; lorazepam 2 mg IM every 30 minutes until resolution
   E. None of the above

3. Negative symptoms in schizophrenia could include all of the following *except*

   A. flat affect.
   B. anhedonia.
   C. avolition.
   D. persecutory delusions.
   E. poverty of thought.

4. A 48-year-old black male arrives at the emergency department seeking his "nerve pill." He has a 27-year history of paranoid schizophrenia with multiple hospitalizations. In recent years, he has been effectively maintained on fluphenazine 10 mg po bid. He now states that he feels "really bad today." His arms and jaws are stiff, his temperature is 104°F, his blood pressure is 176/110, and his WBC is 19,000. LFTs and CPK are ordered STAT. While you await the test results, you should do which of the following?

   A. Discontinue oral fluphenazine and begin quetiapine.
   B. Discontinue oral fluphenazine.
   C. Continue oral fluphenazine and add bromocriptine.
   D. Discontinue oral fluphenazine and give fluphenazine decanoate 25 mg IM STAT.
   E. Do nothing; labs need to be evaluated first.

For questions 5–8, one or more of the answers given may be correct. Answer each question as follows:

   A. I only
   B. II only
   C. I and III only
   D. II and III only
   E. I, II, and III

A 25-year-old white male has been increasingly disruptive at home. He has been claiming that he is the president of the United States and has been staying awake all night planning bills for Congress. He has been argumentative and threatening with his friends and family. Though he appears extremely tired physically, he is constantly active.

5. The psychiatrist has decided to initiate Eskalith CR 450 mg bid in this patient. Which of the following lab tests will need to be performed for this patient before starting this drug therapy regimen?

   I.   Pregnancy test
   II. Thyroid function tests
   III. SCr

6. As the pharmacist on the treatment team, you alert the patient's family to the common side effects of lithium, which include

   I. polyuria.
   II. alopecia.
   III. elevated hepatic enzymes.

7. Which of the following statements are correct regarding the treatment of bipolar disorder?

   I. Lithium and divalproex sodium are considered first-line therapy options for mood stabilization.
   II. When treating a patient with lithium, one must monitor the WBC and ANC because of lithium's propensity to cause agranulocytosis.
   III. Patients diagnosed with bipolar I disorder exhibit intermittent cycles of mania and major depression.

8. Which of the following therapies have been used for the treatment of bipolar disorder?

   I. Olanzapine
   II. Topiramate
   III. Calcium channel blockers

Select the single best response for questions 9–11.

9. Insomnia, GI upset, and headache are common side effects of which of the following antidepressants?

   A. Phenelzine
   B. Amitriptyline
   C. Fluoxetine
   D. Trazodone
   E. Both B and C

10. A 29-year-old depressed black female has shown little improvement with fluoxetine treatment, so the psychiatrist decides to change her medication to tranylcypromine. What is your recommendation for the switch?

    A. Gradually decrease fluoxetine dosage over a 4-week period, and then start tranylcypromine.
    B. Wait 2 weeks after stopping fluoxetine, and then begin tranylcypromine.
    C. Over 6 weeks, gradually decrease fluoxetine dosage as you gradually increase the tranylcypromine dosage.
    D. Wait 5 weeks after stopping fluoxetine before initiating tranylcypromine.

    E. Maintain fluoxetine dosage, and start tranylcypromine; stop the fluoxetine when the tranylcypromine has achieved a therapeutic level.

11. Which of the following has been shown to induce or worsen depression?

    A. Oral contraceptives
    B. Amoxicillin
    C. Thiamine
    D. Methylphenidate
    E. Phenelzine

The following case should be used to answer questions 12 and 13.

K. Y. is a 36-year-old female admitted to your mental health facility for the fifth time in the past 3 years for major depressive disorder. She presents with lack of appetite, avolition, anhedonia, and suicidal ideations with a plan. Vitals include BP 127/76, P 82, R 18, T 98.6°F. Labs include TSH 4, FBG 135, (−) UDS, BAL 0. Her current medications are fluoxetine 40 mg daily, metformin 1,000 mg bid, and hydroxyzine 25 mg tid. K. Y. states compliance and denies side effects. Past medications include citalopram and venlafaxine.

12. What axis diagnosis is major depressive disorder?

    A. I
    B. II
    C. III
    D. IV
    E. V

13. The psychiatrist asks for your recommendation for this patient with refractory depression. What is the best option?

    A. Discontinue fluoxetine, and initiate Pristiq.
    B. Discontinue fluoxetine, wait 2 weeks, and start Selegiline.
    C. Add Abilify to current regimen.
    D. Discontinue fluoxetine, and start Lexapro.
    E. Add Serax to current regimen.

14. Which of the following is correct regarding electroconvulsive therapy (ECT)?

    A. For maximum effectiveness, seizures should last 5–10 minutes.
    B. ECT is contraindicated in patients with COPD.

C. ECT is effective treatment for pregnant females with major depression.

D. Memory loss lasting 1–2 weeks is common.

E. ECT may cause amenorrhea in female patients.

15. A 33-year-old waitress is experiencing symptoms of anxiety, including night terrors and mood lability. She reports no past psychiatric history but admits that these symptoms started about 2 weeks after armed and masked gunmen robbed her restaurant. She is most likely experiencing which of the following?

    A. LSD
    B. PTSD
    C. GAD
    D. OCD

16. A new patient presents to your clinic. He reports that it took him 3 hours to get ready for this appointment and that he returned home several times to check to see if the door was locked. During the interview, he straightens up your desk, making sure all square items are at right angles to each other. He would most likely be diagnosed with which of the following?

    A. PTSD
    B. PCP
    C. OCD
    D. GAD

17. Which of the following statements regarding the use of SSRIs in anxiety disorders is most accurate?

    A. SSRIs are not usually effective in the treatment of anxiety.
    B. SSRI doses for anxiety should be started lower than initial doses for depression.
    C. SSRIs should be used only after a failed treatment trial with benzodiazepines.
    D. SSRIs may be used on a prn basis when anxiety symptoms emerge.

18. Which of the following characteristics is *not* correct regarding benzodiazepines?

    A. They potentiate the effect of γ-aminobutyric acid.
    B. They are highly lipophilic.
    C. They are cross-tolerant with alcohol.

D. Their pharmacologic action is similar to that of buspirone.

E. There is risk of seizure if they are abruptly discontinued.

For questions 19–22, one or more of the following answers given are correct. Answer each question as follows:

A. I only
B. II only
C. I and III only
D. II and III only
E. I, II, and III

19. Which of the following is true regarding anorexia nervosa (AN)?

    I. AN is characterized by recurrent and inappropriate compensatory behavior to prevent weight gain.
    II. Patients with AN generally appear to be of normal weight for age and height.
    III. AN patients have an intense fear of gaining weight or becoming fat, although they are underweight.

20. What DSM-IV criteria for AN are diagnostic for this type of eating disorder?

    I. Absence of at least three consecutive menstrual cycles
    II. Sunken eyes with dark circles underneath
    III. A binge eating–purging episode that occurs at least once in the past 6 months

21. Which of the following is true regarding bulimia nervosa?

    I. The individual may consume 5,000–20,000 calories in a single binge episode that may last as long as 2–8 hours.
    II. The two specific types of bulimic patients are purging type and nonpurging type.
    III. There is an average of two binges per week for 3 consecutive months.

22. Patients with AN may demonstrate which of the following characteristics?

    I. Kleptomania
    II. Laxative or diuretic abuse
    III. Amenorrhea

23. Which of the following is the most appropriate treatment for bulimia nervosa?

A. Insight-oriented therapy
B. Fluoxetine 20 mg qd
C. Fluoxetine 60 mg qam + cognitive behavioral therapy
D. Olanzapine 10 mg qhs
E. Olanzapine 20 mg qhs + family therapy

25-9. Answers

1. **D.** The patient is on haloperidol 10 mg bid. Therefore, to convert to the decanoate injection, the total oral daily dose is multiplied by 10. The dose would be Haldol-D 200 mg IM every 4 weeks.

2. **B.** The patient is experiencing a dystonic reaction, which can be treated with either benztropine 1–2 mg IM or diphenhydramine 25–50 mg IM every 30 minutes until resolved. The dystonic reaction is thought to occur because of an imbalance in dopamine and acetylcholine in the nigrostriatal region of the brain.

3. **D.** Delusions are false beliefs or wrong judgments held with conviction despite incontrovertible evidence to the contrary. Such symptoms are referred to as positive for patients with schizophrenia.

4. **B.** The symptoms that the patient is displaying appear to be the result of neuroleptic malignant syndrome. All neuroleptics have the propensity to cause this rare but deadly adverse effect. The first steps in treating NMS are to discontinue the offending agent, offer supportive therapy, and prescribe a dopamine agonist and (commonly) a skeletal muscle relaxant.

5. **D.** Initiation of lithium requires several baseline lab tests: pregnancy test (if patient is female and of childbearing age), ECG and BP to assess cardiovascular status, thyroid function tests to rule out euthyroid goiter or hypothyroidism, SCr/BUN (lithium is 100% renally eliminated), and CBC with differential to evaluate for leukocytosis. Electrolytes should also be evaluated (decreased sodium can increase lithium levels). Hence, only the pregnancy test should not be performed, because the patient is male.

6. **A.** Common side effects that occur with the initiation of lithium include polyuria, polydipsia, tremor, and GI upset. Common side effects that may occur later in therapy include weight gain and mental dulling. Elevated hepatic enzymes and alopecia are side effects that may occur with divalproex sodium.

7. **C.** Agranulocytosis is a side effect that is monitored weekly with clozapine therapy for 6 months. After 6 months, monitoring can be done every 2 weeks for the duration of therapy.

8. **E.** All of the therapies listed have been used for mood stabilization in bipolar disorder.

9. **C.** SSRIs commonly cause insomnia, GI upset, anxiety, headache, and sexual dysfunction. Phenelzine, amitriptyline, and trazodone cause sedative effects.

10. **D.** Because of fluoxetine's long half-life, 5 weeks should pass before initiating MAOI therapy. If fluoxetine is not cleared from the body by the time the MAOI is started, there is a risk of developing serotonin syndrome.

11. **A.** Many medications can cause or worsen depression, such as antihypertensives (reserpine, methyldopa, propranolol, clonidine); antiparkinsonian agents (levodopa, carbidopa, amantadine); hormonal agents (estrogens, progesterone); corticosteroids; cycloserine; and the anticancer agents vinblastine and vincristine.

12. **A.** Axis I is for clinical disorders.

13. **C.** Abilify (aripiprazole) is approved as adjunct treatment for refractory depression. The patient has already failed a trial with venlafaxine; therefore, initiating therapy with its isomer Pristiq (desvenlafaxine) may not be the best option. MAOIs are a viable fourth-line treatment option. However, you would wait 5 weeks after discontinuing fluoxetine before initiating an MAOI. Lexapro (escitalopram) is an isomer of citalopram, which the patient had already failed. Benzodiazepines are not recommended for treatment of depression.

14. **C.** ECT is a safe and effective therapy for pregnant females and patients with COPD. Relative contraindications include increased intracranial pressure, recent MI, recent intracerebral hemorrhage, and cerebral lesions. Memory loss is a common side effect, but it usually occurs only on the day of treatment and perhaps the following day. The induced seizure lasts 30–90 seconds and is monitored by an EEG. Additionally, ECT does not cause amenorrhea in female patients.

15. **B.** The patient experienced a violent and frightening episode 2 weeks before her symptoms appeared. The symptoms of reexperiencing of the event, night terrors, and mood lability are common in patients with PTSD.

16. **C.** The patient is displaying signs and symptoms of OCD (e.g., a long time is spent getting

ready, and there is repeated checking behavior and preoccupation with rearranging items to 90-degree angles). These activities are time consuming and limit his social and occupational functioning.

17. **B.** Because SSRIs can be activating and may initially cause symptoms of anxiety, it is important to "start low and go slow" with these agents when used for anxiety disorders.

18. **D.** Buspirone's mechanism of action is agonism of 5-HT$_{1A}$ receptors. Buspirone also possesses moderate affinity for D$_2$ receptors. It does not interact with the BZD-GABA receptor complex like the BZDs do. The BZDs cross the blood–brain barrier and are cross-tolerant with alcohol. If BZDs are abruptly discontinued, seizures can result.

19. **C.** Patients with AN refuse to maintain body weight at or above a minimal, normal weight for age and height (less than 15% of expected body weight). Patients with AN may respond to antidepressants, but psychotherapy is usually more effective. AN is most commonly seen in Caucasian, middle- to upper-class females.

20. **A.** DSM-IV criteria list the refusal to maintain body weight at or above a minimal, normal weight for age and height (85% or less of expected body weight and an intense fear of gaining weight or becoming fat although underweight); disturbance in self-perception of body weight (i.e., size, proportion, attractiveness); and amenorrhea for at least three consecutive cycles.

21. **E.** All of the answers are correct regarding bulimia nervosa.

22. **D.** Patients with AN commonly reduce weight by reducing food intake. Many patients use other methods to lose weight such as excessive exercise, laxative or diuretic use, substance abuse, and self-induced vomiting. Amenorrhea ensues as a result of estrogen deficiency; it may occur before weight loss.

23. **C.** Fluoxetine is approved for treating bulimia nervosa; 60 mg is the most common dose. A combination of psychotherapy and pharmacotherapy is preferred.

25-10. References

American Diabetes Association, American Psychiatric Association, American Association of Clinical Endocrinologists, North American Association for the Study of Obesity. Consensus development conference on antipsychotic drugs and obesity and diabetes. *Diabetes Care.* 2004;27:596–601.

American Psychiatric Association. *Diagnostic and Statistical Manual of Mental Disorders.* 4th ed. Text rev. Washington, D.C.: American Psychiatric Association; 2000.

American Psychiatric Association. Practice guideline for the treatment of patients with bipolar disorder (revision). *Am J Psychiatry.* 2002;159(suppl):1–50.

American Psychiatric Association. *Practice Guideline for the Treatment of Patients with Eating Disorders.* 3rd ed. Washington, D.C.: American Psychiatric Association; 2006.

American Psychiatric Association. Practice guideline for the treatment of patients with major depressive disorder (revision). *Am J Psychiatry.* 2000; 157(suppl 4):1–45.

American Psychiatric Association. Practice guideline for the treatment of patients with schizophrenia. *Am J Psychiatry.* 1997;154(suppl 4):1–63.

Bennett JA, Dunayevich E, McElroy SL, et al. The new mood stabilizers and the treatment of bipolar disorder. *Drug Benefit Trends.* 2000;12:3–16.

Botts SR, Raskind J. Gabapentin and lamotrigine in bipolar disorder. *Am J Health-Syst Pharm.* 1999; 56:1939–44.

Canales PL, Cates M, Wells BG. Anxiety disorders. In: Herfindal ET, Gourley DR, eds. *Textbook of Therapeutics: Drug and Disease Management.* 7th ed. Philadelphia: Lippincott Williams & Wilkins; 2000:1185–1202.

Cohen LJ, Jermain DM, Clarke SO, et al. Psychiatric pharmacy practice specialty certification examination review course. Course presented at American Society of Health-System Pharmacists Psychiatric Clinical Specialists Meeting, Denver, Colo., 2001, March 31–April 1.

Crismon ML, Buckley PF. Schizophrenia. In: DiPiro JT, Talbert RL, Yee GC, et al., eds. *Pharmacotherapy: A Pathophysiologic Approach.* 6th ed. New York: McGraw-Hill; 2005:1209–33.

DeVane CL. Keeping depression at bay. *Drug Topics.* 2001;15:49–58.

Easson WM, Rock NL. *Psychiatry Specialty Board Review.* New York: Brunner/Mazel; 1991.

Emsam [package insert]. Princeton, N.J.: Bristol-Myers Squibb; 2006.

Fuller MA, Sajatovic M, eds. *Drug Information for Mental Health.* 1st ed. Cleveland, Ohio: Lexi-Comp; 2001.

Gutierrez MA, Stimmel GL. Mood disorders. In: Helms RA, Quan DJ, Herfindal ET, et al., eds. *Textbook of Therapeutics: Drug and Disease Management.* 8th ed. Philadelphia: Lippincott Williams & Wilkins; 2006:1416–31.

Gutierrez MA, Stimmel GL. Schizophrenia. In: Helms RA, Quan DJ, Herfindal ET, et al., eds. *Textbook of Therapeutics: Drug and Disease Management.* 8th ed. Philadelphia: Lippincott Williams & Wilkins; 2006:1432–42.

Jacobson JL, Jacobson AM, eds. *Psychiatric Secrets.* Philadelphia: Hanley & Belfus; 1996.

Kane JM. Drug therapy: Schizophrenia. *N Engl J Med.* 1996;334:34–41.

Kane JM, McGlashan TH. Treatment of schizophrenia. *Lancet.* 1995;346:820–25.

Keck PE, Perlis RH, Otto MW, et al. The expert consensus guideline series: Treatment of bipolar disorder 2004. 2004 (December):1–120.

Lamictal [package insert]. http://dailymed.nlm.nih.gov/dailymed/drugInfo.cfm?id=10270.

Lieberman JA, Stroup TS, McEvoy JP, et al. Effectiveness of antipsychotic drugs in patients with chronic schizophrenia. *N Engl J Med.* 2005; 353:1209–23.

Mandl DL, Iltz JL. Obesity and eating disorders. In: Herfindal ET, Gourley DR, eds. *Textbook of Therapeutics: Drug and Disease Management.* 7th ed. Philadelphia: Lippincott Williams & Wilkins; 2000:1271–87.

McElroy SL, Keck PE. Pharmacologic agents for the treatment of acute bipolar mania. *Biol Psychiatry.* 2000;48:539–57.

McElroy SL, Shapira NA, Arnold LM, et al. Topiramate in the long-term treatment of binge-eating disorder associated with obesity. *J Clin Psychiatry.* 2004;65(suppl 11):1463–69.

McEvoy JP, Lieberman JA, Stroup TS, et al. Effectiveness of clozapine versus olanzapine, quetiapine, and risperidone in patients with chronic schizophrenia who did not respond to prior atypical antipsychotic treatment. *Am J Psychiatry.* 2006:163:600–10.

McEvoy JP, Scheifler PL, Frances A. The expert consensus guideline series: Treatment of schizophrenia. *J Clin Psychiatry.* 1999;60(suppl 11):3–80.

National Institute of Mental Health. Anxiety disorders. NIH publication no. 00-3879. National Institutes of Health, Bethesda, Md.; 2000.

National Institute of Mental Health. Pamphlet on eating disorders. NIH publication no. 94-3477. Department of Health and Human Services, Washington, D.C.; 1994.

Newcomer JW, Nasrallah HA, Loebel AD. The atypical antipsychotic therapy and metabolic issue national survey. *J Clin Psychopharmacology.* 2004; 24(suppl 1):S1–S6.

Norton J. Oxcarbazepine in mood disorders. *Hosp Pharm.* 2001;36:1254–56.

Post RM. Rapid cycling: Clinical presentation and treatment approaches. New research presented at the 155th Annual Meeting of the American Psychiatric Association. Philadelphia; May 2002.

Ray WA, Chung CP, Murray KT, et al. Atypical antipsychotic drugs and the risk of sudden cardiac death. *N Engl J Med.* 2009;360(3):225–35.

Risby E, Donnigan D, Nemeroff CB. Pharmacotherapeutic considerations for psychiatric disorders: Depression. *Formulary.* 1997;32:46–59.

Risperdal Consta [package insert]. Titusville, N.J.: Ortho-McNeil-Janssen; 2009

Sachs GS, Nierenberg AA, Calabrese JR, et al. Effectiveness of adjunctive antidepressant treatment for bipolar depression. *N Engl J Med.* 2007; 356: 1711–22.

Sachs GS, Printz DJ, Kahn DA, et al. The expert consensus guideline series. Medication treatment of bipolar disorder 2000. *Postgraduate Med.* 2000; 4:1–104.

Schneider LS, Tariot PN, Dagerman KS, et al. Effectiveness of atypical antipsychotic drugs in patients with Alzheimer's disease. *N Engl J Med.* 2006; 355:1525–38.

Stahl SM. *Psychopharmacology of Antidepressants.* London: Martin Dunitz; 1998.

Stahl SM. *Psychopharmacology of Antipsychotics.* London: Martin Dunitz; 1999.

Stroup TS, Lieberman JA, McEvoy JP, et al. Effectiveness of olanzapine, quetiapine, risperidone, and ziprasidone in patients with chronic schizophrenia following discontinuation of a previous atypical antipsychotic. *Am J Psychiatry.* 2006:163: 611–22.

Substance Abuse and Mental Health Services Administration and National Institute of Mental Health. *Mental Health: A Report from the Surgeon General.* Available at: www.surgeongeneral.gov/library/mentalhealth/chapter3/sec6.html.

Trivedi H, Rush AJ, Wisniewski SR, et al. Evaluation of outcomes with citalopram for depression using measurement-based care in STAR*D: Implications for clinical practice. *Am J Psychiatry.* 2006;163: 28–40.

U.S. Food and Drug Administration. FDA proposes new warnings about suicidal thinking, behavior in young adults who take antidepressant medications. Available at: www.fda.gov/News Events/Newsroom/PressAnnouncements/2007/ucm108905.htm.

U.S. Food and Drug Administration. FDA public health advisory: Deaths with antipsychotics in elderly patients with behavioral disturbances. Available at www.fda.gov/Drugs/DrugSafety/PublicHealthAdvisories/ucm053171.htm.

Common Dermatologic Disorders

Shaunta' M. Ray, PharmD, BCPS

26-1. Acne (Acne Vulgaris)

Acne is an inflammatory disorder of the pilosebaceous glands that occurs most commonly during the teenage years, at or soon after puberty. It may reappear later or begin in adults who had clear skin in their teens, more commonly in women than in men.

Classification and Clinical Presentation

- *Type I (comedonal):* A mild form, with primarily noninflammatory lesions (open and closed comedones), relatively few superficial inflammatory lesions, and no scarring
- *Type II (papular):* A moderate form, with multiple papules on the face and trunk and minimal scarring
- *Type III (pustular):* An advanced form that can lead to moderate scarring
- *Type IV (nodulocystic):* The most severe and destructive form, with multiple deep inflammatory lesions or nodules (often called *cysts*) that lead to extensive scarring

Pathophysiology

- Increased sebum production by androgenic hormones at the onset of puberty
- Obstruction of hair follicle opening because of increasing adherence to and production of epithelial cells, producing closed comedones (whiteheads) that progress ultimately to open comedones (blackheads)
- Increased growth of a primary microorganism on the skin and in the sebaceous ducts, *Propionibacterium acnes* (*P acnes*), a gram-positive anaerobic rod that produces enzymes (including lipases)
- Inflammation caused by the enzymatic breakdown of triglycerides into free fatty acids, which causes the influx of polymorphonuclear leukocytes, ultimately resulting in pustule formation

Treatment Principles

- *Type I (comedonal):* Topical nonprescription medications such as benzoyl peroxide, which is usually the first line of therapy
- *Type II (papular):* Topical antibiotics, topical retinoids, or both
- *Type III (pustular):* Oral antibiotics in addition to topical medications
- *Type IV (nodulocystic):* Isotretinoin

Topical Therapy

Nonprescription agents

Benzoyl peroxide is the most effective over-the-counter (OTC) agent. Benzoyl peroxide products 2.5, 5, and 10% are as follows:

- Clean and Clear Gel
- Clearasil maximum strength vanishing cream
- Clearplex
- Exact Acne Medication
- Fostex
- Neutrogena On the Spot Acne Treatment
- Noxzema antiacne lotion
- Oxy-10 Balance Spot Treatment and Face Wash
- Panoxyl Bar
- Stridex Power Pads
- Zapzyt gel

Mechanism of action

These agents destroy the anaerobic *P acnes* through the release of oxygen. An exfoliant effect occurs, causing peeling of the outer layers of the skin.

P acnes does not become resistant to benzoyl peroxide; therefore, it can be used concurrently with topical antibiotics to prevent resistance (e.g., using benzoyl peroxide for one course of therapy, alternating with a course of topical antibiotic therapy).

Patient counseling

- Use with caution with sensitive skin.
- Do not allow contact with eyes, lips, or mouth.
- Avoid unnecessary sun exposure and use sunscreen.

Adverse effects

- These agents may cause redness, dryness, burning, itching, peeling, and swelling.
- They may bleach hair or dyed fabrics.

Other products

- *Sulfur (1–10%):* Products include Bye Bye Blemish—sulfur 10% (keratolytic and antibacterial action)
- *Salicylic acid (0.5–2.0%):* Products include Clearasil Clearstick, Neutrogena Rapid Defense, Noxzema, and Stridex—irritant effect, keratolytic action, and increase in rate of turnover of epithelial cells
- *Resorcinol:* Keratolytic action (usually combined with sulfur)
- *Combinations such as sulfur and resorcinol:* Clearasil and Acnomel
- *Medicated soaps and cleansers:* Alcohol, acetone, and other degreasing lotions

Topical antimicrobial therapy

Topical antimicrobials are outlined in Table 26-1.

Table 26-1. Topical Antimicrobials

Generic name	Trade name	Form
Clindamycin	Cleocin-T	Liquid
Erythromycin	Theramycin Z	Liquid
	Benzamycin 2%	Gel
	Emgel 2%	Gel

Clindamycin

Mechanism of action

Clindamycin suppresses growth of *P acnes*. It may directly reduce free fatty acid concentrations on the skin.

Patient counseling

- Contact physician if no improvement is seen within 6 weeks.
- Discontinue medication and contact physician if severe diarrhea or abdominal cramps or pain develop.

Adverse effects

- Contact dermatitis or hypersensitivity
- Dry or scaly skin or peeling
- Rarely, pseudomembranous colitis (severe abdominal cramps, pain, bloating, and severe diarrhea)

Erythromycin

Mechanism of action

Erythromycin suppresses growth of *P acnes*.

Patient counseling

- Wait at least 1 hour before applying any other topical acne medication.
- Avoid contact with eyes, mouth, nose, and other mucous membranes.
- Although improvement is generally expected within 4 weeks, some patients do not respond for 8–12 weeks.

Adverse effects

- *More common:* Dry or scaly skin, irritation, and itching
- *Less common:* Stinging sensation, peeling, and redness

Retinoids

See Table 26-2 for information about retinoids.

Mechanism of action

- Retinoids are chemically related to vitamin A.
- Retinoids normalize follicular keratinization, heal comedones, decrease sebum production, and decrease inflammatory lesions.

Patient counseling

- Do not use astringents, drying agents, abrasive scrubs, or harsh soaps concurrently, and use mild soap only once or twice daily.

Table 26-2. Retinoids

Generic name	Trade name	Form and strength
Tretinoin	Retin-A	0.025%, 0.05%, 0.1% cream; 0.1% gel; 0.025% lotion
	Retin-A Micro	0.04%, 0.1% gel
	Renova	0.02% cream
	Avita	0.025% cream and gel
Adapalene	Differin	0.1% cream
Tazarotene	Tazorac	0.1%, 0.3% alcohol-free gel; 0.5%, 0.1% gel and cream
Alitretinoin	Panretin	0.1% gel

- Apply every other night to adjust to drying effect for the first 2 weeks.
- Apply nightly after 2 weeks.
- Expect that it may take up to 2–3 months for skin to improve.
- Use sunblock on face before sun exposure because of increased sensitivity.

Adverse drug effects
- These agents may irritate skin and cause redness, dryness, and scaling.
- Tazarotene is the most irritating retinoid.
- Adapalene appears to be least irritating and is preferred for sensitive skin.

Azelaic acid 20%

Trade names are Azelex and Finacea.

Mechanism of action
Axelaic acid 20% suppresses growth of *P acnes*. It improves inflammatory and noninflammatory lesions. It normalizes keratinization, leading to an anticomedonal effect.

Patient counseling
- If sensitivity develops, discontinue use.
- Keep away from mouth, eyes, and mucous membranes.
- Other topical medications must be used at different times during the day.

Adverse drug effects
- Temporary dryness and skin irritation (pruritus and burning) may occur on initiation of therapy.
- Hypopigmentation may occur (caution in dark-skinned individuals).

Systemic Therapy

Antimicrobials

Antimicrobials are useful for type II (papular) acne and type III (pustular) acne.

Dosing
See Table 26-3 for information about dosage. After 6–8 weeks, dosage may be increased if necessary. If the first antibiotic was ineffective after increasing the dosage, a second antibiotic is prescribed.

After 6 months to 1 year of therapy, the antibiotic dose may be tapered if continued at all.

Mechanism of action
Antimicrobials suppress growth of *P acnes* in sebaceous ducts. These agents possibly have a direct anticomedonal effect.

Patient counseling, adverse drug effects, and drug interactions
See chapter on anti-infective agents.

Isotretinoin

Isotretinoin is available in 10, 20, and 40 mg capsules. Trade names are Accutane, Amnesteem, Claravis, and Sotret.

Isotretinoin is for patients with severe, nodulocystic, draining acne who have not responded to systemic antibiotic therapy or who have required more than 3 years of systemic antibiotic therapy.

This agent is over 90% effective in producing an acne-free state for years following a 4- to 5-month course of therapy. Originally held in reserve for severe cases of nodulocystic acne, it may also be indicated as first-line treatment for severe acne that results in scarring.

Table 26-3. Oral Antimicrobials

Generic name	Trade name	Dosage and form
Tetracycline	Achromycin, Sumycin	500 mg qd or bid capsules
Erythromycin	E.E.S., Erythrocin	250–500 mg qd or bid tablets
Doxycycline	Vibramycin	100 mg qd capsules or tablets
Minocycline	Minocin	50 mg bid capsules

iPLEDGE program

The U.S. Food and Drug Administration (FDA) has approved an enhanced risk management program designed to minimize fetal exposure to isotretinoin known as iPLEDGE, which replaced the S.M.A.R.T. (System to Manage Accutane Related Teratogenicity) Program on December 30, 2005. iPLEDGE requires mandatory registration of prescribers, patients, wholesalers, and pharmacies to further the public health goal of eliminating fetal exposure to isotretinoin.

Pharmacies are not able to dispense isotretinoin to people with severe acne who do not enroll in the iPLEDGE program through a physician who is also enrolled. After a pharmacy registers for iPLEDGE at www.ipledgeprogram.com, the "Responsible Site Pharmacist" is sent a follow-up mailing, which contains instructions on how to activate the pharmacy.

The iPLEDGE program requires that all patients meet qualification criteria and monthly program requirements. Before the patient receives his or her isotretinoin prescription each month, the prescriber must counsel the patient and document in the iPLEDGE system that the patient has been counseled about the risks of isotretinoin.

Mechanism of action

Isotretinoin reduces sebum production (up to 90% inhibition). It decreases production of microcomedones, possibly by decreasing cohesiveness of follicular epithelial cells. It can have an anti-inflammatory effect.

Patient counseling

- Isotretinoin should be taken with food and is best absorbed with a fatty meal.
- Patients can take the dose divided twice daily or the entire dose with the evening meal.
- Effects are gradual, and acne may worsen during the first month of therapy; however, improvement usually begins by the sixth week of therapy.
- Use lip balm to treat cheilitis and moisturizers to treat dry skin.

Adverse drug effects

Isotretinoin is teratogenic. It is absolutely contraindicated in pregnancy because it causes significant birth defects. Females of childbearing potential must take measures to avoid pregnancy during the course of isotretinoin therapy.

Females should be tested for pregnancy before initiation of therapy and told to use two methods of contraception for at least 1 month prior to initiation of therapy and for 1 month after discontinuation of therapy.

Side effects and toxicity

- Most common (90–100%):
  - Cheilitis (chapped lips)
  - Dry mouth
  - Dry skin
  - Pruritus
- Common (30–40%):
  - Dry nose, leading to nasal crusting and epistaxis
  - Dry eyes, leading to conjunctivitis and problems with contact lenses
  - Muscular soreness or stiffness
- Less common (10–25%):
  - Headaches
  - Hyperlipidemia (primarily elevation of triglycerides, which may lead to attack of pancreatitis)
- Rare (less than 5%):
  - Decreased night vision
  - Thinning of hair
  - Easily injured skin
  - Peeling of palms and soles
  - Skin rash and skin infections
- Very rare (< 1%):
  - Acute depression (very rare, but reversible if detected early)
  - Pseudotumor cerebri (benign intracranial hypertension with visual disturbances)
- Treatment of most common side effects:
  - *Cheilitis:* Frequent use of lip balm
  - *Dry skin:* Skin lubrication with moisturizers
  - *Nosebleeds:* Lubrication of the nostrils with petrolatum
  - *Muscular soreness or stiffness:* Use of mild OTC analgesic and anti-inflammatory agents

Monitoring parameters

- Lipid panel
- Liver function tests (elevations common during initiation of therapy; usually return to normal during treatment).
- Complete blood counts
- Pregnancy testing for women prior to use of drug

Dosing

The dosage is 1 mg/kg once or twice daily with food; however, the patient may start out with 0.5 mg/kg/d for the first month before increasing. The drug is best absorbed with a fatty meal.

The goal is a total dose of 120–150 mg/kg over 4–5 months. Longer courses of 6–8 months may be required.

Other aspects

Approximately 20% of patients relapse within 1 year, and up to 40% relapse within 3 years after discontinuation of therapy. Repeat therapy for 4–6 months is acceptable and effective.

Oral corticosteroids

Oral corticosteroids are commonly known as *prom pills*. These agents can temporarily suppress acne with a 7- to 10-day course of prednisone 20 mg daily. They are rapidly effective when a brief course is necessary to cause prompt improvement (e.g., important social event such as wedding, prom, and so forth).

Systemic corticosteroids used continuously may actually cause or worsen acne. Topical corticosteroids have no value in the treatment of acne, and the high-potency topical corticosteroids will aggravate acne and should never be used on the faces of acne patients.

26-2. Fungal Skin Infections

Tinea are skin infections known as *dermatomycoses* caused by the fungi *Trichophyton, Microsporum,* and *Epidermophyton.*

Classification

- Tinea pedis (athlete's foot)
- Tinea capitis (ringworm of the scalp)
- Tinea cruris (jock itch)
- Tinea corporis (ringworm of the skin)
- Tinea unguium (onychomycosis; fungal infection of toenails and fingernails)

Pathophysiology

The fungi invade dead cells of the stratum corneum of skin, hair, and nails, digesting keratin. Unlike *Candida,* they cannot exist on unkeratinized mucous membranes.

This condition is more common in immunosuppressed patients.

Treatment Principles and Goals

- *Tinea pedis:* Self-treat topically initially; if ineffective, add orals.
- *Tinea capitis:* Use oral systemic therapy.
- *Tinea cruris:* Self-treat topically initially; if ineffective, add orals.
- *Tinea corporis:* Self-treat topically initially; if ineffective, add orals.
- *Tinea unguium:* Use oral systemic therapy.

Drug Therapy

OTC treatment

- Terbinafine 1% (Lamisil AT) cream, gel, and spray (most effective OTC antifungal agent)
- Miconazole 2% (Micatin, Cruex Spraypowder)
- Clotrimazole 1% (Lotrimin AF lotion, solution, and cream; Desenex AF)
- Tolnaftate 1% (Tinactin, Blis-To-Sol, Ting)
- Undecylenic acid 10–25% (Desenex)

Prescription treatment

See Table 26-4 for a description of prescription drugs.

Topicals

Newer antifungals are initially applied only once daily, and recurrences can be prevented by once- or twice-weekly applications.

Systemic therapy

Occasionally, topical therapy is not effective for tinea pedis, tinea cruris, and tinea corporis, and systemic antifungal therapy is required. Systemic therapy is also required for tinea capitis (ringworm of the scalp) and tinea unguium (fungal infection of the toenails and fingernails). Medications are as follows:

- Griseofulvin
- Ketoconazole
- Fluconazole
- Itraconazole
- Terbinafine

See chapter on anti-infective agents for discussion of systemic antifungals.

Table 26-4. Prescription Topical Antifungals

Generic name	Trade name
Econazole	Spectazole cream
Naftifine	Naftin gel, cream
Ciclopirox	Loprox gel, cream, lotion; Penlac solution
Butenafine	Mentax cream, Lotrimin Ultra

26-3. Hair Loss (Alopecia)

Male pattern baldness (androgenic alopecia) is the gradual and progressive loss of hair in males as they age.

Clinical Presentation

- Onset and progression vary greatly.
- A distinct pattern of progressive hair loss develops in the frontotemporal areas and crown with sparing of the occiput.
- Hair loss is limited to the scalp.
- Miniaturization of hair is seen, where normal thick terminal hairs are converted to very fine vellus hairs.

Pathophysiology

Alopecia is primarily due to two factors:

- Heredity (genetic)
- Testosterone

Testoterone, which promotes growth of hair in the beard, axillae, pubis, and other parts of the body, does not promote the growth of scalp hair. It actually contributes to premature loss because it is converted by the enzyme 5-α-reductase to dihydrotestosterone, which binds preferentially to receptors in the hair follicles on the scalp and causes them to produce progressively thinner hair until the follicles eventually cease activity altogether.

Treatment Principles and Goals

Although there is no cure for androgenic alopecia, two drugs are available for its treatment:

- Minoxidil (Rogaine, available OTC)
- Finasteride (Propecia, by prescription only)

In alopecia's early stages, topical minoxidil or oral finasteride may reverse the gradually decreasing diameter of the hair shaft.

Any hair growth stimulation is temporary and lasts only as long as therapy continues. If therapy is discontinued, new hair growth is lost within 1 year.

Early hair loss occurring recently in younger men is more likely to respond than later hair loss at an older age or when hair loss is not recent.

Alopecia of the crown in males responds better than does hair loss in the frontotemporal area.

Drug Therapy

Minoxidil

OTC trade names are Rogaine 2% and Rogaine Extra Strength 5%.

Mechanism of action

Minoxidil probably increases cutaneous blood flow directly to hair follicles due to vasodilation. It possibly stimulates resting hair follicles (telogen phase) into active growth (anagen phase). It possibly stimulates hair follicle cells.

Patient counseling

- Apply 1 mL twice daily (approximately one 60 mL bottle each month).
- Minoxidil may be applied without shampooing hair.
- Use at least 4 hours before bedtime to avoid oil on pillows and bed linens.
- The drug is absorbed over a 4-hour period, so do not swim, shampoo, or walk in rain for 4 hours.
- Wash hands immediately after application to prevent unwanted absorption.
- Do not inhale mist because systemic absorption is possible.
- Do not use on infected, irritated, inflamed, or sunburned skin.
- Discontinue use immediately and contact physician if chest pain, increased heart rate, faintness or dizziness, or swollen hands or feet occur.
- Women should avoid 5% strength (which has no better results than 2%); they have greater incidence of increased growth of facial hair with the 5% solution.
- Generally, treatment takes 4–6 months before any benefit occurs.
- No effects within 8 months for females and 12 months for males indicate therapeutic failure, and treatment should be discontinued.
- Patients must continue using minoxidil to maintain new hair growth.

Adverse drug effects

- Scalp dermatitis is common, producing dryness, pruritus, and flaking or scaling.
- Hypertrichosis (excessive hair growth) can occur on areas other than scalp (chest, forearms, ear rim, back, face, arms, and so forth).
- Some women report unwanted facial hair growth when minoxidil is applied to scalp, primarily with the 5% solution.

- Use may rarely produce systemic side effects (chest pain, increased heart rate, and faintness or dizziness).
- Use is contraindicated in patients less than age 18.
- Use is contraindicated in women who are pregnant or breastfeeding.

Finasteride

The trade name of finasteride is Propecia 1 mg. It was originally approved in 1992 for the treatment of enlarged prostate glands (benign prostatic hypertrophy) in a 5 mg dose (Proscar). A 1 mg daily dose is approved for males only as prescription treatment for androgenic alopecia.

Over a 2-year period, it may halt the progressive hair loss of androgenic alopecia.

Mechanism of action
Finasteride inhibits the enzyme 5-α-reductase, which is responsible for the conversion of testosterone to the more powerful dihydrotestosterone—the main androgen responsible for androgenic hair loss.

Patient counseling
- Take with or without food.
- Take for at least 3 months to see if the drug is effective.
- Improvement lasts only as long as treatment continues (new hair will be lost within 1 year of stopping treatment).

Adverse drug effects
- Gynecomastia (breast enlargement and tenderness) has been reported from 2 weeks to 2 years following initial therapy, but it is usually reversible when therapy is discontinued.
- Hypersensitivity (skin rash, swelling of lips)
- Decreased libido, erectile dysfunction, and ejaculatory dysfunction occur, which are reversible when the drug is discontinued.
- Use is contraindicated in females of childbearing age, because of abnormalities of the external genitalia in male fetuses; it is also not effective in postmenopausal females.

26-4. Dry Skin

This condition refers to lack of moisture or sebum in the stratum corneum. It most commonly occurs in the winter (also known as *winter rash*). It is more commonly present in older adults.

Clinical Presentation

- Flaking and scaling
- Xerosis and roughness
- Pruritus
- Loss of skin elasticity

Pathophysiology

Dry skin is due to inadequate moisture retention in the stratum corneum, which is caused by the following factors:

- Decreased sebum production and decreasing moisture-binding capacity of skin in elderly patients
- Low humidity, which causes the skin to lose water and become dry and hardened
- Overexposure to sunlight
- Excessive cleansing and bathing, which removes lipids and other skin components
- Chronic skin diseases that impair moisture retention of skin (psoriasis, scleroderma, ichthyosis, contact dermatitis)

Treatment Principles and Goals

The goal of treatment is to increase the moisture level of the stratum corneum by increasing cell hydration and binding capacity, which improves skin permeability and restores elasticity.

Drug Therapy
Emollients and moisturizing agents

Emollients and moisturizing agents include petrolatum and mineral oil (Lubriderm Bath and Shower Oil). They increase the relative moisture content of the stratum corneum and produce a general soothing effect by reducing frictional heat and perspiration.

Humectants

Humectants include glycerin (Corn Husker's Lotion), propylene glycol, and phospholipids. They are hygroscopic agents that increase hydration of the stratum corneum.

Keratin-softening agents

Keratin softening agents include the following:

- Urea (10–30%) (Aquacare and Carmol)
  - Improves the skin's moisture-binding capacity

- Provides keratolytic effect at higher concentrations
- May cause irritation and burning
■ Lactic acid (2–5%) (LactiCare)
  - Increases skin hydration by controlling the rate of keratinization
  - Is markedly hygroscopic
■ Allantoin (Alphosyl, Psorex, Tegrin)
  - Relieves dry skin by disrupting keratin structure (less effective than urea)
  - Desensitizes many skin-sensitizing drugs as a protectant

Antipruritic agents

Antipruritic agents include the following:

■ Camphor and menthol, which provide a cooling sensation
■ Local anesthetics (e.g., benzocaine, pramoxine)
■ Systemic antihistamines (H$_1$-receptor antagonists), which have limited effectiveness
■ Colloidal oatmeal (Aveeno)

Caution: Colloidal oatmeal can cause an extremely slippery bathtub.

Hydrocortisone

Hydrocortisone reduces the inflammatory response that accompanies dry skin conditions. Although it does not directly increase skin hydration, it does prevent itching associated with dry skin and inhibits dehydration.

Ointment is better than cream for dry skin. Patients should be counseled as follows.

■ Use sparingly.
■ Do not use more than 5–7 days for dry skin pruritus.

Astringents

Astringents include aluminum acetate 0.1–0.5% (Burow's solution) and hamamelis water (witch hazel).

Protectants

Zinc oxide is a protectant.

Nondrug Recommendations and Therapy

■ Bathe less frequently.
■ Reduce use of soap to a minimum and use only where necessary.

■ Lubricate skin immediately after bathing (i.e., apply bath oil after bathing and before drying).
■ Use extrafatted soaps such as Basis.

Combination products to treat dry skin

■ *Alpha Keri Moisture Rich Cleansing Bar:* Mineral oil, lanolin oil, and glycerin
■ *Aveeno Bath Treatment Moisturizing Formula:* Colloidal oatmeal and mineral oil
■ *Jergens Advanced Therapy Ultra Healing Lotion:* Dimethicone, lanolin, cetyl alcohol, isopropyl myristate, and glycerin
■ *Keri Original Dry Skin Lotion:* Mineral oil, lanolin oil, glyceryl stearate, and propylene glycol
■ *Moisturel Cream and Lotion:* Petrolatum, dimethicone, cetyl alcohol, and glycerin
■ *Neutrogena Body Oil:* Isopropyl myristate and sesame oil
■ *Pacquin Plus Dry Skin Hand and Body Cream:* Lanolin anhydrous, cetyl alcohol, and glycerin
■ *Vaseline Dermatology Formula Lotion:* White petrolatum, mineral oil, dimethicone, glyceryl stearate, cetyl alcohol, and glycerin

26-5. Dermatitis

Dermatitis is a nonspecific term describing a variety of inflammatory dermatologic conditions characterized by erythema. It is a general term describing any eczematous rash of unknown etiology that cannot be classified among the major endogenous dermatoses. *Eczema* and *dermatitis* are often used interchangeably.

Types and Classification

Several of the major classifications or types of dermatitis are

■ Atopic dermatitis (atopic eczema)
■ Chronic dermatitis (hand dermatitis)
■ Contact dermatitis (irritant and allergic)

Clinical Presentation

Atopic dermatitis (atopic eczema)

Atopic dermatitis occurs primarily in infants and children. It may disappear before adulthood. The cause is unknown but is possibly genetic.

Atopic dermatitis is usually seen on the face, knees, elbows, and neck. It is frequently seen with asthma, allergic rhinitis, and urticaria. Exacerbating factors include soaps, detergents, chemicals, temperature changes, molds, and allergens.

Chronic dermatitis (hand dermatitis or hand eczema)

Chronic dermatitis is a stubborn itchy rash referred to as *eczema* that occurs in certain persons with sensitive or irritable skin. The skin is very dry and easily irritated by overuse of soaps or detergents and by rough woolen clothing.

The condition is exacerbated by very hot or very cold weather. It is probably genetically determined. No permanent cure exists.

The condition usually can be controlled by enhancing skin hydration with emollients and moisturizers and by using hydrocortisone cream to relieve itching.

Contact dermatitis

Irritant contact dermatitis (chemical contact dermatitis)

The condition is caused by exposure to irritating substances producing mechanical or chemical trauma. Examples include soap, solvents, paints, abrasive cleansers, cosmetics, lubricants, antiseptics, cacti, rose hips, thorns, peppers, and tobacco.

Irritant contact dermatitis is not a sensitization, but direct toxicity to skin tissue.

Allergic contact dermatitis

The condition is a process of sensitization with reaction on elicitation. Over 50% of all dermatitis is allergic contact dermatitis.

Examples of reactive elements include benzocaine, zinc pyrithione (ZPT), neomycin, sodium bisulfite, perfumes, many cosmetics, skin lubricants, antiseptic creams, rubber and epoxy glues, poison ivy and oak, and many other common substances.

Treatment Principles and Goals

Treat dermatitis by applying a corticosteroid, according to the following principles:

- Ointments and creams are more lubricating than solutions, lotions, or gels.
- Ointments should be recommended if skin is dry.
- Lotions or gels should be recommended for a weeping, eczematous dermatitis.
- Lotions, solutions, and gels are also easier to use in hairy areas of the body.
- Apply small amounts of corticosteroid cream or ointment, and massage in gently but thoroughly.
- Apply the moderate- and high-strength cortisones only once daily.

- Improvement should begin within 1 week.
- Avoid excess soap, and keep skin lubricated with moisturizers.
- Treat itching with camphor, menthol, phenol, or local anesthetics.
- Occasionally with severe cases (less than 5%), patients may have to use systemic corticosteroids for 1–2 weeks.

Drug Therapy

Topical corticosteroids

See Table 26-5 for information about topical corticosteroids.

Adverse effects

- Striae may result in skin folds.
- Thinning of epidermis occurs where subcutaneous vessels become visible.
- The more potent types can cause or aggravate acne or rosacea on the face.
- Percutaneous absorption can lead to systemic effects (see Chapter 14 on endocrine drugs for complete list of systemic adverse effects).
  - Hyperglycemia
  - Glycosuria
  - Hypothalamic-pituitary-adrenal axis suppression, which could pose a threat in case of surgery, systemic illness, or trauma or injury
- Percutaneous absorption leads to systemic effects most likely with the following:
  - The higher potency types of agents
  - Inflamed skin (also in infants and children)
  - Long-term use or use over a large area of the skin
  - *Caution:* Occlusion markedly increases absorption of topical corticosteroids and should therefore be used cautiously in limited areas and reserved for severe, resistant lesions.

Topical antipruritics

Topical antipruritics include the following:

- Local anesthetics (benzocaine up to 20%, pramoxine 1%)
- Benzyl alcohol
- Colloidal oatmeal (Aveeno)
- Others (camphor, menthol, phenol)

Emollients

- Petrolatum
- Lanolin
- Mineral oil

Table 26-5. Typical Pharmaceutical Ingredients

Relative potency	Generic name	Trade name	Strength
Low	Hydrocortisone (OTC)	Cortaid, Cortizone	1% (OTC)
		Allercort, Hytone, Synacort, Emo-Cort	2.5% (prescription only)
Medium	Desonide	Tridesilon Des Owen	0.05%
	Fluocinolone acetonide	Synalar	0.01–0.025%
	Flurandrenolide	Cordran	0.025–0.05%
	Hydrocortisone butyrate	Locoid	0.1%
	Hydrocortisone valerate	Westcort	0.2%
	Triamcinolone acetonide	Aristocort	0.025%
High	Betamethasone valerate	Valisone, Dermabet	0.1%
	Fluocinolone	Synalar, Synemol	0.025%
	Triamcinolone acetonide	Aristocort	0.1%
Very high	Desoximetasone	Topicort	0.25%
	Diflorasone diacetate	Maxiflor	0.05%
	Fluocinonide	Lidex	0.01–0.05%
	Halcinonide	Halog	0.1%
Ultra-high	Betamethasone dipropionate	Diprosone, Maxivate	0.05%
	Betamethasone dipropionate (in optimized vehicle)	Diprolene AF	0.05%
	Clobetasol propionate	Temovate	0.05%
	Diflorasone diacetate	Psorcon	0.05%
	Halobetasol propionate	Ultravate	0.05%

Topical immunomodulators

Topical immunomodulators are approved for atopic dermatitis. They inhibit activation of T-cells and release of certain inflammatory mediators (cytokines).

The medication is applied bid, with onset in 1–3 weeks. Side effects include stinging, burning, pruritus, and rare flu-like symptoms. Patients should be cautioned to use sunscreen.

Immunomodulator products are as follows:

- Tacrolimus (Protopic) 0.03% and 0.1% ointment
- Pimecrolimus (Elidel) 1% cream

Oral corticosteroids

Corticosteroids are the only systemic anti-inflammatory agents that are effective.

Oral antihistamines

Oral antihistamines have very limited effectiveness but are possibly antipruritic.

26-6. Poison Ivy, Poison Oak, and Poison Sumac Allergy (*Rhus* Dermatitis)

Allergic reaction occurs to sap (urushiol) of some plants of the genus *Rhus* (poison ivy, poison oak, poison sumac). *Rhus* dermatitis is the most common form of allergic contact dermatitis.

Direct contact with leaves, roots, or branches is not required to get a rash. Sap can reach skin indirectly from clothing, a pet, or burning (volatilization).

A *Rhus* allergy is acquired; individuals are not born with it. Most persons are sensitized to *Rhus* because it is such a common plant; however, some people are never allergic to it. No effective way exists to desensitize a person with an allergy to *Rhus* plants.

Types and Classification

- *Mild:* Localized patches of pruritus and erythema develop, followed by appearance of vesicles and papules on the upper or lower extremities.

- **Moderate:** Extensive pruritus and irritation develop, with severe vesicles and appearance of bullae and edematous swelling.
- **Severe:** Extreme pruritus, irritation, and severe vesicle and bullae formation appear. Extensive involvement occurs, widespread over the body, face, or both. Extensive edema of the extremities or face develops. Eye, genitalia, or mucous membrane are involved.

Clinical Presentation

- *Rhus* dermatitis is not contagious.
- Fluid in blisters does not spread rash.
- Rash appears after a latent period that varies from 4 hours to 10 days, depending on an individual's sensitivity and the amount of plant contact.
- When more rash appears after treatment has begun, these are areas with a longer latent period.
- Symptoms may last from 5 to 21 days following initial rash.
- Secondary infections can occur if scratching excoriates the skin and the abrasions become infected.

Treatment Principles and Goals

Rhus dermatitis is self-limited. Mild cases will clear without treatment within 7–14 days.

The goal of treatment is to prevent itching and excessive scratching and possible secondary skin infections.

Treatment options

- *Mild cases:* Use topical antipruritics, such as calamine, camphor, menthol, phenol, or local anesthetics to prevent itching and topical hydrocortisone cream or ointment.
- *Moderate cases:* Use topical high-potency corticosteroids for small areas.
- *Severe cases:* Use systemic corticosteroids daily up to 2 weeks. Severe rash needs systemic corticosteroids to ease the misery and disability. Systemic corticosteroids are usually needed during early severe stages because remedies applied to skin may not penetrate deeply enough.

Therapy
OTC topical therapy

Astringents and protectants
Compresses, soaks, or wet dressings will dry the oozing, reduce the weeping, aid in removal of crusts, and soothe the skin. They include

- Aluminum acetate solution 1:40 ratio (Burow's solution)
- Aluminum sulfate (Domeboro powder)
- Calamine lotion
- Other products such as aluminum hydroxide gel, kaolin, zinc acetate, zinc carbonate, and zinc oxide

Local anesthetics
These products may contain benzocaine up to 20%, pramoxine 1%, and benzyl alcohol. They include

- *Caladryl lotion:* Calamine and pramoxine 1%
- *Ruli calamine spray:* Calamine, benzocaine, and camphor
- *Ivarest 8-Hour Medicated Cream:* Calamine and diphenhydramine 2%
- *Ivy Dry Cream:* Benzyl alcohol, camphor, menthol, and zinc acetate

Other products
Other products include

- Hydrocortisone 1% products
- Colloidal oatmeal (Aveeno) for temporary skin protection from exposures
- Cool compresses

Prescription topical therapy

Use topical medium- to high-potency corticosteroids (see discussion on allergic contact dermatitis in Section 26-5).

Prescription systemic corticosteroid therapy

Use of systemic corticosteroids is the only therapy that will actually reduce the severity and duration of the allergic response. See the discussion on allergic contact dermatitis in Section 26-5 and the discussion on endocrine disorders in Chapter 14 for complete details.

Effects of oral corticosteroids are dramatic (patients can take up to 40–100 mg prednisone for 2 or 3 weeks if necessary); however, many patients clear up quickly with a corticosteroid dosepak (e.g., Decadron or Medrol). Extremely severe cases or large-scale rash may require parenteral dose of corticosteroid (100 mg prednisone equivalent).

Other recommendations

Prevention
- *Avoidance:* Identify the plants—"leaves of three, let it be."
- *Removal:* Washing with soap and water within 15 minutes of exposure may reduce the extent and duration of dermatitis.

■ *Use of bentoquatam 5% solution:* Marketed under the trade name Ivy Block, this lotion is an organoclay. It is the only barrier product approved by the FDA. Patient instructions are to apply the lotion 15 minutes before possible plant contact and reapply every 4 hours.

26-7. Scaly Dermatoses

There are three common forms of scaly dermatoses: dandruff, seborrhea, and psoriasis.

Dandruff

Dandruff is a chronic, noninflammatory scalp condition resulting in excessive scaling of the scalp epidermis. It is a common condition affecting 20% of the population. Though not a serious disorder, dandruff can be cosmetically unsightly.

Clinical presentation

Scaling and pruritus occur, causing white flakes to accumulate on the scalp.

Pathophysiology

Increased epidermal cell turnover rate of approximately twice normal (time reduced from 25–30 days to 13–15 days) prevents complete keratinization of desquamated cells due to unknown processes. Dandruff may be related to increased *Pityrosporum ovale* (*P ovale*), a fungal scalp organism.

Treatment

Routine shampooing with mild hypoallergenic shampoo is essential.

Cytostatic agents

Cytostatic agents suppress cell turnover. The goal is to reduce the epidermal rate of turnover of scalp cells. Agents and their mechanisms of action are as follows:

■ *ZPT (0.3–2%):* Products include Denorex, Head and Shoulders, Sebulon, X-Seb, and Zincon. ZPT has antifungal effect and reduces cell turnover rate.
■ *Selenium sulfide 1%:* Products include Head and Shoulders Intensive Treatment, Selsun Blue 1%, and Selsun 2.5%. Selenium sulfide reduces the cell rate turnover and inhibits growth of *P ovale*.

■ *Coal tar:* Products include Balnetar, Denorex, DHS Tar, Ionil T, Neutrogen T, Pentrax, and Polytar. Coal tar reduces the number and size of epidermal cells.

Patient should be counseled that contact time with cytostatic agents is very important for effectiveness. Advise patients to rub shampoo in well and leave it in up to 5 minutes before rinsing it out.

Keratolytic agents

Keratolytic agents include the following:

■ *Salicylic acid (1.8–3%):* Products include Ionil, Neutrogena, Scalpicin, and Sebucare. Salicylic acid can lower the pH of tissues, thereby increasing the water concentration of epidermal cells, which softens and destroys the stratum corneum. It causes the upper skin layer to become inflamed and soft, followed by desquamation. This keratolytic action removes the scales of dandruff.
■ *Sulfur (2–5%):* Products include Sulfoam, Sulray, and Exsel. Sulfur possibly exerts an antifungal effect. Sulfur is usually found in combinations with salicylic acid.
■ *Combination of sulfur and salicylic acid:* Products include Meted and Sebulex.

Antifungals

Antifungals include the following:

■ Ketoconazole (1%) shampoo (Nizoral AD)
■ Ciclopirox 1% shampoo (Loprox)

Ciclopirox is active against *P ovale*. Patients should be counseled to use it twice weekly or every 3 or 4 days. Stress adequate contact time for a minimum of 3 minutes. Adverse effects include itching, stinging, or irritation.

Seborrhea (Seborrheic Dermatitis)

Seborrhea is a chronic inflammatory skin disease in areas of greatest sebaceous gland activity—on the scalp and other hairy areas such as the face, trunk, armpits, and groin. Seborrhea is not contagious. It persists for life, but it can be controlled.

Clinical presentation

■ Scaling rash accompanied by pruritus
■ Yellowish, greasy scales unlike the dry scales of dandruff
■ Inflammation, often accompanied by erythema

- Fluctuation in severity, characterized by exacerbations and remissions
- Most common on the face, eyebrows, and eyelashes, but not on the extremities
- Aggravated and worsened by nervous stress and poor health

Pathophysiology

- Accelerated cell turnover rate is approximately three times normal rate, probably as few as 9–10 days.
- Seborrhea has a higher cell turnover rate than dandruff, but less than psoriasis.
- *P ovale* may be causative, but this is not universally accepted.

Treatment

Treatment is similar to that for dandruff, but seborrhea is more difficult to treat. Overuse of selenium can make the scalp oily and actually exacerbate seborrhea.

Topical corticosteroids (e.g., Cortaid) are used to control itching and inflammation (up to 7 days) Add the topical antifungal ketoconazole 1% shampoo (Nizoral AD) or ciclopirox 1% shampoo (Loprox). The combination is active against *P ovale*. Patients should be counseled to use it twice weekly, every 3 or 4 days. Stress adequate contact time; leave it in for at least 3 minutes. Adverse effects include itching, stinging, or irritation.

"Cradle cap" (infantile seborrheic dermatitis)

Cradle cap is seborrhea of the scalp in newborns or infants. It is most common in the first few months of life. It is usually on top of head and may be due to poor washing.

Cradle cap is probably not related to fungal infection. It is treated as follows:

- Massage with oils.
- Use nonmedicated shampoos.
- Use milder keratolytics (Meted and Sebulex) two or three times per week.

Psoriasis

Psoriasis is a chronic inflammatory papulosquamous erythematous skin disease. It is marked by the presence of silvery scales with sharply delineated edges. Lesions are usually localized, but can gradually grow to cover large areas.

Psoriasis can have significant physiological and psychological effects. It affects 1–3% of the population, 98% Caucasian.

Classification

- *Type I:* Characterized by early age of onset, family history, and increased frequency of human lymphocyte antigen
- *Type II:* Characterized by development later in life and no family history

Pathophysiology

A hyperproliferative skin condition results from skin cell turnover rate of approximately 10–20 times normal. Skin cells of psoriatic plaque reach the outermost layer in 3–4 days.

A genetic predisposition contributes, as well as exposure of the skin to trauma or triggering factors such as stressful incidents.

Clinical presentation

- Plaque is most common and is known as *psoriasis vulgaris.*
- Plaque is known also as *scales*—silvery on top and pink to red beneath.
- Plaque may be found anywhere on the body, but more likely on scalp, sacral area, and extensor surfaces of knees and elbows (less common on face).
- Borders of plaque are sharp with inflammation surrounding the plaque.
- Psoriasis is a chronic condition and varies from mild forms of the disease to very severe, with such extensive coverage that it hinders social and work life.
- It is marked by spontaneous exacerbations and remissions.

Treatment

Topicals
Topical treatments are as follows:

- Topical corticosteroids
- Coal tar (contained in Denorex, DHS, Ionil T, MG217, Neutrogena T, Pantene Pro-V, Polytar, Tegrin, and X-Seb T Plus)
- Keratolytics (salicylic acid, sulfur)
- Combinations of salicylic acid, sulfur, and coal tar (Sebutone)

- Retinoids (tretinoin, adapalene, tazarotene, alitretinoin)
- Anthralin (Anthraforte, Anthranol, Dritho-Scalp)
- Calcipotriene (Dovonex ointment, cream, and solution—a vitamin D_3 analog)

Caution: If used in conjugation with PUVA (psoralens with ultraviolet-A) therapy, calcipotriene should be applied after light treatment, because PUVA inactivates this product.

Systemic treatment
Systemic treatment may involve the following:

- Oral corticosteroids
- Antimetabolites, such as methotrexate and cyclosporine
- Psoralens (combined with ultraviolet light therapy)
- Immunosuppressants, such as alefacept (Amevive) and etanercept (Enbrel)
- Retinoids, such as acitretin (Soriatane)

Vitamin A analogs are reserved for severe and extensive psoriasis. Their effectiveness approaches that of methotrexate or cyclosporine when combined with ultraviolet light therapy. Adverse effects include dry lips, skin, nail changes, dry eyes, hair loss, hyperlipidemia, pancreatitis, hepatotoxicity, myalgias, and arthralgias. Such drugs are teratogenic. The above listed AE are primarily with systemic therapy; however, topical therapy may also be teratogenic.

Other therapy
Ultraviolet light therapy is also used, often following coal tar applications or concurrent with oral psoralens.

26-8. Pediculosis

Head lice is the primary or most common form of pediculosis. Lice are very common, especially in schoolchildren. They are transmitted by direct contact with the head of an infected individual or through fomites (inanimate objects capable of transmitting disease, such as shared combs, brushes, or headwear). Lice are most common in August and September, after long holidays or summer camps.

Body lice are a less common form that usually occur in individuals who do not change clothing often (e.g., the homeless).

Pubic lice (crab lice) are transferred through sexual contact and are found primarily in pubic areas, but they can also affect armpits.

Classification
There are three types of human pediculosis:

- *Head lice: Pediculus humanus capitis*
- *Body lice: Pediculus humanus corporis* (same species as head lice)
- *Pubic lice: Pthirus pubis* (different species)

Clinical Presentation

- Pruritus is the most common symptom.
- Because lice are often symptomatic, diagnosis is made visually by seeing live lice.
- The flat, gray-brown adult lice are difficult to locate or visualize; the nits (larvae) firmly attached to hair shafts may be more visible.

Drug Therapy
Synergized pyrethrins (0.17–0.33%)

This drug is a natural chemical derived from chrysanthemums that is synergized by addition of 2–4% piperonyl butoxide (petroleum derivative). Trade names include A-200, End-Lice, Lice-Enz, Pronto, R&C shampoo, and Rid.

Mechanism of action
Transmission of nerve cell impulses is blocked in lice, causing paralysis.

Patient counseling
- Wash and dry hair and apply for 10 minutes.
- Use a lice–nit combination to remove dead lice and nits following rinsing.
- Treat all family members.
- Avoid contact with the eyes, mouth, and nose
- Do not use on irritated or inflamed scalp.
- Repeat treatment in 1 week to 10 days.

Adverse drug effects
Adverse effects include irritation, erythema, and itching.

Permethrin 1% and 5%

Permethrin is a synthetic chemical derivative of pyrethrin. Permethrin 1% is available under the trade name Nit Cream Rinse. Permethrin 5%, at prescription-only strength, is available under the trade names Acticin and Elimite Cream.

The 1% OTC-strength treatment is approved for head lice only; however, it is effective against pubic lice. The 5% prescription-strength treatment is approved for scabies l (mites) infestation.

Patients prefer these treatments because of single-application effectiveness.

Mechanism of action
- Transmission of nerve cell impulses is blocked in lice, causing paralysis.

Patient information
- Apply to washed hair and scalp.
- Leave on hair for 10 minutes, and then rinse.
- After rinsing, comb hair with lice comb to remove lice and nits.
- This is a one-time treatment; do not repeat for 10 days.
- All family members should be treated.

Adverse effects
Scalp irritation, pruritus, and stinging may occur. This medication is contraindicated in patients who are allergic to chrysanthemums and in children under age 2.

Lindane (Kwell shampoo, cream, and lotion; prescription only)

Formerly named gamma benzene hexachloride, lindane is effective against head lice and public lice and against scabies (caused by *Sarcoptes scabiei*).

Adverse effects
Lindane is absorbed significantly through the skin and has been reported to have significant neurotoxic effects, especially in infants and children. Central nervous system effects reported include convulsions, dizziness, lack of coordination, restlessness, and irritability. Other effects include rapid heartbeat, muscle cramps, and vomiting.

The OTC medications are considered much safer, especially in children.

Nondrug recommendations

- Change clothing daily.
- Treat infested clothes, and shower daily.
- All household contacts should be inspected and treated if necessary.
- All bed linens and clothes should be dry cleaned or washed in the hot water cycle and dried on the heated-air cycle for at least 20 minutes.
- Wash hairbrushes, combs, and toys in hot water for at least 10 minutes.

- Treat surrounding environment (bedding, pillows, carpets, draperies, and furniture) with A-200 Control Spray or Rid Control Spray.

26-9. Warts

Warts (verrucae) are harmless skin growths resulting from an infectious disease caused by the human papillomavirus.

Classification

- Common warts (verruca vulgaris) are on fingers, hands, and knees.
- Common flat warts (verruca plana) are on face, hands, and legs.
- Plantar warts (verruca plantaris) are on the soles of the feet.
- Anogenital warts (verruca genitalia) are on the anogenital area.

Clinical Presentation

- Warts are contagious, and may spread on the body.
- Warts are more common in children and immunocompromised patients.
- Warts on the face or hands protrude.
- Warts occurring on pressure areas such as the bottom of the feet (plantar warts) grow inward from the pressure of standing and walking, are often painful, and may be confused with corns.

Treatment Principles and Goals

Warts can be eliminated by the following:

- Direct application of caustics, such as salicylic acid, formalin, lactic acid, trichloroacetic acid, and podophyllin
- Freezing (cryotherapy) with liquid nitrogen or with dimethyl ether and propane
- Surgery

OTC drug therapy

Salicylic acid
Patients should be counseled as follows:

- Use topical salicylic acid preparations on a daily basis until the wart is removed.
- Because warts are contagious, use special care in washing hands before and after treatment, and

use a separate towel for drying other parts of the body.

- Do not use salicylic acid on irritated, broken, or infected skin.
- If the wart remains after 12 weeks of continuous treatment, see a dermatologist or podiatrist.

Salicylic acid products are contraindicated in patients with diabetes and other patients with poor circulation because reduced sensation in the foot delays awareness of skin breakdown, allowing possible development of infection that can lead to sepsis. Diabetic patients should see a physician or podiatrist for removal of warts.

OTC salicylic acid products are as follows:

- *Salicylic acid 17% in flexible collodion vehicle:* Compound W gel and liquid, Dr. Scholl's Fast Acting Liquid, Duofilm, Wart-Off, and Off-Ezy Wart Remover Kit
- *Salicylic acid 40% embedded in pads or discs:* Compound W One Step Pads, Dr. Scholl's Clear Away, DuoFilm, and Dr. Scholl's Clear Away Wart Remover Patch

Cryotherapy

Dimethyl ether and propane is FDA approved for OTC removal of common warts and plantar warts.

Cryotherapy irritation leads the host to produce an immune response against the causative virus (similar to liquid nitrogen, which can be administered only by a primary care provider). As a result of freezing, a blister will form under the wart. After about 10 days, the frozen skin and wart fall off, revealing newly formed skin underneath.

Cryotherapy products are as follows:

- *Dimethyl ether and propane:* Dr. Scholl's Freeze Away Wart Remover and Wartner Wart Removal System are approved for removal of common warts.
- *Dimethyl ether, propane, and isobutane:* Compound W Freeze Off is approved for removal of common warts and plantar warts.

Patient instructions are as follows:

- Place the applicator in the spray can, which becomes very cold (−55°C)
- After the applicator is saturated, hold it on the wart for a product-specific time period to freeze the wart (20 seconds for Wartner; 40 seconds for Compound W).
- The process may be repeated after 10 days as many as three or four times for persistent warts.

- *Caution:* Do not use in children under age 4, diabetics, or pregnant or breastfeeding females; on the face, armpits, breasts, buttocks or genitals; on irritated skin; or on mucous membranes (e.g., mouth, nose, and anus).

26-10. Corns and Calluses

Corns and calluses are excessive growth of the upper keratinized layer of the skin. They are more common in women than in men.

Diabetics have an increased incidence of calluses on their feet because of the loss of sensation, preventing them from noticing the pressure that would otherwise be uncomfortable.

Classification

- *Hard corns (heloma durum):* Corns overlying a bony prominence such as the toes or bottom of the heel
- *Soft corns (heloma molle; interdigital corns):* Corns between the toes (especially the fourth and fifth)
- *Calluses (callosities):* Superficial patches of hornified epidermis; flattened, but thickened with no central core

Clinical Presentation and Pathophysiology

Corns and calluses are caused by excessive growth of the upper keratinized layer of the skin (hyperkeratosis), resulting from friction or pressure, usually from improper or tight-fitting shoes.

Treatment

The only FDA-approved OTC medication is salicylic acid formulated in flexible collodion, plasters, disks, or pads.

Mechanism of action

Salicylic acid produces a keratolytic action, which increases hydration and lowers the pH of the outer skin, initially softening and then destroying the outer layer of skin.

Patient counseling

- Do not apply to irritated, infected, or reddened skin.

- If discomfort persists after using for 14 days, see a physician or podiatrist.
- Salicylic acid products are contraindicated in diabetics.

Adverse drug effects

Salicylic acid products are contraindicated in patients with diabetes and other patients with poor circulation because reduced sensation in the foot delays awareness of skin breakdown, allowing possible development of infection that can lead to sepsis. Refer diabetics to a physician or podiatrist for removal of corns or calluses.

OTC salicylic acid (SA) corn and callus products

- Freezone Corn and Callus Remover 13.6% SA
- Freezone One Step Corn Remover 40% SA
- Mediplast 40% SA plaster, cut to size
- Mosco Corn and Callus Remover 17.6% SA
- Off Ezy Corn and Callus Remover 17% SA
- One Step Callus Remover 40% SA
- Dr. Scholl's Corn and Callus Remover Liquid 12.6% SA
- Dr. Scholl's Corn or Callus Cushion Gel 40% SA
- Dr. Scholl's One Step Corn or Callus Remover Disc 40% SA

26-11. Key Points

Acne

- Acne occurs primarily in the teenage years because of the increase of androgens during puberty that produces increased activity of the sebaceous glands.
- Isotretinoin (Accutane) is the drug of choice for nodulocystic acne (type IV acne), which, if left untreated, will lead to extensive scarring.
- Isotretinoin is contraindicated in pregnancy because of the high incidence of serious birth defects.
- The most common side effects of isotretinoin are cheilitis (dry, chapped lips), dry skin, and dry eyes.

Fungal Infections of the Skin

- The most efficacious nonprescription topical antifungal is terbinafine (Lamisil).
- Systemic antifungal therapy is required for treatment of tinea capitis (ringworm of the scalp) and tinea unguium (fungal infection of the toenails and fingernails).

Hair Loss

- Androgenic alopecia—predominantly seen in males—is due to the conversion of testosterone to dihydrotestosterone, which binds to the hair follicles and causes them to produce progressively thinner hair.
- In the treatment of androgenic alopecia, minoxidil (Rogaine) should be applied and left on the scalp for 4 hours for maximum effects.
- Finasteride (Propecia) decreases the effect of androgens on hair follicles by inhibiting 5-α-reductase, which prevents the conversion of testosterone to dihydrotestosterone.

Dry Skin

- Dry skin occurs primarily in older adults because of decreased sebum production and decreased moisture-binding capacity of the skin.
- Products containing urea and lactic acid improve the skin's moisture-binding capacity, thereby increasing skin hydration.

Dermatitis

- Contact dermatitis, whether irritant or allergic, is initially treated with topical corticosteroid products.
- The absorption and subsequent adverse systemic effects of topical corticosteroids are increased in infant skin and with occlusion, the use of high-potency agents, and long-term use.

Poison Ivy, Poison Oak, and Poison Sumac

- Poison ivy, poison oak, and poison sumac are examples of causes of allergic contact dermatitis, which are the result of contact with the sap of plants of the genus *Rhus*.
- Severe cases of poison ivy, poison oak, or poison sumac require systemic corticosteroids to relieve symptoms, decrease the severity of the rash, and shorten the course of the disorder.

Scaly Dermatoses

- The cytostatic agents that suppress cell rate turnover—zinc pyrithione (Head and Shoulders) and selenium sulfide (Selsun Blue)—are the primary agents of choice for treatment of dandruff.
- Seborrhea usually requires topical corticosteroids or the topical antifungal ketoconazole for effective treatment.

- Psoriasis is a chronic inflammatory disease characterized by inflammation and silvery scales (known as *plaques*) with sharp delineated edges.
- Treatment of advanced psoriasis may require systemic corticosteroids or antimetabolites in addition to topical treatments for effective management of the disease.

Pediculosis

- Head lice (*Pediculus humanus capitis*) occur most commonly in elementary schoolchildren in the months of August and September.
- Permethrin (Nix) is the nonprescription agent of choice for treatment of head lice because it usually does not have to be repeated in 7–10 days as do other available nonprescription pediculicidal agents (synergized pyrethrins).

Corns and Warts

- Nonprescription products for the treatment of corns and warts contain salicylic acid.
- Self-treatment for corns or warts with over-the-counter agents is not recommended for diabetic patients because of reduced sensation in their feet that delays awareness of possible development of infections and can lead to sepsis.
- Warts result from an infection of the human papilloma virus and, therefore, are contagious and may spread on the body.
- Warts may be eliminated by surgery, freezing with liquid nitrogen (cryotherapy), or the direct application of caustics (e.g., salicylic acid, formalin, lactic acid, trichloroacetic acid, or podophyllin).

26-12. Questions

1. Initial treatment of mild to moderate acne would include which of the following?

   I.   Topical antimicrobials
   II. Topical retinoids
   III. Isotretinoin

   A. I only
   B. II only
   C. III only
   D. I and II
   E. I, II, and III

2. Acne is due to which of the following?

   I.   Increased sebum production
   II. Obstruction of hair follicle openings
   III. Inflammation

   A. I only
   B. II only
   C. III only
   D. I and II
   E. I, II, and III

3. Patients using topical retinoids such as tretinoin (Retin-A) should be counseled to do which of the following?

   I.   Use sunblock before exposure to sunlight.
   II. Do not use tretinoin with astringents, drying agents, or abrasive soaps.
   III. Expect rapid improvement within 2 or 3 days of starting therapy.

   A. I only
   B. II only
   C. III only
   D. I and II
   E. I, II, and III

4. The most common side effects of isotretinoin (Accutane) include which of the following?

   I.   Cheilitis (dry chapped lips)
   II. Acute depression
   III. Decreased night vision

   A. I only
   B. II only
   C. III only
   D. I and II
   E. I, II, and III

5. Which of the following is an important contraindication and precaution to the use of isotretinoin?

   A. Hypertension
   B. Migraines
   C. Allergic rhinitis
   D. Pregnancy
   E. Streptococcal infections

6. Which of the following is the most efficacious nonprescription topical antifungal?

   A. Tolnaftate (Tinactin)
   B. Terbinafine (Lamisil)
   C. Miconazole (Micatin)

D. Undecylenic acid (Desenex)

E. Clotrimazole (Lotrimin AF)

7. Which of these fungal infections may be treated effectively with the use of topical antifungal agents?

   I.   Tinea capitis (ringworm of the scalp)

   II. Tinea unguium (fungal infection of the toenails and fingernails)

   III. Tinea corporis (ringworm of the skin)

A. I only

B. II only

C. III only

D. I and II

E. I, II, and III

8. Tinea pedis is also known as

A. athlete's foot.

B. jock itch.

C. onychomycosis.

D. ringworm of the scalp.

E. ringworm of the skin.

9. The treatment of choice for tinea unguium would be

A. clotrimazole.

B. miconazole.

C. undecylenic acid.

D. griseofulvin.

E. tolnaftate.

10. All of the following are true regarding androgenic alopecia *except*

A. it is predominantly seen in males.

B. it is caused by the conversion of testosterone to dihydrotestosterone, which binds to the hair follicles, causing them to produce progressively thinner hair.

C. hair growth stimulation is temporary and lasts only as long as therapy continues.

D. hair loss in the frontotemporal area responds to treatment better than hair loss on the crown.

E. Early hair loss occurring recently in young males is more likely to respond than later hair loss at an older age.

11. All of the following are true regarding the patient instructions for the proper use of minoxidil *except*

A. it should be applied on the scalp and left for 4 hours for maximum effect.

B. the patient should not swim, shampoo, or walk in rain soon after the application of minoxidil.

C. do not use on infected, irritated, inflamed, or sunburned skin.

D. the patient must continue therapy to maintain effectiveness.

E. women with alopecia should use the 5% strength of minoxidil rather than the 2% strength.

12. Adverse effects of minoxidil include which of the following?

   I.   Hypertrichosis

   II. Dermatitis and pruritus of the scalp

   III. Hepatic damage

A. I only

B. II only

C. III only

D. I and II

E. I, II, and III

13. The mechanism of action of finasteride (Propecia) to reduce male baldness is

A. a direct effect on hair follicles to deepen hair roots.

B. inhibition of the enzyme 5-α-reductase, which blocks the conversion of testosterone to dihydrotestosterone.

C. increased cutaneous blood flow to the hair follicles on the scalp because of vasodilation.

D. increased cutaneous blood flow to the hair follicles on the scalp because of opening the potassium channel.

E. increased development of new hair follicles on the scalp.

14. All of the following are true regarding finasteride *except*

A. it is contraindicated in females of childbearing age.

B. it was originally approved for treatment of benign prostatic hypertrophy.

C. improvement lasts only as long as treatment continues (new hair will be lost within 1 year of stopping treatment).

D. it must be taken on an empty stomach for complete absorption.

E. 2% of males report reversible sexual dysfunction while taking it.

15. All of the following regarding dry skin are true *except*

   A. it occurs primarily in older adults.
   B. it occurs most commonly in the summer months.
   C. it is caused by decreasing sebum production and decreased moisture-binding capacity of the skin.
   D. flaking, scaling, xerosis, and pruritus are common manifestations of dry skin.
   E. excessive cleansing and bathing removes lipids and worsens dry skin.

16. All of the following statements are true regarding the treatment of dry skin *except*

   A. hydrocortisone should be used only for short-term therapy of dry skin to relieve itching.
   B. urea-containing products improve the skin's moisture-binding capacity.
   C. lactic acid is a keratolytic agent that removes the upper epidermal skin cells and relieves the itching of dry skin.
   D. emollients and moisturizers are helpful in the treatment of dry skin, especially when applied immediately after bathing.
   E. although colloidal oatmeal may be helpful in the treatment of dry skin, patients should be cautioned about the possibility of falling because of a slippery bathtub.

17. The agents of choice for the initial treatment of contact dermatitis, whether irritant or allergic, are

   A. topical antihistamines.
   B. oral antihistamines.
   C. topical corticosteroids.
   D. local anesthetics.
   E. coal tar products.

18. An increase in topical corticosteroid systemic absorption with subsequent systemic side effects may be seen in which of the following?

   I.   Occlusion
   II. Infant's skin
   III. Long-term use of high-potency agents

   A. I only
   B. II only
   C. III only
   D. I and II
   E. I, II, and III

19. All of the following are true regarding poison ivy *except*

   A. it is an example of allergic contact dermatitis.
   B. it is the result of contact with the sap of plants of the genus *Rhus*.
   C. the treatment of choice is desensitization.
   D. it may be caused by direct or indirect contact (e.g., with clothing or pets).
   E. skin eruptions may occur from several hours up to 10 days following contact with the plants.

20. The treatment of choice for severe or extensive cases of poison ivy or poison oak is

   A. a local anesthetic such as benzocaine.
   B. bentoquatam (Ivy Block).
   C. a camphor and menthol antipruritic.
   D. colloidal oatmeal.
   E. a systemic corticosteroid.

21. Which of the following agents for treatment of dandruff are cytostatic agents that suppress cell rate turnover?

   I.   Zinc pyrithione (Head and Shoulders)
   II. Selenium sulfide (Selsun Blue)
   III. Salicylic acid (Ionil)

   A. I only
   B. II only
   C. III only
   D. I and II
   E. I, II, and III

22. All of the following statements are true regarding seborrhea *except*

   A. it is a chronic inflammatory skin disease seen in areas of greatest sebaceous gland activity.
   B. it fluctuates in severity and is worsened by stress and poor health.
   C. moderate to severe cases require topical corticosteroids or the topical antifungal ketoconazole for effective treatment.

D. it is called *cradle cap* when it occurs in infants.

E. it most commonly occurs on the legs and arms.

23. Which of the following are characteristic of psoriasis?

    I.   Chronic inflammation
    II. Silvery scales (known as *plaques*) with sharply delineated edges
    III. Spontaneous exacerbations and remissions

    A. I only
    B. II only
    C. III only
    D. I and II
    E. I, II, and III

24. Treatment of advanced psoriasis may require topical therapy combined with which of the following systemic agents?

    I.   Corticosteroids
    II. Antimetabolites such as methotrexate
    III. Anthralin

    A. I only
    B. II only
    C. III only
    D. I and II
    E. I, II, and III

25. All of the following are true statements regarding head lice (*Pediculus humanus capitis*) *except*

    A. it occurs most commonly in elementary schoolchildren.
    B. it occurs most commonly in the spring months of April and May.
    C. it is transmitted by direct contact.
    D. pruritus is the most common symptom.
    E. head lice is the most common type of pediculosis infestation.

26. All of the following statements are true regarding treatment of pediculosis with synergized pyrethrins (piperonyl butoxide and pyrethrins) *except*

    A. inspect all family contacts, and treat if necessary.
    B. apply after washing and drying the hair, and leave on overnight.

C. remove dead lice and nits after treatment with a lice or nit comb.
D. repeat treatment in 7–10 days.
E. avoid contact with the eyes, nose, and mouth.

27. The most effective nonprescription agent for treatment of head lice is which of the following agents?

    A. Permethrin (Nix)
    B. Synergized pyrethrins (A-200)
    C. Lindane (Kwell)
    D. Ketoconazole
    E. Salicylic acid

28. Nonprescription products for the treatment of corns and warts contain which of the following agents?

    A. Salicylic acid
    B. Ketoconazole
    C. Lactic acid
    D. Acetylsalicylic acid
    E. Hydrocortisone

29. All of following are true statements regarding corns *except:*

    A. They are excess growth of the upper keratinized layer of skin.
    B. Salicylic acid is available in pads, disks, or flexible collodion for removal of corns.
    C. Self-treatment for corns or warts with OTC agents is not recommended for diabetic patients because of the reduced sensation in their feet, which delays awareness of development of infections and may lead to sepsis.
    D. They are contagious and may spread on the body.
    E. They are usually caused by pressure or friction from improper or tight-fitting shoes.

30. All of the following are true statements regarding warts *except*

    A. they result from infection with the human papillomavirus.
    B. they are contagious.
    C. they may spread on the body.
    D. plantar warts are located on the fingers, hands, and knees.
    E. they are more common in children and immunocompromised patients.

31. Warts may be eliminated by which of the following procedures?

    I.   Surgery
    II. Freezing with liquid nitrogen (cryotherapy)
    III. The direct application of caustics (e.g., salicylic acid)

    A. I only
    B. II only
    C. III only
    D. I and II
    E. I, II, and III

26-13. Answers

1. **D.** Topical antimicrobials and topical retinoids are the agents of choice for mild to moderate acne. Isotretinoin (Accutane) is reserved for nodulocystic acne (type IV acne), which, if left untreated, will lead to extensive scarring.

2. **E.** Acne is primarily due to (a) hormonal changes occurring at or near puberty that increase sebum production and obstruct the hair follicle opening and (b) the breaking down of triglycerides to free fatty acids caused by enzymes from *Propionibacterium acnes*, which causes inflammation.

3. **D.** Topical retinoid therapy will sensitize skin to ultraviolet light rays; therefore, patients should use sunblock prior to sun exposure. Patients using topical retinoids should use only mild soaps for cleansing the face and avoid astringents, drying agents, and abrasive soaps. Improvement will usually occur within 2–3 weeks after initiation of therapy.

4. **A.** Cheilitis (dry chapped lips), together with dry skin and dry eyes, are the most common side effects of isotretinoin therapy.

5. **D.** Isotretinoin is contraindicated in pregnancy because of the high incidence of serious birth defects.

6. **B.** Terbinafine (Lamisil) is the most effective nonprescription topical antifungal.

7. **C.** Topical antifungal agents are the first line of therapy against tinea corporis (ringworm of the skin). However, systemic antifungal therapy is usually required for treatment of tinea capitis (ringworm of the scalp) and tinea unguium (fungal infection of the toenails and fingernails).

8. **A.** Tinea pedis is also known as athlete's foot.

9. **D.** The treatment of choice for tinea unguium (fungal infection of the toenails and fingernails) is a systemic antifungal agent such as griseofulvin. Topical therapy is generally not effective for fungal infections of the nails.

10. **D.** Hair loss in the crown responds to treatment better than hair loss of the frontotemporal areas.

11. **E.** Women with alopecia should use only the 2% strength of minoxidil. Studies indicate that there is no greater degree of effectiveness with the 5% strength and the incidence of adverse effects (including increased growth of facial hair) is much greater in women using the 5% preparation.

12. **D.** Common adverse effects of minoxidil include hypertrichosis (increased hair growth in areas other than the scalp) and dermatitis and pruritus of the scalp. Systemic side effects with topical minoxidil are rare and do not include hepatic damage.

13. **B.** The mechanism of action of finasteride to reduce male baldness is blocking of the conversion of testosterone to dihydrotestosterone by inhibiting the enzyme 5-α-reductase.

14. **D.** Finasteride does not have to be taken on an empty stomach. It may be taken with or without food. Finasteride was originally approved for treatment of benign prostatic hypertrophy. Improvement of alopecia lasts only as long as treatment continues, finasteride is contraindicated in females of childbearing age, and 2% of males report reversible sexual dysfunction.

15. **B.** Dry skin occurs most commonly in the winter months and is often referred to as *winter rash*.

16. **C.** Lactic acid is used in the treatment of dry skin, not as a keratolytic agent, but as an agent that increases skin hydration.

17. **C.** Topical corticosteroids are the agents of choice for the initial treatment of irritant or allergic contact dermatitis. If the condition is severe or widespread, oral corticosteroids may be useful. Oral or topical antihistamines have minimal effect in the course of the treatment of contact dermatitis, possibly producing some antipruritic effect, but not affecting the course of the disorder.

18. **E.** Topical corticosteroid systemic absorption is increased on an infant's skin and with occlusion, long-term use, and use of high-potency agents. Systemic corticosteroids' adverse effects may be severe and include adrenocortical suppression.

19. **C.** Desensitization has no place in the treatment of poison ivy, and most studies indicate desensitization is not an effective method to prevent poison ivy.

20. **E.** Systemic corticosteroids are the treatment of choice for severe or extensive cases of poison ivy or poison oak. Topical agents are limited in effectiveness and do not alter the course of the disease.
21. **D.** Zinc pyrithione (Head and Shoulders) and selenium sulfide (Selsun Blue) are cytostatic agents used in the treatment of dandruff that suppress cell rate turnover. Salicylic acid is a keratolytic agent.
22. **E.** Seborrhea most commonly occurs on the face, especially eyebrows and eyelashes, but not on the extremities.
23. **E.** Psoriasis is a chronic inflammatory disease marked by silvery scales (known as *plaques*) with sharp delineated edges and characterized by spontaneous exacerbations and remissions.
24. **D.** Treatment of advanced psoriasis may require topical therapy combined with either oral corticosteroids or antimetabolites such as methotrexate.
25. **B.** Head lice occur most commonly in the months of August and September.
26. **B.** Synergized pyrethrins should be applied after washing and drying the hair and left on for 10 minutes, not overnight.
27. **A.** Permethrin (Nix) does not have to be repeated in 7–10 days as does the other available nonprescription pediculicidal agent, synergized pyrethrins (A-200). Lindane (Kwell) is not available over the counter, and significant neurologic toxicities have been reported with its use.
28. **A.** Nonprescription products for the treatment of corns and warts contain salicylic acid as the active therapeutic agent.
29. **D.** Corns are not contagious and may not spread on the body. Corns are an excess growth of the upper keratinized layer of skin, usually caused by pressure or friction from improper or tight-fitting shoes. Salicylic acid is available OTC for removal of corns in pads, disks, or flexible collodion. Self-treatment for corns or warts with OTC agents is not recommended for diabetic patients because of the reduced sensation in their feet, which delays awareness of the development of infections and could lead to sepsis.
30. **D.** Plantar warts are not located on the fingers, hands, or knees; they are located on the soles of the feet.
31. **E.** Warts may be eliminated by surgery, freezing with liquid nitrogen (cryotherapy), or direct application of caustics (e.g., salicylic acid).

26-14. References

Arndt KA. *Manual of Dermatologic Therapeutics.* 5th ed. Boston: Little, Brown; 1995.

Arndt KA, Wintroub BU, Robinson JK, et al., eds. *Primary Care Dermatology.* Philadelphia: WB Saunders; 1997.

Berardi RR, Ferreri SP, Hume AL, et al., eds. *The Handbook of Nonprescription Drugs.* 16th ed. Washington, D.C.: American Pharmaceutical Association; 2009.

Burnham TH, ed. *Drug Facts and Comparisons.* Baltimore: Lippincott Williams & Wilkins; 2005.

Champion RH, Burton JL, Burns DA, eds. *Textbook of Dermatology.* 6th ed. Oxford, U.K.: Blackwell Scientific Publications; 1998.

Covington, TR. *Nonprescription Drug Therapy: Guiding Patient Self-Care.* Baltimore: Lippincott Williams & Wilkins; 2003.

DiPiro JT, Talbert RL, Yee GC, et al., eds. *Pharmacotherapy: A Pathophysiologic Approach.* 5th ed. Stamford, Conn.: Appleton & Lange; 2004.

Epstein E. *Common Skin Disorders.* 6th ed. Philadelphia: WB Saunders; 2008.

Fitzpatrick JE. *Dermatology Secrets in Color.* 2nd ed. Philadelphia: Hanley and Belfus; 2001.

Freedberg IM, Eisen AZ, Wolff K, et al., eds. *Fitzpatrick's Dermatology in General Medicine.* 5th ed. New York: McGraw-Hill; 1999.

Habif TP, Campbell JL, Quitadamo MJ. *Skin Disease: Diagnosis and Treatment.* St. Louis, Mo.: Mosby; 2001.

Herfindal T, Gourley D, eds. *Textbook of Therapeutics.* 6th ed. Baltimore: Lippincott Williams & Wilkins; 2000.

Odom RB, James WD, Berger TG, eds. *Andrew's Diseases of the Skin: Clinical Dermatology.* Philadelphia: WB Saunders; 2000.

Pray WS. *Nonprescription Product Therapeutics.* Hagerstown, Md.: Lippincott Williams & Wilkins; 1999.

Top OTC/HBC brands in 2002. *Drug Topics.* 2003; 145:33–34.

Wolverton SE, ed. *Comprehensive Dermatologic Drug Therapy.* Philadelphia: WB Saunders; 2001.

Nonprescription Medications

27

Amanda Howard-Thompson, PharmD, BCPS

27-1. Cough, Cold, and Allergy

The Consumer Health Care Products Association announced in October 2008 that manufacturers were voluntarily updating all cough and cold products to state "do not use" in children under age 4. These actions have not changed the official U.S. Food and Drug Administration (FDA) monograph for these drug products. The American Academy of Pediatrics would like the age limit increased to age 6 because of lack of clear evidence of efficacy. The FDA is currently investigating the use of these products in children age 4–6 to determine if further restriction is needed.

Cough

Selected cough products are shown in Table 27-1.

Etiology

- Upper respiratory infection (viral or bacterial)
- Sinusitis
- Rhinitis
- Asthma and chronic obstructive pulmonary disease
- Gastroesophageal reflux disease
- Congestive heart failure
- Drug-induced cough

Cough characteristics

- Productive
- Nonproductive

Pathophysiology

A cough is an important defense mechanism to rid the airways of mucus and foreign bodies. A cough may be acute (< 3 weeks duration) or chronic (> 3 weeks duration).

Nonprescription treatment

Antitussives and cough suppressants
Antitussives and cough suppressants may be narcotic or nonnarcotic.

Codeine
Codeine, a narcotic, is the gold standard of antitussives:

- *Availability:* Without prescription in some states
- *Mechanism of action:* Centrally mediated suppression of cough
- *Adult dose:* 10–20 mg q4–6h (120 mg/d maximum)
- *Role in therapy:* Primarily for night cough
- *Side effects:* Sedation, nausea, and constipation

Dextromethorphan
Dextromethorphan is only category I over-the-counter (OTC) nonnarcotic antitussive:

- *Mechanism of action:* Centrally mediated suppression of cough
- *Adult dosage:* 10–30 mg q4–8h (120 mg/d maximum)
- *Role in therapy:* Nonproductive cough
- *Side effects:* Drowsiness and gastrointestinal (GI) effects
- *Drug interactions:* Monoamine oxidase (MAO) inhibitors

Diphenhydramine
Diphenhydramine is a category II antitussive:

- *Mechanism of action:* Centrally mediated suppression of cough center and anticholinergic
- *Adult dosage:* 25 mg q4h (75 mg/d maximum)

Table 27-1. Selected Examples of Nonprescription Cough Products

Type of product	Generic name	Action	Trade name
Expectorant	Guaifenesin	Immediate release	Robitussin Syrup (100 mg/5 mL)
		Extended release	Mucinex (600 or 1,200 mg)
			Humibid sprinkle (30 mg)
Cough suppressant	Dextromethorphan	Immediate release	Benylin Adult Cough Formula Liquid (15 mg/mL)
		Extended release	Delsym Suspension (30 mg/5 mL)
Combination expectorant and cough suppressant	Guaifenesin and dextromethorphan		Robitussin DM (guaifenesin 100 mg and dextromethorphan 10 mg/5 mL)
Combination expectorant and decongestant	Guaifenesin and pseudoephedrine		Robitussin PE (guaifenesin 100 mg and pseudoephedrine 30 mg/5 mL)

Expectorant

Guaifenesin (Robitussin, Mucinex, Humibid) is the only category I OTC expectorant:

- *Mechanism of action:* Thinning of mucus to enhance clearance
- *Adult dosage:*
  - Immediate-release 200–400 mg q4h (maximum 2,400 mg/d)
  - Extended-release: 600–1,200 mg q12h (maximum 2,400 mg/d)
- *Role in therapy:* Productive cough
- *Side effects:* GI discomfort
- *Patient education:* Increase fluid intake.

Topical antitussives

Of the volatile oils, only camphor and menthol are FDA approved:

- *Mechanism of action:* Local anesthetic effect in nasal mucosa
- *Product availability:* Lozenge, ointment, and steam inhalation
- *Patient education:* Ointment and solution are toxic if ingested.

Sore throat remedies

Sore throat remedies include the following:

- Saline gargle
- Sprays and lozenges:
  - *Benzocaine:* Chloraseptic lozenges and Cepacol lozenges
  - *Dyclonine:* Cepacol Spray
  - *Phenol:* Chloraseptic Gargle
  - *Menthol:* Halls

Common Cold

Etiology

- Usually viral, most commonly rhinoviruses
- Transmitted through hand-to-hand contact followed by touching eyes or nasal mucosa

Pathophysiology

A cold results in the release of numerous inflammatory mediators, primarily cytokines.

Clinical presentation

- Sore throat, nasal symptoms, watery eyes, sneezing, cough, malaise, and low-grade fever occur.
- High fever and myalgias are more characteristic of influenza.
- There is a gradual onset with slow progression.
- Duration is 1–2 weeks.

Treatment

Nonpharmacologic therapy
- Humidifiers
- Increase fluid intake
- Rest

Nonprescription medication treatment (symptomatic)
- Decongestants for nasal congestion
- Antihistamines for excess nasal discharge
- Analgesics for related pain or headaches
- Local anesthetic lozenges or sprays for sore throat (pharyngitis)

Allergic Rhinitis

Etiology

Allergic rhinitis results from exposure to perennial or seasonal allergens, which lead to the development of nasal symptoms.

Pathophysiology

The pathophysiology of allergic rhinitis is complex, involving numerous mediators (primarily histamine) and cell types (mast cells).

Clinical presentation

- *Nasal:* Congestion, rhinorrhea, nasal pruritus, sneezing, and postnasal drip
- *Ocular:* Itching, lacrimation, redness, and irritation
- *General:* Headache, malaise, mood swings, and irritability

Treatment

Nonpharmacologic therapy
Patients should avoid the offending allergens:

- Limit outside exposure during periods of high pollen.
- Avoid indoor and outdoor mold.
- Avoid dust, especially in the bedroom.
- Avoid pet dander, especially cats.

Pharmacotherapeutic options
- *Mild allergies:* Patients should use antihistamines as needed.
- *Moderate allergies:* Patients should use an antihistamine plus decongestant for nasal symptoms and an ophthalmic antihistamine for ocular symptoms.
- *Chronic allergies:* Use cromolyn sodium (Nasalcrom) nasal spray and scheduled nonsedating antihistamine.

Table 27-2. Selected Nonprescription Antihistamine Products

Generic name	Trade name	Adult dosage (maximum daily dose)
Chlorpheniramine	Chlor-Trimeton	4 mg q4–6h (24 mg)
Brompheniramine	Lodrane	4 mg q4–6h (24 mg)
Diphenhydramine	Benadryl	25–50 mg q6h (200 mg)
Clemastine	Tavist	1.34 mg bid (2.68 mg)
Triprolidine	Zymine	2.5 mg q6h (10 mg)
Loratadine	Claritin, Alavert	10 mg qd
Cetirizine	Zyrtec	10 mg qd

Nonprescription Therapy for Treatment of the Common Cold and Allergies

Selected products for treating the common cold and allergies are shown in Tables 27-2, 27-3, and 27-4.

Antihistamines

Selected antihistamines are described in Table 27-2.

Pharmacology
- Antihistamines are H_1-receptor antagonists.
- First-generation antihistamines are nonselective and sedating.
- Second-generation antihistamines are peripherally selective, have low incidence of sedation, and have no anticholinergic effects.

Side effects
- Sedation
- Anticholinergic effects (primarily with first-generation antihistamines)
- Dry mouth
- Dry eyes
- Urinary retention

Table 27-3. Selected Nonprescription Oral Decongestant Products

Generic name	Products	Comments	Side effects	Adult dosage (maximum daily dose)
Phenylephrine	Combination products	Weakest oral decongestant	+	10 mg q4h (60 mg)
Pseudoephedrine	Sudafed	Less central nervous system stimulation	++	60 mg q4–6h (240 mg)

Note: + and ++ indicate the amount of side effects.

Table 27-4. Selected Nonprescription Cold, Allergy, and Sinus Combination Products

Product	Trade name	Primary ingredients
Decongestant and analgesic	Alka-Seltzer Plus Cold and Sinus	Phenylephrine 5 mg + acetaminophen 250 mg
	Aleve-D Sinus & Cold	Pseudoephedrine 120 mg + naproxen 220 mg
	Sudafed Sinus & Cold	Pseudoephedrine 30 mg + acetaminophen 325 mg
Antihistamine, decongestant, and analgesic	Vicks Dayquil Liquicaps	Phenylephrine 5 mg + acetaminophen 325 mg + dextromethorphan 10 mg
	Advil Allergy Sinus Caplets	Chlorpheniramine 6 mg + pseudoephedrine 30 mg + ibuprofen 200 mg
Antihistamine and decongestant	Actifed Cold and Allergy	Chlorpheniramine 4 mg + phenylephrine 10 mg
	Drixoral Cold and Allergy	Dexbrompheniramine 6 mg + pseudoephedrine 120 mg
	Zyrtec D	Cetirizine 5 mg + pseudoephedrine 120 mg
	Claritin-D 24 hour	Loratadine 10 mg + pseudoephedrine 240 mg

- Constipation
- Paradoxical stimulation in some children and elderly patients

Precautions and contraindications
- Do not drive or operate heavy machinery.
- Avoid use with alcohol.
- Prostatic hyperplasia can occur.
- Narrow-angle glaucoma is possible.

Oral decongestants

Selected oral decongestant products are described in Table 27-3.

Pharmacology
- α-adrenergic agonists and vasoconstrictors
- Constriction of blood vessels to decrease blood supply to nasal mucosa and decrease mucosal edema
- No effect on histamine or allergy-mediated reaction

Regulation
The 2005 Combat Methamphetamine Epidemic Act has the following requirements:
- Pseudoephedrine must be kept either behind the counter or in a locked cabinet.
- Quantity is limited to 3.6 g/d and 9 g/month per patient.

- Pharmacists must maintain a logbook with the following information: product name, quantity sold, patient's name and address, and time and date of sale.
- Patients must show valid identification and sign a logbook.

Side effects
These products are relatively safe with no dependence. They can be used long term. The most common side effects are as follows:
- Nervousness
- Irritability
- Restlessness
- Insomnia

Less common side effects include the following:
- Increased heart rate
- Increased blood pressure
- Irregular heartbeat
- Palpitations

Precautions and contraindications
- ***Hypertension:*** These agents are generally accepted with mild or well-controlled hypertension; they should not be used with uncontrolled hypertension.
- ***Heart disease (arrhythmias and ischemic heart disease):*** They increase the heart rate.

- *Diabetes:* They have a minimal effect on blood sugar level.
- *Hyperthyroidism:* This condition is more sensitive to sympathomimetics.
- *Enlarged prostrate:* Benign prostatic hyperplasia (BPH) is exacerbated by constricting smooth muscle of the bladder neck.
- *Narrow-angle glaucoma:* Dilation increases intraocular pressure.
- *Blood pressure:* MAO inhibitors interact with decongestants to increase blood pressure.

Topical decongestants

Pharmacology
- α-adrenergic agonists act locally as vasoconstrictors.
- These agents constrict blood vessels, decrease blood supply to nose, and decrease mucosal edema.
- They have no effect on histamine or allergy-mediated reaction.

Side effects
Minimal systemic absorption results in few side effects. Local effects may include burning, nasal irritation, and sneezing.

Precautions and contraindications
Rhinitis medicamentosa (rebound congestion) may occur if duration of use is > 3–5 days.

Dosage forms
Sprays
Sprays are the simplest dosage delivery. A large surface area is covered. Imprecise dosing and contamination of the bottle are possible. Products include the following:

- *Short-acting:* Phenylephrine (Neo-Synephrine and Vicks Sinex)
- *Longest-acting:* Oxymetazoline (Afrin and Mucinex)

Drops
Drops are preferred for use in small children. They cover a small surface area. They pass to the larynx, where they may be swallowed and result in systemic effects.

Nasal inhaler
A nasal inhaler requires an unobstructed airway to deliver drug to the nasal mucosa. Nasal inhalers contain sympathomimetic amines, as well as camphor and menthol. Medications lose efficacy after 2–3 months. Products include the following:

- Propylhexedrine (Benzedrex inhaler)
- Levodesoxyephedrine (Vicks inhaler)

Nasal saline solution

This solution is very safe and is good for use in infants and children. It can be used with oral decongestants. Products include the following:

- Saline drops (Ayr)
- Saline sprays (Ayr, Ocean Nasal Spray, and HuMist)

Cromolyn (Nasalcrom)
Cromolyn is used to prevent and treat allergic symptoms:

- *Pharmacology:* Mast cell stabilizer; prevention of the mast cells from releasing inflammatory mediators
- *Dosage:* One spray per nostril q4–6h up to four to six times daily
- *Onset of action:* Approximately 1 week; 2–3 weeks for maximal effect
- *Efficacy:* Not efficacious if taken prn; must be taken on a scheduled basis
- *Side effects:* Nasal irritation, nasal burning, stinging, sneezing, cough, unpleasant taste

Analgesics
Analgesics treat the pain, fever, and headaches associated with cold, flu, or allergies. Medications include the following:

- Aspirin (mostly replaced now by acetaminophen and nonsteroidal anti-inflammatory drugs [NSAIDs])
- Acetaminophen (N-acetyl-para-aminophenol, or APAP)
- NSAIDs
  - Ibuprofen
  - Ketoprofen
  - Naproxen

27-2. Constipation

Clinical Presentation

- Patient has difficult or infrequent passage of stools.

■ Patient may complain of abdominal or rectal fullness.

Etiology

Table 27-5 shows the common causes of constipation.

Treatment

Nonpharmacologic therapy

■ Increase fluid intake.
■ Increase dietary fiber.
■ Exercise.
■ Establish good bowel habits.

Nonprescription medication therapy

Bulk-forming laxatives
Selected bulk-forming laxative products are described in Table 27-6.

Mechanism of action
Natural or semisynthetic hydrophilic polysaccharide derivatives are present in bulk-forming laxatives. They absorb water to soften stool, increase bulk, and facilitate peristalsis and elimination. Effects may not be seen for 2–3 days.

Role in therapy
Bulk-forming laxatives are the safest, most natural therapy for constipation. They are the most often recommended medication for chronic use.

Table 27-5. Common Causes of Constipation

Daily habits	Diseases	Medications
Inadequate fluid intake	Parkinson's Disease	Antacids containing Al or Ca
Inadequate fiber intake	Multiple sclerosis	Anticholinergics
Lack of physical exercise	Cerebrovascular disease	Phenothiazines
	Irritable bowel syndrome	Tricyclic antidepressants
	Hemorrhoids	Opiates
	Polyps and tumors	Antihistamines
	Diabetes	ACE inhibitors
	Hypothyroidism	CCB (especially Verapamil)
		Sucralfate
		Iron

Table 27-6. Additional Nonprescription Treatments of Constipation Not Listed in Text

Medication class	Generic name	Brand name
Bulk-forming laxatives	Psyllium seed	Metamucil
	Methylcellulose	Citrucel
	Calcium polycarbophil	FiberCon
	Barley malt extract	Maltsupex
Emollient laxatives	Docusate sodium	Colace, Correctol
	Docusate calcium	Surfak
	Docusate potassium	Dialose
Saline laxatives	Magnesium hydroxide	Milk of Magnesia
	Magnesium citrate	Citroma
	Magnesium sulfate	Epsom salts
	Sodium phosphate	Fleet Phospho-Soda
Combination products	Senna + psyllium	Perdiem
	Senna + docusate	Senokot-S

Drug interactions
■ These laxatives may bind with digoxin, warfarin, and other drugs.
■ Calcium complexes may bind with tetracycline, inhibiting its absorption.
■ Recommend separating doses from other medications.

Side effects
■ Potential exists for allergic reaction or anaphylaxis.
■ Inhalation of powder is reported to cause bronchospasm.
■ Caution diabetics about sugar content of some products.

Emollient laxatives (stool softeners)
Emollient laxatives act as surfactants, absorbing water into the stool. Effects may take 2–3 days. Emollient laxatives may cause systemic absorption of mineral oil; therefore, concurrent use is contraindicated.

Emollient laxatives are often used in combination products. They are useful for patients who should avoid straining during the following:

■ Rectal surgery
■ Postpartum time period
■ Recent myocardial infarction

Selected emollient laxative products are described in Table 27-6.

Stimulant laxatives

Stimulant laxatives stimulate bowel motility through localized mucosal irritation. They increase secretion of fluids into bowel. They can cause cramping. Impaired colon function occurs with chronic use.

Dangers of chronic stimulant laxative use include the following:

- Laxative habit
- Cathartic colon
- Melanosis coli
- Loss of fluids on electrolytes
- Cramping pains

Anthraquinones

Senna (Senokot and Ex-Lax) is an anthraquinone:

- *Pharmacology:* Anthraquinones are absorbed into bloodstream with action on the large intestines. Onset of effects is 6–12 hours. This medication should be taken at bedtime.
- *Side effects:* Such effects include discoloration of urine, stimulant habituation, and melanosis coli (i.e., dark pigmentation of colonic mucosa).
- *Precautions and contraindications:* Do not take while breast-feeding.

Diphenylmethanes

Bisacodyl (Dulcolax tablets or suppositories) is a diphenylmethane. Minimal systemic absorption occurs with this drug. Bisacodyl is the only stimulant compatible with breastfeeding. This medication is enteric coated: do not crush or take with antacids. The onset of effects varies with route of administration:

- *Oral:* 6–8 hours
- *Rectal:* 15–60 minutes

Stimulant oils

Castor oil is a stimulant oil that acts on small intestine. It is a strong cathartic and may induce fluid or electrolyte disturbances. Onset is rapid: 2–6 hours. Castor oil is contraindicated in pregnancy because it may induce labor.

Hyperosmotic laxatives

Glycerin

Glycerin has an osmotic effect and is a local irritant that stimulates bowel movement. Onset of action is usually within 30 minutes. Glycerin suppositories are safe for infants.

Products include Fleets Babylax Liquid and Fleet Glycerin Suppository.

Polyethylene glycol 3350

Polyethylene glycol 3350 was approved for OTC status in October 2006. Its mechanism of action is similar to that of glycerin. This agent is meant for short-term therapy for constipation. Onset of action is usually within 1–3 days. The adult dosage is 17 grams of powder in 4–8 ounces of water. Side effects are as follows:

- Bloating
- Abdominal discomfort
- Cramping
- Flatulence

Products include MiraLAX.

Saline laxatives

With saline laxatives, nonabsorbable cations create osmotic gradient to pull water into intestine. Onset varies depending on the route of administration:

- *Rectal:* 5–30 minutes
- *Oral:* 30 minutes to 4 hours

Twenty percent of magnesium may be absorbed systemically.

Saline laxatives are contraindicated in patients with impaired renal function (magnesium- or phosphate-containing), congestive heart failure, or hypertension (sodium-containing).

Selected saline laxative products are described in Table 27-6.

Lubricant laxatives

Selected lubricant laxative products are as follows:

- *Mineral oil:* Liquid petrolatum
- *Olive oil:* "Sweet oil"

Lubricant laxatives soften the feces by emulsifying the contents of the intestinal tract. Onset of action is 6–8 hours.

These agents may decrease absorption of fat-soluble vitamins and some drugs. They are contraindicated in children and elderly patients because of the risk of aspiration and lipid pneumonitis. Do not administer with stool softeners.

Enemas

Enemas include Fleet Enema (monobasic and dibasic sodium phosphates). They have the following characteristics:

- Oil retention
- Soap suds
- Warm tap water

Special patient populations

Care must be taken with patients who are pregnant:

- Hormonal changes cause smooth muscle relaxation early in pregnancy.
- An enlarged uterus compresses the colon.
- Recommend only bulk-forming laxatives or stool softeners.

27-3. Diarrhea

Clinical Presentation

Diarrhea is the abnormal increase in frequency of stools and stool looseness. It may be acute (< 14 days) or chronic (> 4 weeks).

Etiology

Common causes of diarrhea are shown in Table 27-7.

Complications

- Dehydration (especially in infants and elderly patients)
- Electrolyte abnormalities

Nonpharmacologic Treatment

- Administer oral rehydration therapy, such as Pedialyte.
- Avoid fatty and spicy foods and those with high sugar content.

Table 27-7. Common Causes of Diarrhea

Common Causes

Infection	Medications	Diet
Viral:	Antibiotics	Allergies
Norwalk	Laxatives	Spicy foods
Rotavirus	Magnesium-containing antacids	High carbohydrate load
Bacterial:		Lactose intolerance
Food-borne illness	Cytotoxic agents	
Contaminated water		
Traveler's diarrhea		
Protozoal		

Nonprescription Medication Therapy

Loperamide (Imodium AD)

Loperamide is a synthetic opioid agonist that slows GI motility. The dosage is 4 mg initially and then 2 mg after each loose stool. For OTC use, maximum dose is 8 mg/d, but it can be increased to 16 mg/d with medical supervision.

The medication is well tolerated, but side effects are as follows:

- Constipation
- Dizziness
- Dry mouth

Precautions and contraindications are as follows:

- Loperamide is not recommended for children under age 6 without medical supervision.
- It should not be used if the patient has bloody or black stool; consult physician before use if the patient has a fever, mucus in stool, or a history of liver disease.
- Antiperistaltic action could worsen effects of invasive or inflammatory bacterial infection.

Bismuth subsalicylate

Bismuth subsalicylate (Pepto-Bismol) reacts with stomach acid to form salicylic acid and bismuth oxychloride. It reduces frequency of diarrhea and improves stool consistency. It has a direct antimicrobial effect; therefore, it is effective in traveler's diarrhea.

Side effects include the following:

- Salicylate toxicity (tinnitus)
- Bismuth toxicity (neurotoxicity)
- Gray-black discoloration of tongue or stool

The medication is contraindicated in the following:

- Aspirin allergy
- Children and teens with viral illness (Reye's syndrome)
- Patients having a history of GI bleeding, or using warfarin

New labeling recommends a physician should be consulted prior to use in patients younger than age 12.

27-4. Nausea and Vomiting

Definitions

- *Nausea:* The sensation that one is about to vomit.
- *Vomiting:* The forceful expulsion of gastric contents through the mouth.

Physiology

Vomiting is coordinated by the vomiting center in the medulla. Stimuli from the peripheral nervous system and within the central nervous system (CNS) act on the vomiting center. Responding to these impulses, the vomiting center stimulates the abdominal muscles, stomach, and esophagus to induce vomiting.

Etiology

Common causes of nausea and vomiting are shown in Table 27-8.

Complications

- Dehydration
- Electrolyte imbalance
- Aspiration
- Malnutrition
- Acid-base disturbances

Nonprescription Medication Therapy

In addition to the medications described in this section, Table 27-9 describes drugs of choice for the nausea or vomiting associated with motion sickness.

Antihistamines

Antihistamines cross the blood-brain barrier to depress vestibular excitability.

Phosphorated carbohydrate solution (Emetrol)

This agent is a hyperosmolar solution. It is a mixture of levulose (fructose), dextrose (glucose), and phosphoric acid. It is buffered to a pH of 1.5. It reduces gastric muscle contraction through an unknown direct effect. It must not be diluted (which raises the pH).

Bismuth salts (Pepto-Bismol)

Bismuth salts are available as nonprescription suspension, caplet, and chewable tablet. See Section 27-3 for additional information.

Histamine 2–receptor antagonists

Histamine 2–receptor antagonists (H2RAs) may provide symptomatic relief by inhibiting gastric acid secretion. Potential drug interactions occur with cimetidine.
Side effects are as follows:

- Headache
- Constipation
- Diarrhea

See Section 21-1 on peptic ulcer disease in Chapter 21 for additional information on H2RAs.

Antacids

Antacids may treat nausea, dyspepsia, and stomach upset associated with excessive intake of food or drink. They are combinations of magnesium hydroxide, sodium salts, aluminum hydroxide, calcium carbonate,

Table 27-8. Common Causes of Nausea and Vomiting

Irritation of chemoreceptor trigger zone	Vestibular disorders	CNS disorders	GI disorders
Chemotherapy	Motion sickness	Psychogenic vomiting	Obstruction
Narcotics	Otitis interna	Migraines	Gastroparesis
Theophylline	Meniere's syndrome	Increased intracranial pressure	Gastroenteritis
Digoxin		Psychogenic vomiting	Infection
Antibiotics		Migraines	
Drug withdrawal		Increased intracranial pressure	
Alcohol			
NSAIDs			
Antibiotics			
Ketoacidosis			
Uremia			
Pregnancy			
Electrolyte imbalances			

Table 27-9. Nonprescription Drugs of Choice for Prevention of Motion Sickness

Generic name	Trade name	Dosage		
		Adults (maximum daily dose)	Children age 6–12 (maximum daily dose)	Children age 2–6 (maximum daily dose)
Dimenhydrinate	Dramamine	50–100 mg q4–6h (400 mg)	25–50 mg q6–8h (150 mg)	12.5–25 mg q6–8h (75 mg)
Diphenhydramine	Benadryl	25–50 mg q4–6h (300 mg)	12.5–25 mg q4–6h (150 mg)	6.25 mg q4–6h (37.5 mg)
Cyclizine	Marezine	50 mg q4–6h (200 mg)	25 mg q6–8h (75 mg)	Not recommended
Meclizine	Bonine	25–50 mg qd (50 mg)	Not recommended	Not recommended

and magnesium carbonate. The usual adult dosage is 15 mL 30 minutes after meals and at bedtime.

Side effects include the following:

- Constipation
- Diarrhea
- Sodium overload

Antacids may decrease absorption of some medications. Therefore, administer other medications 1–2 hours before or after antacids.

Nausea may be associated with pregnancy, especially during the first trimester. Nonpharmacologic therapy is recommended in such cases:

- Eat small, frequent meals.
- Avoid rich, fatty foods.
- Snack on salty crackers or pretzels.

Refer the patient to the primary care provider if pharmacologic therapy is being considered.

27-5. Pain and Fever

Pathophysiology of Pain

Nociceptors are peripheral pain receptors. They send pain stimuli to the spinal cord through afferent, nociceptive nerves. Impulses then pass to the brain through dorsal root ganglia.

Pathophysiology of Fever

The core temperature is the temperature of the blood surrounding the hypothalamus. The thermoregulatory center in the anterior hypothalamus controls body temperature through physiologic and behavioral mechanisms. Pyrogens—fever-producing substances—increase the thermoregulatory set point, raising the body temperature.

Nonprescription Medication Therapy

Selected analgesic and antipyretic products are shown in Table 27-10.

Acetaminophen

Acetaminophen exerts analgesic and antipyretic activity through central inhibition of prostaglandin synthesis. It does not have peripheral anti-inflammatory activity.

Acetaminophen is generally well tolerated; however, hepatotoxicity is a possible side effect.

Table 27-10. Selected Analgesic and Antipyretic Products

Generic name	(Trade name)	Dosage	
		Adults (maximum daily dose)	Children (maximum daily dose)
Acetaminophen	Tylenol, Tempra	325–1,000 mg q4–6h (4,000 mg)	10–15 mg/kg q4–6h (5 doses)
Aspirin	Bayer	650–1,000 mg q4–6h (4,000 mg)	10–15 mg/kg q4–6h (80 mg/kg)
Ibuprofen	Motrin, Advil	200–400 mg q4–6h (1,200 mg OTC)	5–10 mg/kg q6–8h (40 mg/kg)
Naproxen sodium	Aleve	220 mg q8–12h (660 mg)	Not recommended < 12 years of age; ≥ 12 years of age: use adult dosage

Drug interactions can occur as follows:

- *Alcohol:* Risk of hepatotoxicity is increased.
- *Warfarin:* Higher doses may enhance hypoprothrombinemic effect of warfarin.

Patients should be aware of the following precautions and contraindications:

- Increased risk of hepatotoxicity
- Dose > 4 g/d
- Preexisting liver disease
- Alcohol use
- Fasting

Use is accepted during pregnancy and breast-feeding.

Salicylates

Salicylates inhibit peripheral prostaglandin synthesis. They reduce pain, inflammation, and fever. Acetylated salicylates (e.g., aspirin) inhibit platelet aggregation. Nonacetylated salicylates (e.g., prescription salsalate, choline magnesium salicylate) do not have significant antiplatelet activity.

Several side effects are associated with salicylates:

- Gastritis
- Gastric ulcers and bleeding
- Allergy and hypersensitivity:
  - Rare (< 1%) in the general population
  - Higher risk in individuals with asthma and nasal polyps
- Reye's syndrome, a potentially fatal illness associated with salicylate use in children and teens with concurrent viral illness (influenza, varicella-zoster)

Drug interactions may occur:

- *Alcohol:* Gastrointestinal toxicity is enhanced.
- *Methotrexate:* Salicylates displace methotrexate from protein-binding sites.
- *Warfarin:* Salicylates enhance hypoprothrombinemic effects of warfarin.

Patients should be aware of the following precautions and contraindications:

- Bleeding disorders
- Hemophilia
- Peptic ulcer disease
- Children or teenagers with viral illness (Reye's syndrome)
- Gout

Salicylates should be avoided in the third trimester of pregnancy.

Nonsteroidal anti-inflammatory drugs

NSAIDs provide peripheral inhibition of prostaglandin synthesis. They offer analgesic, antipyretic, and anti-inflammatory activity.

The ketoprofen (Orudis KT) OTC formulation was discontinued by the manufacturer because of lack of consumer demand.

Side effects include the following:

- Gastrointestinal effects, including bleeding
- Rash
- Photosensitivity
- High incidence of cross-reactivity in individuals with aspirin allergy

Drug interactions may occur as follows:

- *Warfarin:* Increased bleeding risk
- *Alcohol:* Increased risk of gastrointestinal bleeding
- *Methotrexate:* Decreased methotrexate clearance
- *Antihypertensives:*
  - Angiotensin-converting enzyme (ACE) inhibitors: Decreased hypotensive effects, hyperkalemia
  - β-blockers: Decreased hypotensive effects
  - Potassium-sparing diuretics: Hyperkalemia
- *Digoxin:* Decreased renal clearance, risk of digoxin toxicity

Precautions and contraindications are as follows:

- Alcohol (increased risk of GI bleeding)
- Renal impairment
- Congestive heart failure

Special patient populations should be aware of the following:

- Ibuprofen and naproxen are compatible with breastfeeding.
- Avoid NSAIDs in third trimester of pregnancy.

27-6. Ophthalmic Disorders

Dry Eye

- *Definition:* Tear film instability caused by a deficiency of any component of the tear film
- *Clinical presentation:* Ocular discomfort, blurred vision, desire to rub the eyes, and burning or redness

Etiology

- Aqueous tear deficiency
- Exposure to dry air

- Keratoconjunctivitis sicca
- Sjögren's syndrome
- Blepharitis
- Vitamin A deficiency
- Allergic conjunctivitis
- Contact lenses
- Drug-induced (anticholinergic agents and antihistamines) condition

Nonpharmacologic treatment

- Avoid known irritants.
- Use a cool-mist humidifier or warm-steam vaporizer.

Nonprescription medication therapy

Table 27-11 describes the pharmacologic treatment of dry eyes.

Loose Foreign Material in the Eye

Symptoms

Symptoms include irritation, inflammation, involuntary tearing, uncontrollable blinking, and discomfort.

Etiology

Foreign materials may include dirt, an eyelash, or particles suspended by the tears.

Nonprescription treatment

Eyewashes are isotonic, buffered solutions of sterile water. They should not be used if the patient has open wounds near the eye. Contact lens wearers should remove their lenses prior to using eyewashes. Use of eye cups should generally be avoided.

Redness Caused by Minor Irritation

Etiology

Eye redness can be caused by airborne pollutants (gases or smoke), chlorinated water, infectious diseases, or glaucoma.

Nonprescription treatment

Ophthalmic vasoconstrictors, as described in Table 27-12, are used to treat eye redness.

The medications constrict blood vessels of the conjunctiva. Instill 1–2 drops in the affected eye up to four times daily. Minimize systemic absorption by closing the eye after instillation and occluding the tear duct with a finger (punctual occlusion).

These agents are contraindicated in patients with narrow-angle glaucoma because they cause mydriasis. Contact lens wearers also should avoid ophthalmic vasoconstrictors.

A rebound hyperemia can occur, especially with overuse. Tachycardia and aggravate arrhythmias can occur if absorbed systemically.

Table 27-11. Pharmacologic Treatment of Dry Eyes

Product	Common preparations	Comments
Artificial tears a		
Cellulose derivatives (carboxymethylcellulose)	Bion Tears, Celluvisc, Clear Eyes CLR	Has enhanced duration compared to other products; tends to form dry crusts, which may be easily washed off with warm water
Polyvinyl alcohol (glycerin, propylene glycol, polyethylene glycols, polysorbate 80)	Moisture Eyes, Hypo Tears, Murine Tears, Tears Plus	Has shorter duration; has no crust formation
Povidone and dextran 70	AquaSite	Can cause transient stinging or burning
Ocular emollients b		
Lanolin, mineral oil, petrolatum, white ointment, white wax, or yellow wax	Moisture Eyes PM, Lacri-Lube SOP, Refresh PM	

a. Artificial tears act as demulcents to mimic mucin. Use twice daily as suggested.
b. Ointments have longer contact and are more likely to cause blurred vision.

Table 27-12. Ophthalmic Vasoconstrictors

Product	Common preparations	Key points
Phenylephrine	Prefrin Liquifilm Relief	Can precipitate angle-closure glaucoma
Naphazoline	Clear Eyes, Clear Eyes ACR, Allerest, All Clear, All Clear AR	Is ocular decongestant of choice
Tetrahydrozoline	Visine, Vision Clear, Visine Advanced Relief, OptiClear	Is less likely to alter pupil size; may cause stinging on instillation
Oxymetazoline	Visine LR	Is relatively free of ocular or systemic side effects

Ocular decongestants should be avoided in patients with heart disease, high blood pressure, an enlarged prostate, or narrow-angle glaucoma.

Allergic Conjunctivitis

Symptoms

Symptoms include chronic and recurring itching. Eyes are slightly red and tear and burn, but they have little discharge.

Etiology

Animal hair, pollen, ragweed, or plants are possible allergens.

Nonprescription treatment

Antihistamine and mast cell stabilizer
Ketotifen fumarate 0.025% (Zaditor and Alaway), an antihistamine and mast cell stabilizer, may be used to treat allergic conjunctivitis. Instill 1 drop q8–12h in the affected eye. Use in patients ≥ 3 years of age. Relief is provided within minutes, and effects may last up to 12 hours.

Combination products
The following combination products containing an ophthalmic vasoconstrictor and an ocular antihistamine may be used:

- Naphazoline + pheniramine (Naphcon A, Visine A, and Opcon-A)
- Naphazoline + antazoline (Vasocon-A)

Instill 1–2 drops in the affected eye up to four times daily.

Combination products containing ocular decongestants should be avoided in patients with heart disease, high blood pressure, enlarged prostate, or narrow-angle glaucoma.

Conditions Requiring Referral to a Physician or Eye Care Specialist

Corneal edema

Symptoms
Symptoms include foggy vision, haloes around lights, photophobia, irritation, sensation of a foreign body, and extreme pain.

Etiology
Prolonged contact lens wearing, infection, glaucoma, and iritis are possible causes.

Nonprescription treatment
Sodium chloride (2–5%) can be used to treat corneal edema. Instill 1–2 drops in the affected eye every 6 hours. If eye drops do not provide relief, add ointment to therapy.

Foreign body in the eye

Foreign bodies include metal shavings, wood splinters, and dust. Improper removal may lead to permanent damage.

Ocular trauma

Automobile accidents and sports injuries can result in ocular trauma.

Chemical exposure

If chemical exposure occurs, follow these steps:

- Remove contact lenses.
- Flush eye immediately with lukewarm water for at least 15 minutes.
- Do not place drops in the eyes.

27-7. Otic Disorders

Impacted Cerumen

Cerumen-softening agents

Cerumen-softening agents are used as follows:

- Instill in ear.
- Follow with warm water irrigation using otic syringe.

Various types of agents are available:

- *Carbamide peroxide 6.5% in anhydrous glycerin:* Products include Debrox and Murine Earwax Removal System. This agent softens ear wax and facilitates its removal.
- *Hydrogen peroxide and water:* A 1:1 solution of warm water and 3% hydrogen peroxide is used. This mixture is not an effective drying agent.
- *Glycerin:* This emollient and humectant may facilitate the removal of ear wax.
- *Olive oil:* Sometimes called sweet oil, olive oil can also be used.

Water-Clogged Ears

A solution of 95% isopropyl alcohol in 5% anhydrous glycerin (Swim Ear or Auro Dri Drops) may be used to treat water-clogged ears. This solution is the only FDA-approved ear-drying aid.

A compounded solution 50:50 acetic acid (5%) + isopropyl alcohol (95%) may also be used. This combination is recommended by the American Academy of Otolaryngology.

Boils

Boils occur when hair follicles in the ear canal become infected. They are usually self-limiting. They are treated by applying a warm compress.

27-8. Home Monitoring and Test Devices

Fertility Prediction Tests

Basal thermometry

Temperatures can be taken orally, rectally, and vaginally. Temperatures are taken every morning before arising.

Resting temperatures are usually below normal for first part of the reproductive cycle. Temperatures are closer to normal after ovulation.

Temperature results are plotted graphically against time to assess spikes (ovulation). Tests are very user dependent.

Bioself, Fertility Indicator

This device is used to take digital temperature readings. The user must input the first day of menses into the device. The device calculates user's average cycle length and predicts the user's most fertile period.

Each morning, the indicator displays a prediction (90% effective). The device indicates if the user is in a nonfertile phase, if conception is possible, or if the user is in the most fertile phase. The user can obtain a printout through modem download.

Ovulation prediction kits

This test contains antibodies that bind to the lutenizing hormone (LH) in urine. An LH surge is detected by a difference in color or color intensity from one day to the next.

Early morning urine collection is recommended. The user must know the length of the past three cycles before using. Testing usually begins 2–4 days prior to ovulation (based on the average of the past three cycles).

Pregnancy detection

Early testing is very important. Tests detect levels of human chorionic gonadotropin (hCG) in urine (within 1–2 weeks after conception). Antibodies designed to react with hCG form the shape of a straight line, check, or plus sign. If the user is pregnant, color is produced.

Pregnancy tests are 98–100% accurate; however, human error decreases that rate to 50–75% (see Table 27-13).

Important tips for patients using pregnancy tests follow:

- Use of first morning urine to test is encouraged because hCG is more concentrated.
- If use of first morning urine is not possible, the patient should restrict fluids 4–6 hours before urine collection.
- Use only supplied collection devices.
- Try to test the sample immediately after collection. If this is not possible, allow refrigerated samples to come to room temperature.

Table 27-13. Causes of Error in Home Pregnancy Testing

False positives	False negatives
Miscarriage within previous 8 weeks	Test performed first day of a missed cycle
Childbirth within previous 8 weeks	Refrigerated urine not allowed to come to room temperature
Use of fertility medications (Pergonal, Profasi)	Wax cups or household containers with soap residues used for test

- If the test is negative, wait 1 week and retest if the cycle has not yet started.
- If the test is positive, contact an obstetrician–gynecologist immediately and start prenatal vitamins.

Urinary Tract Infection Tests

Two categories are available:

- Tests for nitrites in urine (UTI Bladder Infection Test)
- Tests for nitrites and leukocyte esterase (AZO strips)

Both are specific only for gram-negative organisms.
Inaccurate results are possible in the following circumstances:

- *False-negative result:* Vegetarian diet, vitamin C, or tetracycline
- *False-positive result:* Phenazopyridine

Hypertension
Mercury column devices

These devices use a blood pressure reference standard. Routine home use is discouraged because the devices are cumbersome.

Aneroid devices

Aneroid devices are light, portable, and affordable. Many come with an attached stethoscope. They require good eyesight and hearing for effective use (large-print devices are available).

Digital devices

Digital devices are less accurate than aneroid devices.

Hypercholesterolemia
CholesTrak Home Cholesterol Test

This test checks for total cholesterol only. Results are available without the need for a lab.

Biosafe Total Cholesterol Panel

Fingerstick blood is placed on a small collection card. The sample is mailed to Biosafe Lab. Results for a whole lipid profile are given. A licensed doctor reviews the results before they are sent to the patient.

Cardiocheck

Cardiocheck has the potential to test for TC (total cholesterol), HDL (high-density lipoprotein), and TG (triglycerides). LDL (low-density lipoprotein) must be calculated.
The unit stores results. It is reusable.

Fecal Occult Blood Tests

Three categories are available:

- Toilet tests (EZ-Detect Stool Blood Test), which use biodegradable paper that is placed in the toilet bowl after a bowel movement
- Stool wipes (LifeGuard)
- Manual stool application tests (Colon-Test-Sensitive)

A colorimetric assay is used for hemoglobin. A blue-green color indicates a positive test.
Tests are more likely to detect lower GI problems. False-positive test can occur with the ingestion of red meat or vitamin C.

Acquired Immune Deficiency Syndrome (AIDS)

Home Access and Home Access Express HIV-1 tests check for antibodies to HIV (human immunodeficiency virus). Patients should be aware that it can take 3 weeks to 6 months before antibodies are detectable following infection.
A fingerstick blood sample is placed on the specimen card. The card is mailed to the lab within 10 days. Home Access provides results in 7 days. Home Access Express provides results in 3 days.

27-9. Smoking Cessation

Unless the patient has contraindications, pharmacotherapy should be offered to all patients attempting to quit smoking (Table 27-14).
First-line agents double long-term smoking abstinence rates:

- Nicotine replacement therapy (NRT):
  - Nicotine gum (Nicorette and generic): OTC
  - Nicotine patch (Nicotrol, Nicoderm CQ, and generic): OTC
  - Nicotine lozenge (Commit): OTC
  - Nicotine inhaler (Nicotrol inhaler): prescription only
  - Nicotine nasal spray (Nicotrol NS): prescription only

Table 27-14. The "5 A's" Clinicians Should Use to Assist Patients in Smoking Cessation

Ask about tobacco use.	Identify and document tobacco use status for every patient at every visit.
Advise to quit.	In a clear, strong, and personalized manner, urge every tobacco user to quit.
Assess willingness to make a quit attempt.	Is the tobacco user willing to make a quit attempt at this time?
Assist in quit attempt.	For the patient willing to make a quit attempt, use counseling and pharmacotherapy to help him or her quit.
Arrange follow-up.	Schedule follow-up contact, preferably within the first week after the quit date.

- Bupropion SR (Zyban): prescription only
- Varenicline (Chantix): prescription only

Second-line agents are available if patients fail or cannot tolerate first-line agents:

- Clonidine
- Nortriptyline

Combination NRT

Combining the nicotine patch with a self-administered form of NRT (either the nicotine gum or nicotine nasal spray) is useful for some patients. Combined treatment should be recommended if the patient is unable to quit using a single type of first-line pharmacotherapy.

Side Effects

NRT can have various side effects:

- Gum
  - Patients may experience an unpleasant taste, mouth irritation, jaw muscle soreness, hypersalivation, hiccups, and dyspepsia.
  - Gum can stick to dental work.
  - Warn patients against chewing the gum too fast.
  - Patients with temporomandibular joint pain may want to avoid gum.
- Lozenge
  - Mouth irritation, nausea, hiccups, cough, heartburn, headache, flatulence, and insomnia can occur.
  - Do not use more than one lozenge at a time.
- Patch
  - Local skin reactions (erythema, burning, pruritis) can occur. Treat by rotating sites or applying hydrocortisone or triamcinolone cream.
  - Vivid or abnormal dreams, insomnia, and headache can arise. These effects are more common

in the 24-hour patch. Patients can minimize the effects by using the 16-hour patch or by removing the patch at night before bed.

Contraindications and Precautions

Cardiovascular disease is a contraindication in the following cases:

- < 2 weeks following myocardial infarction
- Serious arrhythmias
- Serious or worsening angina

Esophagitis and peptic ulcer disease is contraindicated with the gum form.

NRT patients should seek medical advice if they are pregnant or breast-feeding.

Patients should not smoke while using NRT.

Allergies, asthma, and sinus conditions are contraindicated with the nasal spray.

27-10. Natural and Herbal Products

Complementary and Alternative Medicine Definitions

- *Conventional treatment:* Medical practices widely accepted and practiced by the mainstream medical community
- *Complementary therapy:* Therapy used in addition to conventional treatments.
- *Alternative therapy:* Therapy used instead of conventional treatments.
- *Dietary supplement:* According to the Dietary Supplement and Health Education Act of 1994, "a product intended to supplement the diet that . . . contains one or more of the following dietary ingredients: a vitamin, mineral, herb, or other botanical, amino acid; a dietary substance for use by man to supplement the diet by increasing the total daily intake; or a concentrate, metabolite, constituent, extract, or combination of these ingredients"

Regulation of Dietary Supplements

Dietary supplements are not regulated as closely as drugs. Table 27-15 provides a comparison.

The following agencies are responsible for regulation:

- *U.S. Food and Drug Administration:* Regulates labeling, safety, and manufacturing
- *U.S. Federal Trade Commission:* Regulates advertising

Table 27-15. Drugs versus Dietary Supplements

Drug	Dietary supplement
Active ingredient is identified.	Active ingredient may not be identified.
Safety and efficacy are proven by manufacturer.	No proof of efficacy is required; FDA must provide proof if unsafe.
Purity and contents are regulated.	No standards exist for quality or purity.
Claims to treat, cure, or prevent disease are made.	No claims to treat, cure, or prevent specific disease are made.

Herbal Products

Alpha lipoic acid

Common uses
Alpha lipoic acid is used for diabetic peripheral neuropathy.

Proposed mechanisms
This product is thought to be a cofactor for several enzymes required for glucose metabolism. It is believed to allow for increased glucose uptake and is considered a chelating and antioxidant agent.

Dosage
The dosage is 600 mg tid orally, taken on an empty stomach and separated at least 2–3 hours from the ingestion of antacids.

Side effects
Side effects include headache, nausea, allergic rash, and hypoglycemia.

Contraindications
Patients with thyroid disease should not take this product.

Asian ginseng *(Panax ginseng)*

Common uses
Asian ginseng is taken to decrease fatigue and enhance concentration.

Proposed mechanisms
This product is thought to suppress and stimulate the CNS. Corticosteroid activity and hypoglycemic activity are considered to occur.

Dosage
The dosage is 1–2 g of crude root or 100–400 mg of ginseng extract tid.

Side effects
Side effects are hypertension; euphoria, restlessness, nervousness, and insomnia; rash; edema; and diarrhea.

Contraindications
Contraindications are as follows:

- Renal failure
- Acute infection
- Pregnancy and lactation
- Active bleeding (peptic ulcer)

Ginseng should be stopped 7–10 days prior to surgery to avoid potential bleeding complications.

Precautions
Caution is warranted in the following circumstances:

- Cardiovascular disease
- Hypertension with or without medical treatment
- Diabetes (specifically with patients receiving medications that may cause hypoglycemia or having diagnosis of hypoglycemia unaware)
- History of hypotension

Interactions
- Risk with anticoagulants and antiplatelet agents (aspirin, ticlopidine, clopidogrel, dipyridamole, warfarin) and other herbs (ginkgo, garlic)
- Stimulants (including caffeine)
- Antipsychotics

Coenzyme Q10 (Ubiquinone)

Common uses
Coenzyme Q10 (CoQ10) is commonly used for cardiovascular conditions.

Proposed mechanisms
CoQ10 is a cofactor for many functions associated with energy production. It is a powerful antioxidant that helps in the regeneration of other antioxidants. It also stabilizes membranes and may have vasodilatory and inotropic effects.

Dosage
For heart failure, cardiomyopathy, and hypertension, the dosage is 100 mg qd bid.

Side effects
Side effects include nausea, GI distress, headache, irritability, and dizziness.

Interactions
- CoQ10 has a similar structure to synthetic vitamin K, which may cause a decrease in

international normalized ratio (INR) levels if used concomitantly with warfarin.

■ HMG CoA (3-hydroxy-3-methylglutaryl-coenzyme A) reductase inhibitors reduce serum levels of CoQ10.

Echinacea purpurea

Common uses
Echinacea purpurea is used for colds and other respiratory tract infections. It is used topically for poorly healing wounds and chronic ulcerations.

Proposed mechanisms
This product is thought to stimulate the immune system. It is believed to increase white blood cells and provide antiviral, antifungal, and anti-inflammatory action.

Dosage
Dosing should begin at the onset of viral symptoms. On day 1, take 50–100 mg tid. Then take 250 mg qid. Continue treatment until 24–48 hours after symptoms abate.

Side effects
Allergic reactions can occur. Limit use to 6–8 weeks at a time.

Contraindications
This product should not be taken by patients with severe systemic illness (HIV/AIDS, multiple sclerosis, tuberculosis) or autoimmune disorders (rheumatoid arthritis).

Interactions
Potentially severe allergic response, including anaphylaxis, may occur in individuals with asthma or allergies to members of the daisy family (ragweed, daisies, chrysanthemums, marigolds). Immunosuppressive agents may interact with this product.

Fish oil

Common uses
Fish oil is often taken to improve cardiovascular health and by patients with hypertriglyceridemia, rheumatoid arthritis, or psoriasis.

Proposed mechanisms
Fish oil provides a source of omega-3 fatty acids (docosahexaenoic acid and eicosapentaenoic acid). It is considered to increase anti-inflammatory cytokines and decrease pro-inflammatory cytokines. It is thought to decrease the intestinal absorption of cholesterol and inhibit the synthesis and degradation of very-low-density lipoprotein particles.

Dosage
■ *General use:* 1–2 g daily
■ *Hypertriglyceridemia:* 2–4 g daily
■ *Rheumatoid arthritis:* 4 g daily
■ *Psoriasis:* 3–4 g daily

Side effects
Side effects include GI distress and fish burp, which may be avoided by using enteric-coated products, taking with meals, or keeping the capsules in the freezer.

Interactions
At doses > 4 g daily, increased bleeding risk is present; therefore, patients on anticoagulation or antiplatelet therapy should be limited to 3 g daily.

Garlic (*Allium sativum*)

Common uses
Garlic is taken to lower cholesterol, prevent atherosclerosis, treat bacterial and fungal infections, and prevent various cancers.

Proposed mechanisms
Garlic is considered to exhibit antimicrobial action through sulfur-containing compounds, inhibit platelet aggregation, act as a free radical scavenger, stimulate fibrinolysis, and lower cholesterol and lipid levels by inhibition of HMG-CoA reductase.

Dosage
Dosage is as follows:

■ 4 g fresh minced garlic bulb
■ 600–900 mg/d (100 mg garlic powder tablets)
■ 3–5 mg allicin daily

Side effects
Side effects include malodorous breath and smell of garlic that may permeate the skin; GI discomfort, heartburn, and gas; and dermatitis and allergic reactions.

Contraindications
Active bleeding (peptic ulcer) can occur. Garlic should be stopped 7–10 days prior to surgery to avoid potential bleeding complications.

Interactions

- *Anticoagulants and antiplatelet agents:* Aspirin, ticlopidine, clopidogrel, dipyridamole, warfarin, ginkgo, ginseng
- *Saquinavir AUC (area under curve):* 50% decrease in healthy volunteers

Ginger

Common use
Ginger is used as an antiemetic.

Proposed mechanism
It is thought to stimulate gastric secretions and peristalsis.

Dosage

- *Pregnancy-induced nausea or vomiting:* Dried ginger 250 mg qid
- *Motion sickness:* Two 500-mg capsules of dried powdered ginger root taken 30 minutes prior to travel, followed by one to two more 500-mg capsules as needed every 4 hours

Side effects
Heartburn and dermatitis may occur.

Interactions
Ginger may increase the risk of hypoglycemia. It alters platelet function at doses > 1 g/d. Use with caution in patients receiving antiplatelet and anticoagulation therapy.

Ginkgo biloba

Common uses
Ginkgo biloba is used to enhance memory and concentration. It is used to treat or prevent Alzheimer's disease and vascular dementias. It is also used to treat intermittent claudication, vertigo, and tinnitus.

Proposed mechanisms
Ginkgo biloba is thought to increase blood flow, act as an antioxidant, and inhibit platelet aggregation.

Dosage
Recommend a standardized product, 120–240 mg/d divided bid or tid.

Side effects

- *Mild:* GI distress, headache, and dizziness can occur.
- *Serious:* Spontaneous bleeding has been reported (e.g., subdural hematomas and subarachnoid hemorrhage).

Interactions
This product may interact with both medications (aspirin, ticlopidine, clopidogrel, dipyridamole, warfarin) and herbs (garlic, ginseng). Interactions are due to antiplatelet or anticoagulant activity.

Contraindications
Ginkgo should be stopped 7–10 days prior to surgery to avoid potential bleeding complications.

Glucosamine and chondroitin sulfate

Common uses
Glucosamine and chondroitin sulfate products are used for osteoarthritis.

Proposed mechanisms
This product serves as a precursor to glycosaminoglycans, which make up cartilage and synovial fluid. It may help regenerate cartilage and replete synovial fluid.

Dosage
Dosage is as follows:

- *Glucosamine:* 500 mg tid (with meals) glucosamine sulfate
- *Chondroitin:* 400 mg tid

These agents are often in a combination product; however, glucosamine has more evidence supporting its use. Full effects may not be seen for 6–8 weeks.

Side effects
Mild GI effects such as nausea and heartburn may occur. Little is known about the long-term use of this product.

Contraindications
Patients with severe shellfish allergy should not take this product.

Green tea

Common uses
Green tea is taken as a performance enhancer and to protect from the development of cardiovascular disease and cancer.

Proposed mechanisms
Green tea contains caffeine, which has a stimulant effect, and antioxidants (EGCG [Epigallocatechin gallate]), which protect against oxidative damage.

Dosage
The common consumption in Asian countries is 3 cups daily. Dosage varies from 1–10 cups daily.

Side effects

GI irritation and both CNS and cardiac stimulation can occur because of caffeine content. Green tea can contain a range of 8–30 mg of caffeine per tea bag.

Drug interactions

Large doses may decrease INR levels, although brewing destroys most of the vitamin K content.

Kava-kava

Common uses

Kava-kava is used for anxiety or stress.

Proposed mechanisms

Kava-kava possibly binds at GABA (γ-aminobutyric acid) receptors. It possibly acts as a dopamine antagonist.

Dosage

The dosage is 100 mg two to three times daily.

Side effects

Side effects are similar to those that occur with alcohol (i.e., it adversely affects motor reflexes and judgment for driving or operating heavy machinery), but kava-kava does not act as a CNS depressant.

Mydriasis and extrapyramidal symptoms may occur.

Yellow, flaking, and scaly skin and eye redness are possible effects.

Liver failure, leading to transplantation or death, is a serious concern (Table 27-16).

Contraindications

Patients who have preexisting liver disease or who regularly ingest alcohol should not take this product.

Precautions

Patients should be counseled as follows:

- Do not take for > 4 weeks.
- Discontinue immediately if jaundice occurs.

Interactions

- *L-dopa:* Decreased effectiveness
- *Barbiturates, benzodiazepines, and alcohol:* Additive sedative effects

Melatonin

Common uses

Melatonin is commonly used for sleep disorders and to reset the sleep–wake cycle (jet lag).

Proposed mechanisms

Melatonin mimics endogenous release of melatonin from the pineal gland. Concentrations increase significantly 1–2 hours before sleep.

Dosage

Dosages are as follows:

- *Insomnia:* 0.3–5 mg 30 minutes prior to bedtime
- *Jet lag:* 2–5 mg in the evening between 5:00 pm and 10:00 pm on the day of arrival and at bedtime for 2–5 days after arrival

Long-term administration is not recommended.

Table 27-16. Natural Products Associated with Serious Toxicity

Common name	Promoted benefit or ailment helped	Associated conditions
Blue cohosh	Uterotonic, diuretic	Vasoconstriction, GI spasms
Comfrey	Gout, arthritis, infections	Obstruction of blood flow to the liver possibly resulting in death
Chinese weight-loss preparations (*Aristolochia fangchi* mistaken for *Stephania tetrandra*)	Primarily weight loss	Kidney cancer (referred to as *Chinese-herb nephropathy*)
Ephedra (ma huang)	Weight loss, energy, decongestion	Hypertension, arrhythmias, seizures, stroke, myocardial infarction, death
Kava-kava	Stress reduction	Liver failure
Licorice root	Peptic ulcers, expectorant	Pseudoaldosteronism
Yohimbe	Aphrodisiac	Weakness, paralysis, anxiety, death (overdose)

Side effects

Melatonin may worsen depression. Other side effects include headache and confusion. Melatonin is possibly an immune stimulant.

Interactions

When melatonin is taken with benzodiazepines, anxiolytic effects are enhanced.

Probiotics

Common uses

Probiotics are taken for antibiotic-induced diarrhea, GI disorders, atopic dermatitis, and allergies.

Proposed mechanisms

Probiotics contain *Lactobacillus* sp, *Bifidobacteria* sp, or *Sacchromyces boulardii*. They are thought to decrease intestinal permeability, normalize gut flora, and decrease inflammatory responses. They possess immunomodulating activity.

Dosage

Lactobacillus sp and *Bifidobacteria* sp are dosed at 1 billion to 10 billion colony-forming units per day. *Sacchromyces boulardii* is dosed at 250–500 mg bid–qid.

Side effects

Bloating, flatulence, and diarrhea may occur.

Contraindications

Because of reports of systemic infection, immunocompromised patients should avoid use.

Interactions

Probiotics may decrease antibiotic absorption; therefore, antimicrobial agents should be administered several hours apart from taking probiotics.

Saw palmetto (*Serenoa repens*)

Common uses

Saw palmetto is used for benign prostatic hyperplasia.

Proposed mechanism

It inhibits 5α-reductase and dihydrotestosterone binding to androgen receptors.

Dosage

For a product with 80–90% fatty acids, the dose is 160 mg bid or 320 mg qd. Take with morning and evening meals to decrease GI upset. Treatment usually lasts for 3 months.

Side effects

Rarely, GI upset, headache, or hypertension may occur. Urinary tract symptoms (urine retention, dysuria) are possible. Impotence may occur.

Precautions

Recommend a thorough prostate exam and discussion with physician before starting treatment to rule out prostate cancer.

St. John's wort (*Hypericum perforatum*)

Common uses

St. John's wort is used to treat depression and anxiety.

Proposed mechanisms

This product is thought to inhibit dopamine, serotonin, and norepinephrine reuptake and to decrease IL-6 (interleukin-6) concentrations.

Dosage

This product is standardized to 0.3% hypericin or 5% hyperforin. The recommended dose is 300–600 mg tid.

Side effects

Mild GI distress, paresthesias, dizziness, fatigue, insomnia, itching, dry mouth, and loss of libido can occur. Photosensitivity can occur: recommend sun avoidance or sunscreen.

Interactions

Interactions are well documented and clinically significant.

Antidepressants (SSRIs [selective serotonin reuptake inhibitors] and TCAs [tricyclic antidepressants]) interact with this product because of a similar mechanism of action resulting in serotonin syndrome.

St. John's wort is an inducer of CYP (cytochrome) 450-3A4, 1A2, and 2C9, causing decreased levels of medications and possibly resulting in reduced therapeutic effects. Medications affected include the following:

- Cyclosporine
- Indinavir
- Digoxin
- Oral contraceptives (Estradiol component)

27-11. Sleep Aids and Stimulants

Insomnia

Nonpharmacologic treatment of insomnia

Nonpharmacologic treatments include the following:

- Establish regular waking and sleeping schedule.
- Exercise regularly.
- Do not nap during the daytime.
- Avoid caffeine, especially after noon.
- Avoid large meals close to bedtime.
- Participate in a relaxing activity at bedtime (e.g., reading or hot bath).

Nonprescription medication treatment

Selected nonprescription products are described in Table 27-17.

Antihistamines

Administer diphenhydramine 25–50 mg 30–60 minutes before bedtime (elderly patients, 25 mg).

Antihistamines block histamine$_1$ and muscarinic receptors. They should be used for short-term management of occasional insomnia in conjunction with good sleep hygiene. Do not exceed 14 days of therapy (to avoid tolerance).

Side effects

Sedation, especially the next morning, may occur. Anticholinergic effects may occur as follows:

- Dry mouth or eyes
- Constipation
- Urinary retention
- Confusion (elderly patients)

Contraindications and precautions

Patients with benign prostatic hyperplasia, dementia, or narrow-angle glaucoma should not use this medication.

Table 27-17. Selected Nonprescription Products for Insomnia

Drug or drug combination	Trade name
Diphenhydramine	Compoz, Sominex
Diphenhydramine + acetaminophen	Tylenol PM, Excedrin PM
Diphenhydramine + aspirin	Bayer PM
Diphenhydramine + ibuprofen	Advil PM

Drowsiness

Nonpharmacologic treatment of drowsiness

Good sleep hygiene is preferable to drug therapy (see previous discussion of insomnia).

Nonprescription medication treatment

Caffeine is the only FDA-approved nonprescription stimulant. It acts as a CNS stimulant.

Physical dependence can develop. Taking 50–200 mg results in increased alertness and decreased fatigue. Taking > 200 mg can result in nervousness, insomnia, and irritability.

Precautions exist with patients with peptic ulcer disease, cardiac dysrhythmias, and anxiety disorders.

Patients who are pregnant should restrict their caffeine intake to < 300 mg daily. Patients who are breast-feeding should be aware that 1% of caffeine crosses into breast milk; peak effect is 1 hour after consumption.

27-12. Overweight and Obesity

Clinical Indicators

The National Heart Lung and Blood Institute of the National Institutes of Health (NHLBI) and World Health Organization definition is based on body mass index (BMI):

- Overweight = BMI 25–29.9
- Obese I = BMI 30–34.9
- Obese II = BMI 35–39.9
- Obese III = BMI ≥ 40

NHLBI also assesses a patient's morbidity and mortality risk with regard to waist circumference:

- Males with a waist circumference > 40 inches
- Females with a waist circumference > 35 inches

These persons are at increased risk of developing type 2 diabetes and cardiovascular disease.

Nonpharmacologic Therapy

Nonpharmacologic therapy involves lifestyle modification.

Caloric restriction

Usually restriction of calories sufficient to create a deficit of 800–100 kcal/d is recommended. A low calorie diet results in a typical weight loss of 1–2 lbs/week. Portion control is essential.

Altered proportions of food groups is an important lifestyle modification:

- *Fat:* < 30% of total calories from fat and < 8–10% of total calories from saturated fat
- *Carbohydrates:* 45–65% of total calories
- *Protein:* 10–35% of total calories

Use of food additives

Artificial sweeteners and fat substitutes can be helpful.

Physical Activity

Increasing physical activity is recommended:

- *For reduction of chronic disease:* Engage in 30 minutes of moderate intensity exercise most days of the week.
- *For prevention of body weight gain over time:* Engage in 60 minutes of moderate to vigorous intensity exercise most days of the week.
- *For sustaining weight loss:* Engage in 60 minutes of moderate intensity exercise most days of the week.

Behavioral therapy

Behavioral therapy involves environmental modification, modified thinking patterns, maintenance of a healthy attitude, and social support.

Nonprescription medication therapy

Orlistat (Alli)

The FDA approved orlistat for nonprescription status in 2007. Orlistat decreases the absorption of dietary fats and inhibits gastric and pancreatic lipases.

Indication

Orlistat is indicated for use in patients ≥ 18 years of age who are overweight (BMI ≥ 25) in conjunction with lifestyle modification.

Dose

Patients should take one 60 mg capsule before meals. They do not have to take the medication if the meal does not contain fat.

Side effects

Side effects include the following:

- Flatulence with oily spotting
- Loose and frequent stools
- Fatty stools
- Fecal urgency
- Incontinence

Decreasing the amount of ingested fat can minimize these effects. Effects generally resolve within a few weeks of initiating therapy.

Contraindications

Patients on cyclosporine and patients with malabsorption disorders should not use this medication. Patients with a history of thyroid disease, cholelithiasis, nephrolithiasis, or pancreatitis should consult a primary care physician prior to use.

Interactions

Decreased absorption of fat-soluble vitamins (especial D & E) occurs. Take a multivitamin at bedtime or separate it from orlistat dose by at least 2 hours.

Concern exists over Vitamin K absorption and possible effects on warfarin; therefore, recommend increased monitoring.

27-13. Key Points

Cough, Cold, and Allergy

- Cough and cold products are not to be used in children < 4 years of age.
- Nonprescription drug therapy for the common cold includes symptomatic management using decongestants (nasal congestion), antihistamines (excess nasal discharge), analgesics (headache), and local anesthetic lozenges or sprays (pharyngitis).
- Nonprescription treatment of allergies includes systemic antihistamines (sedating or nonsedating), ocular antihistamines, decongestants (if nasal congestion), and cromolyn (scheduled, not as needed).
- Cough can be relieved by a product containing a cough suppressant (dextromethorphan). An expectorant (guaifenesin) should be recommended to enhance clearance of mucus.

Constipation

- Diet and lifestyle changes should always be recommended to prevent or treat constipation (exercise and an increase in fiber and fluid intake).
- Bulk-forming laxatives and stool softeners are the safest products to prevent and treat constipation and can be used chronically.
- Stimulant laxatives should be used only occasionally to prevent laxative dependence or other complications.

Diarrhea

- Loperamide or bismuth subsalicylate may be recommended to treat diarrhea.
- Maintaining adequate hydration is very important, especially in young children and elderly patients.

Nausea and Vomiting

- Nonprescription treatment options for nausea and vomiting include antihistamines (meclizine, dimenhydrinate) and phosphorated carbohydrate solution (Emetrol).
- H2RAs (cimetidine, ranitidine); antacids; or bismuth salts (Pepto-Bismol) may relieve gastric discomfort or indigestion.

Pain and Fever

- Pain and fever may be treated with aspirin and other salicylates, NSAIDs, or acetaminophen.
- Aspirin and NSAIDs inhibit platelet aggregation. Nonacetylated salicylates and acetaminophen do not have antiplatelet activity.
- Salicylates and NSAIDs can cause gastropathy, including gastritis, gastric ulcers, and gastric bleeding. They may decrease the effectiveness of some antihypertensives and may have deleterious effects on kidney function.
- Acetaminophen does not have anti-inflammatory activity and can be hepatotoxic in excessive doses (> 4 g/d) or when used concurrently with alcohol.

Ophthalmic Disorders

- Dry eyes can be treated with artificial tears or ocular emollients.
- Ophthalmic vasoconstrictors (ocular decongestants) cause vasoconstriction in the conjunctiva to treat redness. Naphazoline is the ocular decongestant of choice. Ocular decongestants are contraindicated in patients with narrow-angle glaucoma because of the potential to cause rebound.
- Ketotifen fumarate is the safest and most effective product for the treatment of allergic conjunctivitis. Twice daily dosing and safety of this product for children ≥ 3 years of age make it the primary therapy for patients with this condition.

Otic Disorders

- Impacted cerumen can be treated with cerumen-softening agents (carbamide peroxide in anhydrous glycerin + alcohol; hydrogen peroxide + water).

- Water-clogged ears may be managed with the commercial preparation of isopropyl alcohol + anhydrous glycerin or with compounded acetic acid + isopropyl alcohol.

Home Monitoring and Testing Devices

- Other testing devices that were not discussed in detail in this chapter include diabetic meters, male fertility tests, illicit drug use tests, and the hepatitis C test.
- When counseling patients on the use of these devices, it is important to ensure that they understand the directions for use (appropriate timing and causes of false-positive and false negative results), check for expiration dates, and make certain the product is developed to give them the results they are seeking.

Smoking Cessation

- First-line agents for pharmacotherapy in smoking cessation are as follows:
  - Nicotine gum (Nicorette, generic) OTC
  - Nicotine patch (Nicotrol, Nicoderm CQ) OTC
  - Nicotine inhaler (Nicotrol inhaler)
  - Nicotine nasal spray (Nicotrol NS)
  - Bupropion SR (Zyban)
  - Varenicline (Chantix)
- Contraindications and precautions for nicotine replacement therapy are as follows:
  - Cardiovascular disease
    - < 2 weeks post–myocardial infarction
    - Serious arrhythmias
    - Serious or worsening angina
  - Esophagitis and peptic ulcer disease (gum)
- Patients should seek medical advice if pregnant or breast-feeding.
- Patients should not smoke while using nicotine replacement therapy.

Natural and Herbal Products

- Herbal products that should be stopped 7–10 days prior to surgery include ginkgo, garlic, and ginseng.
- St. John's Wort takes several weeks to see effect and has the potential for serious drug interactions.

Sleep Aids

- Diphenhydramine should be used for short-term management of occasional insomnia in conjunction with good sleep hygiene.

Stimulants

■ Caffeine, a CNS stimulant, is the only nonprescription stimulant approved by the FDA.

■ The recommended dosage of 50–200 mg may increase alertness and decrease fatigue.

■ Doses exceeding 200 mg may cause nervousness, insomnia, and irritability.

Overweight and Obesity

■ Overweight and obese persons in the United States have reached epidemic proportions. This condition is significant because it is associated with increased morbidity from cardiovascular disease, diabetes, gall bladder disease, osteoarthritis, respiratory problems, and several different types of cancer.

■ Orlistat (Alli) is an FDA-approved nonprescription medication used for the treatment of overweight patients ≥ 18 years of age. This medication has many side effects that patients may find unpleasant, and as a result, patients should be counseled on these side effects and ways to avoid them. The use of this medication may decrease the absorption of fat-soluble vitamins from the GI tract.

27-14. Questions

1. Which of the following is the primary advantage of recommending dextromethorphan instead of codeine?

   A. It is twice as effective as codeine in suppression of cough.
   B. It has less dependence potential.
   C. It has peripheral rather than central action.
   D. It is less expensive.
   E. It is much longer acting than codeine.

2. All of the following statements regarding guaifenesin are correct *except*

   A. it is the only OTC expectorant approved by the U.S. Food and Drug Administration (FDA).
   B. it requires large amounts of water to be effective.
   C. it is available OTC as Robitussin.
   D. it may cause a decrease in platelet aggregation and an increase in bleeding time.
   E. it is available in some prescription cough and cold formulations.

3. All of the following statements regarding diphenhydramine are true *except*

   A. it is less likely to cause drowsiness than other OTC antihistamines.
   B. it is the active ingredient in some OTC products for insomnia.
   C. it is available OTC under the trade name of Benadryl.
   D. a small percentage of children may exhibit a paradoxical CNS stimulant effect.
   E. elderly patients may experience delirium or confusion with diphenhydramine.

4. All of the following statements about the routine use of oral decongestants in treating the common cold are true *except*

   A. They cannot be used in patients on MAO inhibitor antidepressants.
   B. They are relatively safe, with no dependence.
   C. They are absolutely contraindicated in patients with controlled diabetes and mild hypertension.
   D. The most common side effects are nervousness and insomnia.

5. All of the following are correct generic and trade name combinations *except*

   A. Chlor-Trimeton = chlorpheniramine
   B. Tavist = diphenhydramine
   C. Claritin = loratadine
   D. Nasalcrom = cromolyn
   E. Zyrtec = cetirizine

6. Which of the following is *not* a side effect of loperamide?

   A. Sedation
   B. Dizziness
   C. Dry mouth
   D. Drowsiness
   E. Insomnia

7. Which of the following is *not* an adverse effect of Pepto-Bismol?

   A. Anticholinergic effects, dry mouth, and dry eyes
   B. Tinnitus
   C. Cross-sensitivity to aspirin allergy
   D. Grayish-black tongue
   E. Dark stools

8. Which of the following drugs exhibits analgesic and antipyretic properties, but not peripheral anti-inflammatory properties?

    A. Ibuprofen
    B. Sodium salicylate
    C. Acetaminophen
    D. Magnesium salicylate
    E. Naproxen

9. Which drug does *not* interact with NSAIDs?

    A. Methotrexate
    B. Warfarin
    C. Antihypertensive agents
    D. Diphenhydramine
    E. None of the above

10. Mary is a 32-year-old female with asthma and serious aspirin sensitivity. She comes to the pharmacist seeking assistance in selecting a nonprescription product for aches and pains. Which of the following should the pharmacist recommend for Mary?

    A. Ibuprofen
    B. Naproxen
    C. Acetaminophen
    D. A and B only
    E. All of the above

11. Nonprescription antiemetics are primarily useful for preventing which type of nausea?

    A. Nausea caused by alterations in the vestibular apparatus
    B. Nausea caused by drugs acting centrally on the chemoreceptor trigger zone
    C. Nausea caused by visceral pain
    D. Nausea caused by cortical stimulation from smells or sight
    E. Nausea caused by afferent impulses from the gastrointestinal tract

12. A mother requests advice for her 6-month-old child, who has been constipated for the past 2 days after beginning cereal feedings. Which of the following agents would be the best laxative agent to recommend?

    A. Dulcolax
    B. Fletcher's Castoria
    C. Mineral oil
    D. Glycerin suppositories
    E. Milk of magnesia

13. All of the following statements about stool softeners are true *except*

    A. they are not safe to use in pregnancy.
    B. the onset of action is usually within 1–2 days.
    C. they are useful in patients with constipation who have hemorrhoids.
    D. extra water helps their effectiveness.
    E. they are often combined with mild stimulant laxatives.

14. All of the following statements about bisacodyl are true *except*

    A. it should not be taken concurrently with antacids.
    B. it can be crushed or chewed if needed.
    C. it should not be recommended in pregnancy.
    D. it is available in oral tablet and suppository dosage forms.
    E. it is the active ingredient in Dulcolax.

15. Which of the following antihistamines are available in OTC products for insomnia?

    A. Diphenhydramine
    B. Cetirizine
    C. Loratadine
    D. B and C
    E. All of the above

16. Baby Matthew is 1 year old and weighs 24 lb. He has a fever of 102°F, is irritable, seems uncomfortable, and is not sleeping well. His mother is confused by the assortment of fever relief products. You recommend acetaminophen. Which product and dosage do you recommend?

    A. Tylenol Infant Drops 80 mg/0.8 mL; give 1.6 mL q4–6h
    B. Tylenol Children's Liquid 160 mg/5 mL; give 2 tsp. q6–8h
    C. Advil Infant Drops 50 mg/1.25 mL; give 1.25 mL q4–6h
    D. Motrin Children's Suspension 100 mg/5 mL; give 2.5 mL q6–8h
    E. Tylenol Infant Drops 80 mg/0.8 mL; give 3.2 mL q4–6h

17. The next morning, baby Matthew's mother returns to your pharmacy. Her pediatrician recommended alternating the maximum dose of ibuprofen with the acetaminophen, and she

is asking for help selecting an ibuprofen product and dosage. Which do you recommend?

A. Advil Infant Drops 50 mg/1.25 mL; give 0.625 mL q8h
B. Motrin Children's Suspension 100 mg/5 mL; give 2 tsp q4h
C. Motrin Infant Drops 50 mg/1.25 mL; give 2.5 mL q6h
D. Advil Children's Chewable Tablet 50 mg; give one tablet q8h
E. Advil Children's Chewable Tablet 50 mg; give one-half tablet q4h

18. Which of the following tests does not require a blood sample?

A. Cholesterol test
B. Ovulation prediction tests
C. HIV tests
D. Hepatitis C test
E. Accu-Chek Advantage

19. B. R. is a 62-year-old obese male who has been diagnosed by his physician with benign prostatic hyperplasia. Which of the following herbal remedies might be used to treat his symptoms?

A. Ginseng
B. Echinacea
C. DHEA
D. Garlic
E. Saw palmetto

20. Which of the following products should be discontinued prior to surgery?

A. Ginkgo biloba
B. Gentian root
C. Glutamine
D. Glucosamine
E. Folic acid

21. Cough and cold products are not to be used in children less than _____ years of age.

A. 2
B. 4
C. 6
D. 8
E. 12

22. When a patient is considering the use of nonprescription orlistat, which of the fol-

lowing vitamins may the patient need as additional supplementation because of decreased absorption?

A. B_{12}
B. B_6
C. D
D. C

27-15. Answers

1. B. Although there have been reports of limited recreational abuse of dextromethorphan, its potential for dependence and addiction is significantly less than that of codeine.
2. D. Guaifenesin does not have any effects on platelet aggregation or bleeding time. It is the only FDA-approved OTC expectorant, works better with increased fluid intake, and is included in Robitussin products.
3. A. Diphenhydramine, an ethanolamine, is the most sedating OTC antihistamine.
4. C. Systemic decongestants are not recommended in individuals with uncontrolled diabetes or hypertension because of their sympathomimetic effects. They are contraindicated with MAO inhibitors and can commonly cause nervousness or insomnia.
5. B. Tavist contains clemastine.
6. E. Sedation, dizziness, dry mouth, and drowsiness are common side effects of loperamide. Insomnia is not.
7. A. Common adverse effects of Pepto-Bismol include tinnitus and grayish-black tongue or stools. Pepto-Bismal does contain a salicylate and, therefore, should not be used in individuals with aspirin allergy.
8. C. Acetaminophen is a centrally acting antipyretic and analgesic, but it does not exhibit peripheral anti-inflammatory activity. Salicylates and other NSAIDs do.
9. D. NSAIDs can significantly decrease methotrexate clearance, enhance the effect of warfarin, and blunt the hypotensive effect of hypertensive medications. There is no known interaction with diphenhydramine.
10. C. All NSAIDs and aspirin-containing products should be avoided in individuals with aspirin sensitivity. Acetaminophen can be recommended in this setting.
11. A. Nonprescription antiemetics are antihistamines that exert their effect by inhibiting

histamine in neural centers controlling vomiting, salivation, and vestibular excitability, making them especially well suited for motion sickness.

12. **D.** Glycerin suppositories are safe for infants. The other agents should not be used in this patient population.

13. **A.** Stool softeners are safe to use in pregnancy and usually exert their effect within 1–2 days. Stool softeners are recommended for individuals in whom hard stools or straining could cause pain or complications (e.g., hemorrhoids, postoperative or postpartum time periods, or post–myocardial infarction). Increased fluid intake enhances their effectiveness. They are frequently used in combination products containing stimulant laxatives.

14. **B.** Because bisacodyl is an enteric-coated product, it should not be taken with antacids or be crushed, chewed, or broken. It should not be used in pregnancy. It is available in both oral tablets and rectal suppositories.

15. **A.** Diphenhydramine is an ethanolamine used in sleeping aids. Cetirizine and loratadine are nonsedating antihistamines.

16. **A.** The pediatric dosage of acetaminophen is 10–15 mg/kg q4–6h:

$$24 \text{ lb} \times \text{kg}/2.2 \text{ lb} = 10.9 \text{ kg} \times 10\text{–}15 \text{ mg/kg} = 109.0\text{–}163.5 \text{ mg}$$

Tylenol Infant Drops 80 mg/0.8 mL;
1.6 mL = 160 mg acetaminophen

17. **C.** The pediatric dosage of ibuprofen is 5–10 mg/kg q6–8h:

$$24 \text{ lb} \times \text{kg}/2.2 \text{ lb} = 10.9 \text{ kg} \times 5\text{–}10 \text{ mg/kg} = 54.5\text{–}109.0 \text{ mg}$$

Motrin Infant Drops 50 mg/1.25 mL;
2.5 mL = 100 mg ibuprofen

18. **B.** Cholesterol, HIV, hepatitis C, and blood glucose tests all require a blood sample. Most ovulation prediction tests use urine.

19. **E.** Saw palmetto may have some efficacy in treating benign prostatic hyperplasia, although the patient should be evaluated by a physician to rule out prostate cancer.

20. **A.** Ginkgo biloba has antiplatelet activity and should, therefore, be withheld prior to surgical procedures.

21. **B.** The Consumer Health Care Products Association announced in October 2008 that manufacturers were voluntarily updating all cough and cold products to state "do not use" in children under 4 years of age.

22. **C.** Vitamin D is a fat-soluble vitamin that may have decreased absorption with concomitant orlistat use despite multivitamin supplementation. A multivitamin is best taken at bedtime or separate from an orlistat dose by at least 2 hours.

27-16. References

Berardi RR, ed. *Handbook of Nonprescription Drugs: An Interactive Approach to Self Care*. 16th ed. Washington, D.C.: American Pharmacists Association; 2009.

Fiore MC, Bailey WC, Cohen SJ, et al. *Treating Tobacco Use and Dependence: Clinical Practice Guideline*. Rockville, Md.: U.S. Department of Health and Human Services; 2008.

Pray WS. *Nonprescription Product Therapeutics*. 2nd ed. Baltimore: Lippincott Williams & Wilkins; 2006.

Robbers JE, Tyler VE. *Tyler's Herbs of Choice: The Therapeutic Use of Phytomedicinals*. New York: Hayworth Herbal Press; 1999.

Scott GN, Elmer GW. Update on natural product-drug interactions. *Am J Health-Syst Pharm*. 2002; 59:339–47.

Asthma and Chronic Obstructive Pulmonary Disease

Timothy H. Self, PharmD

28-1. Asthma

Asthma is a chronic inflammatory disorder of the airways in which many cells and cellular elements play a role, in particular mast cells, eosinophils, T-lymphocytes, neutrophils, and epithelial cells. In susceptible individuals, this inflammation causes recurrent episodes of wheezing, breathlessness, chest tightness, and cough, particularly at night and in the early morning. Asthma affects about 22 million Americans and is the most common cause of missed school days for children. Morbidity and mortality caused by asthma are unacceptably high; death rates are greatest in inner-city African Americans and Hispanics.

Types and Classifications

- *Childhood-onset (atopic):* Positive family history of asthma, allergy to tree or grass pollen, house dust mites, cockroaches, household pets, and molds
- *Adult-onset:* Frequently a negative family history and negative skin tests to common aeroallergens

Classification of severity for children over 12 and adults is shown in Figure 28-1. This classification is extremely important in defining treatment options (see Figures 28-2 to 28-4). Classification of severity is taken from the National Institutes of Health (NIH) National Asthma Education and Prevention Program, Expert Panel Report 3, 2007 (EPR-3). See EPR-3 for classification of severity for ages 0–4 years and 5–11 years.

Clinical Presentation

- Episodic wheezing, coughing, chest tightness, and shortness of breath that is worse at night, in the early morning, and with exercise

Pathophysiology

- Asthma is an inflammatory airway disease and also a disease with bronchospasm.
- Common triggers of symptoms include aeroallergens; respiratory viral illness; exercise (especially in cold, dry air); environmental smoke; and fumes.
- Drug-induced asthma includes that caused by aspirin, nonsteroidal anti-inflammatory drugs (NSAIDs), and β-blockers. Low to moderate-dose β_1-selective agents such as atenolol or metoprolol XL can be used if the patient has concurrent post–myocardial infarction or congestive heart failure and does not have severe asthma; COX-2 inhibitors can be used in aspirin-sensitive asthma.
- There is a complex interaction among inflammatory cells (e.g., mast cells, eosinophils, Th2-type lymphocytes); mediators (e.g., leukotrienes); and cytokines (e.g., IL-4, IL-5).
- The result is airway inflammation (mucus and swelling in the lining of the airways) and airway hyperreactivity.
- Early-phase response to inhaling an aeroallergen occurs immediately; late-phase response occurs 4–12 hours later.
- Asthma is commonly worsened by poorly controlled concurrent allergic rhinitis, sinusitis, and gastroesophageal reflux disease (GERD); it may also worsen in the premenstrual or perimenstrual period.

Diagnostic Criteria

- The main basis for diagnosis is a detailed history of episodic symptoms that are typically worse at night and in the early morning and that are associated with common triggers.

Figure 28-1. Classification of Asthma Severity (Ages ≥ 12 and Adults)

Assessing severity and initiating treatment for patients who are not currently taking long-term control medications

Components of Severity		Classification of Asthma Severity ≥12 years of age			
			Persistent		
		Intermittent	Mild	Moderate	Severe
Impairment Normal FEV$_1$/FVC: 8–19 yr 85% 20–39 yr 80% 40–59 yr 75% 60–80 yr 70%	Symptoms	≤2 days/week	>2 days/week but not daily	Daily	Throughout the day
	Nighttime awakenings	≤2x/month	3–4x/month	>1x/week but not nightly	Often 7x/week
	Short-acting beta$_2$-agonist use for symptom control (not prevention of EIB)	≤2 days/week	>2 days/week but not daily, and not more than 1x on any day	Daily	Several times per day
	Interference with normal activity	None	Minor limitation	Some limitation	Extremely limited
	Lung function	• Normal FEV$_1$ between exacerbations • FEV$_1$ >80% predicted • FEV$_1$/FVC normal	• FEV$_1$ >80% predicted • FEV$_1$/FVC normal	• FEV$_1$ >60% but <80% predicted • FEV$_1$/FVC reduced 5%	• FEV$_1$ <60% predicted • FEV$_1$/FVC reduced >5%
Risk	Exacerbations requiring oral systemic corticosteroids	0–1/year (see note)	≥2/year (see note) → ← Consider severity and interval since last exacerbation. → Frequency and severity may fluctuate over time for patients in any severity category. Relative annual risk of exacerbations may be related to FEV$_1$.		
Recommended Step for Initiating Treatment		Step 1	Step 2	Step 3	Step 4 or 5 and consider short course of oral systemic corticosteroids
		In 2–6 weeks, evaluate level of asthma control that is achieved and adjust therapy accordingly.			

Key: FEV$_1$, forced expiratory volume in 1 second; FVC, forced vital capacity; ICU, intensive care unit

Notes:

■ The stepwise approach is meant to assist, not replace, the clinical decisionmaking required to meet individual patient needs.

■ Level of severity is determined by assessment of both impairment and risk. Assess impairment domain by patient's/caregiver's recall of previous 2–4 weeks and spirometry. Assign severity to the most severe category in which any feature occurs.

■ At present, there are inadequate data to correspond frequencies of exacerbations with different levels of asthma severity. In general, more frequent and intense exacerbations (e.g., requiring urgent, unscheduled care, hospitalization, or ICU admission) indicate greater underlying disease severity. For treatment purposes, patients who had ≥2 exacerbations requiring oral systemic corticosteroids in the past year may be considered the same as patients who have persistent asthma, even in the absence of impairment levels consistent with persistent asthma.

Note: PEF, peak expiratory flow; FEV$_1$, forced expiratory volume in 1 second.
Reproduced from NIH *Expert Panel Report 3*.

Figure 28-2. Stepwise Approach for Managing Infants and Young Children (0–4 Years of Age)

Intermittent Asthma	**Persistent Asthma: Daily Medication** Consult with asthma specialist if step 3 care or higher is required. Consider consultation at step 2.

Step 1
Preferred:
SABA PRN

Step 2
Preferred:
Low-dose ICS
Alternative:
Cromolyn or Montelukast

Step 3
Preferred:
Medium-dose ICS

Step 4
Preferred:
Medium-dose ICS + either LABA or Montelukast

Step 5
Preferred:
High-dose ICS + either LABA or Montelukast

Step 6
Preferred:
High-dose ICS + either LABA or Montelukast
Oral systemic corticosteroids

Step up if needed
(first, check adherence, inhaler technique, and environmental control)

Assess control

Step down if possible
(and asthma is well controlled at least 3 months)

Patient Education and Environmental Control at Each Step

Quick-Relief Medication for All Patients

- SABA as needed for symptoms. Intensity of treatment depends on severity of symptoms.
- With viral respiratory infection: SABA q 4–6 hours up to 24 hours (longer with physician consult). Consider short course of oral systemic corticosteroids if exacerbation is severe or patient has history of previous severe exacerbations.
- Caution: Frequent use of SABA may indicate the need to step up treatment. See text for recommendations on initiating daily long-term-control therapy.

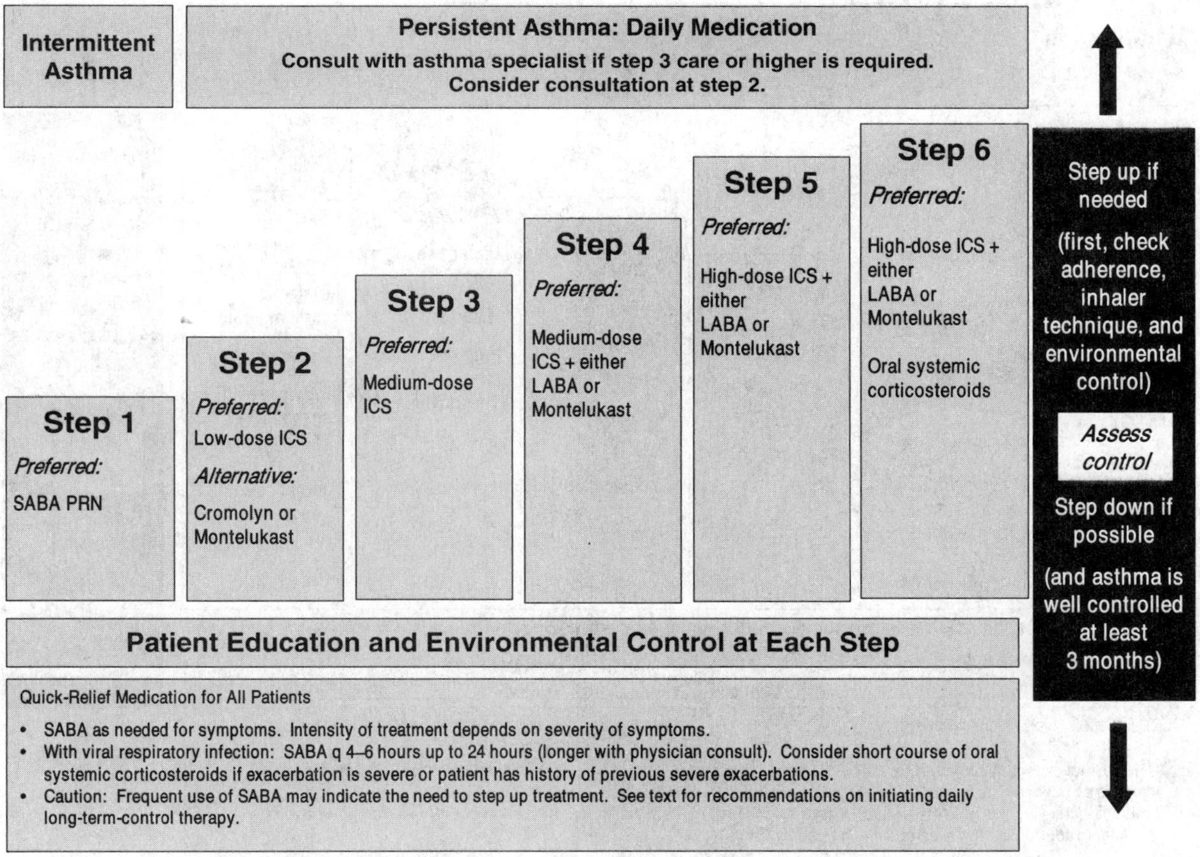

Key: **Alphabetical order is used when more than one treatment option is listed within either preferred or alternative therapy.** ICS, inhaled corticosteroid; LABA, inhaled long-acting beta$_2$-agonist; SABA, inhaled short-acting beta$_2$-agonist

Notes:

- The stepwise approach is meant to assist, not replace, the clinical decisionmaking required to meet individual patient needs.

- If alternative treatment is used and response is inadequate, discontinue it and use the preferred treatment before stepping up.

- If clear benefit is not observed within 4–6 weeks and patient/family medication technique and adherence are satisfactory, consider adjusting therapy or alternative diagnosis.

- Studies on children 0–4 years of age are limited. Step 2 preferred therapy is based on Evidence A. All other recommendations are based on expert opinion and extrapolation from studies in older children.

Reproduced from NIH *Expert Panel Report 3*.

- Reversible airway obstruction (improvement in pulmonary function tests [FEV$_1$] of > 12% after inhaling a short-acting β$_2$ agonist) is often detected.
- Exclude alternate diagnoses (e.g., chronic obstructive pulmonary disease, vocal cord dysfunction).

Treatment Principles and Goals

- Optimal long-term management of asthma includes four major areas: objective assessment and monitoring, environmental control, pharmacologic therapy, and patient education as a partnership.

Figure 28-3. Stepwise Approach for Managing Asthma in Children 5–11 Years of Age: Treatment

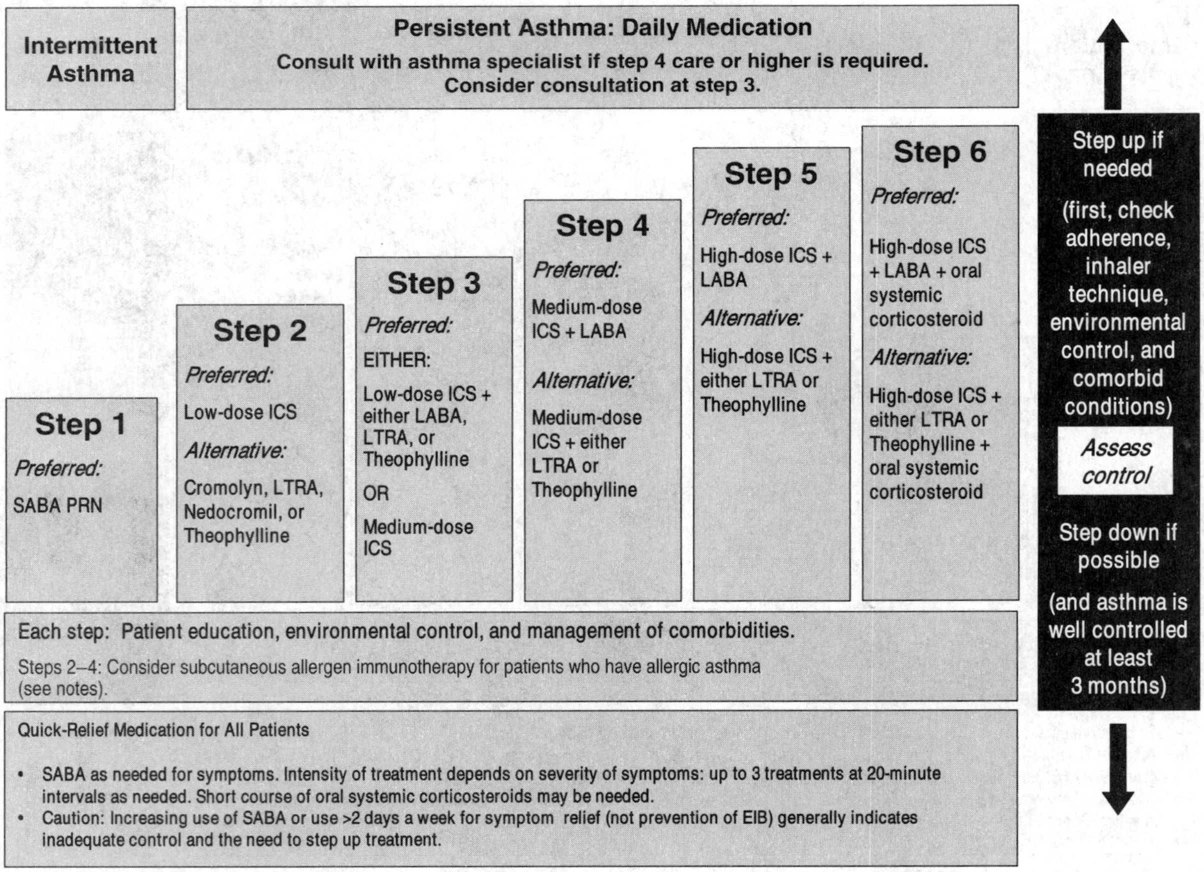

Key: **Alphabetical order is used when more than one treatment option is listed within either preferred or alternative therapy.** ICS, inhaled corticosteroid; LABA, inhaled long-acting beta$_2$-agonist, LTRA, leukotriene receptor antagonist; SABA, inhaled short-acting beta$_2$-agonist

Notes:

- The stepwise approach is meant to assist, not replace, the clinical decisionmaking required to meet individual patient needs.

- If alternative treatment is used and response is inadequate, discontinue it and use the preferred treatment before stepping up.

- Theophylline is a less desirable alternative due to the need to monitor serum concentration levels.

- Step 1 and step 2 medications are based on Evidence A. Step 3 ICS + adjunctive therapy and ICS are based on Evidence B for efficacy of each treatment and extrapolation from comparator trials in older children and adults—comparator trials are not available for this age group; steps 4–6 are based on expert opinion and extrapolation from studies in older children and adults.

- Immunotherapy for steps 2–4 is based on Evidence B for house-dust mites, animal danders, and pollens; evidence is weak or lacking for molds and cockroaches. Evidence is strongest for immunotherapy with single allergens. The role of allergy in asthma is greater in children than in adults. Clinicians who administer immunotherapy should be prepared and equipped to identify and treat anaphylaxis that may occur.

Reproduced from NIH *Expert Panel Report 3.*

Figure 28-4. Stepwise Approach for Managing Asthma ≥ 12 Years of Age and Adults: Treatment

Intermittent Asthma	Persistent Asthma: Daily Medication Consult with asthma specialist if step 4 care or higher is required. Consider consultation at step 3.

Step 1

Preferred:

SABA PRN

Step 2

Preferred:

Low-dose ICS

Alternative:

Cromolyn, LTRA, Nedocromil, or Theophylline

Step 3

Preferred:

Low-dose ICS + LABA

OR

Medium-dose ICS

Alternative:

Low-dose ICS + either LTRA, Theophylline, or Zileuton

Step 4

Preferred:

Medium-dose ICS + LABA

Alternative:

Medium-dose ICS + either LTRA, Theophylline, or Zileuton

Step 5

Preferred:

High-dose ICS + LABA

AND

Consider Omalizumab for patients who have allergies

Step 6

Preferred:

High-dose ICS + LABA + oral corticosteroid

AND

Consider Omalizumab for patients who have allergies

Step up if needed

(first, check adherence, environmental control, and comorbid conditions)

Assess control

Step down if possible

(and asthma is well controlled at least 3 months)

Each step: Patient education, environmental control, and management of comorbidities.

Steps 2–4: Consider subcutaneous allergen immunotherapy for patients who have allergic asthma (see notes).

Quick-Relief Medication for All Patients

- SABA as needed for symptoms. Intensity of treatment depends on severity of symptoms: up to 3 treatments at 20-minute intervals as needed. Short course of oral systemic corticosteroids may be needed.
- Use of SABA >2 days a week for symptom relief (not prevention of EIB) generally indicates inadequate control and the need to step up treatment.

Key: **Alphabetical order is used when more than one treatment option is listed within either preferred or alternative therapy.** EIB, exercise-induced bronchospasm; ICS, inhaled corticosteroid; LABA, long-acting inhaled beta$_2$-agonist; LTRA, leukotriene receptor antagonist; SABA, inhaled short-acting beta$_2$-agonist

Notes:

- The stepwise approach is meant to assist, not replace, the clinical decisionmaking required to meet individual patient needs.
- If alternative treatment is used and response is inadequate, discontinue it and use the preferred treatment before stepping up.
- Zileuton is a less desirable alternative due to limited studies as adjunctive therapy and the need to monitor liver function. Theophylline requires monitoring of serum concentration levels.
- In step 6, before oral systemic corticosteroids are introduced, a trial of high-dose ICS + LABA + either LTRA, theophylline, or zileuton may be considered, although this approach has not been studied in clinical trials.
- Step 1, 2, and 3 preferred therapies are based on Evidence A; step 3 alternative therapy is based on Evidence A for LTRA, Evidence B for theophylline, and Evidence D for zileuton. Step 4 preferred therapy is based on Evidence B, and alternative therapy is based on Evidence B for LTRA and theophylline and Evidence D for zileuton. Step 5 preferred therapy is based on Evidence B. Step 6 preferred therapy is based on (EPR⊠ 2 1997) and Evidence B for omalizumab.
- Immunotherapy for steps 2–4 is based on Evidence B for house-dust mites, animal danders, and pollens; evidence is weak or lacking for molds and cockroaches. Evidence is strongest for immunotherapy with single allergens. The role of allergy in asthma is greater in children than in adults.
- Clinicians who administer immunotherapy or omalizumab should be prepared and equipped to identify and treat anaphylaxis that may occur.

Reproduced from NIH *Expert Panel Report 3.*

■ Treatment goals are to achieve asthma control by *reducing impairment*:
- Prevent chronic and troublesome symptoms (e.g., coughing or breathlessness in the daytime, during the night, or after exercise).
- Require infrequent use (< 2 days/week) of inhaled SABA for quick relief of symptoms.
- Maintain (near) "normal" pulmonary function.
- Maintain normal activity levels (including exercise and other physical activity and attendance at work or school).
- Meet patients' and families' expectations of and satisfaction with asthma care.

■ Treatment goals are to achieve asthma control by *reducing risk*:
- Prevent recurrent exacerbations of asthma and minimize the need for ED visits or hospitalization.
- Prevent progressive loss of lung function; for children, prevent reduced lung growth.
- Provide optimal pharmacotherapy with minimal or no adverse effects.

■ A stepwise approach to managing asthma is shown in Figure 28-2 (ages 0–4), Figure 28-3 (ages 5–11), and Figure 28-4 (ages ≥12 and adults). These treatment guidelines are from EPR-3. See Table 28-1 for long-term control medications.

■ Inhaled corticosteroids are the most efficacious drugs for long-term management of persistent asthma. Addition of a long-acting inhaled β_2 agonist is recommended for patients with moderate or severe persistent asthma.

■ Omalizumab (Xolair): Anti-IgE therapy is primarily indicated for severe persistent asthma patients who have frequent emergency department visits and hospitalizations despite optimal therapy. It is given subcutaneously every 2–4 weeks.

■ Drug therapy is used for acute exacerbations of asthma. See Table 28-2 for quick-relief medications and Figure 28-5 for management of asthma exacerbations.

Monitoring

■ Optimal management for the great majority of patients will result in a dramatic reduction in symptoms (including nocturnal and early morning symptoms), as well as reduced acute care visits, fewer lost work or school days, and reduced need for quick-relief medications.

■ Monitoring peak expiratory flow (PEF) using a peak flow meter at home is required. *Green zone* is 80–100% of personal best value. *Yellow zone*

is 50–79% of personal best and indicates that consultation with a health care professional is advisable. *Red zone*, or < 50% of personal best, indicates that a written action plan should be implemented, and if there is no quick response, immediate medical attention should be sought.

■ Spirometry is performed in the physician's office

Mechanism of Action

For more details, see the section on mechanism of action in EPR-3.

Long-term control medications

Corticosteroids

■ Corticosteroids are anti-inflammatory. They block late reaction to allergen and reduce airway hyperresponsiveness. They inhibit cytokine production, adhesion protein activation, and inflammatory cell migration and activation.

■ Corticosteroids reverse β_2-receptor downregulation and inhibit microvascular leakage.

Cromolyn and nedocromil

(Note: Since the release of EPR-3, cromolyn nebulizer solution and nedocromil MDI became unavailable in the United States in 2008. Cromolyn MDI may be available in the United States through the end of 2009. These drugs are included here for completeness.)

■ Cromolyn and nedocromil are anti-inflammatory. They block early and late reaction to allergen, interfere with chloride channel function, stabilize mast cell membranes, and inhibit activation and release of mediators from eosinophils and epithelial cells.

■ Cromolyn and nedocromil inhibit acute response to exercise, cold dry air, and SO_2.

Long-acting β_2 agonists

■ With bronchodilation, smooth muscle relaxation follows adenylate cyclase activation and an increase in cyclic adenosine monophosphate (AMP), producing functional antagonism of bronchoconstriction.

■ In vitro, long-acting β_2 agonists (LABAs) inhibit mast cell mediator release, decrease vascular permeability, and increase mucociliary clearance.

■ Compared with short-acting inhaled β_2 agonist, salmeterol has a slower onset of action (15–30 minutes). Formoterol has an onset of action within 3 minutes. Both LABAs have a duration of action ≥ 12 hours.

Table 28-1. Long-Term Asthma Control Medications

Generic name	Trade name	Usual dosage range	Dosage form	Schedule[a]
Inhaled corticosteroids				
Beclomethasone HFA 40 mcg/puff; 80 mcg/puff	QVAR	80–480 mcg/d	MDI	Twice daily
Budesonide 200 mcg/inhalation	Pulmicort	1–3 inhalations/d	DPI (Flexhaler)	Twice daily
Budesonide–formoterol combination (each inhalation 4.5 mcg formoterol + budesonide 80.0 mcg or 160.0 mcg)	Symbicort	2 puffs	MDI	Twice daily
Budesonide 0.25 and 0.50 mg	Respules	0.5–2.0 mg/d	Nebulized	Twice daily
Flunisolide 250 mcg/puff	Aerobid	1–8 puffs/d	MDI	Twice daily
Fluticasone 44, 110, 220 mcg/puff	Flovent	88–660 mcg/d	MDI	Twice daily
Fluticasone 50, 100, 250	Flovent Diskus	100–500 mcg/d	DPI	Twice daily
Fluticasone–salmeterol combination (each dose 50 mcg salmeterol + 100, 250, or 500 mcg fluticasone)	Advair Diskus (Advair 100, 250, 500)	1 inhalation	DPI (Diskus)	Twice daily
Fluticasone–salmeterol combination (each puff 21 mcg salmeterol + 45, 115, or 230 mcg fluticasone)	Advair HFA (Advair HFA 45, 115, 230)	2 inhalations/dose	MDI	Twice daily
Mometasone 220 mcg/inhalation	Asmanex Twisthaler	1–2 inhalations/d	DPI	At bedtime
Triamcinolone 75 mcg/puff	Azmacort	4–20 puffs/d	MDI/spacer	Twice daily
Leukotriene modifiers				
Montelukast	Singulair	4 mg (12–23 months)	Oral granules	Every night
		4 mg (age 2–5 years)	Chewable tab	Every night
		5 mg (age 6–14 years)	Chewable tab	Every night
		10 mg (adult) tablet	Tablet	Every night
Zafirlukast	Accolate	20–40 mg/d tablet	Tablet	Twice daily
Zileuton	Zyflo	600 mg/tablet	Tablet	Four times daily
	Zyflo CR	600 mg controlled release tablet (2 tablets/dose)	Controlled release tablet	Twice daily
Mast cell stabilizers				
Cromolyn[b]	Intal	1–4 puffs MDI	MDI	Four times daily
	Intal	20 mg	Nebulizer solution	Four times daily
Long-acting inhaled β₂ agonists				
Formoterol[c]	Foradil Aerolizer	1 inhalation	DPI	Twice daily
Salmeterol[c]	Serevent Diskus	1 inhalation	DPI	Twice daily
Methylxanthines				
Theophylline (numerous products)	Uniphyl	10 mg/kg/d up to 300 mg maximum in adults to start; aim for 5–15 mcg/mL steady state	Tablet	Daily; 5:00 or 6:00 pm

Note: MDI, metered dose inhaler; DPI, dry powder inhaler (breath activated). See EPR-3 and FDA-approved product literature for pediatric doses for each drug product.

a. Usual schedule (some patients do well on once-daily dosing).

b. Since the release of EPR-3, cromolyn nebulizer solution and nedocromil MDI became unavailable in the United States in 2008. Cromolyn MDI may be available in the United States through the end of 2009.

c. Use only in combination with ICS.

d. Complex, high-risk drug to dose; see references cited for details; do not use unless competent in dosing and monitoring serum theophylline concentrations. See EPR-3 for pediatric doses (<1 year of age and >1 year of age).

Table 28-2. Quick-Relief Asthma Medications

Generic name	Trade name	Usual dosage[a]	Dosage form	Schedule
Short-acting inhaled β_2 agonists[b]				
Albuterol HFA	Ventolin, Proventil, Proair	2 puffs	MDI	Every 4 hours as needed
		2.5 mg	Nebulizer solution	Every 4 hours as needed
Pirbuterol	Maxair Autohaler	2 puffs	MDI	Every 4 hours as needed
Anticholinergics				
Ipratropium	Atrovent	2 puffs	MDI	Every 6 hours
		0.25 mg	Nebulizer solution	Every 6 hours
Ipratropium with albuterol	Combivent	2 puffs	MDI	Every 6 hours
		3 mL	Nebulizer solution	Every 6 hours
Systemic corticosteroids[c]				
Methylprednisolone	Medrol	1 mg/kg/d	Tablets	Daily
Prednisone		1 mg/kg/d	Tablets or liquid	Daily
Prednisolone		1 mg/kg/d	Tablets	Daily

Note: See EPR-3 and FDA-approved product literature for pediatric doses for each drug product.
a. Usual dosage for routine home use. (Dose in emergency department is higher and more frequent.)
b. For prevention of exercise-induced asthma, inhale 2 puffs 5–15 minutes before exercise. Increasing use indicates poor asthma control; increase anti-inflammatory therapy and reassess environmental control. (Good asthma control is indicated by infrequent need for quick-relief therapy.)
c. Short courses are used for < 2 weeks.

Methylxanthines
- With bronchodilation, smooth muscle relaxation results from phosphodiesterase inhibition and possibly adenosine antagonism.
- Methylxanthines may affect eosinophilic infiltration into bronchial mucosa as well as decrease T-lymphocyte numbers in epithelium.
- Methylxanthines increase diaphragm contractility and mucociliary clearance.

Leukotriene modifiers
- Leukotriene receptor antagonist; selective competitive inhibitor of $CysLT_1$ receptors
- 5-Lipoxygenase inhibitor

Anti-IgE therapy
- Omalizumab (Xolair) is a humanized monoclonal anti-IgE antibody that binds circulating IgE, thus inhibiting the allergic inflammatory cascade that results when aeroallergens bind to IgE on mast cells.

Quick-relief medications

Short-acting inhaled β_2 agonists
- With bronchodilation, smooth muscle relaxation follows adenylate cyclase activation and an increase in cyclic AMP, producing functional antagonism of bronchoconstriction.

Anticholinergics
- With bronchodilation, there is competitive inhibition of muscarinic cholinergic receptors.
- Anticholinergics reduce intrinsic vagal tone to the airways. They may block reflex bronchoconstriction secondary to irritants or to reflux esophagus.
- Anticholinergics may decrease mucus gland secretion.

Patient Instructions and Counseling

- Patient education is absolutely essential for optimal asthma management.
- Emphasize the need to take controller–preventer medications *every day,* even when the patient feels well and is having no breathing problems.
- Instruct the patient regarding the dangers of overuse of short-acting inhaled β_2 agonists. (The patient should contact a physician if the usual dose does not give quick relief or start the written action plan given by physician.)
- Demonstrate the correct use of the metered dose inhaler (MDI), the MDI plus spacer, and the dry powder inhaler (DPI), and then observe the patient using the devices. Most patients do not perform well initially; the devices can be difficult to use at first (see Figure 28-6 for MDI or MDI

Figure 28-5. Management of Asthma Exacerbations: Emergency Department and Hospital-Based Care

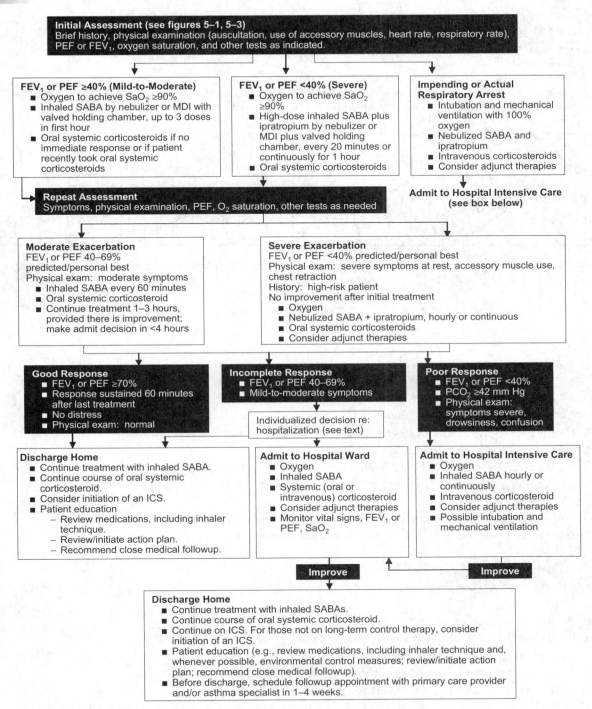

Key: FEV₁, forced expiratory volume in 1 second; ICS, inhaled corticosteroid; MDI, metered dose inhaler; PCO₂, partial pressure carbon dioxide; PEF, peak expiratory flow; SABA, short-acting beta₂-agonist; SaO₂, oxygen saturation

Figure 28-6. Steps for Using an Inhaler

Please demonstrate your inhaler technique at every visit.

1. Remove the cap and hold inhaler upright.
2. Shake the inhaler.
3. Tilt your head back slightly and breathe out slowly.
4. Position the inhaler in one of the following ways (A or B is optimal, but C is acceptable for those who have difficulty with A or B. C is required for breath-activated inhalers):

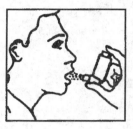 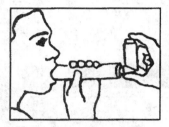 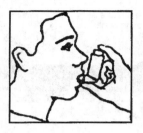 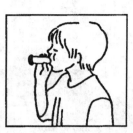

A. Open mouth with inhaler 1 to 2 inches away.

B. Use spacer/holding chamber (that is recommended especially for young children and for people using corticosteroids).

C. In the mouth. Do not use for cortico-steroids.

D. NOTE: Inhaled dry powder capsules require a different inhalation technique. To use a dry powder inhaler, it is important to close the mouth tightly around the mouthpiece of the inhaler and to inhale rapidly.

5. Press down on the inhaler to release medication as you start to breathe in slowly.
6. Breathe in slowly (3 to 5 seconds).
7. Hold your breath for 10 seconds to allow the medicine to reach deeply into your lungs.
8. Repeat puff as directed. Waiting 1 minute between puffs may permit second puff to penetrate your lungs better.
9. Spacers/holding chambers are useful for all patients. They are particularly recommended for young children and older adults and for use with inhaled corticosteroids.

Avoid common inhaler mistakes. Follow these inhaler tips:
- Breathe out *before* pressing your inhaler.
- Inhale *slowly*.
- Breathe in through your mouth, not your nose.
- Press down on your inhaler at the *start* of inhalation (or within the first second of inhalation).
- Keep inhaling as you press down on inhaler.
- Press your inhaler only *once* while you are inhaling (one breath for each puff).
- Make sure you breathe in evenly and deeply.

NOTE: Other inhalers are becoming available in addition to those illustrated above. Different types of inhalers may require different techniques.

Source: *Expert Panel Report 2: Guidelines for the Diagnosis and Management of Asthma.* National Asthma Education and Prevention Program, National Heart, Lung, and Blood Institute, 1997.

Table 28-3. Directions for Use of Peak Flow Meter

1. Stand while using the meter.
2. Position the indicator at the bottom of the scale.
3. Hold the peak flow meter so your fingers do not block the opening.
4. Inhale as deeply as possible, place the mouthpiece well into your mouth, and make sure your lips form a tight seal around it.
5. Blow out as fast and as hard as possible![a] BLAST! (Emphasize to the patient that the maneuver is highly effort dependent.)
6. Repeat steps 2–5 two more times, and record the highest of the three readings along with the date and time.

Note: If a short-acting inhaled β_2 agonist is required in the early morning, remember to check the peak expiratory flow before using the drug and record the value; then repeat PEF testing 15 minutes later.

a. Do not accelerate air with your tongue (i.e., use a spitting motion). This incorrect maneuver will give false elevation in PEF.

spacer use). For DPIs, remember to stress that inhalation must be rapid and deep.

- Demonstrate correct use of peak flow meters, and observe the patient using them (Table 28-3). Explain about the green, yellow, and red zones (including the written action plan).
- Teach how to prevent exercise-induced asthma.
- Be sure patients receive an influenza vaccination every fall.

Adverse Drug Effects

For more details, see the section on adverse drug effects in EPR-3.

Long-term control medications

Inhaled corticosteroids
- Inhaled corticosteroids may cause coughing, dysphonia, and oral thrush (candidiasis).
- In high doses, systemic effects may occur, although studies are not conclusive, and the clinical significance of these effects (e.g., adrenal suppression, osteoporosis, growth suppression, skin thinning, and easy bruising) has not been established.

Cromolyn and nedocromil
- Approximately 15–20% of patients complain of an unpleasant taste from nedocromil. Cromolyn is quite safe with very few side effects.

Long-acting inhaled β_2 agonists
- Tachycardia, skeletal muscle tremor, hypokalemia, or prolongation of QTc interval can occur in an overdose.
- Always use in combination with inhaled corticosteroid in long-term management of asthma. (Use

alone could mask inflammation and increase risk of severe exacerbations.)

Methylxanthines
- Dose-related acute toxicities include tachycardia, nausea and vomiting, tachyarrhythmias (supraventricular), central nervous system stimulation, headache, seizures, hematemesis, hyperglycemia, and hypokalemia.
- Adverse effects at usual therapeutic doses include insomnia, gastric upset, aggravation of ulcer or reflux, increase in hyperactivity in some children, and difficulty in urination in elderly males with prostatism.

Leukotriene modifiers
- Montelukast and zafirlukast are usually well tolerated.
- Zileuton can cause liver dysfunction.

Quick-relief medications

Short-acting inhaled β_2 agonists
- Tachycardia, skeletal muscle tremor, hypokalemia, increased lactic acid, headache, and rarely hyperglycemia can occur.
- In general, the inhaled route causes few systemic adverse effects; patients with preexisting cardiovascular disease, especially the elderly, may have adverse cardiovascular reactions with inhaled therapy.

Anticholinergics
- Drying of mouth and respiratory secretions, increased wheezing in some individuals, and blurred vision if sprayed in eyes can occur.

Systemic corticosteroids
- With short-term use, reversible abnormalities in glucose metabolism, increased appetite, fluid retention, weight gain, mood alteration, hypertension, peptic ulcers, and rarely aseptic necrosis of the femur can occur.
- Consideration should be given to coexisting conditions that could be worsened by systemic corticosteroids, such as herpes virus infections, varicella, tuberculosis, hypertension, peptic ulcer disease, and strongyloidiasis.

Drug–Drug and Drug–Disease Interactions

- For zafirlukast, administration with meals decreases bioavailability. Take at least 1 hour before or 2 hours after meals.

■ Zileuton and zafirlukast may increase the effect of warfarin and increase theophylline levels.

■ Well-known inducers of cytochrome P450 (carbamazepine, phenobarbital, phenytoin, and rifampin) are documented to decrease the effect of systemic corticosteroids.

■ Examples of drugs that may increase the effect of systemic corticosteroids include erythromycin, clarithromycin, itraconazole, oral contraceptives, and conjugated estrogen.

Parameters to Monitor

■ Refill record for daily controller–preventer medications and quick-relief medications

■ Reduction in symptoms (including nocturnal and early morning symptoms)

■ Emergency department visits, hospitalizations, and unscheduled office visits

■ Need for "bursts" of systemic corticosteroids

■ Lost work or school days and the need for quick-relief medications

■ PEF using a peak flow meter at home

In addition, if the patient also has rhinitis or GERD, monitor refills to ensure optimal control. (If rhinitis and GERD are not well controlled, asthma control will likely suffer.)

Kinetics

■ Theophylline is no longer used extensively in asthma, but when it is used, knowledge of its kinetics is essential because of its high risk.

■ Other drugs, disease states, smoking, age, and diet can all affect theophylline kinetics and dose requirements (see Table 28-4).

■ Therapeutic serum theophylline concentrations are 5–15 mcg/mL (*not* the old recommendation of 10–20 mcg/mL; see EPR-3).

■ Elimination half-life in an otherwise healthy nonsmoking adult is about 8 hours. In a smoker, it is about 4 hours, and in a small child (1 year or older), it is about 4 hours.

■ Neonates have greatly prolonged elimination half-life.

■ Elimination half-life in decompensated heart failure or cirrhosis is about 24 hours.

■ Volume of distribution is about 0.5 L/kg.

■ High-fat meals may cause "dose dumping" for some products (check product literature).

Other

■ MDIs should be stored at room temperature, between 59°F and 86°F; if left in a car in freezing or near-freezing temperatures, aerosol particles will be too large to inhale into the lungs.

■ MDIs should be "primed" (one dose released) only with first use or in the case of a prn agent used only once every 2 weeks. (Frequent priming is unnecessary and wastes expensive medications.)

■ HFA MDIs need special attention regarding weekly cleaning of the actuator (see manufacturers' instructions)

■ MDI dust cap should be left on inhaler when not in use. Check mouthpiece for foreign objects before inhaling.

Nondrug Therapy

■ An essential component of optimal asthma management is environmental control.

■ Without good control of the environment at home, school, and work, drug therapy will often be inadequate.

■ Have the patient identify known asthma triggers, and help the patient identify potential triggers not yet realized. (Do not forget someone smoking at home or work!)

28-2. Chronic Obstructive Pulmonary Disease (COPD)

COPD is characterized by airflow limitation that is not fully reversible. The airflow limitation is usually both progressive and associated with an abnormal inflammatory response of the lungs to noxious particles or gases. COPD is a major cause of death and suffering in the United States and around the world. It is the fourth leading cause of chronic morbidity and mortality in the United States.

Types and Classifications

Some clinicians still refer to chronic bronchitis and emphysema in characterizing different levels of COPD (e.g., emphysema patients have destructive damage to the alveolar walls, whereas chronic bronchitis is associated with chronic productive cough). According to the Global Initiative for Chronic Obstructive Lung Disease (GOLD) 2008 update, COPD severity classification is as follows:

Table 28-4. Factors Affecting Serum Theophylline Levels

Factor	Decreases Theophylline Concentrations	Increases Theophylline Concentrations	Recommended Action
Food	↓ or delays absorption of some sustained-release theophylline (SRT) products	↑ rate of absorption (fatty foods) products	Select theophylline preparation that is not affected by food.
Diet	↑ metabolism (high protein)	↓ metabolism (high carbohydrate)	Inform patients that major changes in diet are not recommended while taking theophylline.
Systemic, febrile viral illness (e.g., influenza)		↓ metabolism	Decrease theophylline dose according to serum concentration level. Decrease dose by 50 percent if serum concentration measurement is not available.
Hypoxia, cor pulmonale, and decompensated congestive heart failure, cirrhosis		↓ metabolism	Decrease dose according to serum concentration level.
Age	↑ metabolism (1 to 9 years)	↓ metabolism (< 6 months, elderly)	Adjust dose according to serum concentration level.
Phenobarbital, phenytoin, carbamazepine	↑ metabolism		Increase dose according to serum concentration level.
Cimetidine		↓ metabolism	Use alternative H₂ blocker (e.g., famotidine or ranitidine).
Macrolides: TAO, erythromycin, clarithromycin		↓ metabolism	Use alternative antibiotic or adjust theophylline dose.
Quinolones: ciprofloxacin, enoxacin, pefloxacin		↓ metabolism	Use alternative antibiotic or adjust theophylline dose. Circumvent with ofloxacin if quinolone therapy is required.
Rifampin	↑ metabolism		Increase dose according to serum concentration level.
Ticlopidine		↓ metabolism	Decrease dose according to serum concentration level.
Smoking	↑ metabolism		Advise patient to stop smoking, increase dose according to serum concentration level.

*This list is not all-inclusive; for discussion of other factors, see package inserts.
Reproduced from NIH Expert Panel Report 2.
TAO, triacetyloleandomycin.

- *I. Mild:* $FEV_1/FVC < 0.7$ and $FEV_1 \geq 80\%$ predicted
- *II. Moderate:* $FEV_1/FVC < 0.7$ and $50\% < FEV_1 < 80\%$ predicted
- *III. Severe:* $FEV_1/FVC < 0.7$ and $30\% \leq FEV_1 < 50\%$ predicted
- *IV. Very severe:* $FEV_1/FVC < 0.7$ and $FEV_1 < 30\%$ predicted *or* $FEV_1 < 50\%$ predicted plus chronic respiratory failure.

In addition, examples of factors affecting the severity of this disease include frequency of exacerbations, presence of other disease states, overall health status, and severity of symptoms.

Clinical Presentation

- Shortness of breath
- Cough and sputum production
- Usually, a history of cigarette smoking for several years
- In the more severe form, respiratory failure and heart failure

Pathophysiology

- COPD is usually caused by long-term smoking; it may also be caused by exposure to other noxious particles and gases.
- Chronic inflammation is found throughout the airways but via different inflammatory cells and mediators than those that cause asthma. Thus, the response to inhaled corticosteroids is much less than that seen with asthma.
- An imbalance of proteinases and antiproteinases is found in the lung.
- A rare hereditary cause of emphysema is α_1-antitrypsin deficiency.
- Pathologic changes are found in the central and peripheral airways as well as the alveoli and pulmonary vasculature.
- The following pathological changes are also found:
  - Mucus hypersecretion
  - Ciliary dysfunction
  - Airflow limitation
  - Lung hyperinflation
  - Gas exchange abnormalities
  - Secondary pulmonary hypertension
  - Cor pulmonale

Diagnostic Criteria

- History of cigarette smoking or exposure to other noxious particles or fumes
- Chronic cough and sputum production
- Spirometry (e.g., reduced FEV_1)
- Other lung diseases ruled out

Treatment Principles and Goals

- Management of COPD includes the following principles and goals: prevent progression of disease, relieve symptoms, enhance health status, increase exercise tolerance, prevent and treat exacerbations and complications, and decrease mortality.
- Bronchodilators are central to the symptomatic treatment of COPD; these agents will increase exercise capacity without necessarily improving the FEV_1.
- Inhaled bronchodilators are preferred to oral bronchodilators for initial therapy; the specific choice of agent depends on patient response.
- Long-acting inhaled bronchodilators are more effective and convenient but more expensive. Examples of long-acting bronchodilators include the once-daily anticholinergic tiotropium (Spiriva) and twice-daily LABAs (formoterol and salmeterol—discussed in Section 28-1).

- Short-acting inhaled β_2 agonists are preferred for prn use in patients already receiving LABAs and anticholinergics.
- Inhaled corticosteroids are reserved for COPD patients with severe or very severe disease (Stage III or IV) and frequent exacerbations.
- Theophylline is an option for maintenance therapy in patients who are not optimally controlled with β_2 agonists and anticholinergics.

Therapy at each stage

(See the GOLD 2008 update.)

For each stage, patients should avoid risk factors (e.g., cease smoking) and receive an influenza vaccine each autumn. Also, pneumococcal vaccine should be administered per current guidelines.

- Stage I: Mild COPD
  - Use short-acting bronchodilator as needed.
- Stage II: Moderate COPD
  - Add scheduled therapy with one or more long-acting bronchodilators and rehabilitation.
- Stage III: Severe COPD
  - Use scheduled therapy with one or more long-acting bronchodilators.
  - Add inhaled corticosteroids if patient has recurrent exacerbations.
- Stage IV: Very severe COPD
  - Same treatments as for stage III, and consider surgical treatment.
  - Long-term O_2 therapy if patient experiences chronic respiratory failure.

Drug therapy for acute exacerbations of COPD

- Inhaled albuterol, ipratropium, or both
- Systemic corticosteroids (e.g., prednisolone 30 mg/d for 14 days)
- O_2
- Oral antibiotics for purulent sputum as well as increased sputum volume and increased dyspnea
- Choice of oral antibiotic depends on severity:
  - *Mild exacerbation:* Use amoxicillin, doxycycline, or trimethoprim-sulfamethoxazole (alternatives include β-lactam plus β-lactamase inhibitor, azithromycin, or second- or third-generation cephalosporins).
  - *Moderate exacerbation:* Use a β-lactam plus β-lactamase inhibitor (alternatives are respiratory fluoroquinolones such as moxifloxacin or levofloxacin).
  - *Severe exacerbation with risk factors for Pseudomonas aeruginosa infection:* Use ciprofloxacin or levofloxacin (high dose,

750 mg). If parenteral treatment is needed, use the same fluoroquinolones or an anti-pseudomonal β-lactam.

Monitoring

- Spirometry: FEV_1
- Symptoms of dyspnea, cough, sputum production, and change in sputum color and volume
- PaO_2
- Exercise tolerance or fatigue

Long-term drug therapy

- See content under Section 28-1 for specific drugs.
- Tiotropium is a once-daily anticholinergic bronchodilator that is an option for step 1 treatment of moderate to severe COPD. It is administered by a DPI (HandiHaler). Each dose must be loaded, and deep inhalation does not have to be forceful but must be sufficient to hear the capsule vibrate. Another tiotropium delivery device, Respimat Soft Mist Inhaler (multidose), is available outside the United States.

Nondrug therapy

- Smoking cessation—nicotine replacement therapy, bupropion (Zyban), varenicline (Chantix), support groups, and counseling
- Oxygen therapy
- Nutritional support
- Psychosocial support
- Pulmonary rehabilitation

Smoking cessation is the most important of these therapies.

28-3. Key Points

Asthma

- Asthma is primarily an inflammatory airway disease.
- It is commonly undertreated, resulting in much unnecessary suffering and economic loss.
- Managing patients via the principles of the National Institutes of Health guidelines (EPR-3) has been clearly shown to reduce emergency department visits and hospitalizations and to improve patient quality of life.
- Optimal long-term management includes objective assessment, environmental control, drug therapy, and patient education working in a partnership.

- Patients with persistent asthma need daily controller therapy (anti-inflammatory agents).
- Inhaled corticosteroids are the most efficacious agents to control asthma and are the preferred first-step drug treatment for all ages of mild persistent asthma.
- Inhaled long-acting inhaled β_2 agonists are the preferred treatment to add to inhaled corticosteroids for patients with moderate persistent or severe persistent asthma.
- Short-acting inhaled β_2 agonists are the agents of choice for quick relief of symptoms.
- Pharmacists should teach patients how to use inhalers (MDI, MDI-spacer, and DPI) by demonstrations and *observation* of the patient.
- Pharmacists should instruct patients on how to use peak flow meters, including color-coded zone management with a written action plan. Written action plans may be peak flow based, symptom based, or both.
- Patients must clearly understand the purpose of daily controller or preventer medications versus quick-relief medications. Show patients airway models or colored pictures of normal versus inflamed airways.

Chronic Obstructive Pulmonary Disease

(See the GOLD 2008 update.)

- The overall approach to managing stable COPD should be characterized by a stepwise increase in treatment and should be tailored to reduce symptoms and enhance quality of life.
- Health education can play a role in improving skills, ability to cope with COPD, and health status. It is effective in accomplishing certain goals, including smoking cessation in some patients.
- None of the existing medications for this disease has been shown to modify the long-term decline in pulmonary function that is the hallmark of this COPD. Drug treatment for COPD is used to improve symptoms or decrease complications.
- Bronchodilators are central to the symptomatic management of this disease. They include β_2 agonists, anticholinergics, and theophylline.
- Inhaled therapy with long-acting agents is preferred for reasons of efficacy and convenience.
- Combining bronchodilators may improve efficacy and decrease the risk of side effects compared with increasing the dose of a single bronchodilator.
- Regular treatment with inhaled corticosteroids should be prescribed only for symptomatic

patients with severe or very severe COPD and recurrent exacerbations.

- Chronic treatment with systemic corticosteroids should be avoided because risks outweigh benefits.
- The long-term administration of oxygen (> 15 hours per day) to COPD patients with chronic respiratory failure has been shown to increase survival.
- Patients with COPD benefit from exercise training programs; they show improvement with respect to both exercise tolerance and symptoms of fatigue and dyspnea.
- Influenza vaccine can reduce serious illness in COPD patients. Pneumocococcal polysaccharide vaccine is recommended for patients with COPD who are 65 years of age or older and for patients under 65 years of age who have an $FEV_1 < 40\%$ predicted.

28-4. Questions

1. Asthma is primarily due to which underlying problem?

    A. Pulmonary fibrosis
    B. Infection
    C. Inflammation
    D. Bronchospasm
    E. Granulomas

2. Which objective measure for routine monitoring of asthma is available at home?

    A. PEF
    B. FEV_1
    C. FVC
    D. O_2 saturation
    E. PD20

3. Which device requires slow inhalation?

    A. Diskus
    B. Turbuhaler
    C. Aerolizer
    D. MDI
    E. Rotadisk

4. How many seconds is optimal for breath holding after inhaling from an MDI?

    A. 4
    B. 5

C. 15
D. 2
E. 10

5. When a peak flow meter is used, what percentage of the personal best value is the yellow zone?

    A. < 50
    B. < 60
    C. 50–79
    D. 60–89
    E. 40–60

6. What are the trade names for long-acting inhaled β_2 agonists?

    A. Foradil and Serevent
    B. Pulmicort and Flovent
    C. Aerobid and Combivent
    D. Maxair and Atrovent
    E. Flovent and Ventolin

7. Which disease states decrease theophylline elimination and often result in reduced dosage requirements?

    A. Hepatitis
    B. Heart failure (decompensated)
    C. Hypertension
    D. A, B, and C
    E. A and B

8. Which drugs are preferred for long-term treatment of moderate persistent asthma?

    A. Budesonide + formoterol
    B. Fluticasone + salmeterol
    C. Beclomethasone + ipratropium
    D. A or B
    E. B or C

9. Which drug is a once-daily anticholinergic bronchodilator?

    A. Atrovent
    B. Serevent
    C. Foradil
    D. Spiriva
    E. Proventil

10. For patients with asthma or COPD exacerbations who are not responding adequately to inhaled bronchodilators, what is the

agent of choice to add to manage the acute exacerbation?

A. Fluticasone
B. Budesonide
C. Cromolyn
D. Theophylline
E. Prednisone

11. Which drug may increase serum theophylline concentrations?

A. Clarithromycin
B. Hydrochlorothiazide
C. Carbamazepine
D. Rifampin
E. Phenytoin

12. Which side effect of inhaled corticosteroids is reduced by spacer devices?

A. Hoarseness
B. Decreased bone density
C. Thinning of skin
D. Oropharyngeal candidiasis
E. Cataracts

13. The therapeutic range for theophylline per the NIH guidelines for asthma management is

A. 5–15 mcg/mL
B. 8–12 mcg/mL
C. 10–20 mcg/mL
D. 15–25 mcg/mL
E. 10–15 mcg/mL

14. Which asthma controller drug is given qhs?

A. Accolate
B. Singulair
C. Xolair
D. Intal
E. Medrol

15. Which disease state may worsen asthma?

A. Coronary artery disease
B. GERD
C. Diabetes
D. Hypertension
E. Arthritis

16. Which class of drugs is indicated only in severe COPD patients who have frequent exacerbations?

A. Long-acting inhaled β_2 agonists
B. Anticholinergics
C. Short-acting inhaled β_2 agonists
D. Inhaled corticosteroids
E. Methylxanthines

The next two questions relate to Case Study 28-1.

17. Which class of drugs is preferred in Mr. Johnson for optimal control of asthma?

A. Anticholinergics
B. Inhaled corticosteroids
C. Methylxanthines
D. Mast cell stabilizers
E. Oral corticosteroids

Case Study 28-1 Medication Profile

Patient name	Thomas Johnson
Address	5689 Washington St.
Date of birth	9-15-55
Drug allergies	Aspirin sensitivity
Height	5'10" Weight 75 kg
Diagnosis	(1) Asthma (childhood onset, moderate persistent)
	(2) Allergic rhinitis
	(3) Hypertension

Medications

Date	Rx #	MD	Drug and strength	Quantity	Sig	Refills
3/16	94385	Betts	Accolate 20 mg	60	1 bid	3
3/16	94386	Betts	Albuterol MDI	1	2 puffs q4h	6
3/16	94387	Betts	Flonase	1	bid as dir.	3
3/25	95523	T. Jones	Lopressor 50 mg	60	1 bid	6
3/27	95734	Betts	Albuterol MDI	1	2 puffs q4h	5

Pharmacist notes: 3/16—discussed proper use of MDI and observed patient use. Coached Mr. Johnson to inhale slowly (he was inhaling fast); he used the MDI correctly for the other steps.

18. What is an appropriate alternative to Lopressor in Mr. Johnson?

    A. An ACE inhibitor
    B. Propranolol 40 mg bid
    C. Clonidine
    D. Hydralazine
    E. Atenolol 200 mg daily

The next two questions relate to Case Study 28-2.

19. What concerns should the pharmacist have in this situation regarding theophylline?

    A. Cirrhosis is well documented to decrease elimination of theophylline.
    B. The milligrams per kilogram dose is too low.
    C. Mrs. Adams should be on a q12h product.
    D. Theophylline SR should be dosed in the morning, not evening.
    E. Long-acting inhaled β_2 agonists increase theophylline clearance.

20. The patient has a friend who has COPD and has told her about Spiriva. Mrs. Adams wants to know the opinion of the pharmacist. You would say:

    A. I'll call your doctor and suggest a new prescription for Spiriva.
    B. Spiriva is a third-line drug for COPD; I would not use it now.
    C. Spiriva is a good drug, but I want to talk to your doctor about starting a medicine called Flovent.
    D. Since you have a prescription for Atrovent, I will call your doctor and suggest changing from Atrovent to Spiriva.
    E. I think Symbicort would be better for you.

21. Which drug is best for long-term management of mild persistent asthma?

    A. Cromolyn
    B. Montelukast
    C. Nedocromil
    D. Theophylline
    E. Budesonide

22. Which total daily dose of prednisone is best for home management of an acute exacerbation of asthma in a 60-kg adult?

    A. 5.0 mg
    B. 60.0 mg
    C. 10.0 mg
    D. 20.0 mg
    E. 7.5 mg

23. Which drug is most likely to cause an asthma exacerbation in a patient sensitive to aspirin?

    A. Ibuprofen
    B. Acetaminophen
    C. Celecoxib
    D. Salsalate
    E. Sodium salicylate

24. Which type of inhaler does not work well in very cold temperatures?

    A. Diskus
    B. Turbuhaler
    C. Aerolizer
    D. MDI
    E. Rotahaler

Case Study 28-2 Medication Profile

Patient name	Mrs. S. T. Adams
Address	7129 James Ave.
Date of birth	1-16-37
Drug allergies	Sulfonamides
Height	5'3" **Weight** 55 kg
Diagnosis	(1) COPD—53 pack/year Hx smoking (quit 2 years ago) (2) Cirrhosis

Medications

Date	Rx #	MD	Drug and strength	Quantity	Sig	Refills
2/18	84389	Jones	Serevent Diskus	1	1 bid	6
2/18	84390	Jones	Albuterol MDI	1	2 puffs q4h prn	6
2/18	84391	Jones	Atrovent MDI	1	2 puffs q6h	6
2/18	84392	Jones	Uniphyl 600 mg	30	1 qd 6 PM	2

Pharmacist Notes: 2/18—discussed proper use of Diskus and observed patient use; taught Mrs. Adams to inhale deeply and rapidly (she was inhaling slowly for < 2 seconds). Also observed use of MDI (she forgot to exhale gently before pressing down on MDI).

28-5. Answers

1. C. Although asthma certainly does have a bronchospastic component, it is primarily due to inflammation, so good control of inflammation dramatically reduces bronchospasm. A good indicator of disease control is the rare need for short-acting inhaled β_2 agonists.

2. A. Peak flow meters are inexpensive and relatively easy to use. Good measurement of peak expiratory flow requires appropriate technique, and if good technique is used, patients have valuable objective evidence of asthma control (or exacerbation).

3. D. Dry powder inhalers for asthma therapy that are currently available require rapid inhalation. MDIs require slow inhalation to minimize impaction of aerosol in the mouth and throat.

4. E. Ten seconds is best; there is no need to hold longer. If 10 seconds is uncomfortable, 4–5 seconds is acceptable.

5. C. The yellow zone is 50–79%, which indicates suboptimal control. (The red zone is < 50%, which indicates that the crisis action plan should be started and medical attention should be sought.)

6. A. Foradil (formoterol) and Serevent (salmeterol).

7. E. Hepatitis and decompensated heart failure both can dramatically reduce theophylline clearance.

8. D. (A. budesonide + formoterol *or* B. fluticasone + salmeterol.) See Figures 28-2 and 28-3.

9. D. Atrovent is also a quick-relief agent, but it is not as efficacious in asthma and has a slower onset than albuterol and other short-acting inhaled β_2 agonists.

10. E. Prednisone or other systemic corticosteroids (e.g., methylprednisolone) are well documented to be efficacious in asthma and acute exacerbations of COPD.

11. A. Clarithromycin is documented to increase serum concentrations. Hydrochlorothiazide does not affect serum theophylline concentrations, and the remaining choices are all documented to decrease serum theophylline concentrations.

12. D. Oropharyngeal candidiasis or thrush is correct. The other side effects are not reduced by spacers.

13. A. The currently accepted range for asthma is 5–15 mcg/mL (*not* the old range of 10–20 mcg/mL). There is no benefit in exceeding

15 mcg/mL, and many patients receive benefit at lower doses.

14. B. Because asthma is a disease of circadian rhythm and is worse between 2:00 am and 6:00 am, it is best to give this once-daily drug at bedtime.

15. B. GERD can worsen asthma if it is not properly treated. The exact mechanisms are debated, but there is excellent documentation that asthma improves if this condition is well managed.

16. D. This class of drugs should *not* be used routinely in COPD patients with mild disease. In severe disease, inhaled corticosteroids are indicated, especially if there are frequent exacerbations. Remember that in asthma, inhaled corticosteroids are the best agents for long-term control, but in COPD their role is limited.

17. B. Inhaled corticosteroids are the preferred treatment (see Figures 28-2 and 28-3 for treatment choices). The pharmacist should share the NIH guidelines with Mr. Johnson's prescriber to help ensure optimal care. In addition, the pharmacist should educate the patient regarding the purpose of the medications and proper use of inhalers (e.g., the pharmacist should observe the patient using the device).

18. A. An ACE inhibitor should be efficacious with few side effects (monitor for cough); β-blockers should be avoided in Mr. Johnson unless he is post–myocardial infarction or had congestive heart failure (in which case, use a low dose of a β_1-selective blocker and monitor carefully).

19. A. Cirrhosis is well documented to decrease elimination of theophylline. Ensure a check of a steady-state theophylline level (peak) and anticipate dose reduction (usually 50% dose reduction in liver disease).

20. D. Because the patient has prescriptions for Atrovent and Serevent, a logical change here would be to discontinue the short-acting anticholinergic Atrovent and add the long-acting once-daily anticholinergic tiotropium (Spiriva).

21. E. Budesonide is an inhaled corticosteroid, the class of drugs recommended to treat even mild persistent asthma.

22. B. Sixty milligrams is an appropriate dose. If it is started as soon as the patient is in the red zone and not responding quickly to short-acting inhaled β_2 agonists, usually only a few days of treatment will be required (usually < 1 week).

23. A. Ibuprofen has the same mechanism of action as aspirin and will predictably trigger symptoms

in an aspirin-sensitive patient (i.e., increased production of leukotrienes). COX-2 inhibitors are safe (celecoxib). Acetaminophen is the choice agent for minor pain in these patients.

24. **D.** MDIs release large aerosol particles that do not penetrate deeply into the lungs in cold temperatures. Dry powder inhalers are acceptable.

28-6. References

Asthma

Berger WE, Qaquandah PV, Blake K, et al. Safety of budesonide inhalation suspension in infants aged six to twelve months with mild to moderate persistent asthma or recurrent wheeze. *J Pediatr.* 2005; 146:91–95.

Dolovich MB, Ahrens RC, Hess DR, et al. Device selection and outcomes of aerosol therapy: Evidence-based guidelines: American College of Chest Physicians/American College of Asthma, Allergy, and Immunology. *Chest.* 2005;127:335–71.

Fanta CH. Asthma. *N Engl J Med.* 2009;360: 1002–14. (Drug Therapy Review)

Hendeles L, Jenkins J, Temple R. Revised FDA labeling guideline for theophylline oral dosage forms. *Pharmacotherapy.* 1995;15:409.

National Institutes of Health (NIH). *Expert Panel Report 3: Guidelines for the Diagnosis and Management of Asthma, 2007.* NIH Publication 07-4051. Bethesda, Md.: NIH. Available at: www.nhlbi.nih.gov/guidelines/asthma/asthsumm.htm.

Self TH, Chrisman CR, Mason DL, Rumbak MJ. Reducing emergency department visits and hospitalizations in African American and Hispanic patients with asthma: A 15-year review. *J Asthma.* 2005;42:807–12.

Shannon M. Life-threatening events after theophylline overdose: A 10-year prospective analysis. *Arch Intern Med.* 1999;159:989–94.

Strunk RC, Bloomberg GR. Omalizumab for asthma. *N Engl J Med.* 2006;354:2689–95.

Weiss KB, Sullivan SD. The health economics of asthma and rhinitis: I. Assessing the economic impact. *J Allergy Clin Immunol.* 2001;107:3–8.

Chronic Obstructive Pulmonary Disease

Calverley P, Pauwels R, Vestbo J, et al. Combined salmeterol and fluticasone in the treatment of chronic obstructive pulmonary disease: A randomised controlled trial. *Lancet.* 2003;361:449–56.

Global Initiative for Chronic Obstructive Lung Disease (GOLD). *Global Strategy for the Diagnosis, Management, and Prevention of Chronic Obstructive Pulmonary Disease.* Gig Harbor, Wash.: Medical Communications Resources. Available from: www.goldcopd.org.

Gross NJ. Tiotropium bromide. *Chest.* 2004;126: 1946–53.

Pauwels R, Lofdahl CG, Laitinen LA, et al. Long term treatment with inhaled budesonide in persons with mild COPD who continue smoking. *N Engl J Med.* 1999;340:1948–53.

Rigotti NA. Treatment of tobacco use and dependence. *N Engl J Med.* 2002;346:506–12.

Tashkin DP, Celli B, Senn S, et al. A 4-year trial of tiotropium in chronic obstructive pulmonary disease. *N Engl J Med.* 2008;359:1543–54.

Wedzicha JA, Calverley PMA, Semungal TA, et al. The prevention of chronic obstructive pulmonary disease exacerbations by salmeterol/fluticasone propionate or tiotropium bromide. *Am J Respir Crit Care Med.* 2008;177:19–26.

Infectious Disease 29

Joyce E. Broyles, PharmD, BCNSP

29-1. General Principles of Infectious Disease

Several infectious disease topics are addressed in other chapters of this review, including common colds in Chapter 27, HIV (human immunodeficiency virus) and acquired immune deficiency syndrome (AIDS) in Chapter 31, and otitis media in Chapter 33. For additional information about specific anti-infective agents, see Chapter 30.

Diagnosis

Diagnosis of most infectious diseases consists of isolation and identification of microorganisms, assessment of patient signs and symptoms, and analysis of other laboratory data.

Isolation of organisms

To identify the causative agent of a disease, samples should be taken from appropriate body sites prior to the initiation of anti-infective therapy. Organisms isolated from body sites that normally are sterile (blood, urine, and spinal fluid) yield higher predictive value than do organisms isolated from body sites that normally are bacteriologically colonized (skin or fecal material).

Identification of organisms

To determine the infectious organism's cell morphology and to guide empiric therapy, one must Gram stain body sites for organisms as soon as possible. After the species of organism has been determined, one should expose it to standardized concentrations of antibiotics to determine the concentrations that inhibit growth. The lowest concentration that prevents microbial growth after 18–24 hours is called the *minimum inhibitory concentration* (MIC). The three breakpoint concentrations of antibiotics are susceptible, intermediate, and resistant. An antibiotic's breakpoint concentration is determined by considering (1) tissue concentrations with normal dosing and (2) the organism's population distribution. The breakpoint concentration determines whether the antibiotic can be used for therapy.

Physical signs and symptoms of infection (such as fever, redness, swelling, pain, and cough) must be considered both for initial diagnosis and for assessment of antibiotic effectiveness.

Laboratory tests

In the initial stage of infection, the patient's neutrophil count may increase above normal, and immature neutrophil forms (bands) may appear; therefore, a white blood cell (WBC) count should be taken. Later in the course of illness, the neutrophil count may fall to below normal levels.

Inflammatory markers, such as C-reactive protein, erythrocyte sedimentation rate, and tumor necrosis factor, may increase during infection.

Laboratory tests may not be reliable in patients who are elderly, malnourished, neonatal, or severely infected.

Treatment Strategies

Anti-infective agents should be used only when a significant infection has been diagnosed, when one is strongly suspected, or when prophylactic therapy is indicated.

In situations where multiple organisms could be the infecting agent (e.g., pneumonia), empiric therapy should cover the majority of possible organisms, with de-escalation of antimicrobial therapy when the causative agent is discovered.

Prophylactic therapy

Anti-infective therapy is aimed at preventing infection. Prophylactic therapy commonly is used after exposure to infection (e.g., tuberculosis) or before surgical intervention in areas of high bacterial inoculum (e.g., bowel surgery).

Empiric therapy is directed toward all common pathogens associated with a disease state.

Culture-guided therapy, which usually is narrower spectrum than empiric therapy, covers only the specific organism that is sensitive to the therapy. Culture-guided therapy is preferred because it is more cost-effective and because it decreases bacterial resistance from unnecessary antibiotic exposure.

Choice of Anti-infective Agent

To determine optimal anti-infective therapy or to review the appropriateness of other decisions, a clinician must answer several questions:

■ Is an antibiotic indicated on the basis of the clinical findings?

■ Have appropriate specimens been obtained, examined, and sent for culture?

■ What organisms most likely are causing the infection?

■ If several antibiotics are available to treat the likely or known organism, which agent is best for the patient? (Patient allergies and concurrent disease states should be considered.)

■ Is an antibiotic combination appropriate? (A combination of drugs should be given only when clinical experience has shown such therapy to be more effective than single-agent therapy in a particular setting. Such multiple agent regimens can increase the risk of toxic drug effects; occasionally, they may result in drug antagonism and loss of effectiveness. However, some combinations of anti-infective agents have demonstrated increased effectiveness that is greater than their individual effectiveness combined, a phenomenon known as *synergy*. An example of synergy is the combination of aminoglycosides with cell wall inhibitors, such as penicillin, in many Gram-positive organisms.)

■ What is the best route of administration? (This decision will depend on the overall plan for the patient. Oral therapy is preferred for outpatient therapy; many intravenous anti-infectives have oral forms with similar pharmacokinetic profiles.)

■ What is the appropriate dose and dose interval? (Regimen design should take into account patient size, renal or hepatic function, the disease state to be treated, and pharmacodynamic considerations of the agents used.)

■ Will initial therapy need modification after culture data are returned?

■ What is the optimal duration of therapy, and is the development of resistance during prolonged therapy likely to occur?

Lack of Therapeutic Effectiveness

When anti-infective therapy fails, careful analysis of possible causes should be made prior to changing the regimen. Factors associated with therapeutic failure include misdiagnosis of the infection, improper drug regimen, inappropriate choice of antibiotic agent, and resistance of the infecting agent, as well as situations in which antibiotic therapy may not be effective without additional interventions (e.g., surgical drainage).

29-2. Common Bacterial, Fungal, and Viral Infections

Meningitis

Meningitis is defined as an inflammation of the meninges that is identified by an abnormal number of white blood cells in the cerebrospinal fluid (CSF).

Causative agents

A wide variety of organisms is associated with this disease, including many Gram-positive and Gram-negative organisms.

Clinical presentation

Patients may present with fever, headache, photophobia, neck rigidity, diarrhea, vomiting, and altered mental status. Infants may present with a bulging anterior fontanel.

Diagnostic criteria

Analysis of the cerebrospinal fluid may be diagnostic of the infective agent. Bacterial agents are associated with a large increase in systemic WBCs, presence of WBCs in the CSF, increased CSF protein, and decreased CSF glucose. Fungal and viral agents exhibit smaller increases in CSF WBCs, smaller increases in CSF protein, and limited decreases in CSF glucose.

Treatment

Empiric treatment is usually determined by the age of the patient. Because of limited antibiotic penetration by many agents, the highest safe antibiotic doses are generally used. Table 29-1 summarizes empiric therapy for meningitis.

Endocarditis

Endocarditis is an infection of the endocardium, the membrane lining the heart chamber and valves.

Causative agents

Most patients have previous damage to the heart (e.g., artificial valve placement) prior to infection. The most common organisms are *Streptococcus* and *Staphylococcus* species.

Clinical presentation

Patients present with low-grade fever, fatigue, and weakness. A diagnostic finding is the presence of splinter hemorrhages and petechiae.

Diagnostic criteria

There are no specific laboratory tests for this infection. Most patients present with an elevated erythrocyte sedimentation rate or C-reactive protein. Visualization of the vegetations on the surface of the heart is often diagnostic of the disease.

Treatment

According to American Heart Association guidelines, treatment varies depending on the causative organism and whether or not prosthetic devices are present (which would require longer therapy, if present). Table 29-2 describes therapy for endocarditis.

Acute or Chronic Bronchitis

Bronchitis is an inflammation of the bronchioles, often associated with bronchopneumonia. Chronic bronchitis is mainly associated with heavy smoking.

Causative agents

Viral infections account for half of all cases. *Mycoplasma pneumoniae, Streptococcus pneumoniae, Haemophilus influenzae, Moraxella catarrhalis,* and *Chlamydia pneumoniae* are common bacterial pathogens.

Clinical presentation

Patients present with a history of acute productive cough, a low-grade fever, and a clear chest x-ray.

Diagnostic criteria

Sputum cultures typically are not useful in diagnosis because of multiple etiologies; therefore, most physicians prescribe anti-infectives on the basis of physical findings.

Treatment

Treatment is controversial for most acute illnesses because of the large percentage of viral cases. Chronic cases are treated, but bacterial resistance can easily

---

Table 29-1. Empiric Treatment of Meningitis

Age of patient	Most likely organism	Empiric treatment
Newborn to 1 month	Gram-negative enterics (*Escherichia coli*), group B streptococci, or *Listeria monocytogenes*	Ampicillin and aminoglycoside, cefotaxime, or Ceftriaxone
1 month to 4 years	*Haemophilus influenzae, Neisseria meningitidis,* or *Streptococcus pneumoniae*	Cefotaxime or ceftriaxone, plus vancomycin
5–29 years	*N. meningitidis, S. pneumoniae,* or *H. influenzae*	Cefotaxime or ceftriaxone, plus vancomycin
30–60 years	*S. pneumoniae* or *N. meningitidis*	Cefotaxime or ceftriaxone, plus vancomycin
> 60 years	*S. pneumoniae,* Gram-negative enterics (*E. coli*), or *L. monocytogenes*	Cefotaxime, ceftriaxone, or ampicillin and aminoglycoside-vancomycin

Table 29-2. Therapy for Endocarditis

Organism	Therapy	Duration (weeks)
Penicillin-susceptible streptococci	Penicillin G alone	4
	Penicillin G with gentamicin	2
	Ceftriaxone alone	4
	Vancomycin (if allergic to penicillin)	4
Streptococci relatively resistant to penicillin	Penicillin G alone	4
	Penicillin G with gentamicin	2
	Vancomycin (if allergic to penicillin)	4
Staphylococcus without prosthetic material (methicillin sensitive)	Nafcillin or oxacillin (3–5 days of gentamicin may be added)	4–6
	Cefazolin (with or without gentamicin)	4–6
	Vancomycin (if allergic to penicillin)	4–6
Staphylococcus without prosthetic material (methicillin resistant)	Vancomycin (if allergic to penicillin)	4–6

develop from the use of multiple antibiotic treatments. Table 29-3 describes treatment for acute and chronic bronchitis.

Pneumonia

Pneumonia is an inflammation of the lung parenchyma characterized by consolidation of the affected part, as well as filling of the alveolar air spaces with exudates, inflammatory cells, and fibrin. Distribution may be lobar, segmental, or lobular. If pneumonia is associated with bronchitis (see the previous discussion of bronchitis), it is termed *bronchopneumonia*.

Causative agents

Multiple bacterial etiologies are possible, depending on predisposing conditions (Table 29-4).

Table 29-3. Treatment of Acute and Chronic Bronchitis

Illness	Treatment (7–10 days usual duration)
Acute (rare; for severe disease only)	Erythromycin, clarithromycin, azithromycin (drugs used for treatment of chronic disease may be used)
Chronic	Amoxicillin, amoxicillin-clavulanate, TMP-SMX, erythromycin, clarithromycin, azithromycin, doxycycline, cefuroxime, cefaclor, cefprozil

Clinical presentation

Typically, the onset of illness is abrupt or subacute, with fever, chills, dyspnea, and productive cough predominating. On physical examination, the patient is tachypneic and tachycardic, frequently with chest wall retractions and grunting respirations. The complete blood count usually reflects a leukocytosis with a predominance of polymorphonuclear cells.

Diagnostic criteria

Sputum culture may be useful in identifying some pathogens. However, difficulty in obtaining a deep sputum culture and problems in culturing some organisms (e.g., *Legionella*) make positive identification of the organism difficult.

Treatment

Treatment varies by age group.

Tuberculosis

Tuberculosis is a communicable infectious disease caused by *Mycobacterium tuberculosis*. It can produce silent, latent infection as well as active infection. Although infection of any tissue or organ with *M. tuberculosis* is possible, the usual site of infection is pulmonary.

Table 29-4. Empiric Treatment of Pneumonia

Age or type	Usual organisms	Empiric treatments
Neonatal	Group B streptococci, *Listeria monocytogenes, Escherichia coli*	Ampicillin and gentamicin *or* cefotaxime and gentamicin
1–3 months	*Chlamydia trachomatis, Bordetella* spp.	Erythromycin, clarithromycin, or cefuroxime
3 months to 5 years	*Streptococcus pneumoniae, C. trachomatis*	Clarithromycin, cefuroxime, or cefotaxime
5–18 years	*Mycoplasma pneumoniae, S. pneumoniae, Chlamydia pneumoniae*	Clarithromycin, erythromycin, or cefuroxime
Adult, community-acquired	*S. pneumoniae, Haemophilus influenzae, Klebsiella pneumoniae, M. pneumoniae*	*Ambulatory:* oral macrolide (azithromycin, clarithromycin, erythromycin) or fluoroquinolone (levofloxacin, gatifloxacin or moxifloxacin)
		Hospitalized: cefotaxime or ceftriaxone with or without macrolide *or* fluoroquinolone alone (levofloxacin, gatifloxacin, moxifloxacin)
Adult, hospital-acquired	*K. pneumoniae, Enterobacter aerogenes, Serratia* spp., *Acinetobacter* spp., *Pseudomonas aeruginosa, Staphylococcus aureus*	Aminoglycoside (tobramycin, amikacin, gentamicin) plus one of the following: cefotaxime, ceftriaxone, cefepime, ticarcillin–clavulanic acid, piperacillin-tazobactam, meropenem, or imipenem; vancomycin to be added if methicillin-resistant *S. aureus* suspected
Adult, aspiration	Mouth anaerobes	*Uncomplicated:* penicillin G, clindamycin
		Hospital-acquired: ticarcillin–clavulanic acid, piperacillin-tazobactam

Clinical presentation

Tuberculosis can present with generalized symptoms of weight loss, fever, and night sweats, along with persistent cough productive of sputum. In the absence of other symptoms, latent disease is defined by a positive PPD (purified protein derivative) test.

Diagnostic criteria

Diagnosis often is made by a combination of chest x-ray (which often shows patchy or nodular infiltrates in the apical areas of the upper lobes or the superior segment of the lower lobes) and positive PPD skin test. Patients with severe HIV disease may not react to the standard PPD skin test. Sputum or lung biopsy may be acid-fast stained to reveal the organism. Because of the extended time period needed to grow the organism, sensitivities to anti-infective agents may take weeks to months to determine.

Treatment

See Table 29-5 for a summary of treatments.

Infectious Diarrhea

Diarrhea is defined as an increase in frequency or liquidity of stool (or both) compared to a patient's normal stool.

Table 29-5. Treatment of Tuberculosis

Disease stage	Treatment	Duration
Latent (probably isoniazid sensitive)	Isoniazid	9 months (6 months possible except for children and HIV-positive persons)
Latent (probably isoniazid resistant)	Rifampin + pyrazinamide	2 months
Active disease	Isoniazid + rifampin + pyrazinamide	2–4 months

Causative agents

Many disease states, drugs, and infectious organisms have been associated with diarrhea.

Clinical presentation

The patient may present with several of the following symptoms: fever, chills, nausea, vomiting, and abdominal cramping.

Diagnostic criteria

Etiology often is determined by patient history and physical examination. Because of the nature of the disease, cultures often are not diagnostic, except for determination of carrier states.

Treatment

Supportive care (hydration, antipyretics, and antiemetics) is useful. Antimotility agents are discouraged because of the potential to cause toxic megacolon.

Antibacterial therapy is reserved for severe presentations or for patients with risk factors.

Table 29-6 provides an overview of treatments.

Skin and Soft Tissue Infections

Bacterial infection of the skin can be classified as direct infection of the skin (cellulitis) or secondary infection of a wound or incision.

Causative agents

Cellulitis usually is infection caused by a single organism. The most common organisms are *Streptococcus pyogenes* and *Staphylococcus aureus*. Secondary infections may be polymicrobial, including both anaerobic and aerobic organisms.

Clinical presentation

Skin and soft tissue infections are characterized by erythema and edema of the skin.

Table 29-6. Treatment of Infectious Diarrhea

Symptoms	Organism	Treatment
Violent presentation 1–6 hours after eating high-protein foods (eggs)	*Staphylococcus aureus*	Supportive
Indolent presentation with mild fever after eating meat, vegetables, or eggs	*Bacillus cereus*	Supportive
Mild to severe presentation 8–16 hours after eating canned products	*Clostridium perfringens*	Supportive
Mild to severe presentation with mild fever; may be associated with meat or egg contamination or other foods contaminated with contaminated water	*Escherichia coli*	Supportive, if outpatient; if hospitalized, fluoroquinolones or TMP-SMX
Mild to severe presentation with mild fever, chills, and cramping; associated with other foods contaminated with contaminated water; carrier state possible	*Salmonella* spp.	Treatment only if febrile (fluoroquinolones or TMP-SMX)
Bloody mucoid diarrhea with fever and cramps	*Shigella* spp.	TMP-SMX
Mild indolent presentation, often thought to be "flu"; transmitted by contaminated water	*Campylobacter*	Macrolides or fluoroquinolones
Severe presentation with fever and abdominal pain associated with seafood ingestion	*Yersinia enterocolitica*	Fluoroquinolones
Mild presentation with fever and abdominal pain associated with seafood ingestion	*Vibrio parahaemolyticus*	Tetracycline or fluoroquinolones
Severe, explosive presentation associated with contaminated water	*Vibrio cholerae*	Tetracycline or fluoroquinolones
Mild to severe presentation associated with travel, 6–10 days after exposure, with cramping and low-grade fever	*Escherichia coli*	Mostly supportive; severe prophylactic regimens

Table 29-7. Treatment of Skin and Soft Tissue Infections

Infection	Organisms	Treatments
Cellulitis	Group A streptococcus; *Staphylococcus aureus*	*Outpatient:* dicloxacillin, cefadroxil, cephalexin, erythromycin
		Inpatient: cefazolin, erythromycin
		Severe cases: vancomycin
Diabetic foot infections	*Proteus* spp., *Escherichia coli, S. aureus, Bacteroides fragilis,* anaerobic streptococci	Clindamycin or cephalexin
		Severe cases: ticarcillin–clavulanic acid or other β-lactamase inhibitor; vancomycin may be needed if methicillin-resistant *S. aureus* suspected
Decubitus ulcers	Gram-negative bacilli, *Pseudomonas aeruginosa,* anaerobes	Same as for diabetic foot infections

Diagnostic criteria

Diagnosis is usually made from physical examination. Cultures usually are not diagnostic.

Treatment

Treatment is empiric, based on likely organisms (Table 29-7).

Urinary Tract Infections

Urinary tract infections (UTIs) represent a wide variety of clinical syndromes, including urethritis, cystitis, prostatitis, and pyelonephritis.

Causative agents

The most common agents are Gram-negative facultatively anaerobic rods (coliforms). Hospitalized, catheterized patients also may acquire *Pseudomonas* and *Staphylococcus* species.

Clinical presentation

Lower urinary tract infections tend to present with dysuria, urgency, frequency, nocturia, and suprapubic heaviness or pain. Fever is rare. Upper urinary tract infections tend to present with flank pain and fever.

Diagnostic criteria

Key to the diagnosis of UTIs is the ability to demonstrate significant numbers of organisms present in an appropriately drawn urine sample. In general, higher numbers of organisms ($>10^5$ cells/mL) are needed to diagnose UTIs in females than in males ($>10^3$ cells/mL), because more organisms are able to ascend the shorter female urethra. In addition, the presence of WBCs in the urine sample may be a significant clue for infection.

Treatment

A variety of antibacterials may be useful for the treatment of urinary tract infections (Table 29-8), including

Table 29-8. Treatment of Urinary Tract Infections

Diagnosis	Organisms	Treatments
Acute uncomplicated cystitis	*Escherichia coli, Staphylococcus saprophyticus*	TMP-SMX × 3 days *or* quinolone × 3 days
Acute pyelonephritis	*E. coli, Proteus mirabilis, Klebsiella pneumoniae, Enterococcus* spp.	Quinolone × 14 days *or* TMP-SMX × 14 days; if severe, parenteral therapy with quinolone and extended-spectrum penicillin plus aminoglycoside should be used
Prostatitis	*E. coli, Proteus* spp., *K. pneumoniae*	Quinolone × 4–6 weeks *or* TMP-SMX × 4–6 weeks

fluoroquinolones, cephalosporins, trimethoprim-sulfamethoxazole (TMP-SMX), and doxycycline. Fluoroquinolones are especially useful for the treatment of prostatitis. Length of therapy varies according to the severity of disease.

Bacterial Venereal Diseases (Gonorrhea and Syphilis)

Venereal diseases are diseases that can be transmitted via sexual intercourse. This section covers only the major bacterial venereal diseases, which are gonorrhea and syphilis. Viral venereal diseases (e.g., herpes and hepatitis) will follow in this chapter or other chapters (for HIV, see Chapter 31).

Causative agents

Syphilis is caused by an infection with the spirochete *Treponema pallidum,* whereas gonorrhea is caused by the Gram-negative coccus *Neisseria gonorrhoeae.*

Clinical presentation

Primary syphilis presents as painless lesions or chancres appearing at the site of infection around 21 days after exposure. The lesions persist for about 8 weeks before disappearing spontaneously.

Secondary syphilis develops 2–6 weeks after the onset of the primary stage and is characterized by a variety of rashes and flu-like symptoms. These symptoms disappear without treatment within 4–10 weeks. Untreated patients will develop symptoms of tertiary syphilis within 2–25 years after infection. These symptoms include general paresis, nerve deafness, progressive dementia, and aortic insufficiency.

Gonorrhea, in contrast, presents as a urethritis within 2–3 days of exposure. Dysuria, urinary fre-quency, and purulent discharge are common. The majority of infected patients become asymptomatic without treatment within 6 months. About 15% of infected women will develop pelvic inflammatory disease, which can be an indirect cause of future infertility.

Diagnostic criteria

Because *T. pallidum* cannot be grown in culture, dark-field or indirect fluorescent antibody microscopic examination is used in conjunction with serologic testing for diagnosis. The most common tests used are the Venereal Disease Research Laboratory (VDRL) test and the rapid plasma reagin (RPR) test. Gonorrhea is diagnosed by Gram stain and culture of infected secretions. Alternative methods of diagnosis include enzyme immunoassay and DNA (deoxyribonucleic acid) probes. Patients testing positive for any sexually transmitted disease should be screened for the presence of other venereal diseases.

Treatment

Because of the significant both diseases can potentially cause significant morbidity in infants born to infected mothers, diagnosis and treatment of pregnant women is of concern. The two organisms differ sharply in resistance to anti-infective agents. *T. pallidum* is sensitive to penicillin and has not developed any significant resistance. *N. gonorrhoeae* has developed significant resistance not only to penicillin but also to fluoroquinolones, leaving third-generation cephalosporins as the major treatment modality (Table 29-9). Patients diagnosed with gonorrhea should also receive therapy against chlamydia infection (usually doxycycline 100 mg bid for 7 days or azithromycin 1 g once). All sexual partners must also be treated.

Table 29-9. Treatment of Gonorrhea and Syphilis

Type	Gonorrhea	Syphilis
Uncomplicated adult presentation	Ceftriaxone 125 mg IM × 1 dose *or* spectinomycin 2 g IM q12h × 2 doses	Benzathine penicillin G 2.4 million units IM × 1 dose
Infant born of untreated mother	Cefotaxime 25 mg/kg q12h × 7 days	Penicillin G 50,000–75,000 units/kg q12h × 10–21 days
Disseminated infections	Ceftriaxone 1 g qd × 10 days	*Secondary or latent disease:* benzathine penicillin G 2.4 million units IM q week × 3 doses
		Tertiary disease: penicillin G 2 million to 4 million units q4h for 10–14 days

Sepsis

Sepsis has been defined by the American College of Chest Physicians as the systemic inflammatory response syndrome (SIRS) produced in response to infection. SIRS has been defined as requiring two of the following criteria: temperature > 38°C or < 36°C; heart rate > 90 bpm; respiratory rate >20 breaths/min or $PaCo_2$ <32 torr; WBC >12,000 cells/mm^3 or <4,000 cells/mm^3; or >10% immature (band) forms.

Causative agents

Sepsis may be caused by a variety of organisms, including Gram-negative and Gram-positive organisms, as well as fungi. Most cases occur in a hospital setting and reflect the institution's organisms and resistance patterns.

Clinical presentation

In the early phase, the patient may have fever or hypothermia, rigors, chills, tachycardia, tachypnea, hyperglycemia, and lethargy. The condition progresses to hypotension, hypoglycemia, myocardial depression, oliguria, leukopenia, and pulmonary edema, leading to multisystem organ failure.

Diagnostic criteria

In addition to physical signs and symptoms, cultures of blood, urine, and sputum may yield clues for antibacterial therapy.

Treatment

Local organisms and sensitivities will determine anti-infective therapy. Initial therapy should be broad, covering all likely organisms, until culture results are obtained. *The Medical Letter* suggests the following regimens for life-threatening sepsis in adults: cefotaxime, ceftriaxone, cefepime, ticarcillin-clavulanic acid, piperacillin-tazobactam, meropenem, or imipenem with an aminoglycoside (tobramycin, gentamicin, or amikacin). If Gram-positive organisms are suspected, vancomycin or linezolid may be added to the regimen.

Tick-Borne Systemic Febrile Syndromes (Lyme Disease, Rocky Mountain Spotted Fever, Ehrlichiosis, and Tularemia)

Tick-borne illnesses are similar in transmission and natural history. The organisms responsible for these infections are *Rickettsia,* known for their intracellular growth in host cells. As such, they cannot be grown in culture media, and serologic tests are used for diagnosis. Patients present with fever, rash, and flu-like symptoms, as well as a history of tick exposure.

Treatment

See Table 29-10 for treatment options.

Systemic Fungal Infections

Fungal infections fall into two categories: *primary* (able to cause infection in both healthy and immunocompromised patients) and *opportunistic* (able to cause infection only in immunocompromised patients). Many fungal infections have a pulmonary focus because of the aerosol spread of mold spores. The incidence of fungal infection is rising as a result of increased use of antibacterial agents and the increase in immunocompromised patients.

Clinical presentation

Patients present with a gradual onset of general malaise, fever, and weakness, which are unrelieved by antibacterial therapy. Pulmonary infection usually presents with pneumonia-like symptoms.

Table 29-10. Treatment of Tick-Borne Systemic Febrile Syndromes

Disease	Causative agent	Primary treatment	Alternative treatment
Lyme disease	*Borrelia burgdorferi*	Doxycycline	Cefuroxime
Rocky Mountain spotted fever	*Rickettsia rickettsii*	Doxycycline	Chloramphenicol
Ehrlichiosis	*Ehrlichia phagocytophila*	Doxycycline	Tetracycline
Tularemia	*Francisella tularensis*	Gentamicin or tobramycin	Chloramphenicol; possibly ciprofloxacin

Table 29-11. Treatment of Systemic Fungal Infections

Disease	Organism	Treatments
Invasive pulmonary disease	*Aspergillosis* spp.	Amphotericin B, itraconazole, caspofungin, voriconazole
Cutaneous, pulmonary, or extrapulmonary disease	*Blastomyces dermatitidis*	Itraconazole, amphotericin B, fluconazole
Bloodstream infection	*Candida albicans*	Fluconazole, amphotericin B
Primary pulmonary disease	*Coccidioides immitis*	Itraconazole, fluconazole
Meningitis	*Cryptococcus neoformans*	Amphotericin B + flucytosine, fluconazole
Pulmonary, disseminated, or localized	*Histoplasma capsulatum*	Itraconazole (moderate disease), amphotericin B (severe disease)

Diagnostic criteria

Diagnosis is made from patient history; cultures (usually blood, sputum, and biopsy of lesions); and serologic tests.

Treatment

Treatment often is empiric until the organism is isolated (Table 29-11). Because of the relatively slow growth of most fungi and the lack of commercial testing against antifungal agents, patient response is used to determine resistance to therapy.

Viral Infections (Hepatitis, Influenza, and the Herpes Simplex Family)

Antiviral therapy is not curative in viral infections but decreases the level of virus so that a patient's immune system can handle the infection.

Hepatitis

Hepatitis is a general term referring to a generalized inflammation of the liver. Etiologies may be viral or chemical.

Causative agents
Five viruses (hepatitis types A–E) have been identified as causative agents for hepatitis. Syndromes may be either acute or chronic.

Clinical presentation
Patients present with a history of anorexia, nausea, fatigue, and malaise, which usually progresses to fever, right upper quadrant pain, dark urine, light-colored stools, and worsening of systemic symptoms. Some patients have no symptoms and little hepatic damage.

Diagnostic criteria
In addition to physical signs, laboratory tests are remarkable for elevations in AST (aspartate aminotransferase), ALT (alanine aminotransferase), and serum bilirubin.

Treatment
Treatment depends on the viral strain and type of presentation (Table 29-12). Standard therapies have not been established for hepatitis A, D, or E.

Influenza

Influenza is an acute respiratory viral infection.

Causative agents
Three viruses, influenza A, B, and C, are responsible for most infections.

Clinical presentation
Patients present with sudden onset of chills, fever, severe prostration, headache, muscle aches, and a

Table 29-12. Treatment of Hepatitis

Organism	Presentation	Therapy
Hepatitis B	Chronic	Lamivudine + interferon alfa-2b
Hepatitis C	Chronic	Interferon alfa-2b + ribavirin
Hepatitis C	Acute	Interferon alfa-2b

cough that usually is dry. The primary viral infection may be followed by secondary bacterial infections.

Diagnostic criteria
Diagnosis is from patient physical signs and symptoms.

Therapy
Therapy may be either prophylaxis or treatment and is determined by viral strain in the community (Table 29-13). Currently, no therapies exist for influenza C infections.

Herpes simplex family (herpes, cytomegalovirus, chickenpox or shingles)

The herpes simplex family is responsible for three serious viral infections: herpes genital infections, cytomegalovirus (CMV) infections in the immuno-compromised, and varicella zoster infections (chickenpox and shingles).

Causative agents
Each disease is caused by a slightly different herpes virus.

Clinical presentation
Clinical presentation varies by disease:

- Genital herpes presents with flu-like symptoms of fever, headache, malaise, and myalgias, in addition to development of painful pustular or ulcerative lesions on the external genitalia.
- CMV usually presents as retinitis, colitis, or esophagitis.
- Varicella zoster presents with flu-like symptoms with a pustular rash located on body dermatomes.

Diagnostic criteria
Diagnosis is mostly from signs and symptoms, although tissue samples may be examined for the presence of the virus using immunofluorescence.

Table 29-13. Treatment of Influenza

Organism	Treatment type	Therapy
Influenza A	Prophylaxis	Oseltamivir, rimantadine, amantadine
Influenza A	Treatment	Zanamivir, oseltamivir, rimantadine, amantadine
Influenza B	Prophylaxis	Oseltamivir
Influenza B	Prophylaxis	Zanamivir, oseltamivir

Table 29-14. Treatment of Herpes Virus Infections

Organism	Disease	Treatment
Herpes simplex	Initial episode	Acyclovir
	Recurrence	Famciclovir
	Chronic suppression	Valacyclovir
	Immunocompromised	Acyclovir
	Resistant to acyclovir	Foscarnet
Cytomegalovirus	Retinitis, colitis, esophagitis	Ganciclovir, valganciclovir, foscarnet, cidofovir, fomivirsen
Varicella zoster	Chickenpox, shingles	Acyclovir
Varicella zoster	Immunocompromised, resistant to acyclovir	Foscarnet

Treatment
Treatment depends on viral and disease state. Treatment is summarized in Table 29-14.

29-3. Key Points

- The hallmark of initial anti-infective therapy is to target the specific organisms associated with the disease.
- Conversely, after the identification of the organism causing the disease, anti-infective therapy should be narrowed to cover that specific organism.
- Therapy should reflect not only the best anti-infective agent for the organism but also aspects of the patient's condition (e.g., renal function and concurrent disease states).
- Combination anti-infective therapy should be reserved for documented clinical efficacy, therapeutic failure of monotherapy, and polymicrobial infection.
- Clinical signs of infection should be followed to determine patient response to therapy.
- Empiric therapy of meningitis is age specific, reflecting the age-specific nature of the common pathogens.
- Endocarditis therapy is specific to the organism isolated. The presence of a prosthetic valve increases the time of therapy.
- Many cases of bronchitis are viral in etiology, making routine antibiotic therapy controversial.

- Empiric pneumonia therapy reflects coverage of both age-related organisms and organisms associated with patient-specific risk factors.
- Diarrhea therapy mainly should be supportive, with careful use of anti-infectives and antimotility agents.
- Diagnosis of urinary tract infections varies by numbers of organisms found in the urine. Higher numbers (>10^5 cells/mL) are needed to diagnose UTIs in females than in males (>10^3 cells/mL) because of the higher numbers of organisms able to ascend the shorter female urethra.
- A frequently overlooked aspect of the treatment of bacterial venereal diseases is the treatment of sexual partners.
- Initial therapy of sepsis should be broad in scope, covering all likely organisms, until results of cultures are obtained.
- Because of the long doubling time of most fungi and the difficulty in obtaining sensitivity to specific antifungal agents, patient response is used to determine resistance to therapy.
- Antiviral therapy is not curative but decreases the level of virus so that a patient's immune system can handle the infection.

29-4. Questions

1. The lowest concentration of anti-infective that prevents microbial growth is called the

    A. minimum bactericidal concentration.
    B. minimum bacteriostatic concentration.
    C. minimum inhibitory concentration.
    D. minimum inhibiting concentration.
    E. minimum Schillings concentration.

2. Laboratory markers of infections, such as C-reactive protein, white blood cell count, and erythrocyte sedimentation rate, may not be accurate in which patient populations?

    I.   Elderly patients
    II. Patients with chronic obstructive pulmonary disease
    III. Malnourished patients

    A. I only
    B. II only
    C. I and III only
    D. II and III only
    E. I, II, and III

3. The hallmark of empiric therapy is

    A. coverage of the most common pathogen associated with the infection.
    B. coverage of the common pathogens associated with the infection.
    C. coverage of all possible pathogens associated with the infection.
    D. coverage of polymicrobial pathogens associated with the infection.
    E. coverage of all viral organisms associated with the infection.

4. When two anti-infective therapies together produce a greater effect than the effects of each used alone, this phenomenon is termed

    A. commensalism.
    B. synergy.
    C. antagonism.
    D. additive.
    E. interacting.

5. Analysis of the cerebrospinal fluid may give valuable clues to the identity of the pathogen in meningitis. Given the following results, what would be indicative of a fungal infection?

    I.   Increase in WBCs
    II. Decreased glucose
    III Increased protein

    A. I only
    B. II only
    C. I and III only
    D. II and III only
    E. I, II, and III

6. Empiric therapy for meningitis for patients up to 1 month of age includes

    A. vancomycin and ampicillin.
    B. aminoglycoside and ampicillin.
    C. ceftriaxone and vancomycin.
    D. vancomycin and aminoglycoside.
    E. ampicillin and ceftriaxone.

7. When treating penicillin-allergic patients for endocarditis, _____ may be used for therapy.

    A. vancomycin
    B. erythromycin
    C. cefazolin
    D. meropenem
    E. nafcillin

8. Patients presenting with acute bronchitis without risk factors should be treated empirically with

   A. supportive care.
   B. clarithromycin.
   C. cefuroxime.
   D. ciprofloxacin.
   E. erythromycin.

9. The most common organisms associated with community-acquired pneumonia in adults are

   A. *Chlamydia pneumoniae, Mycoplasma pneumoniae,* and *Haemophilus influenzae.*
   B. *Streptococcus pneumoniae, Haemophilus influenzae,* and *Chlamydia pneumoniae.*
   C. *Mycoplasma pneumoniae, Chlamydia pneumoniae,* and *Streptococcus pneumoniae.*
   D. *Mycoplasma pneumoniae, Streptococcus pneumoniae,* and *Haemophilus influenzae.*
   E. *Chlamydia pneumoniae, Staphylococcus aureus,* and *Haemophilus influenzae.*

10. Empiric therapy for patients with hospital-acquired pneumonia should include

    A. tobramycin and gentamicin.
    B. cefotaxime and cefepime.
    C. vancomycin and gentamicin.
    D. gentamicin and cefepime.
    E. cefepime and vancomycin.

11. Treatment of latent tuberculosis infections in which isoniazid-resistant strains of *Mycobacterium tuberculosis* are predominant should include

    A. rifabutin and pyrazinamide.
    B. rifampin and pyrazinamide.
    C. isoniazid, rifampin, and pyrazinamide.
    D. isoniazid, rifabutin, and pyrazinamide.
    E. ethambutol and rifampin.

12. The use of antimotility agents in infectious diarrhea is

    A. discouraged because of the potential to cause toxic megacolon.
    B. encouraged because of increased cure rates.
    C. discouraged because of increased reinfections.
    D. encouraged because of decreased reinfections.
    E. discouraged because of lack of efficacy.

13. Cellulitis usually is associated with

    A. *Staphylococcus aureus.*
    B. *Streptococcus bovis.*
    C. *Peptostreptococcus boydii.*
    D. *Escherichia coli.*
    E. *Klebsiella pneumoniae.*

14. The best empiric regimen to treat prostate infection is

    A. ciprofloxacin for 10 days.
    B. TMP-SMX for 10 days.
    C. ciprofloxacin and TMP-SMX for 10 days.
    D. ciprofloxacin for 4–6 weeks.
    E. TMP-SMX for 4–6 weeks.

15. Tertiary syphilis in adults should be treated with

    A. benzathine penicillin 2.4 million units × 1 day.
    B. penicillin 50,000 units/kg q12h × 10–21 days.
    C. penicillin 4 million units q4h × 10–14 days.
    D. benzathine penicillin 2.4 million units q week × 3 weeks.
    E. penicillin 150,000 units/kg q12h × 10–21 days.

16. *Candida albicans* infections may be treated with

    A. itraconazole.
    B. amphotericin B.
    C. voriconazole.
    D. caspofungin.
    E. ketoconazole.

17. The antiviral agent with the widest spectrum of activity against influenza is

    A. zanamivir.
    B. rimantadine.
    C. amantadine.
    D. oseltamivir.
    E. acyclovir.

18. Herpes infections resistant to acyclovir may be treated with

    A. famciclovir.
    B. valacyclovir.
    C. foscarnet.
    D. ganciclovir.
    E. high-dose acyclovir.

19. In the list that follows, the only organism that can be cultured easily is

    A. *Treponema pallidum.*
    B. *Mycobacterium tuberculosis.*
    C. *Rickettsia rickettsii.*
    D. *Ehrlichia phagocytophila.*
    E. *Francisella tularensis.*

20. Anti-infective therapy always should be used to treat infectious diarrhea caused by which organism?

    A. *Escherichia coli*
    B. *Vibrio cholerae*
    C. *Staphylococcus aureus*
    D. *Salmonella*
    E. *Bacillus cereus*

21. J. B. is an 18-year-old white female who just gave birth to her first child. Because she presented without any prenatal care or history, a full prenatal panel of tests was taken, including a vaginal swab. Two days after giving birth, she complained of a purulent vaginal discharge and a low-grade fever. Blood cultures were negative, but the vaginal swab revealed the presence of Gram-negative cocci. WBCs were elevated at 13,000 cells/mm^3. What is J. B.'s probable infection?

    A. Herpes simplex
    B. Gonorrhea
    C. Syphilis
    D. Urinary tract infection
    E. Food poisoning

22. What should be done for J. B. and her baby?

    A. Both mother and child should be treated.
    B. Neither mother nor child should be treated.
    C. The child should be treated, but the mother should not.
    D. The mother should be treated, but the child should not.
    E. Mother, child, and partner should be treated.

23. L. B. is a 45-year-old white female presenting to the emergency department with a fever of 103°F, flank pain, dysuria, urgency, and frequency. Her laboratory tests are significant for an increased WBC count of 18,000 cells/mm^3 and 3% immature forms (bands). Her urinalysis revealed >10^5 cells/mL of Gram-negative rods. What does L. B. have?

    A. Herpes simplex
    B. Gonorrhea
    C. Syphilis
    D. Urinary tract infection
    E. Food poisoning

24. What therapy would be useful for L. B.?

    A. Oral quinolone
    B. IV quinolone
    C. Oral penicillin
    D. IV carbapenem
    E. IV vancomycin

29-5. Answers

1. **C.** The minimum inhibitory concentration determines the level of anti-infective to which dosing regimens may be set.
2. **C.** Elderly and malnourished patients may not be able to respond with appropriate laboratory markers of infections because of limited reserves or deletion of inflammatory factors.
3. **B.** Coverage of common pathogens associated with the infection increases the probability of curing the infection without increasing anti-infective exposure to other organisms, which increases the possibility of resistance.
4. **B.** *Synergy* is the correct term.
5. **E.** Although fungal CNS infections show relatively slight changes in WBCs, protein, and glucose compared to bacterial infections, the trend is similar.
6. **B.** This regimen covers the most likely organisms for meningitis in this age group: Gram-negative enterics (e.g., *Escherichia coli*), group B streptococci, and *Listeria monocytogenes*.
7. **A.** Vancomycin covers all Gram-positive organisms associated with endocarditis, with no cross-sensitivity to penicillin.
8. **A.** Because half of bronchitis infections are caused by a viral etiology, antibacterial therapy for low-risk patients should not be attempted, with the exception of severe presentation.
9. **D.** *Chlamydia pneumoniae* is not a pathogen associated with adult pneumonia.
10. **D.** Empiric therapy for hospital-acquired pneumonia should have an aminoglycoside and one other Gram-negative agent, such as cefepime. Vancomycin can be added if methicillin-resistant *Staphylococcus aureus* is suspected.

11. **B.** Latent infections are usually treated with isoniazid alone. In the case of isoniazid-resistant tuberculosis, rifampin and pyrazinamide are effective at treating latent infections. The three-drug regimens are used to treat active disease.

12. **A.** Use of such agents increases the chance of intestinal perforation and increases the length of symptoms.

13. **A.** Most cellulitis infections are associated with *Staphylococcus aureus* and *Streptococcus pyogenes.*

14. **D.** Prostate infections are difficult to treat, requiring 4–6 weeks of therapy. Although TMP-SMX is a reasonable choice for treating most prostate infections, ciprofloxacin is preferred because of its ability to concentrate in prostate fluid.

15. **C.** Because of the organism load of tertiary syphilis, high doses of penicillin G are needed for clinical cure. Responses B and E are congenital syphilis doses for neonates.

16. **B.** Voriconazole and caspofungin have activity against *Candida* but have not yet been tested in a variety of settings. Ketoconazole and itraconazole should not be used for serious *Candida* infections. Amphotericin B and fluconazole are currently recommended for *Candida.*

17. **D.** Oseltamivir may be used for either treatment or prophylaxis against both influenza A and influenza B.

18. **C.** Foscarnet has activity against acyclovir-resistant herpes.

19. **B.** *Mycobacterium tuberculosis,* although very slow growing, can be grown on culture media. The remaining organisms cannot be grown without the use of cell culture techniques, forcing the clinician to rely on serum testing and direct staining for identification of the organism.

20. **B.** *Staphylococcus* and *Bacillus* diarrheas are an intoxication not caused by a living organism. Both *Salmonella* and *E. coli* diarrheas should be treated only if severe or if signs of systemic infection are present. *Vibrio cholerae* causes a severe diarrhea requiring anti-infective treatment.

21. **B.** Given the lack of prenatal care, J.B.'s physical signs and symptoms, and the presence of Gram-negative cocci, J. B. most likely has gonorrhea.

22. **E.** Mother, partner, and child should be treated. J. B. and her partner should receive ceftriaxone 125 mg IM × 1 dose and treatment for concurrent chlamydia infection (doxycycline 100 mg bid × 7 days). The child should receive cefotaxime 25 mg/kg q12h × 7 days. Both mother and child should be screened for additional sexually transmitted diseases.

23. **D.** Given the clinical presentation and laboratory test results, L. B. has a severe urinary tract infection. The presence of systemic symptoms (fever and chills) suggests an upper urinary tract infection or pyelonephritis.

24. **B.** Given the severity of disease, parenteral therapy would be reasonable for initial therapy. Because the Gram stain of the urine revealed Gram-negative rods, either a quinolone or extended-spectrum penicillin in combination with an aminoglycoside would be reasonable empiric therapy until the organism is identified and sensitivities obtained.

29-6. References

Many general references will provide basic information concerning anti-infective therapy. *The Medical Letter* (www.medletter.com) publishes a good yearly review of antibacterial and antiviral therapies in brief. A list of recent practice guidelines in areas of infectious disease follows.

Meningitis

Tunkel AR, Hartman BL, Kaplan SL, et al. Practice guidelines for the management of bacterial meningitis. *Clin Infect Dis.* 2004;39:1267–84.

Endocarditis

Baddour LM, Wilson WR, Bayer AS, et al. Complications: A statement for healthcare professionals from the Committee Infective Endocarditis: Diagnosis, Antimicrobial Therapy, and Management of Complications. *Circulation.* 2005;111: e394–434.

Pneumonia

American Thoracic Society and the Infectious Diseases Society of America. Guidelines for the management of adults with hospital-acquired, ventilator-associated, and healthcare-associated pneumonia. *Am J Respir Crit Care Med.* 2004;171:388–416.

Bartlett JG, Dowell SF, Mandell LA, et al. Practice guidelines for the management of community-acquired pneumonia in adults: Infectious Diseases Society of America. *Clin Infect Dis.* 2000;31: 347–82.

Tuberculosis

Horsburgh CR, Feldman S, Ridzon R. Practice guidelines for the treatment of tuberculosis. *Clin Infect Dis.* 2000;31:633–39.

Infectious diarrhea

Diagnosis and management of food-borne illnesses: A primer for physicians. *MMWR Recomm Rep.* 2001;50(RR-2):1–69.

Guerrant RL, Van Gilder T, Steiner TS, et al. Practice guidelines for the management of infectious diarrhea. *Clin Infect Dis.* 2001;32:331–51.

Soft tissue infections

Lipsky BA, Berendt BA, Deery HG, et al. Diagnosis and treatment of diabetic foot infections. *Clin Infect Dis.* 2004;39:885–910.

Urinary tract infections

Warren JW, Abrutyn E, Hebel JR, et al. Guidelines for antimicrobial treatment of uncomplicated acute bacterial cystitis and acute pyelonephritis in women: Infectious Diseases Society of America (IDSA). *Clin Infect Dis.* 1999;29:745–58.

Bacterial venereal diseases (gonorrhea and syphilis)

Centers for Disease Control and Prevention. Diseases characterized by genital ulcers: Sexually transmitted diseases treatment guidelines. *MMWR Recomm Rep.* 2002;51(RR-6):11–25.

Centers for Disease Control and Prevention. Diseases characterized by urethritis and cervicitis. Sexually transmitted diseases treatment guidelines. *MMWR Recomm Rep.* 2002;51(RR-6):30–42.

Centers for Disease Control and Prevention. Vaccine preventable STDs. Sexually transmitted diseases treatment guidelines. *MMWR Recomm Rep.* 2002;51(RR-6):59–64.

Sepsis

American College of Chest Physicians–Society of Critical Care Medicine Consensus Conference. Definitions for sepsis and organ failure and guidelines for the use of innovative therapies in sepsis. *Crit Care Med.* 1992;20:864–74.

O'Grady NP, Barie PS, Bartlett JG, et al. Practice guidelines for evaluating new fever in critically ill adult patients. *Crit Care Med.* 1998;26:1042–59.

Tick-borne systemic febrile syndromes

Wormser GP, Nadelman RB, Dattwyler RJ, et al. Practice guidelines for the treatment of Lyme disease. *Clin Infect Dis.* 2000;31(suppl 1):1–14.

Systemic fungal infections

Chapman SW, Bradsher RW, Campbell GD, et al. Practice guidelines for the management of patients with blastomycosis. *Clin Infect Dis.* 2000; 30:679–83.

Pappas PG, Rex JH, Sobel JD, et al. Guidelines for the treatment of candidiasis. *Clin Infect Dis.* 2004; 38:161–89.

Saag MS, Graybill RJ, Larsen RA, et al. Practice guidelines for the management of cryptococcal disease. *Clin Infect Dis.* 2000;30:710–18.

Stevens DA, Kan VL, Judson MA, et al. Practice guidelines for diseases caused by *Aspergillus*. *Clin Infect Dis.* 2000;30:696–709.

Viral infections (hepatitis, influenza, and the herpes simplex family)

Association for Genitourinary Medicine, Medical Society for the Study of Venereal Disease. *2002 National Guideline for the Management of Genital Herpes.* London: AGUM, MSSVD; 2002.

Association for Genitourinary Medicine, Medical Society for the Study of Venereal Disease. *2002 National Guideline on the Management of the Viral Hepatitides A, B, and C.* London: AGUM, MSSVD; 2002.

Bridges CB, Fukuda K, Uyeki TM, et al. Prevention and control of influenza: Recommendations of the Advisory Committee on Immunization Practices (ACIP). *MMWR Recomm Rep.* 2002;51 (RR-03):1–31.

Anti-infective Agents · 30

Ronald L. Braden, PharmD
W. Andrew Bell, PharmD

30-1. Aminoglycosides

Aminoglycosides are antibiotics active against most aerobic Gram-negative bacteria and select aerobic Gram-positive bacteria, but they are not effective against most anaerobic bacteria. Aminoglycosides are primarily used in serious infections because of their significant toxicity. The most commonly used aminoglycosides include amikacin, gentamicin, kanamycin, neomycin, netilmicin, streptomycin, and tobramycin.

Mechanism of Action

Aminoglycosides inhibit bacterial protein synthesis through binding to the 30S ribosomal subunit, thereby irreversibly inhibiting bacterial RNA (ribonucleic acid) synthesis. Aminoglycosides are bactericidal.

Spectrum of Activity

Amikacin is a semisynthetic parenteral aminoglycoside with the broadest antimicrobial activity of the class, and it frequently possesses activity against bacteria resistant to other aminoglycosides.

Gentamicin is a parenteral aminoglycoside that is more active against *Acinetobacter, Serratia,* and enterococci than is tobramycin.

Kanamycin and neomycin are minimally absorbed oral aminoglycosides used to decrease bacterial content of the bowel. They have been used for preoperative bowel preparation and as an adjunct in hepatic encephalopathy.

Netilmicin is a parenteral aminoglycoside that may be the least ototoxic aminoglycoside.

Streptomycin is a parenteral aminoglycoside active against enterococci, streptococci, mycobacteria, and some Gram-negative anaerobes. It is used as an adjunct agent only because many bacterial isolates are resistant to streptomycin monotherapy. Streptomycin should be administered only by intramuscular (IM) injection.

Tobramycin is a parenteral aminoglycoside that is more active against *Pseudomonas* than is gentamicin.

Adverse Drug Events

Nephrotoxicity is demonstrated by an increase in blood urea nitrogen (BUN) and serum creatinine. It usually manifests as nonoliguric renal failure and may cause potassium, calcium, and magnesium wasting. Nephrotoxicity may occur in 10–25% of patients receiving aminoglycosides and is usually reversible on discontinuation of the agent. Risk factors include the following:

- Preexisting renal dysfunction
- Prolonged duration of therapy
- Concomitant use of other nephrotoxic agents
- Possibly elevated trough concentrations:
  - Gentamicin and tobramycin > 2 mcg/mL
  - Amikacin > 8 mcg/mL

Neuromuscular blockade is an uncommon but potentially serious toxicity. Risk factors include the following:

- Concomitant use of neuromuscular blocking agents
- Myasthenia gravis
- Hypocalcemia
- Elevated peak serum concentrations

Ototoxicity is due to eighth cranial nerve damage demonstrated by auditory and vestibular symptoms. Auditory symptoms include tinnitus and loss of high-frequency hearing. Vestibular toxicity is demonstrated by dizziness, nystagmus, vertigo, and ataxia. The incidence of ototoxicity is not clearly known because profound high-frequency hearing loss can occur prior to detection.

Pharmacokinetics

Aminoglycosides are renally eliminated:

- $t_{1/2}$ = 2.5–2.7 hours (normal renal function)
- $t_{1/2}$ = ~69 hours (anephric clearance)
- V_d = 0.27–0.3 L/kg (ideal body weight, or IBW)

Target serum concentrations

Traditional dosing is described in Table 30-1.

- Amikacin peak = 15–30 mcg/mL
- Amikacin trough ≤ 5 mcg/mL
- Gentamicin and tobramycin peak = 4–10 mcg/mL
- Gentamicin and tobramycin trough ≤ 2 mcg/mL

Extended interval dosing

- Amikacin trough ≤ 3 mcg/mL (< 5 mcg/mL for VAP [ventilator-associated pneumonia] or HCAP [health care–associated pneumonia])
- Gentamicin and tobramycin ≤ 1 mcg/mL

30-2. Penicillins

Mechanism of Action

Penicillin-binding proteins make up the cell wall. When penicillin binds to these proteins, it is able to inhibit cell wall synthesis in the bacteria, causing cell wall lysis and ultimately cell death.

Penicillins are bactericidal; they inhibit bacterial cell wall synthesis. They are known as β-lactam antibiotics because their chemical structure consists of a β-lactam ring adjoined to a thiazolidine ring.

Penicillinase-resistant penicillins have substitutions to the β-lactam ring that sterically inhibit penicillinase.

Spectrum of Activity and Dosing

See Tables 30-2 and 30-3 for information about the spectrum of activity and dosing of penicillins.

Adverse Drug Events

Allergic or hypersensitivity reaction occurs in 3–10% of patients. Rash (4–8% of patients) or anaphylaxis (0.01–0.05% of patients) can occur within 10–20 minutes and is more common in intravenous (IV) than in oral administration.

Neurologic reactions (seizures) are seen with high doses of penicillin given to patients with renal insufficiency.

Gastrointestinal (GI) effects, including nausea and vomiting, may occur with oral use.

Hypokalemia and hypernatremia may occur with carboxypenicillins.

Increased transaminases occur with oxacillin and nafcillin.

Cholestatic jaundice may occur with ureidopenicillins.

Hematologic reactions (hemolytic anemia) are possible.

Interstitial nephritis is possible.

Drug–Drug Interactions

Probenecid competitively inhibits tubular secretion of penicillins, thus increasing plasma levels. This interaction is employed in serious central nervous system (CNS) infections to increase drug concentrations.

Aminoglycosides are either incompatible or synergistic.

Table 30-1. Aminoglycosides

Generic name	Trade name	Dosage forms	Normal dose	Elimination
Amikacin	Amikin	IV, IM	15–20 mg/kg/d	Renal
Gentamicin	Garamycin	IV, IM	3 mg/kg/d conventional dose, 7 mg/kg/d extended interval	Renal
Kanamycin		IV, po	15 mg/kg/d	Renal
Neomycin		po	50–100 mg/kg/d	Renal
Streptomycin		IM	15 mg/kg/d	Renal
Tobramycin		IV, IM	3 mg/kg/d conventional dose, 7 mg/kg/d extended interval	Renal

Note: Use ideal or adjusted body weight for all aminoglycoside dosing.

Table 30-2. Spectrum of Activity of the Penicillins

Category	Spectrum
Natural penicillins	Natural penicillins are effective against all viridans streptococci and *Streptococcus pyogenes* and against 60% of *S. pneumoniae,* mouth anaerobes, and *Clostridium perfringens* (gas gangrene).
	Because natural penicillins are readily hydrolyzed by penicillinases (β-lactamases), they are ineffective against *Staphylococcus aureus* and other organisms that resist penicillin.
	Penicillin G is 5–10 times more active than penicillin V against Gram-negative organisms and some anaerobic organisms.
Penicillinase-resistant penicillins	These agents are used to treat methicillin-sensitive staphylococci, streptococci (not enterococci species).
Aminopenicillins	Aminopenicillins have greater penetration of the outer membrane of Gram-negative rods and higher affinity for penicillin-binding proteins.
	They cover most enterococci, *Listeria,* and *Proteus mirabilis.*
	They cover 60% of *Streptococcus pneumoniae, Haemophilus influenzae, Escherichia coli,* and some *Salmonella* and *Shigella.*
Carboxypenicillins and ureidopenicillins	The spectrum is like that of ampicillin, but these drugs provide less Gram-positive coverage. They cover *Proteus* (including *P. vulgaris*), *Klebsiella* (not ticarcillin), *Enterobacter,* and *Pseudomonas* (piperacillin > ticarcillin). Add an aminoglycoside for synergy for serious Gram-negative infections.
	Ureidopenicillins possess better in vitro activity against *Pseudomonas* and other Gram-negative organisms. Ureidopenicillins have in vitro activity against streptococci, enterococci, most *Enterobacteriaceae, Pseudomonas,* and many anaerobes, including *Bacteroides fragilis, Fusobacterium, Clostridium,* and peptostreptococci; β-lactamase-producing staphylococci and *Haemophilus influenzae* are resistant to the ureidopenicillins.
β-lactamase inhibitors (clavulanic acid, sulbactam, and tazobactam)	β-lactamase inhibitors are active against some chromosomally produced β-lactamases of *Staphylococcus aureus, Haemophilus influenzae, Moraxela catarrhalis, Bacteroides, Escherichia coli,* and other *Enterobacteriaceae.*
	They are not active against the chromosomally produced β-lactamases of *Enterobacter, Citrobacter, Serratia,* and *Pseudomonas.*
Amoxicillin–clavulanic acid	This combination is active against *Haemophilus influenzae, Moraxela catarrhalis, Klebsiella pneumoniae,* methicillin-sensitive *Staphylococcus aureus,* and anaerobes.
Ticarcillin–clavulanic acid	This combination has more activity against *Haemophilus influenzae, Moraxela catarrhalis, Klebsiela pneumoniae,* methicillin-sensitive *Staphylococcus aureus,* and anaerobes.
Piperacillin-tazobactam	This combination provides more Gram-positive, Gram-negative, and anaerobic coverage than ticarcillin–clavulanic acid; monotherapy treatment fails against *Pseudomonas.*

Concomitant use with an oral contraceptive may decrease the effectiveness of the oral contraceptive and increase incidence of breakthrough bleeding.

Other Characteristics

Nafcillin and oxacillin are eliminated primarily by biliary excretion; therefore, there is no need to adjust dosage for patients with renal dysfunction.

Penicillin G benzathine is a repository drug formulation. When it is given IM, insoluble salt allows slow drug absorption from the injection site, and therefore, penicillin G has a longer duration of action (12–24 hours).

30-3. Cephalosporins

Cephalosporins are β-lactam antibiotics that are structurally and pharmacologically similar to penicillins.

Mechanism of Action

Cephalosporins are bactericidal agents. Antimicrobial activity is achieved through inhibition of mucopeptide

Table 30-3. Dosing of Penicillins

Type and generic name	Trade name	Elimination route	Administration route	Common doses
Natural penicillins				
Penicillin G	Pfizerpen	Renal	IV, IM, po	2 million to 4 million units IV q4h
Penicillin G procaine	Wycillin	Renal	IM	300,000–600,000 units/d
Penicillin G benzathine	Bicillin LA	Renal	IM	Strep throat: 1.2 million units; syphilis: 2.4 million units
Penicillin V (phenoxymethyl penicillin)	Pen-Vee-K, Veetids	Renal	po	250–500 mg po bid–qid (250 mg bid for prophylaxis)
Penicillinase-resistant penicillins				
Oxacillin	Prostaphlin, Bactocill	Hepatic	po, IV, IM	1–2 g IV q4–6h
Nafcillin	Nafcil, Unipen	Hepatic	IV, IM	1–2 g IV q4–6h
Cloxacillin	Cloxapen	Renal	po	200–500 mg q6h
Dicloxacillin	Dynapen, Dycill	Renal	po	250–500 mg po q6h
Aminopenicillins				
Ampicillin	Omnipen, Principen	Renal	po, IM, IV	1–2 g IV q6h
Amoxicillin	Amoxil, Trimox, Moxatag	Renal	po	250–500 mg po q8h 775 mg (ER) po q24h
Ureidopenicillins				
Piperacillin	Pipracil	Renal	IV, IM	3–4 g IV q4–6h
Penicillin plus β-lactamase inhibitors				
Amoxicillin–clavulanic acid	Augmentin	Renal	po	250–500 mg po tid, 500–875 mg po bid
Ampicillin-sulbactam	Unasyn	Renal	IV, IM	1.5 g or 3 g IV q6–8h
Piperacillin-tazobactam	Zosyn	Renal	IV	2.25 to 4.5 g IV q6h
Ticarcillin–clavulanic acid	Timentin	Renal	IV	3.1 g IV q4–6h

synthesis in the bacterial cell wall, which results in the formation of defective cell walls and subsequent cell lysis and cell death.

Spectrum of Activity

Cephalosporins are broad-spectrum antimicrobial agents; however, the spectrum of activity varies greatly among the individual agents. Thus, cephalosporins are grouped into four broad classes, or generations, according to their antimicrobial coverage (Table 30-4).

First-generation agents (cefadroxil, cefazolin, cephalexin)

Gram-positive activity is extensive, including many strains of *Staphylococcus aureus* and *Staphylococcus epidermidis* in addition to *Streptococcus pyogenes* (group A betahemolytic streptococci), *Streptococcus agalactiae* (group B streptococci), and *Streptococcus pneumoniae*. First-generation agents are inactive against enterococci, methicillin-resistant staphylococci (methicillin-resistant *Staphylococcus aureus* [MRSA] and methicillin-resistant *Staphylococcus epidermidis* [MRSE]), and *Listeria monocytogenes*.

Table 30-4. Cephalosporins

Generic name	Trade name	Dosage forms	Dose	Elimination	Notes
First-generation					More Gram-positive than Gram-negative activity
Cefadroxil	Duricef, Ultracef	po	1–2 g/d	Renal	
Cefazolin	Ancef, Kefzol	IV	250–1,000 mg q8h	Renal	
Cephalexin	Keflex	po	250–500 mg q6h	Renal	
Second-generation					Enhanced Gram-negative activity versus first-generation drugs
Cefaclor	Ceclor	po	250–500 mg q8h	Renal	
Cefotetan	Cefotan	IV, IM	1–2 g q12h	Renal	Anaerobic activity, N-methyl-thiotetrazole side-chain
Cefoxitin	Mefoxin	IV	1–2 g q6–8h	Renal	Anaerobic activity
Cefprozil	Cefzil	po	250–500 mg q12–24h	Renal	Anaerobic activity
Cefuroxime	Ceftin, Zinacef	IV, IM	750–1,500 mg q8h	Renal	
Third-generation					More Gram-negative than Gram-positive activity; cerebrospinal fluid penetration
Cefdinir	Omnicef	po	300 mg q12h	Renal	
Cefixime	Suprax	po	400 mg/d	Renal	
Cefotaxime	Claforan	IV	1–2 g q6–8h	Renal	
Cefpodoxime	Vantin	po	100–400 mg q12h	Renal	Anaerobic activity
Ceftazidime	Fortaz, Tazicef	IV, IM	1–2 g q8–12h	Renal	Antipseudomonal activity
Ceftibuten	Cedax	po	400 mg/d	Renal	
Ceftriaxone	Rocephin	IV, IM	1–2 g/d	Renal or biliary	
Fourth-generation					Gram-positive and Gram-negative activity
Cefepime	Maxipime	IV, IM	1–2 g q12h	Renal	Antipseudomonal activity

Gram-negative activity is limited, although some strains of *Escherichia coli*, *Klebsiella pneumoniae*, *Proteus mirabilis*, and *Shigella* may display susceptibility. First-generation agents are inactive against *Haemophilus influenzae*, *Pseudomonas*, *Enterobacter*, *Citrobacter*, *Serratia*, other *Proteus* spp., and anaerobes such as *Bacteroides fragilis*.

Second-generation agents (cefaclor, cefotetan, cefoxitin, cefprozil, cefuroxime)

Gram-positive activity is similar to that of first-generation agents.

Gram-negative activity of second-generation agents is generally more extensive than that of first-generation agents, including some strains of *Acinetobacter*, *Citrobacter*, *Enterobacter*, *Neisseria*, *Proteus*, and *Serratia*, in addition to *Escherichia coli* and *Klebsiella*. Second-generation agents are active against *Haemophilus influenzae*, and some (cefotetan and cefoxitin) also have anaerobic activity. Second-generation agents are inactive against *Pseudomonas*.

Third-generation agents (cefdinir, cefixime, cefotaxime, cefpodoxime, ceftazidime, ceftibuten, ceftriaxone)

Gram-positive activity is decreased versus first- and second-generation agents.

Gram-negative activity is extensive, including *Enterobacter*, *Citrobacter*, *Serratia*, *Neisseria*, and *Haemophilus*. Some third-generation agents are active against *Pseudomonas* (ceftazidime). Anaerobic coverage varies among individual agents.

Fourth-generation agent (cefepime)

Gram-positive activity is increased versus third-generation agents. Cefepime is inactive against MRSA, enterococci, and *Listeria*.

Gram-negative activity is extensive, including enhanced activity against *Pseudomonas* and *Enterobacteriaceae* that produce inducible β-lactamases.

The extended spectrum of activity of cefepime is attributed to a more rapid penetration of the outer membrane of Gram-negative bacteria. Cefepime is also more resistant to inactivation by β-lactamases.

Adverse Drug Events

- Hypersensitivity, including fever, rash, pruritus, urticaria, anaphylaxis, and hemolytic anemia
- GI effects, such as nausea, vomiting, and diarrhea
- Nephrotoxicity (rare)
- Seizures (potential risk with high doses in patients with renal impairment)
- *Clostridium difficile* colitis
- Bleeding or hypoprothrombinemia (cefotetan), which is attributable to the presence of an N-methylthiotetrazole (NMTT) side chain in the structure of these agents (possible prevention or reversal with administration of vitamin K)
- Blood dyscrasias (rare)

Drug–Drug Interactions

Disulfiram-like reactions have been reported with ingestion of alcohol during treatment with cephalosporin antibiotics.

Probenecid competitively inhibits tubular secretion of cephalosporins, resulting in higher serum concentrations.

Drug–Disease Interactions

All cephalosporins (except ceftriaxone) require dosage adjustments in patients with renal insufficiency.

Monitoring Parameters

Serum concentration monitoring is not necessary. Patients should be monitored for clinical response and resolution of infection.

Patient Instructions and Counseling

Verify that the patient is not allergic to penicillins. Cross-sensitivity with penicillins has been reported in up to 10% of patients receiving cephalosporins.

Obtain a thorough history of any patient with a previous hypersensitivity reaction to any β-lactam antibiotic. In general, cephalosporins should be avoided in these patients.

Other

Bacterial resistance to cephalosporins may result through production of β-lactamases.

30-4. Carbapenems

Carbapenems are β-lactam-like antibiotics that are structurally and pharmacologically similar to penicillins.

Mechanism of Action

Carbapenems bind to penicillin-binding proteins in a manner similar to that of β-lactams, thereby inhibiting peptidoglycan synthesis. Carbapenems are bactericidal in susceptible isolates.

Spectrum of Activity

Carbapenems are very broad-spectrum antibiotics with activity against most Gram-positive and Gram-negative aerobes and anaerobes, as well as activity against some *Mycobacterium* and *Chlamydia* spp. Carbapenems other than ertapenem cover *Pseudomonas* and *Acinetobacter* and are the drug of choice for ESBL (extended spectrum β-lactamases)–producing *Entreobactereacea* species.

Adverse Drug Events

GI adverse effects are the most common events reported with imipenem. The effects include nausea, vomiting, diarrhea (including *Clostridium difficile* enterocolitis), gastroenteritis, abdominal pain, glossitis, papillary hypertrophy, staining of the teeth, heartburn, pharyngeal pain, and taste abnormalities.

Eosinophilia, leukopenia, neutropenia, agranulocytosis, hemolytic anemia, and thrombocytopenia have been reported.

Seizures have been reported in approximately 0.4% of patients receiving imipenem. Risk factors include the following:

- History of seizures or head trauma
- High doses
- Renal dysfunction

Imipenem-Cilastatin

Imipenem is a semisynthetic carbapenem β-lactam antibiotic. Cilastatin prevents renal metabolism of imipenem by dehydropeptidases.

Cilastatin competitively inhibits dehydropeptidase—an enzyme present on the brush border of the proximal renal tubule—which hydrolyzes imipenem. Cilastatin has no antibacterial activity.

Meropenem and Doripenem

These agents are similar to imipenem with the following differences:

- Decreased CNS toxicity
- No hydrolysis by dehydropeptidases

Ertapenem

Ertapenem is dosed once daily and does not cover *Pseudomonas*.

30-5. Monobactam

Monobactam antibiotics are cell wall–active antibiotics like the β-lactams, but they do not have a β-lactam ring, thereby decreasing cross-reactivity with penicillins and cephalosporins.

Aztreonam

Aztreonam is the only monobactam antibiotic currently available.

Mechanism of action

Aztreonam inhibits synthesis of bacterial cell walls through binding to penicillin-binding protein 3 of susceptible Gram-negative bacteria, thereby inhibiting peptidoglycan synthesis. This action results in cell wall lyses and cell death.

Spectrum of activity

Aztreonam is active against many aerobic Gram-negative bacteria, but is not active against Gram-positive or anaerobic bacteria. Though some strains of *Pseudomonas* are susceptible, resistance is increasing.

Adverse drug events

- *Hypersensitivity:* Rash, injection site reactions, and eosinophilia
- *GI effects:* Nausea, vomiting, and diarrhea
- *Rare effects:* Hepatotoxicity, neutropenia, and pancytopenia

30-6. Gram-Positive Antibiotics

Linezolid

Linezolid is a synthetic oxazolidine antibiotic (Table 30-5).

Mechanism of action

Linezolid binds to the 23S ribosomal subunit of the 50S RNA subunit that inhibits bacterial translation.

Spectrum of activity

Linezolid is bacteriostatic against enterococci and staphylococci and bactericidal against streptococci. Linezolid is active against *Enterococcus faecium* isolates, including vancomycin-resistant *Enterococci* (VRE), while most *Enterococcus faecalis* isolates are resistant.

Table 30-5. Gram-Positive Antibiotics

Generic name	Trade name	Dosage forms	Dose	Elimination	Notes
Linezolid	Zyvox	IV, po	600 mg q12h	Renal	
Quinupristin-dalfopristin	Synercid	IV	7.5 mg/kg q8h	Hepatic	
Vancomycin	Vancocin	IV, po	15–20 mg/kg q12h IV; 125–250 mg po q6h	Renal	Adjust dose per serum concentrations; only po for *Clostridium difficile*.
Daptomycin	Cubicin	IV	4–6 mg/kg q24h IV	Renal	Monitor creatine phosphokinase weekly.

Adverse drug events

Hematologic effects, including myelosuppression (anemia, leukopenia, pancytopenia, and thrombocytopenia), have been reported. Hematologic effects appear to be reversible on discontinuation of the agent.

Monoamine oxidase (MAO) inhibition may occur. Linezolid is a weak MAO inhibitor and caution should be exercised in patients receiving vasopressors or serotonergic agents (SSRI [selective serotonin reuptake inhibitor], TCA [tricyclic antidepressant], meperidine, and triptans).

Quinupristin-Dalfopristin

Quinupristin-dalfopristin is a semisynthetic streptogramin antibiotic. The combination acts synergistically against Gram-positive bacteria.

Mechanism of action

Quinupristin inhibits late-phase protein synthesis, while dalfopristin inhibits early-phase protein synthesis through binding to the 50S subunit of bacterial RNA.

Spectrum of activity

Quinupristin-dalfopristin is bactericidal against staphylococci and streptococci and bacteriostatic against *Enterococcus faecium,* including VRE. Quinupristin-dalfopristin is not active against *Enterococcus faecalis.*

Adverse drug events

Thrombophlebitis and severe injection site reactions are common, and some sources recommend administration through a central venous catheter only.

Hyperbilirubinemia has been reported in up to 25% of patients receiving the agent.

Arthralgias and myalgias are common, some requiring discontinuation of the agent.

Daptomycin

Daptomycin is a cyclic lipopeptide antibiotic.

Mechanism of action

Daptomycin binds to bacterial cell membranes, causing rapid depolarization, which results in loss of membrane potential. The loss of membrane potential inhibits protein, DNA (deoxyribonucleic acid), and RNA synthesis, resulting in cell death.

Spectrum of activity

Daptomycin is bactericidal against Gram-positive bacteria including staphylococci, streptococci, enterococcus, and *Corynebacterium.* Daptomycin is active against MRSA, as well as enterococci that are resistant to vancomycin, linezolid, or quinupristin-dalfopristin.

Adverse drug events

Dermatologic reactions include injection site reaction, rash, and pruritis. Musculoskeletal effects include increased CPK (creatine phosphokinase), which can progress to rhabdomyolysis (weekly monitoring recommended). Nephrotoxicity and hepatotoxicity have been reported.

Other

Daptomycin is inactivated by the surfactant in the lung and cannot be used to treat pneumonia.

Daptomycin interacts with some PT (prothrombin time) and INR (international normalized ratio) assays, resulting in a false elevation.

Vancomycin

Vancomycin is a glycopeptide antibiotic.

Mechanism of action

Vancomycin binds to the bacterial cell wall, inhibiting peptidoglycan synthesis. This binding occurs at a site different from that of the penicillins. Vancomycin may also inhibit RNA synthesis.

Spectrum of activity

Vancomycin is active against most Gram-positive bacteria, such as staphylococci (including MRSA), streptococci, enterococci, *Corynebacterium,* and *Clostridium* (including *Clostridium difficile*). It is bactericidal against all susceptible isolates except enterococci (bacteriostatic). Vancomycin acts synergistically with aminoglycosides against enterococci.

Adverse drug events

Nephrotoxicity is manifested by an increase in serum creatinine and BUN. The incidence of nephrotoxicity is not well described, but it appears to be low in the absence of concomitant nephrotoxic agents. Renal dysfunction is normally reversible on discontinuation of the agent but may be irreversible.

Ototoxicity is induced by eighth cranial nerve damage and has been reported to cause permanent hearing loss. Vancomycin rarely causes vestibular toxicity. The incidence of ototoxicity appears to be low in the absence of concomitant ototoxic agents.

Thrombophlebitis is common and requires frequent IV site rotation.

Histamine release, or "red-man syndrome," is a reaction most commonly associated with rapid IV infusion. Histamine reactions can be minimized by slow IV infusion, not to exceed 500 mg/30 min.

Monitoring parameters

Vancomycin trough concentrations should be monitored in patients with preexisting renal dysfunction or patients with increased serum creatinine or BUN during therapy. Monitoring of vancomycin peak concentrations is not routinely required, except in patients with serious infections, those with CNS infections, or those not responding to therapy.

Pharmacokinetics

Vancomycin is renally eliminated:

- $t_{1/2}$ = 6 hours (normal renal function)
- $t_{1/2}$ = 7–10 days (anephric patients)
- V_d = 0.7 L/kg (total body weight [TBW])
- Dose = 15–20 mg/kg (TBW)
- Interval = q12h to pulse dosing (based on renal function and pharmacokinetic monitoring)
- Peak concentration = 20–40 mcg/mL
- Trough concentration = 10–20 mcg/mL

30-7. Fluoroquinolones

Quinolones are broad-spectrum antibacterial agents (Table 30-6).

Mechanism of Action

Fluoroquinolones are bactericidal agents. The mechanism of action of these agents is not understood entirely, but antimicrobial activity is known to involve

Table 30-6. Fluoroquinolones and Nonfluorinated Quinolones

Generic name	Trade name	Dosage forms	Normal dose	Elimination	Notes
Fluoroquinolones					
Ciprofloxacin	Cipro	IV	400 mg q12h	Renal	Ciprofloxacin has less Gram-positive activity and enhanced antipseudomonal activity versus other fluoroquinolones.
		po	500 mg q12h		
Levofloxacin	Levaquin	IV, po	500 mg q24h	Renal	
Moxifloxacin	Avelox	po	400 mg bid	Hepatic	
Norfloxacin	Noroxin	po	400 mg qd	Hepatic	
Ofloxacin	Floxin	po, IV	100–400 mg/d	Renal	
Gemifloxacin	Factive	po	320 mg qd	Renal or biliary	Decrease dose if creatinine clearance < 40 mL/min.
Nonfluorinated quinolones					
Nalidixic acid	NegGram	po	1 g q6h	Renal	Nalidixic acid has no Gram-positive activity and is effective only in the genitourinary and GI tracts.

inhibition of bacterial DNA topoisomerase and subsequent disruption of bacterial DNA replication.

Spectrum of Activity

Gram-positive activity includes many strains of staphylococci. Streptococcal activity is variable, and streptococcal resistance to quinolones is increasingly common. Newer fluoroquinolones (moxifloxacin and gemifloxacin) generally demonstrate superior Gram-positive coverage versus older agents (ciprofloxacin, ofloxacin, and levofloxacin). Fluoroquinolones have limited enterococcal activity and are inactive against MRSA.

Gram-negative activity is extensive, including *Escherichia coli, Klebsiella, Enterobacter, Citrobacter, Proteus, Salmonella,* and *Shigella,* in addition to *Moraxella catarrhalis* and *Haemophilus influenzae.* Activity against *Pseudomonas aeruginosa* and *Stenotrophomonas maltophilia* varies among individual agents.

Anaerobic coverage is poor.

Atypical coverage varies among individual agents. All fluoroquinolones are highly active against *Legionella.* Newer agents have more reliable coverage of *Mycoplasma pneumoniae* and *Chlamydia pneumoniae.*

Adverse Drug Events

- *GI effects:* Nausea and dyspepsia
- *CNS effects:* Headache, dizziness, and insomnia
- *Cardiovascular effects:* QT prolongation (avoid use in patients with preexisting QT prolongation)
- *Endocrine effects:* Hypoglycemia or hyperglycemia (reason for withdrawal of gatifloxacin from market)
- *Genitourinary effects:* Crystalluria (at high doses with alkaline pH)
- *Other effects:* Tendinitis and photosensitivity
- *Rare effects:* Rash, urticaria, leukopenia, and hepatotoxicity (reason for withdrawal of trovafloxacin)

Drug–Drug Interactions

Ciprofloxacin increases theophylline levels. Concomitant use should be avoided, or theophylline levels should be monitored during treatment. The risk of theophylline toxicity is lower with other fluoroquinolones.

Antacids, sucralfate, and divalent or trivalent cations (calcium, magnesium, and iron) significantly decrease the absorption of fluoroquinolones. These agents should not be administered for at least 2 hours after each dose of a fluoroquinolone.

Fluoroquinolones may enhance the effects of oral anticoagulants. Monitor PT and INR if concomitant therapy cannot be avoided.

Agents that increase the QT interval (cisapride and class IA or III antiarrhythmics) increase the risk of torsades de pointes. Concomitant use of fluoroquinolones with these agents should be avoided.

Drug–Disease Interactions

Dosage adjustments should be made for renally cleared fluoroquinolones when CrCl (creatinine clearance) is < 40 mL/min.

Monitoring Parameters

Serum concentrations are not monitored. The patient should be monitored for clinical response and resolution of infection.

Kinetics

Quinolones display concentration-dependent activity and have a postantibiotic effect against most susceptible organisms.

Fluoroquinolones have a large volume of distribution and achieve high tissue concentrations in the lung, gallbladder, kidney, prostate, and genitourinary tract.

Patient Instructions and Counseling

- Fluoroquinolones should be avoided in children or pregnant or nursing females because of the risk of cartilage erosion in tendons and growing bone tissue.
- Do *not* take antacids; multivitamins; or other calcium, magnesium, or iron supplements for at least 2 hours after each dose.

30-8. Macrolides and Ketolides

Mechanism of Action

Macrolides are bacteriostatic against susceptible organisms (Table 30-7). The agents bind to the 50S RNA subunit, thereby inhibiting RNA synthesis.

Ketolides are similar to the macrolides. Telithromycin is a derivative of 14-membered ring macrolides and is the first ketolide antibiotic.

Table 30-7. Macrolides and Ketolide

Generic name	Trade name	Dosage forms	Normal dose	Elimination	Notes
Macrolides					
Azithromycin	Zithromax	po, IV	250 mg/d	Hepatic	po dose = IV dose
Clarithromycin	Biaxin, Biaxin XL	po	250 mg bid	Renal	XL = qd dosing
Erythromycin	Various	po	250–500 mg q6h	Hepatic	Erythromycin base, ethyl succinate, and stearate
		IV	500–1,000 mg q6h	Hepatic	Erythromycin lactobionate
Ketolides					
Telithromycin	Ketek	po	800 mg/d	Hepatic	Treatment duration: 5 days for bronchitis, 7–10 days for community-acquired pneumonia; hepatotoxicity

Spectrum of Activity

Macrolides, or erythromycins, are active principally against Gram-positive organisms, including penicillin-resistant streptococci. The macrolides are also effective against *Chlamydia, Mycoplasma, Ureaplasma,* spirochetes, and mycobacteria.

Macrolides are the drugs of choice in atypical pneumonia and *Chlamydia* sexually transmitted diseases.

Telithromycin possesses greater in vitro activity against multidrug-resistant Gram-positive organisms and *Haemophilus influenzae* than do the erythromycins.

Adverse Drug Events

- *GI effects:* Erythromycins stimulate GI motility, leading to abdominal pain and cramping, nausea, vomiting, and diarrhea. Clarithromycin appears to be the least stimulating to the GI tract.
- *Local effects:* Erythromycin lactobionate is reported to cause venous irritation and thrombophlebitis. The agent should be diluted in at least 250 mL and infused over 30–60 minutes to decrease the venous irritation.
- *Cardiac effects:* QT interval prolongation and torsades de pointes have been rarely reported with erythromycins. Adequate dilution and slow IV infusion appear to decrease this reaction.
- *Ototoxicity:* Erythromycin has been rarely reported to be ototoxic in doses of 4 g/d or more.
- *Hepatotoxicity:* Telithromycin appears comparable to the macrolides but carries a black box warning for hepatotoxicity.

30-9. Tetracyclines and Glycylcyclines

Mechanism of Action

Tetracyclines and glycylcyclines are bacteriostatic. They inhibit bacterial protein synthesis by reversible binding on the 30S ribosomal subunit and by blocking of the attachment of transfer RNA to an acceptor site on the messenger RNA ribosomal complex (Table 30-8).

Glycylcyclines (tigecycline) share the same mechanism of action as tetracyclines but have a structural modification that increases affinity and binding to the bacterial ribosome and decreases efflux from the cell. These properties give tigecycline in vitro advantages when compared to tetracycline.

Spectrum of Activity

Tetracyclines are used to treat the following infections:

- *Respiratory infections:* Atypical pneumonia (*Mycoplasma pneumoniae, Chlamydia pneumoniae*)
- *Genital infections:* *Chlamydia trachomatis,* granuloma inguinale
- *Systemic infections:* Relapsing fever (*Borrelia recurrentis*) and *Vibrio* (*V. cholerae, V. vulnificus,* and *V. parahaemolyticus*)
- *Other infections:* MRSA and MRSE (minocycline) when vancomycin or other agents are not considered appropriate; *Pasteurella multocida,*

Table 30-8. Tetracyclines and Glycylcyclines

Generic name	Trade name	Dosage forms	Common doses	Primary mode of elimination
Tetracyclines				
Demeclocycline	Declomycin	po	300–1,000 mg/d	Renal
Doxycycline	Vibramycin and others	po	100–200 mg q12h	Renal
Minocycline	Minocin	po, IV	100–200 mg q12h	Hepatic
Tetracycline	Achromycin V, Sumycin, Tetracyn, and others	po, IV, IM	1–2 g/d	Renal
Glycylcyclines				
Tigecycline	Tygacil	IV	100 mg once, then 50mg q12h IV	Hepatic

Mycobacterium marinum, Yersinia pestis, and *Helicobacter pylori* (in combination with bismuth subsalicylate and metronidazole or clarithromycin)

- **Prophylaxis:** Mefloquine-resistant *Plasmodium falciparum* malaria

Doxycycline is used to treat infections caused by the following organisms:

- *Mycobacterium fortuitum* and *Mycobacterium chelonae*
- *Streptococcus pneumoniae*

Pseudomonas and *Proteus* organisms are now resistant to tetracyclines.

Tetracyclines are used in the treatment of *Propionibacterium acnes.*

Patient Instructions and Counseling

Administering the drug with food can minimize GI distress.

Adverse Drug Events

Photosensitivity reactions can occur, but may be less frequent with doxycycline and minocycline.

Tetracyclines and glycylcyclines are generally contraindicated during pregnancy and breast-feeding and in children younger than age 8 because of their association with tooth discoloration and interference with bone growth.

Hepatotoxicity—specifically acute fatty necrosis—may occur in pregnant women and in patients with renal impairment.

Minocycline use can cause the following:

- Vestibular side effects (dizziness, ataxia, nausea, and vertigo)
- Skin and mucous membrane pigmentation
- Lupus-like symptoms

GI intolerance includes diarrhea, nausea, vomiting, and anorexia.

Cross-sensitivity within the tetracycline group is common.

IV tetracyclines may cause phlebitis.

Drug–Drug and Drug–Disease Interactions

Milk, antacids, iron supplements, and probably other substances with calcium, magnesium, aluminum, and iron decrease tetracycline GI absorption considerably and should be ingested at least several hours before or after administration of tetracycline.

Although doxycycline and minocycline absorption may be less affected by these divalent and trivalent cations, avoiding administration within 1 to 2 hours after ingestion of interfering foods is recommended.

Anticonvulsants (e.g., barbiturates, carbamazepine, and phenytoin) induce hepatic microsomal metabolism of tetracyclines and therefore decrease tetracycline serum concentrations.

If tetracycline is given with cholestyramine or colestipol, these drugs may bind tetracycline and reduce GI absorption.

Oral contraceptive efficacy may be decreased with concurrent use of tetracyclines.

Tetracyclines and glycylcyclines may potentiate warfarin-induced anticoagulation; therefore, monitor PT and INR.

Table 30-9. Sulfonamides

Generic name	Trade name	Dosage forms	Dose	Elimination	Notes
Sulfadiazine		IV, po	2–4 g/d	Renal	
Sulfamethoxazole	Septra	IV, po	1–3 g/d	Hepatic	Combined with trimethoprim (Septra)
Sulfisoxazole	Gantrisin	IV, po	2–8 g/d	Renal	

Demeclocycline antagonizes the action of antidiuretic hormones.

30-10. Sulfonamides

Sulfonamides are synthetic derivatives of sulfanil-amide (Table 30-9). Their usefulness has decreased over time because of the development of resistance.

Mechanism of Action

Sulfonamides interfere with bacterial folic acid synthesis by competitively inhibiting para aminobenzoic acid (PABA) utilization. Sulfonamides are bacteriostatic.

Spectrum of Activity

- *Gram-positive bacteria:* Staphylococci (methicillin-sensitive *Staphylococcus aureus* [MSSA] and MRSA), streptococci (not enterococci), *Bacillus anthracis, Clostridium perfringens,* and *Nocardia*
- *Gram-negative bacteria:* Enterobacter, Escherichia coli, Klebsiella, Proteus, Salmonella,* and *Shigella*
- *Other organisms:* Chlamydia trachomatis, Toxoplasma gondii,* and *Plasmodium*

Adverse Drug Events

Hypersensitivity reactions appear to be cross-reactive with other sulfonamides, diuretics (including acetazol-amide and thiazides), and sulfonylurea antidiabetic agents.

Dermatologic reactions include rash, urticaria, and Stevens–Johnson syndrome.

30-11. Miscellaneous Antibiotics

Clindamycin

Clindamycin is a semisynthetic antibiotic derived from lincomycin (Table 30-10).

Mechanism of action

Clindamycin inhibits the 50S subunit, thereby inhibiting RNA synthesis. Clindamycin is either bacteriostatic or bactericidal, depending on the serum concentration of the agent and the minimum inhibitory concentration (MIC) of the organism.

Spectrum of activity

Clindamycin is active against most aerobic Gram-positive and most anaerobic Gram-negative bacteria. It has no activity against aerobic Gram-negative bacteria.

Adverse drug events

Adverse GI effects occur frequently with all forms of clindamycin, and include nausea, vomiting, diarrhea, abdominal pain, and tenesmus. Clindamycin has induced *Clostridium difficile* enterocolitis.

IV administration can lead to thrombophlebitis, erythema, and pain and swelling at the IV site. IM administration can cause pain, induration, and sterile abscesses.

Clindamycin can cause transient leukopenia, neutropenia, eosinophilia, thrombocytopenia, and agranulocytosis. These effects are usually reversible on discontinuation of the drug.

Other Miscellaneous Antibiotics

See Table 30-10 for information about other miscellaneous antibiotics.

30-12. Antifungal Agents

Amphotericin B

Amphotericin B is a polyene antifungal agent used in the treatment of potentially life-threatening systemic fungal infections (Table 30-11).

Table 30-10. Miscellaneous Antibiotics

Generic name	Trade name	Dosage forms	Dose	Elimination	Notes
Clindamycin	Cleocin	IV, po	300 mg q6h po; 600–900 mg q8h IV	Hepatic	
Carbapenems					
Imipenem-cilastatin	Primaxin	IV, IM	250 mg q6h; 500 mg or 1 g q6h or q8h, depending on whether the organism is fully or moderately susceptible	Renal	
Doripenem	Doribax	IV	500mg q8h	Renal	
Meropenem	Merrem	IV	500–2,000 mg q8h	Renal	
Ertapenem	Invanz	IV, IM	1,000 mg q24h	Renal	
Monobactams					
Aztreonam	Azactam	IV, IM	1–2 g q6h to q12h, depending on the severity of infection	Renal	Not for *Pseudomonas*

Table 30-11. Antifungal Agents

Generic name	Trade name	Dosage forms	Dose	Elimination	Notes
Amphotericin B	Fungizone	IV	0.5–1 mg/kg/d	Unknown	Dose should not exceed 1.5 mg/kg/d.
Amphotericin B (Liposomal, lipid, and cholesterol complex)	Ambisome, Abelcet, Amphotec	IV	3–7 mg/kg/d	Unknown	Drug is 20–30% less nephrotoxic than conventional amphotericin B.
Caspofungin	Cancidas	IV	70 mg once and then 50 mg/d	Hepatic	Dose adjustment is needed for patients with hepatic dysfunction.
Micafungin	Mycamine	IV	100 mg/d	Hepatic	
Anidulafungin	Eraxis	IV	200 mg once and then 100 mg/d	Chemical degradation	
Fluconazole	Diflucan	IV, po	100–800 mg/d	Renal	
Flucytosine	Ancobon	po	50–150 mg/kg/d	Renal	
Griseofulvin	Fulvicin P/G	po	500 mg	Hepatic	
Itraconazole	Sporanox	po	200–600 mg/d	Hepatic	Capsules require acid environment for dissolution and absorption.
Ketoconazole	Nizoral	po, topical	200–400 mg bid	Hepatic	Drug requires acidic environment for dissolution and absorption.
Nystatin	Mycostatin	Topical		Fecal	
Terbinafine	Lamisal	po	250 mg/d	Hepatic	Pulse therapy is also effective.
Voriconazole	Vfend	IV, po	200 mg q12h po; 4–6 mg/kg q12h IV	Renal	
Posaconazole	Noxafil	po	200 mg qid initially and then 400mg bid	Hepatic	Dose limits absorption.

Amphotericin B lipid formulations

Amphotericin B cholesterol sulfate complex (Amphotec), amphotericin B lipid complex (Abelcet), and amphotericin B liposomal (AmBisome) formulations are available for the treatment of severe fungal infections in patients who fail or are intolerant of conventional amphotericin B. The lipid formulations may decrease toxicity by 20–30%.

Mechanism of action

Amphotericin B binds to ergosterol in the fungal cell wall, leading to increased permeability and cell death. Amphotericin B is fungistatic.

Spectrum of activity

- *Aspergillus, Coccidioides, Cryptococcus, Histoplasma,* and *Mucor*
- *Candida,* including C. *albicans,* C. *dubliniensis,* C. *glabrata,* C. *krusei,* C. *parapsilosis,* and C. *tropicalis* (C *lusitaniae* exhibits variable sensitivity)

Adverse drug events

- *Infusion reactions:* Fever, chills, hypotension, rigors, pain, thrombophlebitis, and anaphylaxis can occur.
- *Renal and electrolyte effects:* Nephrotoxicity is the major dose-limiting toxicity, but Hypokalemia, hypocalcemia, and hypomagnesemia can occur. Effects are usually reversible on discontinuation of the agent. Renal tubular acidosis and nephrocalcinosis are possible.
- *Hematologic effects:* Normocytic and normochromic anemia secondary to decreased erythropoietin production may occur.
- *Hepatic effects:* Increased aspartate aminotransferase (AST), alanine aminotransferase (ALT), alkaline phosphatase, and bilirubin are possible.

Echinocandins

Echinocandins (caspofungin, micafungin, and anidulafungin) are a new class of IV antifungal agents.

Mechanism of action

Echinocandins inhibit β-(1,3) glucan synthase, thereby preventing fungi from forming an essential component of their cell wall. This loss of cell wall integrity results in cell lysis and death.

Spectrum of activity

Echinocandins are active against most *Candida* and *Aspergillus* species, but they lack activity against other invasive molds. *Candida Parapsilosis, C. guilliermondii,* and *C. famata* have increased MICs to echinocandins, which may result in an inadequate response to treatment.

Caspofungin

Caspofungin is approved for the treatment of aspergillosis in patients refractory to or intolerant of other therapies and in the treatment of invasive *Candida* infections. Caspofungin is dose adjusted in severe liver dysfunction.

Micafungin and Anidulafungin

Micafungin and anidulafungin are approved for the treatment of invasive *Candida* infections. Micafungin and anidulafungin do not require dose adjustment for renal or hepatic dysfunction.

Adverse drug events

- *Hepatic effects:* Increased AST and ALT
- *Sensitivity reactions:* Histamine-release reactions such as rash, pruritus, and anaphylaxis
- *Infusion reactions:* Fever, thrombophlebitis, nausea, vomiting, and myalgias

Azole Antifungals

Mechanism of action

The azole antifungals appear to inhibit fungal cytochrome P450 14-β-demethylase, thereby decreasing ergosterol concentrations in susceptible fungi.

Drug interactions

All azole antifungals are inhibitors of the cytochrome P450 system and have many critical drug interactions attributable to decreased metabolism and, thus, toxicity.

The azole antifungals have also been shown to prolong the QT interval; thus, coadministration with other drugs that prolong the QT interval is not advised.

Fluconazole

Fluconazole is a synthetic triazole antifungal and is fungistatic.

Spectrum of activity

Candida krusei, C. glabrata, and *C. lusitaniae* are commonly resistant.

Adverse drug events

- *GI effects:* Nausea, vomiting, abdominal pain, and diarrhea
- *Hepatic effects:* Cholestasis, increased AST, ALT, and GGTP (gamma-glutamyl transpeptidase); hepatic necrosis; and, rarely, severe hepatic dysfunction
- *Hemolytic effects:* Eosinophilia, anemia, leukopenia, neutropenia, and thrombocytopenia
- *Nervous system effects:* Rarely, dizziness, headache, somnolence, coma, and seizures

Itraconazole

Itraconazole is a synthetic triazole antifungal.

Spectrum of activity

Itraconazole is effective in aspergillosis, blastomycosis, histoplasmosis, oropharyngeal and esophageal candidiasis, sporotrichosis, onychomycosis, coccidioidomycosis, and cryptococcosis.

Adverse drug events

- *GI effects:* Nausea, vomiting, diarrhea, abdominal pain, dyspepsia, dysphagia, flatulence, gastritis, and ulcerative stomatitis
- *Dermatologic and sensitivity reactions:* Rash, pruritus, urticaria, angioedema, and Stevens–Johnson syndrome
- *Nervous system effects:* Headache, dizziness, tremor, and neuropathy
- *Cardiovascular effects:* Congestive heart failure, peripheral edema, pulmonary edema, prolonged QT interval, ventricular dysrhythmias, and death
- *Hepatic effects:* Increased AST and ALT
- *Electrolyte and metabolic effects:* Hypokalemia, adrenal insufficiency, and gynecomastia

Ketoconazole

Ketoconazole is a synthetic imidazole antifungal.

Spectrum of activity

The spectrum of activity includes blastomycosis, candidiasis, coccidioidomycosis, histoplasmosis, and dermatophytosis.

Adverse drug events

- *GI effects:* Nausea, vomiting, abdominal pain, and GI bleeding
- *Hepatic effects:* Increased AST, ALT, and alkaline phosphatase
- *Endocrine and metabolic effects:* Gynecomastia and decreased cortisol production
- *Dermatologic and sensitivity reactions:* Pruritus, rash, dermatitis, and purpura
- *Nervous system effects:* Headache, dizziness, lethargy, photophobia, and abnormal dreams

Voriconazole

Voriconazole is a synthetic triazole antifungal.

Spectrum of activity

The spectrum of activity includes aspergillosis and *Candida* species (even fluconazole-resistant isolates).

Adverse drug events

- Hepatic effects such as hepatitis, cholestasis, and fulminant hepatic failure
- Visual disturbances and hallucinations
- Dermatologic and sensitivity reactions, including anaphylactoid reactions, pruritus, rash, Stevens–Johnson syndrome, and photosensitivity

Posaconazole

Posaconazole is a synthetic triazole antifungal.

Spectrum of activity

Posaconazole is approved for use in aspergillus and invasive *Candida* infections. It has a broad in vitro spectrum of activity and has been effective against fungi such as zygomycetes and aspergillus strains that are highly resistant to other azoles and amphotericin.

Adverse drug events

- *GI effects:* Nausea, vomiting, diarrhea, and abdominal pain
- *Dermatologic and sensitivity reactions:* Rash and pruritus
- *Nervous system effects:* Headache, dizziness, and confusion
- *Cardiovascular effects:* Hypertension, hypotension, edema, prolonged QT interval, and ventricular dysrhythmias

- *Hepatic effects:* Cholestasis and increased AST and ALT

Flucytosine

Mechanism of action

Flucytosine appears to enter fungal cells, where it is converted to 5-fluorouracil. Flucytosine is either fungistatic or fungicidal, depending on the concentration of the agent.

Spectrum of activity

Flucytosine is active against most strains of *Candida* and *Cryptococcus.*

Adverse drug events

- *GI effects:* GI hemorrhage, ulcerative colitis caused by the antiproliferative effects, anorexia, abdominal pain, nausea, vomiting, and diarrhea
- *Hepatic effects:* Increased AST, ALT, and bilirubin
- *Renal effects:* Increased serum creatinine, BUN, and crystalluria
- *Nervous system effects:* Confusion, hallucinations, psychosis, headache, parkinsonism, paresthesias, peripheral neuropathy, hearing loss, and vertigo
- *Sensitivity reactions:* Erythema, pruritus, urticaria, rash, and toxic epidermal necrolysis

Griseofulvin

Mechanism of action

Griseofulvin disrupts the fungal cell's mitotic spindle structure, thereby inhibiting the metaphase of cell division. Griseofulvin is fungistatic.

Spectrum of activity

The spectrum of activity includes *Trichophyton, Microsporum,* and *Epidermophyton.*

Adverse drug events

- *Nervous system effects:* Headache, fatigue, dizziness, and paresthesias of the hands and feet after prolonged therapy
- *GI effects:* Epigastric pain, nausea, vomiting, flatulence, and diarrhea
- *Renal effects:* Proteinuria and nephrosis

- *Sensitivity reactions:* Rash, urticaria, erythema multiforme, angioedema, serum sickness, photosensitivity, and lupus-like reactions

Nystatin

Mechanism of action

Nystatin binds to fungal sterols. It is fungistatic.

Spectrum of activity

The spectrum of activity includes cutaneous and mucocutaneous candidiasis.

Adverse drug events

Mild nausea and diarrhea may occur.

Terbinafine

Terbinafine is a synthetic allylamine antifungal.

Mechanism of action

Terbinafine interferes with sterol biosynthesis.

Spectrum of activity

The spectrum of activity includes *Trichophyton, Microsporum, Epidermophyton, Aspergillus,* blastomycosis, and yeasts.

Adverse drug events

- *Hepatic effects:* Hepatitis and hepatic failure
- *Dermatologic and sensitivity reactions:* Anaphylactoid reactions, Stevens–Johnson syndrome, and erythema multiforme

30-13. Antitubercular Agents

Aminosalicylic Acid

Mechanism of action

Aminosalicylic acid (para aminosalicylate, or PAS) inhibits folic acid synthesis in a manner similar to that of sulfonamides and is bacteriostatic (Table 30-12).

Spectrum of activity

Aminosalicylic acid is active against *Mycobacterium tuberculosis* only.

Table 30-12. Antitubercular Agents

Generic name	Trade name	Dosage forms	Normal dose	Elimination	Notes
Aminosalicylic acid	Paser	po	150 mg/kg/d	Renal	Maximum dose: 12 g/d
Capreomycin	Capastat	IM	15 mg/kg/d	Renal	Maximum dose: 1 g/d
Cycloserine	Seromycin	po	15–20 mg/kg/d	Renal	Maximum dose: 1 g/d
Ethambutol	Myambutol	po	15–25 mg/kg/d	Hepatic	
Ethionamide	Trecator-SC	po	500–1,000 mg/d	Hepatic	
Isoniazid	Various	po	5–10 mg/kg/d	Hepatic	Maximum dose: 300 mg/d
Pyrazinamide	Various	po	15–30 mg/kg/d	Hepatic	Maximum dose: 2 g/d
Rifampin	Various	po, IV	10–20 mg/kg/d	Hepatic	Maximum dose: 600 mg/d

Adverse drug events

- *GI effects:* Nausea, vomiting, abdominal pain, diarrhea, and anorexia can occur.
- *Vitamin and mineral absorption:* Vitamin B_{12}, folic acid, and iron malabsorption have been rarely reported.
- *Hypersensitivity reactions:* Fever, skin eruptions, joint pain, and leukopenia have been reported.

Capreomycin

Mechanism of action

The exact mechanism of action of capreomycin is unknown. The agent is bacteriostatic against susceptible isolates.

Spectrum of activity

Capreomycin is active against the following *Mycobacterium* species: *M. tuberculosis, M. bovis, M. kansasii,* and *M. avium.*

Adverse drug events

- *Renal effects:* Nephrotoxicity is exhibited in up to 30% of patients receiving the agent. It manifests as acute tubular necrosis, which is usually reversible on discontinuation of the agent.
- *Ototoxicity:* This problem is experienced by up to 30% of patients and is caused by eighth cranial nerve damage, which can produce irreversible hearing loss.
- *Hepatic effects:* Elevated liver function tests have been noted when capreomycin is used in conjunction with other hepatotoxins.
- *Hypersensitivity reactions:* Fever, urticaria, and skin eruptions have been noted.

Cycloserine

Mechanism of action

Cycloserine is structurally similar to D-alanine and inhibits cell wall synthesis by competing for incorporation into the bacterial cell wall.

Spectrum of activity

Cycloserine is active against the following *Mycobacterium* species: *M. tuberculosis, M. bovis, M. avium,* and some *M. kansasii* isolates.

Adverse drug events

CNS effects may occur, including headache, vertigo, confusion, psychosis, and seizures.

Ethambutol

Mechanism of action

Ethambutol appears to inhibit bacterial cellular metabolism and is bacteriostatic.

Spectrum of activity

Ethambutol is active against the following *Mycobacterium* species: *M. tuberculosis, M. bovis,* and some isolates of *M. kansasii* and *M. avium.*

Adverse drug events

Ocular effects may occur. Optic neuritis with decreased visual acuity, central and peripheral scotomas, and loss of red–green color discrimination have been noted. These effects are usually reversible on discontinuation of the agent.

Ethionamide

Mechanism of action

Ethionamide appears to inhibit cell wall synthesis by an unidentified mechanism. It is bactericidal or bacteriostatic, depending on tissue concentrations of the agent.

Spectrum of activity

Ethionamide is active against the following *Mycobacterium* species: *M. tuberculosis, M. bovis, M. kansasii,* and some *M. avium* isolates.

Adverse drug events

Hepatitis is a rare complication.

Isoniazid

Mechanism of action

Isoniazid (INH) appears to inhibit the bacterial cell wall of susceptible isolates and, therefore, is active against actively dividing cells only. It is bactericidal or bacteriostatic, depending on tissue concentrations of the agent.

Spectrum of activity

INH is active against the following *Mycobacterium* species: *M. tuberculosis, M. bovis,* and some strains of *M. kansasii.*

Adverse drug events

- *CNS effects:* Peripheral neuritis and rarely seizures, encephalopathy, and psychosis have been reported.
- *Hepatic effects:* Increases in bilirubin, AST, and ALT are noted in up to 20% of patients receiving this agent. INH has led to fulminant hepatitis and death.
- *Hematologic effects:* Agranulocytosis, eosinophilia, thrombocytopenia, and hemolytic anemia have been reported.

Pyrazinamide

Mechanism of action

Mycobacterium tuberculosis converts pyrazinamide (PZA) to pyrazinoic acid, which possesses antitubercular activity.

Spectrum of activity

PZA is active against *Mycobacterium tuberculosis* only.

Adverse drug events

- *Hepatic effects:* Increased liver enzymes are common, and fulminant hepatitis has been reported.
- *Gout:* PZA inhibits renal excretion of uric acid and may induce or worsen gout.

Rifampin

Mechanism of action

Rifampin inhibits RNA synthesis in susceptible isolates.

Spectrum of activity

Rifampin is active against the following *Mycobacterium* species: *M. tuberculosis, M. bovis, M. kansasii,* and some *M. avium* isolates. Rifampin also has activity against many Gram-positive and Gram-negative organisms.

Adverse drug events

- *GI effects:* Nausea, vomiting, diarrhea, and abdominal pain may require discontinuation of the agent. *Clostridium difficile* colitis has been reported with rifampin.
- *CNS effects:* Headache, dizziness, mental confusion, and psychosis have been reported.
- *Hepatic effects:* Increased bilirubin, AST, and ALT are common. Fulminant hepatitis has been reported.
- *Hematologic effects:* Thrombocytopenia, leukopenia, and hemolytic anemia have been reported rarely.
- *Renal effects:* Renal insufficiency and interstitial nephritis have been reported.

30-14. Key Points

Aminoglycosides

- Aminoglycoside antibiotics exhibit concentration-dependent bacterial killing.
- Aminoglycoside antibiotics are reserved for severe infections or for use against multidrug-resistant bacteria.

- Aminoglycoside antibiotic dosing should be pharmacokinetically tailored for each patient to optimize the therapeutic effect and minimize toxicity.

Antifungal Agents

- Amphotericin B, caspofungin, micafungin, anidulafungin, fluconazole, itraconazole, posaconazole, and voriconazole are effective against systemic fungal infections.
- Imidazole antifungal antibiotics are potent inhibitors of hepatic metabolism, thereby decreasing the elimination of numerous agents.

Gram-Positive Antibiotics

- Daptomycin, linezolid, and quinupristin-dalfopristin are clinically effective against MRSA, MRSE, and VRE.
- Daptomycin cannot be used to treat pneumonia.
- Vancomycin is a broad-spectrum Gram-positive antibiotic that should be pharmacokinetically tailored for each patient to maximize therapeutic benefit and minimize toxicity.

Miscellaneous Antibiotics

- Clindamycin is an effective anaerobic antibiotic and an effective Gram-positive aerobic antibiotic with activity against many MRSA isolates.
- The carbapenem antibiotics possess a very broad spectrum of activity and should be restricted to appropriate indications to minimize development of resistance.

Penicillins

- Penicillin antibiotics exhibit time-above-MIC-dependent bacterial killing.
- All penicillins, except nafcillin and oxacillin, are renally eliminated and require dosage adjustments in patients with renal dysfunction.

Cephalosporins

- Cephalosporin antibiotics exhibit time-above-MIC-dependent bacterial killing.
- In first-generation cephalosporins, Gram-positive activity is extensive, but Gram-negative activity is limited.
- In second-generation cephalosporins, Gram-positive activity is similar to that of first-

generation agents, but Gram-negative activity is generally more extensive than that of first-generation agents.
- In third-generation cephalosporins, Gram-positive activity is decreased compared to that of first- and second-generation agents, but Gram-negative activity is extensive.

Fluoroquinolones

- Quinolone antibiotics exhibit concentration-dependent bacterial killing similar to that of the aminoglycosides.
- The later-generation quinolones possess improved Gram-positive activity, including resistant streptococci.

Sulfonamides

- Sulfonamides are primarily urinary anti-infectives whose usefulness has decreased because of the development of resistance.

Tetracyclines

- Tetracyclines are drugs of choice for Lyme disease and Rocky Mountain spotted fever.

Macrolides

- Macrolides are primarily active against Gram-positive bacteria, including penicillin-resistant streptococci.
- Macrolides are the drugs of choice in atypical pneumonia.
- Telithromycin possesses greater in vitro activity against multidrug-resistant Gram-positive organisms and *Haemophilus influenzae* than do the macrolides but has a black box warning for hepatotoxicity.

Antitubercular Agents

- Isoniazid, rifampin, and streptomycin exhibit the lowest incidence of resistance.
- Isoniazid, rifampin, and pyrazinamide are the agents of first choice.

30-15. Questions

1. Which of the following are true regarding aminoglycoside antibiotics?

I. Aminoglycoside antibiotics are bactericidal against most susceptible isolates.
II. Aminoglycoside antibiotics exhibit concentration-dependent bacterial killing.
III. Aminoglycoside antibiotics should be reserved for serious infections.

A. I only
B. I and II
C. I and III
D. II and III
E. I, II, and III

2. Which of the following most accurately characterize aminoglycoside toxicity?

I. Ototoxicity because of eighth cranial nerve damage
II. Nephrotoxicity exhibited as acute tubular necrosis
III. Bone marrow suppression

A. I only
B. II only
C. III only
D. I and II
E. II and III

3. Which of the following best characterize aminoglycoside antimicrobial activity?

I. Active against most aerobic Gram-negative bacteria
II. Active against most anaerobic Gram-negative bacteria
III. Active against most fungal isolates

A. I only
B. II only
C. III only
D. I and II
E. II and III

4. Which of the following antifungals are effective against systemic infections?

I. Amphotericin B
II. Fluconazole
III. Nystatin

A. I only
B. II only
C. III only
D. I and II
E. I and III

5. Which of the following are true about amphotericin B–induced nephrotoxicity?

I. Nephrotoxicity is the major dose-limiting toxicity.
II. Nephrotoxicity is usually reversible on discontinuation of the drug.
III. Amphotericin B lipid formulations decrease nephrotoxicity by 20–30%.

A. I only
B. II only
C. I and II
D. II and III
E. I, II, and III

6. Which of the following best describe the drug interactions noted with the imidazole antifungals?

I. Increased elimination of warfarin
II. Decreased elimination of warfarin
III. Increased metabolism of the oral contraceptives

A. I only
B. II only
C. III only
D. II and III
E. I, II, and II

7. Linezolid is best described by which of the following?

I. Linezolid is bacteriostatic against staphylococci.
II. Linezolid is bactericidal against staphylococci.
III. Linezolid is a weak MAO inhibitor.

A. I only
B. II only
C. I and III
D. II and III
E. I, II, and III

8. Linezolid possesses activity against which of the following bacteria?

I. MRSA
II. *Enterococcus faecium*
III. *Enterococcus faecalis*

A. I only
B. II only
C. III only
D. I and II
E. I and III

9. Quinupristin-dalfopristin is best described by which of the following?

   I. Quinupristin-dalfopristin exhibits activity against MSSA.
   II. Quinupristin-dalfopristin exhibits activity against MRSA.
   III. Quinupristin-dalfopristin exhibits activity against streptococci.

   A. I only
   B. II only
   C. III only
   D. I and II
   E. I, II, and III

10. Vancomycin is best described by which of the following?

    I. Vancomycin exhibits activity against MRSA.
    II. Vancomycin exhibits activity against *Enterobacter*.
    III. Vancomycin exhibits activity against *Clostridium difficile*.

    A. I only
    B. II only
    C. III only
    D. I and II
    E. I and III

11. Vancomycin toxicity is best described by which of the following?

    I. Nephrotoxicity exhibited as acute tubular necrosis that is seldom reversible
    II. Ototoxicity that is commonly exhibited as vestibular toxicity
    III. Histamine release, or "red-man syndrome," which is associated with rapid IV infusion

    A. I only
    B. II only
    C. III only
    D. I and II
    E. II and III

12. Which of the following best describe appropriate vancomycin monitoring?

    I. Trough serum concentrations should be routinely monitored in patients with preexisting renal dysfunction.

    II. Peak serum concentrations should be routinely monitored in patients with preexisting renal dysfunction.
    III. Serum concentration monitoring is of no benefit in vancomycin monitoring.

    A. I only
    B. II only
    C. III only
    D. I and II
    E. II and III

13. Clindamycin exhibits antibacterial activity against which of the following microorganisms?

    I. Aerobic Gram-positive bacteria
    II. Anaerobic Gram-negative bacteria
    III. Aerobic Gram-negative bacteria

    A. I only
    B. II only
    C. III only
    D. I and II
    E. I and III

14. Which of the following best describe the carbapenem antibiotics?

    I. Carbapenem antibiotics exhibit activity against most Gram-positive and Gram-negative aerobes and anaerobes.
    II. Meropenem induces seizures more commonly than imipenem.
    III. Cilastatin exhibits activity against most Gram-positive aerobes.

    A. I only
    B. II only
    C. III only
    D. I and II
    E. II and III

15. Which of the following best describe the penicillins?

    I. Penicillins exhibit concentration-dependent bacterial killing.
    II. Penicillins exhibit time-above-MIC-dependent bacterial killing.
    III. Penicillins exhibit excellent MRSA activity.

    A. I only
    B. II only
    C. III only
    D. I and II
    E. II and III

16. Which of the following penicillins require dosage adjustment in patients with renal dysfunction?

    I.   Ampicillin
    II. Nafcillin
    III. Oxacillin

    A. I only
    B. II only
    C. III only
    D. I and II
    E. II and III

17. Which of the following best describe the cephalosporins?

    I.   Cephalosporins exhibit concentration-dependent bacterial killing.
    II. Cephalosporins exhibit time-above-MIC-dependent bacterial killing.
    III. Cephalosporins exhibit excellent MRSA activity.

    A. I only
    B. II only
    C. III only
    D. I and II
    E. II and III

18. Which of the following best describe the antibacterial activity of the cephalosporins?

    I.   In first-generation cephalosporins, Gram-positive activity is extensive, but Gram-negative activity is limited.
    II. In second-generation cephalosporins, Gram-positive activity is similar to that of first-generation agents, but Gram-negative activity is generally more extensive than that of first-generation agents.
    III. In third-generation cephalosporins, Gram-positive activity is decreased compared with that of first- and second-generation agents, but Gram-negative activity is extensive.

    A. I only
    B. II only
    C. III only
    D. All of the above
    E. None of the above

19. Which of the following best describe the antibacterial activity of the quinolones?

    I.   Quinolones exhibit concentration-dependent bacterial killing.
    II. Quinolones exhibit time-above-MIC-dependent bacterial killing.
    III. Quinolones exhibit extensive anaerobic activity.

    A. I only
    B. II only
    C. III only
    D. I and III
    E. II and III

20. Which of the following best describe the important patient counseling points for the quinolones?

    I.   Avoid use in children and pregnant or nursing women because of the risk of cartilage erosion in growing bone tissue.
    II. Do not take within 2 hours of taking antacids, multivitamins, calcium, magnesium, or iron supplements.
    III. Take with a full glass of water and remain sitting or upright for 2 hours to avoid esophageal irritation.

    A. I only
    B. II only
    C. III only
    D. I and II
    E. II and III

21. Which of the following best describe the sulfonamides?

    I.   Drugs that interfere with vitamin B_{12} synthesis by competitively inhibiting PABA utilization
    II. Drugs of choice for *Clostridium difficile* colitis
    III. Primarily urinary anti-infectives whose usefulness has decreased because of the development of resistance

    A. I only
    B. II only
    C. III only
    D. I and II
    E. I, II, and III

22. Which of the following best describe the tetracyclines?

    I.   Tetracyclines exhibit bacteriostatic activity.

II. Tetracyclines are the drugs of choice for Lyme disease.

III. Tetracyclines are contraindicated in children under age 8.

A. I only
B. II only
C. III only
D. I and II
E. I, II, and III

23. Which of the following best describe the macrolides?

I. Primarily effective against Gram-positive aerobic bacteria

II. Effective against penicillin-resistant streptococci

III. Ineffective against penicillin-resistant streptococci

A. I only
B. II only
C. III only
D. I and II
E. I and III

24. Which antitubercular agents exhibit the lowest incidence of resistance?

I. Isoniazid
II. Rifampin
III. Streptomycin

A. I only
B. II only
C. III only
D. I and II
E. I, II, and III

25. Which of the following drug combination regimens are considered the agents of first choice for empiric treatment of TB?

I. Isoniazid, rifampin, and streptomycin
II. Isoniazid, rifampin, and pyrazinamide
III. Isoniazid, ethambutol, and cycloserine

A. I only
B. II only
C. III only
D. All of the above
E. None of the above

30-16. Answers

1. **E.** Aminoglycoside antibiotics are bactericidal against most susceptible isolates, exhibit concentration-dependent bacterial killing, and are usually reserved for serious infections due to toxicity.

2. **D.** Ototoxicity is due to eighth cranial nerve damage and may be irreversible. Nephrotoxicity is exhibited as an acute tubular necrosis that is usually reversible and seldom requires dialysis. Neuromuscular blockade is the third most common toxicity noted with the aminoglycosides.

3. **A.** Aminoglycosides are active against most aerobic Gram-negative and selected aerobic Gram-positive bacteria. They have no activity against anaerobic bacteria or fungi.

4. **D.** Amphotericin B, caspofungin, fluconazole, itraconazole, and voriconazole are effective against systemic fungal infections.

5. **E.** Acute renal dysfunction is the most common dose-limiting amphotericin B toxicity, the renal dysfunction is usually reversible and seldom requires dialysis, and lipid formulations decrease toxicity by 20–30%.

6. **B.** The imidazole antifungals decrease hepatic clearance of numerous hepatically metabolized medications, thereby increasing their activity and risk for toxicity.

7. **C.** Linezolid is bacteriostatic against staphylococci and enterococci. It is bactericidal against *Streptococcus* species only. The agent is a weak MAO inhibitor.

8. **D.** Linezolid is active against MSSA, MRSA, and *Enterococcus faecium* (VRE). *Enterococcus faecalis* isolates are resistant.

9. **E.** Quinupristin-dalfopristin is active against MSSA, MRSA, streptococci, and VRE. *Enterococcus faecalis* isolates are commonly resistant.

10. **E.** Vancomycin is active against aerobic Gram-positive bacteria only; it has no clinically significant Gram-negative activity. Vancomycin is the second-line drug of choice for *Clostridium difficile* colitis.

11. **C.** Vancomycin nephrotoxicity is uncommon and is exhibited as acute tubular necrosis, which is commonly reversible and seldom requires dialysis. Ototoxicity is due to eighth cranial nerve damage, which manifests as high-frequency hearing loss, seldom affecting the vestibular system. The histamine, or "red-man syndrome," reaction is most commonly related to the infusion rate.

12. **A.** Vancomycin serum concentration monitoring is not required in patients responding well to therapy and with normal renal function. Vancomycin trough concentrations should be assessed in patients with preexisting or worsening renal function or those not responding to therapy.

13. **D.** Clindamycin exhibits activity against aerobic Gram-positive bacteria and anaerobic Gram-positive and Gram-negative bacteria. It has no clinically significant aerobic Gram-negative activity.

14. **A.** Carbapenems are active against most aerobic and anaerobic Gram-positive and Gram-negative bacteria. Imipenem is more likely to induce seizures, and cilastatin inhibits the metabolism of imipenem but has no antibacterial activity.

15. **B.** Penicillins exhibit time-dependent bacterial killing and have no activity against MRSA.

16. **A.** All penicillins—with the exception of nafcillin and oxacillin—require dosage adjustment in patients with renal dysfunction.

17. **B.** Cephalosporins exhibit time-dependent bacterial killing and have no activity against MRSA.

18. **D.** First-generation cephalosporins exhibit extensive Gram-positive activity but limited Gram-negative activity. Second-generation cephalosporins maintain Gram-positive activity similar to that of the first-generation agents, but their Gram-negative activity is generally improved. Third-generation cephalosporins exhibit decreased Gram-positive activity, but Gram-negative activity is significantly improved.

19. **A.** Quinolones exhibit concentration-dependent bacterial killing similar to that of the aminoglycosides. They possess good aerobic Gram-positive and Gram-negative activity, but have limited anaerobic activity.

20. **D.** Quinolones have been shown to decrease cartilage formation in beagle pups, but this effect in humans is somewhat controversial. Their use in children should be reserved for serious infections to avoid the risk. Quinolones are bound to divalent cations and should not be coadministered. They do not cause significant esophageal irritation.

21. **C.** Sulfonamides interfere with folic acid metabolism by inhibiting PABA utilization. They have no activity against *C. difficile* colitis and are primarily relegated to urinary anti-infectives because of resistance.

22. **E.** Tetracyclines are bacteriostatic. They are drugs of choice for Lyme disease, and they should not be administered to children under age 8 to avoid permanent tooth staining and potential deposition into bone.

23. **D.** Erythromycins are primarily Gram-positive aerobic antibiotics with good activity against most penicillin-resistant *Streptococcus* isolates.

24. **E.** Isoniazid, rifampin, and streptomycin exhibit the lowest incidence of *Mycobacterium tuberculosis* resistance.

25. **B.** Isoniazid, rifampin, and pyrazinamide are considered agents of first choice for empiric treatment of tuberculosis (TB) because of a low incidence of resistance and acceptable tolerability profile. Ethambutol is commonly added to the regimen in areas of increased resistance.

30-17. References

Alvarez-Elcoro S, Enzler MJ. The macrolides: Erythromycin, clarithromycin, and azithromycin. *Mayo Clin Proc.* 1999;74:613–34.

Cappelletty D, Eiselstein-McKitrick K. The echinocandins. *Pharmacotherapy.* (2007) 27: 369–88.

Cunha BA, ed. *Antibiotic Therapy, Part I.* The Medical Clinics of North America. Philadelphia: WB Saunders; 2000.

Cunha BA, ed. *Antibiotic Therapy, Part II.* The Medical Clinics of North America. Philadelphia: WB Saunders; 2001.

Doribax (doripenem IV injection) [product information]. Raritan, N.J.: Ortho-McNeil; 2009.

Edson RS, Terrell CL. The aminoglycosides. *Mayo Clin Proc.* 1999;74:519–28.

Factive (gemifloxacin mesylate tablets) [product information]. Waltham, Mass.: Oscient Pharmaceuticals; 2004.

Hardman JG, Limbird LE, Molinoff PB, et al., eds. *Goodman and Gilman's The Pharmacological Basis of Therapeutics.* 9th ed. New York: McGraw-Hill; 1996.

Hellinger WC, Brewer NS. Carbapenems and monobactams: Imipenem, meropenem, and aztreonam. *Mayo Clin Proc.* 1999;74:420–34.

Kasten MJ. Clindamycin, metronidazole, and chloramphenicol. *Mayo Clin Proc.* 1999;74: 825–34.

Kucers A, Bennett NM, eds. *Use of Antibiotics: A Comprehensive Review with Clinical Emphasis.* 4th ed. Philadelphia: Lippincott Williams & Wilkins; 1998.

Lentino JR, Narita M, Yu VL. New antimicrobial agents as therapy for resistant Gram-positive cocci. *Eur J Clin Microbiol Infect Dis.* 2008;27: 3–15.

Mandell GL, Bennett JE, Dolin R, eds. *Principles and Practice of Infectious Diseases.* 5th ed. Philadelphia: Churchill Livingstone; 2000.

Marshall WF, Blair JE. The cephalosporins. *Mayo Clin Proc.* 1999;74:187–95.

Noxafil (posaconazole) [prescribing information]. Kenilworth, N.J.: Schering; 2006.

Patel R. Antifungal agents: Part I—Amphotericin B preparations and flucytosine. *Mayo Clin Proc.* 1998;73:1205–25.

Pfaller MA, Boyken L, Hollis RJ, et al. In vitro susceptibility of invasive isolates of *Candida* spp. to anidulafungin, caspofungin, and micafungin: Six years of global surveillance. *J Clin Microbiol.* 2008; 46(1): 150–56.

Reese RE, Betts RF, eds. *A Practical Approach to Infectious Diseases.* 4th ed. Boston: Little, Brown; 1996.

Shain CS. Telithromycin: The first of the ketolides. *Ann Pharmacother.* 2002;36:452–64.

Smilack JD. The tetracyclines. *Mayo Clin Proc.* 1999;74:727–30.

Smilack, JD. Trimethoprim-sulfamethoxazole. *Mayo Clin Proc.* 1999;74:730–34.

Terrell CL. Antifungal agents: Part II—The azoles. *Mayo Clin Proc.* 1999;74:78–100.

Tygacil (tigecycline IV injection) [prescribing information]. Philadelphia: Wyeth Pharmaceuticals; 2009.

Van Scoy RE, Wilkowske CJ. Antimycobacterial therapy. *Mayo Clin Proc.* 1999;74:1038–48.

Walker RC. The fluoroquinolones. *Mayo Clin Proc.* 1999;74:1030–37.

Wilhelm MP. Vancomycin. *Mayo Clin Proc.* 1999; 74: 928–35.

Wright AJ. The penicillins. *Mayo Clin Proc.* 1999;74: 290–308.

Human Immunodeficiency Virus and the Acquired Immune Deficiency Syndrome

31

Camille W. Thornton, PharmD

31-1. Overview

Human immunodeficiency virus (HIV) is a retrovirus that depletes the helper T-lymphocytes (CD4 cells), resulting in continued destruction of the immune system and subsequent gradual development of opportunistic infections and malignancies.

Acquired immune deficiency syndrome (AIDS) is HIV with a CD4 count lower than 200 cells/mm^3 or a history of opportunistic infection (e.g., unexplained fever for more than 2 weeks, thrush, *Pneumocystis jiroveci* pneumonia, toxoplasmosis, cryptococcal meningitis, histoplasmosis, *Mycobacterium avium*).

Epidemiology

At the end of 2007, global estimates of children and adults with HIV/AIDS were as follows:

- People living with HIV/AIDS: 33 million
- New HIV infections in 2007: 2.7 million
- Deaths attributable to HIV/AIDS in 2007: 2 million
- Cumulative number of deaths attributable to HIV/AIDS: 33 million

Complete current world epidemiology can be found at www.unaids.org.

At the end of 2006, estimates of children and adults with HIV/AIDS in the United States were as follows:

- People living with HIV/AIDS: 850,000–950,000
- New HIV infections in 2006: 56,300
- Deaths attributable to HIV/AIDS in 2006: 19,454
- Cumulative number of deaths attributable to HIV/AIDS: 549,594
- People who do not know they are infected with HIV: 180,000–280,000

Complete current U.S. epidemiology can be found at www.cdc.gov/hiv/topics/surveillance/resources/slides/epidemiology/index.htm.

HIV has two common subtypes:

- HIV-1: most commonly found in the United States
- HIV-2: most commonly found in Africa

Clinical Presentation

- Patient has an opportunistic infection.
- Patient is not ill but has tested positive for HIV.
- Patient has acute retroviral syndrome:
  - 50% to 90% of patients acutely infected with HIV experience some of the symptoms.
  - Symptoms generally appear 2–4 weeks after virus exposure.
  - Duration of the clinical syndrome is about 14 days (the range is a few days to > 10 weeks).
  - The disease is not readily recognized in the primary care setting because its symptoms are similar to those of the flu, mononucleosis, and other common illnesses.

Testing Recommendations

The U.S. Centers for Disease Control and Prevention recommend the following HIV testing in health care settings:

- Routine, voluntary, opt-out HIV screening for all persons 13–64 years of age in health care settings. Testing is not based on risk factors.
- HIV screening of pregnant women as part of the routine panel of prenatal screening tests. Testing is not based on risk factors.

- Repeat HIV screening of persons with known risk at least annually:
  - Injection drug users and their sex partners
  - Persons who exchange sex for money or drugs
  - Sex partners of HIV-infected persons
  - Men who have sex with men
  - Heterosexual persons who themselves or whose sex partners have had more than one sex partner since their most recent HIV test

Pathophysiology

HIV is a retrovirus that replicates in and destroys CD4 cells. The result is a chronically deteriorating immune system leading to opportunistic infections and eventual death. Seroconversion typically occurs about 3 weeks after the acute infection (the range is from 2 weeks to 6 months). Antibodies generally appear within 3 months of infection (the range is from 2 weeks to 6 months).

Transmission is through infected blood or hazardous body fluids, which can occur during the following activities:

- Unprotected sexual contact with an infected person
  - Multiple partners increase risk.
  - Ongoing or past medical history of sexually transmitted disease increases risk.
- Sharing needles or syringes with an infected person
- Transfusions of infected blood or blood clotting factors (the United States began screening the blood supply in 1985)
- Vertical transmission (infected mother to infant)
- Breast-feeding

Occupational exposure and household contact are rare.

Diagnostic Criteria

Enzyme-linked immunosorbent assay

Enzyme-linked immunosorbent assay (ELISA) is the initial screening test for detection of anti-HIV antibodies. False-positive results can occur in patients with

- Collagen vascular diseases
- Chronic hepatitis
- Other chronic diseases

Western blot

All positive ELISA tests must be confirmed by a Western blot. Specificity and sensitivity of the Western blot is > 99%. The Western blot tests for anti-HIV antibodies.

Other tests

Other diagnostic tests are available. All should be confirmed by a Western blot.

Rapid diagnostic tests can give results from a finger stick or swab of oral fluid in 5–20 minutes.

Monitoring Tools

Viral load

Viral load testing measures the amount of virus in blood. It can assess disease progression and evaluate efficacy of antiretroviral therapy. Its lower limit of detection is less than 50 copies/mL for ultrasensitive assays (less than 400 copies/mL for nonultrasensitive assays). A minimally significant change in viral load is considered to be a threefold or $0.5_{\log 10}$ increase or decrease.

Acute illness and immunizations can cause increases in viral load for 2–4 weeks. Testing should not be performed during this time.

Baseline viral loads are established by averaging two viral loads (that do not differ by > $0.5_{\log 10}$) taken 2–4 weeks apart.

Monitoring of viral load in patients not on antiretroviral therapy should occur every 3–4 months. Monitoring of viral load in patients starting a new regimen should occur 2–8 weeks after treatment initiation and then every 3–4 months.

CD4 cell count

CD4 cell count indicates the extent of immune system damage and the risk of developing opportunistic infections. Normal CD4$^+$ cell counts are 800–1,200 cell/mm^3.

CD4$^+$ cell counts should be measured every 3–4 months in patients on or off antiretroviral therapy. A 30% increase or decrease in CD4$^+$ cells from baseline is considered significant.

Treatment Principles and Goals

Goals of therapy

Therapy has the following goals:

- Maximal and durable suppression of viral load
- Restoration or preservation of immunologic function

- Improvement in quality of life
- Reduction of HIV-related morbidity and mortality

Factors involved in achieving goals of therapy are as follows:

- Adherence to the antiretroviral regimen
- Rational sequencing of drugs
- Preservation of future treatment options
- Use of resistance testing in selected clinical settings

See Table 31-1 for indications for the initiation of antiretroviral therapy in the chronically HIV-1 infected patient.

Guidelines for prevention and treatment and medications used for the treatment of HIV can be located as a living document at www.aidsinfo.nih.gov, which is updated three or four times a year.

Indications for Consideration of Changing Antiretroviral Therapy

Consider changing antiretroviral therapy (ART) with failure to suppress plasma HIV RNA (ribonucleic acid) to undetectable levels (< 50 copies/mL) within 4–6 months of initiating a therapy.

Consider changing ART if virus is detected in plasma repeatedly following initial suppression to undetectable levels.

Table 31-1. Indications for the Initiation of Antiretroviral Therapy in the Chronically HIV-1 Infected Patient

Clinical category	Recommendation
History of AIDS-defining illness	Antiretroviral therapy should be initiated.
CD4 count < 200 cells/mm^3	
CD4 count 200–350 cells/mm^3	
Pregnant women	
Persons with HIV-associated nephropathy	
Persons co-infected with hepatitis B virus (HBV), when HBV treatment is indicated	
Patients with CD4 count > 350 cells/mm^3 who do not meet any of the specific conditions listed above	The optimal time to initiate therapy in asymptomatic patients with CD4 cell counts > 350 cells/mm^3 is not well defined. Patient scenarios and comorbidities should be taken into consideration.

Consider genotyping or phenotyping to assist in identifying drugs for the next regimen if

- Adherent to failing regimen for at least the previous 4–6 weeks or within 4 weeks after regimen discontinuation
- Viral load above 1,000 copies/mL

Consider changing ART if CD4$^+$ T cell numbers persistently decline, as measured on at least two separate occasions.

Consider changing ART if patient evidences clinical deterioration.

Never change just one medication in a failing regimen (i.e., use at least two new drugs, and preferably an entirely new regimen).

Change one medication in a successful regimen if a patient is experiencing intolerable side effects or if the medication has overlapping toxicity with other medications.

Use the treatment history and past and current resistance test results to identify active agents (preferably two or more) to design a new regimen.

31-2. Drug Therapy

See Table 31-2 for antiretroviral agents recommended by the U.S. Department of Health and Human Services for initial treatment of established HIV infection.

Nucleoside Reverse Transcriptase Inhibitors

Nucleoside reverse transcriptase inhibitors (NRTIs) are described in Table 31-3. The mechanism of action of NRTIs is to interfere with HIV viral RNA-dependent DNA (deoxyribonucleic acid) polymerase, resulting in chain termination and inhibition of viral replication.

Didanosine, stavudine, and lamivudine are dosed on the basis of weight. Most NRTIs are not affected by food (except didanosine). NRTIs have a low pill burden as a class and few drug interactions. All are prodrugs requiring two or three phosphorylations for activation.

Four combination products are available:

- Combivir (zidovudine 300 mg + lamivudine 150 mg) every 12 hours
- Trizivir (zidovudine 300 mg + lamivudine 150 mg + abacavir 300 mg) every 12 hours
- Truvada (tenofovir 300 mg + emtricitabine 200 mg) every 24 hours
- Epzicom (lamivudine 300 mg + abacavir 600 mg) every 24 hours

Table 31-2. Antiretroviral Regimens for Treatment of HIV Infection in Antiretroviral-Naive Patients

Type of regimen	NNRTI-PI treatment	NRTI combinations
Preferred	■ Efavirenz[a] ■ Atazanavir[b]-ritonavir once daily ■ Darunavir-ritonavir once daily ■ Fosamprenavir-ritonavir twice daily ■ Lopinavir-ritonavir (coformulated) once or twice daily	■ Tenofovir + emtricitabine (coformulated)
Alternative	■ Nevirapine[c] ■ Atazanavir[b] (unboosted) once daily ■ Fosamprenavir (unboosted) twice daily ■ Fosamprenavir-ritonavir once daily ■ Saquinavir-ritonavir twice daily	■ Abacavir[d]-lamivudine (coformulated) ■ Didanosine + lamivudine or emtricitabine ■ Zidovudine-lamivudine (coformulated)

Note: Combine one PI or one NNRTI with two NRTIs to complete a highly active regimen from the table.
a. Efavirenz is not recommended for use in first-trimester pregnancy or in women with a high pregnancy potential.
b. Atazanavir must be boosted with ritonavir if used with tenofovir.
c. Use caution in women with CD4 cell counts > 250 cells/mm^3 and men with CD4 cell counts > 400 cells/mm^3 because of increased risk of nevirapine-associated toxicity.
d. Only use abacavir in patients who have tested negative for HLA-B*5701.

No special storage requirements are necessary for drugs in this class.

Usually, two NRTIs are used in combination with one non-nucleoside reverse transcriptase inhibitor (NNRTI) or one protease inhibitor (PI).

Monitor for signs and symptoms of the following class toxicities:

■ Lactic acidosis
■ Severe hepatomegaly with steatosis

The following precautions should be kept in mind regarding NRTIs:

■ Most patients should be dose-adjusted for renal impairment (exception: abacavir).
■ Lamivudine and emtricitabine are chemically similar and should not be used in the same regimen.
■ Do not use zidovudine with stavudine because of antagonism (both require thymidine for activation).
■ Do not use didanosine with stavudine during pregnancy because of increased risk of lactic acidosis and liver damage.
■ Tenofovir increases didanosine levels and decreases atazanavir levels. Dosage adjustments are required.
■ Patients should be tested for HLA-B*5701 to determine risk for hypersensitivity reaction to abacavir. Only negative patients should start abacavir.

■ The "D" drugs (ddI [didanosine] and d4T [stavudine]) can cause pancreatitis and peripheral neuropathy; when used together, this effect can be additive.
■ The "D" drugs are more closely associated with lactic acidosis.

Non-nucleoside Reverse Transcriptase Inhibitors

NNRTIs are described in Table 31-4. Their mechanism of action is to competitively inhibit reverse transcriptase, thereby resulting in inhibition of HIV replication.

One-step mutation (K103N) confers resistance to all NNRTIs but etravirine. All should be dose-adjusted for hepatic impairment.

Most are not affected by food (except efavirenz). Efavirenz is contraindicated in pregnancy.

Usually, one NNRTI should be used in combination with two NRTIs.

No special storage requirements are necessary for drugs in this class. Class toxicities include rash and hepatic toxicity.

Drug interactions can occur (see Tables 31-5 and 31-6). All are cytochrome P450 (CYP450)-3A4 inducers or inhibitors.

Table 31-3. Nucleoside Reverse Transcriptase Inhibitors

	Zidovudine (AZT, ZDV)	Lamivudine (3TC)	Abacavir (ABC)	Didanosine (ddl)	Stavudine (d4T)	Tenofovir (TDF)	Emtricitabine (FTC)
Trade name	Retrovir	Epivir	Ziagen	Videx EC, Videx	Zerit	Viread	Emtriva
Form	100 mg caps; 300 mg tabs; also available in combination products[a]; available as generic	150, 300 mg tabs; 10 mg/mL oral solution; also available in combination products[a]	300 mg tabs; 20 mg/mL oral solution; also available in combination products[a]	Videx EC caps: 125, 200, 250, 400 mg; Videx buffered tabs: 25, 50, 100, 150, 200 mg; Videx buffered powders: 100, 167, 250 mg; available as generic: didanosine DR	15, 20, 30, 40 mg caps	300 mg tabs; also available in combination products[b]	200 mg tabs; also available in combination products[b]
Dosing recommendations	300 mg twice daily; 200 mg every 8 hours	150 mg twice daily; 300 mg daily (pediatric dosage based on weight)	300 mg twice daily; 600 mg daily	> 60 kg: 400 mg daily; with tenofovir DF ↓ddl to 250 mg; < 60 kg: 250 mg daily; with tenofovir DF: appropriate ddl dose not known	> 60 kg: 40 mg twice daily; < 60 kg: 30 mg twice daily	300 mg once daily	200 mg once daily
Food effect	Take without regard to meals	Take without regard to meals	Take without regard to meals	Take 0.5 hour before or 2.0 hours after meals	Take without regard to meals	Take without regard to meals	Take without regard to meals
Adverse events	Bone marrow suppression (macrocytic anemia or neutropenia); gastrointestinal intolerance, headache, insomnia, asthenia	Minimal toxicity	Hypersensitivity reaction testing for HLA-B*5701 should be done before start to evaluate patients risk for hypersensitivity; only negative patients should start abacavir. Hypersensitivity symptoms include rash, fever, nausea and vomiting, malaise or fatigue, loss of appetite; respiratory symptoms include sore throat, cough, shortness of breath	Pancreatitis, peripheral neuropathy, nausea, diarrhea	Pancreatitis; peripheral neuropathy; lipodystrophy, hyperlipidemia; rapidly progressive ascending neusomuscular weakness (rare)	Renal insufficiency, asthenia, headache, diarrhea, nausea, or vomiting	Minimal toxicity; hyperpigmentation of palms of hands and soles of feet (rare)

(continued)

Table 31-3. Nucleoside Reverse Transcriptase Inhibitors (*Continued*)

	Zidovudine (AZT, ZDV)	Lamivudine (3TC)	Abacavir (ABC)	Didanosine (ddI)	Stavudine (d4T)	Tenofovir (TDF)	Emtricitabine (FTC)
Drug interactions	Ribavirin, stavudine, methadone; with high dose: ganciclovir, TMP-SMX, other medications that can cause bone marrow suppression	No clinically significant drug interactions	Alcohol increases abacavir levels by 41%.	Methadone, ribavirin, tenofovir, ganciclovir, alcohol; medications that need acidic environment for absorption—buffered forms; use caution with other medications that can cause peripheral neuropathy.	Use with caution with other medications that can cause peripheral neuropathy	Didanosine, atazanavir, cidofovir, ganciclovir, valganciclovir	No clinically significant drug interactions
Monitoring[c]	Complete blood count, liver function tests	None necessary	Signs and symptoms of hypersensitivity reaction	Complete blood count, liver function tests, amylase, uric acid; signs and symptoms of above side effects	Signs and symptoms of above side effects	Renal function	None necessary

a. Combivir: zidovudine 300 mg + lamivudine 150 mg; 1 tablet twice daily. Trizivir: zidovudine 300 mg + lamivudine 150 mg + abacavir 300 mg; 1 tablet twice daily. Epzicom: abacavir 600 mg + lamivudine 300 mg; 1 tablet daily.

b. Truvada: tenofovir 300 mg + emtricitabine 200 mg; 1 tablet daily. Atripla: tenofovir 300 mg + emtricitabine 200 mg + efavirenz 600 mg; 1 tablet at or before bedtime.

c. Monitor all for signs and symptoms of NRTI class toxicities, lactic acidosis, and hepatic steatosis; incidence is higher with stavudine than with other NRTIs.

Table 31-4. Non-nucleoside Reverse Transcriptase Inhibitors

	Efavirenz (EFV)	Nevirapine (NVP)	Etravirine[a] (ETR)	Delavirdine (DLV)
Trade name	Sustiva	Viramune	Intelence	Rescriptor
Form	50, 100, 200 mg caps; 600 mg tabs; also available in combination product[b]	200 mg tab; 10 mg/mL oral suspension	100 mg tabs	100, 200 mg tabs
Dosing recommendations	600 mg at or before bedtime	200 mg daily × 14 days, then 200 mg twice (note CD4 cell count)[c]	200 mg twice daily as tablets or dissolved in water to form a slurry to drink	400 mg every 8 hours as tablets or dissolved in water to form a slurry to drink
Food effect	Take on an empty stomach	Take without regard to meals	Take following a meal	Take without regard to meals
Adverse events	Central nervous system (CNS) side effects,[d] rash,[e] ↑ liver function tests (LFTs), false-positive cannabinoid test, teratogenic in monkeys	Rash,[f] symptomatic hepatitis, including fatal hepatic necrosis	Rash,[e] nausea	Rash,[e] ↑ LFTs, headaches
Drug interactions	CYP450-3A4, CYP450-2C19 inhibitor; CYP450-3A4 inducer (see Tables 31-5 and 31-6)	CYP450-3A4 inducer (see Tables 31-5 and 31-6)	CYP450-3A4, CYP450-2C9, CYP450-2C19 substrate; CYP450-3A4 inducer; CYP450-2C9, CYP450-2C19 inhibitor (see Tables 31-5 and 31-6)	CYP450-3A4, CYP450-2D6 inhibitor (see Tables 31-5 and 31-6); separate dosing with buffered didanosine or antacids by 1 hour
Monitoring[f]	CNS side effects, LFTs, rash	LFTs 2, 4, and 6 weeks, and then monthly for the first 18 weeks	LFTs, rash, nausea	LFTs, rash

a. Etravirine effective in patients with resistance (K103N) to other NNRTIs.
b. Atripla: tenofovir 300 mg + emtricitabine 200 mg + efavarenz 600 mg; one tablet at or before bedtime.
c. Because of the increased risk of symptomatic hepatic events, nevirapine should not be started in women with baseline CD4 cell counts of greater than 250 cells/mm³ or men with baseline CD4 cell counts greater than 400 cells/mm³; it is not recommended in patients with moderate-to-severe hepatic impairment (Child–Pugh B or C).
d. CNS side effects include dizziness, somnolence, insomnia, abnormal dreams, confusion, abnormal thinking, impaired concentration, amnesia, agitation, depersonalization, hallucinations, and euphoria. Use caution in patients with a psychiatric history or previous addictions.
e. Rare cases of Stevens–Johnson syndrome have been reported with the use of NNRTIs; the highest incidence is seen with nevirapine use.
f. Monitor all for signs and symptoms of NNRTI class toxicities, rash, and hepatic toxicity.

Table 31-5. Drugs That Should Not Be Used with NNRTIs

Drug category	Efavirenz	Nevirapine	Etravirine	Delavirdine
Calcium channel blockers	None	None	None	None
Cardiac	None	None	None	None
Lipid-lowering agents	None	None	None	Simvastatin, lovastatin
Antimycobacterials	Rifapentine	Rifapentine	Rifampin, rifapentine	Rifampin, rifapentine, rifabutin
Antihistamines	Astemizole, terfenadine	None	None	Astemizole, terfenadine
Gastrointestinal drugs	Cisapride	None	None	Cisapride, histamine-2 blockers, proton pump inhibitors
Psychotropics	Midazolam, triazolam	None	None	Alprazolam, midazolam, triazolam
Ergot alkaloids (vasoconstrictor)	Ergotamine derivatives	None	None	Ergotamine derivatives
Herbs	St. John's wort	St. John's wort	St. John's wort	St. John's wort
Other	Voriconazole at standard doses	Ketoconazole	Unboosted protease inhibitors, ritonavir-boosted atazanavir, fosamprenavir or tipranavir, other NNRTIs, carbamazepine, phenobarbital, phenytoin	Fosamprenavir, carbamazepine, phenobarbital, phenytoin

Table 31-6. Drug Interactions with NNRTIs Requiring Dose Modifications or Cautious Use

Drug class	Drug
Antiarrhythmics (etravirine only)	Quinidine (delavirdine only)
Antifungals	Itraconazole, ketoconazole, posaconazole, voriconazole
Anticoagulants	Warfarin
Anticonvulsants	Carbamazepine, phenobarbital, phenytoin
Antimicrobials	Clarithromycin, rifabutin, rifampin
Benzodiazepines	Alprazolam, diazepam, midazolam, triazolam
Erectile dysfunction agents	Various
Hormonal contraceptives	Various
HMG-CoA reductase inhibitors	Atorvastatin, lovastatin, simvastatin, pravastatin, rosuvastatin
Narcotic analgesics	Methadone

Protease Inhibitors

Protease inhibitors (PIs) are described in Table 31-7.

Their mechanism of action is to inhibit protease, which then prevents the cleavage of HIV polyproteins and subsequently induces the formation of immature noninfectious viral particles.

All should be dose-adjusted for hepatic impairment. Most should be taken with food (except fosamprenavir, tipranavir, lopinavir-ritonavir tablets, and indinavir). Atazanavir and indinavir require normal acid levels in the stomach for absorption.

Ritonavir is the most potent inhibitor in the class and is primarily used for intensification of other PIs. Ritonavir and tipranavir should be refrigerated.

Goals of intensification are as follows:

- Decrease pill burden
- Decrease frequency of doses (i.e., decrease from q8h to q12h)
- Increase drug levels, resulting in decreased resistance

Table 31-7. Protease Inhibitors

	Lopinavir + ritonavir (LPV/r)	Nelfinavir (NFV)	Atazanavir (ATV)	Fosamprenavir (FPV)	Saquinavir (SQV); SQV-hard gel capsule (HGC)	Darunavir (DRV)	Tipranavir (TPV)	Ritonavir (RTV)	Indinavir (IDV)
Trade name	Kaletra	Viracept	Reyataz	Lexiva	Invirase	Prezista	Aptivus	Norvir	Crixivan
Form	200 mg lopinavir + 100 mg ritonavir tabs; 400 mg lopinavir + 100 mg ritonavir per 5 mL oral solution	250, 625 mg tabs; 50 mg/g oral powder	100, 150, 200, 300 mg caps	700 mg tabs, 50 mg/mL oral suspension	200 mg caps, 500 mg tabs	300, 400, 600 mg tabs	250 mg caps	100 mg caps; 80 mg/mL oral solution	200, 333, 400 mg caps
Dosing recommendations	400 mg lopinavir + 100 mg ritonavir twice daily; 800 mg lopinavir + 200 mg ritonavir once daily (once daily only in treatment-naive patients)	1,250 mg twice daily; 750 mg every 8 hours	ATV 300 mg + RTV 100 mg once daily or 400 mg once daily (unboosted only for PI-naive patients)	ART-naive patients: FPV 1,400 mg twice daily; or FPV 1,400 mg + RTV 100–200 mg once daily; or FPV 700 mg + RTV 100 mg twice daily. PI-experienced patients: FPV 700 mg + RTV 100 mg twice daily	SQV 1,000 mg + RTV 100 mg twice daily	ART-naive patients: DRV 800 mg + RTV 100 mg once daily. ART-experienced patients: DRV 600 mg + RTV 100 mg twice daily	TPV 500 mg + RTV 200 mg twice daily	RTV 100–400 mg 1 or 2 times daily with other PIs for boosting; RTV 600 mg twice daily as single PI	IDV 800 mg every 8 hours or IDV 800 mg + 100–200 mg RTV every 12 hours

(continued)

Table 31-7. Protease Inhibitors (*Continued*)

	Lopinavir + ritonavir (LPV/r)	Nelfinavir (NFV)	Atazanavir (ATV)	Fosamprenavir (FPV)	Saquinavir (SQV); SQV-hard gel capsule (HGC)	Darunavir (DRV)	Tipranavir (TPV)	Ritonavir (RTV)	Indinavir (IDV)
Food effect	Tablet: no food effect Liquid: take with food	Take with food	Take with food	Take with or without food	Take within 2 hours of a meal	Take with food	Take with or without food	Take with food	Unboosted, take 1 hour before or 2 hours after meals; may take with skim milk or low-fat meal; when boosting can take with or without food
Adverse events[a]	GI intolerance, asthenia, ↑LFTs	Diarrhea, ↑LFTs	Increased indirect hyperbilirubinemia, prolonged PR interval (some patients experienced asymptomatic first-degree atrioventricular block); use with caution in patients with underlying conduction defects or on concomitant medications that can cause PR prolongation, nephrolithiasis	Skin rash, GI intolerance, headache, ↑LFTs	GI intolerance, headache, ↑LFTs	Rash, hepatotoxicity, GI intolerance, headache, ↑LFTs	Hepatotoxicity, skin rash, intracranial hemorrhage (rare); patients with risk factors for intracranial hemorrhages are at highest risk	GI intolerance, paresthesias, hepatitis, pancreatitis, asthenia, taste perversion	Nephrolithiasis, GI intolerance, ↑bilirubinemia, headache, asthenia, blurred vision, dizziness, rash, metallic taste, thrombocytopenia, alopecia, hemolytic anemia

Drug interactions	CYP450-3A4 inhibitor and substrate (see Tables 31-10 and 31-11)	CYP450-3A4 inhibitor and substrate (see Tables 31-10 and 31-11)	CYP450-3A4 inhibitor and substrate (see tables 31-9 and 31-10)	CYP450-3A4 inhibitor, inducer, and substrate (see Tables 31-10 and 31-11)	CYP450-3A4 inhibitor and substrate (see Tables 31-10 and 31-11)	CYP 450-3A4 inhibitor and substrate	CYP450 3A4 inducer and substrate; net effect when combined with RTV; CYP-3A4 and CYP-2D6 inhibitor	CYP450 3A4 and 2D6 inhibitor; CYP450 3A4 substrate (CYP-3A4 greater than CYP-2D6)	CYP450 3A4 inhibitor
Storage	Tablets: room temperature; Refrigerated liquid stable until date on label; stable for 2 months at room temperature	Room temperature	Room temperature	Room temperature	Room temperature	Room temperature	Refrigerated capsules stable until date on label; stable for 60 days at room temperature	Refrigerated capsules stable until date on label; stable for 1 month at room temperature	Room temperature
Additional information	Oral solution contains 42% alcohol	Needs 500 kcal of food for absorption; take after eating; boosting with RTV not effective	Reduced incidence of hyperlipidemia; must use boosted regimen with tenofovir or efavirenz; needs normal GI acid concentrations for absorption; drug interactions with proton pump inhibitors, histamine-2 blockers, and antacids	Sulfonamide, caution in patients with history of sulfa allergy	Unboosted SQV not recommended	DRV has a sulfonamide moiety; use with caution in patients with known sulfonamide allergy. Unboosted DRV not recommended.	Clinical hepatitis including hepatic decompensation has been reported; monitor closely, especially in patients with underlying liver diseases. TPV has a sulfonamide moiety; use with caution in patients with known sulfonamide allergy.	Primary role is for boosting of other PIs; most potent CYP450 inhibitor in the class; when used as a single PI, dose should be titrated to above target dose	Patients should drink ≥ 48 oz of water daily to reduce incidence of kidney stones; boosted indinavir increases incidence of kidney stones and requires additional monitoring for signs and symptoms of kidney stones, indirect bilirubin, and platelets

a. PI class side effects: fat maldistribution, hyperglycemia, hyperlipidemia, hypertriglyceridemia, possible increased bleeding episodes in hemophiliacs.

Class toxicities are as follows:

- Fat maldistribution
- Hyperglycemia
- Hyperlipidemia
- Hypertriglyceridemia
- Possible increased bleeding episodes in patients with hemophilia

Baseline PI monitoring is done 4–6 weeks after starting the PI. Monitoring should then take place every 3–6 months thereafter. The following tests are required:

- Glucose test
- Liver function tests (LFTs)
- Total cholesterol panel (particularly triglycerides)
- Signs and symptoms of gastrointestinal (GI) side effects
- Signs and symptoms of fat redistribution

Usually, one PI (boosted PIs preferred) is used in combination with two NRTIs.

All are CYP450-3A4 inhibitors, and drug interactions are typical of CYP450-3A4 inhibitors. See Tables 31-8 and 31-9 for more information about drug interactions.

Entry inhibitors

Entry inhibitors include enfuvirtide (T20) and maraviroc. Enfuvirtide is a fusion inhibitor, whereas maraviroc is a CCR5 (chemokine [C-C motif] receptor 5) antagonist. See Table 31-10 for information.

Enfuvirtide (T20) (Fuzeon)

Enfuvirtide's mechanism of action is to bind to glycoprotein 41 on the HIV surface, thus inhibiting HIV binding to the CD4 cell.

The dose is 90 mg subcutaneous every 12 hours. Side effects include injection-site reactions, an increased rate of bacterial pneumonia, and hypersensitivity.

Enfuvirtide is generally reserved for deep salvage regimens. Preferably, it should be used with at least two other active drugs. Resistance develops quickly with less potent regimens and in cases of poor adherence.

No known significant drug interactions have been seen to date. Enfuvirtide can be taken without regard to meals. It should be stored at room temperature; the reconstituted form should be stored in the refrigerator, where it will be stable for 24 hours.

Maraviroc (Selzentry)

Maraviroc's mechanism of action is to bind to CCR5 receptors on the CD4 cell surface, which inhibits HIV binding and entry into the CD4 cell.

Perform Trofile testing before using maraviroc to determine patient's tropism. The patient must be CCR5 tropic only.

Maraviroc is a CYP450-3A4 substrate. The dose depends on drug reactions:

- Use 150 mg po every 12 hours when giving maraviroc with strong CYP3A4 inhibitors (most PIs).
- Use 300 mg po every 12 hours when giving maraviroc with enfuvirtide, tipranavir-ritonavir, nevirapine, or weak CYP3A4 inhibitors.
- Use 600 mg po every 12 hours when giving with CYP3A4 inducers (efavirenz, rifampin, etc.).

Side effects include abdominal pain, cough, dizziness, musculoskeletal symptoms, pyrexia, rash, upper respiratory tract infections, hepatotoxicity, and orthostatic hypotension.

Preferably, use maraviroc with at least two other active drugs. Take it without regard to meals.

Integrase inhibitors

Integrase inhibitors include raltegravir, which is marketed under the trade name Isentress (Table 31-10). Its mechanism of action is to block activity of the integrase enzyme, thereby preventing HIV DNA from meshing with the CD4 cell DNA. Metabolism is through UDP-glucuronosyltransferase 1A1 (UGT1A1) mediated glucuronidation

Drug interactions occur with rifampin and other drugs that effect UGT1A1. The dose is 400 mg po every 12 hours. Side effects include nausea, headache, diarrhea, pyrexia, creatinine phosphokinase (CPK) elevation. Preferably, raltegravir should be used with at least two other active drugs. Take it without regard to meals.

Potential Benefits of Early Therapy

- Maintenance of a higher CD4 count and prevention of potentially irreversible damage to the immune system
- Decreased risk for HIV-associated complications that can sometimes occur at CD4 counts greater than 350 cells/mm^3, including tuberculosis, non-Hodgkin's lymphoma, Kaposi's sarcoma, peripheral neuropathy, human papillomavirus–

Table 31-8. Drugs That Should Not Be Used with PIs

Drug category	Indinavir	Ritonavir	Saquinavir-ritonavir	Darunavir-ritonavir	Tipranavir-ritonavir	Nelfinavir	Fosamprenavir	Lopinavir-ritonavir	Atazanavir
Calcium channel blockers	None	Bepridil	None	None	Bepridil	None	Bepridil	None	Bepridil
Cardiac	Amiodarone	Amiodarone, flecainide, propafenone, quinidine	None	None	Amiodarone, flecainide, propafenone, quinidine	None	None	Flecainide, propafenone	None
Lipid-lowering agents	Simvastatin, lovastatin	Simvastatin, lovastatin	Simvastatin, lovastatin	Simvastatin, lovastatin	Simvastatin, lovastatin	Simvastatin, lovastatin	Simvastatin, lovastatin	Simvastatin, lovastatin	Simvastatin, lovastatin
Antimycobacterials	Rifampin, rifapentine	Rifapentine	Rifampin, rifapentine	Rifampin, rifapentine	Rifampin, rifapentine	Rifampin, rifapentine	Rifampin, rifapentine	Rifampin, rifapentine	Rifampin, rifapentine
Antihistamines	Astemizole, terfenadine	Astemizole, terfenadine	Astemizole, terfenadine	Astemizole, terfenadine	Astemizole, terfenadine	Astemizole, terfenadine	Astemizole, terfenadine	Astemizole, terfenadine	Astemizole, terfenadine
GI drugs	Cisapride	Cisapride	Cisapride	Cisapride	Cisapride	Cisapride	Cisapride	Cisapride	Cisapride
Neuroleptics	Pimozide	Pimozide	Pimozide	Pimozide	Pimozide	Pimozide	Pimozide	Pimozide	Pimozide
Psychotropics	Midazolam, triazolam	Midazolam, triazolam	Midazolam, triazolam	Midazolam, triazolam	Midazolam, triazolam	Midazolam, triazolam	Midazolam, triazolam	Midazolam, triazolam	Midazolam, triazolam
Ergot alkaloids (vasoconstrictor)	Ergot derivatives	Ergot derivatives	Ergot derivatives	Ergot derivatives	Ergot derivatives	Ergot derivatives	Ergot derivatives	Ergot derivatives	Ergot derivatives
Herbs	St. John's wort	St. John's wort	St. John's wort, garlic supplements	St. John's wort	St. John's wort	St. John's wort	St. John's wort	St. John's wort	St. John's wort
Other	Atazanavir	Voriconazole (with RTV ≥ 400 mg bid), fluticasone, alfuzosin	Fluticasone	Carbamazepine, phenobarbital, phenytoin, fluticasone	Fluticasone	Proton pump inhibitors	Delavirdine, fluticasone, oral contraceptives	Fluticasone	Fluticasone, indinavir, irinotecan, proton pump inhibitors (not recommended for unboosted ATV)

Table 31-9. Drug Interactions with PIs Requiring Dose Modifications or Cautious Use

Drug class	Drug
Antacids (ATV, TPV-RTV)	Various
Antiarrhythmics	Quinidine
Antifungals	Itraconazole, ketoconazole, posaconazole, voriconazole
Anticoagulant	Warfarin
Anticonvulsants	Carbamazepine, phenobarbital, phenytoin
Antidepressants	Desipramine (RTV), trazodone (RTV)
Antimicrobials	Clarithromycin, rifabutin
Benzodiazepines	Alprazolam, diazepam
Calcium channel blockers	Dihydropyridines, diltiazem
Corticosteroids	Dexamethasone (SQV)
Erectile dysfunction agents	Various
Histamine-2 receptor antagonists (ATV-RTV, ATV, FPV)	Various
Hormonal contraceptives	Various
HMG-CoA reductase inhibitors	Atorvastatin, pravastatin (DRV/RTV), rosuvastatin
Narcotic analgesics	Methadone
Proton pump inhibitors (ATV-RTV, SQV-RTV, TPV-RTV)	Various
Selective serotonin reuptake inhibitors	Paroxetine (DRV/RTV), sertraline (DRV/RTV)
Xanthine derivatives	Theophylline (RTV)
Other	Grapefruit juice (IDV, SQV), vitamin C > 1 gram daily (IDV)

associated malignancies, and HIV-associated cognitive impairment
- Decreased risk of nonopportunistic conditions, including cardiovascular disease, renal disease, liver disease, and malignancies and infections that are not associated with AIDS
- Decreased risk of HIV transmission to others, which will have positive public health implications

Potential Risks of Early Therapy

- Development of treatment-related side effects and toxicities
- Development of drug resistance because of incomplete viral suppression, resulting in loss of future treatment options
- Less time for the patient to learn about HIV and its treatment and less time to prepare for the need for adherence to therapy
- Increased total time on medication, with greater chance of treatment fatigue
- Premature use of therapy before the development of more effective, less toxic, or better-studied combinations of antiretroviral drugs
- Transmission of drug-resistant virus in patients who do not maintain full virologic suppression

Counseling

All patients should be counseled on the importance of adherence. Greater than 95% adherence is necessary to decrease the incidence of resistance. Patients should be given tools to facilitate adherence to complicated regimens (e.g., pillboxes, calendars, pagers, etc).

Patients should be counseled on class side effects, especially any that are unique or potentially serious.

Antiretroviral Therapy in the HIV-Infected Pregnant Woman

Highly active antiretroviral therapy (HAART) should be offered if the patient is not already receiving treatment:

- Avoid efavirenz.
- Avoid combining stavudine and didanosine.
- Consider starting treatment after the first trimester.

Continue current combination regimens (preferably with zidovudine) if the patient is already receiving therapy. Doing so decreases the risk of transmission from 30.0% to 2.5%.

Zidovudine alone can decrease risk of transmission when taken during pregnancy. The mother should also receive IV zidovudine during labor. The infant should receive 6 weeks of zidovudine (Table 31-11).

Single-dose nevirapine given at onset of labor in women who have had no prior ART and given once to the infant between 48 and 72 hours of age has been shown to decrease the transmission rate. This treatment can also result in resistance to nevirapine, which negatively affects future treatment options for the mother.

Guidelines for prevention of vertical transmission can be located as a living document at www.aidsinfo.nih.gov, which is updated three or four times a year.

Table 31-10. Integrase and Entry Inhibitors

	Raltegravir (RAL)	Maraviroc (MVC)	Enfuvirtide (T20)
Trade name	Isentress	Selzentry	Fuzeon
Classification	Integrase inhibitor	Entry inhibitor: CCR5 antagonist	Entry inhibitor: fusion inhibitor
Form	400 mg tablets	150, 300 mg tablets	Injectable, in lyophilized powder to be reconstituted with sterile water
Dosing recommendations	RAL 400 mg twice daily	MVC 150 mg po every 12 hours when giving with strong CYP3A4 inhibitors (most PIs) MCV 300 mg po every 12 hours when giving with enfuvirtide, tipranavir-ritonavir, nevirapine, or weak CYP3A4 inhibitors MCV 600 mg po every 12 hours when giving with CYP3A4 inducers (efavirenz, rifampin, etc.)	T20 90 mg/mL injected subcutaneously twice daily; powder should be reconstituted with 1.1 mL sterile water for injection
Food effect	Take with or without food.	Take with or without food.	Take with or without food.
Adverse events	Nausea, headache, diarrhea, pyrexia, CPK elevation	Abdominal pain, cough, dizziness, musculoskeletal symptoms, pyrexia, rash, upper respiratory tract infections, hepatotoxicity, orthostatic hypotension	Local injection site reactions, increased bacterial pneumonia, hypersensitivity reactions
Drug interactions	UGT1A1 mediated glucuronidation. Do not give with rifampin. Dose adjustments may be necessary with other medications metabolized by UGT1A1.	CYP540 3A4 substrate. Do not use with St. John's wort. Dose adjustments needed with itraconazole, ketoconazole, voriconazole, carbamazepine, phenobarbital, phenytoin, clarithromycin, rifabutin, rifampin.	Catabolism
Storage	Room temperature	Room temperature	Room temperature; reconstituted solution should be refrigerated and used within 24 hours
Additional information		Trofile testing should be done before using marivoric to determine patient's tropism—must be CCR5 tropic only.	

Postexposure Prophylaxis

General guidelines

Universal precautions should be taken. The most common infectious exposure is needlesticks or cuts (1 in 300 risk). The risk with mucous membrane exposure is much lower (1 in 1,000 risk).

Postexposure prophylaxis (PEP) can reduce HIV infection by about 80%. Start therapy within 1–2 hours of exposure. The length of therapy is 4 weeks.

Guidelines for PEP can be located as a living document at www.aidsinfo.nih.gov, which is updated three or four times a year. See also Tables 31-12 and 31-13.

Nonoccupational PEP

Patients with exposure to HIV from a known positive source, such as sexual exposure or injection drug use, should receive nonoccupational PEP (nPEP) within 72 hours of the exposure. The length of therapy is 28 days. Figure 31-1 provides an algorithm for evaluation and treatment when nonoccupational exposure occurs. Table 31-14 describes nPEP antiretroviral regimens.

Table 31-11. AIDS Clinical Trials Group 076 Guidelines: Dosing of Zidovudine for Prevention of Vertical Transmission

Period	Guideline
Prepartum	Initiation at 14–34 weeks gestation and continued throughout pregnancy
	Preferred regimen: zidovudine 100 mg 5 times daily
	Acceptable alternative regimens:
	■ AZT 200 mg 3 times daily
	■ AZT 300 mg 2 times daily
Intrapartum	During labor, AZT 2 mg/kg IV over 1 hour, followed by a continuous infusion of 1 mg/kg/h IV until delivery
Postpartum	Oral administration of AZT to the newborn: AZT syrup 2 mg/kg every 6 hours for the first 6 weeks of life, beginning 8–12 hours after birth

Opportunistic Infections

Only two opportunistic infections require primary prophylaxis:

■ *Pneumocystis jiroveci pneumonia (PCP):* Treatment is required when CD4+ cells fall below 200/mm^3. The treatment of choice is trimethoprim-sulfamethoxazole (TMP-SMX) DS po qd (see Table 31-15 for alternatives).

■ *Mycobacterium avium complex bacteremia (MAC):* Treatment is required when CD4+ cells fall below 50/mm^3. Azithromycin 1,200 mg po every week is the treatment of choice.

All other primary prophylaxis occurs only if the patient is antigen-positive or at high risk of exposure to the causative factor. All other opportunistic infections are treated when the patient is diagnosed. After treatment, patients receive suppressive therapy.

Some primary and secondary prophylaxis could possibly be discontinued with immune reconstitution (undetectable viral load and an increase in CD4 cells in response to ART; see Table 31-15).

Immune reconstitution inflammatory syndrome in response to existing or indolent opportunistic infections can sometimes occur when ART is started.

Guidelines for prophylaxis and treatment of opportunistic infections can be located as a living document at www.aidsinfo.nih.gov.

31-3. Prevention Guidelines

■ Abstain from sex with an infected person.
■ Ask about the sexual history of current and future sex partners.
■ Reduce the number of sex partners to minimize the risk of HIV infection.
■ Always use a latex condom from start to finish during any type of sex (vaginal, anal, or oral).
■ Use only water-based lubricants.
■ Avoid alcohol, illicit drugs, and sharing of needles (or syringes, cookers, or other drug paraphernalia).
■ Do not share personal items such as toothbrushes, razors, or any devices used during sex. Such items may be contaminated by blood, semen, or vaginal secretions.
■ Do not donate blood, plasma, sperm, body organs, or tissues if you are infected with HIV or have engaged in sex or needle-sharing behaviors that are risk factors for infection with HIV.

31-4. Hematologic Complications

Anemia can occur in HIV-infected patients. Causes include the following:

■ HIV infection of marrow progenitor cells
■ Drug-induced marrow suppression (zidovudine, ganciclovir, amphotericin, ribavirin, pyrimethamine, interferon, TMP-SMX)

Treatment of anemia is described in Figure 31-2.

31-5. Key Points

■ HIV is a virus that destroys the immune system.
■ AIDS is caused by HIV and is defined as a CD4+ cell count less than 200/mm^3 or the presence of an opportunistic infection.
■ Acute retroviral syndrome occurs in 50–90% of patients within the first 2–4 weeks of infection with HIV.
■ The viral load indicates the amount of virus in the body and is an indication of how well antiretroviral medications are working.
■ The CD4+ cell count refers to the status of the immune system and how much a patient is at risk for developing an opportunistic infection.
■ NRTIs, NNRTIs, PIs, entry inhibitors (fusion inhibitors, CCR5 antagonists), and integrase inhibitors are the currently available classes of medications used to treat HIV.

Table 31-12. Recommended HIV PEP Treatment Options

Exposure type	HIV-positive, class 1[a]	HIV positive, class 2[b]	Source of unknown HIV status	Unknown source	HIV negative
Recommended HIV PEP for percutaneous injuries					
Less severe (example: solid needle or superficial injury)	Basic 2-drug PEP is recommended.	Expanded ≥ 3 drug PEP is recommended.	Generally, no PEP is warranted; however, consider basic 2-drug PEP for source with HIV risk factors.	Generally, no PEP is warranted; however, consider basic 2-drug PEP in settings where exposure to HIV-infected persons is likely.	No PEP is warranted.
More severe (example: large-bore hollow needle, deep puncture, visible blood on device, or needle used in patient's artery or vein)	Expanded 3-drug PEP is recommended.	Expanded ≥ 3-drug PEP is recommended.	Generally, no PEP is warranted; however, consider basic 2-drug PEP for source with HIV risk factors.	Generally, no PEP is warranted; however, consider basic 2-drug PEP in settings where exposure to HIV-infected persons is likely.	No PEP is warranted.
Recommended HIV PEP for mucous membrane exposures and nonintact skin exposures					
Small volume (example: a few drops)	Basic 2-drug PEP should be considered.	Basic 2-drug PEP is recommended.	Generally no PEP is warranted.	Generally no PEP is warranted.	No PEP is warranted.
Large volume (example: major blood splash)	Basic 2-drug PEP is recommended.	Expanded ≥ 3-drug PEP is recommended.	Generally, no PEP is warranted; however, consider basic 2-drug PEP for source with HIV risk factors.	Generally, no PEP is warranted; however, consider basic 2-drug PEP in settings where exposure to HIV-infected persons is likely.	No PEP is warranted.

a. HIV-positive class 1 asymptomatic HIV infection or known low viral load ($< 1,500$ copies/mL).
b. HIV-positive class 2 symptomatic HIV infection, AIDS, acute seroconversion, or known high viral load.

Table 31-13. Regimens for PEP

Type of regimen	Basic 2-drug PEP	Expanded 3-drug PEP
Preferred	▪ Zidovudine + lamivudine or emtricitabine	Basic regimen *plus:*
	▪ Tenofovir + lamivudine or emtricitabine	▪ Lopinavir-ritonavir
Alternative	▪ Stavudine + lamivudine or emtricitabine	Basic regimen *plus:*
	▪ Didanosine + lamivudine or emtricitabine	▪ Atazanavir +/− ritonavir
		▪ Fosamprenavir +/− ritonavir
		▪ Indinavir +/− ritonavir
		▪ Saquinavir-ritonavir
		▪ Nelfinavir
		▪ Efavirenz

Figure 31-1. Algorithm for Evaluation and Treatment of Nonoccupational Exposure

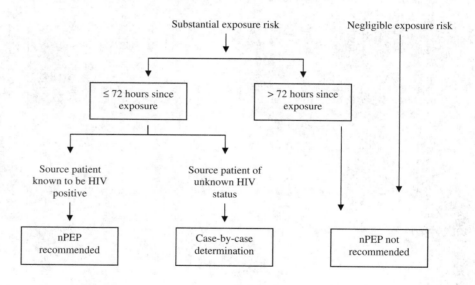

Substantial risk for HIV exposure

Exposure of
vagina, rectum, eye, mouth, other mucous membrane, nonintact skin, or percutaneous contact

With
blood, semen, vaginal secretions, rectal secretions, breast milk, or any body fluid that is visibly contaminated with blood

When
the source is known to be HIV infected.

Negligible risk for HIV exposure

Exposure of
vagina, rectum, eye, mouth, other mucous membrane, intact or nonintact skin, or percutaneous contact

With
urine, nasal secretions, saliva, sweat, or tears if not visibly contaminated with blood

Regardless
of the known or suspected HIV status of the source.

Table 31-14. nPEP Antiretroviral Regimens

Type of regimen	Substantial exposure risk	Negligible exposure risk
Preferred	■ Zidovudine + lamivudine or emtricitabine	■ Lopinavir-ritonavir
	■ Tenofovir + lamivudine or emtricitabine	■ Efavirenz
Alternative	■ Stavudine + lamivudine or emtricitabine	■ Atazanavir +/– ritonavir
	■ Didanosine + lamivudine or emtricitabine	■ Fosamprenavir +/– ritonavir
	■ Abacavir + lamivudine or emtricitabine	■ Indinavir +/– ritonavir
		■ Saquinavir-ritonavir
		■ Nelfinavir
Triple NRTI (only when other regimens cannot be used)	■ Abacavir + lamivudine + zidovudine	

Table 31-15. Opportunistic Infections

Pathogen	Indication	First choice	Alternative regimens	Comments
Pneumocystis jiroveci pneumonia	Prophylaxis: CD4+ < 200/mm³; thrush; unexplained fever ≥ 2 weeks; history of PCP	TMP-SMX	Dapsone, atovaquone, or aerosolized pentamidine	Primary and secondary prophylaxis can be stopped for PCP on immune reconstitution (patients on HAART with CD4+ greater than 200/mm³ for > 3 months).
Pneumocystis jiroveci pneumonia	Acute infection	TMP 15–20 mg/kg/d + SMX 75–100 mg/kg/d po or IV × 21 d in 3–4 divided doses	Pentamidine IV, primaquine + clindamycin, dapsone + TMP, or atovaquone	Patients with PO₂ < 70 mm Hg or A-a gradient > 35 mm Hg should receive a corticosteroid taper; treatment is for 21 days.
Candida	Treatment	Fluconazole, clotrimazole troches, nystatin suspension, itraconazole, posaconazole, amphotericin B, anidulafungin, caspofungin, micafungin, or voriconazole	Any of the preferred regimens	*Thrush:* treat for 10–14 days; CD4+. *Esophagitis:* treat for 2–3 weeks. Chronic use of azoles might promote development of resistance.
Cryptococcal meningitis	Induction therapy (for at least 2 weeks)	Amphotericin B or lipid formulation amphotericin + flucytosine	Amphotericin B + fluconazole, amphotericin B alone, or fluconazole	Condition is spread through inhalation of soil contaminated with bird droppings. It is very important to manage increased intracranial pressures.
Cryptococcal meningitis	Consolidation therapy (for at least 8 weeks)	Fluconazole	Itraconazole	
Cryptococcal meningitis	Maintenance therapy	Fluconazole	Itraconazole	Maintenance therapy is lifelong or until CD4+ ≥ 200/mm³ for > 6 months as a result of ART.

(continued)

Table 31-15. Opportunistic Infections (*Continued*)

Pathogen	Indication	First choice	Alternative regimens	Comments
Toxoplasmosis	Treatment (for at least 6 weeks)	Pyrimethamine + leucovorin + sulfadiazine	Pyrimethamine + leucovorin + clindamycin or atovaquone or azithromycin, TMP-SMX, atovaquone alone, or atovaquone + sulfadiazine	Condition is spread through raw or under-cooked meat (lamb, beef, pork) and by contact with infected cat feces. Dexamethasone may be required if significant cerebral edema is present.
Toxoplasmosis	Chronic maintenance therapy	Pyrimethamine + leucovorin + sulfadiazine	Pyrimethamine + leucovorin + clindamycin or atovaquone	Maintenance therapy is lifelong or until CD4$^+$ ≥ 200/mm^3 for > 6 months as a result of ART and patient is free of signs and symptoms.
Histoplasmosis	Induction therapy (treat for at least 2 weeks)	Liposomal amphotericin B or itraconazole	Amphotericin B, ampho-tericin B lipid complex, or posaconazole	Condition is spread through inhalation of dust particles. Histoplasmosis is found in soils heavily contaminated by avian or bat feces. The Ohio and Mississippi River valleys are endemic areas in the United States.
Histoplasmosis	Maintenance therapy (for at least 12 months)	Itraconazole	Posaconazole	Maintenance therapy can be stopped after 12 months of treatment, CD4$^+$ ≥ 150/mm^3, ART for > 6 months, urine and serum antigen < 4.1 units.
Mycobacterium avium complex	Treatment and mainte-nance therapy	Clarithromycin + ethambutol +/− rifabutin	Azithromycin + ethambutol Alternative third drugs: amikacin, streptomycin, ciprofloxacin, levofloxacin, moxifloxacin	Maintenance therapy may be discontinued after 12 months of treat-ment, CD4 > 100/mm^3 for 6 months on ART after treatment, and patient is asymptomatic.
Mycobacterium avium complex	Primary prophylaxis: generally recommended at CD4 counts < 50/mm^3	Azithromycin or clarithromycin	Rifabutin or azithromycin + rifabutin	It may be possible to dis-continue treatment when CD4 count > 100/mm^3 for > 6 months in patients on ART.
Cytomegalovirus retinitis	Treatment (for 21 days)	Intraocular ganciclovir, valganciclovir, foscarnet, or ganciclovir	Cidofovir	Oral ganciclovir should not be used as sole induction therapy. Optimization of ART is an important part of initial therapy.
Cytomegalovirus retinitis	Maintenance	Valganciclovir or intraocular ganciclovir	Ganciclovir, foscarnet, or cidofovir	Maintenance therapy can be stopped with inactive disease, CD4 > 100–150/mm^3 for 3–6 months in patients on ART.

Figure 31-2. Guidelines for the Treatment of Anemia in the HIV Patient

Goals of therapy:

- Resolution of anemia: Hgb ≥ 12 g/dL or Hct ≥ 36%

- Increased energy, activity, and overall quality of life for patients, prolonged survival

- Reduced need for transfusions

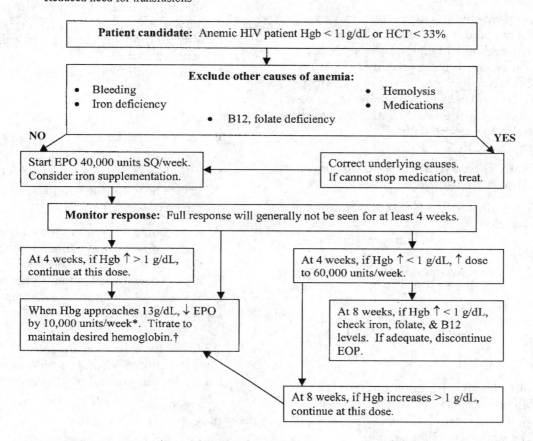

* If Hgb > 15 g/dL at any point, hold EPO and restart when Hgb < 12 g/dL, using dose reduced by
  10,000 units/week.
† During dose adjustment phase, Hgb should be monitored every 2-4 weeks. Allow at least 4 weeks
  to assess response to dose changes.

- Vertical transmission is prevented by treating the mother with HAART (preferred) or zidovudine alone.
- *Pneumocystis jiroveci* pneumonia requires primary prophylaxis at CD4+ cell counts < 200/mm³. TMP-SMX is the preferred treatment.
- *Mycobacterium avium* complex requires primary prophylaxis at CD4+ cell counts < 50/mm³. Azithromycin is the preferred drug.
- All other opportunistic infections require treatment followed by secondary prophylaxis.

31-6. Questions

Use the following case study to answer questions 1–4:

C. T. is a 23-year-old HIV-positive female who presents to the emergency department with shortness of breath and a fever. Physical exam reveals a temperature of 102°F, heart rate of 100 bpm, and decreased breath sounds in the left lower lobe of lungs. Chest x-ray is positive for infiltrates in the left lung. She is diagnosed with PCP. She has no previous history of opportunistic infections and is not on any medications at this time (she has not been seen by a health care provider in over a year). Her CD4$^+$ count is 13 cells/mm^3 and viral load is 170,198 copies/mL.

1. What is the treatment of choice for C. T.'s PCP?

   A. TMP-SMX DS 2 tabs po q8h for 21 days, then 1 tab po daily
   B. Azithromycin 500 mg po on day 1, then 250 mg po daily indefinitely
   C. Doxycycline 100 mg po twice daily for 7 days, then 100 mg po daily
   D. Clarithromycin 500 mg po twice daily for 10 days, then 250 mg po daily
   E. Vancomycin 1 g IV q12h for 10 days, then TMP-SMX DS po daily

2. Should C. T. receive any other prophylaxis against opportunistic infections?

   A. Yes, against MAC: Zithromax 1,200 mg po weekly
   B. Yes, against thrush: Diflucan 100 mg po daily
   C. Yes, against toxoplasmosis: Bactrim DS 1 tab po every Monday, Wednesday, and Friday
   D. Yes, against CMV: Valcyte 450 mg po every Monday, Wednesday, and Friday
   E. No

3. Six weeks later C. T. presents to the HIV clinic for follow-up. Her CD4$^+$ count is 12 cells/mm^3 and viral load is 140,202 copies/mL. Should C. T. be started on HIV therapy?

   A. Yes; her CD4$^+$ cell count is < 200 cells/mm^3 and she has had an opportunistic infection.
   B. Yes; her viral load is greater than 100,000 copies/mL.
   C. Yes; her Western blot was positive for HIV.
   D. Yes; all patients with HIV should be treated as soon as the diagnosis is made.
   E. No.

4. C. T. wishes to be started on HIV therapy. Which of the following would be an appropriate regimen?

   A. Zidovudine + efavirenz + nelfinavir
   B. Zidovudine + stavudine + indinavir
   C. Stavudine + didanosine + fosamprenavir

   D. Tenofovir + emtricitabine + atazanavir-ritonavir
   E. Nelfinavir + indinavir + fosamprenavir

5. HIV can be transmitted by

   A. unprotected sexual contact with an infected person.
   B. sharing needles or syringes with an infected person.
   C. infected mother to infant (vertical transmission).
   D. transfusion of blood (before 1985).
   E. all of the above.

6. M. J. is 13 weeks pregnant and just tested positive for HIV. Her viral load is 22,434 copies/mL and her CD4$^+$ cell count is 425 cells/mm^3. M. J. wishes to receive treatment for her HIV. Which of the following would be an appropriate regimen for M. J.?

   A. Zidovudine + stavudine + indinavir
   B. Zidovudine + lamivudine + lopinavir-ritonavir
   C. Zidovudine + lamivudine + efavirenz
   D. Stavudine + didanosine + nevirapine
   E. No treatment is necessary.

7. Which of the following antiretroviral medications has shown efficacy as monotherapy in decreasing the vertical transmission of HIV?

   A. Efavirenz
   B. Nelfinavir
   C. Zidovudine
   D. Zalcitabine
   E. Stavudine

8. R. C. is a nurse in the emergency department. She has just been stuck with a needle that was used for an HIV-positive patient with a known high viral load. Which of the following is true concerning postexposure prophylaxis?

   I. The regimen should be started within 2 hours of exposure.
   II. R. C. will need to be treated only with zidovudine.
   III. R. C. will need to be treated with a combination of zidovudine + lamivudine + nelfinavir.
   IV. Treatment will continue for 4 weeks.

A. I, III, and IV
B. II only
C. II, III, and IV
D. I and IV
E. I, II, and IV

9. The CD4$^+$ cell count relates to

  I.   the activity of the virus.
  II. the status of the immune system.
  III. how much a patient is at risk for acquiring an opportunistic infection.
  IV. when the patient was infected.
  V.   time to death in treated patients.

  A. IV and V
  B. I, II, and III
  C. II and III
  D. II, III, and IV
  E. I, II, and V

10. The viral load relates to

  A. the activity of the virus and efficacy of antiretroviral therapy.
  B. the status of the immune system.
  C. when the patient was infected.
  D. how much a patient is at risk for acquiring an opportunistic infection.
  E. time to death in a treated patient.

11. S. J. presents to the emergency department with extreme flank pain with nausea and vomiting. He is diagnosed with a kidney stone. His past medical history is positive for HIV and diabetes. His medications include indinavir, lamivudine, didanosine, metformin, and dapsone. Which of his medications might have caused his kidney stone?

  A. Indinavir
  B. Lamivudine
  C. Didanosine
  D. Metformin
  E. Dapsone

12. L. L. comes to the clinic with a chief complaint of burning and tingling in his feet that started about 1 month ago. His current medications include nelfinavir, stavudine, lamivudine, sertraline, and gemfibrozil. Which medication might be causing this problem?

  A. Nelfinavir
  B. Stavudine

  C. Lamivudine
  D. Sertraline
  E. Gemfibrozil

13. S. E. presents to the emergency department with a 2-day history of extreme nausea, vomiting, and abdominal pain. Labs reveal elevations in amylase and lipase, and a diagnosis of pancreatitis is made. His medications include nevirapine, tenofovir, didanosine, and amitriptyline. Which of his medications could have caused his pancreatitis?

  A. Nevirapine
  B. Tenofovir
  C. Didanosine
  D. Amitriptyline
  E. All of the above

14. Which HIV medication should not be used until HLA-B*5701 testing has been performed to assess risk for hypersensitivity?

  A. Efavirenz
  B. Ritonavir
  C. Zidovudine
  D. Abacavir
  E. Lamivudine

15. C. J. is starting efavirenz, tenofovir, lamivudine, and TMP-SMX. What should C. J. be counseled about concerning efavirenz?

  A. Anemia
  B. CNS side effects
  C. Neutropenia
  D. Renal toxicity
  E. Kidney stones

16. Which of the following can cause hepatotoxicity and requires monitoring of liver enzymes at baseline, 2 weeks, 4 weeks, 6 weeks, and then monthly for the first 18 weeks of therapy?

  A. Zidovudine
  B. Zalcitabine
  C. Lopinavir-ritonavir
  D. Fosamprenavir
  E. Nevirapine

17. Which of the following can cause hyperglycemia, hyperlipidemia (particularly elevations in triglycerides), and lipodystrophy?

A. Lopinavir-ritonavir
B. Delavirdine
C. Didanosine
D. Abacavir
E. Lamivudine

18. Lactic acidosis and hepatic steatosis have been reported with which of these antiretroviral medications?

    A. Nevirapine
    B. Efavirenz
    C. Stavudine
    D. Saquinavir
    E. Nelfinavir

19. The mechanism of action of nucleoside reverse transcriptase inhibitors is to

    A. directly inhibit reverse transcriptase.
    B. prevent entry of the proviral DNA into the nucleus of the CD4$^+$ cell.
    C. cause chain termination, resulting in a defective copy of proviral DNA.
    D. prevent entry of HIV into the CD4$^+$ cell.
    E. prevent cleavage of the newly formed polypeptide chains into a viable HIV.

20. The mechanism of action of non-nucleoside reverse transcriptase inhibitors is to

    A. prevent cleavage of the newly formed polypeptide chains into viable HIV.
    B. prevent entry of HIV into the CD4$^+$ cell.
    C. prevent entry of the proviral DNA into the nucleus of the CD4$^+$ cell.
    D. directly inhibit reverse transcriptase.
    E. cause chain termination, resulting in a defective copy of proviral DNA.

21. The mechanism of action of protease inhibitors is to

    A. cause a defective copy of proviral DNA to be made.
    B. prevent entry of the proviral DNA into the nucleus of the CD4$^+$ cell.
    C. prevent cleavage of the newly formed polypeptide chains into a viable HIV.
    D. prevent entry of HIV into the CD4$^+$ cell.
    E. directly inhibit reverse transcriptase.

22. Which of the following medications if used with atazanavir can result in decreased levels and effectiveness of atazanavir?

A. Loratadine
B. Tenofovir
C. Esomeprazole
D. Metoclopramide
E. Glipizide

23. Which of the following opportunistic infections are the only ones requiring primary prophylaxis?

    A. PCP and MAC
    B. PCP and toxoplasmosis
    C. MAC and histoplasmosis
    D. MAC and CMV
    E. PCP and thrush

24. The antifungal of first choice for maintenance therapy after treatment of cryptococcal meningitis is

    A. itraconazole.
    B. fluconazole.
    C. ketoconazole.
    D. amphotericin B.
    E. terbinafine.

25. The first-choice antifungal for treatment of histoplasmosis is

    A. itraconazole.
    B. fluconazole.
    C. ketoconazole.
    D. caspofungin.
    E. terbinafine.

31-7. Answers

1. **A.** The treatment of choice for PCP is TMP-SMX in patients who are not allergic to sulfa medications. Duration of treatment is 21 days. Because this patient's CD4$^+$ cell count is below 200 cells/mm^3 and she has had PCP, she will require secondary prophylaxis once treatment is completed. Preferred prophylaxis is once-daily TMP-SMX DS.

2. **A.** This patient's CD4$^+$ cell count is below 50 cells/mm^3; therefore, she requires primary prophylaxis against MAC. Zithromax is the drug of choice. Prophylaxis against other opportunistic infections is generally not required.

3. **A.** Current guidelines state that any patient who has had an opportunistic infection or a CD4$^+$ cell count less than 200 cells/mm^3 should start treatment for HIV. This patient has had both.

4. **D.** Most regimens contain two NRTIs and either one PI or one NNRTI. A includes one NRTI, one NNRTI, and one PI. E includes three PIs. Zidovudine and stavudine competitively inhibit each other and would not be used in the same regimen (thus, B is incorrect). Didanosine and stavudine should not be used together because of increased toxicity (which makes C incorrect).

5. **E.** All items are important risk factors for transmission of HIV. Breast-feeding, history of sexually transmitted diseases, occupational exposure to HIV-infected fluids (rare), and household exposure to HIV-infected fluids (rare) are also risk factors.

6. **B.** All HIV-positive pregnant women should receive treatment for HIV to decrease the risk of transmission to their offspring. Zidovudine and stavudine competitively inhibit each other and should not be used together. Efavirenz is teratogenic and should not be used in pregnancy. Stavudine and didanosine together are contraindicated in pregnancy because of increased risk of lactic acidosis and liver damage.

7. **C.** Zidovudine and nevirapine are the only HIV medications that can reduce vertical transmission when used as monotherapy. Most practitioners treat with combination therapy because of the increased risk of resistance with monotherapy, which affects future choices of drug regimen.

8. **A.** The approved regimens for postexposure prophylaxis are similar to those for treatment of HIV. Treatment should continue for 4 weeks and should start within 2 hours of exposure.

9. **C.** CD4$^+$ cell count describes the status of the immune system (i.e., how much a patient is at risk for acquiring an opportunistic infection).

10. **A.** Viral load relates to the activity of the virus and efficacy of antiretroviral therapy. The goal of therapy is an undetectable viral load (< 50 copies/mL).

11. **A.** Indinavir can cause kidney stones. Patients should drink at least 48 oz of water a day to decrease the risk of developing a kidney stone.

12. **B.** The "D" drugs, d4T (stavudine) and ddI (didanosine), can cause peripheral neuropathy and pancreatitis.

13. **C.** The "D" drugs, d4T (stavudine) and ddI (didanosine), can cause peripheral neuropathy and pancreatitis.

14. **D.** HLAB5701 testing should be performed prior to use of abacavir to assess risk of hypersensitivity.

15. **B.** Efavirenz can cause central nervous system (CNS) side effects such as dizziness, trouble sleeping, drowsiness, trouble concentrating, and unusual dreams during the first 2–4 weeks of treatment.

16. **E.** All NNRTIs can cause hepatotoxicity. There have been rare reports of hepatotoxicity after just one dose of nevirapine. Liver enzymes should be monitored at baseline, 2 weeks, 4 weeks, 6 weeks, and monthly for the first 18 weeks of therapy.

17. **A.** Class side effects of PIs include hyperglycemia, hyperlipidemia, fat maldistribution, and increased bleeding in hemophiliacs.

18. **C.** Class side effects of NRTIs include lactic acidosis and hepatic steatosis.

19. **C.** NRTIs affect reverse transcriptase by causing chain termination, resulting in a defective copy of proviral DNA.

20. **D.** NNRTIs affect reverse transcriptase by directly inhibiting reverse transcriptase, resulting in less proviral DNA being made.

21. **C.** PIs prevent cleavage of the newly formed polypeptide chains into viable HIV, resulting in an immature virus that is unable to infect other CD4$^+$ cells.

22. **C.** Atazanavir levels are decreased by proton pump inhibitors, H$_2$ blockers, and antacids.

23. **A.** PCP requires primary prophylaxis when the CD4$^+$ cell count falls below 200 cells/mm^3. The preferred medication is TMP-SMX. MAC requires primary prophylaxis when the CD4$^+$ cell count falls below 50 cells/mm^3. The preferred medication is azithromycin.

24. **B.** Generally, cryptococcal meningitis is initially treated with amphotericin B during the induction phase and then fluconazole for the consolidation phase and maintenance therapy.

25. **A.** Histoplasmosis is generally initially treated with amphotericin B or itraconazole for induction therapy and then itraconazole for maintenance therapy.

31-8. References

Bartlett JG, Gallant JE. 2003 *Medical Management of HIV Infection*. Baltimore: Johns Hopkins University Press; 2008:357–60.

Carr A, Miller J, Law M, Cooper DA. A syndrome of lipoatrophy, lactic acidaemia, and liver dysfunction associated with HIV nucleoside analog therapy: Contribution to protease inhibitor–related lipodystrophy syndrome. *AIDS*. 2000; 14:F25–32.

Carr A, Samars K, Thorisdottir A, et al. Diagnosis, prediction, and natural course of HIV-1 protease inhibitor associated lipodystrophy, hyperlipidaemia, and diabetes mellitus: A cohort study. *Lancet*. 1999;353:2093–99.

Centers for Disease Control and Prevention. 1993 revised classification system for HIV infection and expanded surveillance case definition for AIDS among adolescents and adults. *MMWR*. 1992;41:1–19.

Centers for Disease Control and Prevention, Perinatal HIV Guidelines Working Group. Public Health Service Task Force recommendations for the use of antiretroviral drugs in pregnant women infected with HIV-1 for maternal health and for reducing perinatal HIV-1 transmission in the United States. *MMWR*. 1998;47:1–30.

Chaisson RE, Keruly JC, Moore RD. Association of initial CD4 cell count and viral load with response to highly active antiretroviral therapy. *JAMA*. 2000;284:3128–9.

Chesney MA. Factors affecting adherence to antiretroviral therapy. *Clin Infect Dis*. 2000;30(suppl 2): S171–76.

Finzi D, Hermankova M, Pierson T, et al. Identification of a reservoir for HIV-1 in patients on highly active antiretroviral therapy. *Science*. 1997; 278:1295–300.

Furret H, Egger M, Opravil M, et al. Discontinuation of primary prophylaxis against *Pneumocystis carinii* pneumonia in HIV-1 infected adults treated with combination antiretroviral therapy: Swiss HIV Cohort Study. *N Engl J Med*. 1999;340:1301–6.

Hoen B, Dumon B, Harzic M, et al. Highly active antiretroviral treatment initiated early in the course of symptomatic primary HIV-1 infections: Results of the ANRS 053 trial. *J Infect Dis*. 1999;180: 1342–46.

Mellors JW, Munoz A, Giorgi JV, et al. Plasma viral load and CD4+ lymphocytes as prognostic markers of HIV-1 infections. *Ann Intern Med*. 1997;126: 946–54.

National Institutes of Health. Report of the NIH panel to define principles of therapy of HIV infection. *MMWR*. 1998;47(RR-5):1–41.

Sperling RS, Shapiro DE, Coombs RW, et al. Maternal viral load, zidovudine treatment, and the risk of transmission of human immunodeficiency virus type 1 from mother to infant: Pediatric AIDS Clinical Trials Group Protocol 076 Study Group. *N Engl J Med*. 1996;335:1621–29.

U.S. Food and Drug Administration; Health Resources and Services Administration; National Institutes of Health; National Center for HIV, STD, and TB Prevention; National Institute for Occupational Safety and Health; and National Center for Infectious Disease. Notice to readers update: Provisional Public Health Service recommendations for chemoprophylaxis after occupational exposure to HIV. *MMWR*. 1996;45:468–80.

U.S. Public Health Service and Infectious Diseases Society of America. 1999 USPHS/IDSA guidelines for the prevention of opportunistic infections in persons infected with human immunodeficiency virus. *MMWR*. 1999;48(RR-10):1–67.

Vittinghoff E, Scheer S, O'Malley P, et al. Combination antiretroviral therapy and recent declines in AIDS incidence and mortality. *J Infect Dis*. 1999;179: 717–20.

Yeni PG, Hammer SM, Hirsch MS, et al. Treatment for adult HIV infection: 2004 recommendations of the International AIDS Society-USA Panel. *JAMA*. 2004;292:250–65.

Immunization 32

Stephan L. Foster, PharmD

32-1. Introduction

Definitions

- *Immunity:* A naturally or artificially acquired state resulting in an individual being resistant or relatively resistant to the occurrence or effects of a foreign substance. Immunity is the mechanism the body develops for protection from infectious disease. It is usually very specific to a single organism or to a group of closely related organisms.
- *Antigen:* A live or inactivated substance capable of evoking antibody production; antigens can be a live organism, such as bacteria or virus, or an inactivated or killed organism or portion of an organism. A live organism generally evokes the most effective immune response.
- *Antibody:* A protein evoked by an antigen that acts to eliminate that antigen.

Mechanisms for Acquiring Immunity

Active immunity

Active immunity is produced by an individual's own immune system. Immunity acquired in this manner has a delayed onset and is usually permanent. Active immunity may be acquired by having an active disease or by vaccination. B-lymphocytes (B cells) circulate in the blood and bone marrow for many years. Reexposure to the antigen causes the cells to replicate and to produce antibody. These cells are also called *memory B cells.*

Passive immunity

Passive immunity is produced by an animal or human and transferred to another. Immunity acquired in this manner has a rapid onset and usually has a brief duration. An infant receives this type of immunity from his or her mother. All types of blood products contain varying amounts of antibody. Immune globulins and hyperimmune globulins are also used to induce passive immunity. One source of passive immunity is antitoxins, which contain antibodies against a known toxin.

32-2. Vaccines

Vaccination is the process of producing active immunity through the use of vaccines. The immunological response is similar to natural infection, with a lower risk than that of the disease itself.

Classification of Vaccines

Live, attenuated vaccines

Live vaccines are produced by modifying a virus or bacteria to produce immunity. These vaccines usually do not produce disease, but they may. When disease occurs, it is usually much milder than the natural disease. These vaccines must replicate to be effective. They require special handling, such as protection from heat and light, to keep them alive. Circulating antibody from another source may destroy the vaccine virus and cause vaccine failure.

The following live vaccines are available in the United States in 2009:

- Herpes zoster
- Influenza (live attenuated)
- Measles
- Mumps
- Rotavirus

- Rubella
- Typhoid oral
- Varicella
- Vaccinia (smallpox)
- Yellow fever

Inactivated vaccines

Inactivated vaccines are composed of all or a fraction of a virus or bacterium. These fractions include subunits (subvirions), bacterial cell wall polysaccharides, conjugated (attached to a protein carrier) bacteria cell wall polysaccharides, or inactivated toxins (toxoids). The bacteria or virus is inactivated using heat, chemicals, or both. Inactivated vaccines are not alive and cannot replicate; therefore, they are unable to induce disease. Inactivated antigens are not affected by circulating antibody.

The following inactivated vaccines are available in the United States in 2009:

- Anthrax
- Diphtheria
- *Haemophilus influenzae* type B
- Hepatitis A
- Hepatitis B
- Human papillomavirus
- Influenza
- Japanese encephalitis
- Meningococcal A, C, Y, W-135 polysaccharide
- Meningococcal A, C, Y, W-135 conjugate
- Pertussis, acellular
- Pneumococcal polysaccharide
- Pneumococcal conjugate
- Polio
- Rabies
- Tetanus toxoid
- Typhoid injectable

Vaccination Schedules

Vaccination schedules are available for children, adolescents, and adults from the U.S. Centers for Disease Control and Prevention (CDC). These schedules are updated yearly and can be found at www.cdc.gov/vaccines/recs/schedules. The schedules indicate the best times to administer vaccines. Additional catch-up schedules are available for children and adolescents who are behind in their vaccinations.

The CDC schedules describe intervals between doses of the same vaccine in a series. The minimum interval in a series for most vaccines is 4 weeks. Decreasing the interval may interfere with antibody re-

sponse and protection. Usually, the last dose in a series is separated from the previous dose by 4–6 months.

Increasing the interval does not affect vaccine effectiveness. It is never necessary to restart a series except for oral typhoid vaccine.

Administration of Multiple Vaccines

There are no contraindications to the simultaneous administration of any vaccines. Inactivated and live vaccines may be given in any combination at the same time.

Live vaccines must be separated from the administration of antibodies, such as blood products and immune globulins. Inactivated vaccines are not affected by circulating antibody.

If two live vaccines are not given at the same time, a 4-week minimal interval must be observed. The same is not true for two inactivated vaccines or an inactivated plus a live vaccine.

Vaccine Adverse Reactions

Adverse reactions are any untoward side effects caused by a vaccine.

Local reactions are the most common type of adverse reaction. They include pain, swelling, and redness at the site of injection. They usually occur within minutes to hours of the injection and are usually mild and self-limiting. Occasionally, severe local reactions occur that are known as *hypersensitivity reactions*.

Systemic adverse reactions include fever, malaise, myalgias, and headache. Systemic adverse reactions are more common following live vaccines and are similar to a mild case of the disease.

Allergic reactions are reactions to the vaccine antigens or to some component of the vaccine. Although rare, these reactions may be life threatening.

Another type of problem increasingly seen with vaccination is syncope; therefore, it is important to monitor patients for at least 15 minutes following vaccination.

The Vaccine Adverse Events Reporting System is a surveillance system monitored by the CDC, which should be notified within 30 days of an adverse event that requires medical attention.

Contraindications and Precautions

A *contraindication* is a condition that increases the risk of an adverse reaction or decreases the effect of a vaccine.

A *precaution* is a condition that *might* increase the risk of an adverse event or decrease the effect of a vaccine.

Contraindications include the following:

- An anaphylactic reaction to any previous dose of vaccine or to any of its components
- Pregnancy for live vaccines and selected inactivated vaccines
- Immunosuppression for live vaccines and selected inactivated vaccines
- Active, untreated tuberculosis for live vaccines
- In the case of the diphtheria, tetanus, and pertussis (DTaP or Tdap), encephalopathy that occurred within 7 days of a previous DTaP or DTP vaccine

Precautions include the following:

- Acute moderate to severe illness
- Recent administration of antibody-containing blood products and live vaccines
- For the Tdap or DTaP vaccine, unstable or evolving neurological disorder
- For the measles, mumps, and rubella (MMR) vaccine, history of thrombocytopenia or thrombocytopenic purpura
- High fever, shock, persistent crying, seizure caused by a previous dose of DTP, DTaP, or Tdap
- Guillain–Barré syndrome caused by a previous dose of DTP, TDaP, Tdap, or meningococcal conjugate vaccine

Vaccine Management

- Maintain cold chain during shipping.
- Follow manufacturers' recommendation for shipping.
- Keep nonfrozen vaccines from freezing during transport.
- Refrigerate or freeze depending on vaccine immediately on arrival.
- Use proper refrigerators.
  - Monitor temperatures daily.
  - Do not store vaccines in refrigerator door.
  - Store in the middle of the refrigerator.
  - Keep a temperature log.
- Perform proper inventory management.
  - Maintain inventory log.
  - Rotate stock.
  - Follow manufacturers' guidelines for shelf life.
  - Check expiration dates.
  - Designate a person to be responsible for vaccines.
  - Train all staff members to recognize vaccine shipment arrivals.

- Follow manufacturers' directions for reconstitution.

32-3. Diseases and Vaccines

Pneumococcal Disease

There are 90 known serotypes of Gram-positive *Streptococcal pneumonia* bacteria with a polysaccharide capsule. Serious primary diseases associated with *Streptococcal pneumonia* include pneumonia, sepsis, and meningitis.

Rates of disease

Highest rates are seen in children less than 2 years of age. Other children at high risk include those with asplenia, patients with HIV, American Indian and Alaskan Natives, African Americans, and day care attendees. Patients over the age of 50 have fatality rates of 30–60%.

Pneumococcal disease is one of the leading causes of vaccine-preventable diseases, with 20,000–40,000 cases of invasive disease every year. Pneumococcal bacteria are common respiratory tract inhabitants, with estimated asymptomatic carriage rates varying from 5% to 70%. Transmission is through direct person-to-person droplet contamination or autoinoculation by carriers.

Clinical features include abrupt onset, fever, otitis media, shaking chills, productive cough, pleuritic chest pain, dyspnea, hypoxia, tachypnea, headaches, lethargy, vomiting, irritability, nuchal rigidity, seizures, coma, and death.

Resistance to antibiotics is up to 40% in some areas of the United States.

23-valent polysaccharide vaccine (Pneumovax-23 by Merck)

The vaccine is effective against 88% of serotypes causing bacteremic disease; however, it is ineffective in children less than 2 years old.

Indications
- Adults over the age of 65
- Everyone over 2 years of age with chronic disease
- Smokers 19–64 years of age

Dose
The dosage is 0.5 mL intramuscular (IM) or subcutaneous (SC).

Revaccination (two-dose maximum) is recommended in the following cases:

- Patients at high risk of disease if more than 5 years have passed since the previous dose
- Everyone 65 years and older who received an initial dose under the age of 65 and if more than 5 years have passed since the previous dose

Adverse reactions

Adverse reactions include pain, swelling, and redness at the injection site and slight to moderate systemic reactions such as fever and myalgias.

7-valent conjugated polysaccharide vaccine (Prevnar by Wyeth)

The vaccine is effective against 86% of serotypes causing bacteremic disease, 83% of serotypes against meningitis, and 65% of serotypes causing otitis media.

Indications

- All children less than 2 years of age
- Children 24–59 months of age with high-risk medical conditions

Dose

The usual dose is 0.5 mL IM at 2, 4, 6, and 12–15 months of age (see schedules for catch-up recommendations).

Revaccination is not recommended, but high-risk children should receive 23-valent polysaccharide vaccine after 2 years of age.

Adverse reactions

Adverse reactions include pain, swelling, and redness at the injection site, difficulty moving the limb (rare), and slight to moderate systemic reactions such as fever and myalgias.

Influenza

Influenza is an RNA (ribonucleic acid) virus of the orthomyxovirus family.

Antigenic drift, which is frequent minor changes in the antigenic structure of the virus, can reach epidemic proportions, but not every year. For this reason, yearly adjustments in vaccine formulations are required. All three types (A, B, and C) can undergo drifts.

Antigenic shift, which is major changes in one or both of the major antigens in influenza A, resulting in a different subtype, can cause major pandemics in all ages.

Influenza A

Subtypes are based on two surface antigens: hemagglutinin and neuraminidase. Six types of hemagglutinin (H1, H2, H3, H5, H7, and H9) cause disease in humans and cause virus attachment to cells. Two types of neuraminidase cause disease in humans (N1 and N2) and have a role in viral release from cells.

Influenza A causes moderate to severe disease in all ages and can be transmitted in other animals.

Influenza B

Influenza B has no subgroups but has two distinct genetic lineages. It causes milder disease and affects primarily children. It only affects humans.

Influenza C

Influenza C is rarely reported and many cases are subclinical.

Influenza disease

Major serious complications in all types include pneumonia, Reye's syndrome (progressive neurological symptoms associated with aspirin use in children), myocarditis, worsening of chronic bronchitis, and death.

Influenza is one of the leading causes of vaccine-preventable disease, with 20,000–40,000 deaths during epidemics. Pandemics could result in the deaths of millions of people. Rates of disease are highest in the elderly (> 65), children less than 2 years of age, and persons of any age with medical conditions.

Influenza virus penetrates the respiratory epithelial cells and destroys the host. Virus is shed in respiratory secretions for 5–10 days, and transmission is through direct person-to-person droplet contamination or contact. The incubation period is approximately 2 days (range, 1–5 days).

Clinical features include abrupt onset, fever, myalgias, sore throat, nonproductive cough, and headache.

Disease peaks between December and March in the Northern Hemisphere but may occur earlier or later. Year-round cases may be seen in tropical climates.

Resistance to antivirals is increasing.

Inactive influenza vaccine (Fluvirin by Novartis, Fluzone by Sanofi Pasteur, Fluarix and FluLavel by GlaxoSmithKline, Afluria by CSL)

All are inactivated, split-virus vaccines. They contain three vaccine components (two type A viruses and one type B virus).

Vaccines are named according to the virus type/geographic origin/strain sequence number/year of isolation (hemagglutinin neuraminidase for type A only): for example, A/Bisbane/10/2007(H3N2) or B/Florida/4/2006.

Vaccines are effective in up to 90% of healthy adults, 50–60% of the elderly, and 30–40% of the frail elderly.

Indications
- All children 6 months to 18 years of age
- Close contacts of children 0–59 months of age
- Adults 50 years of age or older
- Adults 19 years and older with certain chronic diseases
- Residents of nursing homes or long-term care facilities
- People who may infect others, including contacts of patients with diseases and health care workers
- Pregnant women in all trimesters or women who will become pregnant during the influenza season
- Patients 6 months to 18 years of age on chronic aspirin therapy
- Patients with neurological or neuromuscular disorders
- Anyone who wishes to decrease the likelihood of influenza disease

Contraindications
Contraindications include severe allergic reactions to previous dose and egg allergy.

Adverse reactions
Adverse reactions include pain, swelling, and redness at the injection site and slight to moderate systemic reactions such as fever, myalgias, chills, and malaise. Severe neurologic reactions are rare.

Dose
Normal doses are 6–35 months: 0.25 mL IM (repeat in 1 month if first time); 3–8 years: 0.5 mL (repeat in 1 month if first time); > 8 years: 0.5 mL.

Fluvirin by Novartis is indicated for those ≥ 4 years of age.

Fluarix by GlaxoSmithKline is indicated for those ≥ 3 years of age. FluLaval by GlaxoSmithKline and Afluria by CSL are indicated for those ≥ 18 years of age.

Revaccination yearly is needed.

Intranasal live attenuated influenza vaccine (FluMist by MedImmune)

Intranasal live attenuated influenza vaccine (LAIV) is an attenuated, cold-adapted live influenza vaccine. It has the same vaccine antigens as in inactivated influenza vaccine. Its efficacy is 86–93%. LAIV must be kept refrigerated.

Indications
Indications are similar to those of inactivated vaccine unless contraindications exist:
- Healthy persons 2–49 years of age
- Contacts with high-risk patients, except the severely immunocompromised

Contraindications
With the following contraindications, use inactivated influenza vaccine:
- Children 2–4 years of age with a history of wheezing or asthma
- Persons with chronic medical diseases
- Close contacts of severely immunocompromised persons
- Pregnant women
- Children receiving aspirin therapy
- Persons with a history of Guillain–Barré syndrome

Dose
The dose is 0.1 mL sprayed in each nostril (0.2 mL total). Children age 2–8 who receive influenza vaccine for the first time need two doses 6–8 weeks apart.

Adverse reactions
Adverse reactions are similar to those of the inactivated vaccine and include nasal congestion, headache, and vomiting.

Tetanus

Exotoxin is produced by *Clostridium tetani*, a Gram-positive anaerobic rod that may develop a highly resistant spore. These spores are widely spread in soil, animal intestines and feces, skin surfaces, and infected plants.

The disease is characterized by generalized rigidity and convulsive spasms of skeletal muscles. It usually involves muscles of the face (lockjaw) and neck. Spasms may last 3–4 weeks, and complete recovery may take months.

The bacteria enter the body through contamination of a wound. Spores germinate in an anaerobic environment. Toxins are released and transported through the body.

The incubation period is usually 8 days (range, 3–21 days).

Transmission risk factors include puncture wounds, surgery, burns, minor wounds, dental infections, animal bites, injection drug use, and diabetes. Approximately 10% of cases are of unknown cause. Tetanus is not contagious person to person.

Tetanus occurs in the United States at a rate of 0.02–0.05 per 100,000 persons per year. The case fatality rate is approximately 10–20%.

Complications include laryngospasm, fractures, hypertension, nosocomial infections, pulmonary embolism, aspiration, and death. Wound management recommendations may include tetanus immune globulin (Table 32-1).

Tetanus toxoid vaccine

Tetanus toxoid is usually combined with diphtheria toxoid and pertussis vaccine. Toxoid is formaldehyde-inactivated toxin adsorbed to aluminum. The pediatric version of the vaccine is DT or DTaP. The adult version is Td or Tdap.

Dose

- **Pediatric dose:** A 0.5 mL IM dose of DT or DTaP vaccine is given at 2, 4, 6, and 15–18 months of age. A booster dose should be given at 4–6 years.
- **Adolescent dose:** A 0.5 mL dose of Tdap vaccine is given at 11–12 years.
- **Adult dose:** A 0.5 mL dose of Tdap vaccine is required if tetanus-containing vaccine is indicated.
- **Revaccination:** Every 10 years, revaccination with Td vaccine is required.

Table 32-1. Guidelines for Tetanus Wound Management

Vaccination history	Clean minor wounds Td or Tdap[a]	TIG	All other wounds Td or Tdap[a]	TIG
Unknown or < 3 years since last dose	Yes	No	Yes	Yes
Three or more years since last dose	No[b]	No	No[c]	No

Td, tetanus–diphtheria vaccine; Tdap, tetanus–diphtheria–pertussis vaccine; TIG, tetanus immune globulin.
a. Tdap should be used if the patient has not previously received Tdap and is 10 years or older.
b. Yes, if > 10 years since last dose.
c. Yes, if > 5 years since last dose.

Adverse reactions

Adverse reactions include pain, swelling (nodule may form), and redness at the injection site; systemic reactions are uncommon. An exaggerated (Arthus-type) reaction with extensive, painful swelling from shoulder to elbow can occur at the injection site and is thought to be caused by too-frequent injections.

Diphtheria

Toxin is produced by *Corynebacterium diphtheriae*, an aerobic Gram-positive bacterium. This bacterium must be infected by a virus that carries a genetic code for toxin production.

The most common presentation of diphtheria is characterized by early, nonspecific upper respiratory infection symptoms that develop into pharyngitis. Two to three days later, a bluish-white membrane starts to form that can cover the entire soft palate. The membrane can turn dark if bleeding occurs, and manipulation of the membrane can result in bleeding. Airway obstruction may occur.

Other sites of infection may include the larynx or the skin.

Other complications may include myocarditis, neuritis with paralysis, respiratory failure, and death. The overall case fatality rate is 5–10%.

Asymptomatic human carriers are the source of most infections. The incubation period is usually 2–5 days (range, 1–10 days).

Treatment of acute disease is with antitoxin and antibiotics.

Diphtheria toxoid vaccine

Diphtheria toxoid vaccine is combined with tetanus toxoid and pertussis vaccine. A single-toxoid antigen is not available. Toxoid is formaldehyde-inactivated toxin adsorbed to aluminum.

The pediatric version of the combination (DT or DTaP) contains three or four times as much antigen as the adult version (Td or Tdap).

Dose

- **Pediatric dose:** A 0.5 mL IM dose of DT or DTaP vaccine is given at 2, 4, 6, and 15–18 months of age. A booster dose should be given at 4–6 years.
- **Adolescent dose:** A 0.5 mL dose of Tdap is given at 11–12 years.
- **Adult dose:** A 0.5 mL dose of Tdap vaccine is required if tetanus-containing vaccine is indicated.
- **Revaccination:** Every 10 years, revaccination with Td vaccine is required.

Adverse reactions

Adverse reactions include pain, swelling (nodule may form), and redness at the injection site; systemic reactions are uncommon. An exaggerated (Arthus-type) reaction with extensive, painful swelling from shoulder to elbow can occur at the injection site and is thought to be caused by too-frequent injections of the tetanus antigen component of the combination vaccines.

Pertussis

Pertussis, or whooping cough, is caused by *Bordetella pertussis*, an aerobic, Gram-negative rod. The bacteria produce multiple antigenic products, which are responsible for the clinical disease. The bacteria produce toxin that paralyzes the respiratory cilia and causes inflammation of the respiratory tract.

The presentation of pertussis is in three stages. The first stage is a catarrhal stage with nonspecific upper respiratory infection symptoms. After 1–2 weeks, the paroxysmal stage with the characteristic cough and inspiratory whoop begins and lasts up to 6 weeks. Recovery, the third stage, is gradual, and the cough usually resolves in 2–3 weeks. The presentation in older children and adults may be much milder. They may present with a persistent mild cough that lasts up to 7 days. The illness may appear to be similar to other upper respiratory infections.

Complications may include pneumonia, encephalopathy, seizures, and death. The overall case fatality rate is 0.2%.

Asymptomatic human carriers are the source of most infections. The incubation period is usually 7–10 days (range, 4–21 days). Treatment of acute disease includes supportive care, antibiotics, and prophylaxis of contacts.

Transmission is human to human by the respiratory route. Pertussis is highly contagious, with attack rates of 80% in susceptible contacts.

Pertussis vaccine

Pertussis vaccine is combined with tetanus toxoid and diphtheria toxoid for children. A single-toxoid antigen is not available. A whole-cell vaccine was developed in the 1930s but is no longer available in the United States. Acellular pertussis vaccine was first licensed in 1991 and has fewer side effects than the whole-cell vaccine.

Dose
- **Pediatric dose:** A 0.5 mL IM dose of DTaP vaccine is given at 2, 4, 6, and 15–18 months of age. A booster dose should be given at 4–6 years.

- **Adolescent dose:** A 0.5 mL dose of Tdap of vaccine is given at 11–12 years.
- **Adult dose:** A 0.5 mL dose of Tdap is given one time only.

Adverse reactions
Adverse reactions include pain, swelling (nodule may form), and redness at the injection site; systemic reactions are uncommon. An exaggerated (Arthus-type) reaction with extensive, painful swelling from shoulder to elbow can occur at the injection site and is thought to be caused by too-frequent injections of the tetanus antigen component of the combination vaccines.

Available vaccines
- Tdap (Adacel by Sanofi Pasteur and Boostrix by GSK), indicated for ages 10–64
- DTaP (Tripedia and Daptacel by Sanofi Pasteur and Infanrix by GSK), indicated for age 2 months to 7 years
- Td (various manufacturers), recommended over the age of 7 following one dose of Tdap and for all over the age of 64

Hepatitis B

Hepatitis B is caused by a DNA (deoxyribonucleic acid) virus. It is one of the most common infections worldwide. An estimated 200 million to 300 million chronic carriers of hepatitis B exist worldwide.

The clinical course is similar to that of all other types of viral hepatitis, with symptoms of malaise, weakness, anorexia, nausea, jaundice, abdominal pain, headache, and dark urine. Malaise and fatigue may last for weeks to months after all other symptoms disappear.

Fulminant hepatitis occurs in 1–2% of all cases, with mortality rates of 60–90%.

Complications are usually related to chronic infections with hepatitis B virus and include chronic hepatitis, cirrhosis, liver failure, and hepatocellular carcinoma. Twenty-five percent of all carriers develop chronic, active hepatitis. The risk of becoming a carrier following infection ranges from 6% to 50%.

The incubation period is usually about 90 days (range, 60–150 days). Transmission is human to human by exposure of body fluids by parenteral or mucosal contact. Hepatitis B is a common sexually transmitted disease. Perinatal transmission is a significant mode of infection.

Hepatitis B vaccine

The first vaccine was a plasma-derived vaccine released in 1981 and removed from the market in 1992. The current vaccine is hepatitis B surface antigen (HBsAg), produced using recombinant-DNA technology. It was first released in 1986. Two products are currently marketed: Recombivax HB (Merck) and Engerix-B (GlaxoSmithKline). Although the antigen contents are different, the two vaccines are interchangeable.

Combination vaccines are available.

Dose

The usual pediatric dose is 0.5 mL IM given at birth, 2 months, and 6 months. The usual adult dose is 1.0 mL given at 0, 2, and 6 months. Indications include all infants, all adolescents, and high-risk adults (e.g., those with multiple sex partners or sexually transmitted diseases, those who use injection drugs, those on dialysis, and those with hemophilia).

Adolescents 11–15 years of age may be given a two-dose series separated by 4 months. This dose is approved for only Recombivax HB.

Serological testing may not be accurate after 2 years following vaccination, but immunity continues. Booster doses should not be given.

Adverse reactions

Adverse reactions include pain, swelling (nodule may form), and redness at the injection site; systemic reactions are uncommon.

Haemophilus Influenzae Type B

Haemophilus influenzae is a Gram-negative coccobacillus, whose outer shell consists of a polyribosylribitol phosphate (PRP) polysaccharide capsule. Six distinctly different types of *H. influenzae* exist, labeled a–f; however, *H. influenzae* type b (Hib) is responsible for 95% of human disease.

The organism enters through the nasopharynx and may cause disease or may colonize the nasopharynx, creating an asymptomatic carrier.

The most common clinical infections caused by Hib are meningitis, epiglottitis, pneumonia, arthritis, and cellulitis. Meningitis accounts for 50–65% of all clinical disease and results in a mortality rate of 2–5% and neurological sequelae in 15–30% of cases. Other diseases caused by *H. influenzae* include otitis, sinusitis, and bronchitis; however, these illnesses are usually caused by nontypable (unencapsulated) strains.

Hib is primarily a disease of children, with a peak at age 6–7 months. It rarely attacks after the age of 5 years.

Treatment of acute disease includes hospitalization, intravenous antibiotics, and prophylaxis of contacts. Transmission is human to human by respiratory droplet spread to susceptible individuals.

Haemophilus influenzae vaccine

The incidence of Hib disease has decreased by more than 99% since the introduction of vaccine. The first vaccine licensed (1985–88) was a pure polysaccharide vaccine that was ineffective in children less than 18 months of age. Current vaccines are polysaccharide vaccines conjugated to protein carriers. The specific carriers vary by manufacturer.

PRP-T (ActHIB by Sanofi Pasteur) and PRP-OMB (PedvaxHIB by Merck) are indicated for infants ≥ 6 weeks of age. Doses given before 6 weeks of age may inhibit the production of antibodies to subsequent doses; therefore, the vaccines are contraindicated in children less than 6 weeks of age. PRP-T (Hiberix by GlaxoSmithKline) is indicated only for the booster dose at 15 months to 4 years of age.

Dose

The usual dose for the vaccines approved for infants is 0.5 mL IM given at 2, 4, and 6 months. A booster dose is recommended for children 12–15 months of age. If PRP-OMB (PedvaxHIB) is used for the pediatric series, the 6-month dose should be omitted.

The catch-up series for Hib vaccine varies by age and manufacturer. Consult the package insert for complete dosing information.

Vaccination of children less than 59 months of age is not indicated unless certain medical indications exist. These include persons with asplenia, those with immunodeficiency conditions, and those undergoing immunosuppressive therapy.

Combination vaccines of Hib vaccine and hepatitis B vaccine (COMVAX by Merck) and Hib vaccine and DTaP (TriHIBit by Sanofi Pasteur) are available. TriHIBit is not approved for the initial pediatric series (2, 4, and 6 months) and can be used for a dose only at ≥ 12 months of age when a previous dose of Hib was given ≥ 2 months earlier, and TriHIBit will be the last dose in the Hib series. COMVAX must not be administered before 6 weeks of age. DTaP-Hib-IPV (Pentacel by Sanofi Pasteur) must not be used before the age of 6 weeks.

Adverse reactions

Adverse reactions include pain, swelling, and redness at the injection site; systemic reactions are uncommon.

Hepatitis A

Hepatitis A is caused by an RNA virus and is the most common hepatitis infection in the United States. The clinical course is similar to that of all other types of viral hepatitis, with symptoms of malaise, weakness, anorexia, nausea, jaundice, abdominal pain, headache, and dark urine. Malaise and fatigue usually last for 2 weeks; however, symptoms may last or recur for up to 6 months.

Fulminant hepatitis A is rare but can occur. The incidence increases with age over 40 years. Although serious complications are not as common as with hepatitis B, morbidity and its associated costs (health care costs and lost work days) are significant. There is no risk of the patient becoming a chronic carrier.

The incubation period averages 28 days (range, 15–50 days). Treatment of acute disease is supportive. Transmission is human to human by the fecal–oral route of exposure.

Exposure of an unimmunized person to hepatitis A requires the administration of immune globulin intramuscular (IGIM) as well as beginning the hepatitis A vaccine series, except for healthy persons 1–40 years of age, who may receive the vaccine only.

Hepatitis A vaccine

The available vaccines are Havrix by GlaxoSmithKline and VAQTA by Merck. These are inactivated whole-virus vaccines. Both vaccines are available in pediatric and adult formulations.

Hepatitis A vaccine is indicated for all high-risk patients and routinely for all children 1–2 years of age. Consideration of immunization should be given to all children up to 18 years of age. It is not indicated for children less than 1 year of age. The two vaccines use different potency measurements, but the volume and schedule of the dose is the same.

Dose

Children and adolescents over 1 year of age are given 0.5 mL, repeated in 6–12 months (Havrix) or 6–18 months (VAQTA), for two doses total.

Adults over 18 years old are given 1.0 mL, repeated in 6–12 months, for two doses total.

Combination vaccine

Twinrix, by GlaxoSmithKline, is a combination product with hepatitis B (adult dose) and hepatitis A (pediatric dose).

Dose

The usual dose is 1 mL, given at 0, 1, and 6–12 months. An accelerated schedule can be given at 0, 7 days, and 21–30 days, followed by a booster at 1 year, if protection is needed earlier.

The vaccine is indicated for persons 18 years of age and older.

Adverse reactions

Adverse reactions include pain, redness, and swelling at the injection site. Mild systemic reactions are rare.

Meningococcal Disease

Meningococcal disease is caused by *Neisseria meningiditis,* a Gram-negative bacteria with a polysaccharide capsule. The clinical diseases caused by *N. meningiditis* include meningitis, sepsis, pneumonia, myocarditis, and urethritis. *N. meningiditis* is one of the leading causes of meningitis in the United States. The types of *N. meningiditis* that cause over 95% of disease are serogroups A, B, C, W-135, and Y.

Approximately 2,500–3,000 cases occur per year, with an incidence rate of 2 cases per 100,000 people. The incidence in college freshmen who live in dormitories is approximately 4 cases per 100,000. A carrier state exists that increases in incidence during epidemics.

Parts of the world, including parts of Africa and Asia, have a high rate of disease.

Treatment of acute disease is with antibiotics.

Polysaccharide meningococcal vaccine (Menomune by Sanofi Pasteur)

This polysaccharide vaccine is effective against serogroups A, C, W-135, and Y. The vaccine does not protect against serogroup B, a common cause of infection.

The vaccine is indicated for persons over the age of 2 years. Those who should be vaccinated include military personnel, freshmen college students living in dormitories, those with anatomic or functional asplenia, and travelers to the "meningitis belt" of sub-Saharan Africa. Evidence of immunization is required for religious pilgrimages to Saudi Arabia for the Islamic Hajj. Vaccine may also be useful during an outbreak.

Dose

The dose is 0.5 mL given subcutaneously. A booster dose may be needed after 3–5 years.

Adverse reactions

Adverse reactions include pain, swelling (nodule may form), and redness at the injection site, as well as mild systemic reactions, such as fever, headaches, and malaise.

Conjugated polysaccharide meningococcal vaccine (Menactra by Sanofi Pasteur)

This polysaccharide vaccine that conjugated to diphtheria toxoid. It is effective against serogroups A, C,

W-135, and Y. The vaccine does not protect against serogroup B, a common cause of infection.

Indications

The vaccine is approved for persons 2–55 years of age. The Advisory Committee on Immunization Practices (ACIP) recommends vaccination for persons age 11–12 (catch-up for ages 13–18) and for college freshmen living in dormitories.

Indications are the same as for the polysaccharide vaccine; however, revaccination is recommended for persons who were previously vaccinated and who remain at high risk for the disease. The interval varies based on age at first dose.

Dose

The dose is 0.5 mL given intramuscularly.

Polio

The three poliovirus types are identified as P1, P2, and P3. The virus enters the mouth and replicates in the gastrointestinal tract. From the gastrointestinal tract, the virus enters the bloodstream and infects the cells of the central nervous system.

Up to 95% of all infections are asymptomatic; however, these persons may transmit the infection to others. Approximately 4–8% of infections are mild with nonspecific upper respiratory infection, gastroenteritis, and influenza-like symptoms. Some 1–2% of infections present as nonparalytic aseptic meningitis, which typically resolves in 2–10 days. Flaccid paralysis occurs in less than 1% of those infected.

The incubation period is usually 6–20 days (range, 3–35 days). Treatment of acute disease includes supportive care. Transmission is person to person by the fecal–oral route.

Polio vaccine (IPOL by Sanofi Pasteur)

The current vaccine available in the United States is an inactivated, trivalent injectable vaccine (IPV, or inactivated polio vaccine). Use of oral polio vaccine (OPV) was discontinued in the United States because of the elimination of wild-type polio disease and because yearly cases of vaccine-associated paralytic poliomyelitis (VAPP) were reported.

Dose

The pediatric dose is 0.5 mL IM given at 2, 4, 6–18 months, and 4–6 years of age. Routine vaccine or booster doses for adults are not recommended.

Adverse reactions

Adverse reactions include minor pain, swelling, and redness at the injection site; systemic reactions are uncommon.

Measles, Mumps, and Rubella

Measles

Measles is a viral infection whose main presentation is a maculopapular rash. The virus is shed through the nasopharynx. Ten to 12 days after exposure, the prodrome phase begins, with progressive fever, cough, coryza, and conjunctivitis. Two to 4 days after the prodrome begins, a maculopapular rash begins on the face and head and gradually spreads throughout the body. The rash lasts 3–5 days, then gradually fades.

The incubation period is 10–12 days. Transmission is person to person through large respiratory droplets. Measles is highly contagious.

Complications may include pneumonia, otitis, encephalitis, and death.

Mumps

Mumps is a viral infection with a presentation of parotitis in 30–40% of cases. The virus is shed through the nasopharynx. Fourteen to 18 days after exposure, the prodrome phase begins, with headache, malaise, myalgias, and low-grade fever. Two days after the prodrome begins is when the parotitis begins. Symptoms start to decrease after 1 week and disappear after 10 days.

The incubation period is 14–18 days (range, 14–25 days). Transmission is person to person through large respiratory droplets.

Complications can include orchitis, oophoritis, pancreatitis, and deafness.

Rubella

Rubella is a viral infection with up to 20–50% of cases subclinical and inapparent. The virus is shed through the nasopharynx. A 1–5 day prodrome phase begins after incubation, with headache, malaise, myalgias, lymphadenopathy, low-grade fever, and upper respiratory infection symptoms. This phase is rare in children. Fourteen to 17 days after exposure, a maculopapular rash appears, first on the face and then descending to cover the rest of the body. The rash disappears after about 3 days.

The incubation period is 14 days (range, 12–23 days). Transmission is person to person through large respiratory droplets.

Complications may include arthritis, arthralgias, encephalitis, and hemorrhaging. The major complication is congenital rubella syndrome (CRS), which occurs in the offspring of a woman who had rubella during pregnancy. Babies born with CRS have major birth defects that can affect many organs.

Measles–mumps–rubella vaccine (MMRII by Merck)

The current vaccine available in the United States is a live, attenuated vaccine against all three diseases.

Dose

The usual pediatric dose is 0.5 mL IM given at 12 months of age. A second dose is recommended at 4–6 years of age to produce immunity in those who did not respond to the first dose.

This vaccine is contraindicated in pregnancy. Pregnancy should be avoided for 4 weeks following vaccination.

Serologic testing may be necessary to document immunity.

Vaccination with the combination product should be used when one or more of the vaccines are needed.

Adverse reactions

Adverse reactions include minor pain, swelling, and redness at the injection site and systemic reactions that mimic a mild case of the diseases.

Varicella (Chicken Pox)

Varicella is a viral infection caused by the herpes zoster virus. The primary infection is called *chicken pox*, and the recurrent disease is herpes zoster (called *shingles*).

The virus enters through the respiratory tract and replicates in the nasopharynx and regional lymph glands. The incubation period is 14–16 days (range, 10–21 days).

A prodromal phase may precede the rash with a slight fever and malaise. The rash progresses from a macule to a papule to a vesicle before it crusts over. The rash appears in several waves that last 2–3 days each. The rash first appears on the face and then the trunk (where most of the rash occurs) and the extremities.

Recurrent disease (herpes zoster) appears to be related to aging and immunosuppression. Recurrent disease usually presents as an outbreak of lesions along a dermatome and is usually unilateral. Neuralgia and intense pain may be present.

Transmission of varicella is person to person by infected respiratory secretions. Transmission by patients with herpes zoster is by direct contact with a non-immune person.

Complications may include pneumonia, secondary bacterial infections, central nervous system infections and symptoms, and Reye's syndrome if a child is taking aspirin.

Varicella vaccine (Varivax by Merck)

The current vaccine available in the United States is a live, attenuated vaccine.

Dose

The pediatric dose is 0.5 mL IM, given at 12–18 months of age. A second dose is recommended at 4–6 years of age.

The adult dose (age > 13 years) is two doses of 0.5 mL, each separated by 4–8 weeks.

The vaccine must be stored frozen at +5°F (−15°C) or colder. The diluent used to reconstitute the vaccine should be stored at room temperature or refrigerated.

Contraindications

This vaccine is contraindicated in pregnancy, and pregnancy should be avoided for 4 weeks following vaccination. Other contraindications include immunosuppressive disease or patients receiving immunosuppressive therapy, as well as those receiving antibody-containing blood products.

Adverse reactions

Adverse reactions include minor pain, swelling, and redness at the injection site, and systemic reactions that mimic a mild case of the disease, including a mild generalized rash.

Herpes zoster vaccine (Zostavax by Merck)

This vaccine is same strain of virus as in Varivax but 14 times the dose. It is a live, attenuated vaccine that is 50% effective in preventing herpes zoster.

Indication

It is indicated for all adults over the age of 60 years, regardless of previous zoster outbreak.

Contraindications

Contraindications include immunosuppression, both disease and medically induced.

Dose

The usual dose is 0.65mL subcutaneous (must be reconstituted).

The vaccine must be stored frozen at +5°F (−15°C) or colder. The diluent used to reconstitute the vaccine should be stored at room temperature or refrigerated.

Adverse reactions

Adverse reactions include pain, redness, and swelling at the injection site and an increased incidence of headache.

Rotavirus

Rotavirus is the most common cause of severe gastroenteritis in infants and small children. Symptoms range from mild, watery diarrhea of limited duration to severe diarrhea with vomiting and fever that can result in dehydration.

In the United States, approximately 27 million episodes, 205,000–272,000 emergency visits, 410,000 outpatient visits, 55,000–70,000 hospitalizations, and 20–60 deaths occur each year because of rotavirus infection.

Rotavirus is transmitted by fecal–oral route by close person-to-person contacts and through fomites.

Rotavirus vaccines

Two rotavirus vaccines are available:

- Pentavalent human–bovine reassortant rotavirus vaccine (RotaTeq [RV5] by Merck)
- Monovalent human rotavirus vaccine (Rotarix [RV1] by GlaxoSmithKline)

RV5 is a live, oral vaccine that contains five reassortant rotaviruses and is available as a liquid that requires no reconstitution. RV1 is a live, oral vaccine that contains one human rotavirus strain and is a lyophilized powder that must be reconstituted prior to injection.

Dose

Both vaccines are administered orally. RV5 contains 2 mL per dose, and RV1 contains 1 mL per dose.

RV5 is a three-dose series given at 2, 4, and 6 months of age. RV1 is a two-dose series given at 2 and 4 months of age. The rotavirus series should be started no sooner than 6 weeks of age and must be completed by 8 months, 0 days of age.

Rotavirus vaccine can be administered simultaneously with all other pediatric vaccines indicated at the same age. It should not be given to infants who had a severe reaction to a previous dose.

Precautions include altered immunocompetence, acute gastroenteritis, moderate or severe acute illness, preexisting chronic gastrointestinal disease, and a previous history of intussusception.

Adverse effects

There does not appear to be an increase in the incidence of intussusception with the current vaccines. A previous rotavirus vaccine (Rotashield) was removed from the market in 1999.

Adverse effects may include diarrhea and vomiting.

Human Papillomavirus

Human papillomavirus (HPV) is the most common sexually transmitted disease in the United States. Although most HPV infections are asymptomatic and self-limiting, persistent infection can cause cervical cancer and genital warts.

Approximately 100 HPV types exist, with 40 types affecting the genital area and the remainder associated with skin warts. High-risk viruses can cause low- and high-grade cervical cell abnormalities and anogenital cancers. Approximately 70% of cervical cancers are caused by HPV types 16 and 18. HPV types 6 and 11 cause 90% of all genital warts.

HPV vaccines

Two HPV vaccines are available:

- Quadravalent human papillomavirus vaccine (Gardasil by Merck) protects against HPV types 6, 11, 16, and 18.
- Bivalent human papillomavirus vaccine (Cervarix by GlaxoSmithKline) protects against HPV types 16 and 18.

Indications

Both vaccines are indicated for the prevention of the types of HPV in the specific vaccine, but they are not used for the treatment of HPV infection.

The HPV vaccines are indicated for all women 9–26 years of age and should be given routinely to all 11- to 12-year-old girls. The vaccines are also indicated for the prevention of genital warts in males 9–26 years of age. Vaccination in males is not recommended by the Advisory Committee on Immunization Practices for routine use, but its use is optional.

Contraindications

HPV vaccine is contraindicated in persons who had a reaction to a previous dose.

Dose

The HPV vaccine is inactivated and administered as a three-dose series given at 0, 2, and 6 months. The vaccine must be shaken and 0.5mL administered intramuscularly in the deltoid area.

The HPV vaccine may be given simultaneously with other recommended vaccines.

Adverse reactions

Adverse reactions are primarily local and include pain, redness, and swelling at the injection site. A systemic reaction of fever may occur.

Combination Vaccines

As mentioned in previous sections, several vaccination combinations are on the market:

- Tetanus, diphtheria, and pertussis combinations (various manufacturers): DTaP, DT, Td, Tdap
- Twinrix by GlaxoSmithKline: a combination product with hepatitis B (adult dose) and hepatitis A (pediatric dose)
- Hib vaccine and hepatitis B vaccine: COMVAX by Merck
- Hib vaccine and DTaP: TriHIBit by Sanofi Pasteur
- Pediarix (GlaxoSmithKline)
  - DTaP + hepatitis B + inactivated polio
  - Indicated when all vaccine components indicated
  - Not approved for < 6 weeks or > 7 years of age
  - Efficacy, contraindications, and adverse reactions similar to those of the vaccine components given separately
  - Dose: 0.5 mL IM given at 2, 4, and 6 months of age
  - Must be shaken vigorously prior to drawing up in syringe
  - Can be given even if infant receives birth dose of hepatitis B vaccine
- Pentacel (Sanofi Pasteur)
  - DTaP + Hib + inactivated polio
  - Indicated when all vaccine components indicated
  - Not approved for < 6 weeks or > 4 years of age
  - Efficacy, contraindications, and adverse reactions similar to those of the vaccine components given separately
  - Dose: 0.5 mL IM given at 2, 4, and 6 months of age
  - Must be shaken vigorously prior to drawing up in syringe
  - Can be given even if infant receives birth dose of hepatitis B vaccine
- ProQuad by Merck: a combination vaccine of measles, mumps, rubella, and varicella vaccine
- Kindrix by GlaxoSmithKline: a combination of DTaP and IPV to be given at 4–6 years

32-4. Key Points

- The two types of vaccine antigens are (1) live viruses and (2) inactivated viruses or bacterial components.
- There are two types of immunity: active and passive.
- Adverse effects of inactivated vaccines include pain at the injection site and mild systemic symptoms (mild fever). Adverse effects of live vaccines mimic a mild case of the disease.
- Live vaccines should be avoided during pregnancy.
- Influenza viruses undergo shifts and drifts, which accounts for the need for yearly vaccine changes.
- Wound management must include evaluation for the need for tetanus toxoid and tetanus immune globulin.
- Diphtheria toxoid and tetanus toxoid should always be given together, unless a contraindication to one of the components exists. If there is a need for one, then there is a need for both.
- A combination vaccine of tetanus, diphtheria, and pertussis is available for use in adolescents and adults (Tdap). It is recommended one time for persons 11–64 years of age. Children under the age of 7 years receive DTaP or DT (if unable to tolerate pertussis vaccine). All other ages should receive Td if vaccination is indicated.
- Hepatitis B vaccine is now recommended for all infants, starting at birth, as well as all adolescents. Other indications include adults with high-risk occupations or behaviors.
- Hepatitis A vaccine is recommended for travel to most parts of the world.
- Inactivated polio vaccine is the only polio vaccine recommended for use in the United States. Oral polio vaccine is not recommended because of the high incidence of vaccine-associated paralytic poliomyelitis.
- A second dose of MMR vaccine and varicella vaccine is recommended at 4–6 years of age.
- Combination vaccines are available to decrease the number of injections.

32-5. Questions

1. A 67-year-old patient presents to your pharmacy for a refill of his insulin. It is October, and he asks you to review his immunization

status with him. About which adult vaccine do you need to ask his status?

I.   Influenza vaccine
II. Pneumococcal vaccine
III. Meningococcal vaccine
IV. Hepatitis A vaccine
V.   Diphtheria–tetanus (Td) vaccine

A. I only
B. I and II only
C. III and IV only
D. I, III, and V only
E. I, II, and V only

2. The patient in question 1 states that he received his pneumococcal vaccine 4 years ago. When should he receive another?

A. Never
B. Every year
C. In 5 years
D. When he reaches the age of 68
E. When he reaches the age of 72

3. Which of the following describes the current injectable influenza vaccine used in the United States?

A. Inactivated virus
B. Live attenuated virus
C. Conjugated vaccine
D. Toxoid
E. Toxin

4. Indications for meningococcal conjugate vaccine include

I.   all adolescents 11–12 years of age.
II. travelers to the "meningitis belt" of sub-Saharan Africa.
III. patients with asplenia.
IV. pilgrims to Saudi Arabia for the Islamic hajj.
V.   college freshmen living in dormitories.

A. I only
B. II, III, and V only
C. I, II, and III only
D. II, III, IV, and V only
E. All of the above

5. At what age does one switch from DTaP to Td?

A. 2 years
B. 5 years
C. 7 years
D. 10 years
E. DTaP can be used in all age groups.

6. Which of the following vaccines has *both* a polysaccharide and a conjugated vaccine on the U.S. market?

I.   Influenza
II. Meningococcal vaccine
III. *Haemophilus influenzae* type B vaccine
IV. Hepatitis vaccine
V.   Pneumococcal vaccine

A. IV only
B. II and V only
C. I, II, and III only
D. II, III, and V only
E. All of the above

7. Which polio vaccine schedule is recommended in the United States?

A. Four doses of IPV
B. Four doses of OPV
C. Four doses of IPV plus a booster at 18 years of age
D. Two doses of OPV and 2 doses of IPV
E. Polio vaccine is no longer recommended in the United States.

8. Hepatitis B vaccine is a

A. polysaccharide vaccine.
B. recombinant hepatitis B surface antigen vaccine.
C. live vaccine.
D. conjugate vaccine.
E. a toxoid.

9. An 18-year-old, healthy student is told that she needs to come to the pharmacy for her routine vaccinations prior to starting college. She will be living in the dormitory at school. She has not received any vaccines since grade school. Which of the following vaccines are indicated?

I.   MMR if she has not received a second dose
II. Varicella vaccine if she has not received two doses, has no history of varicella infection, or has negative titers
III. Meningococcal vaccine
IV. Pneumococcal vaccine
V.   Tdap if she has not received one for 10 years

A. All of the above
B. I and II only
C. I, II, III, and IV only
D. I, III, and V only
E. I, II, III, and V only

10. The patient in question 9 is exposed to a patient with hepatitis A 1 month later. She should receive which of the following vaccines?

    A. Hepatitis A vaccine series only
    B. Hepatitis B vaccine series only
    C. Hepatitis A vaccine series plus IGIM
    D. Hepatitis A vaccine plus hepatitis B vaccine series
    E. IGIM only

11. Which of the following is a high-risk group that should be targeted for annual influenza vaccination?

    A. Persons 18–49 years of age
    B. Persons with diabetes
    C. Patients 21–49 years of age with hypertension
    D. Construction workers
    E. Healthy patients 21–49 years of age

12. Which complication of rubella infection is the most significant health problem?

    A. Congenital rubella syndrome
    B. Secondary infection
    C. Patent ductus arteriosus
    D. Diarrhea
    E. Arthritis

13. Which of the following is a valid contraindication to the receipt of a live-virus vaccine?

    A. Taking antibiotics
    B. Recent administration of antibody-containing blood products
    C. Age over 12 months
    D. Allergies to penicillin
    E. A parent or sibling with a cold who is living in the same household

14. The most common adverse reaction to an inactivated vaccine is

    A. Rash
    B. Severe headache
    C. Injection-site reaction
    D. Rhinorrhea
    E. Stomach pain

15. The only vaccine recommended at birth is

    A. DTaP.
    B. IPV.
    C. Hib.

D. pneumococcal conjugate vaccine.
E. hepatitis B.

16. A 32-year-old female is injured in an automobile accident and her spleen is removed. Which of the following vaccines is *not* routinely recommended for asplenic adult patients?

    A. Pneumococcal vaccine
    B. Meningococcal vaccine
    C. IPV
    D. *Haemophilus influenzae* type B vaccine
    E. Yearly influenza vaccines

17. If a second dose of a vaccine were given too soon (before the minimal interval time has passed), the correct course of action would be

    A. restarting the entire series.
    B. not counting that dose and repeating it after the minimal time has passed since the incorrect dose.
    C. not worrying about it and continuing with the next dose as scheduled.
    D. drawing antibody titers to confirm immunity.
    E. doubling the next dose.

18. Which of the following groups of children are *not* at increased risk for pneumococcal disease?

    A. Obese children
    B. Children of Native Alaskan descent
    C. Children of African American descent
    D. Children with sickle cell disease
    E. Children infected with HIV

19. Which of the following statements are true concerning *Haemophilus influenzae* type b vaccine (Hib)?

    I. One dose of Hib is recommended for all infants over the age of 15 months if they have not received a previous dose.
    II. Standard dosing for Hib vaccine is 2, 4, 6, and 12–15 months of age.
    III. The 6-month dose is omitted if PedvaxHIB is used for the first two doses.
    IV. Hib vaccine is not routinely recommended for children 5 years of age and older.

    A. I only
    B. I, II, and III
    C. II, III, and IV
    D. II and III
    E. All are correct.

=off

20. Which of the following vaccines available in the United States is a live, attenuated virus vaccine?

    A. Polio (IPV)
    B. *Haemophilus influenzae* vaccine (Hib)
    C. DTaP
    D. Varicella vaccine
    E. Pneumococcal vaccine

32-6. Answers

1. **E.** Routine vaccinations in the adult are a yearly influenza vaccine, Td vaccine every 10 years, and a single pneumococcal vaccine for patients with select chronic illnesses (such as diabetes). Meningococcal and hepatitis vaccines are recommended only for certain indications.

2. **D.** Routine revaccination with pneumococcal vaccine is not recommended. Revaccination is recommended for select high-risk groups and everyone 65 years and older who received an initial dose under the age of 65 and if more than 5 years have elapsed since the previous dose.

3. **A.** Injected influenza vaccine is an attenuated, split-virus vaccine. The LAIV is administered intranasally.

4. **E.** With the recent availability of a conjugate meningococcal vaccine, the ACIP recommended including all adolescents ages 11–12 among the other recommendations.

5. **C.** DTaP is indicated for children under the age of 7. Because of adverse effects of DTaP in children 7 years of age and older, Td or Tdap is used.

6. **B.** Polysaccharide pneumococcal vaccine (23-valent) is indicated for those over the age of 2 years and conjugated polysaccharide vaccine (7-valent) is approved for ages 2 months to 7 years. A meningococcal conjugate vaccine has recently been approved, and the polysaccharide vaccine will be removed from the market once supplies of the conjugate vaccine are adequate.

7. **A.** OPV is no longer recommended in the United States, and vaccination with IPV will continue until poliovirus is eradicated worldwide.

8. **B.** Hepatitis B vaccine is a recombinant hepatitis B surface antigen vaccine.

9. **E.** Pneumococcal vaccine is not recommended for a healthy individual until the age of 65.

10. **A.** The hepatitis A vaccine alone will protect a healthy individual between 1 and 40 years of age who has previously been exposed to the virus.

11. **B.** High-risk groups targeted for influenza vaccination include persons age 6 months to 18 years and persons > 50 years old. Also included are persons age > 19 years with chronic pulmonary disease (e.g., emphysema, chronic obstructive pulmonary disease); cardiovascular disease (e.g., congestive heart failure, post–myocardial infarction, heart anomalies); metabolic disease (e.g., diabetes); renal dysfunction; hemoglobinopathies (e.g., sickle cell), and immunosuppression (e.g., HIV infection, chemotherapy). Other groups that should receive the vaccine include residents of long-term care facilities, people 24 months to 18 years old on aspirin chronically, pregnant women in all trimesters, hospital and outpatient employees, nursing home employees with patient contact, home health care providers working with high-risk persons, household members of high-risk persons, and persons desiring to avoid influenza infection.

12. **A.** Complications of rubella may include arthritis, arthralgias, encephalitis, and hemorrhaging; however, the major complication is congenital rubella syndrome, which occurs in the offspring of a woman who had rubella during pregnancy. Babies born with CRS have major birth defects that can affect many organs.

13. **B.** Live-virus vaccines will be killed if antibodies have been administered recently. The length of time that must separate these two products depends on the dose and type of antibody-containing blood product being used.

14. **C.** Local reactions are the most common type of adverse reaction, and include pain, swelling, and redness at the site of injection. These reactions usually occur within minutes to hours of the injection and are usually mild and self-limiting. Systemic adverse reactions include fever, malaise, myalgias, and headache and are more common following live vaccines.

15. **E.** All the other listed vaccines are first given at 2 months of age. Hepatitis B vaccine is recommended at birth to decrease the incidence of hepatitis B in infants of hepatitis B–infected mothers.

16. **C.** Asplenic patients require protection against the encapsulated bacteria (pneumococcus, meningococcus, and *Haemophilus*), as well as common viral infections. Previous series completions of routine vaccines, such as measles, varicella, and polio, are adequate for protection. Td vaccines should be repeated every 10 years.

17. **B.** The minimal interval in a series for most vaccines is 4 weeks. Decreasing the interval may interfere with antibody response and pro-

tection. Usually the last dose in a series is separated from the previous dose by 4–6 months. Increasing the interval does not affect vaccine effectiveness. You never need to restart a series except for oral typhoid vaccine.

18. **A.** Rates of pneumococcal disease are highest in children < 2 years of age, those with asplenia, patients with HIV, American Indian and Alaskan Natives, African Americans, and day care attendees. Obesity is not considered a high-risk disease for pneumococcal infection.

19. **E.** Although all the answers are correct, Hib vaccine may be indicated for children over the age of 5 with certain chronic conditions. This vaccine is relatively complicated to use because recommendations vary among manufacturers. Please consult package inserts before administering.

20. **D.** Varicella vaccine, LAIV, measles–mumps–rubella vaccines, and rotavirus vaccines are the only live vaccines routinely administered in the United States. Other nonroutinely administered live vaccines include oral typhoid vaccine, vaccinia (smallpox) vaccine, and yellow fever vaccine. The majority of vaccines are inactivated or killed vaccines.

32-7. References

Advisory Committee on Immunization Practices. A comprehensive immunization strategy to eliminate transmission of hepatitis B virus infection in the United (Part 1). *MMWR.* 2005;54(RR-16):1–23.

Advisory Committee on Immunization Practices. A comprehensive immunization strategy to eliminate transmission of hepatitis B virus infection in the United (Part 2). *MMWR.* 2006;55(RR-16):1–25.

Advisory Committee on Immunization Practices. General recommendations on immunizations. *MMWR.* 2006;55(RR-15):1–48.

Advisory Committee on Immunization Practices. Poliomyelitis prevention in the United States: Updated recommendations. *MMWR.* 2000;49(RR-5):1–22.

Advisory Committee on Immunization Practices. Preventing pneumococcal disease among infants and young children. *MMWR.* 2000;49(RR-9):1–38.

Advisory Committee on Immunization Practices. Preventing tetanus, diphtheria, and pertussis among adolescents: Use of tetanus, reduced diphtheria toxoid, and acellular pertussis vaccine *MMWR.* 2006; 55(RR-3):1–34.

Advisory Committee on Immunization Practices. Preventing tetanus, diphtheria, and pertussis among adults: Use of tetanus, reduced diphtheria toxoid, and acellular pertussis vaccine *MMWR.* 2006;55 (RR-17):1–33.

Advisory Committee on Immunization Practices. Prevention and control of seasonal influenza with vaccines. *MMWR.* 2009;58(RR-8):1–52.

Advisory Committee on Immunization Practices. Prevention and control of meningococcal disease. *MMWR.* 2005;54(RR-7):1–21.

Advisory Committee on Immunization Practices. Prevention of hepatitis A through active or passive immunization. *MMWR.* 2006;55(RR-7):1–23.

Advisory Committee on Immunization Practices. Prevention of pneumococcal disease. *MMWR.* 1997; 46:1–24.

Advisory Committee on Immunization Practices. Prevention of rotavirus gastroenteritis among infants and children. *MMWR.* 2009;58:1–24.

Advisory Committee on Immunization Practices. Prevention of varicella. *MMWR.* 2007;56 (RR-4): 1–40.

Advisory Committee on Immunization Practices. Quadravalent human papillomavirus vaccine. *MMWR.* 2007;56:1–24.

Advisory Committee on Immunization Practices. Revised ACIP recommendation for avoiding pregnancy after receiving a rubella-containing vaccine. *MMWR.* 2001;50:1117.

Advisory Committee on Immunization Practices. Revised recommendations of the Advisory Committee on Immunization Practices to vaccinate all persons aged 11–18 with meningococcal conjugate vaccine. *MMWR.* 2007;56794–95.

Advisory Committee on Immunization Practices. Update: Vaccine side effects, adverse reactions, contraindications, and precautions. *MMWR.* 1996;45 (RR-12):1–35; errata *MMWR.* 1997;46:227.

Advisory Committee on Immunization Practices. Use of diphtheria toxoid–tetanus toxoid–acellular pertussis vaccine as a five dose series. *MMWR.* 2000;49 (RR-13):1–8; erratum *MMWR.* 2000;49(47):1074.

Centers for Disease Control and Prevention. *Epidemiology and Prevention of Vaccine: Preventable Diseases.* 11th ed. Atlanta, Ga.: CDC; 2009.

Centers for Disease Control and Prevention. Vaccines and immunizations Web site. Available at: www.cdc.gov/vaccines/pubs/pinkbook/default.htm.

Grabenstein JD. *Immunofacts: Vaccines and Immunologic Drugs.* St. Louis, Mo.: Wolters Kluwer Health; 2007.

Plotkin SA, Orenstein WA, Offitt P, eds. *Vaccines.* 5th ed. Philadelphia: WB Saunders; 2008.

Pediatrics

Catherine M. Crill, PharmD, BCPS, BCNSP

33-1. Special Drug Therapy Considerations in Pediatric Patients

Pediatric Age Definitions

- *Preterm:* < 36 weeks gestation
- *Term:* ≥ 36 weeks gestation
- *Neonate:* < 1 month
- *Infant:* 1 month to < 1 year
- *Child:* 1–11 years
- *Adolescent:* 12–16 years

Absorption
Gastric pH

Infants may be considered to be in a relative state of achlorhydria (because of decreased basal acid secretion and total volume of secretions); however, they are capable of producing sufficient gastric acid with stimuli (e.g., in response to histamine or pentagastrin challenge, enteral feeding, or stress).

Gastric acid production reaches adult values by approximately age 3.

Implications for drug therapy
- Increased bioavailability of basic drugs
- Decreased bioavailability of acidic drugs
- Increased bioavailability of acid-labile drugs (e.g., penicillin G)

Gastric emptying time in pediatric patients

Gastric emptying time (GET) is longer for pediatric patients than for adults. GET is inversely related to postconceptional age.

GET is characterized by irregular and unpredictable peristalsis and decreased motility. Premature neonates have longer GET than term neonates and have a greater incidence of gastroesophageal reflux. GET is related to the type of feeding. Formula-fed infants exhibit longer transit time than do breast-fed infants.

Pediatric GET approaches adult function by 7–9 months. Stomach muscles are mature at 7 months. Stomach muscles are completely innervated at 9 months.

Implications for drug therapy
Absorption of sustained-release products (e.g., theophylline) is erratic. The rate of absorption in the small intestine, where most drugs are absorbed, is slower; peak drug concentrations are lower for children than for adults.

Pancreatic enzymes and bile salts

- Low levels of amylase and lipase
- Low intraluminal bile acid concentrations and synthesis
- Decreased proteolytic ability

Implications for drug therapy
- Erratic absorption of drugs requiring pancreatic enzymes for hydrolysis (e.g., chloramphenicol)
- Decreased absorption of lipid-soluble drugs
- Decreased fat absorption from enteral feedings
- Decreased absorption of fat-soluble vitamins

Gastrointestinal mucosa

- Functional integrity of intestinal mucosa is decreased.
- The surface area of the gastric mucosa is small compared to that of intestinal mucosa (most drugs are absorbed from the small intestine).

■ Changes in splanchnic blood flow in the neonatal period may alter the concentration gradient across the intestinal mucosa.

Other absorption routes

Skin

Absorption through the skin is inversely related to the thickness of the stratum corneum and directly related to hydration of the skin. Neonates (particularly premature) have increased skin hydration. The stratum corneum of preterm infants is immature and ineffective as an epidermal barrier.

Premature neonates may develop drug toxicity if a drug is administered through the dermal route.

Buccal route

The buccal route is not typically used in pediatric patients.

Intramuscular route

Drug delivery is restricted by volume of medication and the pain associated with administration. Results are variable in premature neonates because of (1) blood flow and vasomotor instabilities and (2) insufficient muscle mass and tone, contraction, and oxygenation.

Rectal administration

Rectal administration is effective for drug delivery in older infants and children.

Administration through intraosseous route

This vessel-rich marrow (up to age 5) is a great site for drug delivery to the systemic circulation. It may be an acceptable route in emergency situations for children over age 5 (vessel-rich marrow is then replaced by yellow marrow).

Distribution

Protein binding

■ Decreased albumin and α_1-acid glycoprotein concentrations
■ Lower binding capacity
■ Qualitative differences in neonatal plasma proteins
■ Competitive binding by endogenous substances (unconjugated bilirubin, free fatty acids)
■ Risk of kernicterus (hypoalbuminemia, unconjugated hyperbilirubinemia, displacement by highly protein-bound drugs or free fatty acids)
■ Exhibition of adult-like binding by 3–6 months of age; adult concentrations of albumin and α_1-acid glycoprotein at 10–12 months

Differences in body composition

■ Vascular and tissue perfusion are altered.
■ The brain and liver are the largest organs in children.
■ Total body water is greater in neonates and infants.
■ Extracellular fluid volume is greater in neonates and infants.
■ There is a relative lack of adipose tissue in neonates and infants (adipose level increases into adulthood).

Implications for drug therapy in neonates and infants

■ Increased free fraction of drugs can occur.
■ Increased potential of drug displacement by endogenous substances is present.
■ Potential risk of kernicterus with physiologic jaundice (unconjugated hyperbilirubinemia) is present.
■ Hydrophilic drugs, which parallel water in the body (e.g., aminoglycosides), exhibit greater volume of distribution.
■ Lipophilic drugs (e.g., diazepam) parallel body fat and will exhibit a smaller volume of distribution.

Liver Metabolism

Phase I reactions (nonsynthetic): Oxidation, reduction, hydrolysis, and hydroxylation

■ The hepatic cytochrome P450 (CYP450) enzyme system is responsible for most phase I reactions.
■ The capacity of isoenzymes in the CYP450 system at birth is 20–70% of adult capacity and increases with postnatal age.
■ Full capacity for reduction is present at birth.
■ Hydrolysis is most developed at birth, followed by the processes of oxidation and hydroxylation.
■ Benzyl alcohol, a preservative present in certain medications, can accumulate in neonates because of underdeveloped alcohol dehydrogenase. Gasping syndrome (i.e., metabolic acidosis, respiratory failure, seizures, neurologic deterioration, and cardiovascular collapse) can result.

Phase II reactions (synthetic): Conjugation with glycine or glutathione, glucuronidation, sulfation, methylation, and acetylation

■ The sulfation pathway is the most developed pathway at birth.
■ Glucuronidation (i.e., UDP-glucuronosyltransferase [UGT] activity) begins around 2 months of age. It reaches adult capacity by age 2.

Assumptions about substances primarily metabolized by glucuronidation (i.e., morphine, bilirubin, and chloramphenicol) are as follows:
- They are potentially toxic in neonates.
- They may exhibit long half-lives (e.g., toxicity with chloramphenicol).
- They may require greater dosing in infants (e.g., morphine conjugated to its more active metabolite).
- They may be metabolized by another pathway in infants (e.g., acetaminophen is primarily metabolized through sulfation in infants).

Methylation is functional in infants but is not significantly expressed in adults. (Methylation is responsible for the conversion of theophylline to caffeine.)

Implications for drug therapy

- For drugs undergoing phase I and II reactions, the metabolism is reduced and the half-life is prolonged in infants and neonates.
- Insufficiency of one pathway may lead to metabolism through another.
- Adverse drug reactions are more likely in younger children (i.e., five times more likely in children under age 1 and three and one-half times more likely in children age 1–4).
- Drug metabolism, which is slower in the neonate, increases between 1 and 5 years of age and is similar to that in adults after puberty.

Renal Elimination

- Renal blood flow is only 5–6% of cardiac output at birth, compared with 15–25% in adults (12 mL/min versus 140 mL/min).
- Glomerular filtration rate is lower at birth and reaches adult values by 1–5 months of age in term infants.
- Tubular secretion is low at birth and reaches adult values by 7 months of age in term infants.
- Renal elimination is affected by prematurity and postconceptional age. It increases with maturity.

Estimation of creatinine clearance in pediatric patients

- The estimation of creatinine clearance (CrCl) is altered by differences in renal blood flow, glomerular filtration, tubular secretion, and muscle mass.

Table 33-1. Proportionality Constant for Calculation of Creatinine Clearance Using the Schwartz Equation[a]

Age	k
Low birth weight ≤ 1 year	0.33
Full term ≤ 1 year	0.45
1–12 years	0.55
14–21 years (female)	0.55
14–21 years (male)	0.70

a. Schwartz et al. 1987.

- It may be affected by the presence of maternal serum creatinine (SCr) over the first week of life (i.e., false underestimation of CrCl).
- The Schwartz equation may be used for calculation of CrCl:

$$\text{CrCl (mL/min/1.73 m}^2) = k \times (\text{length in cm})/\text{SCr}$$

where k = proportionality constant that changes with age and sex (Table 33-1).

Other Pediatric Drug Issues

- Digoxin-like immunoreactive substance (DLIS) is produced in infants. DLIS may interfere with digoxin assays and falsely elevate concentrations.
- Di(2-ethylhexyl)phthalate (DEHP), a plasticizer contained in intravenous (IV) bags, is shown to have an effect on the male reproductive system. Pediatric patients at highest risk of DEHP exposure are neonates on extracorporeal membrane oxygenation, those receiving parenteral and enteral nutrition, and those receiving plasma exchange transfusions.
- Polyethylene glycol, an additive used to promote stability in certain IV medications, can cause hyperosmolarity in infants.

33-2. Specific Infections and Disease States in the Pediatric Population

Otitis Media

Otitis media is an inflammatory process of the middle ear.

Classification

- *Acute otitis media* is an inflammation of the area behind the eardrum (tympanic membrane) in the chamber called the middle ear. It is accompanied by the presence of fluid in the middle ear (effusion) and by the rapid onset of signs or symptoms of ear infection (also see the American Academy of Pediatrics [AAP] and American Academy of Family Physicians [AAFP] definition in section on diagnostic criteria).
- *Recurrent otitis media* is the diagnosis of three episodes of acute otitis media within a 6-month period or four episodes within a year.
- *Otitis media* with effusion is fluid in the middle ear (effusion) without the associated signs or symptoms of acute infection.

Clinical presentation

Signs and symptoms include fever, otalgia (often manifested as ear tugging or pulling), otorrhea (discharge from the ear), changes in balance or hearing, irritability, difficulty sleeping, lethargy, anorexia, vomiting, and diarrhea. Associated findings may be runny nose, congestion, or cough.

Pathophysiology

Eustachian tube dysfunction

The infant's eustachian tube is shorter and more horizontal than that of the adult, thus preventing drainage of middle ear secretions into the nasopharynx and promoting pooling of secretions in the middle ear. Anatomic abnormalities increase risk (e.g., cleft palate and adenoid hypertrophy). An immature immune system or altered host defenses also increase risk, as well as viral infections and allergies increase risk.

Risk factors include male gender; Native American, Canadian Eskimo, or Alaskan descent; family history of acute otitis media or respiratory tract infection; early age of first episode (earlier age is associated with greater severity and recurrence); day care environment; parental smoking; lack of breast-feeding in infancy; and pacifier use.

Complications include mastoiditis, meningitis, subdural empyema, hearing loss, and delayed speech and language development.

Microbial pathogens

Up to 50% of cases of acute otitis media may be viral in origin. The rest are bacterial:

- *Streptococcus pneumoniae* is responsible for 40–50% of bacterial otitis media. Resistance is becoming an increasing problem; bacterial resistance occurs primarily through alteration in penicillin-binding protein (decreased affinity for binding sites).
- *Haemophilus influenzae* (primarily nonencapsulated or nontypeable strains) is responsible for 20–30% of bacterial otitis media cases. Bacterial resistance occurs through β-lactamase production.
- *Moraxella catarrhalis* is responsible for 10–15% of bacterial otitis media. Almost all strains are β-lactamase producing.

Diagnostic criteria

For diagnosis of otitis media, the clinical presentation must show signs and symptoms consistent with infection.

In 2004, the AAP and AAFP published a clinical practice guideline on the diagnosis and management of acute otitis media. The guideline presented a revised definition of acute otitis media as follows: "diagnosis requires: (1) a history of acute onset of signs and symptoms, (2) the presence of middle ear fluid (by a bulging tympanic membrane, limited/absent mobility of or air-fluid level behind the tympanic membrane, or otorrhea), and (3) signs and symptoms of middle ear inflammation (distinct erythema of the tympanic membrane or distinct otalgia referable to the middle ear that interferes with normal sleep/activity)."

When middle ear disease is present, otoscopic examination determines color, translucency, and position. Redness or opacity of membrane, absence of light reflection, or bulging membrane will be observed.

Pneumatic otoscopic examination determines mobility of the tympanic membrane (i.e., presence or absence of effusion). The membrane will not move briskly with positive and negative pressure if effusion is present.

Tympanocentesis (i.e., a needle is inserted through the tympanic membrane to withdraw fluid) allows for culture and identification of the pathogen.

Treatment principles and goals

- Assess and control pain.
- Eradicate infection.
- Prevent complications.
- Avoid unnecessary antibiotic therapy.
- Improve compliance.
- Eliminate presence of effusion.
- Prevent recurrence.

Drug therapy

Many episodes of otitis media will have spontaneous resolution; however, because there is a risk of developing complications from untreated otitis media, antimicrobials remain the mainstay of therapy. Observation therapy may be appropriate in certain patients, depending on age, diagnostic certainty, and severity of illness and when follow-up can be ensured.

First-line therapy

Amoxicillin is the drug of choice for uncomplicated and nonsevere (mild otalgia and fever < 39°C or 102.2°F) acute otitis media. Amoxicillin has excellent in vitro activity against *Streptococcus pneumoniae* and most *Haemophilus influenzae*. It has the optimal pharmacodynamic profile of the available agents and reaches good concentrations in middle ear fluid.

Amoxicillin has an excellent safety and efficacy profile with narrow spectrum of activity. It is palatable and inexpensive. It may overcome drug-resistant *S. pneumoniae* with higher doses (i.e., achieves greater concentrations in middle ear fluid). It does not eradicate β-lactamase–producing organisms.

For penicillin-allergic patients (non–type I hypersensitivity), cefdinir, cefpodoxime, or cefuroxime may be used. In patients with type I reactions (urticaria or anaphylaxis), azithromycin, clarithromycin, trimethoprim-sulfamethoxazole (6–10 mg/kg/day of trimethoprim), or erythromycin-sulfisoxazole (50 mg/kg/day of erythromycin) may be substituted; however, resistance appears to be increasing with these agents. Depending on the severity of the illness, ceftriaxone therapy may be initiated. Clindamycin may be used when drug-resistant *S. pneumoniae* is suspected.

Amoxicillin-clavulanate should be used as first-line therapy, depending on the severity of illness (moderate to severe otalgia or fever ≥ 39°C or 102.2°F).

Other effective antimicrobial agents include other cephalosporins (cefprozil, cefaclor, and ceftibuten). Fluoroquinolones (ciprofloxacin, ofloxacin, levofloxacin) are thought to be effective, but they are not approved for use in pediatric patients.

Dosing issues and drug resistance

Treatment options are described in Table 33-2.

Dosages are as follows:

- *Amoxicillin:* A high dose is recommended (80–90 mg/kg/day).
- *Amoxicillin-clavulanate:* A high dose is recommended (90 mg/kg/day of amoxicillin with 6.4 mg/kg/day of clavulanate). Maintain daily

Table 33-2. Treatment Options for Otitis Media

Severity of illness	First-line therapy	Therapy for penicillin allergy
Nonsevere illness: At diagnosis (initial antibiotic therapy)	Amoxicillin (80–90 mg/kg/day)	*Non–type I:* Cefdinir (14 mg/kg/day in 1 or 2 doses), cefuroxime (30 mg/kg/day in 2 doses), or cefpodoxime (10 mg/kg/day once daily)
		Type I: Azithromycin (10 mg/kg day 1, 5 mg/kg days 2–5) or clarithromycin (15 mg/kg/day in 2 doses)
Severe illness: At diagnosis (initial antibiotic therapy)	Amoxicillin-clavulanate (90 mg/kg/day amoxicillin, 6.4 mg/kg/day clavulanate)	Ceftriaxone (50 mg/kg/day for 1 or 3 days)
Nonsevere illness: Treatment failure at 48–72 hours (initial observation option)	Amoxicillin (80–90 mg/kg/day)	*Non–type I:* Cefdinir (14 mg/kg/day in 1 or 2 doses), cefuroxime (30 mg/kg/day in 2 doses), or cefpodoxime (10 mg/kg/day once daily)
		Type I: Azithromycin (10 mg/kg day 1, 5 mg/kg days 2–5) or clarithromycin (15 mg/kg/day in 2 doses)
Severe illness: Treatment failure at 48–72 hours (initial observation option)	Amoxicillin-clavulanate (90 mg/kg/day amoxicillin, 6.4 mg/kg/day clavulanate)	Ceftriaxone (50 mg/kg/day for 1 or 3 days)
Nonsevere illness: Treatment failure at 48–72 hours (initial antibiotic therapy)	Amoxicillin-clavulanate (90 mg/kg/day amoxicillin, 6.4 mg/kg/day clavulanate)	*Non-type I:* Cefriaxone (50 mg/kg/day for 3 days) *Type I:* Clindamycin (30–40 mg/kg/day in 3 doses)
Severe illness: Treatment failure at 48–72 hours (initial antibiotic therapy)	Ceftriaxone (50 mg/kg/day for 3 days)	Tympanocentesis: Clindamycin (30–40 mg/kg/day in 3 doses)

AAP/AAFP Clinical Practice Guideline, 2004.
Note: Observation option must have follow-up at 48–72 hours and access to antibiotics if symptoms persist or worsen. Nonsevere illness manifests as mild otalgia and fever < 39°C or 102.2°F. Severe illness manifests as moderate to severe otalgia or fever of ≥ 39°C or 102.2°F.

clavulanate dose < 10 mg/kg/day to prevent diarrhea.

■ *Ceftriaxone:* An intramuscular (IM) dose of 50 mg/kg/day (single dose versus three daily doses) is recommended.

Duration of therapy

Two courses of therapy are possible:

■ Standard 10-day course
■ Shorter course (1–7 days)

Advantages of the shorter course are improved compliance, decreased adverse effects of drug therapy, decreased risk of bacterial resistance, and lower costs. Disadvantages are delayed or no cure, increased risk of complications from untreated acute otitis media, and greater risk of recurrence.

A shorter course is not appropriate for the following:

■ Children under age 2 (AAP and AAFP state under age 6)
■ Children with severe disease
■ Those in day care
■ Those with underlying diseases
■ Those with a history of recurrent otitis media

Other therapy

Antipyretics (acetaminophen and ibuprofen) or analgesics may be used. Use acetaminophen with caution in high doses to avoid hepatotoxicity. Use ibuprofen with caution in patients with vomiting, diarrhea, and poor fluid intake, because dehydration predisposes to ibuprofen-induced renal insufficiency. Avoid alternating antipyretic therapy. Encourage parents to choose one agent, inform them of any adverse effects, and educate them about symptoms of these effects (e.g., hepatotoxicity or renal insufficiency).

Narcotic analgesics may be used for moderate to severe pain not controlled with acetaminophen or ibuprofen.

Topical analgesics include otic solutions, such as antipyrine-benzocaine (Auralgan and Americaine Otic) and naturopathic agents (Otikon Otic Solution).

Topical antimicrobials may have a place in therapy, particularly with ruptured membranes (fluoroquinolone or fluoroquinolone and steroid combination otic suspensions [Floxin, Cipro HC, and Ciprodex]).

Antihistamines and decongestants are ineffective at eliminating effusion or relieving symptoms. Use them only if indicated for other signs or symptoms.

Patient instructions and counseling

■ Complete the entire course of prescribed antibiotics.
■ Shake bottle well before administering dose. Follow labeling regarding temperature for storage of medication.
■ Contact the physician if patient develops a rash or has difficulty breathing, or if symptoms persist after 72 hours of initiating therapy.

Adverse drug events

■ *Gastrointestinal effects:* Nausea and diarrhea; discoloration of stools (with cefdinir)
■ *Hypersensitivity:* Rash and anaphylaxis

Drug interactions

Drug interactions may occur with macrolides, particularly erythromycin and clarithromycin.

Nondrug therapy

Local heat or cold therapy may be used (counsel the caregiver on appropriate use and technique to prevent burn injury).

Tympanostomy tubes decrease recurrent episodes, restore hearing, and relieve discomfort. Risks include anesthesia and permanent tympanic membrane scarring.

Observation therapy

Observation therapy is appropriate only when follow-up at 48–72 hours can be ensured and antimicrobials initiated if symptoms persist or worsen. This therapy is not appropriate for the following:

■ Infants < 6 months of age
■ Infants and children between 6 months and 2 years of age with a certain diagnosis (nonsevere or severe illness) or an uncertain diagnosis (severe illness)
■ Children ≥ 2 years of age with a certain diagnosis and severe illness

A *nonsevere illness* is mild otalgia and fever < 39°C or 102.2°F. A *severe illness* is moderate to severe otalgia or fever ≥ 39°C or 102.2°F.

Immunization and immunoprophylaxis

Pneumococcal conjugate vaccination should provide some protection against strains responsible for a majority of bacterial otitis media.

Haemophilus influenzae type B vaccination is of no benefit in otitis media. Most strains causing otitis media are nontypeable and not prevented by vaccination.

Killed and live-attenuated intranasal influenza vaccine may decrease episodes of acute otitis media during the respiratory season. Most children studied were less than 2 years of age.

Risk reduction

- Alter day care attendance (when possible).
- Adopt exclusive breast-feeding for 6 months.
- Avoid supine bottle feeding.
- Reduce or eliminate pacifier use after 6 months of age.
- Eliminate passive exposure to tobacco smoke.

Recurrent otitis media

Prophylaxis with half therapeutic dosing of amoxicillin or sulfisoxazole has been initiated in high-risk patients; however, this practice is no longer recommended because of concerns over emergence of drug-resistant organisms.

Otitis media with effusion

The AAP, AAFP, and the American Academy of Otolaryngology–Head and Neck Surgery published a clinical practice guideline on otitis media with effusion in 2004. It applies to infants and children (2 months to 12 years of age) with or without developmental disabilities or underlying conditions that predispose patients to otitis media with effusion. Recommendations include the following:

- Use pneumatic otoscopy as the primary diagnostic method.
- Distinguish otitis media with effusion from acute otitis media.
- Determine the risk of speech, language, and learning problems.
  - *At-risk children:* More rapid evaluation and intervention
  - *Children not at risk:* Watchful waiting for 3 months from date of onset or diagnosis
- No role exists for antihistamines, decongestants, antimicrobials, or corticosteroids.
- Hearing testing is recommended with effusion lasting ≥ 3 months or when language delay, learning problems, or hearing loss exists.
- For persistent otitis media with effusion (not at risk), perform evaluations every 3–6 months until

effusion is resolved, hearing loss is identified, structural abnormalities are suspected, or the child becomes a surgical candidate (tympanostomy tube insertion is preferred).

Otitis Externa

Otitis externa is an inflammation of the outer ear canal, also referred to as *swimmer's ear*.

Clinical presentation

Patients present with itching, pain, otic exudate, and hearing impairment

Pathophysiology

Moisture is present in the ear canal and the integrity of the ear canal is disrupted. The most common organisms are *Pseudomonas aeruginosa* and *Staphylococcus aureus*. Other pathogens include fungi and *Bacillus* and *Proteus* species.

Therapy consists of antibiotic or steroid otic preparations such as neomycin, polymyxin, and hydrocortisone (Cortisporin Otic) or neomycin, colistin, and hydrocortisone (Coly-Mycin S Otic). Fluoroquinolone otic preparations such as ciprofloxacin (Cipro HC) and ofloxacin (Floxin) can also be used, as well as acetic acid and hydrocortisone otic preparations (VoSol HC Otic) or oral analgesics.

Preventive measures include drying ears after exposure to moisture; using drops containing isopropyl alcohol, with or without acetic acid to reduce pH; and avoiding cotton swabs.

According to a 1994 special report of the American Pharmaceutical Association, otic drops should be applied as follows:

1. Wash hands before and after administration.
2. Warm otic drops to room temperature by holding bottle in hands for several minutes. Avoid instilling cold or hot drops into the ear canal.
3. Shake the bottle if indicated on the label.
4. Tilt the child's head to the side or have the child lie down.
5. Pull the child's ear backward and upward and instill the drops in the ear canal. Do not put the dropper bottle inside the ear canal. To remain free from contamination it should not come into contact with the ear.
6. Press gently on the small flap over the ear to push the drops into the canal.

7. Have the child remain in the same position for the period of time indicated in the labeling. If this is not possible, place a cotton ball gently into the ear to prevent the drops from draining out of the ear canal.

8. Wipe excess medication from the outside of the ear.

Cystic Fibrosis

Cystic fibrosis is an autosomal recessive disease of exocrine gland function resulting in abnormal mucus production.

Genetic classification

Cystic fibrosis is the result of a gene mutation on the long arm of chromosome 7. The protein encoded by this gene, the cystic fibrosis transmembrane regulator (CFTR), is a channel involved in the transport of water and electrolytes.

Defects in processing

The most common genetic mutation involves a 3-base-pair deletion at position 508 (ΔF508). Patients homozygous for ΔF508 are pancreatic insufficient.

Prognosis is not as good as that for patients who are pancreatic sufficient. Defects exist in protein production, regulation, and conduction.

Clinical presentation

Pulmonary complications
Initial manifestations include chronic cough, wheezing, hyperinflation of lungs, or lower respiratory tract infections. Patients present with hypoxia, clubbing, labored breathing, and acute respiratory exacerbations (fever, sputum production, increased oxygen requirements, and dyspnea); changes in forced vital capacity (FVC), forced expiratory volume in 1 second (FEV_1), and residual volume; and the development of a chronic obstructive picture as the disease progresses.

Gastrointestinal complications
Gastrointestinal complications include poor digestion of proteins and fats, resulting in foul-smelling steatorrhea, and distal intestinal obstruction (commonly manifested as vomiting of bilious material, abdominal distension, and pain).

Infants may have meconium ileus and gastroesophageal reflux.

Other complications
Patients may also have the following complications:

- Cirrhosis and cholelithiasis
- Problems with pancreatic function
- Insulin insufficiency and diabetes mellitus
- Malnutrition
- Nasal polyps and sinusitis, anemia, arthritis, osteopenia, and osteoporosis

Pathophysiology

A defect exists in the chloride transport channel in secretory epithelial cells. Normally, chloride is transported out of blood followed by sodium and water. However, with cystic fibrosis, decreased chloride and water secretion and increased sodium absorption lead to thick, dehydrated secretions and mucus. Exocrine gland involvement includes pancreas, hepatobiliary ducts, gastrointestinal tract, and the lungs (secretions build up and block airways and pancreatic and hepatobiliary exocrine flow).

Pulmonary system
Initial obstruction of small airways with mucus plugging results in bronchiolitis and persistence of bacteria, as follows:

- *Early bacterial pathogens: Staphylococcus aureus* and *Haemophilus influenzae* present in younger patients.
- *Later bacterial pathogens: Pseudomonas aeruginosa* is the primary pathogen in late childhood.
- *Other bacterial pathogens: Proteus* and *Klebsiella* species, *Stenotrophomonas maltophilia,* and *Burkholderia cepacia* can be present.

Viral pathogens can also be present.

Chronic pulmonary infection and inflammation progress to large airway and eventual chronic obstructive disease.

Pancreatic system
Pancreatic enzyme insufficiency (trypsin, chymotrypsin, lipases, and amylase) and decreased bicarbonate secretion (necessary for optimal pancreatic enzyme activity) can occur. Thus, maldigestion of fats and proteins and fat-soluble vitamin deficiency may develop.

Insulin insufficiency (resistance and decreased secretion) leads to glucose intolerance and the development of diabetes mellitus (occurs later in the disease process and may be associated with increased morbidity and mortality).

Biliary system

Biliary cirrhosis or fatty infiltration may lead to portal hypertension, development of bleeding varices, hypersplenism, and cholelithiasis.

Sweat glands

A high concentration of sodium and chloride exists in sweat (representing the failure of sweat glands to reabsorb sodium and chloride).

Reproductive system

Male infertility is common because of bilateral absence of vas deferens. Female infertility is due to abnormal cervical mucus.

Diagnostic criteria

Laboratory confirmation of CFTR dysfunction should be obtained through sweat chloride analysis (i.e., administration of pilocarpine):

- Sweat is collected and electrolytes are measured.
- Chloride of 60 mEq/L or more is diagnostic (values of up to 80 mEq/L have been seen in non–cystic fibrosis patients).
- Levels of 50–60 mEq/L are indeterminate, and tests may need to be repeated.

Presence of clinical characteristics of cystic fibrosis should also be observed.

Treatment goals

- Halt or decrease disease progression.
- Maintain normal growth and development and nutrition status.
- Maintain pulmonary function.
- Optimize drug therapy for pharmacokinetic differences in cystic fibrosis patients.

Drug therapy

Drug therapy for cystic fibrosis is described in Table 33-3.

Antibiotic therapy in acute exacerbations

Empiric therapy should be used initially. The patient should then be treated on the basis of sputum culture and sensitivity. Administer intravenously two antibiotics for 14–21 days in combination with aggressive therapy for clearance of secretions. Provide coverage for *Staphylococcus aureus*, *Haemophilus influenzae*, and *Pseudomonas aeruginosa*.

Double coverage of antibiotics is needed when *Pseudomonas* species are suspected, so typically use an antipseudomonal penicillin (piperacillin, mezlocillin, piperacillin-tazobactam, ticarcillin-clavulanate, ticarcillin, aztreonam, meropenem, or imipenem) or a cephalosporin (ceftazidime) plus an aminoglycoside (tobramycin).

Most *S. aureus* are β-lactamase producers, so use an extended spectrum penicillin—β-lactamase inhibitor combination (e.g., ticarcillin-clavulanate). Use vancomycin for methicillin-resistant *S. aureus*.

Burkholderia and *Stenotrophomonas* species are commonly resistant. Follow culture and sensitivity results. Antibiotics that may be effective include trimethoprim-sulfamethoxazole, chloramphenicol, ceftazidime (*B. cepacia*), doxycycline, and piperacillin (*S. maltophilia*).

Other agents include ciprofloxacin.

Antibiotic therapy and chronic suppression
Chronic inhaled antibiotic therapy with tobramycin

This therapy results in significant improvement in FEV_1, decreased hospitalizations, and decreased need for IV antibiotics. Decreased systemic concentrations (i.e., less resistance) and high pulmonary concentrations appear. However, therapy is expensive.

Oral antibiotic therapy

Fluoroquinolones are the only oral antibiotics with good coverage against *Pseudomonas*.

Patient instructions and counseling

Compliance with therapeutic regimens is important.

Pancreatic enzyme supplementation

- Give immediately before or during snacks and meals.
- Capsule may be opened and contents sprinkled on applesauce or other acidic carrier.
- Contents should not be crushed or chewed.

Aminoglycosides

- Monitor urine output.
- Use ibuprofen with caution if dehydration, diarrhea, or decreased oral intake is present.

Adverse drug events

- ***Aminoglycosides:*** Nephrotoxicity and ototoxicity
- ***Ibuprofen:*** Renal insufficiency
- ***Fluoroquinolones:*** Arthropathy

Table 33-3. Drug Therapy for Cystic Fibrosis

Therapeutic category	Indication and mechanism of action	Comments
Pancreatic enzymes: microencapsulated (Creon, Pancrease, Pancrelipase, Ultrase); Tablet (Viokase); Powder (Viokase)	Supplementation or replacement of pancreatic enzymes (treatment of malabsorption syndrome); aid in digestion of proteins, carbohydrates, and fats	Products differ by enzyme content (units of lipase, protease, and amylase) and dosage form. Primary enzyme component is lipase. Dose is typically whole dose with meals and half dose with snacks. Adequate replacement decreases bowel movements and improves stool consistency.
Fat-soluble vitamins	Supplementation of fat-soluble vitamins A, D, E, and K	Vitamins may be dosed individually, through the use of 1 or 2 multivitamins daily, or with a water-miscible combination preparation.
Nebulization therapy	Liquefaction of pulmonary secretions	Nebulization therapy can be accomplished with normal saline or sterile water with or without other therapies.[a]
N-acetylcysteine (Mucomyst)	Lowered mucus viscosity through sulfhydryl group, which opens the disulfide bond in mucoproteins	Bad taste and odor are present. Significant efficacy has not been documented.
Recombinant human DNase (dornase alfa, Pulmozyme)	Contribution of DNA in mucus to viscosity; mechanism of action through cleavage of DNA (thereby decreasing mucus viscosity)	Product is expensive, reduces viscosity, improves pulmonary function, and may decrease respiratory exacerbations.
Ursodeoxycholic acid (ursodiol, Actigall)	Bile acid that suppresses hepatic synthesis and secretion of cholesterol; inhibits intestinal cholesterol absorption; solubilizes cholesterol	Product aids in dissolution of stones with cholelithiasis.
Bronchodilators (β_2-agonists, theophylline)	Bronchodilator in reversible or obstructive airway disease	Bronchodilators may benefit patients with component of reactive airway disease; patients should use β_2-agonist before theophylline because of pharmacokinetic issues. Response (improvement in FEV_1) should be documented before initiating long-term therapy.
Antibiotics	Treatment of infection	Altered pharmacokinetics may affect and complicate therapy.
Ibuprofen	Nonsteroidal anti-inflammatory; controls airway inflammation	Ibuprofen is not used routinely; it may have an effect on slowing pulmonary disease. High dosages are needed to achieve good concentrations (requires therapeutic drug monitoring).
Corticosteroids	Anti-inflammatory	Corticosteroids are not used routinely; they have positive effects on pulmonary function but negative effects on growth and development, glucose sensitivity, and bone health.

a. Other therapies include N-acetylcysteine and recombinant human DNase.

Drug interactions

Pancreatic enzymes and acid suppression therapy may decrease inactivation of enzymes by gastric acid, thereby reducing dose requirement.

Monitoring parameters

Clinical status should be monitored:

- Fever and activity level
- Pulmonary function (as indicated by FEV_1, FVC, residual volume, and chest radiography)

Pharmacokinetic considerations

Aminoglycosides

- Increased clearance and larger V_d, necessitating greater dosing
- Concentration-dependent killing
- Postantibiotic effect against Gram-negative organisms
- Higher doses (10 mg/kg/day tobramycin)
- Peak concentrations from 8–12 mcg/mL
- Trough concentrations of less than 2 mcg/mL

β-Lactams

- No change or increased clearance
- No change or increased V_d
- No postantibiotic effect or concentration-dependent killing

Fluoroquinolones

- Concentration-dependent killing
- Postantibiotic effect against Gram-negative organisms

Nondrug therapy

Pulmonary percussion therapy and postural drainage

The purpose of this therapy is to clear mucus and secretions from the pulmonary system. Therapy is conducted once or twice per day and up to five times daily or more. Percussion is usually conducted after nebulization therapy with or without bronchodilator or mucolytic. Therapy with handheld devices or oscillatory vests can be done.

Transplantation

Lung transplantation is an option. Liver–lung transplantation can be done if there is liver involvement.

Attention-Deficit/Hyperactivity Disorder

According to the American Psychiatric Association's *Diagnostic and Statistical Manual of Mental Disorders* (DSM-IV), attention-deficit/hyperactivity disorder (ADHD) is a behavioral disorder of childhood onset (by age 7) characterized by symptoms of inattentiveness and impulsive or hyperactive behavior.

Classification

DSM-IV makes the following classifications:

- *Combined type:* Criteria for inattention, hyperactivity, and impulsivity are met.
- *Predominantly inattentive type:* Criteria for inattention are met, but not for hyperactivity and impulsivity.
- *Predominantly hyperactive and impulsive type:* Criteria for inattention are not met, and criteria for hyperactivity and impulsivity are met.
- *ADHD not otherwise specified.*

Clinical presentation

- *Inattention:* The child has difficulty paying attention, daydreams frequently, is easily distracted and disorganized, and loses things frequently.
- *Hyperactivity:* The child has difficulty staying seated and talks too much.
- *Impulsivity:* The child acts and speaks out without thinking, and the child also interrupts others frequently.

Pathophysiology

ADHD results from an imbalance in catecholamine neurotransmission (specifically between dopamine and norepinephrine).

Genetic basis

Genetic studies have primarily evaluated genes involved in neurotransmission. ADHD is likely to be due to the interaction of many genes. Most evidence currently indicates that dopamine transmitter (DAT-1) and dopamine D_2 and D_4 receptors are responsible (dopamine and norepinephrine are potent agonists of the D_4 receptor).

Diagnostic criteria

Diagnostic criteria must be met for accurate diagnosis. Diagnosis is based on DSM-IV criteria that six or more of the criteria for inattention or hyperactivity and impulsivity are met for at least 6 months "to a degree that is maladaptive and inconsistent with developmental level."

Some impairment should be present before age 7. Impairment should be present in at least two settings (e.g., home and school). Evidence of clinically significant impairment in functioning should also be present.

Symptoms must not be related to another illness (e.g., schizophrenia or mood disorder).

Treatment goals

- Educate the patient and family.
- Improve functioning and behavior.
- Achieve effective drug therapy with minimal side effects.

Drug therapy

Table 33-4 describes drug therapy for ADHD.

Patient counseling

Advise patients and caregivers of the need to store medications away from other children or siblings because of the potential for lethal overdose (tricyclic antidepressants) and for abuse (stimulants).

Adverse drug events

Stimulants cause anorexia, abdominal pain, headache, insomnia, jitteriness, social withdrawal, transient motor tics, and weight loss (not height dependent).

Methylphenidate is contraindicated in a seizure disorder according to the package insert (i.e., it lowers the seizure threshold). Canada has suspended marketing of Adderall XR because of concern over reports of sudden death and stroke in patients taking Adderall or Adderall XR.

Tricyclics carry cardiotoxicity risk (sudden death). Patients should undergo electrocardiogram (ECG) testing prior to initiation of therapy and periodically throughout therapy.

Bupropion may lower the seizure threshold. Seizures are associated with high doses and a previous history of seizure disorders. Minimize risk by dividing the daily dose or by using the extended-release formulation.

Labeling for all the stimulants and for atomoxetine includes warnings for an increased risk of psychosis or mania, aggression or violent behavior, and anxiety or panic attacks. Atomoxetine labeling includes warnings for an increased risk of suicidal ideation in children and adolescents and for the potential for severe liver injury.

Drug interactions
Methylphenidate
- Methylphenidate should not be given with monoamine oxidase (MAO) inhibitors (severe hypertension).
- Caffeine may enhance stimulant effects.

- Methylphenidate may inhibit metabolism of phenytoin, phenobarbital, warfarin, and tricyclics.

Tricyclics
- Multiple pharmacodynamic and pharmacokinetic drug interactions exist.
- Increased plasma concentrations of tricyclics could result in potential toxicity when certain antidepressants are added to the regimen (fluoxetine, sertraline, fluvoxamine, paroxetine) as well as with cimetidine, methylphenidate, diltiazem, quinidine, and verapamil.
- Decreased concentrations of tricyclics may be seen with concomitant administration of carbamazepine and phenytoin.
- Increased therapeutic effect and potential toxicity may occur with MAO inhibitors.
- Increased central nervous system depressant effects occur with alcohol and sedatives.

Recommendations for therapy and monitoring
The efficacy of therapy should be monitored. Assess behavior changes and evaluate feedback from teachers and parents.

Stimulants
Begin with a low dose, and titrate upward to optimal functioning ability. The patient may need a decreased dose if side effects occur or if no further improvement is seen with the larger dose.

No therapeutic drug monitoring or ECG monitoring is needed.

If one stimulant fails, try another stimulant for the patient. For children who fail two stimulants, try a third type of stimulant.

Tricyclics
Initial and periodic ECGs are needed.

Pharmacokinetic considerations
Methylphenidate does not distribute well into adipose tissue (dose on milligram basis instead of milligrams per kilogram).

Nondrug therapy

- Behavioral techniques (e.g., positive reinforcement, time out, response cost, and token economy)
- Environmental modifications
- Classroom management

Conjunctivitis

Conjunctivitis is an inflammation of the conjunctiva of the eye.

Table 33-4. Drug Therapy for Attention-Deficit/Hyperactivity Disorder

Therapeutic category	Indication and mechanism of action	Comments
Stimulants (first-line therapy)		
Short-acting: methylphenidate (Ritalin, Methylin); intermediate-acting: methylphenidate (Ritalin SR, Metadate ER, Methylin ER); long-acting: methylphenidate (Concerta, Metadate CD, Ritalin LA, Daytrana); short-acting amphetamine (Dexedrine, Dextrostat); intermediate-acting amphetamine (Adderall, Dexedrine Spansule); long-acting amphetamine (Adderall-XR)	Reuptake blockade of catecholamines (norepinephrine and dopamine) in presynaptic nerve endings	Because of concern of sudden death and stroke, methylphenidate should not be used in children or adults with structural cardiac abnormalities.
		Do not give after 4:00 pm because later doses may cause insomnia.
		Spansules may be opened and contents sprinkled on applesauce.
		Methylphenidate is not labeled for use in children < 6 years of age.
		Daytrana is a transdermal patch and should be applied every morning to alternating hips and worn for 9 hours.
		Amphetamines are not labeled for use in children < 3 years of age.
		Adderall can be crushed.
		Drug holidays are recommended (e.g., summer is a good time to see if patient is outgrowing disease).
		Products are not addictive in children with ADHD, but some parents or siblings may abuse child's medications.
Antidepressants (second-line therapy)		
Tricyclics (imipramine, desipramine)	Reuptake blockade of norepinephrine and serotonin presynaptically	Tricyclics may be used in patients who fail to respond or are intolerant to stimulants.
		Tricyclics are drug of choice in ADHD with depression.
		They have longer duration of action.
		No rebound or wearing-off effect occurs.
		Rapid onset occurs in ADHD; effect can be noticed in 3–4 days. Taper off patient's dosage over 2 to 3 weeks.
		Baseline and follow-up ECGs are needed.
Bupropion (Wellbutrin, Wellbutrin SR, Wellbutrin XL)	Indirect dopamine agonist and nonadrenergic effects	Products may induce seizures.
Other agents (not currently supported by most recent AAP Guidelines, 2001)		
D-threo-enantiomer of racemic methylphenidate, dexmethylphenidate (Focalin)	Blockade of dopamine and norepinephrine in presynaptic nerve endings	D-enantiomer is thought to be the more active enantiomer.
Atomoxetine (Strattera)	Noradrenergic-specific reuptake inhibitor	Product is a nonstimulant agent; discontinue in patients who develop jaundice or laboratory evidence of liver injury.
Clonidine	α_2-noradrenergic agonist	Clonidine is a good drug to use with ADHD and coexisting conditions such as sleep disturbances.
Pemoline (Cylert)	Blockade of dopamine and norepinephrine in presynaptic nerve endings	Product was withdrawn by manufacturer; previously, it was rarely used secondary to association with fatal hepatic failure (not dose or time related).

Classification

Conjunctivitis may be bacterial, viral, or allergic.

Clinical presentation

Conjunctivitis is characterized by redness of the eye, itching, ocular discharge, foreign body sensation, and crusting of the eye and eyelid. Patient may have altered vision because of the presence of discharge.

Pathophysiology

Conjunctivitis of the newborn

Inflammation of the conjunctiva often occurs in the first month of life. Causative agents include topical antimicrobial agents; bacteria (primarily *Neisseria gonorrhoeae, Chlamydia trachomatis, Staphylococcus aureus, Staphylococcus epidermidis, Streptococcus pneumoniae, Escherichia coli,* and other Gram-negative bacteria); and viruses (primarily herpes simplex).

Bacterial conjunctivitis (beyond first month of life)

The most common bacteria are *Staphylococcus aureus, Staphylococcus epidermidis, Streptococcus pneumoniae,* and *Haemophilus influenzae* (also gono-coccal and chlamydial). Treat bacterial conjunctivitis with antibiotic therapy.

Viral conjunctivitis

Viral conjunctivitis, also known as pink eye, is contagious. Adenovirus is the most common causative agent.

This condition is commonly preceded by a cold or sore throat or exposure to another person with viral conjunctivitis.

Herpes simplex (corneal involvement may yield permanent visual damage) may also be seen.

Allergic conjunctivitis

Allergic conjunctivitis is caused by exposure to dander, pollen, or topical eye preparation. Most patients will exhibit itching of the eye.

Diagnostic criteria

Diagnosis is based on the patient's symptoms.

Treatment goals

- Eliminate or avoid the allergen (allergic conjunctivitis).
- Treat the underlying infection (bacterial conjunctivitis).
- Decrease severity and provide symptomatic relief (all forms).

Drug therapy

Neonatal

Preventive medicine includes prophylaxis after delivery with antibacterial ophthalmic ointment (erythromycin, tetracycline, silver nitrate, and povidone-iodine):

- **Onset day 1:** No treatment (secondary to prophylaxis after delivery)
- **Onset days 2–4 (Neisseria gonorrhoeae):** Penicillin G or ceftriaxone for 7 days
- **Onset days 3–10 (Chlamydia trachomatis):** Oral erythromycin + erythromycin ointment for 14 days
- **Onset days 2–16 (herpes simplex):** Possibly IV acyclovir

Bacterial (beyond first month of life)

Topical antibiotic therapy (bacitracin-polymyxin B, trimethoprim-polymyxin B, erythromycin, or fluoroquinolone [ciprofloxacin, gentamicin, or tobramycin]) should be used in combination with an antibiotic ointment (erythromycin or bacitracin) at bedtime for 5–7 days.

Gonococcal

Ceftriaxone should be used for one dose. With corneal ulceration, use systemic IV ceftriaxone therapy. Also treat for *Chlamydia* species.

Chlamydial

For adults, oral tetracycline or doxycycline is administered for 2–3 weeks. Administer a single dose of azithromycin to children.

Viral

Ocular lubricant (artificial tears) should be administered every 3–4 hours while the patient is awake.

Allergic

Remove allergen. Use ocular lubricant (artificial tears); ocular decongestants (phenylephrine, naphazoline, tetrahydrozoline, and oxymetazoline: α-adrenergic activity); antihistamines (olopatadine [Patanol]); antihistamine–decongestant combination products (pheniramine and naphazoline [Naphcon-A, Opcon-A, and Visine-A]); topical mast cell stabilizer (cromolyn sodium); combination mast cell stabilizer and antihistamine; or oral antihistamine therapy.

Adverse drug events

Ocular decongestants can cause rebound congestion of the conjunctiva. This reaction is less common with naphazoline and tetrahydrozoline.

Instilling of eye drops and ointment

Wash hands before and after administration. Tilt head back, grasp lower eyelid and pull away from eye, place dropper or ointment tube over eye, and have the child look up immediately before instilling the drop.

For ointment, use a sweeping motion and instill 0.25 to 0.5 inch of ointment inside eyelid. Close eye after instillation, and wait 1–2 minutes. Blot excess ointment or solution away from around the eye. Vision may be temporarily blurred with ointment administration.

Wait 5 minutes between drops for multiple drop therapy. For suspension, place that drop in the eye last. For use of both ointment and drops, instill drops first and wait 10 minutes before applying ointment.

Patient instructions and counseling

- Wash hands.
- Do not share towels or linens.
- Store products according to labeling instructions.

Nondrug therapy

Cold compresses are a helpful nondrug therapy.

Recent Pediatric Medication Issues and Labeling Changes

In October 2004, the U.S. Food and Drug Administration (FDA) mandated black box warnings for all antidepressants regarding the potential for increased suicidal behavior in children.

In January 2005, the FDA sent out a letter warning health care professionals that the use of promethazine is contraindicated in children under age 2 because of the risk of respiratory depression and death.

In July 2005, the FDA mandated black box warnings for the use of fentanyl. The FDA mandated that fentanyl should not be used in children under age 2 and should only be used in children 2 years of age or older if they are already using other opioid narcotic pain medicines (i.e., they are opioid tolerant).

In January 2006, the FDA requested the addition of boxed warnings to the labeling for Elidel Cream (pimecrolimus) and Protopic Ointment (tacrolimus) to notify patients about the possible risk of cancer.

Use of these drugs in children under age 2 is not recommended.

In May 2006, the FDA requested labeling changes for Serevent Diskus (salmeterol xinafoate inhalation powder), Advair Diskus (fluticasone propionate and salmeterol inhalation powder), and Foradil Aerolizer (formoterol fumarate inhalation powder) to include a warning that these medicines may increase the risk of severe asthma attacks and death when these attacks occur.

In August 2007, a letter was sent out warning health care professionals about the concomitant use of ceftriaxone and IV calcium-containing products and the risk of ceftriaxone and calcium precipitation. Deaths attributable to intravascular and pulmonary precipitates have occurred in neonates. Ceftriaxone should not be used in neonates ($\leq$ 28 days of age) if they are receiving or are expected to receive calcium-containing IV products.

In October 2007, the FDA recommended that over-the-counter cough and cold medicines not be used in infants and children under age 2 because of the risk of serious and potentially life-threatening side effects.

In January 2008, the FDA mandated labeling changes for antiepileptic agents to include a warning about the risk of suicidal thoughts or actions.

33-3. Key Points

- The pharmacokinetics and pharmacodynamics of medications are altered by developmental differences in absorption, distribution, metabolism, and elimination in pediatric patients.
- Pharmacotherapy should be adjusted according to the developmental differences to optimize therapeutic efficacy while minimizing the risk of toxicity.
- Although spontaneous resolution does occur in many cases of acute otitis media, antibiotic therapy is initiated to prevent complications such as meningitis and mastoiditis. The observation option is an acceptable initial treatment for select patients depending on age, certainty of diagnosis, and disease severity.
- The incidence of drug-resistant *Streptococcus pneumoniae* is increasing. Because of its safety profile, cost, and excellent pharmacodynamic profile against sensitive and drug-resistant *S. pneumoniae*, amoxicillin remains the drug of choice for uncomplicated and nonsevere

acute otitis media. Higher doses should routinely be used.

■ Therapy for cystic fibrosis should focus on halting the progression of the disease and maintaining pulmonary function. Appropriate therapies decrease mucus viscosity and increase clearance of secretions; manage acute infectious exacerbations; and by using appropriate pancreatic enzyme supplementation, maintain normal growth and development.

■ Pharmacokinetics of medications in cystic fibrosis patients may be altered; therapeutic drug monitoring and dose alterations should be conducted to ensure efficacy and decrease toxicity.

■ An accurate diagnosis of attention-deficit/hyperactivity disorder, a behavioral disorder of childhood onset characterized by inattentiveness, hyperactivity, and impulsivity, should be obtained prior to initiating drug therapy.

■ Pharmacotherapy for ADHD is with stimulants (first line) and antidepressants (second line).

■ ADHD pharmacotherapy should be titrated to the desired functional effect without increasing the risk of side effects.

■ ADHD therapy should include behavioral modification. Monitoring of drug and nondrug therapy should include input from different environments (i.e., parents and teachers).

■ Bacterial and viral conjunctivitis may occur in the first month of life. Antimicrobial ointment administration should be instituted after delivery for prophylaxis.

■ Bacterial, viral, and allergic conjunctivitis should be treated with antimicrobial therapy (bacterial); symptomatic therapy (bacterial, viral, and allergic); and ocular antihistamines, decongestants, mast cell stabilizers, or combination products (allergic).

33-4. Questions

1. J. S., a 4-day-old infant (37 weeks' gestation, birth weight 3.2 kg, length 52 cm), has been admitted to the hospital secondary to spiking temperatures. J. S. has demonstrated decreased oral intake and irritability since being discharged home from the newborn nursery 2 days ago. J. S. is started on IV fluid at maintenance volume and antimicrobial therapy with ampicillin 165 mg IV q6h and gentamicin 8 mg IV q8h. Cultures have been obtained and are pending from blood, urine, and CSF. Laboratory assessment includes the following: Na 142 mEq/L, K 3.5 mEq/L, Cl 108 mEq/L, HCO_3 22 mEq/L, BUN 15 mg/dL, SCr 0.9 mg/dL, and Glc 88 mg/dL. What is J. S.'s estimated creatinine clearance (in milliliters per minute)?

   A. 100
   B. 80
   C. 60
   D. 50
   E. 25

2. Which of the following may affect the creatinine clearance estimate in this patient?

   I.   The presence of maternal serum creatinine
   I.   Decreased glomerular filtration rate
   II. Increased tubular secretion rate

   A. I only
   B. III only
   C. I and II only
   D. II and III only
   E. I, II, and III

3. Aminoglycosides are hydrophilic compounds. Which of the following is true regarding aminoglycoside pharmacokinetic parameters in premature neonates compared with those in adults?

   A. Increased clearance
   B. Increased V_d
   C. Decreased half-life
   D. Unchanged elimination
   E. Increased liver metabolism

4. Which of the following may complicate phenytoin therapy in a 2-day-old infant with new-onset seizures?

   I.   Hypoalbuminemia
   II. Physiologic jaundice
   III. IV lipid therapy

   A. I only
   B. III only
   C. I and II only
   D. II and III only
   E. I, II, and III

5. A drug metabolized through which of the following reactions is a concern in the neonatal population?

A. Hydrolysis
B. Reduction
C. Sulfation
D. Glucuronidation
E. Methylation

6. M. J., a 7-month-old female, is brought to your pharmacy by her mother, who describes the infant as having new onset of fever (102.5°F) and increased irritability in the past 24 hours. The mother states that she stayed home with M. J. today instead of sending her to day care. M. J. has been bottle-fed since birth. Family history is significant for an older sibling with a recent upper respiratory tract infection. Examination of her ear canal using a pneumatic otoscope reveals a bulging, red tympanic membrane with no mobility on negative or positive pressure. Computer records reveal she has been treated for acute otitis media twice since birth (at 3 and 5 months of age). Decisions for antimicrobial therapy in this patient should be based on coverage for which of the following pathogens?

A. *Staphylococcus epidermidis, Streptococcus pneumoniae,* and *Pseudomonas aeruginosa*
B. *Streptococcus pneumoniae, Haemophilus influenzae,* and *Moraxella catarrhalis*
C. *Haemophilus influenzae, Streptococcus pyogenes,* and *Pseudomonas aeruginosa*
D. *Streptococcus pneumoniae, Staphylococcus aureus,* and *Moraxella catarrhalis*
E. *Staphylococcus epidermidis, Pseudomonas aeruginosa,* and *Burkholderia cepacia*

7. The drug of choice for M. J.'s current episode of acute otitis media is

A. amoxicillin.
B. amoxicillin-clavulanate.
C. IM ceftriaxone.
D. cefixime.
E. trimethoprim-sulfamethoxazole.

8. When the pharmacist is counseling M. J.'s mother about the antibiotic suspension prescribed by M. J.'s physician, which of the following should be discussed?

I. Risk factors for otitis media
II. Whether the suspension should be refrigerated
III. The need to shake the suspension vigorously prior to administration

A. I only
B. III only
C. I and II only
D. II and III only
E. I, II, and III

9. Which of the following is a common side effect of amoxicillin-clavulanate therapy?

A. Hemolytic anemia
B. Liver function test abnormalities
C. Pancreatitis
D. Diarrhea
E. Headache

10. Which of the following is a side effect that should be a concern in a child with acute otitis media and nausea and vomiting who is receiving ibuprofen for fever?

A. Stevens–Johnson syndrome
B. Renal insufficiency
C. Hyponatremia
D. Oral candidiasis
E. Liver failure

11. How is otitis externa, or swimmer's ear, best treated?

A. Instill an antimicrobial and steroid solution into the ear canal.
B. Apply antimicrobial ointment into the ear canal with a cotton swab.
C. Instill an antihistamine solution into the ear canal.
D. Increase pH of the ear canal with administration of Burow's solution.
E. Decrease pH of ear canal with administration of dilute HCl solution.

12. R. E., age 15, weighs 40 kg and has cystic fibrosis. R. E. is admitted to the hospital secondary to an acute pulmonary exacerbation. Home medications include Ultrase as directed, TOBI nebulization, ADEK qd, and dornase alfa (qd nebulization). She is started on ceftazidime 2 g IV q8h and tobramycin 130 mg IV q8h. Which of the following should be ordered in this patient?

A. Serum tobramycin peak concentration
B. Serum tobramycin trough concentration
C. Serum tobramycin peak and trough concentrations
D. Sputum ceftazidime concentration
E. Sputum ceftazidime and tobramycin concentrations

13. Sputum cultures taken from R. E. shortly after hospital admission are positive for *Staphylococcus aureus* (non–methicillin sensitive). Which of the following agents should be initiated at this time?

    A. Oxacillin
    B. Ticarcillin
    C. Piperacillin
    D. Vancomycin
    E. Amikacin

14. Which of the following is a pancreatic enzyme supplement?

    A. Actigall
    B. Beractant
    C. Creon
    D. Diabinese
    E. Pulmozyme

15. Which of the following can be used to decrease the viscosity of pulmonary secretions?

    A. Exosurf
    B. Mucomyst
    C. Protilase
    D. Liquaemin
    E. Serevent

16. Counseling a patient on the use of pancreatic enzyme supplementation should include which of the following?

    A. Capsules may be opened and sprinkled over any food.
    B. Capsule contents should not be crushed or chewed.
    C. The total daily dose may be given at one time in the evening.
    D. Adequate supplementation will increase bowel movement frequency.
    E. The supplementation dose should not change with diet changes.

17. N. G., age 8, has newly diagnosed attention-deficit/hyperactivity disorder. Which of the following is *not* considered first-line therapy for N. G.?

    A. Ritalin
    B. Dexedrine
    C. Wellbutrin
    D. Adderall
    E. Methylin

18. Atomoxetine is associated with which of the following serious adverse effects?

    A. Hepatic injury
    B. Renal failure
    C. Cardiovascular collapse
    D. Anaphylaxis
    E. Toxic epidermal necrolysis

19. T. S., age 9, is being started on imipramine therapy after failing therapy for ADHD with several different stimulants. T. S. has two other siblings, a 15-year-old brother and a 3-year-old sister. The pharmacist instructs T. S.'s parents to keep the medicine away from siblings and in a safe place. What is the most likely reason for the pharmacist's concern?

    I.   Toxicity of imipramine with overdose
    II. Abuse potential of imipramine
    III. Stability of imipramine product

    A. I only
    B. III only
    C. I and II only
    D. II and III only
    E. I, II, and III

20. A decrease in seizure threshold is a side effect of which of the following agents used for ADHD?

    I.   Methylphenidate
    II. Bupropion
    III. Clonidine

    A. I only
    B. III only
    C. I and II only
    D. II and III only
    E. I, II, and III

21. Every spring, M. S. develops itchy, red eyes, which are often swollen and draining. Which of the following is the most likely cause of this ocular disorder?

    A. Viral conjunctivitis
    B. Bacterial conjunctivitis
    C. Allergic conjunctivitis
    D. Blepharitis
    E. Episcleritis

22. Which of the following therapies is *not* an appropriate recommendation for M. S.'s symptoms?

A. Ocular lubricant
B. Ocular decongestant
C. Ocular antihistamine
D. Ocular mast cell stabilizer
E. Ocular antimicrobial

23. Which of the following is *not* commonly associated with conjunctivitis?

    A. *Chlamydia*
    B. *Neisseria*
    C. *Staphylococcus*
    D. *Streptococcus*
    E. *Clostridium*

24. Which of the following is a side effect of the prolonged use of ocular decongestants?

    A. Peripheral vasodilation
    B. Rebound conjunctival congestion
    C. Development of arrhythmias
    D. Development of tolerance
    E. Development of allergy to product

33-5. Answers

1. **E.** Using the Schwartz equation, J. S.'s estimated creatinine clearance is 26 mL/min (CrCl = 0.45 × 52/0.9).

2. **C.** The presence of maternal serum creatinine that decreases in neonates over the first week of life may cause a false underestimate of creatinine clearance to be calculated during this time. If one assumes that by the end of the first week of life, J. S.'s SCr has decreased to within the normal infant range to 0.4 mg/dL, the estimated CrCl would be 59 mL/min (CrCl = 0.45 × 52/0.4). Other factors that affect creatinine clearance in the neonate and infant include a decreased glomerular filtration rate and a decreased tubular secretion rate.

3. **B.** Aminoglycosides are hydrophilic compounds; they will exhibit larger volumes of distribution in patients with greater total body water. Neonates and infants have greater total body water, greater extracellular fluid volume, and a relative lack of adipose tissue.

4. **E.** Phenytoin is a highly plasma protein-bound drug. The total and free concentrations of highly protein-bound drugs may be altered because of developmental differences in protein binding (decreased protein concentrations and altered binding capacity) and displacement by endogenous substances (e.g., free fatty acids and unconjugated bilirubin). Physiologic jaundice, as exhibited by increasing total and unconjugated bilirubin concentrations, may occur in the neonatal period. Unconjugated bilirubin may displace drugs from albumin binding sites. Additionally, one of the by-products of lipid metabolism, free fatty acids, may also displace drugs from albumin binding sites (thereby increasing the free drug concentration). Kernicterus (also known as *yellow brain*) may occur when unconjugated bilirubin displaced by drugs or other endogenous substances (i.e., free fatty acids) crosses the blood–brain barrier, where it can deposit in the brain and cause neurologic complications.

5. **D.** UDPG (uridine diphosphoglucose)–glucuronyl transferase is responsible for conjugation of endogenous substances (bilirubin) and medications (morphine and chloramphenicol). The capacity for glucuronidation metabolism does not begin until around 2 months of age and reaches adult capacity by 2 years of age. Medications metabolized through this system are potential toxins in the neonatal population. An example would be the use of chloramphenicol in neonates and the development of "gray-baby syndrome" because of drug accumulation. Hydrolysis, reduction, sulfation, and methylation are functional in the neonatal period and should not pose drug therapy complications in this population.

6. **B.** The most common pathogens in acute otitis media are *Streptococcus pneumoniae* (40–50%), *Haemophilus influenzae* (20–30%), and *Moraxella catarrhalis* (10–15%).

7. **B.** Despite the emergence of drug–resistant *Streptococcus pneumoniae*, amoxicillin—because of its excellent pharmacodynamic profile, side effect profile, and cost—remains the drug of choice in uncomplicated and nonsevere acute otitis media. However, amoxicillin-clavulanate is now considered first-line therapy in patients with severe illness. This patient is considered to be in the high-risk group (age < 2 years, day care attendance, and recurrent otitis media) and should be treated with antibiotics. High-dose therapy with amoxicillin-clavulanate (90 mg/kg/day amoxicillin and 6.4 mg/kg/day clavulanate) should be used first line in this patient because of symptoms consistent with severe illness

(moderate or severe otalgia or fever of 39°C or 102.2°F or greater).

8. **E.** Counseling should include specific information about the antibiotic, its side effect profile, storage information, information about administering the medicine, dosage instructions, the importance of taking the full course, and the need to shake the bottle prior to administering the dose. In addition, a discussion of risk factors for acute otitis media and preventive measures (pneumococcal and flu immunization) is appropriate in a counseling session.

9. **D.** The most common side effects with amoxicillin-clavulanate therapy include rash, urticaria, nausea, vomiting, and diarrhea. Although the other listed side effects may be seen with other antibiotic therapies, they do not typically occur with amoxicillin-clavulanate therapy.

10. **B.** Dehydration, which may develop in a child who is vomiting, is a risk factor for ibuprofen-induced renal insufficiency. If ibuprofen is used as an antipyretic or analgesic in pediatric patients, the parents or caregivers should be counseled regarding this risk and the need to follow intakes and outputs during the period of acute illness (i.e., gastroenteritis) when the child may be receiving ibuprofen therapy.

11. **A.** The treatment of otitis externa includes the instillation of an antibiotic and steroid otic solution into the ear canal. Cotton swabs should be avoided to prevent otitis externa. Antihistamine solutions are not indicated in the treatment of otitis externa. Otic solutions containing acetic acid may also be of benefit in otitis externa by decreasing (not increasing) the pH of the ear canal and lowering its bacteria-harboring potential. Hydrochloric acid in any form should not be used in the ear canal.

12. **C.** Therapeutic drug monitoring is a critical part of the overall therapeutic plan in patients with cystic fibrosis. Patients with cystic fibrosis exhibit altered pharmacokinetic parameters of aminoglycosides, primarily increased clearance and greater volumes of distribution. Tobramycin peak concentrations should be obtained to make sure the dose being given is sufficient to reach concentrations of 8–12 mcg/mL, and trough concentrations should be obtained to ensure adequate renal clearance (cystic fibrosis patients receive higher milligram/kilogram doses).

13. **D.** *S. aureus* is a common pathogen in cystic fibrosis patients. Methicillin–sensitive *S. aureus*

may be treated with a number of agents (e.g., oxacillin); however, methicillin–resistant *S. aureus* should be treated with vancomycin.

14. **C.** Creon is the brand name for a pancreatic enzyme supplement. Creon is available as a microencapsulated formulation.

15. **B.** Mucomyst is the brand name for N-acetylcysteine, which lowers mucus viscosity (the sulfhydryl group opens the disulfide bond in mucoproteins).

16. **B.** Pancreatic enzyme products are available in powder, tablet, and microencapsulated formulations. The microencapsulated formulations may be opened and the contents sprinkled over acidic foods (e.g., applesauce). Contents should not be crushed or chewed. Additionally, the dose should be based on the amount and type of food (i.e., full doses with meals or half-doses with snacks and light meals). Adequate replacement will actually decrease bowel movements and improve stool consistency (i.e., decrease steatorrhea).

17. **C.** All of the listed products are stimulants, with the exception of Wellbutrin. Stimulants are considered first-line therapy for ADHD; antidepressants may be considered second-line agents.

18. **A.** Atomoxetine's labeling has a warning about the potential for severe liver injury. Atomoxetine should be discontinued in any patient who develops jaundice or laboratory evidence of liver injury.

19. **A.** Overdose of tricyclic antidepressants may be fatal because of the development of arrhythmias. Because T. S. has a younger sibling in the house, there is a potential for the child to get into her older brother's medicine. Stimulants may have the potential for abuse in patients who do not have ADHD (i.e., the 15-year-old brother), but tricyclic antidepressants are not associated with a high abuse potential. There are no stability issues with imipramine.

20. **C.** Both bupropion and methylphenidate may lower the seizure threshold. Clonidine is not associated with seizure occurrence.

21. **C.** Allergic conjunctivitis occurs after exposure to allergens, primarily dander or pollen. Patients suffering from allergic conjunctivitis will typically complain of eye itching.

22. **E.** Antimicrobial therapy has no place in therapy for allergic conjunctivitis. Ocular lubricants, decongestants, antihistamines, mast

cell stabilizers, or combinations of these products are appropriate options for allergic conjunctivitis.

23. **E.** The most common pathogens in neonatal bacterial conjunctivitis are *Neisseria gonorrhoeae*, *Chlamydia trachomatis*, *Staphylococcus aureus*, *Staphylococcus epidermidis*, *Streptococcus pneumoniae*, and *Escherichia coli*. Bacterial conjunctivitis beyond the first month of life is most commonly caused by *Staphylococcus aureus*, *Staphylococcus epidermidis*, *Streptococcus pneumoniae*, and *Haemophilus influenzae*. *Clostridium*, an anaerobe, is not a common bacterial pathogen in conjunctivitis.

24. **B.** Not unlike reactions from prolonged use of nasal decongestants, prolonged use of ocular decongestants may cause rebound congestion of the conjunctiva. This effect is less pronounced with naphazoline and tetrahydrozoline.

33-6. References

American Academy of Child and Adolescent Psychiatry. Practice parameter for the use of stimulant medication in the treatment of children, adolescents, and adults. *J Am Acad Child Adolesc Psychiatry*. 2002;41(suppl 2):26S–49S.

American Academy of Family Physicians, American Academy of Otolaryngology–Head and Neck Surgery, American Academy of Pediatrics Subcommittee on Otitis Media with Effusion. Otitis media with effusion. *Pediatrics*. 2004;113: 1412–29.

American Academy of Pediatrics, Committee on Quality Improvement and Subcommittee on Attention-Deficit/Hyperactivity Disorder. Clinical practice guideline: Treatment of the school-aged child with attention-deficit/hyperactivity disorder. *Pediatrics*. 2001;108:1033–44.

American Academy of Pediatrics, Committee on Quality Improvement and Subcommittee on Attention-Deficit/Hyperactivity Disorder. Diagnosis and evaluation of the child with attention-deficit/hyperactivity disorder. *Pediatrics*. 2000; 105:1158–70.

American Academy of Pediatrics, Subcommittee on Management of Acute Otitis Media. Diagnosis and management of acute otitis media. *Pediatrics*. 2004;113:1451–65.

American Pharmaceutical Association. *Special Report: Medication Administration Problem-Solving in Ambulatory Care*. Washington, D.C.: American Pharmaceutical Association; 1994:9.

American Psychiatric Association. *Diagnostic and Statistical Manual of Mental Disorders* (DSM-IV), 4th ed. Washington, D.C.: American Psychiatric Association; 1994:78–85.

Beringer P. Cystic fibrosis. In: Herfindal ET, Gourley DR, eds. *Textbook of Therapeutics: Drug and Disease Management*. 7th ed. Baltimore: Lippincott Williams & Wilkins; 2000:781–94.

Clinical Practice Guidelines for Cystic Fibrosis Committee. *Clinical Practice Guidelines for Cystic Fibrosis*. Bethesda, Md.: Cystic Fibrosis Foundation; 1997.

Dowell SF, Butler JC, Giebink GS, et al. Acute otitis media: Management and surveillance in an era of pneumococcal resistance—A report from the Drug-Resistant *Streptococcus pneumoniae* Therapeutic Working Group. *Pediatr Infect Dis J*. 1999; 18:1–9.

Dowell SF, Marcy SM, Phillips WR, et al. Otitis media—Principles of judicious use of antimicrobial agents. *Pediatrics*. 1998;101:165–71.

Faden H, Duffy L, Boeve M. Otitis media: Back to basics. *Pediatr Infect Dis J*. 1998;17:1105–13.

Fiscella RG, Jensen MK. Ophthalmic disorders. In: Berardi RR, Ferreri SP, Hume AL, et al., eds. *Handbook of Nonprescription Drugs: An Interactive Approach to Self-Care*. 16th ed. Washington, D.C.: American Pharmaceutical Association; 2009: 519–43.

Kearns GL, Abdel-Rahman SM, Alander SW, et al. Developmental pharmacology: Drug disposition, action, and therapy in infants and children. *N Engl J Med*. 2003;349:1157–67.

Krypel L. Otic disorders. In: Berardi RR, Ferreri SP, Hume AL, et al., eds. *Handbook of Nonprescription Drugs. An Interactive Approach to Self-Care*. 16th ed. Washington, D.C.: American Pharmaceutical Association; 2009:569–80.

Leeder JS, Kearns GL. Pharmacogenetics in pediatrics: Implications for practice. *Pediatr Clin North Am*. 1998;44:55–77.

Milavetz G. Cystic fibrosis. In: Dipiro JT, Talbert RL, Yee GC, et al., eds. *Pharmacotherapy: A Pathophysiologic Approach*. 7th ed. New York: McGraw-Hill; 2008:535–46.

Miyagi SJ, Collier AC. Pediatric development of glucoronidation: The ontogeny of hepatic UGT1A4. *Drug Metab Dispos*. 2007;35:1587–92.

Oszko MA. Common ear disorders. In: Herfindal ET, Gourley DR, eds. *Textbook of Therapeutics: Drug and Disease Management*. 7th ed. Baltimore: Lippincott Williams & Wilkins; 2000:1049–56.

Rappley MD. Attention deficit-hyperactivity disorder. *N Engl J Med.* 2005;352:165–73.

Schwartz GJ, Brion LP, Spitzer A. The use of plasma creatinine concentration for estimating glomerular filtration rate in infants, children, and adolescents. *Pediatr Clin North Am.* 1987;34:571–90.

Solomon SD. Common eye disorders. In: Herfindal ET, Gourley DR, eds. *Textbook of Therapeutics:*

Drug and Disease Management. 7th ed. Baltimore: Lippincott Williams & Wilkins; 2000:1037–48.

Stewart CF, Hampton EM. Effects of maturation on drug disposition in pediatric patients. *Clin Pharmacol.* 1987;6:548–64.

Yaffe SJ, Aranda JV. *Pediatric Pharmacology: Therapeutic Principles in Practice.* 2nd ed. Philadelphia: WB Saunders; 1992.

Geriatrics and Gerontology

34

William Nathan Rawls, PharmD

34-1. Overview

Gerontology is the study of the problems of aging and all its aspects. *Geriatrics* focuses on the diseases associated with aging and the treatments for those conditions. Geriatrics is of particular concern for pharmacists.

More than 12% of the U.S. population is older than 65 years of age. By 2050, the percentage is expected to increase to over 20%.

Persons over 65 years of age have more chronic illnesses and take more prescription and nonprescription drugs than persons in younger age groups. The use of herbal or dietary supplements by older adults has increased significantly in the last 10 years, with the increased risk of adverse events and drug interactions.

Age-related physiologic changes and increased medication use contribute to a greater risk of adverse drug events. Changes in vision, hearing, and mental functioning can result in increased problems with medication compliance.

Adverse Drug Events in the Older Adult

Drug-related hospitalizations occur four times more often for older adults than for younger adults.

Older adults receiving multiple medications are at risk of a "prescribing cascade" that occurs when an unrecognized adverse effect of a medication is treated as a new illness and additional medications are prescribed.

Older adults are at increased risk of drug–drug interactions when taking multiple medications, and this potential is decreased by medication simplification.

The possibility that a newly developed medical condition or worsening of an existing illness is related to an older adult's medication or herbal use should be considered when a pharmacist is making medication recommendations.

Changes in Pharmacokinetics Associated with Aging

Decreased absorption of various drugs occurs secondary to decreased stomach acidity and changes in blood flow to the stomach (the least altered by aging).

Altered drug distribution is caused by a decrease in total body water, increased lipid storage, and decreased serum albumin in malnourished elderly persons. These factors can contribute to increased serum levels of drugs.

Decreased hepatic blood flow and reduced hepatic enzyme activity cause slower drug metabolism. Increased levels of drugs require increased metabolism by the liver.

Elimination of drugs by the kidneys is slowed because of decreased renal blood flow and lowered glomerular filtration. Thus, drug accumulation develops.

The Cockcroft–Gault formula for estimating creatinine clearance can be used to predict renal function in the elderly:

$$\text{CrCl}(\text{mL/min}) = \frac{(140 - \text{age}) \times \text{weight in kg}}{72 \times \text{Cr}}$$

Note: Use ideal body weight. The equation above is for males. For females, multiply the result by 0.85.

In dosing the elderly, the general rule is to start with lower doses than those used in younger patients and to increase doses at a slower rate.

34-2. Drugs of Concern

The following drugs can cause psychiatric symptoms:

- Anticholinergics
- Narcotics
- Tricyclic antidepressants
- Central nervous system stimulants
- Antiparkinson drugs

The following drugs can produce anxiety symptoms:

- Theophylline
- Nasal decongestants
- β-agonists
- Antiparkinson drugs
- Appetite suppressants

The following drugs can contribute to nutritional deficiencies:

- Diuretics
- Digoxin, digitalis
- Laxatives (overuse)
- Sedatives (overuse)

These specific drugs pose a risk to geriatric patients:

- Long-acting benzodiazepines (e.g., chlordiazepoxide [Librium] and diazepam [Valium]) should be avoided because of the risk of prolonged sedation and increased risks of falls and fractures.
- Amitriptyline (Elavil) has potent anticholinergic and sedating effects with risk to older patients.
- Digoxin (Lanoxin) at higher doses (> 0.125 mg daily) has an increased risk of toxicity without greater benefits.
- Meperidine (Demerol) taken orally has an increased risk of respiratory and circulatory depression.
- Antipsychotic use may result in the increased risk of heart events and infections.

34-3. Medication Compliance and the Older Adult

Types of noncompliant behavior in the elderly include the following:

- Failure to take medications
- Premature discontinuation of a medication
- Excessive consumption of a medication
- Use of medications not currently prescribed

Several strategies can improve patient medication compliance:

- Limit the number of different medications and decrease the dose frequency.
- Simplify dosage instructions.
- Tailor the regimen to the patient's schedule.
- Use compliance aids and telephone reminders.
- Enlist the assistance of family members and friends.

34-4. Basic Components of Evaluating Drug Therapy in Older Adults

These questions should be answered in an evaluation of drug therapy:

- Why is the drug being used? A diagnosis or reason should be given
- Is the drug being given correctly? The dosage, form, and schedule of administration should be analyzed.
- Are any symptoms or complaints related to drug therapy?
- Is monitoring of treatment ongoing?
- What is the endpoint of therapy?

34-5. Alzheimer's Disease and Related Dementias

Dementia is the decline in intellectual abilities (e.g., impairment of memory, judgment, and abstract thinking) coupled with changes in personality. Dementia patients tend to be described as cognitively impaired.

Cognition is the mental process by which people become aware of objects of thought and perception, including all aspects of thinking and remembering. Impairment of cognition significantly affects the life of the dementia patient, his or her family members, and the community in general.

Types of Dementia

Alzheimer's disease accounts for approximately 70% of dementias. Vascular dementias account for approximately 15% of dementias. Patients may have both Alzheimer's disease and vascular dementia.

Other Causes of Dementia

- Vascular disease, cerebrovascular accidents (strokes)
- Neurologic disorders such as Parkinson's disease, frontotemporal dementia, dementia with Lewy bodies, and Huntington's chorea
- Metabolic disorders such as hypothyroidism, alcoholism, and anemia
- Infectious diseases such as meningitis, syphilis, AIDS (acquired immune deficiency syndrome)

Clinical Presentation

Alzheimer's disease is a progressive neurologic disease that results in impaired memory and intellectual functioning and altered behavior. Alzheimer's disease is characterized by the slow onset of symptoms leading to loss of ability to function independently. Symptoms may include psychoses with hallucinations, illusions, and delusional thinking. As Alzheimer's disease progresses, the brain continues to deteriorate.

Depression can cause cognitive impairment similar to that of Alzheimer's disease and should be identified and treated.

Pathophysiology

Hallmark pathologic changes in the brain are linked to Alzheimer's disease (i.e., neuritic plaques and neurofibrillary tangles increase). Neuritic plaques are composed of amyloid proteins deposited on neurons. Neurofibrillary tangles exist within neurons and disrupt normal function.

Neurotransmitters are also altered in Alzheimer's disease. Acetylcholine concentrations decrease significantly.

Diagnostic Criteria

Diagnosis of Alzheimer's disease requires the presence of memory impairment and one or more of the following:

- Aphasia (language disturbance)
- Apraxia (impaired motor abilities)
- Agnosia (failure to recognize objects)
- Disturbance of executive function (e.g., planning, organizing)

Treatment Principles

When evaluating a patient for treatment of dementia and Alzheimer's disease, review the patient's medications and consider any that might cause mental confusion or worsen underlying disease states. Drugs that block activity of acetylcholine can worsen dementia and decrease the effectiveness of medications used to treat Alzheimer's disease.

Anticholinergic drugs are used for a variety of conditions, ranging from depression to incontinence. Indications should be identified before treating Alzheimer's disease. Anticholinergic effects can be additive (i.e., a combination of anticholinergic drugs can result in toxicity even when each is given at low doses; see Table 34-1).

Provide support to caregivers, and treat the patient's behavioral and mood symptoms.

Table 34-1. Anticholinergic Drugs That Can Worsen Alzheimer's Disease

Class	Drugs
Antidepressants	*Highest effects:* amitriptyline, amoxapine, clomipramine, protriptyline; *moderate effects:* bupropion, doxepin, imipramine, maprotiline, trimipramine
Antiparkinsonian agents	Benztropine, trihexyphenidyl
Antipsychotics	*Highest effects:* clozapine, mesoridazine, olanzapine, promazine, triflupromazine, thioridazine; *moderate effects:* chlorpromazine, chlorprothixene, pimozide
Antispasmodics	Atropine, belladonna alkaloids, dicyclomine, glycopyrrolate, hyoscyamine, methscopolamine, oxyphencyclimine, propantheline, oxybutynin, flavoxate, terodiline
Antihistamines	*Highest effects:* carbinoxamine, clemastine, diphenhydramine, promethazine; *moderate effects:* azatadine, brompheniramine, chlorpheniramine, cyproheptadine, dexchlorpheniramine, triprolidine, hydroxyzine
Antiemetic–antivertigo agents	Meclizine, scopolamine, dimenhydrinate, trimethobenzamide, prochlorperazine
Other agents with some anticholinergic activity	Paroxetine

Consider a trial of a cholinesterase inhibitor and monitor for benefits to memory and cognitive functioning.

Monitoring

Monitor memory and cognitive functions every 6–12 months.

Routinely assess behaviors and ability to perform activities of daily living (e.g., bathing, feeding, toileting, dressing).

Monitor for focal neurologic signs and symptoms that may suggest other causes of changes in cognitive function.

Drug Therapy

The pharmacologic approach to treatment falls into two categories:

- Medications used to control behavioral and emotional symptoms
- Medications used to slow or reverse the disease process

Symptomatic therapy

Medications used to control behavioral and emotional symptoms are used to provide symptomatic improvement and do not affect the outcome of the disease.

Anxiolytics are used to decrease anxiety and possibly agitation, motor restlessness, and insomnia. Such medications include lorazepam (Ativan), oxazepam (Serax), and buspirone (Buspar). The benzodiazepines can increase the risk of falls and injury.

Antidepressants improve depression, which can worsen the cognitive functioning of a patient with Alzheimer's disease. Antidepressants include sertraline (Zoloft) and citalopram (Celexa).

Antipsychotics are used to decrease psychotic symptoms such as hallucinations and delusions. Antipsychotics such as haloperidol (Haldol), risperidone (Risperdal), and aripiprazole (Abilify) may reduce agitation and aggressiveness in dementia patients. A U.S. Food and Drug Administration (FDA) black box warning concerning the risk of increased mortality (cardiac events and infections) is associated with the use of antipsychotics in demented elderly patients.

Sedative-hypnotics are used for short-term treatment of insomnia but can increase confusion and memory impairment. These medications include trazodone (Desyrel), zolpidem (Ambien), and temazepam (Restoril).

Cholinesterase inhibitors

Medications used to slow or reverse the symptoms of Alzheimer's (see Table 34-2) affect acetylcholine activity in the brain. Acetylcholine levels may be decreased by as much as 90% in Alzheimer's disease. These levels can be increased by inhibiting the enzyme acetylcholinesterase.

Acetylcholinesterase inhibitors increase acetylcholine but do not replace lost cholinergic neurons or change the underlying pathology. This class of medications is used to prevent or slow deterioration in cognitive functioning.

The first cholinesterase inhibitor approved to treat Alzheimer's disease was tacrine (Cognex), which proved beneficial but may cause hepatotoxicity (damage to the liver). Thus, tacrine requires regular liver function testing and is rarely prescribed.

Table 34-2. Drugs Used to Treat Alzheimer's Disease

Generic name	Trade name	Usual dosage	Dosage forms	Adverse effects
Tacrine	Cognex	10–20 mg bid	Capsules	Nausea and vomiting, hepatotoxicity
Donepezil	Aricept	5–10 mg at bedtime	Tablets, oral solution, disintegrating tablets	Nausea and vomiting
Rivastigmine	Exelon	1.5–6 mg bid	Capsules, transdermal patch	Nausea and vomiting, anorexia, weight loss
Galantamine	Razadyne	4–12 mg bid	Tablets, extended-release capules, oral solution	Nausea and vomiting
Memantine	Namenda	10 mg bid	Tablets, oral solution	Headache, constipation, dizziness, hypertension

Safer cholinesterase inhibitors include the following:

- Donepezil (Aricept) is selective for acetyl-cholinesterase in the brain (i.e., not in peripheral tissues) and is approved for mild to moderate and moderate to severe dementia.
- Rivastigmine (Exelon), a nonselective cholinesterase inhibitor, decreases both acetylcholinesterase and butyrylcholinesterase. It is approved for mild to moderate Alzheimer's disease and dementia associated with Parkinson's disease.
- Galantamine (Razadyne) is a selective acetyl-cholinesterase inhibitor that activates nicotinic receptors, which may increase acetylcholine. It is approved for mild to moderate Alzheimer's disease dementia.

Patient instructions and counseling
Donepezil
Give orally, 5 mg daily for 4–6 weeks. Increase dosage to 10 mg daily at bedtime. Take with or without food.

Rivastigmine
Oral doses are given with a gradual dosage increase. Begin at 1.5 mg twice daily and then 3.0 mg twice daily, 4.5 mg twice daily, and 6.0 mg twice daily, with a minimum of 2 weeks between dose increases. If rivastigmine is discontinued because of adverse effects, restart at beginning dose. Take with meals in divided doses. Transdermal patch dosing begins with 4.6 mg every 24 hours, once daily for 4 weeks. It then increases to 9.5 mg every 24 hours, once daily.

Galantamine
Doses begin with 4 mg twice daily for 4 weeks, 8 mg twice daily for 4 weeks, and then 12 mg twice daily. If galantamine is discontinued for more than a few days, restart at the beginning dose. In hepatic or renal dysfunction, doses should not exceed 16 mg per day. Do not use in instances of severe dysfunction. Take with meals in divided doses. Initiate therapy with extended-release capsules at 8 mg daily with a morning meal for 4 weeks. Increase the dose to 16 mg daily for 4 weeks and then 24 mg daily.

Adverse drug events
- ***Donepezil:*** Side effects include nausea, vomiting, and gastrointestinal (GI) symptoms. These side effects may be minimized by increasing the dose at 6 weeks.
- ***Rivastigmine:*** Side effects include nausea, vomiting, GI upset, and possibly significant weight loss. Adverse effects are dose related and may be lessened by increasing the dose at a slower rate.
- ***Galantamine:*** Adverse effects include nausea, vomiting, and GI upset. Slow dose titration will decrease side effects.

NMDA-receptor antagonists

Blocking the excitotoxicity effects of the neurotransmitter glutamate at N-methyl-D-aspartate (NMDA) receptors has been reported to be beneficial in Alzheimer's disease. Memantine (Namenda) is an NMDA-receptor antagonist used for moderate to severe Alzheimer's disease dementia. Doses begin with 5 mg daily for 1 week, increasing to 5 mg twice daily, with weekly increases to 10 mg twice daily.

The dose should be reduced to 5 mg twice daily in patients with renal impairment (creatinine clearance less than 30mL/min).

Side effects include drowsiness, dizziness, headache, blood pressure elevations, and motor restlessness.

Drug–drug interactions

Anticholinergic drugs will reduce the effectiveness of cholinesterase inhibitors and cause dry mouth, blurred vision, constipation, and mental confusion (i.e., conditions that are more problematic in the elderly).

Cytochrome P450 enzyme inhibitors of 2D6 and 3A4 increase levels of galantamine and donepezil by inhibiting their metabolism.

Dextromethorphan (Robitussin DM), a potent NMDA-receptor antagonist, should be used cautiously with memantine. Smoking and nicotine products may alter levels of memantine. Concurrent use of amantadine increases the potential for adverse effects.

Parameters to monitor

- Monitor cognitive function (e.g., poor results on mini–mental state exam, decline in performance of activities of daily living, incidence of behaviors that indicate cognitive decline).
- Watch for signs and symptoms of toxicity.
- Discontinue treatment with active peptic ulcer disease, severe bradycardia, and acute medical illness.
- Perform periodic complete blood cell count and basic chemistries.
- Look for expected benefits with the use of cholinesterase inhibitors and NMDA-receptor antagonists. Such benefits include improvement in memory, some stabilization of behaviors or

mood, and possible slowing of the progression of the disease.

Nonprescription agents

High-dose vitamin E (2,000 units daily) has been recommended as an antioxidant to slow progression of Alzheimer's disease. Vitamin E may interfere with vitamin K absorption and result in increased risk of bleeding. Increased mortality has been reported with high-dose vitamin E. The potential toxicity of high-dose vitamin E may outweigh the benefits.

Ginkgo biloba, an herb, has been used to treat symptoms of Alzheimer's disease with reports of modest benefits. Ginkgo biloba is associated with increased risk of bleeding and hemorrhage, especially when combined with daily aspirin use, and is not recommended.

Nondrug Therapy

The treatment of Alzheimer's disease includes nonpharmacologic and pharmacologic therapies. Patients need to live in an environment that permits safe activities while minimizing risk.

Caregivers need training and support to deal with the behavioral and functional issues associated with this disease. Caregivers are at risk for depression and stress-related medical illnesses. Caregivers may also neglect their own health care needs and should be encouraged to maintain a healthy lifestyle.

34-6. Parkinson's Disease

Parkinson's disease (PD) is a chronic progressive neurologic disorder with symptoms that present as a variable combination of rigidity, tremor, bradykinesia, and changes in posture and ambulation. An estimated 1 million persons in the United States suffer from PD. Approximately 60,000 new cases are diagnosed each year.

The risk of developing PD increases with age, and a substantial increase in the U.S. population of persons over 60 years of age is predicted.

Because medications are the primary treatment for PD, pharmacists play an important role in the care of these patients.

Classification

The two classes of PD are primary parkinsonism and secondary parkinsonism. Primary parkinsonism has no identified cause. Secondary parkinsonism can be the result of drug use (e.g., reserpine, metoclopramide, antipsychotics); infections; trauma; or toxins.

Clinical Presentation

Clinical signs and symptoms of PD develop insidiously, progress slowly, may fluctuate, and worsen with time despite pharmacologic therapy.

Symptoms

Tremors at rest may begin unilaterally and are present in 70% of PD patients. Tremors that do not occur during sleep may worsen with stress.

Rigidity of limbs and trunk may develop. The face may have a masklike expression. Patients may have difficulty dressing or standing from a seated position.

Akinesia (the absence of movement) and bradykinesia (slowed movements) can occur. Postural instability with abnormal gait and an increased risk of falls are often experienced.

Depression and possibly dementia are possible nonmotor symptoms of PD.

Other symptoms include micrographia (small writing), drooling, decreased blinking, constipation, and incontinence.

Pathophysiology

PD involves a progressive degeneration of the substantia nigra in the brain with a decrease in dopaminergic cells (more than the typical decrease that accompanies normal aging). The most significant neurotransmitter in PD is dopamine, but other neurotransmitters may play a role (e.g., acetylcholine, glutamate, GABA, serotonin, norepinephrine).

The etiology is unknown, but genetic susceptibility is possible. Environmental toxins combined with aging may also be responsible for the development of PD.

Diagnostic Criteria

Clinical diagnosis is based on the presence of bradykinesia and either rest tremor or rigidity. The stages of the disease are described in Table 34-3.

Treatment Principles and Goals

The goal for treating PD is to relieve symptoms and maintain or improve quality of life for the patient. Treatment should be initiated when functional impairment and discomfort for the patient or caregiver occurs.

Table 34-3. The Stages of Parkinson's Disease

Stage	Characteristics
1	Only unilateral involvement, with minimal or no functional impairment
2	Bilateral involvement without impairment of balance
3	Mild to moderate bilateral disease, with some postural instability (patient can maintain independence)
4	Severe disability (patient is unable to live alone independently)
5	Inability to walk or stand without assistance

A safe environment and caregiver support programs in addition to medications will often allow patients to remain in the community.

Drug Therapy

Mechanism of action

Medications increase dopamine or dopamine activity by directly stimulating dopamine receptors or by blocking acetylcholine activity, which results in increased dopamine effects (Table 34-4).

Selection of an initial medication to treat PD may vary with the prescriber. Some choose to begin

Table 34-4. Drugs for Treating Parkinson's Disease

Generic name	Trade name	Mechanism of action	Dosage and available strengths and forms
Carbidopa-levodopa	Sinemet	Increases dopamine (levodopa); prevents metabolism (carbidopa)	Give 25/100 mg/d at breakfast; increase to 25/100 mg tid. Dosage may be increased to 25/250 mg qid. Sustained-release 25/100 mg and 50/200 mg tablets are available.
Bromocriptine	Parlodel	Directly stimulates dopamine receptors	Give 1.25 mg bid with meals; increase by 2.5 mg/d every day, up to 100 mg/d. 2.5 mg and 5 mg tablets are available.
Pramipexole	Mirapex	Directly stimulates dopamine receptors	Give 0.125 mg tid; increase weekly to 0.5–1.5 mg tid. 0.125, 0.25, 1, and 1.5 mg tablets are available.
Ropinirole	Requip	Directly stimulates dopamine receptors	Give 0.25 mg tid; increase gradually to a maximum of 24 mg/d. 0.25, 0.5, 1, 2, 4, and 5 mg tablets are available.
Apomorphine		Directly stimulates dopamine receptors	Give 0.2–0.6 ml (2–6 mg) SC for acute attacks. Oral antiemetic (trimethobenzamide) given concurrently.
Selegiline	(Eldepryl, Carbex, Atapryl, Zelapar)	Inhibits monoamine oxidase B; increases dopamine and serotonin	Initially give 5 mg at breakfast; increase to 5 mg at breakfast and lunch. 5 mg capsules, 5 mg tablets, and 1.25 mg oral disintegrating tablets (Zelapar) are available.
Rasagiline	(Azilect)	Inhibits monoamine oxidase B; increases dopamine and serotonin	Initial monotherapy is 0.5 mg once daily, as adjunct to levodopa 0.5 mg to 1 mg daily. 0.5 mg and 1 mg tablets are available.
Entacapone	(Comtan)	Inhibits catecholamine *O*-methyl transferase (COMT), increasing dopamine	Give 200 mg with each dose of carbidopa-levodopa; maximum is 1,600 mg/d. 200 mg tablets are available.
Tolcapone	(Tasmar)	Inhibits COMT, increasing dopamine	Give 100 mg tid; discontinue if no benefits in 3 weeks. 100 and 200 mg tablets are available.
Amantadine	Symmetrel	May increase presynaptic release of dopamine; blocks reuptake	Give 100 mg bid; maximum is dose 400 mg/d. 100 mg tablets, 100 mg capsules, and 50 mg/5 mL syrup are available.
Benztropine	Cogentin	Blocks acetylcholine; may balance dopamine	Give 1–2 mg po, IM, or IV at bedtime or 0.5–6 mg/d in divided doses. 0.5, 1, and 2 mg tablets and 1 mg/mL injection are available.
Trihexyphenidyl	Artane	Blocks acetylcholine; may balance dopamine	Give 1 mg/d up to 5 mg/d (divided doses); 2 and 5 mg tablets and 2 mg/5 mL elixir are available.
Carbidopa-entacapone-levodopa	Stalevo	Combined effects of all three agents	Dosage is individualized, up to 8 tablets per day. Three dosage combinations are available.

IM, intramuscular; IV, intravenous; SC, subcutaneous.

therapy with selegiline (Eldepryl), which offers possible neuroprotection; others prescribe carbidopa-levodopa (Sinemet), which has proven benefits. Some experts will initiate therapy with a dopamine agonist in patients younger than 60 years of age.

Levodopa

Levodopa is the most effective drug in the treatment of PD and is converted to dopamine in the body. It is given with carbidopa, a decarboxylase inhibitor that prevents the peripheral conversion of levodopa to dopamine, thereby reducing nausea and vomiting while allowing more drug to pass through the blood–brain barrier.

Generally, doses are increased gradually to minimize the risk of side effects. Doses are given before meals to facilitate absorption. Carbidopa effectively inhibits peripheral conversion of levodopa at doses of 100 mg per day.

Levodopa provides benefits to all stages of PD, but chronic use is associated with adverse effects. Patients may have periods of good mobility alternating with periods of impaired motor function.

Dopamine agonists

Dopamine agonists work directly on dopamine receptors and do not require metabolic conversion. They may be used as monotherapy or as adjunctive therapy, allowing lower doses of carbidopa-levodopa.

Selective monoamine oxidase type B inhibitors

Monamine oxidase (MAO)-B inhibitors may be used as initial therapy in early PD and as adjunct treatment for more advanced disease. They may have neuroprotective properties.

With doses used for PD, adverse effects from consuming tyramine-containing foods would not be expected.

Catechol-O-methyl transferase inhibitors

Catechol-O-methyl transferase (COMT) inhibitors are ineffective when given alone and should always be given with carbidopa-levodopa. They are most often used to treat patients during end-of-dose wearing-off periods and patients experiencing motor fluctuations.

Treatment complications and strategies for improving patient response

- *No initial response:* If the patient does not initially respond to levodopa (carbidopa-levodopa combination), gradually increase the dose to at least 1,000–1,500 mg of levodopa.
- *Suboptimal response:* After increasing levodopa, add another drug (e.g., a dopamine agonist, selegiline, or a COMT inhibitor).
- *"On and off" phenomenon:* This type of response is associated with advancing disease and loss of benefits from a dose of medication. Use more frequent doses or sustained-release levodopa.
- *Acute intermittent hypomobility "off" episodes:* Such episodes are seen in advanced disease. They can be treated with subcutaneous injections of apomorphine, a direct-acting dopamine agonist.
- *End-of-dose or "wearing-off" period:* A decreased duration of benefit after a dose is experienced during a wearing-off period. Levodopa wanes after less than 4 hours; therefore, use combination therapy (two or more drugs), give levodopa more frequently, or use sustained-release levodopa (Sinemet CR).

Patient instructions and counseling

- Usually take medications on an empty stomach. Eat shortly afterward to avoid upset stomach.
- Take a missed dose as soon as possible. Skip the missed dose if the next scheduled dose is within 2 hours.
- Dizziness, drowsiness, and stomach upset may occur and make operating equipment dangerous.
- Report any confusion, mood changes, and uncontrolled movements to the prescriber as soon as possible.
- If taking a sustained-release product, do not crush.

Adverse effects and drug–drug interactions

Adverse effects of medications used to treat PD are described in Table 34-5. See Table 34-6 for information concerning drug–drug interactions.

Parameters to monitor

- Liver function, complete blood count, basic chemistries (periodically)
- Blood pressure, pulse, ECG (periodically)
- Reduction of rigidity, tremor, slowed movements
- Examination for mental confusion, mood changes, psychotic thinking

Nondrug Therapy for Parkinson's Disease

Educate the patient and caregiver about the benefits and side effects of PD medications. Provide aids for

Table 34-5. Adverse Effects of Medications Used to Treat Parkinson's Disease

Drug	Adverse effects
Dopaminergics: levodopa, pramipexole, bromocriptine, ropinirole, amantadine	Nausea and vomiting, agitation, confusion, depression, psychoses, orthostatic hypotension, dyskinetic movements, "sleep attacks," and "pathologic gambling" (dopamine agonists)
MAO-B inhibitors: selegiline, rasagiline	Nausea and vomiting, insomnia, dizziness, agitation, confusion, dyskinetic movements, anorexia
Amantadine	Confusion, dizziness, depression, anxiety, psychoses, insomnia
COMT inhibitors: tolcapone, entacapone	Nausea and vomiting, diarrhea, dyskinesia, urine coloration, liver toxicity (tolcapone)
Anticholinergics: benztropine, trihexyphenidyl	Dry mouth, blurred vision, constipation, urinary retention, confusion, agitation, psychoses

compliance to enable the patient to participate in medication use as long as he or she is physically capable.

Physical therapy or occupational therapy may be important in maintaining physical activity and improving safety of working and living quarters. As PD progresses, speech therapy may be necessary to maintain communication ability.

Dietary consultation may assist the patient in nutritional concerns related to swallowing difficulties and food selections.

34-7. Glaucoma

Glaucoma is a group of eye diseases characterized by an increase in intraocular pressure (IOP), which causes pathologic changes in the optic nerve and typical visual-field defects. Glaucoma affects over 4 million Americans, and as many as 15 million more people may have increased IOP but no clinical signs and symptoms of glaucoma.

The prevalence of glaucoma increases with age and is most often seen in those 65 years of age or older. The number of persons with glaucoma is expected to increase with the aging of the American population. With improved screening programs to identify those with increased IOP, an increase in the number of those diagnosed with glaucoma is expected.

Classification

Open-angle glaucoma is a form of primary glaucoma. The angle of the anterior chamber remains open in an eye, but filtration of aqueous humor is gradually diminished because of the tissues of the angle. Open-angle glaucoma accounts for approximately 80–90% of cases.

Angle-closure (narrow-angle) glaucoma is a form of primary glaucoma in an eye characterized by a shallow anterior chamber and a narrow angle. The filtration of aqueous humor is compromised because of the iris blocking the angle.

Table 34-6. Drug–Drug Interactions with Medications Used to Treat Parkinson's Disease

Medication	Interacting drug	Outcome
Dopamine agonists (e.g., bromocriptine, ropinirole)	Dopamine antagonists (e.g., haloperidol, metoclopramide)	Inhibition of benefits with worsening parkinsonism
Levodopa	Dopamine antagonists	Inhibition of benefits with worsening parkinsonism
Apomorphine	Ondansetron, other serotonin-receptor antagonists	Severe hypotension and loss of consciousness
Selegiline	Serotonergics, selective serotonin reuptake inhibitors, buspirone, mirtazapine	Serotonin syndrome (confusion, agitation, tremor, seizures, coma)
COMT inhibitors	Nonselective MAO inhibitors: phenelzine	Serotonin syndrome; hypertensive crisis secondary to increased catecholamines

Congenital glaucoma results from defective development of the structures in and around the anterior chamber of the eye and results in impairment of aqueous humor.

Clinical Presentation

Clinical signs and symptoms of open-angle glaucoma develop slowly and may present with only minor symptoms, such as headache and mild eye pain. Optic nerve damage results from chronic elevations in IOP. Hence, early and consistent treatment is important to prevent loss of vision.

Acute angle-closure glaucoma presents with blurred vision, severe ocular pain, and possible nausea and vomiting. It should be considered a medical emergency, and immediate care should be recommended.

Chronic angle-closure glaucoma may have symptoms similar to those of open-angle glaucoma.

Tonometry is used to screen for IOP, but direct ophthalmoscopy (slit-lamp examination) is necessary to accurately evaluate the eye for changes in the optic nerve.

Pathophysiology

The pathogenesis of glaucoma results from changes in aqueous humor (the fluid filling the eye and in front of the lens) outflow that result in increased IOP. This increase in pressure leads to optic nerve atrophy and progressive loss of vision.

Increased IOP can result from decreased elimination or increased production of aqueous humor. Aqueous humor is secreted by the ciliary processes into the posterior chamber of the eye. It then flows through the trabecular meshwork and the canal of Schlemm.

Open-angle glaucoma is the result of decreased elimination of aqueous humor as it passes through the trabecular meshwork, thereby resulting in elevated IOP.

Angle-closure glaucoma is caused by papillary blockage of aqueous humor outflow. This blockage can result when a patient has a narrow anterior chamber in the eye or a dilated pupil where the iris comes into greater contact with the lens. With the blocking of outflow, aqueous humor accumulates in the posterior chamber, presses the lens forward, and further decreases drainage, with possible complete blockage as the outcome.

Diagnostic Criteria

- Elevated IOP as determined by tonometry
- Funduscopic assessment to identify characteristic changes in the optic disc and retina

Treatment Principles

Figure 34-1 illustrates the treatment of open-angle glaucoma. Treatment principles of glaucoma are as follows:

- Reduce IOP to prevent optic nerve damage and visual field loss.
- Use topical medications as first-line treatment.
- Consider acute angle-closure glaucoma as a medical emergency.

Monitoring

Periodic screening for increased IOP should be done, with yearly examinations for those over 65 years of age and as part of a routine eye examination.

Drug Therapy

Mechanism of action

Medications are considered the mainstay of therapy for the treatment of glaucoma (Table 34-7). β-adrenergic

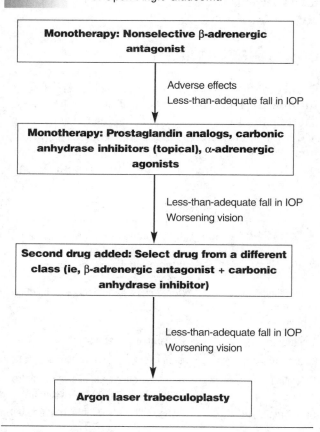

Figure 34-1. Algorithm for the Treatment of Open-Angle Glaucoma

Table 34-7. Medications for the Treatment of Glaucoma

Generic name	Trade name	Form	Usual dosage	Comments
Nonselective β antagonists				Nonselective β antagonists are often the first choice for open-angle glaucoma.
Timolol	Timoptic	0.25% and 0.50% solution and gel-forming solution	1 drop twice daily; gel solution used once daily	
Carteolol	Ocupress	1% ophthalmic solution	1 drop twice daily	
Levobunolol	Betagen	0.25% and 0.50% solution	1 or 2 drops 1–4 times daily	
Metipranolol	Optipranolol	0.3% solution	1 drop twice daily	
Selective β₁ antagonists				
Betaxolol	Betoptic	0.25% and 0.50% solution	1 or 2 drops twice daily	Drug is cardioselective. It has less effect on heart rate and blood pressure.
Levobetaxolol	Betaxon	0.50% solution	1 drop twice daily	Drug is cardioselective.
Carbonic anhydrase inhibitors				
Acetazolamide	Diamox	125 and 250 mg tablets, 500 mg extended-release capsules	250 mg 1–4 times daily; extended-release 1 or 2 times daily	Do not use with sulfa allergy.
Dorzolamide	Trusopt	2.0% solution	1 drop 3 times daily	Do not use with sulfa allergy.
Brinzolamide	Azopt	1.0% solution	1 drop 3 times daily	Do not use with sulfa allergy.
Methazolamide	Neptazane	25 and 50 mg tablets	15–50 mg 1–3 times daily	Do not use with sulfa allergy.
Prostaglandin analogues				
Latanoprost	Xalatan	0.005% solution, refrigerated	1 drop at bedtime	Drug can change blue eyes to brown.
Bimatoprost	Lumigan	0.03% solution	1 drop at bedtime	Drug can cause darkening of eyelids and eyelashes.
Travoprost	Travatan	0.004% solution	1 drop at bedtime	Ocular hyperemia frequently occurs.
Unoprostone	Rescula	0.15% solution	1 drop twice daily	If used with another drop, wait 5 minutes.
α₂-adrenergic agonists				
Brimonidine	Alphagan	0.15% solution	1 drop 3 times daily	Wait at least 15 minutes after using before placing soft contacts.
Dipivefrin	Propine	0.1% solution	1 drop twice daily	Dipivefrin is a prodrug of epinephrine.
Cholinergics (miotics)				
Pilocarpine	Pilocar	0.5%, 1%, 2%, 3%, 4%, 6%, 8% solution, 4% gel	1 or 2 drops 3–4 times daily; ½ inch gel at bedtime	A once weekly dose form called Ocuserts is available.

blocking drugs (β-blockers) are considered first-line treatment for open-angle glaucoma. β-adrenergic antagonists can be nonselective (i.e., they block both β₁ and β₂ receptors) or selective (i.e., they block only β₁ receptors). Drugs that block only β₁ receptors are considered cardioselective and cause less decrease in blood pressure and heart rate.

β-adrenergic antagonists

Nonselective β antagonists include timolol, carteolol, levobunolol, and metipranolol. β₁-selective antagonists include betaxolol and levobetaxolol.

Therapy is initiated with a single topical ophthalmic solution, and additional agents are added if decrease in IOP is less than acceptable. The effects of therapy on IOP should be apparent after a week of treatment.

Prostaglandin analogues are also used as first-line treatment (or in combination with β-blockers). Topical carbonic anhydrase inhibitors and α₂ agonists may be used in treatment.

Medications such as epinephrine, pilocarpine, and oral carbonic anhydrase inhibitors are prescribed less often, but they are considered to be effective adjunctive drugs.

Patient instructions and counseling

Multiple factors present obstacles that can interfere with good compliance. Patients are often asymptomatic and do not feel treatment is necessary. Because decreased vision is associated with glaucoma, patients may have difficulty with written instructions.

Adequate glaucoma therapy often requires two or more types of eye drops that may have to be given more than once daily. Correct administration of eye drops requires coordination and reasonable cognitive functioning.

Glaucoma is more common in the elderly, who may have more difficulty complying with prescribed medications.

Patient guidelines concerning the use of eye drops to treat glaucoma follow:

- Wash hands before administering eye drops, and avoid touching the dropper tip.

- Confirm that the medication is not outdated and has been stored properly.
- Looking upward, pull the lower lid down and instill the correct number of drops.
- Close the eye to allow the medication to have maximal effect.
- In most cases, wait 5 or more minutes between different medications.

Adverse drug events

Table 34-8 describes the adverse effects that may be seen with glaucoma medications.

Drug–drug interactions

Drug interactions between topical medications and systemic drugs are unlikely.

Acetazolamide interacts with the following:

- Aspirin to cause increased aspirin levels and possible toxicity
- Cyclosporine to cause increased cyclosporine levels
- Lithium to cause either increased or decreased lithium levels
- Phenytoin to cause an increased risk of osteomalacia

Parameters to monitor

Medication use is critical to the successful treatment of glaucoma and should be monitored by the health professional.

Table 34-8. Classification, Mechanism of Action, and Adverse Effects of Glaucoma Medications

Medication class	Mechanism of action	Adverse effects
β-adrenergic antagonists (timolol, metipranolol, carteolol, levobunolol, etc.)	Decrease in aqueous humor formation with slight increase in outflow (β selective)	Adverse cardiac effects, worsening pulmonary disease, depression, dizziness
Miotics (cholinergics) (pilocarpine, carbachol)	Increase in aqueous humor outflow	Miosis, brow ache, dizziness, nausea, flushing, itching, sweating, confusion
Carbonic anhydrase inhibitors (dorzolamide, brinzolamide)	Decrease in aqueous humor formation	Lethargy, decreased appetite, GI upset, urinary frequency
Prostaglandin analogues (latanoprost, travoprost, bimatoprost)	Increased uveoscleral outflow without effect on aqueous humor formation	Iris pigmentation, eyelid darkening, macular edema
α₂-adrenergic agonists (apraclonidine, brimonidine)	Decrease in aqueous humor formation	Tachycardia, dry mouth, eyelid elevation, central nervous system effects in the old and very young
Other α-adrenergic agonists (epinephrine, dipivefrin)	Increase in aqueous humor outflow	Tachycardia, increased blood pressure, allergic responses

Other aspects

A combination is available of timolol 0.5% and dorzolamide 2% (Cosopt). This combination effectively lowers IOP and requires only twice-daily doses. This simplified dosing should improve compliance with treatment. This combination (i.e., using two drugs from different categories) represents a sound treatment approach. Poor response to therapy may result in the prescribing of multiple medications, which may negatively affect the patient's ability to successfully use the more complex regimen.

Nondrug Therapy

Laser surgery

Argon laser trabeculoplasty has proven effective as adjunctive therapy that increases the flow of aqueous humor.

Surgery

A surgical procedure involves creating new means of drainage for aqueous humor to leave the anterior chamber.

34-8. Key Points

Alzheimer's Disease

- Alzheimer's disease is a progressive neurologic disease that results in impaired memory, intellectual functioning, and behavior.
- Alzheimer's disease has no cure, but therapies exist to decrease memory impairment as well as improve behavior and patient functioning.
- Other forms of dementia that are potentially reversible should be identified and treated accordingly.
- New drug therapies may slow the progression of Alzheimer's disease and allow patients to remain in the least restrictive environment possible.
- Caregiver support and education are important measures to ensure patient safety and well-being.

Parkinson's Disease

- Parkinson's disease is a chronic, progressive neurologic disease for which no cure exists; medications are available to slow the progression of symptoms.
- The etiology of Parkinson's disease is unknown but may involve genetic susceptibility combined with environmental toxins and age-related changes in the brain.
- Dopamine, the central neurotransmitter, is decreased in Parkinson's disease, and current drug therapy is primarily directed at increasing dopamine levels.
- Drug therapy monitoring in Parkinson's disease requires an understanding of a variety of different medications that may cause significant adverse effects.
- Physical therapy, occupational therapy, dietary considerations, and support counseling for caregivers are necessary components of treating Parkinson's disease.

Glaucoma

- Glaucoma, a group of eye diseases, is characterized by increased intraocular pressure resulting in damage to the optic nerve and possible blindness.
- Open-angle glaucoma is the most common form of this disease; angle-closure glaucoma can be a medical emergency.
- The goal of therapy is to reduce intraocular pressure with the simplest medication regimen possible.
- Drug therapy for glaucoma usually begins with a topical β-adrenergic antagonist; patients often require combination therapy.
- Medication compliance is essential in the control of glaucoma. Education of the patient and caregiver is required to overcome treatment barriers.

34-9. Questions

1. Of the following pharmacokinetic processes, which is the least altered by aging?

    A. Absorption
    B. Distribution
    C. Metabolism
    D. Elimination
    E. Excretion

2. Which of the following is given as a once-daily oral dose?

    A. Buspirone
    B. Donepezil
    C. Memantine
    D. Rivastigmine
    E. Tacrine

3. Galantamine increases levels of which neuro-transmitter?

   A. Acetylcholine
   B. Dopamine
   C. Melatonin
   D. Norepinephrine
   E. Serotonin

4. Weight loss is most often associated with which of the following?

   A. Donepezil
   B. Galantamine
   C. Mirtazapine
   D. Rivastigmine
   E. Tacrine

5. Which of the following statements concerning donepezil are correct?

   I. It inhibits acetylcholinesterase but not butyrylcholinesterase.
   II. It should be taken with meals in divided doses.
   III. Side effects include tachycardia and blood pressure alterations.

   A. I only
   B. III only
   C. I and II only
   D. II and III only
   E. I, II, and III

6. Of the following medications used to treat behavioral and emotional symptoms in Alzheimer's patients, which has an FDA black box warning of increased mortality?

   A. Buspirone
   B. Citalopram
   C. Lorazepam
   D. Risperidone
   E. Zolpidem

7. The maximum daily dose of galantamine in patients with renal impairment is

   A. 8 mg/d.
   B. 12 mg/d.
   C. 16 mg/d.
   D. 24 mg/d.
   E. 32 mg/d.

8. All of the following could worsen cognition in Alzheimer's disease patients *except*

   A. dicyclomine.
   B. dimenhydrinate.

C. meclizine.
D. trazodone.
E. trihexyphenidyl.

9. Memantine's reported benefit in treating the symptoms of Alzheimer's disease is thought to be the result of

   A. increasing serotonin receptor activity.
   B. blocking the effect of glutamate on receptors.
   C. direct blocking of acetylcholine receptors.
   D. decreasing intracellular dopamine activity.
   E. decreasing amyloid deposits in the brain.

10. Which works by direct stimulation of dopamine receptors?

    A. Amantadine
    B. Benztropine
    C. Entacapone
    D. Ropinirole
    E. Selegiline

11. Which of the following has a risk of causing a significant drug interaction if taken with ondansetron?

    A. Amantadine
    B. Apomorphine
    C. Carbidopa-levodopa
    D. Pramipexole
    E. Entacapone

12. What would be the most likely outcome if a Parkinson's patient on levodopa were also prescribed haloperidol?

    A. Excessive nausea and vomiting
    B. Hypertensive crisis
    C. Tachycardia and possible chest pain
    D. Worsening symptoms of Parkinson's disease
    E. Excessive somnolence

13. Which inhibits monoamine oxidase (MAO)?

    A. Benztropine
    B. Bromocriptine
    C. Pramipexole
    D. Rasagiline
    E. Tolcapone

14. How does carbidopa affect levodopa?

    A. It slows the release from presynaptic neurons.
    B. It prevents the excretion of dopamine.

C. It increases stimulation of dopamine receptors.

D. It decreases tolerance to normal doses.

E. It inhibits the peripheral conversion to dopamine.

15. A patient with Parkinson's disease currently taking selegiline has been prescribed mirtazapine (Remeron). What would be the most likely outcome of this combination?

A. Inhibition of benefits with worsening parkinsonism

B. No significant drug interaction

C. Risk of serotonin syndrome

D. Increased benefits with improved parkinsonism

E. Hypertensive episode

16. Which of the following statements are true concerning the treatment of Parkinson's disease?

I. Entacapone is not used as monotherapy except for patients with end-of-dose wearing-off periods and for those experiencing motor fluctuations.

II. Pramipexole has been reported to cause "sleep attacks."

III. Food–drug interactions would not be expected with selegiline when given at doses of 10 mg daily.

A. I only

B. III only

C. I and II only

D. II and III only

E. I, II, and III

17. Timolol ophthalmic drops would be more likely to cause which adverse effect as compared to levobetaxolol ophthalmic drops?

A. Agitation and restlessness

B. Nausea and vomiting

C. Confusion

D. Change in heart rate and blood pressure

E. Altered intraocular pressure

18. Which of the following would *not* be considered for monotherapy of glaucoma?

A. Latanoprost

B. Dorzolamide

C. Carteolol

D. Methazolamide

E. Brimonidine

19. Which of the following can cause iris pigmentation changes?

A. Acetazolamide

B. Betaxolol

C. Brimonidine

D. Latanoprost

E. Pilocarpine

20. Which of the following is available as a fixed combination product?

A. Dorzolamide and timolol

B. Betaxolol and bimatoprost

C. Bimatoprost and levobunolol

D. Latanoprost and timolol

E. Methazolamide and latanoprost

21. All of the following are available as an ophthalmic solution *except*

A. brimonidine.

B. dipivefrin.

C. dorzolamide.

D. methazolamide.

E. metipranolol.

22. Which should *not* be used if a patient has a sulfa allergy?

A. Betaxolol

B. Bimatoprost

C. Brimonidine

D. Brinzolamide

E. Unoprostone

23. Which of the following is true about α_2-adrenergic agonists?

A. They cause an increase in aqueous humor synthesis.

B. They cause a decrease in aqueous humor formation.

C. They cause an increase in uveoscleral outflow.

D. They cause an increase in aqueous humor outflow.

E. They cause a decrease in uveoscleral outflow.

24. Which of the following statements concerning glaucoma therapy is correct?

I. Carteolol is available as an ophthalmic solution and as a gel-forming solution.

II. Latanoprost and metipranolol ophthalmic solutions should be stored in the refrigerator.

III. Prostaglandin analogues, β-adrenergic antagonists, and α-adrenergic agonists can be used as monotherapy.

A. I only
B. III only
C. I and II only
D. II and III only
E. I, II, and III

34-10. Answers

1. **A.** Of all the age-related changes of the pharmacokinetic process, absorption is the least altered, perhaps because most drugs are passively absorbed.

2. **B.** All of these drugs except donepezil require at least twice-daily dosing. Donepezil has a long half-life, which allows once-daily doses. None of these agents is available in sustained-release forms, although rivastigmine has a once-daily patch. Buspirone is an antianxiety drug that is dosed twice or three times daily.

3. **A.** Galantamine is a cholinesterase inhibitor, and all cholinesterase inhibitors increase levels of acetylcholine, the neurotransmitter that appears to be involved with memory function.

4. **D.** Weight loss, probably because of nausea and vomiting, is a warning for rivastigmine. In controlled trials, approximately 26% of women on doses of 9 mg/d or greater had weight loss of equal to or greater than 7% of their baseline weight.

5. **A.** Donepezil is selective for acetylcholinesterase and does not inhibit butyrylcholinesterase. Donepezil does not have to be taken with meals and is given once daily. Donepezil does not increase heart rate, and this class of medications that increase acetylcholine should be used with caution in patients with bradycardia.

6. **D.** Risperidone, as well as other atypical antipsychotics, increases mortality risk when given to dementia patients with agitation or aggressive behaviors. This is probably a class effect, and any antipsychotic should be used only if no alternative medication is effective.

7. **C.** With renal or hepatic dysfunction, galantamine doses should not exceed 16 mg/d. With severe renal or hepatic dysfunction, galantamine should not be used.

8. **D.** All of the drugs listed—with the exception of trazodone—have anticholinergic activity. Decreasing the activity of acetylcholine could worsen dementia and block benefits of cholinesterase inhibitors. Trazodone is an antidepressant with sedating properties but little anticholinergic activity. It may be given at bedtime to help with sleep. Trazodone does have a side effect of orthostatic hypotension.

9. **B.** Glutamate is the main excitatory neurotransmitter in the central nervous system, and one theory states that blocking the effects of glutamate on NMDA receptors will decrease symptoms of Alzheimer's disease.

10. **D.** Ropinirole directly stimulates dopamine receptors; the other drugs increase dopamine activity by different mechanisms.

11. **B.** Apomorphine can cause severe hypotension and loss of consciousness when taken with ondansetron and other serotonin-receptor antagonists.

12. **D.** Haloperidol and other antipsychotics block dopamine activity and can worsen PD. They can also block the benefits of PD medications, which increase dopamine activity.

13. **D.** Rasagiline is an MAO inhibitor that is selective for MAO-B, which decreases the potential for drug–drug and drug–food interactions. At higher doses, this selectivity lessens.

14. **E.** Carbidopa inhibits the peripheral conversion of levodopa to dopamine, thus allowing more levodopa to cross the blood–brain barrier, and decreases adverse effects from dopamine.

15. **C.** The combination of two drugs that increase serotonin levels can result in serotonin syndrome, which can cause confusion, agitation, tremor, seizures and coma.

16. **D.** Entacapone should always be given with carbidopa-levodopa because benefits depend on carbidopa inhibiting the peripheral conversion of levodopa.

17. **D.** Timolol is a nonselective β-adrenergic antagonist that causes a reduction in heart rate and blood pressure. There is enough absorption from eye drops to produce these cardiac effects.

18. **D.** All of the other choices could be considered as monotherapy for glaucoma. Methazolamide is an oral carbonic anhydrase inhibitor and is used in conjunction with ophthalmic drops.

19. **D.** Latanoprost, a prostaglandin analogue, is known to change iris pigmentation and to darken eyelashes.

20. **A.** Dorzolamide plus timolol (Cosopt) is the only combination ophthalmic solution for treating glaucoma. An advantage for using a combination product would be increased compliance.

21. **D.** Methazolamide and acetazolamide are both available only as oral tablets or capsules. Topical carbonic anhydrase inhibitors are brinzolamide and dorzolamide.

22. **D.** Patients with sulfa allergy should not be given a carbonic anhydrase inhibitor.

23. **B.** Brimonidine and other α_2-adrenergic agonists cause a decrease in aqueous humor formation.

24. **B.** All of these drugs can be used as monotherapy in glaucoma. Timolol and pilocarpine are available as gel forms. Latanoprost (but not metipranolol) should be stored in a refrigerator before dispensing.

34-11. References

Chen JJ, Shimomua SK. Parkinsonism. In: Herfindal ET, Gourley DR, eds. *Textbook of Therapeutics*. 8th ed. Philadelphia: WB Saunders; 2006:839–54.

Grutzendler J, Morris JC. Cholinesterase inhibitors for Alzheimer's disease. *Drugs*. 2001;61:41–52.

Khaw P, Shah P, Elkington A. Glaucoma-1 treatment. *BMJ*. 2004;328(7432):156–8.

Olanow CW, Watts RL, Koller WC. An algorithm for the management of Parkinson's disease. *Neurology*. 2001;56:872–91.

Rawls WN. Alzheimer's disease. In: Herfindal ET, Gourley DR, eds. *Textbook of Therapeutics*. 8th ed. Philadelphia: WB Saunders; 2006:1811–28.

Scarpini E, Scheltens P, Felman H. Treatment of Alzheimer's disease: Current status and new perspectives. *Lancet Neurol*. 2003;2:539–47.

Steinman MA, Landefeld C, Rosenthal GE, et al. Polypharmacy and prescribing quality in older people. *J Am Geriatr Soc*. 2006;54:1516.

Toxicology and Chem-Bioterrorism

35

Peter A. Chyka, PharmD, FAACT, DABAT

35-1. Overview of Poisoning and Toxicology

Poisoning in America

Poisoning exposures and overdoses affect more than 2.5 million people annually, and more than 37,000 deaths occur yearly. A large number of poisonings occur in young children (< 1% of deaths are in preschool-age children), but most fatalities occur in adults.

Any chemical can become toxic if the exposure is too great in relation to body weight and tolerance. Medications are the most common cause of poisoning morbidity and mortality (Table 35-1).

Most poisonings in preschool-age children are unintentional or accidental. Unintentional poisonings can also occur in adolescents and adults; however, intentional (suicide and drug abuse) poisonings and overdoses are common.

Toxicology is the study of the adverse effects of chemicals and other xenobiotics on living organisms. There are several specialized areas of toxicology, including basic science, clinical, analytical, forensic, regulatory, and occupational settings, that have a unique focus and purpose.

In general, toxicity occurs when too much of a substance is taken in relation to a normally tolerable dose. Different mechanisms by which a chemical can produce toxicity include the following:

- Exaggeration of pharmacologic effects
- Formation of reactive toxic metabolites
- Formation of intracellular free radicals
- Interference with enzyme action
- Interference with DNA (deoxyribonucleic acid) or RNA (ribonucleic acid) synthesis
- Inactivation of biochemical cofactors
- Initiation of premature cell aging (apoptosis)
- Tissue destruction on contact

Poison Prevention Approaches and Pharmacy

Poison Prevention Packaging Act of 1970: Safety caps

This act was issued to prevent preschool-age children from opening and ingesting harmful substances or to delay the opening of packaging containing such substances (to limit the amount of harmful substance that may be ingested within a reasonable amount of time).

Drugs requiring safety caps include aspirin, ibuprofen, acetaminophen, and oral prescription drugs with certain exceptions (e.g., birth control pills and nitroglycerin).

Use of poison control centers

A poison control center determines if a true poisoning exists, recommends first aid, refers poisoning victims to health care facilities for further evaluation and treatment, monitors the progress and outcome of each poisoning case, and documents poisoning experiences. Programs and materials on poison prevention are also available.

Nationwide access is available by calling 1-800-222-1222 for 24-hour poison center services for the area from which the call is placed in the United States.

The contributions of Adrianne Y. Butler, PharmD; Billie J. Holliman, PharmD; and C. Renee Adams-McDowell, PharmD, to the first edition of this chapter are acknowledged.

Table 35-1. Ranking of Most Frequent Poisonings from U.S. Poison Centers and Emergency Departments, 2006

Cases from poison centers[a]	Cases from emergency departments[b]
Analgesics	Alcohol, alone or in combination
Cosmetics and personal care products	Cocaine
	Marijuana
Cleaning substances	Anxiolytics and sedatives
Sedative drugs	Opioid analgesics
Foreign bodies	Nonopioid analgesics
Cough and cold drugs	Heroin
Topical drugs	Antidepressant drugs
Pesticides	Amphetamines
Antidepressant drugs	Antipsychotic drugs
Bites and envenomations	Muscle relaxant drugs
Cardiovascular drugs	Cardiovascular drugs
Alcohols	

a. Categories are listed in decreasing order of frequency and are based on 2,403,539 poison exposures. Source: Bronstein AC, Spyker DA, Cantelina LR, et al. 2006 annual report of the American Association of Poison Control Centers' National Poison Data System (NCDS). *Clin Toxicol.* 2007;45:815–917.
b. Categories are listed in decreasing order of frequency and are based on cases of substance abuse, poisoning, overmedication, and attempted suicide in 2006. Source: Office of Applied Studies, Substance Abuse and Mental Health Services Administration. *Drug Abuse Warning Network, 2006.* DHHS publication SMA 08-4339. Rockville, Md.: Substance Abuse and Mental Health Services Administration; 2008.

Poison prevention tips for consumers

- Store all drugs and chemicals out of the reach of children.
- Never put chemicals in food containers.
- Choose products with safety caps when there is a choice, and use them properly.
- Read and follow all label directions carefully.
- Never call medicine "candy."
- Use safety latches.

Pharmacy Requirements of the Joint Commission on Accreditation of Healthcare Organizations

- Maintain and keep available the medical staff–approved stock of antidotes and other emergency drugs in both the pharmacy and patient care areas.

- Maintain authoritative and current antidote information.
- Keep the phone number of the poison control center readily available in areas outside of the pharmacy where drugs are stored.

Emergency Actions

First aid should be administered, if applicable. Table 35-2 describes first-aid techniques.

Other considerations

- Avoid wasting time looking for an "antidote" at home.
- Do not use home remedies such as saltwater, mustard powder, raw eggs, hydrogen peroxide, cooking grease, or gagging.
- Immediately call 911 or an ambulance if the person is not breathing, has had a seizure, or is unresponsive.
- For other situations, contact a poison center immediately to determine whether first aid should be used or whether a poisoning emergency exists.

Decontamination of the Gastrointestinal Tract

The practice of using drugs to decrease the absorption of other drugs from the gastrointestinal tract is in a state of change. For example, ipecac syrup is being

Table 35-2. First Aid for Poisoning Emergencies

Type of emergency	First-aid response
Inhaled poison	Immediately get the person to fresh air. Avoid breathing fumes. Open doors and windows wide.
Poison on the skin	Remove any contaminated clothing, and flood skin with water for at least 15 minutes.
Poison in the eye	Remove contact lenses. Flood the eye with water, pouring it from a large glass 2–3 inches from the eye. Repeat for a total of 15–30 minutes. Do not force the eyelid open.
Swallowed poison	Unless the victim is unconscious, is having convulsions, or cannot swallow, give a small glassful (2–4 oz) of water immediately. Call a poison center for advice about whether other actions are needed.

abandoned by many as a home- or hospital-based therapy, and its use is primarily at the preference of the consulting poison center or health care professional. Current recommendations are described in this section, as well as basic information about the drugs in case they are encountered.

Current recommendations

Ipecac syrup has questionable effectiveness, and its use is generally now avoided.

Gastric lavage involves placing a tube into the stomach through a nostril or the mouth and repetitively washing out the stomach contents with water or a saline solution. This method of gastric decontamination is of questionable effectiveness, particularly if it is performed more than 1 hour after ingestion of toxin.

Cathartics such as magnesium citrate are not routinely used any more.

Activated charcoal given orally is often the only treatment necessary if the toxin is adsorbed and the activated charcoal is used within 1–2 hours of ingestion of the toxin.

Whole bowel irrigation can be considered if the toxin is poorly or slowly adsorbed and its presence in the gastrointestinal tract is likely.

Ipecac syrup

Indications and dosage

Ipecac syrup was previously used for general prophylaxis of selected poisonings of expected minor or moderate severity in alert patients. Many clinicians have abandoned it as a prehospital or hospital treatment. In 2003, the American Academy of Pediatrics recommended that ipecac syrup no longer be used routinely as a home treatment for poisoning.

Contraindications

- The patient is experiencing pronounced sleepiness, coma, or seizures.
- The patient has ingested caustics, aliphatic hydrocarbons, and fast-acting agents that produce coma or seizures (e.g., tricyclic antidepressants, clonidine, calcium channel blockers, beta blockers, and hypoglycemic agents).
- Time since ingestion is believed to be 1 hour or more.

Adverse effects

- *Common:* Diarrhea, sleepiness, and protracted vomiting
- *Uncommon:* Mallory–Weiss tears and tracheal aspiration into the lungs.

Disadvantage

A disadvantage of ipecac syrup is that emesis and the drug's relative lack of efficacy complicate administration of other oral therapies.

Activated charcoal

Indications and dosage

This agent is occasionally used to adsorb poisons in an alert or comatose patient. Administer as a slurry by mouth or through a lavage tube:

- *Children:* 25–50 g
- *Adults:* 25–100 g

Contraindications

- Ingestions of aliphatic hydrocarbons and caustics
- Absence of patient's bowel sounds
- Ingestions of heavy metals (sodium, lithium, iron, or lead) or simple alcohols

Adverse effects

- *Uncommon:* Tracheal aspiration and pneumonitis
- *Common:* Emesis and soiling of clothes and furnishings

Advantages and disadvantages

- *Advantages:* Rapid onset of action, nonspecific action for a wide variety of chemicals, and reasonable effectiveness within 1 hour of ingestion
- *Disadvantages:* Messy and difficult administration and possible removal of beneficial drugs together with the toxin

Cathartics

Cathartics were previously used as an adjunct to activated charcoal administration to decrease gastrointestinal transit time. Their efficacy is unproved. Fluid and electrolyte disturbances are possible with repeated doses.

Cathartics may contribute to emesis following activated charcoal use.

Agents previously used include magnesium citrate, magnesium sulfate, sodium sulfate, and sorbitol. Some activated charcoal products contain sorbitol mixed in the preparation. The sorbitol concentration varies from brand to brand.

Whole bowel irrigation

Indications and technique

Whole bowel irrigation is generally used to wash out the gastrointestinal tract when using charcoal may be inappropriate (e.g., if iron or lithium was ingested) and the toxin is suspected to be present in the gastro-intestinal tract (e.g., when drugs are sustained-release formulations or when the patient ingested illicit drugs packed in condoms).

Use larger volumes of polyethylene glycol electrolyte solutions (e.g., Colyte, GoLYTELY) than the amounts conventionally used for bowel preparation. Administer by mouth or through a gastric or duodenal tube for treatment of poisoning:

- *Children:* 25 mL/kg/h (approximately 500 mL/h) up to 2–5 L
- *Adults:* 2 L/h up to 5–10 L

Contraindications
- Ingestion of caustics or aliphatic hydrocarbons
- Patients with absent bowel sounds or gastro-intestinal tract obstruction

Adverse effects
Few adverse effects have been reported, but limited results are available from which to draw conclusions. Some nausea and vomiting have been reported.

Advantages and disadvantages
- *Advantages:* Prompt whole-bowel evacuation within 2 hours
- *Disadvantages:* Messy procedure because of rectal effluent

Other hospital-based therapies

These therapies include supportive and symptomatic care, multiple doses of activated charcoal (to enhance systemic elimination when appropriate), hemodialysis (to enhance systemic elimination when appropriate), and use of antidotes (to antagonize or reverse toxic effects when indicated).

35-2. Substance Abuse and Toxicology

Substance abuse often leads to acute and chronic toxicity. Table 35-3 shows selected drugs of abuse.

During 2007, 35.7 million Americans age 12 and older (14.4% of the population) admitted using an illicit drug in the past year, and 9.9 million (4.0%) reported driving under the influence of an illicit drug during the past year.

Approximately 1.4 million adults are treated in emergency departments annually for abuse and misuse of drugs not including alcohol, with one-third involving alcohol in combination with other drugs.

Management of the acute condition generally follows the same guidelines as those for management of poisonings and overdoses. A challenge in treating patients during acute drug overdose is determining the possible agents taken and possible adulterants (e.g., talc, strychnine, other drugs) or contaminants.

Chronic abuse can foster dependence, which often leads to withdrawal symptoms when the patient stops using the drugs. Detoxification programs, long-term behavioral counseling, and drugs to produce aversion or substitution to drug-taking behaviors are often needed.

35-3. Antidotes

Role of Antidotes

An antidote counteracts or changes the nature of a poison. Few antidotes are available relative to the large number of potential poisons. Table 35-4 lists antidotes that are commonly used in the treatment of a patient with a poisoning or an overdose.

Many hospitals have an insufficient stock of antidotes. The pharmacy and therapeutics committee of a hospital should regularly review the inventory of antidotes.

Selected Antidotes

Acetylcysteine

Acetylcysteine is available under the trade names Mucomyst (10%, 20% oral solution) and Acetadote (20% for injection).

Uses
Acetylcysteine is used to treat acute acetaminophen overdose. An unapproved indication is to treat adverse reactions to drugs that may produce free radicals as part of the adverse reaction; the dosage regimen is unique to the application.

Mechanism of action
Acetylcysteine protects the liver from the toxic effects of an acetaminophen metabolite by supplying glutathione to aid in metabolism of the reactive metabolite. Other mechanisms are also proposed, which include providing sulfate for acetaminophen metabolism and minimizing the formation of free radicals.

This agent may be useful in minimizing hepatotoxic injury once it has begun. It also may aid in cases of fulminant hepatic failure.

Table 35-3. Selected Drugs of Abuse and Addictive Substances

Substance	Slang names	Methods of abuse	Major or unique health effects
Androgenic anabolic steroids	Roids	These drugs are taken orally or injected, typically in cycles of weeks or months ("cycling"). Users often combine several different types of steroids ("stacking").	Anabolic steroids are synthetic derivatives of testosterone. Abuse can lead to serious health problems, some irreversible.
			Men: Shrinking of the testicles, reduced sperm count, infertility, baldness, gynecomastia, and increased risk for prostate cancer can occur.
			Women: Growth of facial hair, male-pattern baldness, changes in or cessation of the menstrual cycle, enlargement of the clitoris, and deepened voice can occur.
			Adolescents: Stunted growth by premature skeletal maturation and accelerated puberty changes can occur.
			Other major side effects include jaundice, fluid retention, high blood pressure, and severe acne. Extreme mood swings, including manic-like symptoms leading to violence and depression, are often experienced when drugs are stopped, and such symptoms may contribute to dependence.
Barbiturates	Barbs, downers	Barbiturates can be ingested or injected.	Barbiturates are CNS depressants that at high doses can become general anesthetics.
			With high doses, coma, ataxia, depressed reflexes, hypotension, and respiratory depression can occur.
			CNS depressants should not be combined with any medication or substance that causes sedation, including prescription pain medicines, certain over-the-counter cold and allergy medications, or alcoholic drinks. The effects of the drugs can combine to slow breathing or to slow both the heart and respiration, which can be fatal.
			Discontinuing prolonged use of high doses of barbiturates can lead to withdrawal.
Cocaine	Snow, crack (the street name given to cocaine that has been processed from cocaine hydrochloride to the free base for smoking), rock	Cocaine can be sniffed or snorted, injected, or smoked (free-base and crack cocaine). It is poorly absorbed orally.	Cocaine is a CNS stimulant that produces euphoric effects and hyperstimulation such as dilated pupils, increased temperature, tachycardia, and hypertension.
			Prolonged cocaine snorting can result in ulceration of the mucous membranes of the nose and can damage the nasal septum enough to cause it to collapse.
			Cocaine-related deaths are often a result of cardiac arrest or seizures followed by respiratory arrest.
			Tolerance to the euphoric effects develops.
			When addicted individuals stop using cocaine, they often become depressed.

(continued)

Table 35-3. Selected Drugs of Abuse and Addictive Substances *(Continued)*

Substance	Slang names	Methods of abuse	Major or unique health effects
Dextromethorphan	DXM, DM, robo, velvet, rojo	This drug is taken orally by drinking dextromethorphan-containing cough syrups. Availability of the powdered form has led to repackaging as capsules or tablets and to snorting.	Dextromethorphan is the dextro isomer of levomethorphan. It has no analgesic, opiate-like, dependence-producing properties. A behaviorally active metabolite, dextrorphan is structurally related to PCP (phencyclidine) and ketamine and may contribute to its abuse potential.
			The typical clinical presentation of intoxication involves hyperexcitability, lethargy, ataxia, slurred speech, sweating, hypertension, and nystagmus. Abusers report a heightened sense of perceptual awareness, altered time perception, and visual hallucinations.
			The majority of abuse occurs among teenagers and young adults who use dextromethorphan alone or mixed with other drugs. It has been sold as "ecstasy." It has been identified as a filler in confiscated samples of bogus heroin and bogus ketamine.
			Procedures to extract dextromethorphan from cough syrups are described on the Internet, which has led to the availability of powdered forms.
Ethanol	Various names and alcoholic drinks	Ethanol is ingested.	Ethanol is a CNS depressant that at high doses can lead to hypotension, hypoglycemia, respiratory depression, and death. Acute intoxication leads to ataxia, sedation, emesis, and slurred speech.
			Chronic abuse leads to many medical complications such as esophageal varices, hepatic failure with ascites, and malnutrition.
			Tolerance, dependence, and withdrawal develop with chronic abuse.
Gamma-hydroxybutyrate (GHB)	Liquid ecstasy, soap, easy lay, Georgia home boy, somatomax, scoop, grievous bodily harm	GHB is ingested.	GHB is a CNS depressant abused for euphoric, sedative, and anabolic (body-building) effects.
			Coma and seizures are likely; increased risk of seizures occurs when combined with methamphetamine.
			Use with alcohol causes nausea and difficulty breathing.
			GHB and two of its precursors, gamma-butyrolactone (GBL) and 1,4-butanediol (BD) have been involved in poisonings, overdoses, date rapes, and deaths. They are produced by illicit laboratories.
			GHB may produce withdrawal effects.
Heroin	Smack, H, skag, junk	Heroin can be injected, snorted, or smoked.	Abuse is associated with fatal overdose, spontaneous abortion, collapsed veins, and infectious diseases, including HIV/AIDS and hepatitis.
			Effects include euphoria ("rush") followed by an alternately wakeful and drowsy state ("on the nod").
			CNS depression, respiratory depression, miosis (pinpoint pupils), and pulmonary edema can occur.
			Street heroin may have additives.
			With regular use, tolerance develops and withdrawal is possible.

Toxicology and Chem-Bioterrorism** **765**

	Street names	Route	Effects
Inhalants	Various names	Inhalants are sniffed or huffed.	Inhalants include a variety of breathable chemical vapors that produce psychoactive effects. They are found in industrial or household solvents or solvent-containing products, including paint thinners or solvents, degreasers, dry-cleaning fluids, gasoline, and glues. Nearly all abused inhalants produce short-term intoxicating and CNS depressant effects similar to anesthetics. Intoxication usually lasts only a few minutes. Successive inhalations lead to loss of inhibition and control. Continued use can lead to coma. In some cases, heart failure and death occur within minutes of a session of prolonged use ("sudden sniffing death").
Injected drugs	Various names	Such drugs are injected, which is referred to as "shooting up" or "mainlining."	Injecting drug users are at risk for transmitting or acquiring HIV/AIDS, hepatitis, bacterial infections, and fungal infections if needles or other injection equipment are shared. Chronic users may develop collapsed veins, infection of the heart lining and valves, skin abscesses, cellulitis, and liver disease. Because some abusers dissolve the tablets in water and inject the mixture, emboli can form from the insoluble materials in the tablets.
Ketamine	K, special K, cat Valium, vitamin K	Ketamine is injected or snorted.	Ketamine is an anesthetic that has been approved for human and veterinary use. Certain doses can cause dream-like states and hallucinations. At high doses, ketamine can cause delirium, amnesia, impaired motor function, hypertension, depression, and potentially fatal respiratory depression.
Lysergic acid diethylamide (LSD)	Acid, L, blotter, cubes, sugar, dots	LSD is ingested. It is often added to absorbent paper, such as blotter paper, and divided into small decorated squares ("blotter acid") or placed on dot-like candy ("dots") or sugar cubes ("cubes," "sugar").	LSD is a hallucinogen sold on the street in tablets, capsules, and liquid form. Effects are unpredictable. Physical effects include mydriasis (dilated pupils), elevated temperature, tachycardia, hypertension, sweating, loss of appetite, sleeplessness, dry mouth, and tremors. Sensations and feelings change more dramatically than do the physical signs. In sufficient doses, the drug produces delusions and visual hallucinations. Some users experience severe, terrifying thoughts and feelings; fear of losing control; fear of insanity and death; and despair. Fatal accidents have occurred during intoxication. Many users experience flashbacks.

Table 35-3. Selected Drugs of Abuse and Addictive Substances (*Continued*)

Substance	Slang names	Methods of abuse	Major or unique health effects
Marijuana	Pot; herb; weed; grass; widow; ganja; hash; and trademarked varieties of cannabis, such as Bubble Gum, Northern Lights, Juicy Fruit, Afghani #1, and a number of Skunk varieties	Marijuana is smoked as a cigarette ("joint," "nail"), in a pipe ("bong"), or in blunts (cigars that have been emptied of tobacco and refilled with marijuana, often in combination with another drug). It is also ingested when mixed in food or brewed as a tea.	Main active chemical in marijuana is THC (delta-9-tetrahydrocannabinol). Delirium, conjunctivitis, and food craving are typical. Short-term effects include problems with memory and learning, distorted perception, difficulty in thinking and problem solving, loss of coordination, and tachycardia. Risk of heart attack more than quadruples in the first hour after smoking marijuana. Users experience the same respiratory problems as cigarette smokers (see nicotine); burning and stinging of the mouth and throat, often accompanied by a heavy cough, can occur. Drug craving and withdrawal effects can occur.
3-4,-methylene-dioxy-methamphet-amine (MDMA)	Ecstasy, Adam, XTC, hug, beans, love drug	MDMA is ingested, snorted, injected, or used in suppository form.	MDMA is a synthetic, psychoactive drug with both stimulant and hallucinogenic properties. It increases pulse and blood pressure. In high doses, it can cause malignant hyperthermia leading to rhabdomyolysis (muscle breakdown with kidney and cardiovascular system failure). Psychological difficulties, which include confusion, depression, sleep problems, drug craving, severe anxiety, and paranoia, occur during use and sometimes for weeks afterward. Physical symptoms include muscle tension, involuntary teeth clenching, nausea, blurred vision, nystagmus, faintness, chills, or sweating. Content of the MDMA pills also varies widely, and may include caffeine, dextromethorphan, heroin, and mescaline. In some areas, the MDMA-like substance paramethoxyamphetamine (PMA) has led to death when mistaken for true MDMA; deaths were due to complications from hyperthermia.
Methamphetamine	Crank, meth, speed, chalk, ice, crystal, glass	Methamphetamine can be ingested, snorted in the powder form, or injected. The clear, chunky crystals resembling ice can be smoked and are referred to as "ice," "crystal," and "glass."	Methamphetamine is an addictive stimulant chemically related to amphetamine. It produces euphoria, irritability, insomnia, confusion, tremors, convulsions, anxiety, paranoia, and aggressiveness. Higher doses lead to hypertension, tachycardia, stroke, arrhythmias, cardiovascular collapse, and death. Hyperthermia and convulsions can result in death. Prolonged use leads to extreme anorexia and is associated with tooth decay and skin lesions. Methamphetamine is made in illegal laboratories and may contain contaminants and by-products. The potential for abuse and dependence is high.

Nicotine	Various names and products	Nicotine is smoked with tobacco in cigarettes, cigars, and pipes. It also is in chewing tobacco.	Nicotine is a highly addictive CNS stimulant and sedative. Stimulation is followed by depression and fatigue, leading the user to seek more nicotine. Women who smoke and take oral contraceptives are more prone to cardiovascular and cerebrovascular diseases, especially those older than 30. Pregnant women have an increased risk of having stillborn or premature infants or infants with low birth weight. Respiratory problems include daily cough and phlegm production, more frequent acute respiratory illness, a heightened risk of lung infections, and a greater tendency toward obstructed airways and cancer of the respiratory tract and lungs. Tar in cigarettes is associated with a higher rate of lung cancer, emphysema, and bronchial disorders. Carbon monoxide in the smoke increases the chance of cardiovascular diseases. Nicotine tolerance, dependence, and withdrawal symptoms occur.
Opioids	Various names	Opioids are ingested or injected.	Opioids include morphine; codeine; oxycodone (Oxycontin, MS Contin); propoxyphene (Darvon); hydrocodone (Vicodin); hydromorphone (Dilaudid); and meperidine (Demerol). They cause drowsiness and constipation. Large single doses cause coma, hypotension, respiratory depression, and in some cases seizures and death. Mixing with alcohol and other CNS depressants increases the risk of coma and death. Chronic use of opioids produces tolerance, physical dependence, and withdrawal symptoms.
Phencyclidine (PCP)	Angel dust, ozone, wack, rocket fuel; killer joints or crystal supergrass when combined with marijuana	PCP is snorted, smoked, or eaten. For smoking, PCP is often applied to a leafy material such as mint, parsley, oregano, or marijuana	PCP is an addictive hallucinogen and sedative that often leads to psychological dependence, craving, and compulsive PCP-seeking behavior. Users often become violent or suicidal and are very dangerous to themselves and others. At low to moderate doses, effects include slight tachypnea, more pronounced tachycardia and hypertension, shallow respirations, and profuse sweating. Generalized numbness of the extremities and muscular lack of coordination also may occur. Psychological effects include distinct changes in body awareness, similar to those associated with alcohol intoxication. At high doses, effects include decreased blood pressure, pulse, and respirations; nausea and vomiting; blurred vision and nystagmus; drooling; ataxia; and seizures, coma, and death (though death more often results from accidental injury or suicide during PCP intoxication). Psychological effects at high doses include illusions, hallucinations, and effects that mimic the full range of symptoms of schizophrenia. Interactions with other CNS depressants, such as alcohol and benzodiazepines, can lead to coma. PCP is illegally manufactured in illicit laboratories.

(continued)

Table 35-3. Selected Drugs of Abuse and Addictive Substances *(Continued)*

Substance	Slang names	Methods of abuse	Major or unique health effects
Flunitrazepam (Rohypnol)	Rophie, roofies, roche, roach, rope, the date rape drug, forget-me	Rohypnol is ingested.	Rohypnol, a trade name for flunitrazepam, is a benzodiazepine that is not sold in the United States, but is smuggled into it. It produces sedative-hypnotic effects, including muscle relaxation and amnesia. It can also produce physical and psychological dependence.
			When mixed with alcohol, Rohypnol can incapacitate victims, can prevent them from resisting sexual assault, and can produce anterograde amnesia. It may also be lethal when mixed with alcohol or other CNS depressants.
			Clonazepam (Klonopin) and alprazolam (Xanax) are being abused like Rohypnol.
Stimulants, amphetamines, and related compounds	Speed, dexies, uppers	These drugs are ingested. Tablets can also be crushed and snorted.	These substances are CNS stimulants that increase alertness, attention, and energy, as well as increase blood pressure, pulse, and respiration.
			High doses can lead to arrhythmias; hypertension; hyperthermia; and potential for cardiovascular failure, stroke, or lethal seizures.
			Taking high doses of some stimulants repeatedly over a short period of time can lead to hostility or feelings of paranoia in some individuals.
			Stimulants such as dextroamphetamine (Dexedrine) and methylphenidate (Ritalin) can be addictive when misused.

Sources: National Institute on Drug Abuse, National Institutes of Health, 2009; Diversion Control Program, Drug Enforcement Administration, U.S. Department of Justice, 2009. Available at: www.deadiversion.usdoj.gov/drugs_concern/index.html.

Table 35-4. Commonly Used Antidotes

Toxin	Antidote (trade name)	Adult dose	Pediatric dose
Acetaminophen	Acetylcysteine (Mucomyst)	Oral loading dose: 140 mg/kg; maintenance dose: 70 mg/kg every 4 hours for 17 doses	Same as adult dose regimen
	Acetylcysteine (Acetadote)	IV infusion: 150 mg/kg in 200 mL D_5W over 1 hour, then 50 mg/kg in 500 mL 5% dextrose in water (D_5W) over 4 hours, followed by 100 mg/kg in 1,000 mL D_5W over 16 hours	Same as adult dose regimen
Anticholinergic compounds	Physostigmine salicylate (Antilirium)	1–2 mg slow IV infusion over 3–5 minutes titrated to effect	0.02 mg/kg slow IV infusion over 3–5 minutes titrated to effect
Arsenic	Succimer (Chemet)	10 mg/kg orally 3 times per day	Same as adult dose regimen
	Dimercaprol, also called British antilewisite (BAL in Oil), only if unable to tolerate oral succimer	3–5 mg/kg intramuscular every 4–6 hours	3–5 mg/kg intramuscular every 4–6 hours
Benzodiazepines	Flumazenil (Romazicon)[a]	0.2 mg IV bolus titrated to effect or total dose of 3 mg	0.01 mg/kg IV bolus titrated to effect or total dose of 1–3 mg
β-blockers	Glucagon (GlucaGen)	5–10 mg IV bolus, followed by 5–10 mg/h IV infusion titrated to effect	0.15 mg/kg mg IV bolus, followed by 0.1 mg/h IV infusion titrated to effect
Calcium channel blockers	Calcium chloride 10%	10–20 mL IV bolus; repeat doses and IV infusions common	0.1–0.2 mL/kg IV bolus; repeat doses and IV infusions common
	Glucagon (GlucaGen)	5–10 mg IV bolus, followed by 5–10 mg/h IV	0.15 mg IV bolus, followed by 0.1 mg/h IV infusion titrated to effect
Carbamates	Atropine	2–4 mg IV bolus, repeat doses titrated to effect	1 mg/kg IV bolus, repeat doses titrated to effect
Cyanide	Cyanide antidote kit composed of sodium nitrite 3% and sodium thiosulfate	Sodium nitrite: 300 mg slow IV infusion; sodium thiosulfate: 12.5 g IV infusion	Sodium nitrite: 0.15–0.33 mL/kg to maximum of 300 mg slow IV infusion; sodium thiosulfate: 400 mg/kg up to 12.5 g IV infusion
	Hydroxocobalamin (CyanoKit)[b] available since 2007	5 g IV infusion over 15 min; up to 5 g more based on response	70 mg/kg IV infusion based on use outside the United States
Digoxin	Digoxin immune Fab (Digibind, DigiFab)	Empiric dosing: 10–20 vials IV bolus for life-threatening toxicity (see package insert for other dosing regimens)	Empiric dosing: same as adult dose regiment (see package insert for other dosing regimens)
Ethylene glycol, methanol	Ethanol 10%	Loading dose 10 mL/kg IV or orally, followed by maintenance dose 1–2 mL/kg/h IV infusion or oral dose	Same as adult dose regimen
	Fomepizole (Antizol)	15 mg/kg IV bolus; smaller repeat doses may be necessary	Same as adult dose regimen
Iron	Deferoxamine (Desferal)	5–15 mg/kg/h IV infusion titrated to effect	Same as adult dose regimen
Isoniazid	Pyridoxine, also called vitamin B_6	1 g per gram ingested or empiric dosing of 5 g IV bolus	1 g per gram ingested or empiric dosing of 75 mg/kg IV bolus up to 5 g

(continued)

Table 35-4. Commonly Used Antidotes *(Continued)*

Toxin	Antidote (trade name)	Adult dose	Pediatric dose
Lead	Succimer (Chemet)	10 mg/kg orally 3 times per day; repeat doses common	Same as adult dose regimen
	Dimercaprol (also called British antilewisite [BAL]), only for lead encephalopathy (BAL in Oil)	3–5 mg/kg intramuscularly or 50–75 mg/m² intramuscularly	Same as adult dose regimen
	Calcium disodium ethylene-diaminetetraacetic acid (Calcium Disodium Versenate)	20–30 mg/kg diluted in 250 mL IV infusion over 12–24 hours (start 4 hours after BAL administration)	Same as adult dose regimen
Methemoglobinemia	Methylene blue	1–2 mg/kg slow IV infusion; repeat doses common	Same as adult dose regimen
Opioids	Naloxone (Narcan)	0.4–2.0 mg IV titrated to effect	Same as adult dose regimen
Organophosphates	Atropine	2–4 mg IV bolus; repeat doses titrated to effect	0.1 mg/kg IV bolus; repeat doses titrated to effect
	Pralidoxime hydrochloride (Protopam)	1–2 g slow IV infusion followed by 500 mg/h continuous infusion or 1 g every 4 hours	20–40 mg/kg slow IV infusion, followed by 5–10 mg/kg/h continuous infusion or 20 mg/kg every 4 hours
Salicylate	Sodium bicarbonate	150 mEq with 40 mEq KCl in 1 L of D_5W infused to maintain urine output at 1–2 mL/kg/h and a urine pH approximately 7.5	Same as adult dose regimen
Snake envenomation, crotaline[b] (rattlesnakes, cottonmouth, copperhead)	Crotalidae polyvalent immune Fab, ovine (CroFab)	Empiric dose: 4–6 vials IV infusion over 1 hour; additional doses depend on patient response (see package insert for dosing)	Same as adult dose regimen
Tricyclic antidepressants, agents with type 1a antiarrhythmic effects	Sodium bicarbonate	1–2 mEq/kg IV bolus; repeat boluses titrated to QRS duration (do not exceed arterial pH of 7.55)	Same as adult dose regimen
Warfarin, superwarfarins	Fresh-frozen plasma	Fresh-frozen plasma for life-threatening hemorrhage	Same as adult indication
	Vitamin K_1 (Mephyton, AquaMEPHYTON)	10–50 mg slow IV infusion or taken subcutaneously or orally	0.6 mg/kg slow IV infusion or taken subcutaneously or orally

Source: Based on American College of Emergency Physicians. Clinical policy for the initial approach to patients presenting with acute toxic ingestion or dermal or inhalation exposure. *Ann Emerg Med.* 1999;33:735–61.

Note: The table lists common antidotes that may need to be used emergently for patients presenting with acute toxic ingestion or dermal or inhalation exposure. Dosages are derived from standard texts and references and are given as convenience references. These should not be considered specific treatment guidelines; consult appropriate resources.

a. Potential risks may exceed the benefits because of precipitation of intractable seizures.

b. Information updated by author January 2009.

Indications

Acute overdoses of acetaminophen produce a reactive metabolite that leads to hepatotoxicity (jaundice, coagulopathy, hypoglycemia, hepatic failure, hepatic encephalopathy, hepatorenal failure). Symptoms become evident 1–2 days after ingestion.

Acetylcysteine can prevent or minimize hepatic injury if given early. For best results, administer within 10 hours of ingestion of acetaminophen overdose. It is minimally effective when started 24 hours after ingestion.

The need for therapy is determined by obtaining a serum concentration of acetaminophen at least 4 hours after ingestion (and within 24 hours) and plotting it on the acetaminophen nomogram to determine whether there is a risk for hepatotoxicity.

Contraindications

Use of acetylcysteine is contraindicated if there is a known hypersensitivity to the drug.

Adverse effects

With oral administration, nausea and vomiting are common.

With intravenous (IV) administration, anaphylactoid reactions (rash, hypotension, wheezing, and dyspnea) have been reported. Acute flushing and erythema may occur during the first hour of infusion and typically resolve spontaneously.

Dosage

Table 35-4 gives dosage information on drug products for oral or IV administration available in the United States.

Atropine

Indications

Atropine is used in cases of organophosphate (including chem-bioterrorism nerve agents) and carbamate anticholinesterase insecticide poisoning:

- For control of pulmonary hypersecretion, atropine is given in repeated doses intravenously until secretions have dried. Atropinization may have to be maintained for hours to days.
- For control of bradycardia, atropine is given until the heart rate increases or until a need for alternatives is indicated.

Nontoxicologic indications include atropine use for premedication to anesthesia induction (for antisecretory effects) and ophthalmic mydriasis and cycloplegia.

Mechanism of action

Atropine is an anticholinergic agent that competitively inhibits acetylcholine at muscarinic receptors. It has little effect on nicotinic receptors.

Contraindications

There are no contraindications in cases of insecticide poisoning. Contraindications for other indications are as follows:

- Hypersensitivity to atropine or anticholinergics
- Narrow-angle glaucoma
- Reflux esophagitis
- Obstructive gastrointestinal disease
- Ulcerative colitis or toxic megacolon
- Obstructive uropathy
- Unstable cardiovascular status in acute hemorrhage or thyrotoxicosis

- Paralytic ileus or intestinal atony
- Myasthenia gravis

Adverse effects

Exaggeration of anticholinergic effects (e.g., tachycardia, hypertension, sedation, hallucinations, mydriasis, changes in intraocular pressure, warm red skin, dry mouth, urinary retention, ileus, dysrhythmias, and seizures) can occur.

When large doses of atropine are used, the agent should be free of preservatives, because agents such as benzyl alcohol or chlorobutanol can produce their own toxicity.

Dosage

For bronchorrhea and bronchospasm from organophosphates or carbamates, the adult dose is 2–5 mg (pediatric dose is 0.05 mg/kg) slowly administered intravenously. This dose is repeated at 10- to 30-minute intervals until bronchial hypersecretion is resolved. Severe poisonings may require up to 100 mg over a few hours to several grams over several weeks. If atropinization is required for several days, continuous atropine infusion may be used (rates of 0.02–0.08 mg/kg/h are recommended).

For symptomatic bradycardia (for mild poisonings), the adult dose is 1 mg (pediatric dose is 0.01 mg/kg) intravenously. For moderate to severe poisonings, adult doses increase to 2–5 mg (pediatric doses are 0.02–0.05 mg/kg) and should be repeated every few minutes until heart rate increases.

Digoxin immune Fab (Digibind and DigiFab)

Uses

Digoxin immune Fab is used to treat life-threatening acute or chronic digoxin poisoning.

Some cross-reactivity with digitoxin and other digoxin-like compounds (digitalis, foxglove, lily of the valley, and bufadienolide from cane frogs) can occur.

Mechanism of action

Digoxin immune Fab binds digoxin in plasma, promotes redistribution from tissues, and enhances elimination in the urine. The digoxin bound to digoxin immune Fab is inactive. Each 40 mg (1 vial) binds 0.6 mg of digoxin.

Digoxin immune Fab is a monovalent, digoxin-specific, antigen-binding fragment (Fab) that is produced in healthy sheep.

Indications

Chronic digoxin toxicity typically begins with nausea, vomiting, diarrhea, fatigue, confusion, blurred vision, diplopia, and the observation of white borders or halos around dark objects. Deterioration of renal function, hypokalemia, or drug interactions often lead to toxicity.

Acute digoxin poisoning has early symptoms similar to those of chronic poisoning, but the onset is more abrupt. Nausea and vomiting are common, and the serum potassium concentration is typically normal or elevated.

A wide variety of arrhythmias occur with acute or chronic digoxin poisoning.

Digoxin immune Fab is reserved for life-threatening symptoms such as bradycardia, second- and third-degree heart block that is unresponsive to atropine, ventricular arrhythmias, and hyperkalemia (typically in excess of 5 mEq/L).

Contraindications

Digoxin immune Fab is contraindicated in patients with hypersensitivity to sheep.

Adverse effects

Common adverse effects include hypokalemia, allergic reactions (1% of patients), and hypotension. For patients on maintenance digoxin therapy, the abrupt binding of digoxin will lead to loss of therapeutic effect and a prompt decrease in potassium concentrations.

Dosage

Digoxin immune Fab is administered by IV infusion or rapid IV bolus (Table 35-4).

Dosage is determined by one of several approaches, depending on available information, as follows: empiric dosage of 10–20 vials (Table 35-4), dosing based on the dose of digoxin ingested, or dosing based on the serum digoxin concentration.

Flumazenil (Romazicon)

Uses

Flumazenil is used in cases of benzodiazepine overdose and in reversal of conscious sedation and general anesthesia from benzodiazepines.

Mechanism of action

Flumazenil is a competitive antagonist of the benzodiazepine receptor in the central nervous system (CNS).

Indications

Flumazenil should be used adjunctively with supportive care. Sedation can recur following ingestion of a benzodiazepine with a long half-life, requiring additional doses of flumazenil. In a suicidal over-

dose, it is rarely used because of the risk of potential co-ingestants. If no response occurs to a 5 mg cumulative dose, the sedation is probably not related to a benzodiazepine.

Contraindications

Flumazenil is contraindicated in patients with known hypersensitivity to it.

Co-ingestion of tricyclic antidepressants may precipitate ventricular dysrhythmias or seizures. Other mixed overdoses can decrease the seizure threshold (i.e., haloperidol, bupropion, lithium).

Abrupt withdrawal of flumazenil in patients on maintenance therapy, such as for treatment of epilepsy, can precipitate seizures.

Flumazenil is contraindicated in patients with increased intracranial pressure, because the antidote may potentially alter cerebral blood flow.

It can produce withdrawal in the benzodiazepine-dependent patient.

Adverse effects

Flumazenil has a wide margin of safety when not contraindicated.

Side effects include agitation, sweating, headache, abnormal vision, dizziness, and pain at the administration site. Rarely reported side effects include bradycardia, tachycardia, hypotension, and hypertension.

Dosage

Table 35-4 gives dosage information for IV administration.

Naloxone (Narcan)

Uses

Naloxone is used in the following cases:

- Reversal of opioid anesthesia
- Respiratory or CNS depression related to opioid toxicity
- Empiric administration in patients with altered mental status of unknown etiology

Mechanism of action

Naloxone is an opioid antagonist. It competes at three CNS opioid receptors (mu, kappa, and delta) and leads to reversal of the depressive opioid effects.

Indications

Opioids cause sedation, respiratory depression, hypotension, miosis, and analgesia. Because it has no agonist activity, naloxone will not worsen respiratory depression. The goal of therapy is to restore adequate spontaneous respirations.

When being administered naloxone, a patient should be monitored for respiratory rate changes and for opiate withdrawal symptoms (anxiety, hypertension, tachycardia, diarrhea, and seizure). To avoid withdrawal, use the lowest possible dose that maintains proper ventilation. The patient should be observed for respiratory depression once naloxone therapy is discontinued because the half-life of naloxone may be shorter than that of the opioid. If a patient is not responsive to 10 mg of naloxone, it is doubtful that an opioid is causing the respiratory depression.

Contraindications
- Avoid in patients with a known hypersensitivity to it.
- Use with caution in the opiate-dependent patient.
- Use with caution in patients with preexisting cardiovascular disease or those receiving cardiotoxic drugs.

Adverse effects
Use in an opiate-dependent patient can precipitate withdrawal. Withdrawal convulsions in a neonate can be life threatening.

Hypertension and dysrhythmias occur more often with opioid reversal in postoperative patients who have underlying cardiac and pulmonary complications.

Dosage
The IV route is preferred in emergency situations because of the rapid onset of action within 1–2 minutes (Table 35-4).

Naloxone has poor oral bioavailability.

The intramuscular and subcutaneous routes have erratic absorption.

Pralidoxime (Protopam)

Uses
Pralidoxime is used in cases of severe poisoning by an organophosphate anticholinesterase insecticide or chem-bioterrorism nerve agent.

Mechanism of action
Pralidoxime dephosphorylates acetylcholinesterase and regenerates acetylcholinesterase activity.

Indications
Pralidoxime is indicated in severe organophosphate or nerve agent poisoning, in combination with atropine, to resolve nicotinic (muscle and diaphragmatic weakness, fasciculations, muscle cramps) and central (coma, seizures) cholinergic manifestations. It is ineffective for organophosphates without anticholinesterase activity.

Its use in cases of carbamate poisoning is controversial, but some sources do recommend it for severe cases.

Contraindications
Pralidoxime should not be used in patients who are hypersensitive to the drug.

Adverse effects
- Tachycardia, dizziness, hyperventilation, and laryngospasm associated with rapid IV infusion
- Nausea, vomiting, diarrhea, bitter aftertaste, and rash after oral doses
- Blurred vision and diplopia
- Possible neuromuscular blockade (weakness) with high levels or in patients with myasthenia gravis

Dosage
See Table 35-4 for IV doses.

35-4. Terrorism and Disaster Preparedness

The world faces the growing threat of attacks with biological, chemical, explosive, and radiological weapons. Health care professionals should have an awareness of the potential for biological terrorism, an appreciation for epidemiologic clues of a chem-bioterrorist event, and a basic understanding of the classes of agents that can be weaponized and their effects.

Biological Threats

Bioterrorism is the deliberate use of infectious biological agents to cause illness and is categorized for risk by the Centers for Disease Control and Prevention (CDC) as follows:

- *Category A* agents are high-priority agents that can be easily transmitted, can result in high mortality rates, and have the potential for major public health impact. They include smallpox, anthrax, plague, botulism, tularemia, and viral hemorrhagic fevers (filoviruses [e.g., Ebola and Marburg] and arenaviruses [e.g., Lassa and Machupo]).
- *Category B* agents include brucellosis; epsilon toxin of *Clostridium perfringens;* food safety threats (e.g., *Salmonella* species, *Escherichia*

coli O157:H7, *Shigella*); glanders (*Burkholderia mallei*); melioidosis (*B pseudomallei*); psittacosis (*Chlamydia psittaci*); Q fever (*Coxiella burnetii*); ricin; staphylococcal enterotoxin B; typhus fever; viral encephalitis (alphaviruses such as Venezuelan equine encephalitis, eastern equine encephalitis, and western equine encephalitis), and water safety threats (e.g., *Vibrio cholerae, Cryptosporidium parvum*).

- *Category C* agents include emerging infectious disease threats such as Nipah virus and hantavirus.

See Table 35-5 for clinical features and suggested treatment for likely forms of category A diseases and for ricin, a category B agent that has been weaponized and used in terrorism.

The mode of transmission for biological agents is essentially the same as that of all other infectious diseases:

- Aerosol (most common form for biological weapons)
- Dermal contact
- Injection
- Food
- Water

Chemical Threats

Toxic chemicals that may be used in warfare and in a chemical terrorism attack include nerve, vesicant or blister, blood, choking or pulmonary, incapacitating, and tear- and vomit-inducing (riot control) agents. See Table 35-6 for descriptions, symptoms, and treatment of chemicals most likely to be used.

Normally, toxic chemicals used for these purposes are liquids or solids. Often they are dispersed in the air in aerosols.

The CDC also considers several commonly available agents to be threats, including hydrofluoric acid; benzene; ethylene glycol (antifreeze); and various metals such as arsenic, mercury, and thallium. These agents are not detailed in Table 35-6.

Radiological Threats

Radiological weapons involve nuclear radiation or radioactive materials with various radionucleotides. Radionucleotides can produce topical and systemic effects that may be immediate or delayed, depending on the agent, route of exposure, and extent of exposure.

Medical management of radiological emergencies and terrorist attacks is specific for radionucleotides.

Guidance on treatment is available from the Radiation Emergency Assistance Center/Training Site (REAC/TS) at the Oak Ridge Institute for Science and Education (Oak Ridge, Tennessee). The emergency response phone number is 1-865-576-1005; ask for REAC/TS. For program information, visit www.orise.orau.gov/reacts.

The early use of stable iodine, taken as potassium iodide or sodium iodide tablets, can reduce the uptake of radioiodine by the thyroid. Many individuals near nuclear reactors will maintain a stock of stable iodine tablets in the event of a radioactive accident. Ingestion of stable iodine is of little value for other radionucleotide exposures unless the radioactive constituents are unknown, as in a "dirty bomb."

Prussian blue 500-mg capsules are approved for the treatment of patients with exposures to radioactive cesium (Cs-137) and thallium (Tl-201). Prussian blue absorbs the radioactivity that is recirculated in the intestines and thereby enhances its elimination in the stool. The drug is available from the CDC.

Calcium and zinc salts of diethylene triamine pentaacetic acid for IV infusion and aerosol nebulization are approved to treat patients who have been exposed to radionucleotides that may be found in a "dirty bomb" such as plutonium, americium, and curium. The drugs form chelates with the radionucleotides that are excreted in the urine. The drugs are available from the CDC.

Emergency Preparedness

Pharmacists are in a unique position to quickly recognize communitywide patterns of symptoms, illness, and mortality in humans and animals that can be important clues to terrorist events.

The CDC advises that if citizens believe that they have been exposed to a biological or chemical agent, or if they believe an intentional biological threat will occur or is occurring, they should contact their local health or police department or another law enforcement agency (e.g., the Federal Bureau of Investigation). These agencies will notify the state health department and other response partners, through a preestablished notification list that channels to the CDC.

The CDC maintains the Strategic National Stockpile (SNS) to ensure the availability and rapid deployment of life-saving pharmaceuticals, antidotes, and other medical supplies and equipment necessary to counter nerve agents, biological pathogens, and chemical agents. The SNS program stands ready for immediate deployment to any U.S. location in the event of a terrorist attack using a biological toxin or chemical agent

Table 35-5. Biological Agents That May Be Used in a Terrorist Attack

Biological agent and description	Clinical features	Treatment
Smallpox is caused by the *variola* virus and may be spread by aerosol or direct contact with infected persons or fluids.	Early symptoms resemble a mild viral illness, with a 2- to 4-day nonspecific prodrome of fever and myalgias before rash onset. Pustules form, and then scabs form and fall off, leaving pitted scars. When all the scabs have fallen off (in about 3 weeks), patients are no longer contagious. Smallpox rash is typically most prominent on the face and extremities, and lesions form at the same time.[a]	No specific treatment exists. A live-virus vaccine of *vaccinia* virus (Dryvax) is primarily preventive for close contacts, but vaccination within 4 days of exposure *may* prevent or lessen disease.
Anthrax is caused by *Bacillus anthracis,* a Gram-positive spore-forming rod. It has 3 major forms (cutaneous, inhalation, and gastrointestinal), and none are contagious.	*Cutaneous:* This form begins as a small papule and progresses to a vesicle in 1–2 days, followed by a necrotic, normally painless ulcer. Victim may have fever, malaise, headache, and regional lymphadenopathy. *Inhalation:* This form initially resembles a viral illness with sore throat, mild fever, muscle aches, and malaise. It often has minimally productive cough, nausea or vomiting, and chest discomfort, which may progress to respiratory failure and shock, with meningitis frequently developing.[b] *Gastrointestinal:* This form causes severe abdominal or oropharyngeal distress, followed by fever and signs of septicemia, bloody vomit, and diarrhea.	Ciprofloxacin and doxycycline are FDA-approved for postexposure prophylaxis (PEP) of children and adults, while levofloxacin is approved for adults 18 years of age and older. Ciprofloxacin and doxycycline are FDA-approved for treatment. Amoxicillin or penicillin may be used if hypersensitivity or other risks are present. Persons at risk for inhalation anthrax need 60 days of prophylactic antibiotics. Anthrax Vaccine Adsorbed (BioThraxT) given intramuscularly is indicated for active immunization for the prevention of disease caused by *Bacillus anthracis* in persons age 18–65 at high risk of exposure.
Plague, caused by *Yersinia pestis,* has several forms, with pneumonic plague being the most virulent.	Clinical features of aerosolized pneumonic plague include fever, cough with mucopurulent sputum, hemoptysis, and chest pain with signs consistent with severe pneumonia 1–6 days after exposure. Septic shock and high mortality can occur within 2–4 days of symptom onset without early treatment. *Y. pestis*–caused bubonic plague is less likely to be weaponized.	Early treatment for pneumonic plague with streptomycin or gentamicin is advised. Other antibiotics may also be effective. A vaccine is no longer manufactured.
Botulism, caused by *Clostridium botulinum,* may be foodborne or airborne.	Clinical features include acute symmetric descending paralysis in a proximal to distal pattern; prominent bulbar palsies such as diplopia, dysarthria, dysphonia, and dysphagia that typically present 12–72 hours postexposure; and respiratory dysfunction from respiratory muscle paralysis or upper airway obstruction without sensory deficits.	Antitoxin (most effective within 24 hours of exposure) is maintained and dispensed by the CDC. Most patients recover after supportive care, often with mechanical ventilation for weeks to months.
Tularemia, caused by *Francisela tularensis,* is one of the most infectious bacteria known.	Inhalation exposure causes an abrupt onset of a nonspecific febrile illness beginning 3–5 days postexposure, with incipient pneumonia, pleuritis, and hilar lymphadenopathy. Without treatment, respiratory failure, shock, and death are possible. Like botulism and anthrax, tularemia is not contagious, so patients who have tularemia do not need to be isolated.	Prompt treatment with streptomycin, gentamicin, chloramphenicol, doxycycline, or ciprofloxacin is advised, as is early PEP use of doxycycline or ciprofloxacin.

(continued)

Table 35-5. Biological Agents That May Be Used in a Terrorist Attack *(Continued)*

Biological agent and description	Clinical features	Treatment
Viral hemorrhagic fevers (VHFs) include filoviruses, arenaviruses, bunyaviruses, and flaviviruses. (Other VHFs exist but are not considered a serious bioterrorism risk.) Filoviruses and arenaviruses are most virulent, but all viruses listed here are considered serious biological threats; exposure is by all routes, including direct and aerosol.	With filoviruses (Ebola and Marburg types), an abrupt onset of an undifferentiated febrile illness with high fever occurs 2–21 days after exposure. A maculopapular rash, prominent on the trunk, develops about 5 days later, with progressive bleeding symptoms such as petechiae, ecchymosis, disseminated intra-vascular coagulation, and hemorrhages. With arenaviruses (Lassa and multiple New World arenaviruses, including Machupo, which causes Bolivian hemorrhagic fever), symptoms and onset are similar to filoviruses, but with a gradual onset of rash, hemorrhagic diathesis, and shock. Bunyaviruses cause Rift Valley fever (< 1% develop hemorrhagic fever). Flaviviruses cause yellow fever, Omsk hemor-rhagic fever, and Kyasanur Forest disease.	The mainstay of treatment is supportive to maintain fluid and electrolyte balance, circulatory volume, and blood pressure. There are no FDA-approved antiviral drugs or vaccines.
Ricin, from castor beans, is cytotoxic through inhibition of protein synthesis; abrin is a similar toxalbumin agent.	Within a few hours of inhalation, victims develop cough and dyspnea, with the lungs rapidly becoming severely inflamed and filled with fluid. Skin might turn blue from cyanosis or flush red. Ingestion causes internal bleeding of the stomach and intestines. Injection kills the closest muscles and lymph nodes before spreading to other organs. Death can occur within 36–48 hours of all types of exposure from multiple organ failure.	No antidote is available. The mainstay of treatment is supportive, varying with the route of exposure. If victims survive more than 5 days, survival is likely.

a. In contrast, chickenpox rash is prominent on the trunk and develops in groups of lesions over several days.
b. In contrast, influenza patients rarely have a runny nose and usually have an abnormal chest x-ray and high white-blood-cell count.

directed against a civilian population. A limited stock of drugs to treat nerve agents (CHEMPACK) has been deployed to emergency medical services and hospital sites throughout the United States and is maintained by the CDC. For further information, visit the CDC Web site at www.cdc.gov.

Pharmacists should consider volunteering in their communities to assist with emergency preparedness. Roles in mass dispensing and vaccination clinics, SNS deployment, and general disaster medical relief are possible opportunities. Contact the local health department or emergency medical services agency.

Essential steps to volunteering for emergency preparedness include reaching an understanding with one's family and employer, registering as a volunteer and identifying skills to contribute, obtaining security credentials, participating in training, and doing whatever it takes when needed.

35-5. Key Points

■ Medications are the most common cause of poisoning morbidity and mortality. Any chemical can become toxic if too much is taken in relation to body weight and tolerance. A large number of poisonings occur in young children, but most fatalities occur in adults.

■ Several approaches can minimize the risk of unintentional childhood poisonings (e.g., use of safety latches, proper storage of poisonous substances, and adherence to label instructions), but the proper use of child-resistant containers (safety caps) is one of the most effective means.

■ As part of the Poison Prevention Packaging Act of 1970, pharmacists are required to dispense oral prescription drugs (with certain exceptions such as nitroglycerin and oral contraceptives) in

Table 35-6. Chemical Agents That May Be Used in a Terrorist Attack

Chemical agents	Clinical features	Treatment
Nerve agents: G agents: sarin (GB), soman (GD), tabun (GA), cyclohexyl sarin (GF) V agents: VX	These nerve agents are organophosphates that attach to and inhibit acetylcholinesterase at muscarinic and nicotinic receptors, causing cholinergic crisis with miosis; vomiting; diarrhea; excessive bronchial, lacrimal, dermal, nasal, and salivary secretions; bradycardia or tachycardia; skeletal muscle fasciculations; paralysis; seizures; and respiratory failure. They are well absorbed through all routes of exposure. Symptoms occur within minutes after significant exposure and up to 18 hours after liquid exposure.	Rapid, thorough decontamination is needed. Antidotes include atropine to reverse muscarinic symptoms and pralidoxime early to restore acetylcholinesterase before permanent deactivation (aging) of the enzyme. Also give diazepam or lorazepam for seizures.
Blister agents: Mustards and nitrogen mustards Lewisites Chloroarsines Mustard–lewisite combinations Phosgene oxime (CX)	Mustards are vesicants that cause blistering of the skin and mucous membranes on contact, damaging skin, eyes, and lungs. Damage is immediate, but symptoms can be delayed 2–24 hours. Liquid forms are more likely to cause burns and scarring than will gas. All forms are absorbed through the skin and distributed systemically. Nitrogen mustards cause bone marrow suppression in 3–5 days. Sulfur mustards have garlic, onion, mustard, or no odor. Nitrogen mustards can smell fishy, musty, soapy, or fruity. Lewisites and chloroarsines are arsenical vesicants that cause immediate pain and damage to the eyes, skin, and respiratory tract, although lesions may take hours to form. After absorption, they cause increased capillary permeability leading to hypovolemia, shock, and organ damage. Lewisite smells like geraniums. A mustard–lewisite combination is lewisite combined with distilled mustard. Phosgene oxime is readily absorbed—causing immediate, painful corrosive and necrotic tissue damage—and has a disagreeable odor.	Sulfur and nitrogen mustards (thought to be alkylating agents that crosslink DNA strands) have no antidote. Avoiding contact or effecting rapid, thorough decontamination are the only preventions. Treatment is supportive. Exposure is not usually fatal (sulfur type < 5% fatal in World War I). No mustard is in tissue or blister fluids. British antilewisite is specific antidote for lewisite, used intramuscularly for systemic effects or topically as skin or eye ointment. Chloroarsine treatment is similar, except atropine sulfate ointment is used for eyes. No antidote exists for phosgene oxime. Rapid decontamination and supportive treatment are used as for any corrosive agent.
Blood agents: Arsine (SA) Cyanide gases: hydrogen cyanide (AC), cyanogen chloride (CK) Cyanide solids: potassium (KCN), sodium (NaCN) cyanide	Arsine is a gas that causes nausea, vomiting, hemolysis, and secondary renal failure in 1–2 hours to 11 days. It has a garlic-like odor. Inhalation of highly concentrated cyanide causes an increased rate and depth of breathing in 15 seconds, convulsions in 30 seconds, cessation of respiration in 2–4 minutes, and cessation of heartbeat in 4–8 minutes. Progress and severity of symptoms after ingestion or inhalation of lower gas concentrations are slower and dose dependent. Gas may have odor of bitter almonds or peach kernels (AC); no odor; or irritating, lacrimating properties like riot control agents (CK).	For arsines, use symptomatic management of hemolysis, normally without chelation. Cyanides bind to cytochrome oxidase. Two antidote kits are available. Cyanide Antidote Kit has a methemoglobin-forming agent (sodium nitrite) that binds cyanide and a sulfur donor to convert it to excretable sodium thiocyanate (sodium thiosulfate). CyanoKit combines hydroxocobalamin with cyanide to form nontoxic cyanocobalamin (vitamin B_{12}). Fresh air, oxygen, and supportive treatment are essential.

(continued)

Table 35-6. Chemical Agents That May Be Used in a Terrorist Attack *(Continued)*

Chemical agents	Clinical features	Treatment

Choking and pulmonary agents:
 	
  Phosgene (CG)
 	
  Diphosgene (DP)
 	
  Ammonia
 	
  Chlorine (CL)
 	
  Hydrogen chloride
 	
  Nitrogen oxide (NO)
 	
  Perfluoroisobutylene (PHIB)
 	
  Others
	Phosgene gas causes eye, nose, throat, and pulmonary irritation, with serious pulmonary injury and edema delayed up to 48 hours, because it hydrolyzes to hydrochloric acid in moist conditions. It has a new-mown-hay odor. Phosgene is the prototype agent in the group. Other agents cause immediate irritation with potential for more severe delayed effects.
	
	Ammonia hydrolyzes to caustic ammonium hydroxide.
	
	Chlorine (pungent, greenish gas) hydrolyzes to hydrochloric acid.
	
	Perfluoroisobutylene is a toxic pyrolysis product of Teflon.
	
	Nitrogen oxides are components of blast weapons or fire.
	
	Others include red (RP) and white phosphorus, sulfur trioxide-chlorosulfonic acid (FS), titanium tetrachloride (FM), and zinc oxide (HC).
		Phosgene has no antidote. Good decontamination and symptomatic treatment are needed.
		
		Treatment of other agents is similar because all agents in this class are gases with no antidotes. Thorough, rapid decontamination with fresh air is the best initial management, with thorough flushing of exposed eyes and skin and symptomatic treatment.

Incapacitating agents	These agents contain a variety of fast-acting central nervous system and respiratory depressants, often with hallucinogenic properties. The CDC list includes BZ/agent 15 (glycolate anticholinergic), cannabinoids, fentanyls and other opioids, LSD, and phenothiazines.	Management is decontamination with supportive treatment, and antidotes should be used when they exist (physostigmine for anticholinergics; naloxone for opioids).
Riot control and tear gases	Lacrimators include chloroacetophenone (CN) in several solvents and chloropicrin (PS), bromobenzylcyanide (CA), dibenzoxazepine (CR), and 2-chlorobenzalmalononitrile (CS) gases.	Treatment is symptomatic after decontamination. No antidotes are available.
Vomiting agents	These agents include adamsite (DM), diphenyl-chloroarsine (DA), and diphenylcyanoarsine (DC). They are rapidly incapacitating, irritant gases.	Symptomatic measures are used for sneezing, coughing, and vomiting (e.g., antiemetics).

Note: Military names are in parentheses.

child-resistant containers unless the patient or prescriber indicates the desire for a nonsafety cap.

- Immediate first aid for a poison exposure can minimize potential toxic effects and involves water and fresh air, depending on the route of exposure. Contact a poison center immediately through the nationwide access number (1-800-222-1222) to determine whether first aid should be administered or whether a poisoning emergency exists.
- The use of drugs to decrease the absorption of drugs from the gastrointestinal tract after a poisoning or overdose is in a state of change.

- Ipecac syrup—an orally administered emetic—has questionable effectiveness, and its use is now generally avoided. It should not be used when (1) the person exhibits sleepiness, coma, or seizures; (2) agents such as caustics and aliphatic hydrocarbons and fast-acting agents that produce coma or seizures (e.g., tricyclic antidepressants, clonidine, strychnine, hypoglycemic agents) have been ingested; (3) the ingestion was greater than 1 hour ago; or (4) there is an obvious need for hospital referral.
- Cathartics such as magnesium citrate are not routinely used.

- Activated charcoal—an orally administered adsorbent—is often the only treatment necessary if the toxin can be adsorbed and it is used within 1–2 hours of ingestion. It should be avoided in ingestions of aliphatic hydrocarbons and caustics and in patients with absent bowel sounds, and it is not useful with ingestion of heavy metals (sodium, lithium, iron, or lead) or simple alcohols.
- Whole-bowel irrigation, with products such as CoLyte and GoLYTELY, can be considered if the toxin is poorly adsorbed and its presence in the gastrointestinal tract is likely.
- Other hospital-based therapies include supportive and symptomatic care, multiple doses of activated charcoal (to enhance systemic elimination when appropriate), hemodialysis (to enhance systemic elimination when appropriate), and use of antidotes (to antagonize or reverse toxic effects when indicated).
- Substance abuse often leads to acute and chronic toxicity from a variety of medications, commercial products, and illicit agents. The management of acute toxicity from substance abuse typically follows the same general approaches as those for poisoning and overdose. A challenge faced in many acute drug overdose episodes is determining the agents taken and possible adulterants or contaminants. Chronic abuse can lead to dependence and withdrawal symptoms when use is stopped.
- Few antidotes are available relative to the large number of potential poisons. The use of an antidote is usually an adjunct to conventional and supportive therapies. Many hospitals have an insufficient stock of antidotes.
- Acetylcysteine is a glutathione substitute in the metabolism of the acetaminophen-toxic reactive metabolite. It is most effective in preventing hepatotoxicity if given orally within 10 hours of an acetaminophen overdose, and it may also help later to minimize hepatic injury once it has begun. Oral (Mucomyst) and IV (Acetadote) preparations are available.
- Atropine is used to treat the muscarinic effects (bronchorrhea, bradycardia, etc.) produced by organophosphate and carbamate insecticides and anticholinesterase nerve gas agents by competing with acetylcholine for binding at muscarinic receptors in the nervous system.
- Pralidoxime (Protopam) reactivates the enzyme acetylcholinesterase by dephosphorylation and allows metabolism of accumulated amounts of acetylcholine produced by enzyme inhibition from exposures to anticholinesterase nerve gas agents and organophosphate and carbamate insecticides.
- Digoxin immune Fab (Digibind, DigiFab) is a specific antibody for digoxin, but it exhibits some cross-reactivity with other digoxin-like compounds. It is an ovine-derived antigen-binding fragment reserved for the treatment of life-threatening symptoms of digoxin overdose (e.g., bradycardia, ventricular arrhythmias, second- and third-degree heart block, hyperkalemia).
- Flumazenil (Romazicon) is a competitive antagonist of benzodiazepines at the benzodiazepine receptor in the CNS. It is used in the treatment of severe CNS and respiratory depression that may occur when benzodiazepines are used as an anesthetic or taken as an overdose. Seizures may occur when flumazenil is administered to patients with co-ingestants of tricyclic antidepressants—drugs that lower the seizure threshold—and to patients requiring benzodiazepines for seizure control.
- Administration of naloxone (Narcan), a competitive antagonist of opiate binding at the opioid receptors in the CNS, reverses the CNS and respiratory depression of opiate toxicity. Naloxone may precipitate withdrawal symptoms in opiate-dependent patients.
- Bioterrorism is the deliberate use of infectious biological agents to cause illness. High-priority agents can be easily transmitted, result in high mortality rates, and have the potential for major public health impact. They include smallpox (*Variola* virus), anthrax (*Bacillus anthracis*), plague (*Yersinia pestis*), botulism (*Clostridium botulinum*), tularemia (*Francisela tularensis*), and viral hemorrhagic fevers (e.g., Ebola, Marburg, Lassa, Machupo).
- These chemicals can be used in warfare and may be used in a terrorist attack:
  - Substances that act on nerves (e.g., anticholinesterase agents such as sarin)
  - Substances that are blistering or vesicant agents (e.g., mustard agents, lewisites)
  - Substances that act on blood (e.g., arsine, cyanide)
  - Substances that act on the pulmonary system (e.g., phosgene, chlorine, ammonia)
  - Substances that are incapacitating (e.g., fast-acting CNS depressants or hallucinogens)
  - Substances that can also be used in riot control (e.g., various lacrimating agents such as

chloroacetophenone and vomiting agents such as adamsite).

■ Health care providers must have an awareness of the potential for terrorism, an appreciation for epidemiologic clues of a chem-bioterrorist event, and a basic understanding of the classes of agents that can be weaponized and their effects. The CDC maintains the Strategic National Stockpile. The SNS can be rapidly deployed to communities to ensure the availability of life-saving pharmaceuticals, antidotes, other medical supplies, and equipment necessary to counter nerve agents, biological pathogens, and chemical agents.

35-6. Questions

1. Flumazenil is contraindicated in which of the following?

    I. A patient with QRS widening with a known ingestion of Elavil
    II. A patient who was previously given flumazenil and who now complains of abnormal vision and dizziness
    III. A patient with known use of cocaine

    A. I only
    B. II only
    C. III only
    D. I and III
    E. I and II

2. A patient is brought to the emergency department. She is experiencing CNS and respiratory depression, which are suspected to be related to ingestion of her sister's MS Contin. You recommend supportive care and the administration of which of the following?

    A. Flumazenil
    B. Naloxone
    C. Lorazepam
    D. Flumazenil and Narcan
    E. Pyridoxine

3. A police officer presents to the emergency room with a rash. He fears that he was exposed to a biological weapon several days before the rash appeared. You notice the rash is forming pustules and is most prominent on the face and extremities. The patient says the rash developed all at once. He has possibly contracted which of the following?

    A. Smallpox
    B. Chickenpox
    C. Anthrax
    D. Tularemia
    E. None of the above

4. What is the recommended treatment for the likely disease?

    I. Supportive, as there is no specific treatment
    II. Ciprofloxacin
    III. Doxycycline

    A. II or III
    B. II and III
    C. I only
    D. II only
    E. III only

5. Which of the following is the currently available prevention for smallpox?

    I. Dryvax
    II. A live-virus preparation of the vaccinia virus
    III. Avoidance of direct contact with infected persons and their body fluids

    A. I only
    B. I and II only
    C. II and III only
    D. I, II, and III
    E. No vaccine is currently available.

6. A patient presents with a black, necrotic, painless skin lesion on her arm. She also complains of fever, malaise, headache, and swelling of her underarm lymph nodes. Which of the following is the possible biological agent responsible for these symptoms?

    A. Hemorrhagic fever virus
    B. Anthrax
    C. Botulism
    D. Tularemia
    E. Arsine

7. The recommended antibiotic treatment of the infection in question 6 may include which of the following?

    A. Ciprofloxacin
    B. Doxycycline
    C. Amoxicillin
    D. All of the above
    E. Supportive therapy, as there is no specific treatment

8. Inhalation exposure to the agent in question 6 requires which of the following?

 A. Postexposure prophylaxis with ciprofloxacin, doxycycline, or levofloxacin for 60 days
 B. Immediate vaccination of civilian personnel
 C. Early treatment with streptomycin or gentamicin
 D. Early treatment with ribavirin
 E. None of the above

9. A cab driver presents to the emergency department with vomiting, diarrhea, sweating, salivation, moist rales, bradycardia, muscle tremor, and weakness. He reports inhaling a mist dropped from a low-flying plane several hours earlier. You also note that he has miosis and his respiratory difficulty is increasing rapidly. Which of the following is the likely mechanism of toxicity of the poison?

 A. Inhibition of protein synthesis
 B. Binding of the agent to cytochrome oxidase
 C. Inhibition of acetylcholinesterase
 D. An alkylating agent that cross-links DNA strands
 E. None of the above

10. The recommended initial management of the symptoms in question 9 includes all *except* which of the following?

 A. Immediate decontamination of skin and eyes
 B. Disposal of contaminated clothes
 C. British antilewisite
 D. Atropine
 E. Pralidoxime

11. The patient in question 9 deteriorates and develops seizures. Which of the following do you recommend?

 A. Phenytoin
 B. Diazepam
 C. Lithium
 D. Dryvax
 E. All of the above

12. Which of the following conditions or situations is *not* a contraindication to the use of ipecac syrup?

 A. High blood pressure controlled with drug therapy

 B. Seizures shortly before administration
 C. Unresponsiveness to verbal commands
 D. Ingestion of a corrosive agent
 E. A and C

13. Which of the following is an effect of activated charcoal?

 A. Promotes dissolution of tablets
 B. Minimizes drug absorption from the gastrointestinal tract
 C. Increases urinary flow
 D. Enhances systemic elimination of certain drugs
 E. B and D

14. Which of the following is useful in the treatment of acetaminophen poisoning?

 A. Acetylcysteine
 B. Dimercaprol
 C. Pralidoxime
 D. Atropine
 E. Dryvax

15. Digoxin immune Fab is used to treat which of the following signs or symptoms of digoxin poisoning?

 A. Hypokalemia
 B. Diplopia
 C. Ventricular tachycardia
 D. Second-degree heart block unresponsive to atropine
 E. C and D

16. How does crack cocaine differ from pharmaceutical cocaine?

 A. Crack cocaine is more stable under heat and can be smoked.
 B. Pharmaceutical cocaine is the hydrochloride salt.
 C. Crack cocaine is the free-base form of cocaine.
 D. Crack cocaine may be contaminated with other substances.
 E. All of the above.

17. Which of the following mechanisms is associated with the production of hepatic injury from an acute overdose of acetaminophen?

 A. Interference with RNA (ribonucleic acid) synthesis

B. Interference with transaminase enzyme activity

C. Direct toxicity of acetaminophen

D. Formation of a toxic metabolite

E. Exaggeration of its pharmacologic effects

18. Which of the following signs or symptoms is characteristic of an acute exposure to an organophosphate as an insecticide or terrorist weapon?

A. Dry mouth and mucous membranes

B. Excessive bronchial secretions

C. Muscle rigidity

D. Urinary retention

E. All of the above

35-7. Answers

1. **D.** Flumazenil is contraindicated in all patients who have ingested a tricyclic antidepressant and have cardiac symptoms because its use could cause ventricular dysrhythmias. It is not recommended in mixed overdose where the co-ingested drug can cause a seizure (i.e., cocaine). Statement II describes associated adverse effects with that may occur with the administration of flumazenil; they are not contraindications.

2. **B.** Naloxone is an opioid antagonist.

3. **A.** See Table 35-5. Smallpox is the most likely agent. The agent causes formation of a pustular rash that is typically most prominent on the face and extremities. Lesions form at the same time. Chickenpox rash is most prominent on the trunk and develops in successive groups of lesions over several days. Anthrax forms painless necrotic lesions. Tularemia causes a nonspecific febrile illness that rapidly develops into pneumonia.

4. **C.** See Table 35-5. Smallpox has no specific treatment, but the live-vaccine (Dryvax) *may* lessen the disease if given within 4 days of the exposure. Ciprofloxacin and doxycycline are used in the management of anthrax, plague, and tularemia.

5. **D.** See Table 35-5. All options are correct.

6. **B.** See Tables 35-5 and 35-6. Anthrax forms a painless, necrotic ulcer. Hemorrhagic fever viruses cause a rash that develops into petechiae, ecchymosis, hemorrhages, and other bleeding symptoms. Botulism causes a symmetric descending paralysis. Tularemia causes a non-

specific febrile illness that rapidly develops into pneumonia. Arsine is a chemical agent that causes nausea, vomiting, hemolysis, and secondary renal failure. Arsine is produced when water comes into contact with metallic arsenide or when acids come into contact with metallic arsenic or arsenical compounds. The mechanism of hemolysis is not specifically known, but the most recent mechanism postulated involves a direct arsine–hemoglobin interaction that forms arsenic metabolites, causing direct alteration of the erythrocyte cell membrane.

7. **D.** See Table 35-5. Ciprofloxacin, levofloxacin, and doxycycline are approved by the U.S. Food and Drug Administration (FDA) for treatment of anthrax, while amoxicillin can be used when the other drugs are not tolerated or pose patient-specific risks. These agents can be used separately or in combination, depending on the symptoms and the patient's sensitivity to the agents. Antimicrobial resistance to ciprofloxacin has been growing rapidly because of widespread overuse after the anthrax-contaminated mail episodes in 2002.

8. **A.** See Table 35-5. Persons at risk for inhalational anthrax need 60 days of prophylactic antibiotics. Ciprofloxacin and doxycycline are FDA-approved for postexposure prophylaxis (PEP) in adults and children; levofloxacin is used in adults 18 years of age and older. If these drugs are not tolerated, amoxicillin can be used. In 2009, a vaccine (BioThraxT) became available that can be given postexposure in conjunction with antibiotics or as a vaccination for high-risk personnel (e.g., military or lab personnel likely to be in contact with the bacteria). Streptomycin and gentamicin are among the suggested treatments for pneumonic plague. Ribavirin is a potential treatment for some hemorrhagic fever viruses.

9. **C.** See Table 35-6. The symptoms exhibited are classically cholinergic, and the likely chemical agents causing these symptoms are organophosphates such as nerve agents or possibly organophosphate pesticides. Both can be spread by low-flying planes. Inhibition of protein synthesis is the mechanism of toxicity of ricin or abrin. Cyanides bind to cytochrome oxidase, thereby interrupting normal cellular respiration and causing rapid convulsions. Blister agents such as sulfur and nitrogen mustards are thought to be alkylating agents that cross-link DNA

strands, thereby separating dermal layers in the skin and causing fluid-filled blisters to form.

10. **C.** British antilewisite is a specific antidote for lewisite. See Table 35-6. It also is used as a chelator for treatment of acute arsenic, inorganic or elemental mercury, gold, and other heavy metal poisonings. See Table 35-4. The other measures are treatments for organophosphate agents. Good decontamination and disposal of contaminated clothes (especially leather) are needed, because organophosphates are well absorbed across the skin, through the lungs, and through ingestion—essentially all possible routes of exposure. Atropine is used for muscarinic symptoms (miosis; nausea and vomiting; diarrhea; urination; bradycardia; and excessive bronchial, lacrimal, dermal, nasal, and salivary secretions). Pralidoxime is used with atropine to resolve severe organophosphate symptoms (such as those from exposure to nerve agents), including nicotinic symptoms of muscle weakness and cramps, fasciculations, and tachycardia, and CNS symptoms such as coma and seizures.

11. **B.** See Table 35-6. Recommended treatment for seizures attributable to organophosphate agents is either diazepam or lorazepam. Phenytoin is a seizure medication, but benzodiazepines (then barbiturates if benzodiazepines fail) are generally preferred over phenytoin for the control of overdose- or withdrawal-related seizures. Lithium is not a seizure medicine and, in fact, may cause seizures with elevated blood concentrations. Dryvax is a vaccine for smallpox.

12. **A.** Controlled high blood pressure is not a problem with the use of ipecac syrup, but the other situations are clear contraindications because of potential aspiration (seizures and unresponsiveness) and additional esophageal burns on vomiting up gastric contents (corrosive).

13. **E.** Activated charcoal adsorbs chemicals on contact and prevents their absorption into the bloodstream. For certain drugs (e.g., phenobarbital, theophylline), multiple doses of activated charcoal can promote the back diffusion of drugs across the intestinal capillary bed into the lumen of the gut, trap it there, and promote its elimination. The elimination half-life can be decreased by as much as one-half.

14. **A.** Acetylcysteine prevents the development of liver injury from acetaminophen if given early after ingestion and, in some cases, may help minimize the effects of hepatotoxicity after it has occurred.

15. **E.** Digoxin immune Fab is reserved for life-threatening symptoms because of its profound effects, scarcity, and high cost. Most serious cases of digoxin poisoning have normal or high potassium concentrations because of the digoxin's interference with the sodium-potassium ATPase pump.

16. **E.** All are differences between the two forms of cocaine.

17. **D.** Acetaminophen forms a toxic metabolite that has a direct toxic effect within the hepatocyte. It has other proposed mechanisms, but this mechanism is thought to be the inciting event. See the description for acetylcysteine in Section 35-3.

18. **B.** Excessive bronchial secretions are one of the principal causes of death from exposure to organophosphates. The other symptoms are not observed. See the description for atropine and pralidoxime in Section 35-3.

35-8. References

General Toxicology

American College of Emergency Physicians. Clinical policy for the initial approach to patients presenting with acute toxic ingestion or dermal or inhalation exposure. *Ann Emerg Med.* 1999;33:735–61.

Bronstein AC, Spyker DA, Cantelina LR, et al. 2006 annual report of the American Association of Poison Control Centers' National Poison Data System (NCDS). *Clin Toxicol.* 2007;45:815–917.

Chyka PA. Clinical toxicology. In: Dipiro JT, Talbert RL, Yee GC, et al., eds. *Pharmacotherapy: A Pathophysiologic Approach.* 7th ed. New York: McGraw-Hill; 2008:69–90.

Dart RC, ed. *Medical Toxicology.* 3rd ed. Philadelphia: Lippincott Williams & Wilkins; 2004.

Diversion Control Program, Drug Enforcement Administration, U.S. Department of Justice. Drugs and chemicals of concern. Available at: www.deadiversion.usdoj.gov/drugs_concern/index.html.

Flomenbaum NE, Goldfrank LR, Hoffman RS, et al., eds. *Goldfrank's Toxicologic Emergencies.* 8th ed. New York: McGraw-Hill; 2006.

Ford MD, Delaney KA, Ling LJ, Erickson T. *Clinical Toxicology.* Philadelphia: WB Saunders; 2001.

Klaassen CD. Principles of toxicology and treatment of poisoning. In: Brunton LL, Lazo JS, Parker KL, eds. *Goodman and Gilman's The Pharmacological Basis of Therapeutics.* 11th ed. New York: McGraw-Hill; 2006:1739–51.

National Institute on Drug Abuse, National Institutes of Health. NIDA InfoFacts: Science-based facts on drug abuse and addiction. Available at: www.nida. nih.gov/Infofacts/Infofaxindex.html.

Office of Applied Studies, Substance Abuse and Mental Health Services Administration. *Drug Abuse Warning Network, 2006.* DHHS publication SMA 08-4339. Rockville, Md.: Substance Abuse and Mental Health Services Administration; 2008.

Olson KR, ed. *Poisoning and Drug Overdose.* 5th ed. New York: Lange/McGraw-Hill; 2007.

Terrorist Threats

Abramowicz M, ed. Prevention and treatment of injury from chemical warfare agents. *Med Letter.* 2002;44:1–4.

Kales SN, Christiani DC. Acute chemical emergencies. *N Engl J Med.* 2004;350:800–8.

Oak Ridge Institute for Science and Education. Managing radiation emergencies: Guidance for hospital medical management. Available at: www.orise. orau.gov/reacts/.

Setlak P. Bioterrorism preparedness and response: Emerging role for health-system pharmacists. *Am J Health-Syst Pharm.* 2004;61:1167–75.

Shepherd G, Schwartz RB. Emergency preparedness: Identification and management of chemical and radiological exposures. In: Dipiro JT, Talbert RL, Yee GC, et al., eds. *Pharmacotherapy: A Pathophysiologic Approach.* 7th ed. New York: McGraw-Hill; 2008:93.

Terriff CM, Brouillard JE, Costanigro LT, Gruber JS. Emergency preparedness: Identification and management of biological exposures. In: Dipiro JT, Talbert RL, Yee GC, et al., eds. *Pharmacotherapy: A Pathophysiologic Approach.* 7th ed. New York: McGraw-Hill; 2008:91.

U.S. Centers for Disease Control and Prevention. Emergency preparedness and response. Available at: www.bt.cdc.gov.

U.S. Department of Health and Human Services. National disaster medical response. Available at: www.hhs.gov/aspr/opeo/ndms/.

U.S. Food and Drug Administration. Drug preparedness and response to bioterrorism. Available at: www.fda.gov/Drugs/EmergencyPreparedness/BioterrorismandDrugPreparedness/default.htm.

Anemias 36

Trevor McKibbin, PharmD, MS, BCPS

36-1. Disease Overview

Anemia is a reduction in red cell mass that decreases the oxygen-carrying capacity of the blood. This chapter will focus on iron deficiency anemia (IDA), megaloblastic anemias, and anemia of renal failure.

Epidemiology

Approximately 3.4 million Americans have anemia. Anemia is more common in women than men.

Seventy-five percent of anemias result from iron deficiency, anemia of chronic disease, and acute bleeding. The remaining 25% of anemia cases result from bone marrow damage, decreased erythropoiesis, and hemolysis. IDA is the single most common form of anemia, accounting for 25% of all cases.

Kinetic Approach to Anemia

Anemia may be caused by one or more of three mechanisms: decreased red blood cell (RBC) production, increased RBC destruction, and blood loss.

Classification by Morphology

The most common way to classify an anemia is by the morphology (shape and structure) of the RBCs.

Macrocytic (large cell) morphology

Anemias in this class include the following:

- Megaloblastic anemia
- Folic acid deficiency (decreased red blood cell production)
- Vitamin B_{12} deficiency (decreased red blood cell production)
- Pernicious anemia

Normochromic, normocytic morphology

Anemias in this class may result from following:

- Acute blood loss
- Bone marrow failure (decreased RBC production)
- Hemolysis (increased RBC destruction)
- Immunologic destruction, such as occurs in autoimmune diseases and endocrine disorders

In aplastic anemia, marrow fails to produce all three types of blood cells, which results in anemia, neutropenia (decreased white blood cells), and thrombocytopenia (decreased platelets). About half of aplastic anemia cases are believed to be caused by drugs or chemicals. Drugs that cause aplastic anemia include chloramphenicol, felbamate, carbamazepine, and phenytoin.

Genetically inherited enzyme deficiencies such as glucose-6-phosphate dehydrogenase (G6PD) deficiency can lead to hemolysis, because RBCs deficient in G6PD are susceptible to hemolysis when exposed to certain oxidant drugs (e.g., dapsone, sulfamethoxazole, and nitrofurantoin).

RBC membrane abnormalities, such as those caused by hereditary spherocytosis, can cause increased RBC destruction.

Hypochromic (low hemoglobin content) or microcytic (small cell) morphology

Anemias in this class include the following:

- Iron deficiency anemia (decreased red blood cell production)

- Certain genetic anomalies, such as sickle cell anemia and thalassemia

Clinical Presentation

The signs and symptoms of anemia depend on the amount of time during which the anemia has developed and the severity of RBC depletion. An anemia that has developed over a long period of time may be asymptomatic in the beginning stages and then progress to fatigue, malaise, headache, exertional dyspnea, angina, pallor, or loss of skin tone. A patient with acute anemia, such as from recent blood loss, may present with tachycardia, shortness of breath, or lightheadedness.

Many of the signs and symptoms of anemia are secondary to tissue hypoxia. In the case of hypoxia, blood supply is shunted to life-sustaining organs (brain, heart, and kidney) and away from nonvital organs (e.g., extremities or nail beds), which results in pallor of the skin.

The various types of anemia have additional signs and symptoms that will be discussed in further detail in elsewhere in the chapter.

Pathophysiology

Iron deficiency anemia

IDA is the most common anemia, accounting for one-fourth of all anemia cases. It is caused by iron store depletion resulting from

- Inadequate oral intake of iron (especially animal protein)
- Increased iron demands, such as those found in
  - Pregnant or lactating women
  - Infants and adolescents, who experience periods of rapid growth
  - The elderly
- Blood loss as a result of
  - Menstruation or postpartum blood loss
  - Trauma
  - Gastrointestinal (GI) ulcers
- Inadequate absorption as a result of
  - Medications (e.g., tetracyclines)
  - Gastrectomy
  - Enteritis
  - Persistent diarrhea
- Disease states, such as
  - Carcinomas
  - Rheumatoid arthritis

Hemoglobin is composed of iron (heme) and proteins (globin). Lack of iron results in reduced hemoglobin synthesis. The RBCs produced under those conditions are

- Hypochromic (decreased concentration of hemoglobin)
- Microcytic (smaller cells)

Megaloblastic anemias

Megaloblastic anemias either are caused by a deficiency in or an inability to use vitamin B_{12} (cobalamin) or folic acid.

Vitamin B_{12} deficiency can result from

- *Decreased intake:* This problem may occur with patients who are strict vegetarians.
- *Decreased absorption:* Vitamin B_{12} requires gastric intrinsic factor to be absorbed. The lack of intrinsic factor results in pernicious anemia, which can be inherited or acquired by gastrectomy.
- *Achlorhydria:* Vitamin B_{12} requires an acidic environment to be absorbed. Chronic therapy with proton pump inhibitors and H_2 antagonists may contribute to vitamin B_{12} deficiency.
- *Inadequate utilization of vitamin B_{12}:* This problem can be a result of protein deficiencies.

Folic acid deficiency can result from

- *Decreased intake:* This problem is especially found in patients who are alcoholic, indigent, or elderly.
- *Decreased absorption:* This problem occurs in patients with Crohn's disease or celiac disease. It can also be drug induced.
- *Increased demands:* For example, deficiencies may occur during pregnancy or growth spurts or could accompany malignancy or long-term hemodialysis.
- *Use of certain drugs:* Such drugs include methotrexate and phenytoin.

Both vitamin B_{12} and folic acid are necessary for the RNA (ribonucleic acid) and DNA (deoxyribonucleic acid) required for cell division during the development of RBCs. Because RNA and DNA synthesis is impeded when vitamin B_{12} and folic acid levels are deficient, cell divisions are skipped, resulting in abnormally large cells (macrocytic anemia).

Anemia of renal failure

The primary reason that patients with renal failure are anemic is because of the lack of erythropoietin (EPO) production. EPO is a hormone produced primarily (90%) in the kidneys that stimulates the synthesis and differentiation of erythroid progenitor cells (precursors to RBCs).

The uremic environment in patients with chronic renal failure decreases the lifespan of RBCs.

Folic acid deficiency also can develop as a result of increased folic acid demands during synthesis of RBCs. Additionally, folic acid can be removed during hemodialysis.

Patients with chronic renal failure can become iron deficient as a result of iron and blood loss during dialysis.

Diagnostic Criteria

If anemia is suspected, the following blood tests should be performed:

- Complete blood cell count (CBC), which includes
  - Hemoglobin (Hgb)
  - Hematocrit (Hct)
  - RBC count
  - Red cell indices:
    - Mean corpuscular volume (MCV), which is a measure of the size of RBCs
    - Mean corpuscular hemoglobin (MCH), which is a measure of the weight of hemoglobin in a RBC (MCH will be low in the case of microcytosis or hypochromia)
    - Mean corpuscular hemoglobin concentration (MCHC), which is a measure of the weight of hemoglobin, but is more useful than MCH because it can distinguish between low hemoglobin (hypochromia) and a small cell (MCHC will be low only in the case of hypochromia)
    - Platelets
    - Reticulocyte count (pre-RBCs)
  - Red cell morphology
  - Serum iron, total iron binding capacity (TIBC), transferrin saturation, and ferritin
  - Bilirubin, which is a by-product of RBC destruction

Other tests include the following:

- Stool test for presence of blood
- Peripheral blood smear
- Thorough history and physical examination

Iron deficiency anemia

Blood work

The first level to decrease will be ferritin (storage form of iron). However, ferritin may be increased in inflammatory diseases. The iron level will be low. TIBC, which is a measure of the amount of binding space left on transferrin (transport protein of iron), will be increased. (Less iron in the blood means that more space will be available on the transferrin molecule.)

As the iron deficiency progresses, hemoglobin will decrease, because iron is a component of hemoglobin. Decreased hemoglobin indicates a hypochromic anemia. The hematocrit also will eventually fall.

MCV will be decreased, which indicates microcytosis. MCH and MCHC will be decreased, which indicates decreased hemoglobin. The blood smear will show a microcytic, hypochromic cell.

Specific signs and symptoms

In addition to the general signs and symptoms listed previously for anemia, the following additional symptoms may be present in severe IDA:

- Koilonychias (spoon-shaped nails)
- Angular stomatitis or glossitis
- Pica (appetite for nonfood substances such as chalk, soil, or clay)

Megaloblastic anemias

Blood work

Blood work should show the following:

- Decreased Hct and Hgb
- Decreased RBC count
- Elevated MCH, which indicates a macrocytosis
- Normal iron level, TIBC, and reticulocyte count

Vitamin B$_{12}$ deficiency

If the problem is vitamin B$_{12}$, the serum B$_{12}$ level will be decreased. A positive Schilling test will indicate pernicious anemia. (The Schilling test determines absorption of vitamin B$_{12}$ by measuring the amount of radioactive B$_{12}$ excreted in urine.)

Additional signs and symptoms include the following:

- Loss of vibratory sensation in lower extremities
- Ataxia or vertigo
- Glossitis
- Muscle weakness
- Neuropsychiatric abnormalities (e.g., irritability or emotional instability, dementia, psychosis)

Folic acid deficiency

In a case of folic acid deficiency, the folate level will be decreased. Overall, folic acid deficiency anemia is very similar to vitamin B$_{12}$ deficiency anemia, except that the neurological symptoms that may be present with vitamin B_{12} deficiency anemia are absent.

Anemia of renal failure

As the name implies, this anemia occurs in patients with chronic renal failure. Before diagnosis, other causes must be ruled out (e.g., blood loss). CBC will reveal a normochromic, normocytic anemia.

Treatment Principles and Goals

Iron deficiency anemia

In IDA treatment, the goal is to normalize Hgb and Hct:

- Hgb should increase 2 g/dL in 3 weeks.
- Hct should increase 6% in 3 weeks.
- Reticulocytosis usually will occur within 1 week.

If those indices do not improve within their respective time frames, the diagnosis should be reevaluated, and compliance with therapy should be confirmed.

A second goal is to replenish iron stores. Although Hgb and Hct will return to normal within 1–2 months, iron therapy should be continued for 3–6 months after Hgb is normalized to replenish total body iron stores.

Megaloblastic anemias

Goals of vitamin B_{12} replacement
Hgb should increase within 1 week.

If neurologic symptoms were present, they should improve within 24 hours. However, if vitamin B_{12} deficiency is long-standing, symptoms may not be relieved completely for several months.

Maintenance administration of vitamin B_{12} should continue for as long as nutritional intake is a problem.

Goals of folic acid replacement
RBC morphology will correct within 1–2 days. Hgb will start to normalize within 10 days. Hct will return to normal levels within 2 months.

Maintenance administration of folic acid should continue for as long as nutritional intake of folic acid is a problem.

Anemia of renal failure

The initial therapy goal is to reach a target Hgb of 11–12 g/dL through a slow, steady increase (usually within 2–4 months). Medication doses of erythropoiesis-stimulating agents should be titrated to maintain a Hgb level between 11–12 g/dL, not to exceed a Hgb of 13 g/dL.

Because laboratory variability in the measurement of hematocrit is greater than that of hemoglobin, reliance on the Hct measurement alone is not the optimal method for assessing the patient's response to treatment.

36-2. Drug Therapy

Iron Deficiency Anemia

Treatment consists of iron supplementation through therapeutic iron preparations (200 mg of elemental iron per day in 2–3 divided doses) (Table 36-1). Iron is best absorbed in the reduced (ferrous) form. Ferrous sulfate salt, which is 20% elemental iron, is the most common form. Therefore, ferrous sulfate 325 mg tid will treat iron deficiency adequately.

Intravenous (IV) iron preparations should be used only in cases of

- Iron malabsorption
- Oral noncompliance
- Refusal of blood transfusion

IV iron formulations often are used in patients with chronic renal failure who require dialysis along with human recombinant erythropoietin therapy. Four IV iron products are available in the United States:

- Iron dextran (InFeD and Dexferrum)
- Ferric gluconate (Ferrlecit)

Table 36-1. Drugs Used to Treat Iron Deficiency Anemia

Generic name	(trade name)	Elemental Fe (%)	Dose (mg)	Fe content (mg)
Ferrous sulfate	(Feosol, Fer-in-Sol)	20	325	65
Ferrous gluconate	(Fergon)	12	300	35
Ferrous fumarate	(Femiron, Fumerin, Feostat)	33	300	99

- Iron sucrose (Venofer)
- Feraheme (ferumoxytol)

Ferumoxytol was recently approved for iron-deficiency anemia in adult patients with chronic kidney disease.

Mechanism of action

Iron supplementation corrects the iron deficiency and enables Hgb to be synthesized at normal levels.

Patient instructions (for oral supplementation)

- Take iron supplementation 1–2 hours prior to a meal (on an empty stomach).
- If iron is intolerable on an empty stomach, take it with a small snack, but try to avoid dairy products or tea. (Food can decrease the absorption of iron by 50%.) Take it with orange juice if possible (orange juice may increase absorption).
- Keep out of reach of children. Iron is a major cause of ingestion deaths in children.
- Take iron 1 hour before or 3 hours after any antacids.
- Some medications interact with iron. Please ask your physician or pharmacist before taking any new medications in combination with iron.
- If constipation occurs, you may take over-the-counter docusate.

Adverse drug effects

The oral formulation primarily has GI effects:

- Dark-colored stools
- Constipation or diarrhea
- Nausea or vomiting

The IV formulations may have the following effects:

- Injection site reactions
- GI effects (e.g., diarrhea, nausea)
- Hypotension
- Allergic reactions, including anaphylaxis

The risk of anaphylaxis is greatest with iron dextran. Clinicians commonly administer a test dose before infusing the entire dose of this agent. Premedication with antihistamines and corticosteroids also may prevent anaphylaxis.

Drug interactions

- ***Antibiotics (tetracycline and quinolones):*** Iron binds to these antibiotics, preventing absorption.
- ***Antacids:*** Iron needs an acidic environment for optimal absorption.

Monitoring parameters

- Have reticulocytes, Hgb, and Hct increased?
- Is the iron tolerable? (Tolerance will influence compliance.)
- Is the patient improving symptomatically?

Kinetics

Bioavailability is increased in an acidic environment and is decreased by food.

Megaloblastic Anemias

Vitamin B_{12} should be administered orally if absorption is not an issue. The recommended daily intake is 2 mcg. A solution for nasal administration of vitamin B_{12} is also available.

A vitamin B_{12} deficiency that leads to pernicious anemia is usually corrected through intramuscular (IM) vitamin B_{12} (cyanocobalamin) injection as follows:

- Initially 1,000 mcg IM every day for 1 week
- Then 100–1,000 mcg IM every week for 4 weeks
- Then 100–1,000 mcg IM every month thereafter for maintenance

Although IM vitamin B_{12} is used more often, patients with deficiency states may be supplemented orally in very high doses (e.g., 1,000–2,000 mcg per day).

People choosing vegan diets should supplement with vitamin B_{12} daily and may require lower maintenance doses than those with absorption abnormalities. Pregnant women and breast-feeding mothers may have higher daily requirements.

Mechanism of action

Vitamin B_{12} supplementation allows for normal synthesis of the RNA and DNA involved in the synthesis of RBCs.

Patient instructions

If injections are given at home, the patient or family members should be counseled on sterile injection techniques and proper needle disposal.

Adverse drug effects

Vitamin B_{12} supplementation can cause the following adverse effects:

- Hyperuricemia or hypokalemia caused by increased synthesis of reticulocytes

- Sodium retention
- An expansion of the intravascular volume as a result of increased RBC synthesis, which can increase cardiac output and cause angina or dyspnea
- Itching in 1–10% of patients
- Diarrhea in 1–10% of patients
- Anaphylaxis in < 1% of patients

Monitoring parameters

- Monitor CBC. Is there an increase in Hgb?
- Is the patient improving symptomatically (especially neurologic symptoms, if present)?
- Is the potassium level normal?

Kinetics

Intrinsic factor is necessary for vitamin B_{12} absorption. It must be present for vitamin B_{12} to be transported across the GI mucosa.

Vitamin B_{12} is bound in blood to transcobalamin II and converted in tissues to active coenzymes methylcobalamin and deoxyadenosylcobalamin.

Folic Acid Deficiency Anemia

Folic acid deficiency anemia is corrected by supplementing folic acid 1 mg daily for 4 months. Once the underlying cause of the deficiency is corrected, folic acid supplementation may be discontinued. Long-term folate administration is necessary if the cause is not corrected, such as in hemodialysis or alcoholism.

Mechanism of action

Folic acid supplementation allows for normal RNA and DNA synthesis, both of which are involved in the synthesis of RBCs.

Patient instructions

- Stress the importance of compliance with regimen.
- Women of childbearing age should be counseled to take a multivitamin containing folic acid, regardless of whether an anemia is present, to prevent neural tube birth defects.

Adverse drug effects

Fewer than 1% of patients have allergic reactions to folic acid.

Drug interactions

Folic acid may increase phenytoin metabolism.

Phenytoin, primidone, sulfasalazine, para-aminosalicylic acid, and oral contraceptives may decrease folic acid concentrations.

Chloramphenicol may blunt response to folic acid.

Monitoring parameters

- Is the RBC morphology normalizing?
- Are the Hgb and Hct normalizing?
- Is the patient complying?

Kinetics

Folic acid is a water-soluble B vitamin absorbed in the small intestine with C_{max} at 30 minutes to 1 hour.

Anemia of Renal Failure

Recombinant human erythropoietin

The primary cause of anemia in renal failure is decreased EPO synthesis; therefore, the optimal drug for this type of anemia is an erythropoiesis stimulating agent (ESA). Epoetin alfa (Procrit, Epogen) and darbepoetin alfa (Aranesp) are ESAs with similar mechanisms of action, but darbepoetin alfa has a longer half-life.

An ESA is indicated in the treatment of anemia associated with chronic renal failure, including dialysis and nondialysis patients. ESAs are indicated to elevate or maintain the RBCs and to decrease the need for transfusions in these patients. (Nondialysis patients with symptomatic anemia considered for therapy should have an Hct < 30%.) The National Kidney Foundation–Kidney Disease Outcomes Quality Initiative (NKF-K/DOQI) guidelines recommend that epoetin be administered subcutaneously, because that route of administration is as effective (or more effective) than IV administration. However, epoetin often is administered intravenously in patients on dialysis, because the dialysis port offers easy IV access.

Mechanism of action

Human recombinant erythropoietin stimulates erythropoiesis (increased RBC production).

Patient instructions (Epoetin alfa)

- Do not shake the vial because the epoetin may break down, thus decreasing the medication's effectiveness.

- Store the medication in the refrigerator, but do not freeze. Keep it out of direct sunlight.
- Make sure that the solution in the vial is clear and free of particulate matter. Do not use if the solution is cloudy or frothy.
- Monitor your blood pressure at home and alert your physician of any significant increases in blood pressure.
- Single-use vials are intended to be used only once. Discard any remaining solution and vial. If the label is marked with an "M," the vial is a multidose vial, and it may be stored in the refrigerator for 21 days.
- Take your blood pressure medications *exactly* as prescribed while on this medication, and maintain a sodium-restricted diet.
- Avoid hazardous activity in the first 90 days of therapy (e.g., operating heavy machinery).
- As with all medications, watch for signs of possible allergic reaction. Tell your doctor if you experience a local reaction (swelling, itching, redness).
- A very small number of patients may experience an anaphylactic reaction (shortness of breath, wheezing, low blood pressure, rapid heart rate, sweating). If any of those reactions occur, discontinue using the medication immediately and call 911.
- Follow the instructions for correct sterile injection technique and needle disposal (Box 36-1).

Box 36-1. Instructions for Self-Administering Epotein Alfa

Preparing the dose

1. Wash your hands thoroughly with soap and water before preparing the medication.

2. Check the date on the epoetin alfa vial to be sure that the drug has not expired.

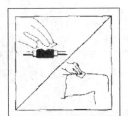

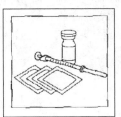

3. Remove the vial of epoetin alfa from the refrigerator and allow it to reach room temperature. **Each epoetin alfa vial is designed to be used only once: do not re-enter the vial.** It is not necessary to shake epoetin alfa. Prolonged vigorous shaking may damage the product. Assemble the other supplies you will need for your injection.

4. Hemodialysis patients should wipe off the venous port of the hemodialysis tubing with an antiseptic swab. Peritoneal dialysis patients should cleanse the skin with an antiseptic swab where the injection is to be made.

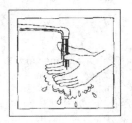

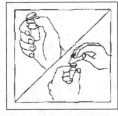

5. Flip off the red protective cap but do not remove the gray rubber stopper. Wipe the top of the gray rubber stopper with an antiseptic swab.

6. Using a syringe and needle designed for subcutaneous injection, draw air into the syringe by pulling back on the plunger. The amount of air should be equal to your epoetin alfa dose.

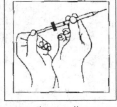

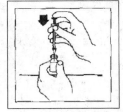

7. Carefully remove the needle cover. Put the needle through the gray rubber stopper of the epoetin alfa vial.

8. Push the plunger in to discharge air into the vial. The air injected into the vial will allow epoetin alfa to be easily withdrawn into the syringe.

9. Turn the vial and syringe upside down in one hand. Be sure the tip of the needle is in the epoetin alfa solution. Your other hand will be free to move the plunger. Draw back on the plunger slowly to draw the correct dose of epoetin alfa into the syringe.

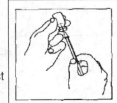

10. Check for air bubbles. The air is harmless, but too large an air bubble will reduce the epoetin alfa dose. To remove air bubbles, gently tap the syringe to move the air bubbles to the top of the syringe, then use the plunger to push the solution and the air back into the vial. Then re-measure your correct dose of epoetin alfa.

11. Double-check your dose. Remove the needle from the vial. Do not lay the syringe down or allow the needle to touch anything.

(continued)

Box 36-1. Instructions for Self-Administering Epotein Alfa *(Continued)*

Injecting the dose
Patients on home hemodialysis using the intravenous injection route:

1. Insert the needle of the syringe into the previously cleansed venous port and inject the epoetin alfa.

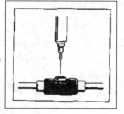

2. Remove the syringe and dispose of the whole unit. Use the disposable syringe only once. Dispose of syringes and needles as directed by your doctor, by following these simple steps:

- Place all used needles and syringes in a hard plastic container with a screw-on cap, or a metal container with a plastic lid, such as a coffee can properly labeled as to contents. If a metal container is used, cut a small hole in the plastic lid and tape the lid to the metal container. If a hard plastic container is used, always screw the cap on tightly after each use. When the container is full, tape around the cap or lid, and dispose of it according to your doctor's instructions.
- Do not use glass or clear plastic containers, or any container that will be recycled or returned to a store.
- Always store the container out of the reach of children.
- Please check with your doctor, nurse, or pharmacist for other suggestions. There may be special state and local laws that they will discuss with you.

Patients on home peritoneal dialysis or home hemodialysis using the subcutaneous route:

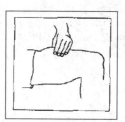

1. With one hand, stabilize the previously cleansed skin by spreading it or by pinching up a large area with your free hand.

2. Hold the syringe with the other hand, as you would a pencil. Double check that the correct amount of epoetin alfa is in the syringe. Insert the needle straight into the skin at a 90° angle. Pull the plunger back slightly. If blood comes into the syringe, do not inject epoetin alfa, as the needle has entered a blood vessel; withdraw the syringe and inject at a different site. Inject the epoetin alfa by pushing the plunger all the way down.

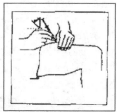

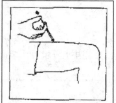

3. Hold an antiseptic swab near the needle and pull the needle straight out of the skin. Press the antiseptic swab over the injection site for several seconds. Use the disposable syringe only once.

4. **Use the disposable syringe only once.** Dispose of syringes and needles as directed in the instructions at left, under step 2.

5. Always change the site for each injection as directed. Occasionally a problem may develop at the injection site. If you notice a lump, swelling, or bruising that does not go away, contact your doctor. You may wish to record the site you just used so you can keep track.

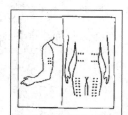

Adverse drug effects
Table 36-2 shows adverse effects of epoetin alfa and the percentage of patients reporting them. The most common adverse effect is elevated blood pressure. ESAs are contraindicated in patients with uncontrolled hypertension.

Pure red cell aplasia (PRCA), in association with neutralizing antibodies to native erythropoietin, has been reported rarely in the literature. If PRCA is suspected, discontinue epoetin immediately.

Drug interactions
No drug interactions have been reported.

Monitoring parameters
Prior to initiation of therapy, the patient's iron stores should be evaluated. Transferrin saturation should be at least 20% and ferritin at least 100 ng/mL. Patients on ESA therapy often require iron supplementation for efficacy of the ESA.

Table 36-2. Percentage of Patients Reporting Adverse Effects of Epoetin Alfa

Event	Patients treated with epoetin alfa (*n* = 200)	Patients on placebo (*n* = 135)
Hypertension	24%	19%
Headache	16%	12%
Arthralgias	11%	6%
Nausea	11%	9%
Edema	9%	10%
Fatigue	9%	14%
Vomiting	8%	5%
Chest pain	7%	9%
Skin reaction at site of administration	7%	12%
Asthenia	7%	12%
Dizziness	7%	13%
Clotted access	7%	2%
Significant adverse events:[a]		
Seizure	1.1%	1.1%
Cerebrovascular accident–transient ischemic attack	0.4%	0.6%
Myocardial infarction	0.4%	1.1%
Death	0.0%	1.7%

a. Significant adverse events of concern in patients with chronic renal failure treated in double-blind, placebo-controlled trials occurred in the percentages of patients shown during the blinded phase of the studies.
Reproduced from Procrit package insert with permission of Ortho Biotech Products.

Monitor Hgb very closely. Once Hct approaches 12 g/dL, the dose of epoetin should be decreased. If Hgb increases more than 1 g/dL within 2 weeks, the dose should be decreased. The dose should be increased if Hgb has not increased 1 g/dL in 8 weeks and Hgb is not in the target Hct range of 11–12 g/dL.

Blood pressure should be adequately controlled prior to initiation of ESA therapy. Blood pressure must be closely monitored and controlled during therapy.

Monitor serum chemistries.

Kinetics
The half-life of epoetin is approximately 4–13 hours. The half-life of epoetin in patients not on dialysis with serum creatinine > 3 is no different than in patients requiring dialysis.

Other aspects
Epoetin alfa is also available in predrawn syringes.

Darbepoetin

Mechanism of action
Darbepoetin has the same mechanism of action as epoetin.

Patient instructions
Counseling points are very similar for both darbepoetin and epoetin, except that all darbepoetin vials are single-use only; therefore, the patient should dispose of the vial as instructed after each dose. Both darbepoetin and epoetin are available in predrawn syringes.

Adverse drug effects
The most common adverse effects are:

- ***Cardiovascular:*** Hypertension, hypotension, edema, arrhythmia
- ***GI:*** Nausea, vomiting, diarrhea, constipation
- ***Central nervous system:*** Fatigue, fever, headache

- *Neuromuscular or skeletal:* Myalgia, arthralgia, limb pain
- *Respiratory:* Infection, dyspnea, cough

Drug interactions

No drug interactions have been reported.

Monitoring parameters

- Monitor patient's iron stores prior to and during therapy.
- Monitor patient's blood pressure.
- Adjust dose by closely monitoring Hgb every week until maintenance dose is established. Target Hgb is 12g/dL. Increase dose if Hgb increases more than 1 g/dL over a 4-week period. Decrease dose by 25% if Hgb increases more than 1 g/dL over 2-week period.

Kinetics

Darbepoetin's half-life is 21 hours when administered intravenously and 49 hours when administered subcutaneously. Its half-life is approximately three times longer than epoetin's. Because of its longer half-life, less frequent dosing options are available with darbepoetin.

36-3. Nondrug Therapy

Iron Deficiency Anemia

Dietary supplementation plays an important role in IDA treatment:

- Increase intake of iron-rich foods, such as meat, fish, and poultry.
- Drink orange juice with meals when possible.
- Limit tea or milk with meals. Only use in moderation between meals.

Folic Acid Deficiency Anemia

Dietary supplementation also is important in treating folic acid deficiency:

- To get as much dietary folate as possible, do not overcook vegetables. Eat them raw or steamed.
- Eat a wide variety of properly prepared vegetables, fruits, and mushrooms.

36-4. Key Points

- Anemia is a reduction in red cell mass, which decreases the blood's oxygen-carrying capacity.

- Iron deficiency anemia is the most common anemia, accounting for 25% of all cases. IDA presents as a microcytic, hypochromic anemia.
- Iron preparations are best absorbed on an empty stomach.
- Iron preparations are hard to tolerate as a result of their numerous GI effects, which may necessitate administration with a small snack.
- Megaloblastic anemias are macrocytic and are the result of a folic acid or vitamin B_{12} deficiency.
- Vitamin B_{12} requires intrinsic factor to be absorbed. Patients deficient in intrinsic factor develop pernicious anemia.
- Because many patients experience difficulties absorbing vitamin B_{12}, it often is administered via an IM injection.
- The primary reason that patients with renal failure are anemic is because of the lack of erythropoietin production.
- Anemia of renal failure is treated with subcutaneous or (SC) IV epoetin.
- Patients receiving epoetin must have their hematocrit and blood pressures monitored routinely.
- Darbepoetin has the same mechanism of action as epoetin, but it is longer acting and can be administered less frequently.

36-5. Questions

Use Patient Profile 1 to answer questions 1–5.

1. Which medication could present a problem with Mr. McBeavy's iron supplement?

   A. Acetaminophen
   B. Ranitidine
   C. Maalox
   D. Docusate
   E. Ranitidine and Maalox

2. Mr. McBeavy admits to you that he is not able to take his iron tablet because it makes him nauseated. What advice can you give him?

   A. Take your iron with some crackers and milk.
   B. Take your iron with some crackers and water.
   C. Don't worry about it. It's only a vitamin.
   D. Start taking iron with the largest meal of the day.
   E. Take iron after breakfast.

Patient Profile 1—SuperPrice Drug Store

Patient name: George M. McBeavy

DOB: 7/11/52

Weight: 193 pounds

Problem list

Gastroesophageal reflux disease

Iron deficiency anemia

Hypertension

Medication record

Ferrous sulfate 325 mg tid

Hydrochlorothiazide 25 mg daily

Address: 1040 Dauberson Ave.

Allergies: NKDA

OTC recommendations

Maalox 1 tbsp q2h prn for "indigestion"

Acetaminophen 325 mg q4–6h prn for headache

Ranitidine 75 mg daily prn for "heartburn"

Docusate 100 mg daily for constipation

---

3. If Mr. McBeavy's anemia progresses to severe stages, what effects may he experience?

    A. Koilonychia (spooning of the nails)
    B. Pica (e.g., craving ice, clay, chalk)
    C. Glossitis (sore, beefy red tongue)
    D. Extreme fatigue
    E. All of the above

4. If you were to examine Mr. McBeavy's blood smear, you would find cells that are

    A. microcytic and hypochromic.
    B. macrocytic and hypochromic.
    C. macrocytic and normochromic.
    D. microcytic and normochromic.

5. When one is examining Mr. McBeavy's iron study results, which of the following would be consistent with iron deficiency anemia?

    A. Elevated TIBC
    B. Elevated ferritin
    C. Elevated MCV
    D. Elevated hemoglobin
    E. Elevated hematocrit

6. Which iron preparation is most likely to cause an anaphylactic reaction?

    A. IV iron dextran
    B. IV iron sucrose
    C. IV sodium ferric gluconate
    D. Extended-release ferrous sulfate po
    E. Immediate-release ferrous sulfate po

7. Why are sustained-release (SR) preparations of iron *not* the ideal formulation?

    A. The incidence of nausea is higher with SR formulations.
    B. They are dosed only once daily, and goal Hgb levels are not attained.
    C. Because SR preparations are dissolved in the small intestines, the alkaline environment results in a lower bioavailability than the acidic environment of the stomach.
    D. Dissolution in the small intestines is not bioavailable, because intrinsic factor is not present in the small intestines.
    E. SR preparations require dosing with food.

8. Which of the following options would you advise a patient to drink with meals to optimize iron absorption from meals?

    A. Orange juice
    B. Coffee
    C. Tea
    D. Milk

9. The most likely regimen to supplement vitamin B_{12} is

    A. 1,000 mcg po every month.
    B. 1,000 mcg IV every month.
    C. 1,000 mcg IM every month.
    D. 1,000 mcg IM every day.
    E. Any one of the above is a reasonable regimen.

10. To be absorbed, vitamin B_{12} requires which of the following?

    A. Pernicious factor
    B. Transcobalamin II

C. Intrinsic factor
D. Vitamin B_{12} absorption factor
E. All of the above

11. Folic acid deficiency could be found in all of the following patients *except*

   A. strict vegetarians.
   B. alcoholics.
   C. the indigent.
   D. people who routinely overcook their vegetables.
   E. a college student whose diet consists only of burgers and potato chips.

12. Folic acid may interact with which of the following medications?

   A. Propranolol
   B. Propoxyphene
   C. Piroxicam
   D. Phenytoin
   E. Prednisone

13. The two macrocytic anemias are

   A. vitamin B_{12} deficiency and iron deficiency anemias.
   B. vitamin B_{12} deficiency and folic acid deficiency anemias.
   C. iron deficiency and folic acid deficiency anemias.
   D. sickle cell anemia and anemia of renal failure.
   E. iron deficiency and pernicious anemias.

14. The best regimen to replace folic acid is

   A. folic acid 1 mg po every day for 3–4 months.
   B. folic acid 10 mg po every day for 3–4 months.
   C. folic acid 10 mg IV for 2 weeks, then 1 mg po every day for 2 months.
   D. folic acid 1 mg po three times weekly for 3–4 months.
   E. folic acid 1 mg po once monthly for 6 months.

15. The most common medication given to treat anemia of renal failure is

   A. vitamin B_{12}.
   B. a solution of citric acid in combination with sodium acetate.

C. epoetin alfa.
D. ferrous sulfate po.
E. folic acid po.

16. What advantage does darbepoetin have over epoetin?

   A. Lower incidence of hypertension
   B. Fewer drug interactions
   C. Lower cost
   D. Longer half-life and less frequent administration
   E. Improved tolerability

17. The most common side effect of epoetin is

   A. anaphylaxis.
   B. hypertension.
   C. pure red cell aplasia.
   D. injection site reaction.
   E. weight gain.

18. Prior to initiation of epoetin therapy, which of the following should be evaluated?

   A. Folic acid and vitamin B_{12} levels
   B. Transferrin and ferritin levels
   C. Erythropoietin receptor level
   D. Presence or absence of intrinsic factor
   E. All of the above

19. In which of the following patients would it be possible to teach self-administration of epoetin at home?

   I. A patient on home hemodialysis taking epoetin via IV administration
   II. A patient on home peritoneal dialysis taking epoetin via SC administration
   III. A patient on home hemodialysis taking epoetin via SC administration

   A. II only
   B. II and III only
   C. III only
   D. I, II, and III
   E. I only

Use Patient Profile 2 to answer questions 20–23.

20. Which of the following will be monitored when Mrs. Wiley starts epoetin therapy?
   A. Blood pressure
   B. Hematocrit
   C. Serum chemistries

Patient Profile 2—Central Dialysis Center

Patient name: Rebecca S. Wiley

Weight: 148 pounds

Diagnosis:

Hypertension

Diabetes mellitus

End-stage renal disease

Hyperlipidemia

Labs:

Ferritin: 80 ng/mL (normal)

Transferrin saturation: 15% (low)

Hct: 32% (low)

Hemoglobin: 8.6 g/dL (low)

Address: 1460 Sawyer Brown Rd.

Allergies: Penicillin (rash)

Dialysis schedule: Monday, Wednesday, Friday

Medications:

Insulin NPH 30 U bid

Simvastatin 20 mg qhs

Atenolol 25 mg after dialysis

Nephrocaps 1 capsule daily

D. Iron profile

E. All of the above

21. The target Hgb range for Mrs. Wiley is

    A. 11–12 g/dL.

    B. 9–11 g/dL.

    C. 11–13 g/dL.

    D. 12–13 g/dL.

    E. 9–14 g/dL.

22. Which of Mrs. Wiley's medications will interact with epoetin?

    A. Insulin

    B. Simvastatin

    C. Atenolol

    D. None of the above

    E. All of the above

23. What medication should be added to Mrs. Wiley's regimen?

    A. Oral propranolol

    B. IV iron

    C. Oral levothyroxine

    D. IM vitamin B_{12}

    E. No additional medications are required at this time.

36-6. Answers

1. E. Iron is best absorbed in an acidic environment. Therefore, antacids dramatically decrease the absorption of iron. Iron supplements should be taken 1 hour before or 3 hours after antacids.

2. B. Many patients are not able to tolerate iron on an empty stomach. Those patients should take iron with a small snack. Milk would not be acceptable in this case, because dairy products decrease the absorption of iron.

3. E. Koilonychia, pica, extreme fatigue, and glossitis all are symptoms of severe iron deficiency anemia.

4. A. Iron deficiency produces a hypochromic (low-hemoglobin) anemia, given that iron is a component of the hemoglobin molecule. The cells are also microcytic (meaning "small cell"), because they spend longer in the marrow awaiting proper hemoglobin synthesis and therefore divide more.

5. A. Total iron-binding capacity is elevated in IDA. TIBC is a measure of the amount of binding space left on transferrin (the transport protein of iron). Less iron in the blood means that more space is available on the transferrin molecule.

6. A. IV iron dextran has the highest incidence of anaphylaxis among the four IV iron preparations available.

7. C. SR preparations are left intact in the stomach and are dissolved in the small intestine. The alkaline environment of the small intestine tends to form insoluble iron complexes that cannot be absorbed.

8. A. Tea and milk can decrease the absorption of iron from a meal by more than 50%. Orange juice, however, can double the absorption of iron from food.

9. **C.** The most common IM dose of vitamin B_{12} is 1,000 mcg per month. However, vitamin B_{12} may be supplemented by the oral route if absorption is not impaired. Additionally, it may be supplemented in very high doses, such as 1,000–2,000 mcg per day in pernicious anemia.

10. **C.** Vitamin B_{12} requires intrinsic factor for absorption.

11. **A.** Folic acid deficiency is found in alcoholics, the indigent, and—rarely—in people who overcook their vegetables routinely. Strict vegetarians do not develop folic acid deficiency because a folate-rich diet includes various types of vegetables.

12. **D.** Phenytoin increases the metabolism of folate, thereby decreasing the effectiveness of folic acid.

13. **B.** Vitamin B_{12} deficiency and folic acid anemias are both macrocytic (large cell) anemias. Iron deficiency anemia and sickle cell anemia are both microcytic and hypochromic anemias.

14. **A.** Folic acid is administered po because it is absorbed easily. The proper dose is 1 mg folic acid po every day, and the deficiency should be corrected after 3–4 months.

15. **C.** Epoetin is the most common medication used to treat anemia of renal failure, because it stimulates erythropoiesis. The lack of erythropoietin production is the primary cause of anemia of renal failure.

16. **D.** Darbepoetin is very similar to epoetin because it has the same mechanism of action and similar side effects. However, it has a longer half-life and can be administered less frequently.

17. **B.** Hypertension is the most common adverse drug effect from epoetin.

18. **B.** Transferrin and ferritin levels should be evaluated prior to epoetin therapy. IDA is a common problem in patients with end-stage renal disease. The patient's transferrin should be at least 20% and ferritin should be at least 100 ng/mL before epoetin therapy is initiated.

19. **D.** Patients on home peritoneal dialysis or hemodialysis can be taught to self-administer SC injections. Additionally, if patients are receiving home hemodialysis, they can be taught to take their epoetin intravenously through the dialysis venous port.

20. **E.** Iron profiles need to be monitored prior to starting epoetin and periodically during therapy because IDA is very common in dialysis patients. Blood pressure needs to be monitored because increased blood pressure is the most common adverse effect of epoetin. Hematocrit levels need to be checked as a measure of response to epoetin, and levels should be maintained at 30–36%. Serum chemistries need to be monitored regularly in any patient with end-stage renal disease, because most electrolytes are regulated by the kidney.

21. **A.** The target range of Hgb for patients receiving epoetin is 11–12 g/dL.

22. **D.** No drugs are known to interact with epoetin.

23. **B.** Mrs. Wiley's ferritin is less than 100 ng/mL, and her transferring saturation is less than 20%. Most hemodialysis patients receiving epoetin will need iron therapy at some point during their treatment.

36-7. References

Agarwal AK. Practical approach to the diagnosis and treatment of anemia associated with CKD in elderly. *J Am Med Dir Assoc.* 2006;7(suppl 1):S7–12.

Alleyne M, Horne MK, Miller JL. Individualized treatment for iron-deficiency anemia in adults. *Am J Med.* 2008;121:943.

Fishbane S. Safety in iron management. *Am J Kid Dis.* 2003;41:S18–26.

Ineck B, Mason BJ, Lyons W. Anemias. In: Dipiro JT, Talbert RL, Yee GC, et al., eds. *Pharmacotherapy: A Pathophysiologic Approach.* 7th ed. New York: McGraw-Hill; 2008:1639–64.

National Kidney Foundation: K/DOQI clinical practice guidelines for anemia of chronic kidney disease, 2000. *Am J Kidney Dis.* 2001;37(suppl 1): S182–238.

Parker KP, Mitch WE, Stivelman JC, et al. Safety and efficacy of low-dose subcutaneous erythropoietin in hemodialysis patients. *J Am Soc Nephrol.* 1999; 8:288.

Procrit [package insert]. Raritan, N.J.: Ortho Biotech Products; 2000.

Thromboembolic Disease

Gale Hamann, PharmD, BCPS, CDE

37

37-1. Venous Thromboembolic Disease

Definition and Epidemiology

Venous thromboembolism (VTE) is a disease process that involves the development of a deep venous thrombosis (DVT), a pulmonary embolism (PE), or both.

A *pulmonary embolism* is a thrombus or foreign substance from the systemic circulation that lodges in the pulmonary artery or its branches and causes a complete or partial occlusion of pulmonary blood flow.

A *deep venous thrombosis* is a thrombus that forms most commonly in the popliteal or femoral veins, the veins of the calf, or the iliac veins of the upper leg. Veins of the upper extremities are less commonly involved.

Approximately 2 million Americans develop VTE each year; 600,000 people in this group have VTE manifested as a PE, and of these, 200,000 die. It is estimated that 1 million Americans will develop a clinically silent PE that goes undiagnosed.

Complications of VTE are postthrombotic syndrome and pulmonary hypertension. *Postthrombotic syndrome* is characterized as swelling in the affected lower extremity after a DVT. *Pulmonary hypertension* is a complication that can occur after a PE and is characterized by elevated arterial pressures in the pulmonary vasculature.

The incidence of VTE increases with age and doubles in each decade of life after age 50. VTE costs an estimated $1.5 billion annually.

Clinical Presentation

The most common symptoms of a PE are dyspnea, cough, hemoptysis, tachypnea, tachycardia, pleuritic chest pain, diaphoresis, and overwhelming anxiety. The patient may be cyanotic and hypoxemic secondary to having a reduced ability to oxygenate the blood. Patients with a massive PE may present with syncope. The mortality rate of a PE ranges from 2.3% to 17%.

The most common symptoms of a DVT are pain, tenderness, edema, and erythema of the affected extremity. Other symptoms may include dilation of the superficial veins, a palpable cord, and a positive Homans' sign.

Pathophysiology

Venous thrombi generally form in areas of the veins where blood flow is slowed or disrupted. Often they begin as small thrombi in the large venous sinuses of a valve cusp pocket in the veins of the calf or thigh. Trauma to the vessel causes the release of tissue factor. Tissue factor, in turn, activates the coagulation cascade. This activity results in the formation of thrombin and ultimately the formation of fibrin to form clots. Other common factors that can precipitate the development of a thrombus include disrupted blood flow from immobility or hypercoagulability.

Risk factors for VTE include the following:

- Age over 40 years
- Prolonged immobility
- Major surgery involving the abdomen, pelvis, and lower extremities
- Trauma, especially fractures of the hips, pelvis, and lower extremities
- Malignancy
- Pregnancy
- Previous VTE
- Congestive heart failure or cardiomyopathy
- Stroke

- Acute myocardial infarction
- Indwelling central venous catheter
- Hypercoagulability
- Estrogen therapy
- Varicose veins
- Obesity
- Inflammatory bowel disease
- Nephrotic syndrome
- Myeloproliferative disease

A PE is the result of a dislodged thrombus that is embolized from a thrombus in the deep venous structures of the legs, pelvis, or arms. The embolus travels to the lungs, where it is trapped in the pulmonary arterial microvasculature. Blood flow is obstructed from the PE, which leads to lung edema and reduced pulmonary compliance. This condition results in inadequate oxygen exchange, leading to hypoxemia. Blood flow in the pulmonary artery increases right ventricular afterload, which may lead to right ventricular dilation, dysfunction, and ischemia.

Diagnosis

A DVT is diagnosed on the basis of a detailed history and clinical symptoms. A duplex ultrasound, which measures both blood flow and compressibility of the affected vessel, confirms the diagnosis.

A PE is diagnosed based on a detailed history and clinical symptoms. A spiral CT (computed tomography) scan or a ventilation-perfusion scan confirms the diagnosis.

VTE Prophylaxis

Table 37-1 shows recommendations for VTE prophylaxis.

VTE Treatment

VTE treatment success with unfractionated heparin (UFH) is related to obtaining therapeutic activated partial thromboplastin time (aPTT) levels as rapidly as possible (Table 37-2). Studies have indicated that the VTE recurrence risk is 20–25% higher if aPTT levels are not within the therapeutic range at 24 hours. The therapeutic range for an aPTT is determined by an antifactor Xa chromogenic assay of 0.3–0.7 IU/mL.

The use of low molecular weight heparin (LMWH) has enabled treatment of a DVT to move from a hospitalization of 5–7 days to either a hospital stay of 1–2 days or outpatient management (Table 37-3).

Table 37-1. Recommendations for VTE Prophylaxis

Medical condition	Recommended therapy
General medical	
General medical patients with risk factors	LMWH, LDUH, or fondaparinux
Acute myocardial infarction	LDUH, IV UFH
Ischemic stroke	LDUH, LMWH; if anticoagulation prophylaxis is contraindicated, GCS or IPC
General surgery	
Low risk:	
Patients undergoing minor procedures with no additional VTE risk factors	Early and frequent ambulation
Moderate risk:	
Major surgery for benign disease	LMWH, LDUH, or fondaparinux
General surgery with multiple VTE risk factors	LMWH, LDUH tid, or fondaparinux
Higher risk:	
Major surgery for cancer	LMWH, LDUH tid, or fondaparinux combined with GCS ± IPC
Major surgery for cancer or previous VTE	LMWH, LDUH tid, or fondaparinux
	LMWH during hospitalization and continue up to 28 days post-discharge
General surgery with high risk of bleeding	Mechanical prophylaxis with GCS or IPC until bleeding risk decreases, then use appropriate pharmacologic thromboprophylaxis

Table 37-1. Recommendations for VTE Prophylaxis *(Continued)*

Medical condition	Recommended therapy
Gynecologic surgery	
Low risk and no VTE risk factors or laparoscopic procedure	Early and frequent ambulation
Laparoscopic procedure with additional VTE risk factors	LMWH, LDUH, IPC, or GCS
Major surgery for benign disease without risk factors	LDUH, LMWH, or IPC starting just before surgery and continued until ambulating
Major surgery for malignancy and for patients with additional VTE risk factors	LMWH, LDUH tid, or IPC started before surgery and continued until ambulating; alternatively, LMWH, LDUH plus GCS or IPC, or fondaparinux
Select high-risk patients with major cancer surgery or a previous VTE	LMWH may be considered for up to 28 days after discharge
Urologic surgery	
Transurethral or low-risk procedure	Early and frequent ambulation
Major or open urologic procedure	LDUH bid to tid, LMWH, fondaparinux, GCS and/or IPC
Highest-risk patients	LMWH or fondaparinux with GCS ± IPC started before surgery and continued until ambulating
Other	
Elective total hip replacement	LMWH, fondaparinux, or warfarin for at least 10 days and up to 35 days; IPC is an alternative option with bleeding risk
Elective total knee replacement	LMWH, fondaparinux, or warfarin for at least 10 days and up to 35 days; IPC is an alternative option with bleeding risk
Hip fracture surgery	Fondaparinux, LMWH, warfarin, or LDUH for at least 10 days and up to 35 days
Neurosurgery	IPC, LDUH, or LMWH when risk of bleeding resolved
Trauma	LMWH, IPC, or GCS if bleeding occurs
Acute spinal cord injury	LMWH ± IPC or ES; convert to warfarin

Adapted with permission from Geerts WH, Bergqvist D, Pineo GF, et al. Prevention of venous thromboembolism: American College of Chest Physicians Evidence-Based Clinical Practice Guidelines (8th edition). *Chest* 2008;133(suppl 6):381S–453S.
Note: LMWH, low-molecular-weight heparin: enoxaparin 30 mg SC q 12 hours, enoxaparin 40 mg SC q 24 hours, dalteparin 5,000 units SC q 24 hours; LDUH, low-dose unfractionated heparin, 5,000 units SC q 8–12 hours; fondaparinux 2.5 mg SC q 24 hours; UFH, unfractionated heparin; GCS, graduated compression stocking; IPC, intermittent pneumatic compression device; warfarin, target INR 2.5, range 2.0–3.0.

Table 37-2. Guidelines for Anticoagulation: IV Unfractionated Heparin

Indication	Guidelines
VTE suspected	Obtain baseline aPTT, PT, and CBC count.
	Check for contraindications to heparin therapy.
	Order imaging study; administer IV bolus of heparin 80 IU/kg or 5,000 IU.
VTE confirmed	Rebolus with IV heparin 80 IU/kg and start maintenance infusion at 18 IU/kg/h.
	Check aPTT at 6 hours to keep aPTT in a range that corresponds to a therapeutic blood heparin level.
	Check platelet count between days 1 and 3.
	Start warfarin therapy on day 1 at 5 mg, and adjust subsequent daily dose according to INR.
	Stop heparin after at least 4–5 days of combined therapy when INR is ≥ 2.0 for 24 hours.
	Anticoagulate with warfarin for at least 3 months at an INR of 2.5; range of 2.0–3.0.

Adapted with permission from Kearon C, Kahn SR, Agnelli G, et al. Antithrombotic therapy for venous thromboembolic disease: American College of Chest Physicians Evidence-Based Clinical Practice Guidelines (8th edition). *Chest.* 2008;133(suppl 6):454S–545S.
Note: For treatment with subcutaneous UFH, give 250 IU/kg SC q 12 hours to obtain a therapeutic aPTT in 6 hours.

Table 37-3. Guidelines for Anticoagulation: LMWH or Fondaparinux

Indication	Guidelines
VTE suspected	Obtain baseline aPTT, PT, and CBC.
	Check for contraindications to LMWH or fondaparinux therapy.
	Order imaging study; administer LMWH or fondaparinux.
VTE confirmed	Continue LMWH or fondaparinux.
	Check platelet count between days 3 and 5.
	Start warfarin therapy on day 1 at 5 mg, and adjust subsequent daily dose according to INR.
	Stop LMWH or fondaparinux after at least 4–5 days of combined therapy when INR is ≥ 2.0 for 24 hours.
	Continue warfarin for at least 3 months at an INR of 2.5; range of 2.0–3.0.

Adapted with permission from Kearon C, Kahn SR, Agnelli G, et al. Antithrombotic therapy for venous thromboembolic disease: American College of Chest Physicians Evidence-Based Clinical Practice Guidelines (8th edition). *Chest.* 2008;133(suppl 6):454S–545S.
Note: Dalteparin sodium 200 anti-Xa IU/kg per day SC; single dose should not exceed 18,000 IU. Enoxaparin 1 mg/kg SC q 12 hours or 1.5 mg/kg SC q 24 hours; single dose should not exceed 180 mg. Fondaparinux 5 mg for < 50 kg; 7.5 mg for 50–100 kg; 10 mg for > 100 kg SC q 24 hours.

With outpatient DVT treatment, the diagnosis may take place in either a physician's office or the emergency department. After a Doppler ultrasound confirms the diagnosis of a DVT, the patient is educated on administration of LMWH and receives the first dose of LMWH at that time. After those steps, LMWH and warfarin are administered on an outpatient basis. Warfarin is monitored with an international normalized ratio (INR) at 1- or 2-day intervals. After two therapeutic INRs, the LMWH may be discontinued; warfarin is continued for at least 3 months, and the patient is evaluated for long-term anticoagulation or as indicated (Table 37-4).

Drug Therapy

Unfractionated heparin

Mechanism of action
UFH binds to antithrombin (AT) and converts it from a slow progressive thrombin inhibitor to a rapid thrombin inhibitor. This, in turn, catalyzes inactivation of factors XIIa, XIa, IXa, Xa, and IIa (thrombin).

Table 37-4. Duration of Anticoagulation Therapy

Indication	Duration of anticoagulation
VTE secondary to transient risk factor	Warfarin therapy for 3 months
First unprovoked VTE	Warfarin therapy for at least 3 months, but consider long-term therapy based on risk–benefit ratio
Second unprovoked VTE	Warfarin therapy long term
VTE and cancer	LMWH for the first 3–6 months of long-term anticoagulation therapy, followed by anticoagulation with LMWH or warfarin therapy long term or until cancer resolves

Adapted with permission from Kearon C, Kahn SR, Agnelli G, et al. Antithrombotic therapy for venous thromboembolic disease: American College of Chest Physicians Evidence-Based Clinical Practice Guidelines (8th edition). *Chest.* 2008;133(suppl 6):454S–545S.

Patient counseling
Patients need to monitor for signs and symptoms of bleeding or bruising, especially at surgical sites.

Therapeutic use
- Prevention and treatment of VTE
- Prevention of VTE in patients with a previous VTE or a known hypercoagulability
- Prophylaxis for VTE in high-risk populations
- Prevention of a mural thrombosis after myocardial infarction (MI)
- Treatment of patients with unstable angina and MI
- Prevention of acute thrombosis after coronary thrombolysis

Parameters to monitor
Heparin is monitored by an aPTT, which is sensitive to the inhibitory effects of heparin on factors IIa (thrombin), Xa, and IXa.

The College of American Pathologists and the American College of Chest Physicians (ACCP) recommend against the use of a fixed aPTT therapeutic range of 1.5–2.5 times a control aPTT. They do recommend that a therapeutic aPTT range be established on the basis of an antifactor Xa concentration of 0.3–0.7 units/mL.

An aPTT should be measured 6 hours after a bolus dose of heparin or after any dosage change and then every 6 hours until a therapeutic aPTT is reached. Once a therapeutic aPTT is achieved, an aPTT may be evaluated every 24 hours.

Platelet count and hematocrit should be evaluated at baseline and every 1–3 days.

Pharmacokinetics

The pharmacokinetics of heparin differs depending on whether an intravenous (IV) or subcutaneous (SC) route of administration is used.

Heparin is cleared from the body by a rapid saturable mechanism that occurs at therapeutic doses. A second, slower unsaturable first-order clearance that is largely by renal means occurs at high doses.

The half-life of heparin varies from approximately 30 minutes after an IV bolus of 25 international units (IU)/kg to 60 minutes after an IV bolus at 100 IU/kg.

Dosing

Heparin should be dosed using a weight-based nomogram. A therapeutic range for heparin is determined by an antifactor Xa chromogenic assay of 0.3–0.7 IU/mL. Weight-based dosing nomograms are effective in achieving a therapeutic aPTT, although they are not universally transferable to every hospital. Published nomograms are specific only for the reagent and instrument used to validate that nomogram.

Determining a therapeutic range by using the calculation of 1.5–2.5 times the mean control aPTT may be erroneous. Previous weight-based nomograms, which use a therapeutic range based on the calculation of 1.5–2.5 times the control aPTT, have been recognized to be accurate only for that aPTT reagent used. Table 37-5 is an example of a weight-based dos-

ing nomogram. Each hospital should develop its own nomogram based on its therapeutic range.

Another approach to heparin therapy is to administer an IV bolus of 5,000 IU followed by a continuous infusion of at least 30,000–35,000 IU over 24 hours. The infusion rate is adjusted to maintain a therapeutic aPTT.

UFH may be administered subcutaneously every 12 hours. The patient should receive an initial dose of 17,500 IU or 250 IU/kg SC q12h. The dose should be adjusted to an aPTT that corresponds to a plasma heparin level of antifactor Xa chromogenic assay of 0.3–0.7 IU/mL. This level should be measured 6 hours after the injection.

Alternatively, UFH may be administered as a fixed dose that is unmonitored. An initial dose of 333 IU/kg is administered, followed by 250 IU/kg SC every 12 hours.

Adverse effects

The most common adverse effects are minor bleeding in the form of gingival bleeding, epistaxis, and ecchymosis. The most common serious adverse effects of heparin are gastrointestinal or urogenital bleeding.

Fatal or life-threatening adverse effects often result from intracranial or retroperitoneal bleeding.

Transient thrombocytopenia may occur within the first 2–4 days of therapy, which will resolve with continued therapy. Heparin-induced thrombocytopenia may also occur, which requires discontinuation of the heparin.

Osteoporosis is a risk with chronic use.

Contraindications

Contraindications include the following:

- Active bleeding
- Severe uncontrolled hypertension
- History of heparin-induced thrombocytopenia

Use epidural or spinal anesthesia with caution because patients are at risk of developing an epidural or spinal hematoma, which can result in long-term or permanent paralysis.

LMWHs and pentasaccharides

Table 37-6 describes LMWH and pentasaccharide dosage forms. The pharmacokinetics of LMWHs and pentasaccharides are described in Table 37-7.

Mechanism of action

LMWHs inhibit factor Xa and, to a much lesser extent, factor IIa.

Table 37-5. Body Weight–Based Dosing of IV Heparin

aPTT	Dose
Initial dose	80 IU/kg bolus, then 18 IU/kg per hour
< 35	80 IU/kg bolus, then 4 IU/kg per hour
35–45	80 IU/kg bolus, then 2 IU/kg per hour
46–70[a]	No change
71–90	Decrease infusion rate by 2 IU/kg per hour
> 90	Hold infusion 1 hour, then decrease infusion rate by 3 IU/kg per hour

Adapted from Raschke RA, Gollihare B, Peirce JC. The effectiveness of implementing the weight-based heparin nomogram as a practice guideline. *Arch Intern Med.* 1996;156:1645–49.

a. The therapeutic aPTT range of 46–70 seconds corresponded to antifactor Xa activity of 0.3–0.7 IU/mL at the time this study was performed. The therapeutic range at any institution should be established by correlation with antifactor Xa levels in this range.

Table 37-6. LMWH and Pentasaccharide Dosage Forms

Generic name	Trade name	Form and dose
LMWH		
Dalteparin	Fragmin	2,500, 5,000, 7,5000 10,000, 12,500, 15,000, 17,500, and 18,000 unit syringe
Enoxaparin	Lovenox	30, 40, 60, 80, 100, 120, and 150 mg syringe
Tinzaparin	Innohep	20,000 anti-Xa IU/mL 2 mL vial
Pentasaccharide		
Fondaparinux	Arixtra	2.5, 5, 7.5, and 10 mg syringe

Fondaparinux is a pentasaccharide. It binds selectively to AT, which potentiates the inactivation of factor Xa in the coagulation cascades, thus inhibiting the formation of thrombin.

Advantages of LMWH and fondaparinux over UFH
- LMWHs and fondaparinux have fewer interactions with plasma proteins; thus, they have a more predictable response at lower doses.
- LMWHs have a much longer half-life, which allows them to be administered subcutaneously every 12–24 hours.
- Fondaparinux has a half-life of 17–21 hours, which allows dosing every 24 hours.
- LMWHs have a lower incidence of osteoporosis and heparin-induced thrombocytopenia. Fondaparinux does not cause heparin-induced thrombocytopenia and can be used as an anticoagulant to treat heparin-induced thrombocytopenia.

Therapeutic use
- Prevention and treatment of VTE
- Prevention of VTE in patients with a previous VTE or a known hypercoagulability

Table 37-7. Pharmacokinetics of LMWHs and Pentasaccharides

Drug	Bioavailability (%)	Half-life (hours)	Xa:IIa binding ratio
Enoxaparin	92	3–6	1.9:1
Dalteparin	87	3–5	2.7:1
Tinzaparin	90	2–6	2:1
Fondaparinux	100	17–21	Only Xa binding

- Prophylaxis for VTE in high-risk populations
- Arterial embolism prevention in patients with mechanical or tissue prosthetic heart valve replacement
- Arterial embolism prevention in patients with atrial fibrillation or atrial flutter
- Arterial embolism prevention in patients with an acute cardioembolic stroke

Parameters to monitor
Monitor platelet counts, hematocrit and hemoglobin, and signs and symptoms of bleeding.

Bone mineral density should be monitored with long-term use.

Anti-Xa heparin levels can be monitored in obese patients or in patients receiving LMWH who have significant renal impairment. Anti-Xa levels should be drawn 4 hours after a dose. Therapeutic levels are 0.6–1.0 IU/mL for twice-daily dosing and 1–2 IU/mL for once-daily dosing. The therapeutic range for dalteparin is 0.5–1.5 IU/mL 4–6 hours after receiving 3–4 doses.

Prothrombin time (PT)/INR and aPTT are not useful in monitoring LMWH.

Currently, fondaparinux has no direct monitoring parameters.

Dosing LMWH and fondaparinux
See Tables 37-8 and 37-9 for dosage requirements.

Patient counseling
- Strict compliance is necessary to ensure a consistent level of anticoagulation.
- Notify a health care provider if an increase occurs in bruising, hematuria, melena, hemoptysis, epistaxis, or gingival bleeding or if any other abnormal bleeding happens.
- Consult a health care provider or pharmacist before taking any over-the-counter medications.
- Avoid aspirin or nonsteroidal anti-inflammatory drugs (NSAIDs).
- The air bubble in the LMWH or fondaparinux syringe should be near the plunger prior to injection. This method ensures that all of the drug is expelled from the syringe and helps minimize the amount of bleeding, bruising, and hematoma formation from the injection site.

Adverse effects
The most common adverse effects are minor bleeding in the form of gingival bleeding, epistaxis, and ecchymosis. The most common serious adverse effects of heparin are gastrointestinal or urogenital bleeding.

Table 37-8. Indications and Recommended Doses of LMWH and Fondaparinux

Indication	Enoxaparin	Dalteparin	Tinzaparin	Fondaparinux
Total hip replacement	30 mg SC q 12 hours *or* 40 mg SC q 24 hours	5,000 units SC 0–14 hours before surgery, then q 24 hours *or* 2,500 units SC 2 hours before surgery, then 5,000 units q 24 hours *or* 2,500 units SC 2 hours before surgery and 4–8 hours after, then 5,000 units q 24 hours		2.5 mg SC q 24 hours starting 6–8 hours after surgery
Total knee replacement	30 mg SC q 12 hours			2.5 mg SC q 24 hours starting 6–8 hours after surgery
Abdominal surgery	40 mg SC q 24 hours	2,500 units SC 1–2 hours before surgery, then 5,000 units q 24 hours		2.5 mg SC q 24 hours starting 6–8 hours after surgery
Hip fracture				2.5 mg SC q 24 hours starting 6–8 hours after surgery
Acute medical illness	40 mg SC q 24 hours	5,000 units SC q 24 hours		
Trauma	30 mg SC q 12 hours			
DVT treatment with or without PE	1 mg/kg SC q 12 hours *or* 1.5 mg/kg SC q 24 hours		175 units/kg SC q 24 hours	5 mg for < 50 kg; 7.5 mg for 50–100 kg; 10 mg for > 100 kg SC q 24 hours
VTE in patients with cancer		200 IU/kg SC daily for 1 month, followed by 150 IU/kg for 5 months		
Unstable angina	1 mg/kg SC q 12 hours	120 units/kg SC q 12 hours		

Fatal or life-threatening adverse effects often result from intracranial or retroperitoneal bleeding.

Heparin-induced thrombocytopenia can occur with LMWH, but its incidence is greater with UFH.

Osteoporosis can occur with chronic use.

Direct thrombin inhibitors

Direct thrombin inhibitors are as follows:

- Lepirudin (Refludan)
- Argatroban

Mechanism of action

Lepirudin is a recombinant DNA–derived polypeptide nearly identical to hirudin. It produces an anticoagulant effect by binding directly to thrombin and does not require AT to yield its effect. Lepirudin does not bind to other plasma proteins as heparin does.

Argatroban is a synthetic molecule that reversibly binds to thrombin.

Therapeutic use

Lepirudin is used for the treatment of DVT and heparin-induced thrombocytopenia.

Argatroban is used for treatment of heparin-induced thrombocytopenia and percutaneous coronary intervention.

Pharmacokinetics

Lepirudin has a half-life of 1–2 hours. Approximately 45% of lepirudin is eliminated by the kidneys.

Argatroban is metabolized in the liver to inactive metabolites. The half-life is 0.5–1 hour.

Parameters to monitor

Lepirudin

Monitor complete blood count (CBC) and signs and symptoms of bleeding.

Monitor the therapeutic effect by measuring the aPTT 4 hours after beginning therapy and after a dosage change. After the aPTT is stable within the therapeutic range, daily monitoring is sufficient.

Table 37-9. Enoxaparin Dosage Regimens for Patients with Severe Renal Impairment (Creatinine Clearance < 30 mL/min)

Indication	Dosage regimen
Prophylaxis in abdominal surgery	30 mg SC once daily
Prophylaxis in hip or knee replacement surgery	30 mg SC once daily
Prophylaxis in medical patients during acute illness	30 mg SC once daily
Prophylaxis of ischemic complications of unstable angina and non-Q-wave myocardial infarction,when concurrently administered with aspirin	1 mg/kg SC once daily
Inpatient treatment of acute DVT with or without PE, when administered in conjunction with warfarin sodium	1 mg/kg SC once daily
Outpatient treatment of acute DVT without PE, when administered in conjunction with warfarin sodium	1 mg/kg SC once daily

Argatroban

Monitor CBC and signs and symptoms of bleeding. The aPTT is used to monitor and adjust argatroban therapy. The aPTT should be drawn 2 hours after an infusion is started and after each dosage change.

Argatroban will also elevate a PT/INR. For patients on concomitant warfarin therapy, this effect may impede monitoring and make proper assessment of the INR difficult. For combination therapy, argatroban may be discontinued after an INR is greater than 4. An INR should be drawn after 4–6 hours. If the INR is in the therapeutic range, continue with warfarin only. If the INR is below the therapeutic range, restart argatroban and increase the dose of warfarin. Repeat this procedure until the INR is within the therapeutic range.

Dosing
Lepirudin

Administer a bolus dose of 0.4 mg/kg IV over 15–20 seconds with an infusion of 0.15 mg/kg/h. Measure an aPTT 4 hours after the infusion. Titrate the infusion to a therapeutic range. The therapeutic range is a target range aPTT ratio of 1.5 to 2.5. If the aPTT is below the therapeutic range, increase the infusion by 20%. If the aPTT is above the therapeutic

range, hold the infusion for 2 hours, and then decrease the infusion by 50%. Four hours after a dosage change, aPTTs should be measured.

Argatroban

Administer a continuous IV infusion at the rate of 2 mcg/kg/min. Adjust infusion rate to maintain an aPTT ratio of 1.5 to 2.5. The usual dose is 2–10 mcg/kg/min.

The dose should be reduced in moderate hepatic insufficiency. A continuous IV infusion should begin at a rate of 0.5 mcg/kg/min. Because of the prolonged elimination half-life, measure an aPTT 4 hours after initiation or a dosage change.

Patient counseling
Monitor symptoms of bruising and bleeding, and report them to a health care provider immediately.

Adverse effects
The most common adverse effects are minor bleeding in the form of gingival bleeding, epistaxis, and ecchymosis. The most common serious adverse effects are gastrointestinal or urogenital bleeding.

Fatal or life-threatening adverse effects often result from intracranial or retroperitoneal bleeding.

There is no known antidote for lepirudin or argatroban. The anticoagulant effect declines rapidly after discontinuation of the drug.

Nonhemorrhagic effects such as fever, nausea, vomiting, and allergic reactions rarely occur.

Warfarin (Coumadin)
Dosage forms
- **Tablets:** 1 mg (pink), 2 mg (lavender), 2.5 mg (green), 3 mg (tan), 4 mg (blue), 5 mg (peach), 6 mg (teal), 7.5 mg (yellow), and 10 mg (white)
- **Injections (IV):** 5 mg powder for reconstitution (2 mg/mL)

Mechanism of action
Warfarin is a vitamin K antagonist that produces its pharmacologic effect by interfering with the interconversion of vitamin K and its 2,3-epoxide (vitamin K epoxide). Warfarin leads to the depletion or reduction in activity of vitamin K–dependent coagulation proteins (factors II, VII, IX, and X) produced in the liver. The level and activity of the vitamin K–dependent clotting factors decline over 6–96 hours. At least 4–5 days of warfarin therapy are necessary before a patient is completely anticoagulated.

Therapeutic use

- Prevention and treatment of VTE
- Prevention of VTE in patients with a previous VTE or a known hypercoagulability
- Prophylaxis for VTE in high-risk populations
- Prevention of arterial embolism in patients with mechanical or tissue prosthetic heart valve replacement
- Prevention of arterial embolism in patients with atrial fibrillation or atrial flutter
- Prevention of arterial embolism in patients with a previous cardioembolic stroke
- Prevention of acute MI in patients with peripheral arterial disease

Patient counseling

- Warfarin should be taken at the same time every day.
- Strict compliance is necessary to ensure a consistent level of anticoagulation.
- Strict compliance with a consistent vitamin K diet is necessary to ensure a consistent level of anticoagulation.
- Notify the health care provider in the event of hematuria, melena, epistaxis, hemoptysis, increased bruising, or any abnormal bleeding.
- Notify all health care providers, including dentists, of warfarin therapy.
- Blood monitoring to determine an adequate level of anticoagulation and compliance is necessary at regular intervals.
- Consult the health care provider or pharmacist before taking any new prescription or over-the-counter medications.
- Avoid aspirin or NSAIDs unless instructed otherwise by a physician.
- Women of childbearing age should use an effective form of birth control because warfarin has teratogenic effects.

Parameters to monitor

Warfarin therapy is monitored by a prothrombin time. The PT responds to a reduction in factors II, VII, and X. The INR is used to standardize the responsiveness of thromboplastin to the anticoagulant effects of warfarin. The INR is calculated by the following equation:

$$INR = (observed\ PT/mean\ normal\ PT)^{ISI}$$

ISI is the International Sensitivity Index, which is a measure of thromboplastin sensitivity. The lower the ISI is, the more responsive the thromboplastin is to the anticoagulant effects of warfarin.

The *ACCP Evidenced-Based Clinical Practice Guidelines* (8th edition) recommends two intensities of anticoagulation: a less intense level with a target INR of 2.5 and a range of 2.0–3.0, and a high-intensity level of anticoagulation with a target INR of 3.0 and a range of 2.5–3.5 (Table 37-10).

Upon initiation of warfarin therapy, the INR should be evaluated daily if the patient is in the hospital and every 2–3 days if the patient is not hospitalized.

Pharmacokinetics

Warfarin is a racemic mixture of two optically active isomers, warfarin S and warfarin R, in roughly equal amounts. The S isomer is five times more potent than the R isomer.

Warfarin is rapidly and completely absorbed from the gastrointestinal tract with peak concentration in approximately 90 minutes. Warfarin is 99% protein-bound with a half-life of 36–42 hours.

The onset of anticoagulation occurs after 4–5 days of therapy and is caused by the depletion of the clotting factors rather than steady-state concentrations of warfarin. Thus, the onset of action is based on the half-life of the clotting factors II, VII, IX, and X.

Dosing

Time in the therapeutic range and intensity of anticoagulation are critical for optimizing the therapeutic efficacy of warfarin and minimizing the risk of hemorrhage.

Warfarin initiation does not require loading. Loading doses can result in an inappropriate increase in the INR, which is not reflective of an anticoagulant effect.

Initiating warfarin at 5 mg daily should result in an INR around 2.0 in 4–5 days for most patients. An alternative method is to administer between 5 and 10 mg for the first 1 or 2 days and then adjust the dose depending on the INR response.

Initiating warfarin at a dose of ≤ 5 mg daily may be appropriate in the elderly; in patients with liver disease, heart failure, or malnutrition; in patients taking drugs known to increase the responsiveness to warfarin; or in patients with a high risk of bleeding.

Initiating warfarin at a dose of 7.5–10 mg daily may be appropriate for young, healthy, or obese patients.

If a rapid anticoagulant effect is indicated, IV heparin, LMWH, or fondaparinux should be administered along with warfarin for at least 4–5 days until a therapeutic INR is reached. Heparin, LMWH, or

Table 37-10. Recommended Therapeutic Ranges for Oral Anticoagulation

Indication	Target INR (INR range)
Prophylaxis of VTE (high-risk surgery)	2.5 (2.0–3.0)
Treatment of VTE	2.5 (2.0–3.0)
Unprovoked VTE in patients who desire less-intensive monitoring after 3 months of conventional therapy	(1.5–2.0) with less frequent monitoring
Prevention of thromboembolic events in patients with antiphospholipid syndrome with a lupus inhibitor	2.5 (2.0–3.0)
Patients with recurrent thromboembolic events with a therapeutic INR and a lupus inhibitor	3.0 (2.5–3.5)
Prevention of arterial embolism in atrial fibrillation	2.5 (2.0–3.0)
Prevention of arterial embolism with a bileaflet or Medtronic Hall tilting disk mechanical prosthetic heart valve in the aortic position who are in sinus rhythm without atrial enlargement	2.5 (2.0–3.0)
Prevention of arterial embolism in tilting disk or bileaflet mechanical prosthetic heart valve in the mitral position; caged ball or caged disk mechanical prosthetic valves	3.0 (2.5–3.5)
Mechanical prosthetic valve with additional risk factors such as atrial fibrillation, MI, left atrial enlargement, low ejection fraction, hypercoagulable state, or atherosclerotic vascular disease	3.0 (2.5–3.5) combined with low doses of aspirin 50–100 mg daily
Mechanical prosthetic valve with system embolism despite a therapeutic INR of 2.0–3.0	3.0 (2.5–3.5) ± low doses of aspirin 50–100 mg daily
Mechanical prosthetic valve with system embolism despite a therapeutic INR of 2.5–3.5	3.5 (3.0–4.0) ± low doses of aspirin 50–100 mg daily

Adapted with permission from Hirsh J, Guyatt G, Albers GW, et al. Executive summary: American College of Chest Physicians Evidence-Based Clinical Practice Guidelines (8th edition). *Chest.* 2008;133(suppl 6):71S–105S

fondaparinux may be discontinued when the INR is within the therapeutic range on two consecutive occasions.

Disease state interaction

Disease states that can increase the response to warfarin are hyperthyroidism, congestive heart failure, liver disease, fever, and genetic warfarin increased sensitivity.

Disease states that can decrease the response to warfarin are hypothyroidism and genetic warfarin resistance. Patient nonadherence can also result in a reduced warfarin response.

Drug–drug interactions

Warfarin is a drug with a narrow therapeutic index. Numerous drugs interact with warfarin to potentiate or reduce its anticoagulant effect. Because the S isomer is five times more active than the R isomer, drugs that inhibit or induce the S isomer will have a more significant effect on warfarin than drugs that inhibit or induce the R isomer (Table 37-11).

Drug–food interactions

Foods that contain high amounts of vitamin K can reduce the anticoagulant effect of warfarin (Table 37-11). It is important that patients be consistent in their consumption of these foods and that they evenly space their consumption over a 7-day period. If a patient suddenly stops eating these foods, the INR may dramatically increase.

Adverse effects

The most common adverse effect is minor bleeding in the form of gingival bleeding, epistaxis, and ecchymosis. The most common serious adverse effects of warfarin are either gastrointestinal or urogenital bleeding.

Warfarin-induced skin necrosis is a rare, but serious adverse effect. Skin necrosis begins within 10 days of warfarin initiation. It is characterized by painful, erythematous lesions on breast, thighs, and buttocks, which may progress to hemorrhagic lesions. It may be associated with protein C deficiency and, to a lesser effect, protein S deficiency. The concomitant use of

Table 37-11. Drugs and Foods That Can Interact with Warfarin

Type of interaction	Interacting substance
Potentiation of anticoagulant effect	Acetaminophen, alcohol (acute use), anabolic steroids, cimetidine, clofibrate, disulfiram, piroxicam, omeprazole, simvastatin, sulfinpyrazone
Highly significant potentiation of anticoagulant effect	Amiodarone, ciprofloxacin, erythromycin, fluconazole, isoniazid, itraconazole, ketoconazole, levothyroxine, metronidazole, phenytoin, trimethoprim-sulfamethoxazole, vitamin E (high doses)
Reduction of anticoagulation effect	Alcohol (chronic use), dicloxacillin, griseofulvin
Highly significant reduction of anticoagulation effect	Barbiturates, carbamazepine, cholestyramine, enteral feeding, nafcillin, rifampin, vitamin K–containing foods (broccoli, brussels sprouts, cabbage, canola oil, cauliflower, coleslaw, collard greens, endive, green kale, lettuce, mayonnaise, mustard greens, soybean oil, spinach)

UFH, LMWH, or fondaparinux with initiation of warfarin can prevent its occurrence.

Purple toe syndrome is a dark blue-tinged discoloration of the feet that occurs rarely 3–8 weeks after warfarin initiation.

Fatal or life-threatening adverse effects are related to intracranial or retroperitoneal bleeding. Box 37-1 outlines the treatment guidelines for the management of elevated INRs or bleeding.

Special precautions must be taken for patients undergoing invasive procedures. Table 37-12 outlines the risk stratifications for perioperative arterial or venous thromboembolism. Box 37-2 outlines the recommendations for managing anticoagulation in these patients.

37-2. Atrial Fibrillation

Definition and Epidemiology

Atrial fibrillation (AF) is a supraventricular tachyarrhythmia characterized by uncoordinated atrial activity up to 300–500 beats per minute that is associated with an irregular ventricular response. Uncontrolled AF can result in a rapid ventricular response, which can affect blood circulation. AF may be chronic or paroxysmal in nature.

Box 37-1. Management of Elevated INRs or Bleeding in Patients Receiving Vitamin K Antagonists

INR Above Therapeutic Range But < 5.0; No Significant Bleeding

Lower dose or omit dose, monitor more frequently, and resume at lower dose when INR is therapeutic. If INR is only minimally above therapeutic range, no dose reduction may be required.

INR ≥ 5.0 But < 9.0; No Significant Bleeding

Omit the next one or two doses, monitor more frequently, and resume at an appropriately adjusted dose when the INR is in the therapeutic range.

Alternatively, omit the dose and give vitamin K (1.0–2.5 mg orally), particularly if the patient is at increased risk of bleeding. If more rapid reversal is necessary because the patient requires urgent surgery, vitamin K (≤ 5 mg orally) can be given with the expectation that a reduction of the INR will occur in 24 hours. If the INR is still high, additional vitamin K (1–2 mg orally) can be given.

INR ≥ 9.0; No Significant Bleeding

Hold warfarin therapy and give higher dose of vitamin K (2.5–5.0 mg orally) with the expectation that the INR will be reduced substantially in 24–48 hours. Monitor more frequently and use additional vitamin K if necessary. Resume therapy at an appropriately adjusted dose when the INR is therapeutic.

Serious Bleeding at Any Elevation of INR

Hold warfarin therapy and give vitamin K (10 mg by slow IV infusion), supplemented with fresh frozen plasma, prothrombin complex concentrate, or recombinant factor VIIa, depending on the urgency of the situation. Vitamin K can be repeated every 12 hours.

Life-threatening Bleeding

Hold warfarin therapy and give fresh-frozen plasma, prothrombin complex concentrate, or recombinant factor VIIa supplement with vitamin K (10 mg by slow IV infusion). Repeat, if necessary, depending on INR.

Reprinted with permission from Ansell J, Hirsh J, Dalen JE, et al. Pharmacology and management of the vitamin K antagonists: American College of Chest Physicians Evidence-Based Clinical Practice Guidelines (8th edition). *Chest.* 2008;133(suppl 6):160S–98S.

Over 2.2 million Americans have AF, which increases in prevalence after age 45 and greatly accelerates after age 65. An estimated 10% of Americans over the age of 80 have AF.

AF is a risk factor for the development of a stroke. It is estimated that 4.5% of patients with nonvalvular

Table 37-12. Suggested Patient Risk Stratification for Perioperative Arterial or Venous Thromboembolism

Risk	Mechanical heart valve	Atrial fibrillation	VTE
High	Any mitral valve prosthesis	CHADS$_2$ score of 5 or 6	Recent (within 3 months) VTE
	Older (caged-ball or tilting disc) aortic valve prosthesis	Recent (within 3 months) stroke or transient ischemic attack	Severe thrombophilia (e.g., deficiency of protein C, protein S, or antithrombin; antiphospholipid antibodies; or multiple abnormities)
	Recent (within 6 months) stroke or transient ischemic attack	Rheumatic valvular heart disease	
Moderate	Bileaflet aortic valve prosthesis and one of the following: atrial fibrillation, prior stroke or transient ischemic attack, hypertension, diabetes, congestive heart failure, age > 75 years	CHADS$_2$ score of 3 or 4	VTE within the past 3 to 12 months
			Nonsevere thrombophilic conditions (e.g., heterozygous factor V Leiden mutation, heterozygous factor II mutation)
			Recurrent VTE
			Active cancer (treated within 6 months) or palliative
Low	Bileaflet aortic valve prosthesis without atrial fibrillation and no other risk factors for stroke	CHADS$_2$ score of 0 or 2 (and no prior stroke or transient ischemic attack)	Single VTE occurred > 12 months ago and no other risk factors

CHADS$_2$, congestive heart failure, hypertension, age, diabetes, stroke.

Box 37-2. Recommendations for Managing Anticoagulation Therapy in Patients Requiring Invasive Procedures

Patients with Low Risk of Thromboembolism

- Discontinue warfarin 5 days prior to procedure.
- Consider bridging with low-dose SC LMWH.
- Suggest therapeutic-dose SC LMWH over other management options.

Patients with Moderate Risk of Thromboembolism

- Discontinue warfarin 5 days prior to procedure.
- Consider bridging with therapeutic-dose SC LMWH or IV UFH or with low-dose SC LMWH over not bridging during interruption of warfarin therapy.
- Suggest therapeutic-dose SC LMWH over other management options.

Patients with High Risk of Thromboembolism

- Discontinue warfarin 5 days prior to procedure.
- Bridge with therapeutic-dose SC LMWH or IV UFH during interruption of warfarin therapy.
- In patients whose INR is still elevated (> 1.5) 1 to 2 days before surgery, administer 1 to 2 mg oral vitamin K to normalize INR.
- Discontinue therapeutic-dose LMWH 24 hours prior to procedure and administer half the total daily dose as the last preoperative dose.
- Discontinue UFH approximately 4 hours before a procedure.
- Suggest LMWH over IV UFH.
- Restart warfarin 12–24 hours after procedure or when hemostasis is adequate.
- Resume therapeutic-dose LMWH approximately 24 hours after the procedure or when hemostasis is adequate.
- In patients at high bleeding risk, delay therapeutic-dose LMWH or UFH for 48–72 hours or administer low-dose LMWH or UFH when hemostasis is secured, or completely avoid LMWH or UFH.
- Individualize treatment plans based on postoperative hemostasis and bleeding risk.

Patients Undergoing Minor Dental or Dermatologic Procedure or Cataract Removal

- Continue warfarin therapy around the time of the procedure.
- Coadminister an oral prohemostatic agent such as tranexamic acid or epsilon amino caproic acid mouthwash for dental procedures.

Adapted with permission from Douketis JD, Berger PB, Dunn AS, et al. The perioperative management of antithrombotic therapy: Antithrombotic and thrombolytic therapy: American College of Chest Physicians Evidence-Based Clinical Practice Guidelines (8th edition). *Chest.* 2008;133(suppl 6):299S–339S.

AF, if untreated, would experience a stroke. If transient ischemic attack and silent stroke are included, the incidence is around 7%.

The Framingham Heart Study demonstrated that patients with rheumatic heart disease and AF had a 17-fold increase in the incidence of stroke compared to age-matched controls.

Clinical Presentation

AF is characterized by an "irregularly irregular" heartbeat, with the possibility of a rapid ventricular response. Common symptoms are palpitations and fatigue. Patients may complain of their heart "fluttering" and feeling weak.

Drug Therapy

Warfarin therapy has demonstrated approximately a 68% (50–70%) relative risk reduction in stroke in patients with AF, whereas aspirin therapy has demonstrated only a 21% (0–38%) relative risk reduction. A meta-analysis of five studies reported a 36% relative risk reduction in all strokes and a 46% reduction in ischemic strokes with warfarin compared to aspirin. Randomized controlled studies have demonstrated that anticoagulation with warfarin, INR 2–3, is highly effective in reducing the risk of stroke. Warfarin therapy with an INR 1.2–1.5 has not been shown to be effective in stroke prevention; in addition, an INR > 4 was associated with a higher rate of intracranial hemorrhage. Conversely, the risk of bleeding and intracranial hemorrhage is higher with warfarin therapy than with aspirin.

Risk stratification for stroke in AF has been developed (Tables 37-13 and 37-14). Table 37-15 gives treatment guidelines for stroke prevention based on risk stratifications.

Table 37-13. Risk Stratification in AF Based on CHADS$_2$ Score

Risk factors	Points
Previous stroke, transient ischemic attack	2
Congestive heart failure	1
Hypertension	1
Diabetes	1
Age > 75	1

Gage BF, Waterman AD, Shannon W, et al. Validation of clinical classification schemes for predicting stroke: Results from the National Registry of Atrial Fibrillation. *JAMA* 2001;285:2864–70.

Table 37-14. Stroke Rate Based on CHADS$_2$ Score

CHADS$_2$ score	Stroke risk[a]
0	1.9%
1	2.8%
2	4.0%
3	5.9%
4	8.5%
5	12.5%
6	18.2%

Gage BF, Waterman AD, Shannon W, et al. Validation of clinical classification schemes for predicting stroke: Results from the National Registry of Atrial Fibrillation. *JAMA* 2001;285:2864–70.
a. Adjusted stroke rate per 100 person-years.

Other Therapy

Cardioversion, described in Box 37-3, is an elective procedure for AF patients.

37-3. Stroke

Definition and Epidemiology

Stroke is defined as a sudden onset of focal neurologic deficit lasting longer than 24 hours.

Table 37-15. Recommendations for Antithrombotic Therapy in AF

Risk category	Recommended therapy
No risk factors, age ≤ 75	Aspirin, 75–325 mg daily
One risk factor, age > 75, hypertension, diabetes, moderate or severe left ventricular systolic dysfunction, or heart failure	Aspirin, 75 to 325 mg daily, or warfarin with a target INR of 2.5 (INR range of 2.0–3.0)
Prior ischemic stroke, transient ischemic attack, or systemic embolism	Warfarin with a target INR of 2.5 (INR range of 2.0–3.0)
Two or more risk factors, age > 75, hypertension, diabetes, moderate or severe left ventricular systolic dysfunction, or heart failure	Warfarin with a target INR of 2.5 (INR range of 2.0–3.0)

Adapted with permission from Singer DE, Alberts GW, Dalen JE, et al. Antithrombotic therapy in atrial fibrillation: American College of Chest Physicians Evidence-Based Clinical Practice Guidelines (8th edition). *Chest.* 2008;133(suppl 6):546S–92S.

Box 37-3. Anticoagulation for Elective Cardioversion in Patients with AF

Patients with AF of ≥ 48 hours, or unknown duration, who are scheduled for elective cardioversion should be anticoagulated with warfarin to a target INR of 2.5 with a range of 2.0–3.0 for 3 weeks prior to direct current or pharmacologic cardioversion and for 4 weeks after successful cardioversion. If AF returns, then continue chronic anticoagulation with warfarin at a target INR of 2.5 (range of 2.0–3.0).

Alternatively, such patients should be anticoagulated with IV UFH with a target aPTT of 60 seconds (range of 50–70 seconds), full dose LMWH, or at least 5 days of warfarin with a target INR of 2.5 (range of 2.0–3.0) at the time of cardioversion. Then undergo transesophageal echocardiography (TEE). If no thrombus is seen on TEE and cardioversion is successful, anticoagulation should be continued with a target INR of 2.5 (range of 2.0–3.0) for at least 4 weeks. If a thrombus is seen on TEE, then cardioversion should be postponed and anticoagulation should be continued indefinitely. The TEE should be repeated before attempting cardioversion later.

For patients with AF for < 48 hours in duration, cardioversion may be performed without anticoagulation. However, in patients without a contraindication to anticoagulation, begin IV UFH (target aPTT of 60 seconds; range of 50–70 seconds) or use full-dose LMWH at presentation. If the patient has risk factors for stroke, then a TEE-guided approach is a reasonable alternative strategy.

For emergency cardioversion in hemodynamically unstable patients, IV UFH (target aPTT of 50 seconds; range of 50–70 seconds) should be started as soon as possible, followed by 4 weeks of anticoagulation with warfarin (target INR of 2.5; range of 2.0–3.0).

Oral anticoagulation at the time of cardioversion in patients with atrial flutter is recommended in a manner similar to that used for AF.

Adapted with permission from Singer DE, Alberts GW, Dalen JE, et al. Antithrombotic therapy in atrial fibrillation: American College of Chest Physicians Evidence-Based Clinical Practice Guidelines (8th edition). *Chest.* 2008(suppl 6);133:546S–92S.

Transient ischemic attack (TIA) is defined as a focal ischemic neurologic deficit usually lasting 2–5 minutes, which resolves completely in less than 24 hours.

After heart disease and cancer, stroke is the third-leading cause of death in America. Approximately 700,000 Americans suffer a stroke each year; 500,000 of these individuals experience their first stroke, and 200,000 experience a recurrent stroke. The incidence of stroke increases with age, and the rate doubles for each decade after age 55.

Hypertension is a factor in 70% of patients who suffer a stroke.

Risk factors for stroke are as follows:

- Hypertension
- Smoking
- Heart disease (coronary heart disease, heart failure, left ventricular hypertrophy, and atrial fibrillation)
- Elevated pulse pressure
- Previous TIA or stroke
- Diabetes
- Hyperlipidemia
- Obesity

Cigarette smoking increases the risk of stroke two to three times compared with the risk in nonsmokers. Atrial fibrillation increases the risk of a stroke six times.

Clinical Presentation

Symptoms of a stroke depend on where the stroke occurred in the brain and the rapidity with which the symptoms develop. One or more TIAs commonly precede a stroke. Symptoms range from focal deficits to more significant deficits, such as hemiplegia or hemiparesthesia, blindness in one eye, or speech difficulties.

Pathophysiology

Fifteen percent of strokes are hemorrhagic in nature. The remaining 85% of strokes are ischemic in nature. In the case of ischemic strokes,

- 20% are cardioembolic.
- 20% are due to atherosclerotic cerebrovascular disease.
- 25% are due to penetrating artery disease or lacunar infarctions.
- 30% are cryptogenic.
- 5% are due to other causes.

Atherosclerosis and plaque formation result in arterial narrowing, which leads to stenosis with reduced blood flow. This condition may enhance platelet aggregation, which can lead to an arterial occlusion. An occlusive clot is present in up to 80% of ischemic strokes.

The Framingham Heart Study indicates that a strong relationship exists between hypertension and the risk of both hemorrhagic and nonhemorrhagic stroke. Atherothrombotic infarctions occur four times more often in patients with hypertension (blood pressure > 165/95 mm Hg) than in patients without hypertension. The treatment of hypertension reduces the incidence of stroke by 35–40%.

Cardioembolic etiology accounts for one-fifth of all ischemic strokes. The most common cause of a cardiac embolism is AF; other factors include valvular heart disease, coronary heart disease, prosthetic heart valves, and dilated cardiomyopathy. A cardioembolic stroke often has an abrupt onset and more commonly involves the middle cerebral artery.

Diagnosis and Prevention

Diagnosis is based on physical examination, medical history, and diagnostic imaging such as CT scan, magnetic resonance imaging (MRI) scan, magnetic resonance angiography (MRA), or cerebral arteriography.
   Preventive measures are as follows:

- Maintain blood pressure < 140/90 mm Hg or < 130/90 mm Hg for patients with diabetes or coronary artery disease.
- Control hyperlipidemia with statin therapy (low-density lipoprotein < 100 mg/dL).
- Maintain glycemic control (hemoglobin A1c < 7%).
- Stop smoking.
- Reduce weight if overweight.
- Exercise (i.e., 30 minutes of moderate exercise daily).
- Implement the DASH (Dietary Approaches to Stop Hypertension) diet (low in sodium and saturated fat; high in fruits, vegetables, whole grains, and fiber).

Drug Therapy

Tissue plasminogen activator

Mechanism of action
Because most strokes are caused by a thromboembolic occlusion in an intracranial artery, thrombolytic therapy is key to restoring or improving perfusion. Tissue plasma activator (t-PA) is a plasminogen activator (serine protease) that enhances the conversion of plasminogen to plasmin in the presence of fibrin. t-PA binds to fibrin in a thrombus and converts bound plasminogen to plasmin. Plasmin, an enzyme responsible for clot dissolution, initiates local fibrinolysis.

Indications
Criteria for use in acute treatment of stroke are as follows:

- Onset of symptoms < 3–4.5 hours
- No indication of intracranial hemorrhage from baseline CT scan of the head
- Blood pressure < 185/110 mm Hg
- Platelets > 100,000/mm^3
- No conditions present that would increase the patient's likelihood of bleeding

- No heparin therapy within 48 hours with an elevated aPTT
- No oral anticoagulants or an INR > 1.7
- No suspicion of subarachnoid hemorrhage on pretreatment evaluation
- No gastrointestinal or urinary tract hemorrhage within 21 days
- No stroke or serious head injury within 3 months
- No recent (within 3 months) intracranial or intraspinal surgery
- No seizure at the onset of stroke
- No active internal bleeding
- No intracranial neoplasm, arteriovenous malformation, or aneurysm
- No major surgery or serious trauma within 2 weeks
- No clinical symptoms suggesting post-MI or pericarditis
- Not currently pregnant or lactating

Specific treatment guidelines are available to evaluate patient characteristics for the use of t-PA in acute stroke.

Dose
t-PA is administered at a dose of 0.9 mg/kg (maximum dose 90 mg) IV, with 10% of the dose given as an initial bolus over 1 minute and the balance infused over 60 minutes.

Parameters to monitor
Monitor hematocrit, mental status, and signs and symptoms of bleeding.

Adverse drug reactions
Bleeding is the most common adverse effect with t-PA. The most common sites of bleeding are gastrointestinal, urogenital, retroperitoneal, and intracranial.

Contraindications
Contraindications include intracranial hemorrhage, recent stroke, blood pressure > 185/100 mm Hg, active internal hemorrhage, platelets < 100,000/mm^3, anticoagulant therapy within 24 hours of t-PA, intracranial neoplasm, arteriovenous malformation, and aneurysm.

Antiplatelet drugs

Aspirin
Mechanism of action
Aspirin produces its antiplatelet effect by irreversibly inactivating the enzyme cyclooxygenase, which prevents the conversion of arachidonic acid to thromboxane A$_2$. Thromboxane A$_2$ stimulates platelet aggregation. The effects of aspirin on platelets occur for

the life of the platelet (i.e., approximately 5–7 days). Aspirin has demonstrated a 27–30% risk reduction of stroke.

Patient counseling

- Notify physician if melena, persistent stomach pain or discomfort, breathing difficulties, increased bleeding or bruising, or skin rashes develop.
- Avoid NSAIDs or warfarin unless instructed otherwise by a physician.
- Avoid over-the-counter medications that contain aspirin.
- Do not crush or chew enteric-coated aspirin.

Dose

Within 24–48 hours of an acute ischemic stroke, patients should receive aspirin 325 mg daily. Aspirin is effective for stroke prevention at a dose of 50–325 mg daily.

Monitoring parameters

Signs and symptoms of bleeding should be monitored.

Adverse drug reactions

Adverse drug reactions include nausea, vomiting, dyspepsia, gastrointestinal ulceration, gastric erosion, duodenal ulcers, gastrointestinal hemorrhage, rash, urticaria, angioedema, bronchospasm, and asthma exacerbation.

Drug–drug interactions

Warfarin, UFH, LMWH, NSAIDs, fondaparinux, and clopidogrel may increase the risk of bleeding if used in combination with aspirin.

Drug–disease interactions

Use enteric-coated aspirin after an acute episode of peptic or gastric ulcer disease.

Avoid aspirin use if there is a risk of aspirin-induced asthma.

Clopidogrel (Plavix)
Mechanism of action

Clopidogrel is a selective and irreversible inhibitor of adenosine diphosphate–induced platelet aggregation that does not affect arachidonic acid metabolism. The effects of clopidogrel on platelets occur for the life of the platelet, approximately 5–7 days.

The CAPRIE (Clopidogrel versus Aspirin in Patients at Risk of Ischemic Event) trial demonstrated an 8.7% relative risk reduction of composite outcomes of ischemic stroke, MI, or vascular death with the use of clopidogrel versus aspirin in patients with a recent stroke or MI or in patients with symptomatic peripheral arterial disease. Clopidogrel was most beneficial for patients with peripheral artery disease and showed a 23.8% relative risk reduction over aspirin.

Dose

Clopidogrel is effective in stroke prevention at a dose of 75 mg daily.

Patient counseling

- Notify physician of melena, persistent stomach pain or discomfort, increased bleeding or bruising, or development of a skin rash.
- Avoid NSAIDs or warfarin unless instructed otherwise by a physician.
- Avoid over-the-counter medications that contain aspirin.

Parameters to monitor

Signs and symptoms of bleeding should be monitored.

Adverse drug reactions

Nausea, dyspepsia, diarrhea, abdominal pain, increased bruising, and bleeding may occur.

Drug–drug interaction

Warfarin, aspirin, NSAIDs, UFH, fondaparinux, and LMWH can increase the risk of bleeding if combined with clopidogrel.

Clopidogrel may inhibit cytochrome isoenzyme CYP450-2C9 substrates, thus creating the potential to inhibit the metabolism of fluvastatin, tolbutamide, and torsemide. Close monitoring may be advisable.

Proton pump inhibitors may inhibit the activation of clopidogrel, thus reducing its effectiveness.

Drug–disease interactions

Use clopidogrel with caution in peptic or gastric ulcer disease.

It may require dosage reduction in moderate to severe hepatic dysfunction.

Extended-release dipyridamole plus immediate-release aspirin (Aggrenox)
Mechanism of action

Dipyridamole is a phosphodiesterase inhibitor that increases cyclic adenosine monophosphate in the platelet, which potentiates the deaggregating effects of prostacyclin on platelets.

The Second European Stroke Prevention Study demonstrated that a combination of dipyridamole 200 mg and aspirin 25 mg bid showed a 37% stroke risk reduction compared to placebo and reduced the risk of nonfatal and fatal stroke by 23% compared to aspirin.

Patient counseling

- Notify physician of melena, persistent stomach pain or discomfort, breathing difficulties, increased bleeding or bruising, or development of a skin rash.
- Avoid NSAIDs or warfarin unless instructed otherwise by a physician.
- Avoid over-the-counter medications that contain aspirin.
- Take this medication on an empty stomach, 1 hour before or 2 hours after meals. If stomach upset occurs, take it with food or milk.
- Do not crush or chew.

Dose

A combination of extended-release dipyridamole 200 mg with immediate-release aspirin 25 mg in a capsule is taken twice daily.

Parameters to monitor

Signs and symptoms of bleeding should be monitored.

Adverse drug reactions

Adverse reactions include headache, nausea, vomiting, dyspepsia, gastrointestinal ulceration, gastric erosion, duodenal ulcers, gastrointestinal hemorrhage, rash, urticaria, angioedema, hypotension, dizziness, flushing, epistaxis, bronchospasm, and asthma exacerbation.

Drug–drug interactions

Warfarin, UFH, LMWH, NSAIDs, fondaparinux, aspirin, and clopidogrel may increase the risk of bleeding if used in combination with this product.

Drug–disease interaction

Use dipyridamole-aspirin with caution in the presence of peptic or gastric ulcer disease.

37-4. Key Points

- Appropriate VTE prophylaxis should be used with all patients who have risk factors for its development. *ACCP Evidenced-Based Clinical Practice Guidelines* (8th edition) has guidelines for VTE prophylaxis specific for at-risk patient populations.
- UFH should be administered as a bolus of 80 IU/kg IV, then a maintenance infusion of 18 IU/kg per hour. Heparin is monitored by aPTT levels. A therapeutic aPTT range should be determined for each hospital or laboratory that corresponds to an antifactor Xa concentration of 0.3–0.7 IU/mL.
- LMWH offers a more predictable response at lower doses without the need to monitor levels, except in patients with severe renal impairment or in obesity. It has a lower incidence of osteoporosis and heparin-induced thrombocytopenia. It can also be administered once or twice daily by SC injection, which allows care to shift from the hospital to the outpatient arena.
- An acute VTE should be treated with IV UFH, LMWH, or fondaparinux to provide immediate anticoagulation, followed by the initiation of warfarin therapy. Warfarin should be initiated at 5.0–7.5 mg daily for most patients. Patients with malnutrition, liver disease, or heart failure; patients who are taking drugs known to increase the responsiveness to warfarin; patients who have a high risk for bleeding; or elderly patients may be started at a lower dose. UFH, LMWH, or fondaparinux should be overlapped with warfarin for at least 4–5 days or until two consecutive INRs are within the therapeutic range.
- Patients with a single VTE with reversible, time-limited risk factors should be anticoagulated for 3 months. Patients with a single idiopathic VTE should be anticoagulated for at least 3 months, but consider long-term therapy depending on the risk–benefit ratio. Patients with a recurrent VTE should be anticoagulated long term.
- Atrial fibrillation is a condition that predisposes a patient to the development of a stroke. Warfarin titrated to a target INR of 2.5 with a range of 2.0–3.0 reduces the risk for stroke by approximately 68% (50–70%). Aspirin is not as effective as warfarin in high-risk patients with AF, with an approximately 21% (0–38%) relative risk reduction.
- Patients with a thromboembolic occlusion in an intracranial artery should receive t-PA, provided that the following conditions are met:
  - Onset of symptoms is less than 3–4.5 hours.
  - CT scan of the head does not indicate an intracranial hemorrhage.
  - Blood pressure < 185/100 mm Hg.
  - Conditions are not present that would increase the patient's likelihood of bleeding.
- t-PA is administered at a dose of 0.9 mg/kg (maximum dose 90 mg) IV with 10% of the dose given as an initial bolus over 1 minute and the balance infused over 60 minutes.

■ The drugs of choice for a noncardioembolic stroke are
  • Aspirin 50–325 mg daily
  • Clopidogrel 75 mg daily
  • Aspirin 25 mg/dipyridamole 200 mg bid

37-5. Questions

1. A 24-year-old female presents to the emergency department with complaints of severe shortness of breath, dyspnea, and chest pain. She is also experiencing tachycardia and tachypnea. Two days prior she noticed pain and swelling in her left lower extremity. Her past medical history is negative for thrombosis. Her current medications include Tri-Levlen daily and ibuprofen 600 mg q6h prn for pain. A duplex ultrasound of the left lower extremity revealed a DVT. Her vital signs are T, 98.4°; P, 124/min; R, 36/min; BP, 162/100 mm Hg; Wt, 100 kg; Ht, 165 cm. The most likely cause of her shortness of breath, dyspnea, and chest pain is

    A. bronchitis.
    B. asthma exacerbation.
    C. pulmonary embolism.
    D. heart failure exacerbation.
    E. atrial fibrillation.

2. This patient is started on heparin therapy. Which dosage regimen is most appropriate?

    A. IV heparin 20,000 IU bolus, then 5,000 IU/h
    B. IV heparin 8,000 IU bolus, then 1,800 IU/h
    C. IV heparin 5,000 IU bolus, then 500 IU/h
    D. IV heparin 5,000 IU q12h
    E. SC heparin 5,000 IU q12h

3. All of the following are risk factors for a DVT *except*

    A. hip replacement surgery.
    B. knee replacement surgery.
    C. hernia repair surgery.
    D. hip fracture surgery.
    E. abdominal surgery.

4. Which diagnostic test would be most helpful with the diagnosis of a pulmonary embolism?

    A. Chest x-ray
    B. Electrocardiogram
    C. Spiral CT of the chest
    D. Bronchoscopy
    E. Echocardiogram

5. A patient is started on warfarin for atrial fibrillation. What is an appropriate starting dose of warfarin?

    A. 1 mg daily
    B. 5 mg daily
    C. 15 mg daily
    D. 20 mg daily
    E. 25 mg daily

6. What laboratory test is used to monitor heparin therapy?

    A. aPTT
    B. PT
    C. INR
    D. Clotting time
    E. Factor XIa

7. A 47-year-old patient is diagnosed with a lower-extremity DVT. The patient's height is 6 feet and weight is 220 lb (100 kg). The physician would like to treat this patient on an outpatient basis with warfarin and low molecular weight heparin. Which dose below would be the most appropriate?

    A. Enoxaparin 30 mg SC q12h
    B. Enoxaparin 40 mg SC q24h
    C. Enoxaparin 100 mg SC q12h
    D. Enoxaparin 200 mg SC q12h
    E. Enoxaparin 220 mg SC q12h

8. How long should enoxaparin be continued in a patient with an acute DVT?

    A. At least 4–5 days until the INR is > 2.0 for 24 hours
    B. At least 42 days until the INR is > 3.0 for 24 hours
    C. At least 24 hours until the INR is > 4.0 for 24 hours
    D. At least 48 hours until the INR is > 4.0 for 24 hours
    E. At least 7–10 days until the INR is > 3.5 for 24 hours

9. All of the following statements are important information to communicate to a patient on warfarin therapy *except*

A. Take warfarin every day without missing any doses.

B. Eat a consistent amount of vitamin K–rich foods per week.

C. Report any symptoms of bleeding to your physician.

D. Take warfarin with meals and remain standing for 30 minutes.

E. Do not take aspirin-containing products unless directed to do so by your physician.

10. Vitamin K–rich foods can affect the anticoagulant effect of warfarin. Which of the following foods can decrease the anticoagulant effects of warfarin?

I.   Lima beans
II. Spinach
III. Broccoli

A. Only I is correct.
B. Only III is correct.
C. I and II are both correct.
D. II and III are both correct.
E. I, II, and III are correct.

11. Drugs can affect the anticoagulant effect of warfarin. Which of the following drugs can increase the effects of warfarin?

I.   Ciprofloxacin
II. Trimethoprim-sulfamethoxazole
III. Fluconazole

A. Only I is correct.
B. Only III is correct.
C. I and II are both correct.
D. II and III are both correct.
E. I, II, and III are correct.

12. What is the most appropriate therapy for a patient with atrial fibrillation, cerebrovascular accident, hypertension, and diabetes?

A. Aspirin 325 mg daily
B. Warfarin 5 mg daily
C. Clopidogrel 75 mg daily
D. t-PA 90 mg daily
E. Aspirin 25 mg/dipyridamole 200 bid

13. A patient presented to the emergency department with symptoms of aphasia and dysarthria, which resolved over the course of 3 days. The patient has a history of hyperlipidemia, type 2 diabetes mellitus, and hypertension.

An echocardiogram showed an ejection fraction of 55%, normal valve function, and normal chamber size. An electrocardiogram showed normal sinus rhythm. Carotid ultrasound indicated moderate stenosis. A CT of the head showed no hemorrhages. Blood pressure was 178/102 mm Hg. Hemoglobin A1c was 10.2%. A lipid profile was as follows: total cholesterol: 294 mg/dL; HDL: 32 mg/dL; LDL: 218 mg/dL; triglycerides: 200 mg/dL. Medications include glipizide 10 mg daily and hydrochlorothiazide 25 mg daily. Which therapy is indicated in this patient?

A. Aspirin 325 mg po daily
B. Clopidogrel 75 mg po bid
C. Aspirin 25 mg/dipyridamole 200 mg po daily
D. Warfarin 5 mg po daily
E. t-PA 90 mg po daily

14. All of the following are other treatment goals for this patient *except*

A. hemoglobin A1c < 7%.
B. blood pressure < 130/80 mm Hg.
C. LDL < 100 mg/dL.
D. aPTT 70–100 seconds.
E. smoking cessation.

15. Fondaparinux is an anticoagulant that inhibits which clotting factor?

A. IIa
B. IXa
C. Xa
D. XIa
E. VIIa

16. A 58-year-old male is scheduled for a total knee replacement tomorrow. He has a medical history of hypertension, for which he is treated with amlodipine 5 mg daily. His height is 6 feet 2 inches and his weight is 176 lb (80 kg). What form of DVT prophylaxis is indicated in this patient?

I.   Enoxaparin 30 mg SC q12h
II. Fondaparinux 2.5 mg SC q24h
III. Aspirin 325 mg daily

A. Only I is correct.
B. Only III is correct.
C. Either I or II are correct.
D. Either II or III are correct.
E. I, II, and III are correct.

17. A 68-year-old male presents to the emergency department with complaints of epistaxis as well as bruising on his arms and legs. He has been taking warfarin 8 mg daily. His INR is 10.2. What is the most appropriate therapy to reverse his warfarin toxicity?

    A. Hold warfarin for 4 days; restart warfarin at a lower dose when his INR is < 3.0.
    B. Hold warfarin and administer vitamin K 0.5 mg IV; restart warfarin at a lower dose when his INR is < 3.0.
    C. Hold warfarin and administer tranexamic acid 10 mg IV; restart warfarin at a lower dose when his INR is < 3.0.
    D. Hold warfarin and administer vitamin K 5 mg po; restart warfarin at a lower dose when his INR is < 3.0.
    E. Hold warfarin and administer prothrombin complex 5 mg po; restart warfarin at a lower dose when his INR is < 3.0.

18. A 63-year-old is receiving warfarin 7.5 mg daily for atrial fibrillation. What therapeutic INR range is indicated for this patient?

    A. 1.0–2.0
    B. 1.5–2.5
    C. 2.0–3.0
    D. 2.0–3.5
    E. 2.5–3.5

19. A 56-year-old female presents to the emergency department with complaints of flank pain, dysuria, and increased urinary frequency. She is diagnosed with a urinary tract infection. Her past medical history includes type 2 diabetes mellitus, hypertension, and atrial fibrillation. Her medications include metformin 1 g bid, quinapril 40 mg daily, and warfarin 5 mg daily. What would be the most appropriate antibiotic to treat this patient's UTI?

    A. Septra DS bid
    B. Ciprofloxacin 500 mg bid
    C. Rifampin 300 mg qid
    D. Doxycycline 100 mg bid
    E. Erythromycin 500 mg qid

20. Which of the following drugs produce action by inhibiting platelet activity?

    I. Clopidogrel
    II. Dipyridamole
    III. t-PA

    A. Only I is correct.
    B. Only III is correct.
    C. I and II are both correct.
    D. II and III are both correct.
    E. I, II, and III are correct.

21. What color is warfarin 7.5 mg?

    A. White
    B. Blue
    C. Yellow
    D. Pink
    E. Green

22. Which of the following is a common side effect associated with unfractionated heparin?

    A. Hypokalemia
    B. Hypoglycemia
    C. Ecchymosis
    D. Nausea
    E. Hyponatremia

23. What is the length of anticoagulation therapy for atrial fibrillation?

    A. 3 months
    B. 6 months
    C. 9 months
    D. 12 months
    E. Long term

24. Advantages of LMWH over UFH include all of the following *except*

    A. SC administration.
    B. no dosage adjustment needed with renal insufficiency.
    C. once- or twice-daily dosing.
    D. predictable response at lower doses.
    E. lower incidence of heparin-induced thrombocytopenia.

37-6. Answers

1. C. Symptoms of shortness of breath, dyspnea, chest pain, tachycardia, and tachypnea, along with a recent history of a DVT, are indications of a pulmonary embolism. A ventilation-perfusion scan or a spiral CT of the chest would confirm the diagnosis.
2. B. Several studies have indicated that weight-based dosing of heparin is more effective in

obtaining therapeutic aPTT than standard heparin titration. A weight-based protocol with an 80 IU/kg IV bolus followed by an infusion of 18 IU/kg per hour should produce aPTTs close to the therapeutic range. The other doses are not appropriate.

3. **C.** High-risk surgeries involve the abdomen and lower extremities; thus, hip and knee replacement as well as hip fracture surgery are major risk factors for the development of a VTE. Hernia repair surgery is considered minor surgery and, unless the patient has other risk factors, would not require DVT prophylaxis other than early ambulation.

4. **C.** A spiral CT of the chest or a ventilation-perfusion scan would be necessary to confirm the diagnosis of a PE. Chest x-ray, electrocardiogram, echocardiogram, or bronchoscopy would not assist with the diagnosis.

5. **B.** Warfarin 5 mg daily should result in an INR around 2.0 within 4–5 days. The other doses are either extremely low or high for the majority of patients. Higher doses of warfarin may elevate an INR, but this increase may not be associated with a level of anticoagulation. A rapid increase in INR is due to depletion of factor VII rather than the anticoagulant effect that is associated with depletion of factors II and X.

6. **A.** An aPTT is the laboratory test used to monitor heparin therapy. An aPTT should be checked 6 hours after a dosage change and every 24 hours if it is within the therapeutic range. A PT/INR is used to monitor warfarin therapy.

7. **C.** Enoxaparin 100 mg SC q12h or 1 mg/kg SC q12h is the dose for treatment of an acute DVT. Enoxaparin 30 mg SC q12h and 40 mg SC q24h are doses used for DVT prophylaxis. Enoxaparin 200 mg SC q12h and 220 mg SC q12h are extremely high doses.

8. **A.** For the treatment of an active DVT or PE, at least 4–5 days of heparin or LMWH overlap with warfarin is needed before an anticoagulant effect is produced by warfarin. Heparin or LMWH should be discontinued after an INR is > 2.0 for 24 hours.

9. **D.** Statements A, B, C, and E are important to discuss with patients on warfarin. Patients should follow strict compliance with warfarin. They should eat vitamin K–rich foods consis-

tently over the course of a week and report any symptoms of bleeding to their physician.

10. **D.** Green, leafy vegetables contain higher amounts of vitamin K; thus, spinach and broccoli can reduce an INR. Lima beans, although green, do not have a large amount of vitamin K.

11. **E.** All of these drugs have the potential to produce a major rise in INR. These drugs should not be combined with warfarin if possible.

12. **B.** In a patient with AF with multiple risk factors for a stroke (hypertension, prior cerebrovascular accident, and diabetes), warfarin is the drug of choice if the patient is a good warfarin candidate. Aspirin and clopidogrel are antiplatelet agents and are not as effective as warfarin in stroke risk reduction. t-PA is used for acute stroke treatment and administered intravenously.

13. **A.** Aspirin 325 mg daily is correct. Clopidogrel is dosed at 75 mg daily rather than bid. Aspirin 25 mg/dipyridamole 200 mg is dosed bid rather than daily. Warfarin is not appropriate in this patient because there is no indication that this was a cardioembolic stroke (the echocardiogram and electrocardiogram were normal). t-PA is not used orally and is used only for acute treatment of stroke to restore perfusion. Moderate stenosis of the carotid artery indicates atherosclerotic disease is present, and antiplatelet therapy is indicated.

14. **D.** All of the goals are correct except aPTT range. Because antiplatelet therapy is indicated in this patient, aPTT monitoring is not indicated.

15. **C.** Fondaparinux inhibits factor Xa.

16. **C.** Enoxaparin 30 mg SC q12h or fondaparinux 2.5 mg SC q24h are correct. Aspirin is not effective for DVT prophylaxis in knee replacement surgery.

17. **D.** Warfarin toxicity with an INR of 10.2 can be effectively reversed by holding the dose of warfarin and administering vitamin K 5 mg orally. Warfarin should be restarted when the INR is < 3.0. The IV route is used only in emergent situations because anaphylactic reactions are possible. Prothrombin complex is administered IV only for severe bleeding situations.

18. **C.** The therapeutic range for oral anticoagulation is an INR of 2.0–3.0, with a target of 2.5. Increased bleeding is associated with an INR > 4.0, and embolic events are more common with an INR < 1.5.

19. **D.** Doxycycline 100 mg bid would be the most appropriate therapy for a UTI. Septra DS, erythromycin, and ciprofloxacin will interact with warfarin to elevate the INR.

20. **C.** Clopidogrel and dipyridamole both inhibit antiplatelet activity, and t-PA is a thrombolytic agent.

21. **C.** Warfarin 7.5 mg is yellow, 1 mg is pink, 10 mg is white, and 4 mg is blue.

22. **C.** Minor bleeding and bruising are common side effects of heparin therapy. Other common areas for bleeding are the urogenital and gastrointestinal tracts.

23. **E.** The duration of anticoagulation therapy for patients with AF is lifelong. The risk for stroke is present as long as AF is present. Patients who undergo direct current cardioversion to normal sinus rhythm require anticoagulation therapy for 4 weeks after conversion because the risk of stroke remains high during this period.

24. **B.** Because LMWHs are renally eliminated, they must be dose-adjusted for creatinine clearance < 30 mL/min. Guidelines have recently been released for enoxaparin dosing in renal impairment. For DVT prophylaxis, enoxaparin should be administered 30 mg SC q24h rather than q12h. For DVT treatment, enoxaparin should be administered 1 mg/kg SC q24h rather than q12h.

37-7. References

Adams HP, Albers G, Albers MJ, et al. Update to the AHA/ASA recommendations for the prevention of stroke in patients with stroke and transient ischemic attaches. *Stroke.* 2008;39:1647–52.

Adams HP, del Zoppo G, Albert MJ, et al. AHA/ASA scientific statement, guidelines for early management of adults with ischemic stroke. *Stroke.* 2007; 38:1655–711.

Albers GW, Amarenco P, Easton JD, et al. Antithrombotic and thrombolytic therapy for ischemic stroke: American College of Chest Physicians Evidence-Based Clinical Practice Guidelines (8th edition). *Chest.* 2008;133(suppl 6):630S–69S.

Ansell J, Hirsh J, Dalen JE, et al. Pharmacology and management of the vitamin K antagonists: American College of Chest Physicians Evidence-Based Clinical Practice Guidelines (8th edition). *Chest.* 2008;133(suppl 6):160S–98S.

Deeb SN, O'Gara PT, Madias C, et al. Valvular and structural heart disease: American College of Chest Physicians Evidence-Based Clinical Practice Guidelines (8th edition). *Chest.* 2008;133(suppl 6): 593S–629S.

del Zoppo GJ, Saver JL, Jauch EC, et al. Expansion of the time window for treatment of acute ischemic stroke with intravenous tissue plasminogen activator: A science advisory from the American Heart Association/American Stroke Association. *Stroke.* 2009;40;2945–48.

Douketis JD, Berger PB, Dunn AS, et al. The perioperative management of antithrombotic therapy: Antithrombotic and thrombolytic therapy: American College of Chest Physicians Evidence-Based Clinical Practice Guidelines (8th edition). *Chest.* 2008;133(suppl 6):299S–339S.

Fagan SC, Hess DC. Stroke. In: Dipiro JT, Talbert RL, Yee GC, et al., eds. *Pharmacotherapy: A Pathophysiologic Approach.* 7th ed. New York: McGraw-Hill; 2008:373–84.

Fuster V, Ryden LE, Asinger RW, et al. ACC/AHA/ESC 2006 guidelines for the management of atrial fibrillation: Executive summary. *Circulation.* 2006; 114:e257–354.

Gage BF, Waterman AD, Shannon W, et al. Validation of clinical classification schemes for predicting stroke: Results from the National Registry of Atrial Fibrillation. *JAMA* 2001;285:2864–70.

Geerts WH, Bergquist D, Pineo GF, et al. Prevention of venous thromboembolism: American College of Chest Physicians Evidence-Based Clinical Practice Guidelines (8th Edition). *Chest.* 2008;133(suppl 6):381S–453S.

Goldstein LB, Adams R, Becker K, et al. Primary prevention of ischemic stroke: A statement for healthcare professionals from the Stroke Council of the American Heart Association. *Circulation.* 2001; 103:163–83.

Haines S, Witt DM, Nutescu EA. Venous thromboembolism. In: Dipiro JT, Talbert RL, Yee GC, et al., eds. *Pharmacotherapy: A Pathophysiologic Approach.* 7th ed. New York: McGraw-Hill; 2008: 331–72.

Hirsh J, Anand SS, Halperin JL, et al. Guide to anticoagulant therapy: Heparin—a statement for healthcare professionals from the American Heart Association. *Circulation.* 2001;103:2994–3018.

Hirsh J, Bauer KA, Donati MB, et al. Parenteral anticoagulants: American College of Chest Physicians Evidence-Based Clinical Practice Guidelines (8th edition). *Chest.* 2008;133(suppl 6):141S–59S.

Hirsh J, Fuster V, Ansell J, et al. American Heart Association/American College of Cardiology Foundation guide to warfarin therapy. *Circulation.* 2003;107:1692–711.

Hirsh J, Guyatt G, Albers, GW, et al. Executive summary: American College of Chest Physicians Evidence-Based Clinical Practice Guidelines (8th edition). *Chest.* 2008;133(suppl 6):71S–105S.

Kearon C, Kahn SR, Agnelli G, et al. Antithrombotic therapy for venous thromboembolic disease: American College of Chest Physicians Evidence-Based Clinical Practice Guidelines (8th edition). *Chest.* 2008;133(suppl 6):454S–545S.

Raschke RA, Gollihare B, Peirce JC. The effectiveness of implementing the weight-based heparin nomogram as a practice guideline. *Arch Intern Med.* 1996;156:1645–49.

Singer DE, Alberts GW, Dalen JE, et al. Antithrombotic therapy in atrial fibrillation: American College of Chest Physicians Evidence-Based Clinical Practice Guidelines (8th edition). *Chest.* 2008; 133(suppl 6):546S–92S.

2009–10 Drug and Data Updates

Katie J. Suda, PharmD, MS
Mina Tadrous, PharmD, MS

This chapter describes U.S. Food and Drug Administration (FDA) new drug approvals, indications, and formulations beginning January 2009 through June 2010.

38-1. Chapter 8: Hypertension

Azor (Amlodipine and Olmesartan)

New indication: First-line treatment for high blood pressure

Exforge HCT (Amlodipine, Valsartan, and Hydrochlorothiazide)

Class: Antihypertensive

Form: Tablets

Formulations: Amlodipine/valsartan/hydrochlorothiazide 5 mg/160 mg/12.5 mg, 10 mg/160 mg/12.5 mg, 5 mg/160 mg/25 mg, 10 mg/160 mg/25 mg, 10 mg/320 mg/25 mg

Dose: Once daily

Mechanism of action: Amlodipine blocks the contractile effects of calcium on cardiac and vascular smooth muscle cells; valsartan blocks the vasoconstriction and sodium-retaining effects of angiotensin II on cardiac, vascular smooth muscle, adrenal, and renal cells; and hydrochlorothiazide directly promotes the excretion of sodium and chloride in the kidneys, thereby leading to reductions in intravascular volume.

FDA-approved indication: Treatment of hypertension, but not approved for initial therapy

Adverse reactions: Dizziness, peripheral edema, headache, dyspepsia, fatigue, muscle spasms, back pain, nausea, nasopharyngitis

Drug interactions: The following reactions are related to hydrochlorothiazide:

- Alcohol, barbiturates, and narcotics may cause a potentiation of orthostatic hypotension.
- Antidiabetic drugs may require dosage adjustment.
- Cholestyramine and colestipol may cause reduced absorption of thiazides.
- Corticosteroids and adrenocorticotropic hormone (ACTH) may cause hypokalemia and electrolyte depletion.
- Reduced renal clearance and high risk of lithium toxicity exist when used with diuretics; these medications should not be used in combination.
- Nonsteroidal anti-inflammatory drugs (NSAIDs) can reduce diuretic, natriuretic, and antihypertensive effects of diuretics.

Monitoring parameters: Blood pressure, electrolyte panel, hepatic function tests, infection, renal function tests, serum cholesterol and triglycerides, serum uric acid levels, signs and symptoms of peripheral edema

Patient counseling: Report dizziness; swelling of the hands, ankles, or feet; and signs or symptoms of hypokalemia. Talk to your doctor about other treatment options to lower your blood pressure if you plan to become pregnant.

Revatio (Sildenafil Citrate)

New formulation: Intravenous (IV) formulation (10 mg/12.5 mL) for the treatment of pulmonary arterial hypertension

Tekturna HCT (Aliskiren and Hydrochlorothiazide)

New indication: Treatment of hypertension in patients unlikely to achieve their blood pressure goals with a single agent

Tekturna (Aliskiren) Tablets

Boxed warning: Discontinue use in pregnancy. See www.fda.gov/Safety/MedWatch/SafetyInformation/ucm192032.htm.

Twynsta (Telmisartan and Amlodipine)

Class: Angiotensin II receptor blocker and a dihydropyridine calcium channel blocker

Form: Tablets

Formulations: Amlodipine/telmisartan 5 mg/40 mg, 5 mg/80 mg, 10 mg/40 mg, 10 mg/80 mg

Dose: Amlodipine 5–10 mg and telmisartan 40–80 mg once daily. Titrate to blood pressure control.

Mechanism of action: Amlodipine inhibits the influx of calcium into smooth and cardiac muscle. Telmisartan blocks the binding of angiotensin II to the angiotensin II type 1 (AT1) receptor.

FDA-approved indication: Treatment of hypertension

Adverse reactions: Orthostatic hypotension, peripheral edema, back pain, dizziness, hyperkalemia, myocardial infarction, decreased renal function

Drug interactions: Although no drug interaction studies have been conducted with the combination drug, studies have been completed with the individual components. Telmisartan drug–drug interactions are as follows:

- Increase in digoxin and lithium levels
- Increase in ramipril and ramiprilat levels; decrease in telmisartan levels
- Possible inhibition of medications metabolized by cytochrome P450 (CYP) 2C19
- Increase in arrhythmias when used in combination with amiodarone

Monitoring parameters: Blood pressure, electrolytes, renal function

Patient counseling: Report signs and symptoms of orthostatic hypotension, angina, or hyperkalemia. Do not use potassium supplements or salt substitutes that contain potassium while on this drug. Do not take while pregnant.

Valturna (Aliskiren and Valsartan)

Class: Antihypertensive

Form: Tablets

Formulations: Aliskiren/valsartan 150/160 mg, 300/320 mg

Dose: Initiate with 150/160 mg once daily. Titrate as needed up to a maximum of 300/320 mg.

Mechanism of action: Aliskiren is a potent, direct inhibitor of renin, causing a decrease in plasma renin activity and inhibiting the conversion of angiotensinogen to angiotensin I. Valsartan is a nonpeptide, specific angiotensin II receptor blocker acting on the AT1 receptor subtype. The combination of aliskiren and valsartan works synergistically to reduce blood pressure by acting on different sites of the renin–angiotensin–aldosterone system.

FDA-approved indication: Treatment of hypertension in patients not controlled with monotherapy or as initial therapy in patients likely to need multiple medications to meet recommended blood pressure goals

Adverse reactions: Angioedema, fatigue, nasopharyngitis

Drug interactions: Cyclosporine, lithium

Monitoring parameters: Blood pressure, serum electrolyte levels, renal function

Patient counseling: Seek immediate medical attention if swelling of the face, lips, tongue, throat, arms, or legs occurs. Report signs or symptoms of hypotension. Maintain adequate hydration, and take consistently with meals.

38-2. Chapter 9: Heart Failure

No new approvals, formulations, indications, or boxed warnings were issued.

38-3. Chapter 10: Cardiac Arrhythmias

Multaq (Dronedarone)

Class: Antiarrhythmic

Form: Tablets

Formulation: 400 mg

Dose: Atrial fibrillation/atrial flutter, paroxysmal or persistent: 400 mg orally twice daily with morning and evening meals

Mechanism of action: Exact mechanism of action is unknown; the drug exhibits antiarrhythmic properties of all four Vaughan-Williams classes.

FDA-approved indications: Atrial fibrillation (paroxysmal or persistent), atrial flutter (paroxysmal or persistent)

Adverse reactions: Heart failure, QT prolongation, bradycardia, photosensitivity, elevated creatinine, diarrhea, asthenia, nausea, pruritus, abdominal pain, vomiting, dyspepsia

Drug interactions: The drug is metabolized by CYP3A and is a moderate inhibitor of CYP3A and CYP2D6:

- *Antiarrhythmics:* Avoid concomitant use.
- *Digoxin:* Consider discontinuation or halve dose of digoxin prior to treatment initiation and monitor.
- *Calcium channel blockers:* Initiate with low dose and increase after electrocardiogram (ECG) verification of tolerability.
- *β-blockers:* Drug may provoke excessive bradycardia. Initiate with low dose and increase after ECG verification of tolerability.
- *CYP3A inducers:* Avoid concomitant use.
- *Grapefruit juice:* Avoid concomitant use.
- *Statins:* Follow label recommendations for concomitant use of certain statins with a CYP3A and P-glycoprotein (Pgp) inhibitor such as dronedarone.
- *CYP3A substrates with a narrow therapeutic index (e.g., sirolimus and tacrolimus):* Monitor and adjust dosage of concomitant drug as needed when used with dronedarone.

Monitoring parameters: Cardiac rhythm

Patient counseling: Medication should be taken with a meal. Do not take with grapefruit juice. If a dose is missed, take the next dose at the regularly scheduled time and do not double the dose. Inform health care provider if signs or symptoms of worsening heart failure develop and if you have any past history of heart failure, rhythm disturbance other than atrial fibrillation or flutter, or predisposing conditions such as uncorrected hypokalemia.

38-4. Chapter 11: Ischemic Heart Disease

Effient (Prasugrel)

Class: Adenosine diphosphate (ADP)–induced aggregation inhibitor; platelet aggregation inhibitor

Form: Tablets

Formulations: 5 mg, 10 mg

Dose: Initiate treatment with a single 60 mg oral loading dose; continue at 10 mg once daily with or without food. Consider 5 mg once daily for patients weighing less than 60 kg. Patients should take aspirin daily in conjunction with prasugrel therapy.

Mechanism of action: Thienopyridine inhibits ADP-induced platelet activation and aggregation by inhibiting the platelet P2Y12 ADP reception.

FDA-approved indication: Reduction of thrombotic cardiovascular events in patients with acute coronary syndrome (unstable angina, non-ST-segment myocardial infarction, ST-segment myocardial infarction) managed with percutaneous coronary intervention

Adverse reactions: Bleeding, including life-threatening and fatal bleeding (boxed warning); atrial fibrillation; leucopenia; bradyarrhythmia

Drug interactions: Prasugrel is metabolized by CYP450 2B6, 3A4, and 2C9/19 (minor). Potentially any medication that alters the CYP450 system can interact with prasugrel. Both warfarin and NSAIDs increase the risk of bleeding.

Monitoring parameters: Bleeding; other specific monitoring not determined

Patient counseling: Do not discontinue without first discussing with the prescriber. Bruising and bleeding will occur more easily, and bleeding will take longer than usual to stop; report any unanticipated, prolonged, or excessive bleeding or any blood in stool or urine. Get prompt medical attention if any of the following symptoms occur and cannot otherwise be explained: fever, weakness, extreme skin paleness, purple skin patches, yellowing of the skin or eyes, or neurological changes.

Micardis (Telmisartan)

New indication: Cardiovascular risk reduction in patients where angiotensin-converting enzyme (ACE) inhibitors are contraindicated

38-5. Chapter 12: Hyperlipidemia

Crestor (Rosuvastatin Calcium)

New indication: Treatment of heterozygous familial hypercholesterolemia in pediatric patients

Livalo (Pitavastatin)

Class: 3-hydroxy-3-methyl-glutaryl-coenzyme A (HMG-CoA) reductase inhibitor

Form: Tablets

Formulations: 1 mg, 2 mg, 4 mg

Dose: 1–4 mg once daily

Mechanism of action: Inhibition of HMG-CoA reductase, which inhibits cholesterol synthesis in the liver

FDA-approved indication: Primary hyperlipidemia and mixed dyslipidemia as adjunctive therapy to diet to reduce elevated total cholesterol, low-density lipoprotein (LDL) cholesterol, apolipoprotein B, and triglycerides and to increase high-density lipoprotein (HDL) cholesterol

Adverse reactions: Myalgia, back pain, diarrhea, constipation, extremity pain, myopathy, rhabdomyolysis

Drug interactions: The following interactions have been noted:

- Lopinavir/ritonavir and cyclosporine should not be used with pitavastatin.
- Erythromycin increases pitavastatin exposure; limit pitavastatin dose to 1 mg once daily.
- Rifampin increases pitavastatin exposure; limit pitavastatin dose to 2 mg once daily.
- Use of pitavastatin with fibrate products may increase the risk of adverse skeletal muscle effects.

Monitoring parameters: Lipid profile and liver function tests

Patient counseling: Take any time of day with or without food. Report any signs or symptoms of unexplained muscle pain, tenderness, or weakness. Adverse effects to a fetus may be caused if female patients receive treatment with this drug; contraception should be used.

Welchol (Colesevelam Hydrochloride)

New indication: To lower LDL cholesterol in pediatric patients with heterozygous familial hypercholesterolemia

38-6. Chapter 13: Diabetes Mellitus

ACTOplus Met (Pioglitazone and Metformin)

New dosage form: Pioglitazone 45 mg/metformin extended-release (ER) 2,000 mg per day

Byetta (Exenatide)

New indication: First-line treatment for type 2 diabetes

Cycloset (Bromocriptine)

Class: An ergot derivative that is a dopamine receptor agonist

Form: Tablets

Formulation: 0.8 mg

Dose: Initial dose is one tablet (0.8 mg) daily, increased weekly by one tablet until maximal tolerated daily dose of 1.6–4.8 mg is achieved.

Mechanism of action: The mechanism by which bromocriptine improves glycemic control is unknown. Morning administration of bromocriptine improves glycemic control in patients with type 2 diabetes without increasing plasma insulin concentrations.

FDA-approved indication: Adjunct to diet and exercise to improve glycemic control in adults with type 2 diabetes mellitus

Adverse reactions: Nausea, fatigue, dizziness, vomiting, headache

Drug interactions: Do not use in patients with hypersensitivity to ergot-related drugs. Bromocriptine may increase the unbound fraction of highly protein-bound therapies, altering their effectiveness and safety profiles. It may increase ergot-related side effects or reduce ergot effectiveness for migraines if coadministered within 6 hours of ergot-related drugs. Bromocriptine is extensively metabolized by CYP3A4; use caution when coadministering strong inhibitors, inducers, or substrates for CYP3A4.

Monitoring parameters: Routine monitoring of fasting plasma glucose and glycosylated hemoglobin

Patient counseling: Take bromocriptine by mouth each day with food within 2 hours after waking in the morning. If you miss your morning dose, wait until the next morning to take your medication; do not take a double dose. During periods of stress on the body, such as fever, trauma, infection, or surgery, your medication needs may change.

Onglyza (Saxagliptin)

Class: Dipeptidyl peptidase-4 (DPP4) enzyme inhibitor

Form: Tablets

Formulations: 2.5 mg, 5 mg

Dose: 2.5 mg or 5 mg by mouth once daily with or without food

Mechanism of action: Inhibits dipeptidyl peptidase-4, slowing incretin metabolism, increasing insulin synthesis or release and decreasing glucagon levels

FDA-approved indication: Adjunct to diet and exercise to improve glycemic control in adults with type 2 diabetes mellitus

Adverse reactions: Reactions include upper respiratory tract infection, urinary tract infection, headache, and hypersensitivity reactions. Peripheral edema was reported more commonly in patients treated with saxagliptin and a thiazolidinedione. Hypoglycemia was reported more commonly in patients treated with saxagliptin and a sulfonylurea.

Drug interactions: Coadministration with strong CYP3A4/5 inhibitors significantly increases saxagliptin concentrations; limit saxagliptin dose to 2.5 mg once daily.

Monitoring parameters: Blood glucose and A1c

Patient counseling: Report signs and symptoms of hypoglycemia, fluid retention, and allergic reactions.

Victoza (Liraglutide)

Class: Peptide

Form: Solution for subcutaneous injection

Formulation: Prefilled, multidose pen that delivers doses of 0.6 mg, 1.2 mg, or 1.8 mg (6 mg/mL, 3 mL)

Dose: Administer subcutaneous injection once daily. Initiate at 0.6 mg for 1 week. After 1 week, increase dose to 1.2 mg as tolerated. If glycemic control is not achieved, increase dose to 1.8 mg if tolerated.

Mechanism of action: Liraglutide is a glucagon-like peptide-1 (GLP-1) receptor agonist.

FDA-approved indication: Improvement of glycemic control in adults with type 2 diabetes mellitus in combination with diet and exercise

Adverse reactions: Headache, nausea, diarrhea, anti-liraglutide antibody formation causing urticaria

Drug interactions: Liraglutide may affect absorption of concomitantly administered oral medications because of delays in gastric emptying caused by liraglutide.

Monitoring parameters: Blood glucose, A1c, and serum calcitonin

Patient counseling: There is a potential risk of benign and malignant thyroid c-cell tumors in mice and rats (human relevance is still unknown). There is a risk of pancreatitis. Never share the pen with other patients.

38-7. Chapter 14: Thyroid, Adrenal, and Miscellaneous Endocrine Drugs

Edluar (Zolpidem Tartrate)

New formulation: 5 mg and 10 mg sublingual tablets

Forteo (Teriparatide [Recombinant DNA Origin])

New indication: Treatment of glucocorticoid-induced osteoporosis

Propylthiouracil (PTU) Tablets

Boxed warning: Potentially fatal cases of severe liver injury and acute liver failure; some required transplantation in adult and pediatric patients. PTU should be used only in patients in whom other treatments are not tolerated or contraindicated. See www.fda.gov/Safety/MedWatch/SafetyInformation/ucm209256.htm.

Vpriv (Velaglucerase Alfa)

Class: Enzyme

Form: Solution for infusion

Formulations: 200- and 400-unit single-use vials

Dose: Administer 60 units/kg every other week as a 60-minute IV infusion.

Mechanism of action: Velaglucerase alfa reduces the amount of accumulated glucocerebroside.

FDA-approved indication: Indicated for long-term enzyme replacement therapy for pediatric and adult patients with type 1 Gaucher disease

Adverse reactions: Infusion-related reactions, headache, dizziness, abdominal pain, nausea, back pain, joint pain, upper respiratory tract infections, activated partial thromboplastin time prolonged, fatigue, pyrexia

Drug interactions: None known

Patient counseling: Medication must be administered under the supervision of a health care provider. There is a risk of infusion-related adverse reactions.

Zenpep (Pancrelipase) Delayed Release

Note: Zenpep was formerly marketed as Zentase

New indication: Pancreatic exocrine dysfunction

38-8. Chapter 15: Women's Health

Lysteda (Tranexamic Acid)

Class: Antifibrinolytic agent

Form: Tablets

Formulation: 650 mg

Dose: 1,300 mg orally three times daily for a maximum of 5 days during monthly menstruation. Adjust dose if serum creatinine is higher than 1.4 mg/dL.

Mechanism of action: In the presence of tranexamic acid, the lysine receptor binding sites of plasmin for fibrin are occupied, preventing binding to fibrin monomers, thus preserving and stabilizing fibrin's matrix structure.

FDA-approved indication: Primary menorrhagia

Adverse reactions: Headache, sinus and nasal symptoms, back pain, abdominal pain, musculoskeletal pain, joint pain, muscle cramps, migraine, anemia and fatigue, visual or ocular adverse events, thromboembolic events, severe allergic reactions

Drug interactions: Hormonal contraceptives, factor IX complex concentrates, anti-inhibitor coagulant concentrates, all-trans retinoic acid (oral tretinoin), tissue plasminogen activators

Monitoring parameters: Visual and ocular signs and symptoms, signs and symptoms of thromboembolic events

Patient counseling: Tell your physician about any hormonal contraceptives you are using. You should not take tranexamic acid if you do not have your period. Report any visual or ocular adverse events to your health care professional. Report any history or signs and symptoms of thromboembolic events.

Natazia (Estradiol Valerate and Estradiol Valerate/Dienogest)

Class: Combination oral contraceptive (COC)

Form: Tablets

Formulations: Consists of 28 film-coated tablets. The tablets vary: two 3 mg estradiol valerate, five 2 mg estradiol valerate/2 mg dienogest, seventeen 2 mg estradiol valerate/3 mg dienogest, two 1 mg estradiol valerate, and two inert tablets.

Dose: Take one tablet daily at the same time every day. Tablets must be taken in order directed in blister pack.

Mechanism of action: COC lowers the risk of pregnancy by suppressing ovulation.

FDA-approved indication: Indicated for use by women to prevent pregnancy

Adverse reactions: Headaches, irregular uterine bleeding, breast tenderness, nausea and vomiting, acne, increased weight

Drug interactions: Drugs that induce CYP3A4 may decrease the effectiveness or increase breakthrough bleeding.

Monitoring parameters: Yearly visit to health care provider for blood pressure and other indicated health care

Patient counseling: There is an increased risk associated with the use of COC and smoking. This medication does not protect against HIV and other sexually transmitted infections. It is important to take the medication daily at the same time.

Plan B One-Step (Levonorgestrel)

Class: Postcoital contraceptives

Form: Tablets

Formulation: 1.5 mg

Dose: One tablet (1.5 mg) orally as soon as possible within 72 hours after unprotected intercourse

Mechanism of action: Tubal transport of ova or sperm is altered, preventing ovulation or fertilization; the drug alters endometrium, possibly preventing implantation.

FDA-approved indication: Postcoital emergency contraception

Adverse reactions: Heavy menstrual bleeding, nausea, abdominal pain, fatigue, headache, dizziness

Drug interactions: Drugs that induce CYP3A4 may decrease the effectiveness of levonorgestrel.

Monitoring parameters: Menstrual bleeding, pregnancy test results

Patient counseling: Do not use this medication if you are already pregnant. It is not intended for use as a routine form of birth control. Take one tablet within 72 hours of unprotected intercourse. Consider repeat dose if vomiting occurs within 2 hours.

Prolia (Denosumab)

Class: Monoclonal antibody

Form: Solution for injection

Formulations: Single-use prefilled syringe containing 60 mg in a 1 mL solution; also available in a single-use vial containing 60 mg in 1 mL solution

Dose: Administer 60 mg every 6 months as a subcutaneous injection.

Mechanism of action: Denosumab binds to protein receptors essential for the formation, function, and survival of osteoclasts, the cell responsible for bone resorption.

FDA-approved indication: Indicated in the treatment of postmenopausal women with osteoporosis at high risk of fracture

Adverse reactions: Back pain, pain in extremity, hypercholesterolemia, bone pain, cystitis, pancreatitis

Drug interactions: None known

Patient counseling: Store medication in the refrigerator. Do not shake before use.

Prometrium (Progesterone, USP)

Boxed warning (updated): There is increased risk of myocardial infarction, stroke, invasive breast cancer, pulmonary emboli, deep vein thrombosis, and dementia in postmenopausal women. See www.fda.gov/Safety/MedWatch/SafetyInformation/ucm171199.htm.

Reclast (Zoledronic Acid)

New dosage regimen: Prevention of postmenopausal osteoporosis for 2 years with a single dose

Vagifem (Estradiol)

New dosage regimen: 10 mcg dose to treat atrophic vaginitis caused by menopause

38-9. Chapter 16: Kidney Disease

Extraneal (Icodextrin) Peritoneal Dialysis Solution

Boxed warning: Drug–device interaction may occur with glucose monitoring devices using glucose dehydrogenase pyrroloquinoline quinone (GDH PQQ)–based or glucose-dye-oxidoreductase (GDO)–based methods. See www.fda.gov/Safety/MedWatch/SafetyInformation/Safety-RelatedDrugLabelingChanges/ucm153519.htm.

Feraheme (Ferumoxytol)

Class: Parenteral mineral–trace mineral

Form: IV injection

Formulation: 510 mg of elemental iron in 17 mL (30 mg/mL)

Dose: 510 mg IV followed by a second dose given 3 to 8 days later

Mechanism of action: Ferumoxytol is a superparamagnetic iron oxide that releases iron in the macrophages to be stored as ferritin for incorporation into hemoglobin.

FDA-approved indication: Treatment of iron deficiency anemia in adult patients with chronic kidney disease

Adverse reactions: Diarrhea, nausea, dizziness, hypotension, constipation, peripheral edema

Drug interactions: None known

Monitoring parameters: Evaluate hematologic response (i.e., hemoglobin, ferritin, iron, and transferrin saturation) at least one month following the second ferumoxytol injection for evidence of efficacy.

Patient counseling: Report any history of reactions to parenteral iron products to your prescriber before taking this medication. Report any signs and symptoms of hypersensitivity that may develop during and following ferumoxytol administration, such as rash, itching, dizziness, lightheadedness, swelling, and breathing problems.

38-10. Chapter 17: Critical Care, Fluids, and Electrolytes

Adcirca (Tadalafil)

Class: Phosphodiesterase 5 (PDE5) inhibitor

Form: Tablets

Formulation: 20 mg

Dose: 40 mg once daily, with or without food

Mechanism of action: Inhibition of PDE5 by tadalafil increases the concentrations of cyclic guanosine monophosphate, resulting in relaxation of pulmonary vascular smooth muscle cells and vasodilation of the pulmonary vascular bed.

FDA-approved indication: Treatment of pulmonary arterial hypertension

Adverse reactions: Headache; myalgia; flushing; nausea and upset stomach; nasal congestion; pain in the arms, legs, or back

Drug interactions: Use with ritonavir requires dosage adjustment. Avoid concomitant administration of tadalafil with potent CYP3A inhibitors and inducers.

Monitoring parameters: Pulmonary arterial hypertension, blood pressure, chest pain, erection lasting more than 4 hours, hearing loss, signs of pulmonary edema, vision loss

Patient counseling: Tadalafil is contraindicated with any use of organic nitrates. Do not take with Cialis or other PDE5 inhibitors. Seek immediate medical attention in the event of a sudden loss of hearing or loss of vision in one or both eyes while taking tadalafil. These events may be accompanied by tinnitus and dizziness.

Berinert (C1 Esterase Inhibitor [Human])

Class: C1 esterase inhibitor

Form: IV injection

Formulation: 500 units in a single-dose vial with 10 mL of diluent

Dose: 20 units/kg slow IV injection at a rate of 4 mL/min

Mechanism of action: Inhibits several of the major cascade systems, including the complement system, the intrinsic coagulation system, the fibrinolytic system, and the coagulation cascade (including C1r, C1s, coagulation factor XIIa, kallikrein, and coagulation factor XIa)

FDA-approved indication: Treatment of acute abdominal and facial attacks of hereditary angioedema

Adverse reactions: Abdominal pain, headache, rash, hypersensitivity reaction, thrombosis, increase in pain associated with hereditary angioedema, muscle spasm, vomiting, diarrhea

Drug interactions: None known

Monitoring parameters: Symptoms of hypersensitivity during or after infusion, signs of thrombosis

Patient counseling: Report signs and symptoms of thrombosis or hypersensitivity. Tell your doctor if you become pregnant or are planning to breastfeed. Berinert is made from human blood and has the risk of transmitting infectious agents.

Ilaris (Canakinumab)

Class: Interleukin (IL)–1β blocker

Form: Injection

Formulation: Sterile, single-use 6 mL, glass vial containing 180 mg of canakinumab as a lyophilized powder for reconstitution

Dose: Dose is based on patient body weight:

- 150 mg for cryopyrin-associated periodic syndromes (CAPS) patients with body weight greater than 40 kg
- 2 mg/kg for CAPS patients with body weight equal to or greater than 15 kg and less than or equal to 40 kg
- In children 15–40 kg with an inadequate response, the dose can be increased to 3 mg/kg

Mechanism of action: Binds to human IL-1β and neutralizes its activity by blocking its interaction with IL-1 receptors, but it does not bind IL-1α or IL-1 receptor antagonist (IL-1ra).

FDA-approved indication: Treatment of CAPS, in adults and children 4 years of age and older, including familial cold autoinflammatory syndrome and Muckle–Wells syndrome

Adverse reactions: Nasopharyngitis, diarrhea, influenza, headache, nausea

Drug interactions: None known

Monitoring parameters: Serum C reactive protein and serum amyloid A levels periodically; improvement in signs and symptoms of CAPS (i.e., fever, urticaria-like rash, arthralgia, myalgia, fatigue, and conjunctivitis); latent tuberculosis test before initiating therapy

Patient counseling: Contact your health care professional immediately if you develop an infection after starting canakinumab. Do not take any IL-1 blocking drug, including canakinumab, if you are also taking a drug that blocks tumor necrosis factor (TNF), such as etanercept, infliximab, or adalimumab. Patients should be cautioned not to initiate treatment with canakinumab if they have a chronic or active infection, including HIV or hepatitis B or C.

Lumizyme (Alglucosidase Alfa)

Class: Enzyme

Form: Injection

Formulation: 5 mg/mL

Dose: Recommended dose of 20 mg/kg administered every 2 weeks by IV infusion

Mechanism of action: Alglucosidase alfa provides an exogenous source of acid α-glucosidase (GAA). Deficiency or lack of GAA is the cause of Pompe disease.

FDA-approved indication: Indicated for use in patients 8 years and older with late-onset Pompe disease (GAA deficiency) with no evidence of cardiac hypertrophy

Adverse reactions: Infusion reactions, anaphylaxis (can be life threatening), urticaria, diarrhea, vomiting, dyspnea, rash, pharyngolaryngeal pain, neck pain, flushing, hypoacusis, chest discomfort

Drug interactions: None known

Monitoring parameters: Close monitoring is highly recommended postinfusion for a prolonged period.

Patient counseling: Because of the risk of infusion reactions, this medication should be administered only under the supervision of trained and certified prescribers. Prescribers must be enrolled and meet all the conditions of the Lumizyme ACE (Alglucosidase Alfa Control and Education) program.

Samsca (Tolvaptan)

Class: Selective vasopressin V2-receptor antagonist

Form: Tablets

Formulations: 15 mg, 30 mg

Dose: 15 mg once daily

Mechanism of action: Tolvaptan antagonizes the effect of vasopressin and causes an increase in urine water excretion that results in an increase in free water clearance (aquaresis), a decrease in urine osmolality, and a resulting increase in serum sodium concentrations.

FDA-approved indication: Treatment of clinically significant hypervolemic and euvolemic hyponatremia (serum sodium < 125 mEq/L or less marked hyponatremia that is symptomatic and has resisted correction with fluid restriction), including patients with heart failure, cirrhosis, and syndrome of inappropriate antidiuretic hormone (SIADH)

Adverse reactions: Thirst, dry mouth, asthenia, constipation, pollakiuria or polyuria, hyperglycemia

Drug interactions: CYP3A inhibitors can lead to a marked increase in tolvaptan concentrations. Do not use tolvaptan with strong inhibitors of CYP3A and avoid concomitant use with moderate CYP3A inhibitors. Avoid coadministration of CYP3A inducers with tolvaptan, which can lead to a reduction in the plasma concentration and decreased effectiveness of tolvaptan treatment. The dose of tolvaptan may have to be reduced when coadministered with Pgp inhibitors.

Monitoring parameters: Pulmonary arterial hypertension, blood pressure, chest pain, erection lasting more than 4 hours, hearing loss, signs of pulmonary edema, vision loss, serum potassium levels

Patient counseling: Because of the potential for interactions, inform your health care provider if you are taking or plan to take any prescription or nonprescription drugs.

Tyvaso (Treprostinil)

Class: Prostaglandin

Form: Inhalation solution

Formulation: 1.74 mg/2.9 mL nebules

Dose: 18 mcg (three breaths) via oral inhalation four times daily (approximately 4 hours apart) during waking hours; increase by three breaths/dose every 1–2 weeks; maximum dose of nine breaths four times daily

Mechanism of action: Medication dilates pulmonary and systemic vessels and inhibits platelet aggregation.

FDA-approved indication: Treatment of pulmonary arterial hypertension (World Health Organization Group I) in patients with New York Heart Association Class III symptoms, to increase walking distance

Adverse reactions: Cough, headache, nausea, dizziness, flushing, throat irritation, pharyngolaryngeal pain, diarrhea

Drug interactions: Concomitant diuretics, antihypertensives, or other vasodilators may increase the risk of systemic hypotension.

Monitoring parameters: Increased walking distance is indicative of efficacy. Worsening of lung disease and loss of drug effect may be observed in patients with acute pulmonary infections.

Patient counseling: Drug may cause symptomatic hypotension and increased risk of bleeding. Advise patient on proper administration technique, to avoid contact with the skin or eyes, and to take missed or interrupted dose as soon as possible.

38-11. Chapter 18: Nutrition

No new approvals, formulations, indications, or boxed warnings were issued.

38-12. Chapter 19: Oncology

Afinitor (Everolimus)

Class: Mammalian target of rapamycin (mTOR) inhibitor

Dose: 10 mg daily

Mechanism of action: Afinitor is an mTOR inhibitor that has been shown to reduce cell proliferation, angiogenesis, and glucose uptake.

FDA-approved indication: Treatment of advanced renal cell carcinoma for patients that have failed treatment with sunitinib or sorafenib

Adverse reactions: Stomatitis, infections, asthenia, fatigue, cough, diarrhea

Drug interactions: Avoid use with strong to moderate Pgp inhibitors, CYP3A4 inhibitors, and strong CYP3A4 inducers.

Monitoring parameters: Serum creatinine, BUN (blood urea nitrogen), fasting lipid panel, complete blood count (CBC), fasting blood glucose

Patient counseling: Take everolimus at the same time every day, with or without food. This medication can cause shortness of breath and lung or breathing problems. Everolimus increases the risk of infection. Do not use if you are allergic to sirolimus or temsirolimus or if you are pregnant, nursing, or plan to become pregnant. Do not use everolimus if you have uncontrolled blood pressure, high cholesterol, or liver problems or if you have received or are going to receive a live vaccine.

Alimta (Pemetrexed)

New indication: Maintenance therapy for nonsquamous, non-small-cell lung cancer

Arzerra (Ofatumumab)

Class: Monoclonal antibody

Form: IV infusion

Formulation: IV solution 20 mg/mL (100 mg/5mL single-use vial)

Dose: 300 mg initial dose, followed 1 week later by 2,000 mg weekly for seven doses, followed 4 weeks later by 2,000 mg every 4 weeks for four doses. Administer as an IV infusion; do not administer as IV push or bolus. Premedicate 30 minutes to 2 hours before each dose with oral acetaminophen, oral or IV antihistamine, and an IV corticosteroid.

Mechanism of action: Ofatumumab binds to the CD20 molecule expressed on normal B-lymphocytes (pre-B- to mature B-lymphocyte) and on B-cell chronic lymphocytic leukemia (CLL) and causes cell-lysis.

FDA-approved indication: CLL refractory to fludarabine and alemtuzumab

Adverse reactions: Infusion reactions, cytopenia, progressive multifocal leukoencephalopathy (PML), hepatitis B reactivation, intestinal obstruction, neutropenia, pneumonia, pyrexia, cough, diarrhea, anemia, fatigue, dyspnea, rash, nausea, bronchitis, upper respiratory tract infections

Drug interactions: None known

Monitoring parameters: Monitor for infusion reactions, CBC and platelet count, signs and symptoms of PML and hepatitis B in carriers

Patient counseling: Contact your health care professional if you experience signs and symptoms of infusion reactions, including fever, chills, rash, or breathing problems within 24 hours of infusion; bleeding; easy bruising; petechiae; pallor; worsening weakness; fatigue; signs of infections; new neurological symptoms; symptoms of hepatitis; and new or worsening abdominal pain or nausea. Talk to your doctor about risks and benefits of therapy if you are pregnant, plan on becoming pregnant, or are breast-feeding.

Avastin (Bevacizumab)

New indications: Most common types of kidney cancer; single-agent therapy for the treatment of glioblastoma with progressive disease following prior therapy

Cysview Kit (Hexaminolevulinate Hydrochloride)

New dosage form: 100 mg/vial solution

Elitek (Rasburicase)

New indication: Management of plasma uric acid levels in adults with leukemia, lymphoma, and solid tumors receiving anticancer therapy

Folotyn (Pralatrexate)

Class: Antimetabolite

Form: Injection

Formulation: 20 mg/mL

Dose: A 30 mg/m^2 IV push is administered over 3–5 minutes once weekly for 6 weeks in 7-week cycles. Treatment interruption or dose reduction to 20 mg/m^2 may be needed to manage adverse drug reactions. All patients should receive vitamin supplementation with folic acid 1–1.25 mg orally daily (10 days before treatment, during treatment, and 30 days after treatment) and vitamin B$_{12}$ 1,000 mcg intramuscular (every 8–10 weeks).

Mechanism of action: Pralatrexate is a dihydrofolate reductase inhibitor and a competitive inhibitor for polyglutamylation via the folylpolyglutamyl synthetase enzyme, which results in depletion of thymidine and other biological molecules, synthesis of which depends on single carbon transfer.

FDA-approved indication: Relapsed or refractory peripheral T-cell lymphoma

Adverse reactions: Edema, constipation, inflammatory disease of mucous membrane, nausea, anemia, neutropenia, thrombocytopenia, cough, fatigue

Drug interactions: Probenecid (probable), NSAIDs, and trimethoprim/sulfamethoxazole may result in delayed renal clearance.

Monitoring parameters: CBC, liver function tests

Patient counseling: Report signs or symptoms of infections or bleeding. Take folic acid and vitamin B_{12} to reduce possible side effects.

Fludara (Fludarabine Phosphate)

Boxed warning (updated): Coma, seizures, agitation, and confusion have been reported at doses recommended for CLL. Review prescribing information for the complete boxed warning. See www.fda.gov/ Safety/MedWatch/SafetyInformation/Safety-Related DrugLabelingChanges/ucm132995.htm.

Istodax (Romidepsin)

Class: Histone deacetylase inhibitor

Form: IV injection

Formulation: 10 mg powder for solution with 2 mL diluents

Dose: 14 mg/m² administered intravenously over a 4-hour period on days 1, 8, and 15 of a 28-day cycle. Cycles should be repeated every 28 days provided that the patient continues to benefit from and tolerates the therapy.

Mechanism of action: Romidepsin inhibits the catalysis of the removal of acetyl groups from acetylated lysine residues in histones, causing the accumulation of acetylated histones and inducing cell-cycle arrest and apoptosis of some cancer cell lines.

FDA-approved indication: Cutaneous T-cell lymphoma

Adverse reactions: QT prolongation, cytopenias, ECG changes, nausea, fatigue, infections, vomiting, anorexia

Drug interactions: Estrogen-containing contraceptives, warfarin, CYP3A4 inhibitors, CYP3A4 inducers, Pgp inhibitors

Monitoring parameters: Potassium and magnesium, hematological parameters, ECG in patients at risk for QT prolongation

Patient counseling: Estrogen-containing birth control may be less effective during therapy. Report excessive nausea and vomiting, abnormal heartbeat, chest pain, or shortness of breath to your health care provider. Seek immediate attention if excessive bleeding occurs. Do not take if you become pregnant.

Jevtana (Cabazitaxel)

Class: Microtubule inhibitor

Form: IV infusion

Formulation: Single-use vial 60 mg/1.5 mL

Dose: Recommended dose of 25 mg/m² administered every 3 weeks as a 1-hour IV infusion in combination with prednisone

Mechanism of action: Cabazitaxel is a microtubule inhibitor. Cabazitaxel binds to tubulin and promotes assembly into microtubules, thereby inhibiting disassembly and leading to stabilization of microtubules and inhibition of miotic and interphase cellular functions.

FDA-approved indication: Indicated for use in patients in combination with prednisone for treatment of hormone-refractory metastatic prostate cancer previously treated with a docetaxel-containing treatment regimen

Adverse reactions: Neutropenia, anemia, leucopenia, thrombocytopenia, diarrhea, fatigue, nausea, vomiting, constipation, asthenia, abdominal pain, hematuria, back pain, anorexia, peripheral neuropathy, pyrexia, dyspnea, dysgeusia, cough, arthralgia, alopecia

Drug interactions: Use with caution in patients taking concomitant medications that induce or inhibit CYP3A.

Monitoring parameters: CBC

Patient counseling: Report signs of hypersensitivity and monitor your temperature frequently. It is important to use oral prednisone prescribed.

Novantrone (Mitoxantrone Hydrochloride)

Boxed warning: The FDA has issued the following boxed warnings.

- Secondary acute myeloid leukemia in patients with multiple sclerosis and cancer (www.fda .gov/Safety/MedWatch/SafetyInformation/ ucm219174.htm)

■ Dose-related risk of potentially fatal congestive heart failure either during treatment or in the long term after treatment was discontinued (www.fda.gov/Safety/MedWatch/Safety Information/Safety-RelatedDrugLabeling Changes/ucm133055.htm)

Prograf (Tacrolimus)

Labeling revision: Prograf (tacrolimus) in conjunction with mycophenolate mofetil in kidney transplant recipients

Sprycel (Dasatinib)

Labeling revision: Treatment of adults in all phases of chronic myeloid leukemia (chronic, accelerated, or myeloid or lymphoid blast phase) with resistance or intolerance to prior therapy including Gleevec (imatinib mesylate)

Tasigna (Nilotinib)

Boxed warning (updated): Decreased dose is recommended in patients with hepatic dysfunction because of potential QT interval prolongation. See www.fda .gov/Safety/MedWatch/SafetyInformation/ucm1822 34.htm.

Temodar (Temozolomide)

New formulation: Temozolomide powder for IV use: 100 mg/vial

Trelstar (Triptorelin Pamoate)

New dosage form: 22.5 mg base/vial for injection

Votrient (Pazopanib)

Class: Tyrosine kinase inhibitor

Form: Tablets

Formulations: 200 mg, 400 mg

Dose: 400 mg initially, titrated to 800 mg (in 200 mg increments) once daily as tolerated

Mechanism of action: Medication inhibits tyrosine kinase, vascular endothelial growth factor receptors, platelet-derived growth factor receptors, fibroblast growth factor receptors, cytokine receptor (kit), IL-2 receptor inducible T-cell kinase, leukocyte-specific protein tyrosine kinase, and transmembrane glycoprotein receptor tyrosine kinase.

FDA-approved indication: Renal cell carcinoma

Adverse reactions: Possible reactions include hepatotoxicity, hypertension, hair color change, hypomagnesemia, hypophosphatemia, increased glucose, diarrhea, loss of appetite, nausea, vomiting, fatigue, myocardial infarction, prolonged QT interval, hypothyroidism, proteinuria, gastrointestinal (GI) perforation or fistula, decreased wound healing. Do not administer pazopanib to patients with arterial thrombotic events, hemoptysis, cerebral, or serious GI hemorrhage in the past 6 months.

Drug interactions: CYP3A4 inhibitors or inducers; substrates of CYP3A4, CYP2D6, or CYP2C8

Monitoring parameters: Liver function tests, ECG, serum electrolytes, thyroid function tests, urinalysis, blood pressure

Patient counseling: Take at least 1 hour before or 2 hours after a meal. If a dose is missed, it should not be taken if less than 12 hours remain until the next dose. Do not take if you are pregnant. Report any signs of hepatotoxicity to a medical provider. Skin or hair may change color during treatment.

Zevalin (Ibritumomab Tiuxetan)

New indication: First-line therapy in treatment of follicular non-Hodgkin's lymphoma

38-13. Chapter 20: Solid Organ Transplantation

Rapamune (Sirolimus)

Boxed warning (revised): Medication is not recommended in liver or lung transplant patients secondary to serious, including fatal, reactions. Review prescribing information for the complete boxed warning: www.fda.gov/Safety/MedWatch/SafetyInformation/ucm187076.htm.

Zortress (Everolimus)

Class: Macrolide immunosuppressant

Form: Tablets

Formulations: 0.25 mg, 0.5 mg, 0.75 mg

Dose: Initiate dose at 0.75 mg twice daily, with adjustment based on target trough everolimus concentrations between 3 and 8 ng/mL.

Mechanism of action: Everolimus inhibits antigenic- and interleukin-stimulated activation and proliferation of T- and B-lymphocytes.

FDA-approved indication: Medication is indicated for use in prophylaxis of organ rejection in adult patients at low to moderate immunologic risk receiving kidney transplant.

Adverse reactions: Peripheral edema, constipation, hypertension, nausea, anemia, urinary tract infection, hyperlipidemia

Drug interactions: Everolimus is metabolized by CYP3A4; possible dose adjustments may be necessary when used in conjunction with inducers and inhibitors.

Monitoring parameters: Everolimus and cyclosporine concentrations and lipids

Patient counseling: There is a risk of increased infection, nephrotoxicity, and possible development of lymphomas. Avoid grapefruit and grapefruit juices. All changes to doses should be made under the supervision of a health care provider.

38-14. Chapter 21: Gastrointestinal Diseases

Cimzia (Certolizumab Pegol)

Boxed warning (revised): There is a risk of serious infections. See www.fda.gov/Drugs/DrugSafety/PostmarketDrugSafetyInformationforPatientsand Providers/ucm109340.htm.

Creon (Pancrelipase)

Class: Pancreatic enzyme

Form: Delayed-release capsules

Formulations: The following formulations are available:

- 6,000 USP units lipase, 19,000 USP units protease, 30,000 USP units amylase
- 12,000 USP units lipase, 38,000 USP units protease, 60,000 USP units amylase
- 24,000 USP units lipase, 76,000 USP units protease, 120,000 USP units amylase

Dose: Begin adults and children 4 years of age and older with 500 lipase units/kg of body weight per meal to a maximum of 2,500 lipase units/kg of body weight per meal (or less than or equal to 10,000 lipase units/kg of body weight per day) or less than 4,000 lipase units/g fat ingested per day.

Mechanism of action: In the duodenum and proximal small intestine, the enzymes catalyze the hydrolysis of fats into monoglycerol, glycerol, and fatty acids; protein into peptides and amino acids; and starch into dextrins and short-chain sugars.

FDA-approved indication: Treatment of exocrine pancreatic insufficiency caused by cystic fibrosis or other conditions

Adverse reactions: Fibrosing colonopathy; distal intestinal obstruction syndrome; recurrence of pre-existing carcinoma; severe allergic reactions, including anaphylaxis, asthma, hives, and pruritus

Drug interactions: None known

Monitoring parameters: CBC and enzyme concentrations; serum uric acid levels in patients with gout, renal impairment, or preexisting hyperuricemia

Patient counseling: Pancrelipase may increase the likelihood of having a rare bowel disorder called *fibrosing colonopathy*. Contact your health care professional immediately if any unusual or severe stomach area (abdominal) pain develops.

Carbaglu (Carglumic Acid)

Class: Enzyme

Form: Tablets

Formulation: 200 mg

Dose: Recommended daily dosing range of 100–250 mg/kg/day. The total dose can be divided into two to four doses daily.

Mechanism of action: Carglumic acid is a structural analogue of N-acetylglutamate, which is an essential activator of carbamoyl phosphate synthase 1 in the liver mitochondria.

FDA-approved indication: Indicated for use in patients with acute hyperammonemia caused by deficiency of the hepatic enzyme N-acetylglutamate synthase (NAGS). It is also indicated for maintenance therapy in the treatment of chronic hyperammonemia in those with a deficiency of NAGS.

Adverse reactions: Infections, vomiting, abdominal pain, pyrexia, tonsillitis, anemia, ear infection, diarrhea, nasopharyngitis, headache

Drug interactions: None known

Monitoring parameters: Plasma ammonia levels

Patient counseling: Tablets should not be swallowed whole and not crushed. The tablets should be dispersed in a minimum of 2.5 mL of water. The tablets do not dissolve completely, and some undissolved particles may remain. Store in the refrigerator until use; once open, store at room temperature.

Kapidex (Dexlansoprazole)

Class: Proton pump inhibitor (PPI)

Form: Capsules

Formulations: 30 mg, 60 mg; delayed release

Dose: The following doses apply:

- *Healing of erosive esophagitis:* 60 mg once daily for up to 8 weeks (recommended)
- *Maintenance of healed erosive esophagitis:* 30 mg once daily (controlled studies have not been extended beyond 6 months)
- *Symptomatic non-erosive gastroesophageal reflux disease (GERD):* 30 mg once daily for 4 weeks

Mechanism of action: Dexlansoprazole is a PPI that suppresses gastric acid secretion by specific inhibition of the (H+, K+)-ATPase in the gastric parietal cell. By acting specifically on the proton pump, dexlansoprazole blocks the final step of acid production.

FDA-approved indications: Medication is indicated for healing of all grades of erosive esophagitis for up to 8 weeks and maintenance of healed erosive esophagitis for up to 6 months, as well as treatment of heartburn associated with non-erosive GERD for 4 weeks.

Adverse reactions: Diarrhea, abdominal pain, nausea, upper respiratory tract infection, vomiting, flatulence

Drug interactions: The following interactions have been observed:

- Dexlansoprazole may interfere with absorption of drugs with pH-dependent absorption (e.g., ampicillin esters, digoxin, iron salts, ketoconazole).
- Dexlansoprazole may decrease systemic concentrations of atazanavir.
- Increased international normalized ratio and prothrombin time may occur with coadministration of PPIs and warfarin.
- Increased blood levels of tacrolimus may occur.

Monitoring parameters: GI symptoms

Patient counseling: Take exactly as prescribed for the full duration with or without food. Swallow capsules whole or open capsules and sprinkle on a tablespoonful of applesauce.

Metozolv ODT (Metoclopramide)

New dosage form: Orally disintegrating tablets

New indications: New indications are as follows:

- Short-term (4–12 weeks) treatment of symptomatic gastroesophageal reflux in adults with symptomatic and documented disease who fail to respond to conventional therapy
- Treatment of acute and recurrent diabetic gastroparesis (diabetic gastric stasis) in adults

Boxed warning: Treatment can lead to tardive dyskinesia; avoid treatment longer than 12 weeks. See www.fda.gov/Safety/MedWatch/SafetyInformation/ucm170934.htm.

OsmoPrep (Sodium Phosphate Monobasic Monohydrate, USP, and sodium phosphate) and Visicol (Sodium Phosphate Monobasic Monohydrate, USP, and Sodium Phosphate Dibasic Anhydrous, USP)

Boxed warning: Acute phosphate nephropathy may occur in patients administered oral sodium phosphate products for colon cleansing before colonoscopy. Some reactions have led to decreased renal function and dialysis. See www.fda.gov/Drugs/DrugSafety/PostmarketDrugSafetyInformationforPatientsandProviders/ucm103354.htm.

Reglan (Metoclopramide)

Boxed warning: Treatment can lead to tardive dyskinesia; avoid treatment longer than 12 weeks. See www.fda.gov/Safety/MedWatch/SafetyInformation/ucm170934.htm.

Remicade (Infliximab)

Boxed warning (updated): Disseminated invasive fungal infections, such as histoplasmosis and tuberculosis, have been reported. Malignancies, lymphomas, and fatal cases of hepatosplenic T-cell lymphomas have also occurred in patients receiving therapy. See www.fda.gov/Safety/MedWatch/SafetyInformation/SafetyAlertsforHumanMedicalProducts/ucm172751.htm.

38-15. Chapter 22: Rheumatoid Arthritis, Osteoarthritis, Gout, and Lupus

Actemra (Tocilizumab)

Class: Monoclonal antibody

Form: IV infusion

Formulations: 80 mg/4 mL, 200 mg/10 mL, 400 mg/20 mL

Dose: Dose once every 4 weeks as a 60-minute single IV drip infusion.

Mechanism of action: Tocilizumab is an IL-6 receptor inhibitor.

FDA-approved indication: Treatment of adult patients with moderately to severely active rheumatoid arthritis who have an inadequate response to one or more TNF antagonist therapies

Adverse reactions: Upper respiratory tract infections, common cold, sinus infections, headache, increased blood pressure, increased alanine aminotransferase

Drug interactions: Tocilizumab may have interactions with CYP450 substrate medications. This issue is more relevant in medications with a narrow therapeutic index. Live vaccines should not be administered.

Monitoring parameters: Monitoring parameters include neutrophils, platelets, lipids, and liver functions tests. Patients should also be monitored for development of infections.

Patient counseling: Instruct patients on the importance of contacting their health care provider when symptoms suggesting infection and persistent abdominal pain develop.

Ampyra (Dalfampridine)

Class: Potassium channel blocker

Form: Tablets

Formulation: 10 mg

Dose: Twice daily

Mechanism of action: Mechanism is still unknown. Dalfampridine is a broad-spectrum potassium channel blocker.

FDA-approved indication: To improve walking in patients with multiple sclerosis

Adverse reactions: Urinary tract infections, insomnia, dizziness, headache, nausea, asthenia, back pain, balance disorder, multiple sclerosis relapse, paresthesia, nasopharyngitis, constipation, dyspepsia, pharyngolaryngeal pain

Drug interactions: None known

Patient counseling: Take with or without food. Notify your health care provider if you experience any signs or symptoms of an allergic reaction.

Cimzia (Certolizumab Pegol)

New indication: Moderate to severe rheumatoid arthritis

Colcrys (Colchicine)

New indication: Prevention of gout flares

Extavia (Interferon Beta-1b)

Class: Interferon

Form: Subcutaneous injection

Formulations: 0.3 mg of interferon beta-1b; 15 mg albumin (human), USP; and 15 mg mannitol, USP

Dose: The recommended dose is 0.25 mg injected subcutaneously every other day. Generally, start at 0.0625 mg (0.25 mL) subcutaneously ever other day, and increase over a 6-week period to 0.25 mg (1 mL) every other day. Instruct patients in the use of aseptic technique when administering interferon beta-1b.

Mechanism of action: Exact mechanism of action is unknown (immunomodulator).

FDA-approved indications: The medication has been approved for treatment of relapsing forms of multiple sclerosis to reduce the frequency of clinical exacerbations. Patients with multiple sclerosis in whom efficacy has been demonstrated include patients who have experienced a first clinical episode and have MRI (magnetic resonance imaging) features consistent with multiple sclerosis.

Adverse reactions: Injection-site reactions and necrosis, rash, leucopenia, lymphopenia, neutropenia, lymphadenopathy, hypertension, increased muscle tone, myalgia, asthenia, headache, insomnia, peripheral edema, fever, pain, shivering, depression, suicidal ideation, increased liver function tests

Drug interactions: None known

Monitoring parameters: CBC, blood chemistries, liver function tests, thyroid function tests

Patient counseling: This medication is an injectable. The medication is packaged as a powder with a liquid and should be mixed according to instructions. Swirl to mix, but do not shake. Use a different body part after each injection. Using aseptic technique, administer the medication within 3 hours of mixing into the upper arm, abdomen, thighs, or buttocks.

Savella (Milnacipran Hydrochloride)

Class: Selective serotonin and norepinephrine reuptake inhibitor

Form: Tablets

Formulations: 12.5 mg, 25 mg, 50 mg, 100 mg

Dose: The following guidelines apply:

- The recommended dose is 50 mg twice daily.
- The dose should be titrated up to the recommended dose of 100 mg/day:
  - Day 1: 12.5 mg once
  - Days 2–3: 12.5 mg twice daily
  - Days 4–7: 25 mg twice daily
  - After day 7: 50 mg twice daily
- The dose may be increased to 200 mg/day depending on individual patient response.
- Dose adjustments are needed with severe renal impairment.

Mechanism of action: Milnacipran is a selective norepinephrine and serotonin reuptake inhibitor. The exact mechanism of the central pain inhibitory action and ability to improve fibromyalgia symptoms is unknown.

FDA-approved indication: Management of fibromyalgia; not approved for use in pediatric patients

Adverse reactions: Nausea, palpitations, headache, constipation, increased heart rate, hyperhidrosis, vomiting, dizziness, hypertension, hot flushes

Boxed warning: Increased risk of suicidal ideation, thinking, and behavior in children, adolescents, and young adults taking antidepressants for major depressive disorder and other psychiatric disorders

Drug interactions: Milnacipran undergoes minimal CYP450-related metabolism, with the majority of the dose excreted unchanged in urine, and low binding to plasma proteins:

- *Lithium:* Coadministration may result in serotonin syndrome.
- *Epinephrine and norepinephrine:* Concomitant use may result in paroxysmal hypertension and possible arrhythmia.
- *Serotonergic drugs:* Coadministration may result in hypertension and coronary artery vasoconstriction.
- *Digoxin:* Concomitant use is associated with potentiation of adverse hemodynamic effects (postural hypotension and tachycardia with IV digoxin).
- *Clonidine:* Coadministration may inhibit clonidine's antihypertensive effect.
- *Clomipramine:* Increase in euphoria and postural hypotension may occur when patient is switched from clomipramine to milnacipran.
- *Central nervous system (CNS)–active drugs:* Given primary CNS effects of milnacipran, caution is advised when used in combination.

- *Monoamine oxidase inhibitors (MAOIs):* Concurrent administration may result in CNS toxicity or serotonin syndrome.

Monitoring parameters: Pain, physical functioning, blood pressure, heart rate, liver function tests, and serum sodium levels

Patient counseling: There is a suicide risk with this medication. Serotonin syndrome may occur. Medication may affect blood pressure and pulse. Abnormal bleeding may occur with concomitant use of NSAIDs, aspirin, and other coagulation-affecting drugs. Ability to operate machinery may be impaired. Avoid alcohol consumption and abrupt discontinuation. Notify your health care provider if you are pregnant or plan to become pregnant or if you are breast-feeding.

Simponi (Golimumab)

Class: TNF blocker

Form: Injection

Formulation: 50 mg/0.5mL in a single-dose, prefilled SmartJect autoinjector

Dose: 50 mg administered by subcutaneous injection once a month

Mechanism of action: Golimumab binds to both the soluble and the transmembrane bioactive forms of human TNFα. This interaction prevents the binding of TNFα to its receptors, thereby inhibiting the biological activity of TNFα (a cytokine protein).

FDA-approved indications: Treatment of moderately to severely active rheumatoid arthritis, active psoriatic arthritis, and active ankylosing spondylitis

Adverse reactions: Immunosuppression, upper respiratory tract infection, nasopharyngitis

Drug interactions: The following interactions have been noted:

- Abatacept poses an increased risk of serious infection.
- Anakinra poses an increased risk of serious infection.
- Live vaccines should not be given with golimumab.

Monitoring parameters: Normalization of serum C-reactive protein levels, evidence of prior hepatitis B virus infection, signs and symptoms of infection, latent or active tuberculosis, patients with congestive heart failure

Patient counseling: Golimumab may lower the ability of your immune system to fight infections. Contact your doctor if you develop any symptoms of infection.

Uloric (Febuxostat)

Class: Xanthine oxidase inhibitor

Dose: Starting dose is 40 mg once daily. If serum uric acid is less than 6 mg/dL after 2 weeks, increase dose to 80 mg daily.

Mechanism of action: Febuxostat decreases serum uric acid by inhibiting xanthine oxidase, the enzyme responsible for converting xanthine to uric acid.

FDA-approved indication: Chronic management of (symptomatic) hyperuricemia in patients with gout

Adverse reactions: Liver function abnormalities, nausea, arthralgia, dizziness, and rash may occur. Febuxostat may increase gout flares during initiation; do not discontinue febuxostat with gout flares. More cardiovascular and thromboembolic events were observed in clinical trials.

Drug interactions: Febuxostat is contraindicated in patients using azathioprine, mercaptopurine, or theophylline. Coadministration could increase their concentration, resulting in toxicity.

Monitoring parameters: Liver function tests, serum uric acid level (less than 6 mg/dL), and signs and symptoms of myocardial infarction and stroke

Patient counseling: Febuxostat may be taken with or without food or antacids. Inform a health care professional if you develop a rash, chest pain, shortness of breath, or symptoms suggestive of a stroke. Do not stop taking febuxostat if a flare develops.

TNF Blockers

TNF blockers in this boxed warning include

- Cimzia (certolizumab pegol)
- Enbrel (etanercept)
- Humira (adalimumab)
- Remicade (infliximab)
- Simponi (golimumab)

Boxed warning (revised): Cases of lymphoma and other malignancies, some fatal, have been reported in pediatric patients. Review prescribing information for complete boxed warning:

- For certolizumab pegol, www.fda.gov/Safety/MedWatch/SafetyInformation/ucm194120.htm
- For etanercept, www.fda.gov/Safety/MedWatch/SafetyInformation/ucm194135.htm
- For adalimumab, www.fda.gov/Safety/MedWatch/SafetyInformation/ucm194134.htm
- For infliximab, www.fda.gov/Safety/MedWatch/SafetyInformation/ucm194136.htm
- For golimumab, www.fda.gov/Safety/MedWatch/SafetyInformation/ucm194137.htm

Vimovo (Esomeprazole Magnesium/Naproxen)

New formulation: 20 mg esomeprazole magnesium and 500 or 375 mg naproxen

38-16. Chapter 23: Pain Management and Migraines

Actiq (Fentanyl Citrate)

Boxed warning (revised): Potential exists for fatal overdose when Actiq is substituted for other fentanyl products (because of differences in the extent of fentanyl absorption). When Actiq is prescribed, the dose should not be converted on a microgram per microgram basis from other fentanyl products. See www.fda.gov/Safety/MedWatch/SafetyInformation/ucm194045.htm.

Acuvail (Ketorolac Tromethamine)

Class: NSAIDS, ophthalmic

Form: Ophthalmic solution

Formulation: 0.45%

Dose: One drop to affected eye twice daily beginning one day before cataract surgery and continued through the first 2 weeks of the postoperative period

Mechanism of action: Medication inhibits prostaglandin biosynthesis.

FDA-approved indication: Treatment of pain and inflammation following cataract surgery

Adverse reactions: Increased intraocular pressure, conjunctival hemorrhage, blurred vision

Drug interactions: None known

Monitoring parameters: Visual changes

Patient counseling: Slow or delayed healing may occur while using NSAIDs. The solution from one individual single-use vial is to be used immediately in the affected eye after opening. The drug should not be administered while you are wearing contact lenses. If you develop an intercurrent ocular condition or have ocular surgery, seek immediate advice from your health care provider.

Alsuma (Sumatriptan Succinate)

New formulation: 6 mg/0.5 mL solution for sub-cutaneous injection

Axert (Almotriptan)

Change in patient population: Approved for treatment of migraine in adolescents

Caldolor (Ibuprofen)

Class: NSAID

Form: IV injection

Formulations: 400 mg/4 mL, 800 mg/8 mL

Dose: The following doses apply to the listed indication:

- *Pain:* 400–800 mg intravenously over 30 minutes every 6 hours as necessary
- *Fever:* 400 mg intravenously over 30 minutes followed by 400 mg every 4–6 hours or 100–200 mg every 4 hours as necessary

Mechanism of action: Ibuprofen's mechanism of action, like that of other NSAIDs, is not completely understood but may be related to prostaglandin synthetase inhibition.

FDA-approved indication: Management of mild to moderate pain, severe pain as an adjunct to opioid analgesics, and reduction of fever

Adverse reactions: Nausea, flatulence, vomiting, headache, hemorrhage, dizziness

Drug interactions: The following interactions have been noted:

- *ACE inhibitors:* NSAIDs may diminish the antihypertensive effect of ACE inhibitors.
- *Aspirin:* Concomitant administration of ibuprofen and aspirin is not generally recommended because of the potential for increased adverse effects.

Monitoring parameters: CBC and chemistry profiles, GI bleeding, fecal occult blood test, blood pressure

Patient counseling: Risk of ulcers, bleeding, myocardial infarction, or stroke may increase. The drug is contraindicated for the treatment of perioperative pain in the setting of coronary artery bypass graft surgery.

Cambia (Diclofenac Potassium)

Class: NSAID

Form: Oral solution

Formulation: Each packet contains buffered diclofenac potassium 50 mg in a soluble powder.

Dose: A single 50 mg dose is given. Mix single packet contents with 1–2 ounces (30–60 mL) of water prior to administration.

Mechanism of action: Mechanism of action is not fully known but may be associated with inhibition of prostaglandin synthetase.

FDA-approved indication: Acute treatment of migraine attacks with or without aura in adults 18 years of age or older

Adverse reactions: Nausea and dizziness

Drug interactions: The following interactions are possible:

- *Aspirin:* Concomitant administration with other NSAIDs is not recommended because of an increased risk of adverse reactions, including GI bleeding.
- *Anticoagulants:* Concomitant use of diclofenac and anticoagulants (e.g., warfarin) increases the risk of serious GI bleeding.

Monitoring parameters: GI bleeding, blood pressure, CBC, chemistry profile, fluid retention or edema, renal and hepatic function tests, symptoms of hepatotoxicity and hypersensitivity reactions

Patient counseling: Be alert for signs and symptoms of chest pain, shortness of breath, weakness, slurring of speech, and ulcerations and bleeding.

Dysport (AbobotulinumtoxinA)

Class: Acetylcholine release inhibitor and a neuromuscular blocking agent

Form: Injection

Formulations: The following formulations are available:

- *Cervical dystonia:* Single-use, sterile 500-unit vial for reconstitution with 1 mL of 0.9% sodium chloride injection USP (without preservative) and a single-use, sterile 300-unit vial for reconstitution with 0.6 mL of 0.9% sodium chloride injection USP (without preservative)
- *Glabellar lines:* Single-use, sterile 300-unit vial for reconstitution with 2.5 mL or 1.5 mL of 0.9% sodium chloride injection USP (without preservative)

Dose:

- *Cervical dystonia:* Initial dose of 500 units is given intramuscularly as a divided dose among the affected muscles; retreatment should be administered every 12–16 weeks or longer.

- *Glabellar lines:* A total dose of 50 units, divided in five equal aliquots of 10 units each, should be administered to affected muscles to achieve clinical effect; retreatment should be administered no more frequently than every 3 months.

Mechanism of action: Medication inhibits release of the neurotransmitter, acetylcholine, from peripheral cholinergic nerve endings.

FDA-approved indication: Treatment of cervical dystonia in adults to reduce the severity of abnormal head position and neck pain and the temporary improvement in the appearance of moderate to severe glabellar lines in adults younger than 65 years of age

Adverse reactions: Possible reactions include the following:

- *Cervical dystonia:* muscular weakness, dysphagia, dry mouth, injection-site pain or discomfort, fatigue, headache, neck pain, musculoskeletal pain, dysphonia, eye disorders
- *Glabellar lines:* nasopharyngitis, headache, injection-site or reaction, upper respiratory tract infection, eyelid edema, eyelid ptosis, sinusitis, nausea

Drug interactions: Aminoglycosides or other agents interfering with neuromuscular transmission (e.g., curare-like agents) or muscle relaxants should be observed closely because the effect of botulinum toxin may be potentiated. Use of anticholinergic drugs may potentiate systemic anticholinergic effects.

Monitoring parameters: Botulism and the associated signs and symptoms, deep dermal scarring, excessive weakened or atrophy in the targeted muscles, distant spread of toxin effect

Patient counseling: Symptomatic improvement may not be seen for a specific amount of time. Cervical dystonia may improve within 2 weeks with a peak improvement in 4 weeks.

Embeda (Morphine Sulfate and Naltrexone Hydrochloride)

Class: Opioid agonist–antagonist

Form: Extended-release capsules

Formulations: morphine sulfate/naltrexone hydrochloride 20 mg/0.8 mg, 30 mg/1.2 mg, 50 mg/2 mg, 60 mg/2.4 mg, 80 mg/3.2 mg, 100 mg/4 mg

Dose: Swallow whole once or twice daily.

Mechanism of action: Morphine sulfate binds to opioid receptors, producing analgesia and sedation (opioid agonist). Naltrexone is added to reduce drug liking and euphoria if crushed, chewed, or dissolved.

FDA-approved indication: The drug is approved for management of moderate to severe pain when a continuous, around-the-clock opioid analgesic is needed for an extended period of time. It is *not* intended for use as a prn analgesic.

Adverse reactions: Constipation, nausea, somnolence

Drug interactions: The following interactions have been observed:

- CNS depressants should be used with caution and in reduced dosage.
- Muscle relaxants may enhance the action and produce an increased degree of respiratory depression.
- Mixed agonist–antagonist opioid analgesics may reduce the analgesic effect and may precipitate withdrawal symptoms.
- MAOIs should not be used concomitantly or within 14 days of discontinuing treatment.

Monitoring parameters: Creatinine, pain-scale results, symptoms of respiratory depression

Patient counseling: Swallow whole or sprinkle the contents of the capsules on applesauce. This medication is *not* intended for use as an "as needed" analgesic. Do not consume alcoholic beverages or use prescription or nonprescription medications containing alcohol.

Exalgo (Hydromorphone Hydrochloride)

New dosage form: Extended-release tablets of 8 mg, 12 mg, and 16 mg; dosed once daily

Lyrica (Ketorolac Tromethamine)

New dosage form: 15.75 mg/spray nasal spray

Lyrica (Pregabalin)

New dosage form: 20 mg/mL oral solution

Onsolis (Fentanyl)

Class: Opioids

Form: Buccal soluble films

Formulations: 200 mcg, 400 mcg, 600 mcg, 800 mcg, 1200 mcg

Dose: The following dosing guidelines apply:

- Give an initial dose of one 200 mcg film strip;

titrate up to a maximum dose of 1,200 mcg/dose *or* four 200 mcg films *or* four doses/day.

- Separate all doses by at least 2 hours.
- For initial titration, increase dose by 200 mcg/episode prn; for maintenance dosing, increase only after several episodes were not adequately managed by prescribed dose; use a single film once dose is established.

Mechanism of action: Mu-receptor agonist

FDA-approved indication: Management of breakthrough pain in patients with cancer, 18 years of age or older, who are already receiving and who are tolerant to opioid therapy for their underlying persistent cancer pain

Adverse reactions: Nausea, vomiting, dizziness, dehydration, dyspnea, somnolence

Drug interactions: CYP3A4 inhibitors and inducers

Monitoring parameters: Respiratory depression, pain-scale results

Patient counseling: All patients should be opioid tolerant and enrolled in the FOCUS Program for Onsolis to receive the medication. Open the foil package immediately before use. This medication is a small film that should be stuck to the inside of the cheek. Multiple films should not be placed on top of each other. Do not drink fluids until 5 minutes after administration. Keep away from children (the dose of fentanyl may be fatal to children).

Pennsaid (Diclofenac Sodium)

Class: NSAID

Form: Topical solution

Formulation: 1.5%

Dose: Apply four times daily. Dispense 10 drops in the hand or on the knee, and spread evenly all over the knee: front, back, and sides. Repeat until a total of 40 drops have been used. Repeat for other knee.

FDA-approved indication: To treat signs and symptoms of osteoarthritis of the knee

Adverse reactions: Application-site reactions

Patient counseling: You should avoid contact of topical solution with the eyes and mucosa. If eye contact occurs, immediately wash out the eye with water or saline, and consult a physician if irritation persists for more than 1 hour.

Qutenza (Capsaicin)

Class: Analgesic and transient receptor potential cation channel V1 agonist

Form: Patch

Formulation: 8% transdermal patch

Dose: A single 60-minute application of up to four patches is given every 3 months as needed on the most painful areas. Do not apply more frequently than every 3 months. Do not use on broken skin. Do not use latex gloves when handling capsaicin. Apply a topical anesthetic before patch application. Do not use near eyes or mucus membranes. After removal of patch, clean with cleansing gel for 1 minute and then dry.

FDA-approved indication: Postherpetic neuralgia

Adverse reactions: Application-site reactions, hypertension

Drug interactions: None known

Monitoring parameters: Blood pressure

Patient counseling: The treated area may be sensitive to heat for a few days following treatment. Inform your health care provider if you are pregnant or breastfeeding or of any recent cardiovascular events.

Ryzolt (Tramadol Hydrochloride)

New formulation: 100 mg, 200 mg, 300 mg capsules, extended release

Sumavel DosePro (Sumatriptan)

Class: Antimigraine, serotonin receptor agonist, 5-HT1

Form: Injection

Formulation: 6 mg/0.5mL

Dose: For acute migraine or cluster headache, give one dose of 6 mg subcutaneously. A second dose may be administered after 1 hour if headache recurs to a maximum dose of two doses (12 mg) in 24 hours.

Mechanism of action: Medication activates vascular serotonin 5-HT1 receptors, producing vasoconstriction (selective serotonin agonist).

Adverse reactions: Possible reactions include injection-site reactions; tingling; discomfort in nasal cavity, sinuses, and jaw; dizziness; drowsiness; headache; and feelings of heaviness, pressure, tightness (head and chest), and numbness. Serotonin syndrome and serious cardiac events have also been reported, including disturbances in cardiac rhythm and myocardial infarction.

FDA-approved indications: Treatment of cluster headaches and migraines (with and without aura)

Drug interactions: MAOIs and selective serotonin reuptake inhibitors or serotonin–norepinephrine reuptake inhibitors are contraindicated; 5-HT1 agonists, ergot alkaloids, ergotamine, or caffeine should not be used within 24 hours of Sumavel DosePro.

Monitoring parameters: Blood pressure, cardiovascular evaluation

Patient counseling: Instruct patients on the use of the device and subcutaneous administration. A loud burst of air will be heard and a sensation will be felt at administration. Injection site should be on the thigh or abdomen (space 2 inches from the navel).

Zipsor (Diclofenac Potassium)

Class: NSAID

Form: Capsules

Formulation: 25 mg liquid-filled capsule

Dose: 25 mg four times a day

Mechanism of action: The mechanism of action is not completely understood. It may involve inhibition of the cyclooxygenase (COX-1 and COX-2) pathways or prostaglandin synthetase inhibition.

FDA-approved indication: Relief of mild to moderate acute pain in adults

Adverse reactions: Abdominal pain, constipation, diarrhea, dyspepsia, nausea, vomiting, dizziness, headache, somnolence, pruritus, increased sweating

Drug interactions: Concomitant administration of diclofenac and aspirin is not generally recommended because of the potential of increased adverse effects, including GI bleeding, which may increase with coadministration of anticoagulants and diclofenac.

Monitoring parameters: GI bleeding, blood pressure, CBC, chemistry profile, fluid retention or edema, hepatic function, renal function testing, symptoms of hepatotoxicity and hypersensitivity reactions

Patient counseling: Patients should be aware of the following:

- *Cardiovascular effects:* Be alert for signs and symptoms of chest pain, shortness of breath, weakness, and slurring of speech and ask for medical advice when observing any indicative sign or symptoms.
- *Gastrointestinal effects:* Be alert for signs and symptoms of ulcerations and bleeding and ask for medical advice when observing any indicative sign or symptoms, including epigastric pain, dyspepsia, melena, and hematemesis.
- *Hepatotoxicity:* Be alert for warning signs and symptoms of hepatotoxicity (e.g., nausea, fatigue, lethargy, pruritus, jaundice, right upper

quadrant tenderness, and flu-like symptoms). If these signs or symptoms occur, stop therapy with diclofenac and seek immediate medical therapy.

38-17. Chapter 24: Seizure Disorders

Lamictal ODT (Lamotrigine)

New dosage form: Orally disintegrating tablets

Lamictal XR (Lamotrigine)

New dosage form: Extended-release tablets: 25 mg, 50 mg, 100 mg, 200 mg

New indication: Once daily as add-on epilepsy therapy for primary generalized tonic-clonic seizures

Sabril (Vigabatrin)

Class: Anticonvulsant, γ-aminobutyric acid (GABA), GABA transaminase inhibitor

Form: Tablets, oral solution

Formulation: 500 mg

Dose: Initiate therapy at 500 mg twice daily, increasing total daily dose per instructions to a recommended dose of 1.5 g twice daily.

Mechanism of action: The exact mechanism of vigabatrin's antiseizure properties is not known but is thought to be primarily the result of its action as an irreversible inhibitor of GABA transaminase, the enzyme responsible for the metabolism of the inhibitory neurotransmitter GABA. This inhibition causes increased levels of GABA in the central nervous system.

FDA-approved indication: Refractory complex partial seizures in adults. Vigabatrin should be used as adjunctive therapy in patients who have responded inadequately to several alternative treatments.

Adverse reactions: Vision loss, fatigue, somnolence, nystagmus, tremor, blurred vision, memory impairment, weight gain, arthralgia, anemia, peripheral neuropathy, edema, abnormal coordination, confused state

Drug interactions: Decreased phenytoin and increased carbamazepine levels have been reported.

Monitoring parameters: Vision tests, seizures

Patient counseling: There is a risk of permanent vision loss, specifically peripheral vision. Report any vision changes immediately. Avoid activities requiring mental alertness or coordination until drug effects are realized, because this medicine may cause dizziness or somnolence.

Vimpat (Lacosamide)

New dosage form: 10 mg/mL oral solution

38-18. Chapter 25: Psychiatric Disease

Butrans (Buprenorphine)

New formulation: 5 mcg/hr, 10 mcg/hr, 20 mcg/hr extended-release transdermal patch

Chantix (Varenicline)

Boxed warning: Serious neuropsychiatric events, such as depression, suicidal ideation, suicide attempt, and completed suicide, have been reported in patients taking this drug. See www.fda.gov/Safety/MedWatch/SafetyInformation/ucm175783.htm.

Cymbalta (Duloxetine)

New indication: Maintenance treatment of generalized anxiety disorder

Fanapt (Iloperidone)

Class: Atypical antipsychotic agent
Form: Tablets
Formulations: 1 mg, 2 mg, 4 mg, 6 mg, 8 mg, 10 mg, 12 mg
Dose: 12–24 mg/day administered twice daily
Mechanism of action: The exact mechanism is unknown, but it may be secondary to dopamine type 2 and serotonin type 2 antagonisms.
FDA-approved indication: Acute treatment of adults with schizophrenia
Adverse reactions: Dizziness, dry mouth, fatigue, nasal congestion, orthostatic hypotension, somnolence, tachycardia, increased weight
Drug interactions: The dose of iloperidone should be reduced when coadministered with a strong CYP2D6 or CYP3A4 inhibitor.

Monitoring parameters: CBC with differential, cerebrovascular events, dizziness, ECG, QTc interval prolongation, neuroleptic malignant syndrome, orthostatic vital signs, serum potassium and magnesium, suicide monitoring, tardive dyskinesia

Patient counseling: Health care professionals are advised to discuss the following issues with patients for whom they prescribe iloperidone: QT interval prolongation, neuroleptic malignant syndrome, orthostatic hypotension, and interference with cognitive and motor performance.

Invega Sustenna (Paliperidone Palmitate)

New dosage forms: Suspension, extended release, intramuscular
New indications: Acute and maintenance treatment of schizophrenia; treatment for schizoaffective disorder

Oleptro (Trazodone Hydrochloride)

New dosage form: Extended-release tablets: 150 mg, 300 mg

Risperdal (Risperidone)

New indication: Monotherapy and adjunctive therapy in the maintenance treatment of bipolar I disorder

Saphris (Asenapine)

Class: Antipsychotics, second generation
Form: Sublingual tablets
Formulations: 5 mg, 10 mg
Dose: For schizophrenia, give 5 mg sublingually twice daily. For bipolar disorder, give 10 mg sublingually twice daily; the dose can be decreased to 5 mg twice daily if adverse effects occur. The maximum dose is 10 mg twice daily.
Mechanism of action: The exact mechanism of action is unknown; it antagonizes dopamine type 2 receptors and serotonin 5-HT2A receptors.
FDA-approved indications: Acute treatment of schizophrenia and manic or mixed episodes associated with bipolar I disorder in adults
Adverse reactions: The following adverse reactions have been observed:

- *Patients with schizophrenia:* Akathisia, oral hypoesthesia, somnolence

■ *Patients with bipolar disorder:* Somnolence, dizziness, extrapyramidal symptoms other than akathisia, increased weight

Drug interactions: In the case of fluvoxamine (strong CYP1A2 inhibitor) and paroxetine (CYP2D6 substrate and inhibitor), approach coadministration cautiously.

Monitoring parameters: The following should be monitored:

■ Fasting glucose at baseline if diabetes risk factors are present

■ CBC for patients with preexisting leukopenia or history of drug-induced leukopenia or neutropenia

■ Orthostatic vital signs in the case of hypotension risk

Patient counseling: You may be more sensitive to temperature extremes such as very hot or cold conditions. This medication should be taken with a full glass of water. The tablet should not be swallowed; the sublingual tablets should be placed under the tongue and left to dissolve completely within seconds. Eating and drinking should be avoided for 10 minutes after administration.

Seroquel XR (Quetiapine)

New indication: Add-on treatment of major depressive disorder

Wellbutrin (Bupropion Hydrochloride) and Zyban (Bupropion Hydrochloride)

Boxed warning: Patients undergoing treatment for smoking cessation should be monitored for neuropsychiatric symptoms, including changes in behavior, hostility, agitation, depressed mood, and suicide-related events. Symptoms may persist after discontinuation of bupropion. See www.fda.gov/Safety/MedWatch/SafetyInformation/ucm176817.htm and www.fda.gov/Safety/MedWatch/SafetyInformation/ucm176815.htm.

Zyprexa (Olanzapine)

New indication: Treatment of schizophrenia and manic or mixed episodes associated with bipolar I disorder in adolescents (ages 13–17)

Zyprexa Relprevv (Olanzapine)

New formulation: Extended-release injectable suspension for treatment of schizophrenia

38-19. Chapter 26: Common Dermatologic Disorders

Asclera (Polidocanol)

Class: Sclerosing agent

Form: Injection

Formulations: 0.5% and 1% solution in 2 mL glass ampoules

Dose: Volume injected depends on extent of varicose veins (spider veins: use 0.5%; reticular veins: use 1%). Use 0.1–0.3 mL for each injection into each varicose vein. The maximum recommended volume for one treatment is 10 mL.

Mechanism of action: Polidocanol induces endothelial damage. Platelets then aggregate at the site of the damage and attach to the venous wall. Eventually, a dense network of platelets, cellular debris, and fibrin occludes the vessel.

FDA-approved indications: Treatment of uncomplicated spider veins and uncomplicated reticular veins in the lower extremity.

Adverse reactions: Local reactions at site of injection

Drug interactions: None known

Patient counseling: Wear compression stockings for 2–3 days continuously on the treated legs after treatment and 2–3 weeks during the daytime after treatment. Walk 15–20 minutes immediately after procedure. Avoid long plane rides, heavy exercise, and hot baths for 2–3 days after treatment.

Botox and Botox Cosmetic (Botulinum Toxin Type A) and Myobloc (Botulinum Toxin Type B)

Boxed warning: Risk of systemic spread of toxin exists. See www.fda.gov/Safety/MedWatch/SafetyInformation/SafetyAlertsforHumanMedicalProducts/ucm164255.htm.

Differin (Adapalene)

New dosage form: 0.1% topical lotion

Evolence (Dermal Filler)

Labeling revision approved: Labeling supplement that includes efficacy and safety data through 12 months

Kalbitor (Ecallantide)

Class: Plasma kallikrein inhibitor

Form: Subcutaneous injection

Formulation: 10 mg/mL

Dose: Administer 30 mg subcutaneously in three 10 mg (1 mL) injections. An additional 30 mg dose may be administered within a 24-hour period if attack persists.

Mechanism of action: Ecallantide inhibits plasma kallikrein and decreases the conversion of high-molecular-weight kininogen to bradykinin.

FDA-approved indication: Treatment of acute attacks of hereditary angioedema in patients 16 years of age and older

Adverse reactions: Anaphylaxis, headache, nausea, diarrhea, pyrexia, injection-site reactions, nasopharyngitis

Drug interactions: None known

Monitoring parameters: Symptoms of hypersensitivity reaction

Patient counseling: Report any signs or symptoms of a hypersensitivity reaction to your health care professional.

Raptiva (Efalizumab)

Note: Voluntarily withdrawn from the U.S. market as of June 2009

Boxed warning: Risk of progressive multifocal leukoencephalopathy exists. See www.fda.gov/Safety/Med Watch/SafetyInformation/SafetyAlertsforHuman MedicalProducts/ucm149675.htm.

Sculptra (Injectable Poly-L-Lactic Acid)

New indication: Correction of nasolabial fold contour deficiencies and other facial wrinkles

Stelara (Ustekinumab)

Class: Monoclonal antibody

Form: Injection

Formulation: 45 mg/0.5 mL, 90 mg/1 mL

Dose: Dosage is determined according to patient weight:

- *100 kg or less:* 45 mg subcutaneously initially and 4 weeks later, followed by 45 mg every 12 weeks
- *Greater than 100 kg:* 90 mg subcutaneously initially and 4 weeks later, followed by 90 mg every 12 weeks

Mechanism of action: Human immunoglobulin G1-kappa monoclonal antibody binds to the p40 sub-units of the IL-12 and IL-23 cytokines, which are involved in inflammatory and immune responses.

FDA-approved indication: Moderate to severe plaque psoriasis in patients who are candidates for phototherapy or systemic therapy

Adverse reactions: Nasopharyngitis, upper respiratory tract infection, headache, fatigue

Drug interactions: Concomitant use of live vaccines with immunosuppressants or phototherapy has not been evaluated.

Monitoring parameters: Tuberculin test prior to initiating therapy

Patient counseling: Do not take live vaccines because of drug-induced immunosuppression, and notify the prescriber if symptoms of headache, seizures, confusion, or vision change occur.

Vectical (Calcitriol)

New formulation: 3mcg/g calcitriol ointment

38-20. Chapter 27: Nonprescription Medications

Advil Congestion Relief (Ibuprofen and Phenylephrine Hydrochloride)

New formulation: 200 mg ibuprofen and 10 mg phenylephrine

Prevacid 24HR (Lansoprazole)

New dosage form: Over-the-counter (OTC) Prevacid 24HR contains 15mg of lansoprazole.

Zegerid OTC (Omeprazole and Sodium Bicarbonate)

New indication: OTC version of Zegerid for the treatment of heartburn

38-21. Chapter 28: Asthma and Chronic Obstructive Pulmonary Disease

Astepro (Azelastine)

New formulation: 0.15% (205.5 mcg base/spray)

Bepreve (Bepotastine)

Class: Antihistamine

Form: Ophthalmic solution

Formulation: 1.5%

Dose: Instill one drop into the affected eye twice daily.

Mechanism of action: Medication acts topically as a histamine-1 receptor antagonist and inhibits the release of histamine from mast cells.

FDA-approved indication: Treatment of itching associated with allergic conjunctivitis

Adverse reactions: Taste disturbances, headache, eye irritation, nasopharyngitis

Drug interactions: None known

Monitoring parameters: Relief of ocular itching associated with allergic conjunctivitis

Patient counseling: The drug may cause a mild taste in the mouth, eye irritation, headache, and nasopharyngitis. Instruct patient on proper instillation technique and not to wear contacts if eyes are red during therapy. Advise patient to remove contact lenses prior to instilling drug; contacts may be reinserted 10 minutes following instillation.

Dulera (Formoterol Fumarate and Mometasone Furoate)

New formulation: Metered-dose inhaler containing 0.005 mg formoterol fumarate and 0.1 mg mometasone furoate per inhalation or 0.005 mg formoterol fumarate and 0.2 mg mometasone furoate per inhalation

Long-Acting Beta Agonists

Long-acting beta agonists include the following:

- Advair Diskus (fluticasone propionate and salmeterol xinafoate) inhalation powder
- Advair HFA (fluticasone propionate and salmeterol xinafoate) inhalation aerosol
- Brovana (arformoterol tartrate) inhalation solution
- Foradil Aerolizer (formoterol fumarate) inhalation powder
- Foradil Certihaler (formoterol fumarate) inhalation powder
- Perforomist (formoterol fumarate) inhalation solution
- Serevent Diskus (salmeterol xinafoate) inhalation powder
- Symbicort (budesonide and formoterol) inhalation aerosol

Boxed Warning: Increased risk of asthma-related deaths has been noted with use of these medications. See www.fda.gov/Safety/MedWatch/Safety Information/ucm218833.htm.

Spiriva HandiHaler (Tiotropium Bromide)

New indication: Reduction of chronic obstructive pulmonary disease exacerbations

38-22. Chapter 30: Anti-infective Agents

Besivance (Besifloxacin)

Class: Quinolone antimicrobial

Form: Ophthalmic suspension

Formulation: 0.6% (6 mg/mL)

Dose: Instill one drop in the affected eye three times a day 4–12 hours apart for 7 days.

Mechanism of action: Medication inhibits bacterial DNA (deoxyribonucleic acid) gyrase and topoisomerase IV, resulting in impaired replication, transcription, and repair of bacterial DNA and impairment of the partitioning of the chromosomal DNA during bacterial cell division.

FDA-approved indication: Bacterial conjunctivitis

Adverse reactions: Conjunctival redness, blurred vision, eye pain, eye irritation, eye pruritus, headache

Drug interactions: None known

Monitoring parameters: Resolution of clinical symptoms of conjunctivitis

Patient counseling: Avoid contaminating the applicator tip with material from the eye, fingers, or other sources. Do not wear contact lenses if you have signs or symptoms of bacterial conjunctivitis during the course of therapy.

Cetraxal (Ciprofloxacin Otic)

Class: Quinolone antimicrobial

Form: 0.2% otic solution

Formulation: Each single-use container of ciprofloxacin otic delivers 0.25 mL of solution equivalent to 0.5 mg of ciprofloxacin.

Dose: For adults, instill the contents of one single-use container (deliverable volume: 0.25 mL) into the affected ear twice daily (approximately 12 hours apart) for 7 days.

Mechanism of action: The bactericidal action of ciprofloxacin results from interference with the enzyme DNA gyrase, which is needed for the synthesis of bacterial DNA.

FDA-approved indication: Treatment of acute otitis externa caused by susceptible isolates of *Pseudomonas aeruginosa* or *Staphylococcus aureus.*

Adverse reactions: Application-site pain, ear pruritus, fungal superinfection, headache

Drug interactions: None known

Monitoring parameters: Cultures may be necessary if infection does not improve after 1 week of treatment. Monitor for reduced earache, reduced swelling of external auditory canal, and reduced outer ear tenderness.

Patient counseling: Ciprofloxacin otic is for otic use only (not for ophthalmic, injection, or inhalation use). Ciprofloxacin otic should be used for as long as it is prescribed, even if the symptoms improve. Directions for use are as follows:

- Wash hands before use.
- Warm the container in your hands for at least 1 minute before use to minimize dizziness that may result from the instillation of a cold solution into the ear canal. Twist off and discard top of container.
- Lie with the affected ear upward, and then instill the contents of one container into the ear. Maintain this position for at least 1 minute to facilitate penetration of the drops into the ear.
- Repeat, if necessary, for the opposite ear.
- Discard used container.
- Store unused containers in pouch to protect from light.

Cleocin HCL (Clindamycin Hydrochloride)

Boxed warning: Clostridium difficile–associated diarrhea has been reported with use of this medication. See www.fda.gov/Safety/MedWatch/Safety Information/ucm194129.htm.

Coartem (Artemether and Lumefantrine)

Class: Antimalarial agent

Form: Tablets

Formulation: Artemether 20 mg and lumefantrine 120 mg

Dose: Adult treatment of uncomplicated malaria is as follows:

- *Patients 25 to < 35 kg:* Three tablets at hour 0 and hour 8 on the first day, followed by three tablets twice daily on days 2 and 3 (total of 18 tablets per treatment course)
- *Patients 35 kg or more:* Four tablets at hour 0 and hour 8 on the first day, followed by four tablets twice daily on days 2 and 3 (total of 24 tablets per treatment course)

Mechanism of action: Artemether and lumefantrine inhibit nucleic acid and protein synthesis during erythrocytic stages of *Plasmodium falciparum.*

FDA-approved indication: Treatment of acute, uncomplicated malaria infections caused by *P. falciparum*

Adverse reactions: Palpitations, headache, dizziness, fever, chills, anorexia, weakness, arthralgia, myalgia, cough

Drug interactions: Multiple drug interactions are possible; refer to prescribing information. Artemether induces CYP3A4. Artemether and lumefantrine are metabolized primarily by CYP3A4. Lumefantrine inhibits CYP2D6. Cisapride and QTc-prolonging agents may enhance the QTc-prolonging effect of dronedarone, phenothiazines, pimozide, and ranolazine.

Monitoring parameters: Assess for current or potential QT prolongation before beginning therapy.

Patient counseling: It is important to complete the course of therapy. Take Coartem with food (a full meal if possible). It may cause upset stomach, nausea, or loss of appetite. Eating small, frequent meals; using frequent mouth care; sucking lozenges; or chewing gum may help. Report chest pain or palpitation, rash, unusual fatigue, muscle weakness or pain, or any other adverse reactions.

Oravig (Miconazole)

New dosage form: 50 mg buccal tablets

Qualaquin (Quinine Sulfate)

Boxed warning: Thrombocytopenia, hemolytic-uremic syndrome and thrombotic thrombocytopenic purpura, and other hematologic reactions are possible. Development of chronic renal impairment in patients experiencing thrombotic thrombocytopenic purpura has been reported. See www.fda.gov/Safety/Med Watch/SafetyInformation/ucm194391.htm.

Sporanox (Itraconazole)

Boxed warning: Sudden death may occur in patients receiving itraconazole with levacetylmethadol (levomethadyl). See www.fda.gov/Safety/MedWatch/SafetyInformation/Safety-RelatedDrugLabelingChanges/ucm133470.htm.

Tobradex ST (Tobramycin and Dexamethasone)

New formulation: Strength has been changed from previous formulation: (0.3% and 0.05%).

Ulesfia (Benzyl Alcohol)

Class: Topical antiparasitic

Form: Lotion

Formulation: 5% in 8-ounce bottles

Dose: Dosing is based on hair length:

- *Short (up to 2 inches):* up to three-fourths bottle
- *Short (2–4 inches):* up to one bottle
- *Medium (4–8 inches):* up to one and one-half bottles
- *Medium (8–16 inches):* up to three bottles
- *Long (16–22 inches):* up to four bottles
- *Long (22 inches or more):* up to six bottles

Mechanism of action: Benzyl alcohol inhibits lice from closing their respiratory spiracles, allowing the vehicle to obstruct the spiracles and causing the lice to asphyxiate.

FDA-approved indication: Treatment of head lice infestation in patients 6 months of age and older

Adverse reactions: Ocular irritation, application-site irritation, application-site anesthesia and hypoesthesia

Drug interactions: None known

Monitoring parameters: None known

Patient counseling: Lice are removed with one treatment, but a second treatment is needed 1 week after the first treatment to remove the eggs.

Valcyte (Valganciclovir)

New dosage form: 50 mg/mL oral solution

Vibativ (Telavancin)

Class: Glycopeptide antibiotic

Form: IV infusion

Formulations: 250 mg, 750 mg

Dose: 10 mg/kg IV over 60 minutes once every 24 hours for 7–14 days

Mechanism of action: Medication inhibits bacterial cell-wall synthesis.

FDA-approved indication: Complicated infection of skin or subcutaneous tissue

Adverse reactions: Nausea, taste disturbances, vomiting, abnormal urine, QT prolongation, increase in serum creatinine, risk of fetal malformation (boxed warning)

Drug interactions: Increased risk of QTc prolongation in drugs known to prolong the QTc interval

Monitoring parameters: Serum pregnancy test (before initiation of therapy), CBC, renal function test

Patient counseling: Women should use effective contraception while taking this medication.

Xerese (Acyclovir and Hydrocortisone)

Note: Initially FDA-approved as Lipsovir

Class: Antiviral

Form: Topical cream

Formulations: 1%, 5%

Dose: Apply topically at first signs and symptoms of herpes to the affected areas on lips or around the mouth five times daily for 5 days.

Mechanism of action: Acyclovir inhibits herpes simplex viral DNA replication; hydrocortisone is an anti-inflammatory.

FDA-approved indication: Early treatment of recurrent herpes labialis (cold sores) to reduce the likelihood of ulcerative cold sores and to shorten the lesion healing time

Adverse reactions: Application-site reactions, including pigment changes, dry skin, and erythema

Drug interactions: None known

Monitoring parameters: Signs and symptoms of cold sores

Patient counseling: Do not use in the eyes, mouth, or nose or on the genital area. Apply a thin layer to the affected area, but do not rub the cream into the cold sore or cover the area with a bandage. Do not wet the area for 30 minutes after application. Use the medication as instructed even if you are feeling better.

Xifaxan (Rifaximin)

New indication: Reduction of risk of overt hepatic encephalopathy recurrence in patients older than 18 years of age

Zirgan (Ganciclovir)

New form: Ophthalmic gel

New indication: Herpes simplex keratitis

38-23. Chapter 31: Human Immunodeficiency Virus and the Acquired Immune Deficiency Syndrome

Epzicom (Abacavir Sulfate and Lamivudine) and Trizivir (Abacavir Sulfate, Lamivudine, and Zidovudine)

Boxed warning (updated): High risk of hypersensitivity exists in patients who carry the HLA-B*5701 allele. All patients should be screened for the HLA-B*5701 allele. Regardless of status, abacavir-containing products should be discontinued and not reintroduced in patients who experience an allergic reaction. See www.fda.gov/Drugs/DrugSafety/DrugSafetyNewsletter/ucm110235.htm#AbacavirMarketedasZiagenandAbacavir-CombinationProductsMarketedasTrizivirandEpzicom:HypersensitivityReactionHLA-B5701andSkinPatchTesting.

Intelence (Etravirine)

Class: Non-nucleoside reverse transcriptase inhibitor (NNRTI)

Form: Tablets

Formulation: 100 mg

Dose: 200 mg orally twice daily following a meal

FDA-approved indication: Treatment of HIV-1 in treatment-experienced adult patients with viral stains resistant to an NNRTI and other antiretroviral agents

Adverse reactions: Rash, peripheral neuropathy, Stevens–Johnson Syndrome, toxic epidermal necrolysis, hypersensitivity characterized by hepatic failure, fat redistribution, immune reconstitution syndrome

Drug interactions: Tipranavir–ritonavir; fosamprenavir–ritonavir; atazanavir–ritonavir; protease inhibitors administered without ritonavir; NNRTIs; inhibitors and inducers of CYP3A, CYP2C9, CYP2C19, and substrates of CYP3A, CYP2C9, CYP2C19, and Pgp

Monitoring parameters: Liver function tests, viral load, CD4 count, viral resistance, signs and symptoms of severe skin reactions or hypersensitivity reactions

Patient counseling: Contact health care professional if rash develops. Take after a meal.

Lamivudine and Stavudine

New dosage forms: 150 mg lamivudine and 30 mg stavudine; 150 mg lamivudine and 40 mg stavudine

Nevirapine

New dosage form: 50 mg tablets for oral suspension

Norvir (Ritonavir)

New dosage form: 100 mg tablets

Reyataz (Atazanavir Sulfate)

New labeling revision: Labeling update to include 96-week data for previously untreated HIV-1 infected adult patients

Stavudine/Lamivudine/Nevirapine

New formulation: 30 mg/150 mg/200 mg; 40 mg/150 mg/200 mg

38-24. Chapter 32: Immunization

Agriflu (Influenza Virus Vaccine, Inactivated)

Class: Viral vaccine

Form: Intramuscular injection

Formulation: 0.5 mL single-dose prefilled syringe

Dose: 0.5 mL

FDA-approved indication: Influenza prophylaxis in adults 18 years of age and older against influenza subtypes A and B

Adverse reactions: Injection-site pain, headache, myalgia, malaise

Drug interactions: Immunosuppressive therapy may reduce efficacy.

Patient counseling: Do not take the vaccine if you have a history of allergy to any of the components of the vaccine, including eggs, kanamycin, or neomycin.

BioThrax (Anthrax Vaccine Adsorbed)

Labeling revision approved: Shelf life of BioThrax extended to 4 years.

Cervarix (Human Papillomavirus Bivalent [Types 16 and 18] Vaccine, Recombinant)

Class: Viral vaccine

Form: Intramuscular injection

Formulations: Single-dose vials (0.5 mL) and prefilled TIP-LOK syringes

Dose: Cervical cancer prophylaxis (10–25 years of age) 0.5 mL IM for three doses at 0, 1, and 6 months

Mechanism of action: Vaccine promotes development of immunoglobulin G–neutralizing antibodies against human papillomavirus (HPV) L1 capsid proteins.

FDA-approved indication: HPV prophylaxis

Adverse reactions: Injection-site reactions, GI symptoms, arthralgia, myalgias, headache, fatigue, syncope, hypersensitivity reaction, angioedema

Drug interactions: Immunosuppressive therapy may reduce efficacy.

Monitoring parameters: Monitor for syncope, tonic-clonic movement, or other seizure-like activity for 15 minutes after administration of vaccine.

Patient counseling: The prefilled syringes contain latex, which may cause allergic reaction if you have latex allergy. The vaccine is not recommended if you are pregnant or are planning to become pregnant during the vaccine course.

Fluarix (Influenza Virus Vaccine, Inactivated)

New indication: Vaccine for the prevention of influenza subtypes A and B in patients 3 years of age and older

Fluzone (Influenza Virus Vaccine, Inactivated)

New formulation: High-dose (180 mcg/0.5 mL) seasonal influenza vaccine intended for people 65 years of age and older

Gardasil (HPV Quadrivalent [Types 6, 11, 16, and 18] Vaccine, Recombinant)

New indication: Use in boys and young men

Hiberix (*Haemophilus influenzae* Type b Conjugate Vaccine [Tetanus Toxoid Conjugate])

Class: Vaccine

Form: Intramuscular injection

Formulation: 10 mcg

Dose: 0.5 mL intramuscular for one to three doses, depending on age

Mechanism of action: The vaccine (meningococcal protein conjugate) is designed to produce antibodies to capsular polyribosylribitol phosphate, which is a component of encapsulated *Haemophilus influenzae* type b.

FDA-approved indication: Active immunization for the prevention of invasive disease caused by *Haemophilus influenzae* type b

Adverse reactions: Injection-site reactions, restlessness, fever

Drug interactions: Do not mix with any other vaccine in the same syringe or vial.

Monitoring parameters: None recommended

Patient counseling: Contact your health care professional immediately if any of the following occur: itching or hives; swelling in the face, hands, or mouth; trouble breathing; fever over 103° F.

Influenza A (H1N1) 2009 Monovalent Vaccine (H1N1 Influenza Virus Vaccine)

Class: Vaccine

Form: Intramuscular injection

Formulation: 15 mcg/0.5 mL

Dose: 0.5 mL single dose injected in deltoid muscle

Mechanism of action: Vaccine induces immunity by forming antibiotics specific to the influenza virus strain.

FDA-approved indication: Active immunization of people 6 months of age and older against influenza disease caused by pandemic (H1N1) 2009 virus

Adverse reactions: Injection-site pain, nausea, myalgia, headache, malaise

Drug interactions: Do not mix with other vaccines in the same syringe or vial. Immunosuppressive agents may reduce the immune response.

Monitoring parameters: No specific monitoring has been determined.

Patient counseling: This vaccine contains killed virus and cannot cause influenza.

38-25. Chapter 33: Pediatrics

Abilify (Aripiprazole)

New indication: Treatment of irritability associated with autistic disorder in pediatric patients (ages 6–17 years)

Cayston (Aztreonam)

New dosage form: 75 mg/mL solution for inhalation

Intuniv (Guanfacine)

Note: Intuniv was formerly marketed as Connexyn.

Form: Extended-release tablets

New indication: Treatment of attention-deficit hyperactivity disorder

Vyvanse (Lisdexamfetamine Dimesylate)

Labeling revision: Includes 13-hour postdose efficacy data for pediatric patients (ages 6–12 years)

Xyzal (Levocetirizine)

New indication: Children 6 months of age and older for the relief of perennial allergic rhinitis and chronic idiopathic urticaria

38-26. Chapter 34: Geriatrics and Gerontology

Azilect (Rasagiline Mesylate)

New labeling revision: Reduced medication and tyramine-containing food restrictions

Gelnique (Oxybutynin Chloride) 10% Gel

New formulation: 1 g unit dose (1.14 mL) 100mg/g oxybutynin chloride gel

Jalyn (Dutasteride and Tamsulosin)

New formulation: 0.5 mg dutasteride and 0.4 mg tamsulosin

Mirapex ER (Pramipexole Dihydrochloride)

New dosage form: Extended-release tablets: 0.375 mg, 0.75 mg, 1.5 mg, 3 mg, 4.5 mg

Namenda XR (Memantine Hydrochloride)

New dosage form: Extended-release capsules: 7 mg, 14 mg, 21 mg, 28 mg

Staxyn (Vardenafil Hydrochloride)

New dosage form: 10 mg oral disintegrating tablets

38-27. Chapter 36: Anemias

Exjade (Deferasirox)

Boxed warning: Renal impairment and failure, hepatic impairment and failure, and GI hemorrhage may occur; all may be fatal. Reactions were more frequently observed in patients with advanced age, myelodysplastic syndromes, previous renal or hepatic impairment, or low platelet counts. See www.fda.gov/Safety/MedWatch/SafetyInformation/SafetyAlertsfor HumanMedicalProducts/ucm200850.htm.

Parenteral Iron Dextran Products

Parenteral iron dextran products include the following:

- DexFerrum (iron dextran) injection
- INFeD (iron dextran) injection

Boxed warning: Anaphylactic-type reactions, including fatal cases, may occur following administration. See www.fda.gov/Safety/MedWatch/Safety Information/ucm181751.htm and www.fda.gov/Safety/MedWatch/SafetyInformation/ucm181990.htm.

Wilate (Von Willebrand Factor/Coagulation Factor VIII Complex [Human])

Class: Antihemophilic agent

Form: IV injection

Formulations: 450 IU von Willebrand factor ristocetin cofactor (VWF:RCo) and 450 IU factor VIII activities in 5 mL, 900 IU VWF:RCo and 900 IU factor VIII activities in 10 mL

Dose: Dosing may need to be modified depending on the location and the severity of the bleed:

- Minor hemorrhage:
  - Loading dose of 20–40 IU/kg
  - Maintenance dose of 20–30 IU/kg every 12–24 hours for up to 3 days
- Major hemorrhage:
  - Loading dose of 40–60 IU/kg
  - Maintenance dose of 20–40 IU/kg every 12–24 hours for up to 5–7 days

Mechanism of action: Medication corrects the low factor VIII levels in the patient and promotes adherence of the platelets to the endothelium at the site of injury.

FDA-approved indication: Treatment of spontaneous and trauma-induced bleeding episodes in patients with severe von Willebrand disease

Adverse reactions: Hypersensitivity, thromboembolic events, urticaria, dizziness

Drug interactions: None known

Monitoring parameters: Bleeding, CBC, plasma levels of VWF:RCo and coagulation factor VIII complex activities

Patient counseling: A risk exists for transmitting infectious agents through blood products. Monitoring is required when using this agent. Counsel patients on symptoms of hypersensitivity reactions.

38-28. Chapter 37: Thromboembolic Disease

Low-Molecular-Weight Heparins

Low-molecular-weight heparins include the following:

- Arixtra (fondaparinux sodium) injection
- Fragmin (dalteparin sodium) injection
- Innohep (tinzaparin sodium) injection
- Lovenox (enoxaparin sodium) injection

Boxed warning: Epidural or spinal hematomas in patients receiving neuraxial anesthesia or undergoing spinal puncture may result in long-term or permanent paralysis. See www.fda.gov/Safety/MedWatch/Safety Information/ucm196983.htm.

Plavix (Clopidogrel)

Boxed warning: Effectiveness is decreased in patients who are poor metabolizers of clopidogrel. Tests are available to identify genetic differences in CYP2C19 genotype function, an indicator for poor metabolizers. In poor metabolizers, alternate treatments or dosing should be used.

38-29. Other Changes

Carpine (Pilocarpine Hydrochloride)

New formulation: 1%, 2%, and 4% ophthalmic solutions

MembraneBlue 0.15% (Trypan Blue Ophthalmic Solution)

Class: Ophthalmic surgical dye

Dosage Form: Solution

Formulation: Trypan blue ophthalmic solution in a volume of 0.5 mL

Dose: Inject into vitreous cavity and remove excess.

Mechanism of action: Selectively stains membranes in the human eye

FDA-approved indication: Medication is used as an aid in ophthalmic surgery to stain epiretinal membranes that are being removed.

Adverse reactions: Staining or discoloration of intraocular lenses

Drug interactions: None known

Monitoring parameters: None known

Patient counseling: Only professionals may administer this drug; it is not for patient use.

Ozurdex (Dexamethasone)

Class: Corticosteroids

Form: Ophthalmic intravitreal injection

Formulation: Dexamethasone 0.7 mg in the Novadur solid polymer drug-delivery system

Dose: Refer to prescribing information; the intravitreal injection procedure should be carried out under controlled aseptic conditions.

Mechanism of action: Medication suppresses inflammation by inhibiting multiple inflammatory cytokines, resulting in decreased edema, fibrin deposition, capillary leakage, and migration of inflammatory cells.

FDA-approved indication: Treatment of macular edema following branch retinal vein occlusion or central retinal vein occlusion

Adverse reactions: Increased intraocular pressure and conjunctival hemorrhage, especially in patients taking steroids

Drug interactions: None known

Monitoring parameters: The following should be monitored:

- *Pulmonary sarcoidosis:* Spirometry tests at onset, during treatment, and after stopping treatment for up to 2 years
- *Intravitreal injection-related effects:* Intraocular pressure routinely with prolonged ophthalmic use
- *Perfusion of optic nerve head immediately after administration:* Tonometry within 30 minutes and biomicroscopy between 2 and 7 days following administration

Patient counseling: If the eye becomes red, sensitive to light, painful, or develops a change in vision, seek immediate care from an ophthalmologist. You may experience temporary visual blurring after receiving an intravitreal injection. Do not drive or use machines until this condition has resolved.

Appendixes

Katie J. Suda, PharmD, MS
Anne M. Hurley, PharmD

Appendix A

Normal Laboratory Values

Test	Conventional units	SI units
Albumin	3.5–5 g/dL	35–50 g/L
Alkaline phosphatase		
Adults	30–120 units/L	0.5–2 nkat/L
Children	< 350 units/L	< 350 units/L
Adolescent males	< 500 units/L	< 500 units/L
Adolescent females	25–100 units/L	25–100 units/L
Amylase	0.58–1.97 mckat/L	35–118 IU/L
Anion gap	7–16 mEq/L	7–16 mmol/L
Arterial blood gases (ABG)		
HCO_3	21–28 mEq/L	21–28 mmol/L
O_2 saturation	94–100%	0.94–1
pH	7.35–7.45	7.35–7.45
P_{O_2}	80–105 mmHg	10.6–14 kPa
P_{CO_2}	35–45 mmHg	4.7–6 kPa
Basal metabolic panel (BMP)		
Bicarbonate	22–29 mEq/L	22–29 mmol/L
Blood urea nitrogen (BUN)		
Adults	8–25 mg/dL	2.9–8.9 mmol/L
Children	5–18 mg/dL	1.8–6.4 mmol/L
Chloride	97–110 mEq/L	97–110 mmol/L
Creatinine		
Males	0.7–1.3 mg/dL	62–115 µmol/L
Females	0.6–1.1 mg/dL	53–97 µmol/L
Glucose (fasting, plasma)	65–109 mg/dL	3.6–6 mmol/L
Potassium	3.5–5 mEq/L	3.5–5 mmol/L
Sodium	136–145 mEq/L	136–145 mmol/L

(continued)

Test	Conventional units	SI units
Blood pressure (mm Hg)		
Normal	< 120/< 80	< 120/< 80
Prehypertension	120–139/80–89	120–139/80–89
Hypertension		
Stage 1	140–159/90–99	140–159/90–99
Stage 2	≥ 160/100	≥ 160/100
Hypertensive crisis	> 180/> 120	> 180/> 120
Isolated systolic	> 140/< 90	> 140/< 90
Calcitonin	< 100 pg/mL	< 100 ng/L
Calcium	8.6–10.3 mg/dL	2.15–2.58 mmol/L
Carbon dioxide	21–30 mEq/L	21–30 mmol/L
Coagulation screen		
Activated partial thromboplastin time (aPTT)	22–37 seconds	22–37 seconds
Antithrombin III (antigenic)	22–39 mg/dL	220–390 mg/L
Antithrombin III (functional)	80–130%	0.8–1.3 units/L
Bleeding time	3–9.5 min	180–570 seconds
Protein C	0.7–1.4 µ/mL	700–1,400 units/mL
Protein S	0.7–1.4 µ/mL	700–1,400 units/mL
Prothrombin time (PT)	10–13 seconds	10–13 seconds
Complete blood count (CBC)		
Hemoglobin (Hb)		
Males	13.8–17.5 g/dL	138–175 g/L
Females	12.1–15.3 g/dL	121–153 g/L
Hematocrit (Hct)		
Males	40.7–50.3%	0.407–0.503
Females	36–46%	0.36–0.46
Mean corpuscular volume (MCV)	80–100 mcm^3	80–100 fL
Mean corpuscular hemoglobin (MCH)	27–33 pg/cell	1.66–2.09 fmol/cell
Mean corpuscular hemoglobin concentrate (MCHC)	33–36 g/dL	20.3–22 mmol/L
Platelet count	150–350 × 10^3/mm^3	150–350 × 10^9/L
Red blood cells (RBC)		
Males	4.5–5.9 × 10^6/mm^3	4.5–5.9 × 10^{12}/L
Females	4–5.2 × 10^6/mm^3	4-5–2 × 10^{12}/L
White blood cells (WBC)	4.5–11 × 10^3 cells/mm^3	4.5–11 × 10^9 cells/L
White blood cell differential		
Basophils	0–0.19 × 10^3 cells/microL	0–0.19 × 10^9 cells/L
Eosinophils	0–0.45 × 10^3 cells/microL	0–0.45 × 10^9 cells/L
Lymphocytes	1.5–4 × 10^3 cells/microL	1.5–4 × 10^9 cells/L
Monocytes	0.2–0.95 × 10^3 cells/microL	0.2–0.95 × 10^9 cells/L
Neutrophils (absolute)	1.8–7.7 × 10^3 cells/microL	1.8–7.7 × 10^9 cells/L
Corticotropin (ACTH) 08:00h	< 60 pg/mL	< 13.2 pmol/L
Cortisol 08:00h	5–30 mcg/dL	138–810 nmol/L

Test	Conventional units	SI units
Creatinine kinase		
Males	30–220 IU/L	0.5–3.67 mckat/L
Females	20–170 IU/L	0.33–2.83 mckat/L
Glucose tolerance test		
Baseline fasting blood glucose	70–105 mg/dL	3.9–5.8 mmol/L
60-minute fasting blood glucose	120–170 mg/dL	6.7–9.4 mmol/L
90-minute fasting blood glucose	100–140 mg/dL	5.6–7.8 mmol/L
120-minute fasting blood glucose	70–120 mg/dL	3.9–6.7 mmol/L
Hematologic tests		
Erythrocyte sedimentation rate (ESR)		
Adult males	0–17 mm/h	0–17 mm/h
Adult females	1–25 mm/h	1–25 mm/h
Children	0–10 mm/h	0–10 mm/h
Ferritin		
Males	30–300 ng/mL	30–300 mcg/L
Females	10–200 ng/mL	10–200 mcg/L
Fibrinogen	150–400 mg/dL	1.5–4 g/L
Hemoglobin A1c	5.3–7.5%	0.053–0.075
Iron		
Males	45–160 mcg/dL	8.1–31.3 mcmol/L
Females	30–160 mcg/dL	5.4–31.3 mcmol/L
Reticulocytes	0.5–1.5%	0.005–0.015
Total iron binding capacity (TIBC)	220–420 mcg/dL	39.4–75.2 mcmol/L
Transferrin saturation		
Males	20–50%	0.20–0.50
Females	15–50%	0.15–0.5
Vitamin B_{12}	223–1,132 pg/mL	165–835 pmol/L
Isoenzymes		
Creatine phosphokinase (MB)	0–7 IU/L	0–0.12 μkat/L
Lipase	10–150 units/L	10–150 units/L
Lipids		
Total cholesterol		
Desirable	< 200 mg/dL	< 5.2 mmol/L
Borderline-high	200–239 mg/dL	< 5.2–6.2 mmol/L
High	> 239 mg/dL	> 6.2 mmol/L
Low-density lipoprotein (LDL)		
Desirable	< 130 mg/dL	< 3.36 mmol/L
Borderline-high	130–159 mg/dL	3.36–4.11 mmol/L
High	> 159 mg/dL	> 4.11 mmol/L
High-density lipoprotein (HDL)		
Low	< 40 mg/dL	< 1.03 mmol/L
Desirable	> 60 mg/dL	≥ 1.55 mmol/L

(continued)

Test	Conventional units	SI units
Triglycerides		
Desirable	< 150 mg/dL	< 1.7 mmol/L
Borderline-high	150–199 mg/dL	1.7–2.25 mmol/L
High	200–499 mg/dL	2.26–5.64 mmol/L
Very high	> 500 mg/dL	> 5.65 mmol/L
Liver function tests (LFTs)		
Alanine aminotransferase (ALT, SGPT)	7–53 IU/L	0.12–0.88 mckat/L
Ammonia (NH4+)	15–45 µg/dL	11–32 µmol/L
Aspartate aminotransferase (AST, SGOT)	11–47 IU/L	0.18–0.78 mckat/L
Bilirubin (adults) (F)		
Conjugated	≤ 0.2 mg/dL	≤ 4 mcmol/L
Total	0.1–1 mg/dL	2–18 mcmol/L
Lactate dehydrogenase (LDH)	100–250 IU/L	1.67–4.17 mckat/L
Magnesium	1.3–2.2 mEq/L	0.65–1.1 mmol/L
Phosphate	2.5–5 mg/dL	0.8–1.6 mmol/L
Prolactin		
Males	0–15 ng/mL	0–15 mcg/L
Females	0–20 ng/mL	0–20 mcg/L
Protein, total	5.5–8 g/dL	55–80 g/L
Thyroid hormone function tests		
Free thyroxine (Free T_4)	0.8–2.7 ng/dL	10–35 pmol/L
Thyroid-stimulating hormone (TSH)	0.35–6.2 mcU/mL	0.35–6.2 mU/L
Thyroxine-binding globulin capacity	10–26 mcg/dL	100–260 mcg/L
Total triiodothyronine (T_3)	60–181 ng/dL	0.92–2.78 nmol/L
Total thyroxine by RIA (T_4)	4.5–10.9 mcg/dL	58–140 nmol/L
Uric acid	3–8 mg/dL	179–476 mcmol/L

References

Dipiro JT, Talbert RL, Yee GC, et al., eds. *Pharmacotherapy: A Pathophysiologic Approach*. 7th ed. New York: McGraw-Hill; 2008.

Facts and Comparisons 4.0. St. Louis, Mo.: Wolters Kluwer Health. Available at: www.factsand comparisons.com. Updated periodically.

Micromedex Healthcare Series. Greenwood Village, Colo.: Thomson Healthcare. Available at: www.thomsonhc.com. Updated periodically.

Appendix B

Drugs in Renal Failure

			Dose adjustment for renal failure			
Generic name	Trade name	Dose for normal renal function	CrCl > 50 mL/min	CrCl = 10–50 mL/min	CrCl < 10 mL/min	Supplement for hemodialysis
Analgesics						
Acetaminophen	FeverAll, Genapap, Tylenol	650 mg po q4h	q4h	q6h	q8h	None
Aspirin	Ascriptin, Aspergum, Aspirtab, Bayer, Easprin, Ecotrin, Ecpirin, Entercote	650 mg po q4h	q4h	q4–6h	Avoid	Dose after dialysis
Butorphanol		2 mg q3–4h	Same	75% of normal dose	50% of normal dose	No data
Codeine		30–60 mg po q4–6h	Same	75% of normal dose	50% of normal dose	No data
Fentanyl	Sublimaze	Anesthetic induction (individualized)	Same	75% of normal dose	50% of normal dose	Not applicable
Hydromorphone	Dilaudid	1–2 mg IV q4–6h	Same	Same	Same	Same
Meperidine	Demerol	50–100 mg IV or po q3–4h	Same	37.5–75 mg IV or po q3–4h	25–50 mg IV or po q3–4h	Avoid
Methadone		2.5–10 mg q6–8h	Same	Same	50–75% of normal dose	Same
Morphine		20–25 mg po q4h	Same	15–18.75 mg po q4h	10–12.5 mg po q4h	Same
Pentazocine		50 mg q4h	Same	75% of normal dose	50% of normal dose	Same
Propoxyphene	Darvon	65 mg po q6–8h	Same	Same	Avoid	Avoid
Antiarrhythmics						
N-acetyl-procainamide		500 mg q6–8h	Same	50% q8–12h	25% q12–18h	Same
Adenosine	Adenocard	3–6 mg IV bolus	Same	Same	Same	Same
Atropine		0.5–1 mg IV push q3–5 min, max 0.04 mg/kg	Same	Same	Same	Same
Class I						
Moricizine	Ethmozine	200–300 mg po q8h	Same	Same	Same	Same
Propafenone	Rythmol	150–300 mg po q8h	Same	Same	Same	Same

(continued)

Generic name	Trade name	Dose for normal renal function	Dose adjustment for renal failure			Supplement for hemodialysis
			CrCl > 50 mL/min	CrCl = 10–50 mL/min	CrCl < 10 mL/min	
Class Ia						
Disopyramide	Norpace	100–200 mg q6h	100–200 mg q8h	100–200 mg q12–24h	100–200 mg q24–48h	Same
Procainamide	Procan, Pronestyl	1,000–2,500 mg q12h	1,000–2,500 mg q4h	1,000–2,500 mg q6–12h	1,000–2,500 mg q8–24h	Maintenance dose post-HD
Quinidine	Quinidex, Quinaglute	300–600 mg po q8–12h	Same	Same	150–300 mg po q4–6h	Dose post-HD
Class Ib						
Lidocaine	Xylocaine	50–100 mg IV over 1–2 min bolus, then 1–4 mg/min IV	Same	Same	Same	Same
Mexiletine	Mexitil	200–400 mg po q8–12h	Same	Same	Same	Same
Tocainide	Tonocard	400–600 mg po q8h	Same	Same	Same	Dose post-HD
Class Ic						
Encainide	Enkaid	25–50 mg po q8–12h	25–50 mg po q12–24h	25 mg po q24h	25 mg po q24h	Same
Flecainide	Tambocor	50–100 mg po q12h	Same	25–50 mg po q12h	25–50 mg po q12h	Same
Class II (see β-blockers in antihypertensives)						
Class III						
Amiodarone	Cordarone	800–2,000 mg load, then 200–600 mg q24h	Same	Same	Same	Same
Bretylium	Bretyol	5–30mg/kg load, then 5–10 mg IV q6h	Same	25–50% of normal dose	25% of normal dose	Same
Class IV (see calcium channel blockers in antihypertensives)						

Antibiotics

Aminoglycosides

Drug	Trade					Post-HD
Amikacin	Amikin	7.5 mg/kg IV q12h	60–90% of normal dose q12h	30–70% of normal dose q12–18h	20–30% of normal dose q24–48h	50% of full dose post-HD
Gentamicin	Garamycin	1.7 mg/kg q8h	1.7 mg/kg q8–24h	1.7 mg/kg q12–48h by levels	1.7 mg/kg IV q48–72h by levels	50% of full dose post-HD
Tobramycin	Nebcin	1.7 mg/kg q8h	1.7 mg/kg q8–24h	1.7 mg/kg q24–48h by levels	1.7 mg/kg IV q48–72h by levels	50% of full dose post-HD

Cephalosporins

Drug	Trade					Post-HD
Cefaclor	Ceclor	250–500 mg po q8h	Same	Same	Same	250–500 mg po post-HD
Cefadroxil	Duricef	0.5–1 g po q12h	500 mg po q12h	500 mg po q12–24h	500 mg po q24–48h	0.5–1 g po post-HD
Cefazolin	Ancef, Kexol	0.25–2g q6h	0.25–2g q8h	0.25–2g q12h	50% of normal dose q24–48h	15–20 mg/kg post-HD
Cefepime	Maxipime	250–2,000 mg q8–12h	Same	125–2,000 mg q24h	25–50% of normal dose q24h	25–50% of normal dose q24h post-HD
Cefixime	Suprax	200 mg po q12h	150–200 mg po q12h	150 mg po q12h	100 mg po q12h	300 mg po post-HD
Cefotaxime	Claforan	1–2 g IV q6–12h	Same	1–2 g IV q8–12h	1–2 g IV q24h	0.5–2 g IV q24h post-HD
Cefotetan	Cefotan	1–2 g IV q12h	Same	50% of normal dose	25% of normal dose	1g post-HD
Cefoxitin	Mefoxin	1–2 g IV q6–8h	1–2 g IV q8–12h	1–2 g IV q24–48h	1–2 g IV q24–48h	1g post-HD
Cefpodoxime	Vantin	100–400 mg q12h	Same	Same	100–400 mg q24h	Dose post-HD
Cefprozil	Cefzil	250–500 mg po q12h	Same	50% q12h	50% q12h	250 mg po post-HD
Ceftazidime	Ceptaz, Fortaz, Tazicef, Tazidime	1 g IV q8–12h	1 g IV q12h	0.5–1 g IV q12–24h	500 mg q24–48h	1g post-HD
Ceftizoxime	Cefizox	1–2 g IV q8h	0.5–1.5 g q8h	0.25–1 g q12h	0.5–1 g q24–48h	1 g post-HD
Ceftriaxone	Rocephin	0.25–2 g IV q12–24h	Same	Same	Same	Same
Cefuroxime	Ceftin, Kefurox, Zinacef	250–500 mg q12h	Same	Same	Same	Dose post-HD
Cephalexin	Keflex	250–500 mg po q6h	250–500 mg po q6–8h	250–500 mg po q12h	250–500 mg po q12h	Dose post-HD

(continued)

Generic name	Trade name	Dose for normal renal function	Dose adjustment for renal failure			Supplement for hemodialysis
			CrCl > 50 mL/min	CrCl = 10–50 mL/min	CrCl < 10 mL/min	
Fluoroquinolones						
Ciprofloxacin	Cipro	500–750 mg po q12h; 400 mg IV q12h	Same	250–500 mg po q18h; 400 mg IV q24h	250–500 mg po q18h; 400 mg IV q24h	250 mg q12h (200 mg if IV)
Gatifloxacin	Tequin	400 mg po or IV q24h	Same	400 mg po or IV × 1, then 200 mg po or IV q24h	400 mg IV or po × 1, then 200 mg po or IV q24h	400 mg po or IV × 1, then 200 mg po or IV q24h post-HD
Levofloxacin	Levaquin	250–500 mg po or IV q24h	Same	500 mg po or IV × 1, then 250 mg po or IV q48h	500 mg po or IV × 1, then 250 mg po or IV q48h	500 mg po or IV × 1, then 250 mg po or IV q48h post-HD
Miscellaneous						
Aztreonam	Azactam	500 mg–2 g q8–12h	Same	250 mg–1 g q8–12h	125–500 mg q8–12h	1–2 g IV loading dose, then 0.5 g IV q6–8h post-HD
Erythromycin	E-Mycin	250–500 mg po q6h	Same	Same	Same	Same
Imipenem	Primaxin	0.25–1 g IV q6h	Same	500 mg IV q12h	250 mg IV q12h	250 mg IV q12h post-HD
Linezolid	Zyvox	600 mg IV q12h	Same	Same	Same	Dose post-HD
Meropenem	Merrem	1–2 g IV q8h	Same	50–100% normal dose q12h	50% normal dose q24h	500 mg IV q24h post-HD
Quinupristin-dalfopristin	Synercid	7.5 mg/kg IV q8h	Same	Same	Same	Same
Rifampin	Rifadin	600 mg po q24h	Same	300–600 mg po q24–48h	300–600 mg po q48h	Same
Trimethoprim-sulfamethoxazole	Bactrim, Septra	8–20 mg/kg/d po q6–12h or IV q12h	Same	4–10 mg/kg/d po or IV q12h	Avoid	2–5 mg/kg/d po or IV q24h post-HD
Vancomycin	Vancocin	500 mg IV q6h or 1 g q12h	1 g IV q12–24h	1 g IV q24–96h	1 g IV q4–7d	1 g IV q4–7d

Penicillins

Drug	Brand					
Amoxicillin-clavulanic acid	Augmentin	250–500 mg po q8h; 875 mg po bid	Same	250–500 mg po q12h	250–500 mg po q24h	250–500 mg po q24h; supplemental dose during and at the end of dialysis
Ampicillin	Principen, Omnipen	250–500 mg q6h	250–500 mg q6h	250–500 mg q6–12h	250–500 mg q12–24h	dose post-HD
Ampicillin-sulbactam	Unasyn	1.5–3 g q6h	1.5–3 g q8h	1.5–3 g q12h	1.5–3 g q24h	dose post-HD
Methicillin	Staphcillin	1–2 g IV q4–6h	Same	1–2 g IV q6–8h	1–2 g IV q8–12h	Same
Nafcillin	Nafcin, Unipen	1–2 g IV q4–6h	Same	Same	Same	Same
Oxacillin	Bactocil	1–2 g IV q4–6h	Same	Same	Same	Same
Penicillin G		1–4 million units IV q4–6h	1–4 million units IV q6–8h	1–4 million units IV q8–12h	1–4 million units IV q12–18h	1–4 million units IV q12–18h
Piperacillin	Pipracil	3–4 g IV q6h	Same	3–4 g IV q6–8h	3–4 g IV q8h	2 g IV q8h plus 1 g post-HD
Piperacillin-tazobactam	Zosyn	3.375–4.5 g IV q6–8h	3.375 g	2.25 g IV q6h (q8h if CrCl < 20 mL/min)	2.25 g q8h	2.25 g IV q8h post-HD
Ticarcillin	Ticar	3 g IV q4h	1–2 g IV q4–8h	1–2 g IV q8h	1–2 g IV q12h	2 g IV q12h; 3 g supplement post-HD
Ticarcillin-clavulanic acid	Timentin	3.1 g IV q4h	2 g IV q4h or 3.1 g IV q4–8h	2 g IV q4–8h	2 g IV q12h	2 g IV q12h post-HD

Anticoagulants

Drug	Brand					
Enoxaparin	Lovenox	30 mg SC q12h	Same	30 mg SC qd	30 mg SC qd	Limited data
		40 mg SC qd	Same	30 mg SC qd	30 mg SC qd	
		1 mg/kg SC q12h	Same	1 mg/kg SC qd	1 mg/kg SC qd	

Anticonvulsants

Drug	Brand					
Carbamazepine	Tegretol	200 mg po bid; second dose: 1,200 mg po q24h	Same	Same	Same	75% of normal dose
Diazepam	Valium	2–10 mg po q6–24h	Same	Same	Same	Same
Ethosuximide	Zarontin	500–1,500 mg po q24h	Same	Same	75% of normal dose	Same
Gabapentin	Neurontin	300–600 mg po tid	400 mg po tid	300 mg po q12–24h	300 mg po qod	300 mg load, then 200–300 mg post-HD

(continued)

Generic name	Trade name	Dose for normal renal function	Dose adjustment for renal failure			Supplement for hemodialysis
			CrCl > 50 mL/min	CrCl = 10–50 mL/min	CrCl < 10 mL/min	
Lamotrigine	Lamictal	50 mg po q12–24h initially, then 100–500 mg po q24h	Same	75% of normal dose	100 mg qod	100 mg postdialysis
Lorazepam	Ativan	1–2 mg q8–12h	Same	Same	Same	Same
Oxcarbazepine	Trileptal	300–600 mg bid	Same	75–100% of normal dose	50% of normal dose	50% of normal dose post-HD
Phenobarbital	Luminal, Solfoton	50–100 mg q8–12h	Same	Same	50–100 mg q12–16h	Dosage supplementation is required post-HD
Phenytoin	Dilantin	100 mg tid	Same	Same	Same	Same
Primidone	Mysoline	250 mg tid or qid	250 mg q8h	250 mg q8–12h	250 mg q12–24h	30% of normal dose post-HD
Sodium valproate	Depakene, Depakote	15–60 mg/kg q24h	Same	Same	Same	No dose adjustment necessary
Topiramate	Topamax	200 mg po q12h	Same	50% of normal dose	25% of normal dose	Same
Antiemetics						
Metoclopramide	Reglan	10–15 mg IV qid	Same	7.5–15 mg IV q6h	5–7.5 mg IV q6h	Same
Antifungals						
Amphotericin B nonlipid	Fungizone	0.25–1 mg/kg IV q24h	Same	Same	0.25–1 mg/kg IV q24–36h	Same
Amphotericin B lipid complex	Abelcet	5 mg/kg IV q24h	Consider dosage adjustment; specific guidelines not available	Consider dosage adjustment; specific guidelines not available	Consider dosage adjustment; specific guidelines not available	Supplemental dose is not necessary
Amphotericin B cholesteryl sulfate complex	Amphotec	3–6 mg/kg/d IV q24h	Same	Same	3–6 mg/kg/d IV q48h	3–6 mg/kg/d IV q48h
Amphotericin B liposome	AmBisome	3–5 mg/kg IV q24h	Same	Same	3–5 mg/kg IV q48h	3–5 mg/kg IV q48h

Appendixes **865**

Drug	Brand	Normal dose				Post-HD
Fluconazole	Diflucan	100–400 mg po or IV q24h	Same	50–200 mg po or IV q24h	50–200 mg po or IV q24h	Same
Itraconazole	Sponanox	100–200 mg po or IV q12h	Same	Same	100–200 mg po q24h (IV contraindicated)	100 mg po q12–24h (oral only)
Ketoconazole	Nizoral	200–400 mg po q24h	Same	Same	Same	Same
Antihistamines						
Cimetidine	Tagamet	400 mg po bid or 400–800 mg qhs	Same	200 mg po bid	300 mg q8–12h	Dose post-HD
Famotidine	Pepcid	20–40 mg po qhs	5–20 mg po qhs	2–10 mg po qhs	2–4 mg po qhs	Supplemental doses are not required post-HD
Nizatidine	Axid	150 mg po q12h or 300 mg po qhs	150 mg po q24h	150 mg po q24–48h	150 mg po q48–72h	150 mg po q48h
Ranitidine	Zantac	150–300 mg po qhs; 50 mg IV q6h; 6.25 mg/h continuous infusion	75–150 mg po qhs; 50 mg IV q12h	150 mg po q12–24h; 50 mg IV q18–24h	75–150 mg po q24h; 50 mg IV q24h	50% of po dose post-HD; 50 mg IV q24h post-HD
Antihypertensives						
Angiotensin-converting enzyme (ACE) inhibitors						
Benazepril	Lotensin	10–40 mg po q12–24h	10–40 mg po q24h	5–20 mg po q24h	5–20 mg po q24h	5–20 mg po q24h
Captopril	Capoten	25–150 mg po q8h	25–150 mg po q8–12h	18.75–75 mg po q12–18h	12.5–50 mg po q24h	Administer dose post-HD or administer 25–35% supplemental dose
Enalapril	Vasotec	5–10 mg po q12h	5 mg po qd titrated upwards to maximum of 40 mg	2.5–10 mg po q12h	2.5–5 mg po q12h	2.5–7.5 po q12h
Enalaprilat	Vasotec	1.25–5 mg IV q6h	1.25–2.5 mg IV q6h	0.625 mg IV × 1, then up to 1.25 mg q6h if response is inadequate	0.625 mg IV × 1, then up to 1.25 mg q6h if response is inadequate	0.625 mg IV q6h
Fosinopril	Monopril	10–40 mg po q12–24h	10–40 mg po q24h	10–40 mg po q24h	7.5–30 mg po q24h	Same

(continued)

Generic name	Trade name	Dose for normal renal function	Dose adjustment for renal failure			Supplement for hemodialysis
			CrCl > 50 mL/min	CrCl = 10–50 mL/min	CrCl < 10 mL/min	
Lisinopril	Zestril	10–40 mg po q24h	Same	2.5–7.5 mg po q24h	1.25–2.5 mg po q24h	2.5 mg initially, then 20% of patient's dose post-HD if patient is on a dosing regimen
Quinapril	Accupril	10–80 mg po q24h	10 mg po qd initially	7.5–60 mg po q24h	7.5–60 mg po q24h	2.5 mg initially, then 25% of patient's dose post-HD if patient is on a dosing regimen
Ramipril	Altace	2.5–20 mg po q24h	Same	1.25–15 mg po q24h	1.25–10 mg po q24h	Supplement 20% of patient's dose post-HD
α-blockers						
Doxazosin	Cardura	1–16 mg po q24h	Same	Same	Same	Same
Prazosin	Minipress	1–15 mg po q12h	Same	Same	Same	Same
Terazosin	Hytrin	1–20 mg po q24h	Same	Same	Same	Same
Angiotensin-receptor blockers						
Candesartan	Atacand	8–32 mg po q24h	Same	Same	Same	Same
Irbesartan	Avapro	150–300 mg po q24h	Same	Same	Same	75 mg initial dose
Losartan	Cozaar	25–100 mg po q12–24h	Same	Same	Same	Same
Valsartan	Diovan	80–320 mg po q24h	Same	Same	Same	Same
β-blockers						
Atenolol	Tenormin	50–100 mg po q24h	Same	25–50 mg po q24h	25 mg po q96h	Administer dose post-HD or administer 25–50 mg supplemental dose
Carvedilol	Coreg	6.25–50 mg po q12h	Same	Same	Same	Same
Labetalol	Normodyne	200–400 mg po bid	Same	Same	Same	Same
Metoprolol	Lopressor	50–400 mg po q24h	Same	Same	Same	Supplement 50 mg po post-HD
Nadolol	Corgard	40–320 mg/d po single or divided doses	40–320 mg/d po q24h	40–320 mg/d po q24–48h	40–320 mg/d po q40–60h	Supplemental dose post-HD

Drug	Brand					
Pindolol	Visken	10–40 mg po q12h	Same	Same	Same	Same
Propranolol	Inderal	80–160 mg po bid	Same	Same	Same	Same
Sotalol	Betapace	80–160 mg po q12h	80–160 mg po q12–24h	80–160 mg po q24–48h	80–160 mg po q4–72h	Same; supplement 80 mg post-HD
Calcium channel blockers						
Amlodipine	Norvasc	2.5–10 mg po q24h	Same	Same	Same	Same
Diltiazem	Dilacor, Cardizem, Tiazac	180–480 mg po q24h	Same	Same	Same	Same
Felodipine	Plendil	2.5–10 mg po q24h	Same	Same	Same	Same
Isradipine	Dynacirc	2.5–5 mg po q12–24h	Same	Same	Same	Same
Nicardipine	Cardene	20–40 mg po tid	Same	Same	Same	Same
Nifedipine	Adalat, Procardia	10–30 mg/d po tid	Same	Same	Same	Same
Nimodipine	Nimotop	30 mg po q8h	Same	Same	Same	Same
Verapamil	Calan, Isoptin, Verelan	80–120 mg po q8h	Same	Same	Same	Same
Diuretics						
Bumetanide	Bumex	1–2 mg IV q8–12h	Same	Same	Same	Same
Furosemide	Lasix	40–80 mg IV q12h	Same	Same	Same	Same
Hydrochlorothiazide	Hydrodiuril	25–200 mg po qd tid	Same	Same	Not effective	Not applicable
Spironolactone	Aldactone	25 mg tid–qid	25 mg q6–12h	25 mg q12–24h	Avoid	Not applicable
Triamterene	Dyrenium	25–150 mg q12–24h	25–150 mg q12h	25–150 mg q12–24h	Avoid	Not applicable
Antivirals						
Acyclovir	Zovirax	5–10 mg/kg po or IV q8h	Same	5–10 mg/kg po or IV q12–24h	2.5–5 mg/kg po or IV q24h	2.5–5 mg/kg po or IV q24h post-HD
Amantadine	Symmetrel	100 mg po q12h	Same	100 mg po q24–48h	200 mg po q7d	200 mg po q7d
Didanosine	Videx	200 mg po q12h; second dose: 250–400 mg q24h	200 mg po q12h	200 mg po q24h	100 mg po q24h	Dose per CrCl < 10 mL/min; no supplemental dosing necessary
Entecavir	Baraclude	0.5–1 mg po qd	0.25–0.5 mg qd	0.15–0.3 mg qd	0.05–0.1 mg qd	Dose post-HD: 0.05 mg po qd for treatment-naïve patients and 0.1 mg po qd for lamivudine-refractory patients

(continued)

Generic name	Trade name	Dose for normal renal function	Dose adjustment for renal failure			Supplement for hemodialysis
			CrCl > 50 mL/min	CrCl = 10–50 mL/min	CrCl < 10 mL/min	
Famciclovir	Famvir	125 mg po q12h or 500 mg po q8h	500 mg q8–12h	125 mg po q12–24h or 500 mg po 12–24h	62.5 mg po q24h or 250 mg po q24h	250 mg following each dialysis session
Ganciclovir	Cytovene	5 mg/kg IV q12h	2.5–5 mg/kg q12h	1.25–2.5 mg/kg q24h	1.25 mg/kg 3 times/week	1.25 mg/kg 3 times/week post-HD
Indinavir	Crixan	800 mg po q8h	No data: same	No data: same	No data: same	No adjustment necessary
Lamivudine	Epivir	150–300 mg po q12–24h	100–300 mg po qd	50–150 mg po q24h	25–50 mg po q24h	Supplemental dosing is not required
Nelfinavir	Viracept	750 mg po q8h; second dose: 1,250 mg bid	Same	Same	Same	Same
Nevirapine	Viramune	200 mg po q24h × 14 d, then q12h	Same	Same	Same	An additional 200 mg dose is recommended following dialysis
Ribavirin	Rebetol	1,000–1,200 mg q24h	Same	Avoid	Avoid	Additional dose recommended after each dialysis session in HIV patients with CrCl < 10 mL/min
Ritonavir	Norvir	600 mg po q12h	Same	Same	Same	Same
Saquinavir	Fortovase, Invirase	600–1,200 mg po q8h	Same	Same	Same	Same
Stavudine	Zerit	30–40 mg po q12h	Same	15–20 mg po q12–24h	15–20 mg po q24h	15–20 mg po q24h
Valacyclovir	Valtrex	500 mg po q12h to 1,000 mg po q8h	Same	500–1,000 mg po q12–24h	500 mg q24h	Dose post-HD
Zalcitabine	Hivid	0.75 mg po q8h	Same	0.75 mg po q12h	0.75 mg po q24h	No data
Zidovudine	Retrovir	200 mg po q8h; second dose: 300 mg po q12h	Same	Same	100 mg po q8h	100 mg po q8h
Bisphosphonates						
Zoledronic acid	Zometa	4 mg IV	3.5 mg IV	3–3.3 mg IV	Avoid	No data

Gout agents

Generic	Brand	Normal dose				
Allopurinol	Zyloprim	300 mg po q24h	150–200 mg po q24h	150 mg po q24h	100 mg po q48h	150 mg supplemental dose
Colchicine	Acetycol, Colsalide	Acute: 2 mg, then 0.5 mg po q6h; chronic: 0.5–1 mg po q24h	Same	Decrease normal dose by 50% to no change	Decrease normal dose by 25%	Same
Probenecid	Benemid	500 mg po bid	Not effective	Not effective	Not effective	Not effective

Hypoglycemic agents

Generic	Brand	Normal dose				
Acarbose	Precose	50–200 mg po tid	25–200 mg po tid	Avoid	Avoid	No data
Acetohexamide	Dymelor	250–1,500 mg po q24h	Avoid	Avoid	Avoid	No data
Chlorpropamide	Diabinese	100–500 mg po q24h	50–250 mg po q24h	Avoid	Avoid	Avoid
Exenatide	Byetta	5–10 mcg SC bid	Same	Avoid	Avoid	Avoid
Glipizide	Glucotrol	2.5–15 mg po q24h	Same	1.25–7.5 mg po	1.25–7.5 mg po	Same
Glyburide	Diabeta, Glynase, Micronase, PresTab	1.25–20 mg po q24h	No data	No data	Avoid	Avoid
Insulin		Variable	100% of normal dose	75% of normal dose	50% of normal dose	No supplement necessary
Metformin	Glucophage	500–850 mg po bid	250–425 mg po bid	125–212 mg po bid	Avoid	No data
Tolazamide	Tolinase	100–250 mg po q24h	Same	Same	Same	No data
Tolbutamide	Orinase	1–2 g q24h	Same	Same	Same	No supplement necessary

Nonsteroidal anti-inflammatory agents

Generic	Brand	Normal dose				
Diclofenac	Voltaren	25–75 mg po bid	12.5–37.5 mg po bid	6.25–37.5 mg po bid	6.25–18.75 mg po bid	No supplement necessary
Etodolac	Lodine	200 mg bid	Same	Same	Same	Same
Ibuprofen	Advil, Motrin	800 mg po tid	Same	Same	Same	Same
Indomethacin	Indocin	25–50 mg po tid	Same	Same	Same	Same
Ketorolac	Toradol	60 mg IM loading dose, then 15–30 mg q6h; 30 mg IV loading dose, then 15 mg q6h	Same	50% of normal dose	25–50% of normal dose	15 mg IM or IV q6h (no bolus dose)
Nabumetone	Relafen		Same	Same	50% of normal dose	

(continued)

Generic name	Trade name	Dose for normal renal function	Dose adjustment for renal failure			Supplement for hemodialysis
			CrCl > 50 mL/min	CrCl = 10–50 mL/min	CrCl < 10 mL/min	
Naproxen	Naprosyn	1–2 g po q24h	Same	0.5–1 g po q24h	0.5–1 g po q24h	No supplement necessary
Oxaprozin	Daypro	1,200 mg po q24h	Same	Same	Same	Same
Tolmetin	Tolectin	400 mg po tid	Same	Same	Same	Same
Proton pump inhibitors						
Esomeprazole	Nexium	20–40 mg po q24h	Same	Same	Same	Same
Lansoprazole	Prevacid	15–60 mg po q24h	Same	Same	Same	Same
Omeprazole	Prilosec	20–60 mg po q24h	Same	Same	Same	Same
Pantoprazole	Protonix	20–80 mg po q24h; 80 mg IV q12h	Same	Same	Same	Same

References

Aronoff GR, Bennett WM, Berns JS, et al. *Drug Prescribing in Renal Failure: Dosing Guidelines for Adults and Children.* 5th ed. Philadelphia, Pa.: American College of Physicians; 2007.

Micromedex Healthcare Series. Greenwood Village, Colo.: Thomson Healthcare. Available at: www.thomsonhc.com. Updated periodically.

UpToDate. Waltham, Mass.: Wolters Kluwer Health. Available at: www.uptodate.com. Updated periodically.

Appendix C

Drugs in Hepatic Failure

Drug	Trade name	Dose
Abacavir	Ziagen	For mild impairment, use 200 mg bid; abacavir is contraindicated in patients with moderate to severe impairment.
Acetaminophen	Cetafen, FeverAll, Silapap, Tylenol	Use with caution; avoid chronic use in patients with impairment.
Amiodarone	Cordarone, Pacerone	Dose adjustment may be necessary in patients with hepatic dysfunction.
Amitriptyline	Elavil	Begin with low initial doses, and increase dose as tolerated and needed.
Amlodipine	Norvasc	Start dose at 2.5 mg po daily.
Amoxicillin–clavulanic acid	Augmentin	Use with caution in patients with impairment, and monitor hepatic function with prolonged use.
Aspirin		Avoid in patients with severe hepatic dysfunction.
Atomoxetine	Strattera	Decrease dose by 50% in patients with moderate hepatic dysfunction; give 25% of normal dose if hepatic dysfunction is severe.
Azathioprine	Imuran	Monitor hepatic transaminases every 2 weeks for 4 weeks, then monthly thereafter.
Azithromycin	Zithromax	Use with caution in patients with impairment because of potential for hepatotoxicity.
Azole antifungals:		
Fluconazole	Diflucan	No adjustments are necessary.
Itraconazole	Sporanox	Adjustments may be necessary, but no guidelines are available.
Ketoconazole	Nizoral	Dose reduction should be considered in patients with severe liver disease.
Posaconazole	Noxafil	Use with caution.
Voriconazole	VFEND	For patients with mild to moderate hepatic dysfunction, use standard loading dose; reduce maintenance dosage by 50% for patients with severe hepatic impairment; use only when benefit outweighs risk; monitor closely for toxicity.
Benzodiazepines:		
Alprazolam	Xanax	Reduce by 50–60% or avoid in patients with cirrhosis.
Chlordiazepoxide	Librium	Avoid or decrease dose in patients with cirrhosis or hepatitis (5 mg po bid–qid).
Diazepam	Valium	Decrease dose by 50% in patients with liver disease.
Lorazepam	Ativan	Use with caution.
Midazolam	Versed	Dose reduction of 50% may be necessary.
Oxazepam	Serax	No dose adjustments are necessary.
Temazepam	Restoril	No dose adjustments are necessary.
Triazolam	Halcion	Dose reduction of 50% may be necessary (0.125 mg po at night).
Bicalutamide	Casodex	No adjustment is needed; use with caution in patients with moderate to severe hepatic dysfunction; discontinue if alanine transaminase > 2 times upper limit of normal or jaundice develops.
Bisoprolol	Zebeta	Decrease initial dose to 2.5 mg in patients with hepatic insufficiency; do not exceed a dose of 10 mg daily.
Bosentan	Tracleer	Liver function should be tested monthly; adjust or discontinue accordingly.
Buspirone	Buspar	Avoid in patients with severe hepatic dysfunction; use lower initial doses, and increase gradually as needed and tolerated.

(continued)

Drug	Trade name	Dose
Bupivacaine	Marcaine, Sensorcaine	Dose adjustment is recommended in patients with severe disease; use with caution.
Carbamazepine	Tegretol	Avoid in patients with hepatic disease.
Celecoxib	Celebrex	Decrease dose by 50% in patients with moderate hepatic dysfunction; avoid in patients with severe hepatic dysfunction.
Chlorambucil	Leukeran	Adjustment may be necessary in patients with impairment.
Chloramphenicol		Use with caution; monitor serum concentrations; dose may be decreased in patients with hepatic impairment.
Chlorpromazine	Thorazine	Use doses in the lower ranges with frequent monitoring and gradual dose adjustment.
Cimetidine	Tagamet	Decrease dose by 50% in patients with severe hepatic dysfunction.
Clindamycin	Cleocin	Decrease dose in patients with severe hepatic dysfunction.
Clomiphene	Clomid, Serophene	Clomiphene is contraindicated in patients with liver disease.
Codeine		Dose adjustment may be necessary; use with caution in patients with severe impairment.
Cyclosporin	Gengraf, Neoral, Restasis, Sandimmune	Dose adjustment may be necessary; monitor levels closely.
Cytarabine	Cytosar	Dose reduction may be necessary; use with caution in patients with hepatic impairment.
Dacarbazine	DTIC	Dacarbazine may cause hepatotoxicity; monitor closely for signs.
Darunavir	Prezista	No dose adjustment is needed for patients with mild to moderate hepatic impairment; avoid in patients with severe impairment; monitor liver function tests at baseline, then periodically thereafter.
Daunorubicin	Cerubidine	If bilirubin is 1.2–3 mg/dL, reduce dose by 25%; if > 3 mg/dL, reduce dose by 50%.
Delavirdine	Rescriptor	Use with caution in patients with hepatic impairment.
Didanosine	Videx	Consider dose adjustment; monitor for toxicity.
Diltiazem	Cardizem, Cartia, Dilacor, Tiazac	Use with caution because diltiazem is extensively metabolized by the liver.
Disulfiram	Antabuse	Use with caution in patients with hepatic cirrhosis or hepatic insufficiency; avoid in patients with advanced or severe hepatic disease.
Doxorubicin	Adriamycin, Rubex	If bilirubin is 1.2–3 mg/dL, reduce dose by 50%; if bilirubin is 3.1–5 mg/dL, reduce dose by 75%.
Efavirenz	Sustiva	Use with caution in patients with hepatic impairment.
Erythromycin	E-Mycin	Dose reduction may be necessary in patients with hepatic dysfunction.
Esomeprazole	Nexium	Do not exceed a dose of 20 mg in patients with severe hepatic dysfunction.
Estrogens		Use with caution in patients with impaired liver function.
Felodipine	Plendil	Initial dose is 2.5 mg/day; monitor blood pressure.
Flecainide	Tambocor	Flecainide has an increased half-life in patients with hepatic impairment; monitor plasma levels; avoid use in patients with significant impairment.
Flumazenil	Romazicon	Use caution with initial and repeated doses in patients with liver disease.
Fluorouracil	Adrucil, Carac, Efudex, Fluoroplex	Use with extreme caution.
Fluphenazine	Prolixin	Use with caution.

Drug	Trade name	Dose
Furosemide	Lasix	Furosemide has a diminished natriuretic effect with increased sensitivity to hypokalemia and volume depletion in patients with cirrhosis; monitor effects, especially with high doses.
Griseofulvin	Grifulvin, Gris-PEG	Griseofulvin is contraindicated in patients with severe liver disease.
Haloperidol	Haldol	Use with caution in patients with hepatic impairment.
3-hydroxy-3-methyl-glutaryl-coenzyme A (HMG-CoA) reductase inhibitors		Avoid in patients with elevated serum transaminases.
Ibuprofen	Addaprin, Advil, Genpril, I-Prin, Midol, Motrin, NeoProfin, Proprinal, Ultraprin	Use with caution in patients with hepatic impairment; avoid in patients with severe impairment.
Indinavir	Crixivan	Decrease dose to 600 mg q8h in patients with mild to moderate hepatic dysfunction.
Interferon beta-1a	Avonex	Consider a dose reduction if serum glutamic pyruvic transaminase > 5 times upper limit of normal; discontinue if jaundice or other symptoms of liver disease develop.
Interferon beta-1b	Betaseron	Test liver function at months 1, 3, and 6, then periodically thereafter.
Isoniazid	Laniazid, Nydrazid	Lower doses may be necessary; defer therapy for treatment of latent tuberculosis infection in patients with acute hepatic disease.
Isotretinoin	Accutane	Empiric dose reductions are recommended in patients with hepatitis; monitor liver function tests at baseline, then at weekly or biweekly intervals until a response to the treatment is established.
Lamivudine-zidovudine	Combivir	Fixed-dose combinations should not be used in patients with impaired hepatic function; lamivudine-zidovudine is contraindicated in patients with hepatic impairment.
Lamotrigine	Lamictal	Reduce initial, escalation, and maintenance doses by 25% in patients with moderate to severe hepatic impairment without ascites; decrease doses by 50% in patients with severe hepatic dysfunction with ascites.
Lansoprazole	Prevacid	Decrease dose in patients with severe hepatic dysfunction.
Leflunomide	Arava	Avoid in patients with moderate to severe hepatic dysfunction; decrease dose to 10 mg/d if liver enzymes are elevated to 2 times the upper limit of normal; discontinue if liver enzymes are elevated to 3 times the upper limit of normal.
Levonorgestrel	Mirena, Plan B	Levonorgestrel is contraindicated in patients with acute liver disease.
Lidocaine	Xylocaine	Dose adjustments may be required.
Losartan	Cozaar	Initiation of therapy at a reduced dosage may be advisable in patients with hepatic impairment.
Medroxyprogesterone	Depo-Provera, Provera	Medroxyprogesterone is contraindicated in patients with severe hepatic impairment.
Mefloquine	Lariam	Mefloquine may have increased half-life and plasma levels.
Mercaptopurine	Purinethol	Dose reduction may be necessary in patients with hepatic impairment.
Metformin	Glucophage	Avoid; liver disease is a risk factor for developing lactic acidosis during therapy.
Methadone	Dolophine	Adjust dose in patients with impairment because of risk of accumulation; avoid in patients with severe disease.

(continued)

Drug	Trade name	Dose
Methotrexate	Folex, Rheumatrex	Decrease dose by 25% when bilirubin is 3.1–5 mg/dL or aspartate transaminase is > 180 IU; avoid if bilirubin is > 5 mg/dL.
Methyldopa	Aldomet	Methyldopa is contraindicated in patients with liver disease.
Metoprolol	Lopressor	Dose adjustment may be necessary in patients with hepatic insufficiency; no recommendations are available.
Metronidazole	Flagyl	Decrease dose in patients with severe disease; no recommendations are available.
Mexiletine	Mexitil	Decrease dose to 25–30% of normal dose.
Morphine	Avinza, DepoDur, Duramorph, Infumorph, Kadian, MS Contin, Oramorph SR, Roxanol	Decrease dose in patients with cirrhosis.
Nabumetone	Relafen	Use with caution in patients with severe hepatic insufficiency; reduce dose if necessary.
Nefazodone	Serzone	Avoid in patients with elevated transaminases.
Nelfinavir	Viracept	No adjustment is necessary for patients with mild impairment; use is not recommended in patients with moderate to severe impairment.
Nevirapine	Viramune	Nevirapine is contraindicated in patients with moderate to severe impairment.
Nifedipine	Adalat, Procardia	Decrease dose by 50–60% in patients with cirrhosis.
Nisoldipine	Sular	Starting dose is not to exceed 8.5 mg/d in patients with liver impairment.
Ofloxacin	Floxin	Do not exceed 400 mg/d in patients with severe liver dysfunction.
Omeprazole	Prilosec	Decrease dose in patients with hepatic dysfunction.
Ondansetron	Zofran	Do not exceed 8 mg/d in patients with severe hepatic insufficiency.
Oxycodone	Oxycontin	Dose should be decreased in patients with severe liver disease.
Pantoprazole	Protonix	Adjustment is not required.
Pioglitazone	Actos	For alanine aminotransferase < 2.5 upper limit of normal, use caution; for active liver disease (alanine aminotransferase > 2.5 upper limit of normal), avoid use.
Phenobarbital	Barbita, Luminal, Solfoton	Dose reduction may be necessary in patients with hepatic dysfunction.
Phenytoin	Dilantin	Monitor levels frequently because dose reduction may be necessary in patients with hepatic insufficiency; increased unbound concentrations may occur.
Prednisolone	Econopred, Orapred, Pediapred, Pred Forte, Pred Mild, Prelone	Prednisolone is contraindicated in patients with cirrhosis; use with caution in patients with severe hepatic impairment.
Procainamide	Procanbid, Promine, Pronestyl, Rhythmin	Lower doses or longer dosing intervals may be required in patients with hepatic failure.
Procarbazine	Matulane	Use with caution in patients with impairment.
Propranolol	Betachron, Inderal	Marked slowing of heart rate may occur in patients with chronic liver disease with conventional doses; low initial dose and slow titration are suggested. Monitor more frequently in patients with hepatic dysfunction; regular heart rate monitoring is recommended.
Pyrazinamide		Pyrazinamide is contraindicated in patients with severe dysfunction.
Quinidine	Cardioquin, Quinaglute, Quinalan, Quinidex, Quinora	Reduction of maintenance doses by 50% may be necessary in patients with hepatic impairment; monitor serum levels closely.

Drug	Trade name	Dose
Ranitidine	Zantac	Ranitidine may have minor changes in half-life, distribution, clearance, and bioavailability; no adjustment is necessary; monitor serum levels and liver function tests.
Ribavirin	Copegus, Rebetol, Ribasphere, Virazole	Ribavirin is contraindicated in patients with hepatic decompensation.
Rifampin	Rifadin, Rimactane	Dose reductions may be necessary to reduce hepatotoxicity; use with caution or avoid in patients with hepatic impairment.
Risperidone	Risperdal	Decrease dose in patients with hepatic dysfunction. For IM, administer titrated oral doses prior to starting IM. For po, start at 0.5 mg bid and titrate.
Ritonavir	Norvir	No adjustments are needed; monitor closely. Decrease dose about 40% in steady state in patients with mild to moderate impairment. No data are available for patients with severe impairment; monitor closely.
Saquinavir	Fortovase, Invirase	Use with caution in patients with mild to moderate hepatic impairment; saquinavir is contraindicated in patients with severe impairment.
Selective serotonin reuptake inhibitors (SSRIs) and serotonin-norepinephrine reuptake inhibitors:		Dose should be decreased or dosing interval increased in patients with hepatic insufficiency.
Citalopram	Celexa	A 20-mg dose is recommended for patients with decreased hepatic function; dosage may be increased to 40 mg/d only in nonresponsive patients.
Fluoxetine	Prozac	A lower or less frequent dose is recommended in patients with hepatic impairment because of a prolonged elimination half-life.
Fluvoxamine	Luvox	Decrease the dose or frequency, and titrate slowly in patients with hepatic insufficiency.
Paroxetine	Paxil	Dose initially at 10 mg qd or at 12.5 mg qd of the controlled-release product; doses should not exceed 40 mg qd or 50 mg qd of the controlled-release product.
Sertraline	Zoloft	Decrease the dose, or increase the interval.
Venlafaxine	Effexor	Decrease the dose by 50% in patients with mild to moderate hepatic impairment.
Sodium nitroprusside	Nipride, Nitropress	Use with caution in patients with hepatic impairment.
Succinylcholine	Anectine, Quelicin	Decrease dose in patients with severe disease.
Sulfamethoxazole-trimethoprim	Bactrim, Setpra, Sulfatrim	Sulfamethoxazole-trimethoprim is contraindicated in patients with marked hepatic damage if not monitored.
Sulfonylureas:		Dose reduction may be necessary in patients with hepatic disease.
Chlorpropamide	Diabinese	Use conservative initial and maintenance doses.
Glimepiride	Amaryl	Use conservative initial and maintenance doses.
Glipizide	Glucotrol	Start dose at 2.5 mg po qd.
Glyburide	Diabeta, Glynase, Micronase	Use conservative initial and maintenance doses; avoid use in patients with severe disease.
Tolazamide	Tolinase	Use conservative initial and maintenance doses.
Tolbutamide	Orinase	Use conservative initial and maintenance doses.
Tacrolimus	Prograf	Dose at the low end of the dosing range in patients with hepatic impairment; consider dose adjustment; monitor closely.

(continued)

Drug	Trade name	Dose
Testosterone	Androderm, Androgel, Delatestryl, Depo-Testosterone, First-Testosterone MC, Striant, Testim, Testopel	Decrease dose in patients with impairment; testosterone is contraindicated in patients with severe hepatic impairment.
Tetracycline	Sumycin	Use with caution in patients with impairment.
Theophylline	Aerolate, Aminophyllin, Aquaphyllin, Asmalix, Bronkodyl, Choledyl, Duraphyl, Respbid, Slo-bid, Slo-Phyllin, Sustaire, Theo-24, Theobid, Theochron, Theoclear, Theo-Dur, Theolair, Theon, Theospan, Theovent, Truphylline	Dose reduction may be necessary in patients with hepatic insufficiency; monitor serum levels frequently.
Tiagabine	Gabitril	Dose adjustments may be necessary in patients with impairment caused by decreased clearance.
Tipranavir	Aptivus	No dose adjustment is necessary for patients with mild impairment. Tipranavir is contraindicated in patients with moderate to severe hepatotoxicity; monitor liver functions at baseline, then periodically thereafter.
Tramadol	Ultram	Immediate release: Dose 50 mg po q12h in patients with cirrhosis. Extended release: This form is not recommended.
Tricyclic antidepressants:		Start low dose initially, and increase as needed and tolerated.
Amitriptyline	Elavil	
Clomipramine	Anafranil	
Desipramine	Norpramin	
Doxepin	Sinequan	
Imipramine	Tofranil	
Nortriptyline	Pamelor	
Protriptyline	Vivactil	
Valproic acid	Depakene, Depakote	Avoid in patients with hepatic disease or significant hepatic insufficiency.
Verapamil	Calan, Covera, Isoptin, Verelan	Decrease dose by 20–50% in patients with impairment.
Vinblastine	Velban	If bilirubin is > 3 mg/100mL, reduce dose by 50%.
Vincristine	Vincasar PFS	If bilirubin is > 3 mg/100mL, reduce dose by 50%.
Warfarin	Coumadin	Use initial dose of 5 mg or less, with adjustments based on international normalized ratio.
Zafirlukast	Accolate	Consider a decreased dose in patients with impairment; monitor for adverse effects.
Zalcitabine	Hivid	Avoid in patients with liver function tests > 5 times the upper limit of normal.
Zidovudine	Retrovir	Decrease daily dose or extend dosing interval.

Reference

Micromedex Healthcare Series. Greenwood Village, Colo.: Thomson Healthcare. Available at: www.thomsonhc.com. Updated periodically.

Appendix D

Top 200 Prescription Drugs

The following list of the top 200 prescriptions for 2007 is ranked by number of U.S. prescriptions dispensed. The list was obtained with permission from RxList at www.rxlist.com with data furnished by Verispan VONA.

Rank	Trade name	Generic name	Rank	Trade name	Generic name
1.	Lipitor	Atorvastatin	37.	Lotrel	Amlodipine-benazepril
2.	Singulair	Montelukast	38.	Actonel	Risedronate
3.	Lexapro	Escitalopram	39.	Ambien CR	Zolpidem
4.	Nexium	Esomeprazole	40.	Cozaar	Losartan
5.	Synthroid	Levothyroxine	41.	Coreg	Carvedilol
6.	Plavix	Clopidogrel	42.	Valtrex	Valacyclovir
7.	Toprol XL	Metoprolol	43.	Lyrica	Pregabalin
8.	Prevacid	Lansoprazole	44.	Concerta	Methylphenidate
9.	Vytorin	Ezetimibe-simvastatin	45.	Ambien	Zolpidem
10.	Advair Diskus	Fluticasone-salmeterol (inhaled)	46.	Risperdal	Risperidone
11.	Zyrtec	Cetirizine	47.	Digitek	Digoxin
12.	Effexor XR	Venlafaxine	48.	Topamax	Topiramate
13.	Protonix	Pantoprazole	49.	Chantix	Varenicline
14.	Diovan	Valsartan	50.	Avandia	Rosiglitazone
15.	Fosamax	Alendronate	51.	Lamictal	Lamotrigine
16.	Zetia	Ezetimibe	52.	Ortho Tri-Cyclen Lo	Ethinyl estradiol–norgestimate
17.	Crestor	Rosuvastatin	53.	Xalatan	Latanoprost ophthalmic
18.	Levaquin	Levofloxacin	54.	Aciphex	Rabeprazole
19.	Diovan HCT	Hydrochlorothiazide-valsartan	55.	Hyzaar	Hydrochlorothiazide-losartan
20.	Klor-Con	Potassium chloride	56.	Spiriva	Tiotropium (inhaled)
21.	Cymbalta	Duloxetine	57.	Wellbutrin XL	Bupropion HCl
22.	Actos	Pioglitazone	58.	Lunesta	Eszopiclone
23.	Premarin Tabs	Estrogens (conjugated)	59.	Benicar	Olmesartan
24.	ProAir HFA	Albuterol (inhaled)	60.	Benicar HCT	Hydrochlorothiazide-olmesartan
25.	Celebrex	Celecoxib	61.	Aricept	Donepezil
26.	Flomax	Tamsulosin	62.	Avapro	Irbesartan
27.	Seroquel	Quetiapine	63.	Detrol LA	Tolterodine
28.	Norvasc	Amlodipine	64.	Trinessa	Ethinyl estradiol and norgestimate
29.	Nasonex	Mometasone nasal	65.	Cialis	Tadalafil
30.	Tricor	Fenofibrate	66.	Combivent	Albuterol-ipratropium (inhaled)
31.	Lantus	Insulin glargine	67.	Budeprion XL	Bupropion HCl
32.	Viagra	Sildenafil	68.	Yaz	Drospirenone–ethinyl estradiol
33.	Altace	Ramipril	69.	Glycolax	Polyethylene glycol 3350
34.	Yasmin 28	Drospirenone–ethinyl estradiol	70.	Imitrex Oral	Sumatriptan
35.	Levoxyl	Levothyroxine	71.	Evista	Raloxifene
36.	Adderall XR	Amphetamine-dextroamphetamine	72.	NuvaRing	Etonogestrel–ethinyl estradiol (vaginal)

(continued)

Rank	Trade name	Generic name	Rank	Trade name	Generic name
73.	Omnicef	Cefdinir	114.	Low-Ogestrel	Ethinyl estradiol–norgestrel
74.	Nisapan	Niacin	115.	Vivelle-DOT	Estradiol (transdermal)
75.	Tri-Sprintec	Ethinyl estradiol–norgestimate	116.	Apri	Desogestrel–ethinyl estradiol
76.	Boniva	Ibandronate	117.	Loestrin 24 Fe	Ethinyl estradiol–norethindrone
77.	Flovent HFA	Fluticasone (inhaled)	118.	Levothroid	Levothyroxine
78.	Avelox	Moxifloxacin	119.	Necon 1/35	Ethinyl estradiol–norethindrone
79.	Abilify	Aripiprazole	120.	Fosamax Plus D	Alendronate-cholecalciferol
80.	Avalide	Hydrochlorothiazide-irbesartan	121.	Byetta	Exenatide
81.	Requip	Ropinirole	122.	Pulmicort Respules	Budesonide (inhaled)
82.	Zyrtex Syrup	Cetirizine	123.	Paxil CR	Paroxetine
83.	Coumadin Tabs	Warfarin	124.	Glipizide XL	Glipizide
84.	Zyprexa	Olanzapine	125.	Provigil	Modafinil
85.	Depakote ER	Divalproex sodium	126.	Trileptal	Oxcarbazepine
86.	Nasacort AQ	Triamcinolone (nasal)	127.	Humulin N	Insulin (NPH)
87.	Skelaxin	Metaxalone	128.	Lumigan	Bimatoprost (ophthalmic)
88.	Allegra-D	Fexofenadine-pseudoephedrine	129.	Alphagan P	Brimonidine (ophthalmic)
89.	Humalog	Insulin lispro	130.	Xopenex HFA	Levalbuterol (inhaled)
90.	Vigamox	Moxifloxacin ophthalmic	131.	Tobradex	Tobramycin-dexamethasone (ophthalmic)
91.	Endocet	Acetaminophen-oxycodone	132.	Trivora-28	Ethinyl estradiol–levonorgestrel
92.	Budeprion SR	Bupropion XL	133.	Atacand	Candesartan
93.	Depakote	Divalproex sodium	134.	Xopenex	Levalbuterol (inhaled)
94.	Namenda	Memantine	135.	Cosopt	Dorzolamide-timolol (ophthalmic)
95.	Lidoderm	Lidocaine topical	136.	Geodeon Oral	Ziprasidone
96.	Strattera	Atomoxetine	137.	Micardis	Telmisartan
97.	Aviane	Ethinyl estradiol–levonorgestrel	138.	Lovaza	Omega-3 acid ethyl esters
98.	Patanol	Olopatadine (ophthalmic)	139.	Micardis HCT	Telmisartan/hydrochlorothiazide
99.	Proventil HFA	Albuterol (inhaled)	140.	Focalin XR	Dexmethylphenidate
100.	Clarinex	Desloratadine	141.	OxyContin	Oxycodone
101.	Thyroid, Armour	Thyroid desiccated	142.	Mirapex	Pramipexole
102.	Astelin	Azelastine (nasal)	143.	Prometrium	Progesterone (micronized)
103.	Zyrtex-D	Cetirizine-pseudoephedrine	144.	Humulin 70/30	Insulin (NPH/regular)
104.	Tussionex	Chlorpheniramine-hydrocodone	145.	Ciprodex Otic	Ciprofloxacin-dexamethasone (otic)
105.	Caduet	Amlodipine-atorvastatin	146.	Restasis	Cyclosporine (ophthalmic)
106.	Avodart	Dutasteride	147.	Suboxone	Buprenorphine-naloxone
107.	Keppra	Levetiracetam	148.	Zymar	Gatifloxacin (ophthalmic)
108.	Januvia	Sitagliptin	149.	Arimidex	Anastrozole
109.	Kariva	Desogestrel–ethinyl estradiol	150.	Sprintec	Ethinyl estradiol–norgestimate
110.	Prempro	Estrogens (conjugated)–medroxyprogesterone	151.	Dilantin Kapseals	Phenytoin
111.	Rhinocort Aqua	Budesonide (nasal)	152.	Fluzone	Influenza vaccine
112.	Levitra	Vardenafil	153.	BenzaClin	Benzoyl peroxide–clindamycin (topical)
113.	Ortho Evra	Ethinyl estradiol–norelgestromin (transdermal)			

Rank	Trade name	Generic name	Rank	Trade name	Generic name
154.	Vesicare	Solifenacin	178.	Sular	Nisoldipine
155.	Asacol	Mesalamine	179.	Lescol XL	Fluvastatin
156.	Avandamet	Metformin-rosiglitazone	180.	Novolin 70/30	Insulin (NPH/regular)
157.	Lanoxin	Digoxin	181.	Epipen	epinephrine
158.	Travantan	Travoprost (ophthalmic)	182.	Actoplus Met	Pioglitazone HCl–metformin HCl
159.	Zoloft	Sertraline	183.	M-Oxy	Oxycodone
160.	Bactroban	Mupirocin (topical)	184.	Rozerem	Ramelteon — *Fall asleep*
161.	Tamiflu	Oseltamivir	185.	Enablex	Darifenacin
162.	Guaifenex PSE	Guaifenesin-pseudoephedrine	186.	Jantoven	Warfarin
163.	Differin	Adapalene (topical)	187.	Catapres-TTS	Clonidine (transdermal)
164.	Premarin Vaginal	Estrogens (conjugated, vaginal)	188.	Junel Fe	Ethinyl estradiol–norethindrone
165.	Pseudovent 400	Pseudoephedrine HCl (extended-release)–guaifenesin	189.	Coreg CR	Carvedilol
			190.	Ortho Tri-Cyclen	Ethinyl estradiol–norgestimate
166.	Vagifem	Estradiol (vaginal)	191.	Primacare One	Prenatal vitamin supplement
167.	Levora	Ethinyl estradiol–levonorgestrel	192.	Zovirax Topical	Acyclovir (topical)
168.	Relpax	Eletriptan	193.	Trilyte	Polyethylene glycol–electrolytes
169.	Allegra-D 24 Hour	Fexofenadine-pseudoephedrine	194.	Aldara	Imiquimod
170.	Methylin	Methylphenidate	195.	Necon 0.5./35E	Norethindrone–ethinyl estradiol
171.	AndroGel	Testosterone (topical)	196.	Arthrotec	Diclofenac sodium–misoprostol
172.	Aggrenox	Aspirin-dipyridamole	197.	Ultram ER	Tramadol
173.	Propecia	Finasteride	198.	Ceron-DM	Chlorpheniramine-dextromethorphan-phenylephrine
174.	Asmanex	Mometasone (inhaled)			
175.	NovoLog Mix 70/30	Insulin aspart protamine–insulin aspart	199.	Ethedent	1.1% sodium fluoride
176.	Uroxatral	Alfuzosin	200.	Elidel	Pimecrolimus (topical)
177.	Estrostep Fe	Ethinyl estradiol–norethindrone			

Reference

RxList. The Top 200 Prescriptions for 2007 by Number of U.S. Prescriptions Dispensed. Available at: www.rxlist.com/script/main/hp.asp.

Appendix E

Top 200 Over-the-Counter Products

The following is a list of the top 200 over-the-counter (OTC) and health and beauty care brands based on dollar amount sold in 2004. The list was obtained with permission from *Drug Topics 2007*.

Rank	Product
1.	Private label cold, allergy, and sinus tablets or packets
2.	Private label internal analgesic tablets
3.	Prilosec OTC antacid tablets
4.	Private label mineral supplements
5.	Always sanitary napkins or liners
6.	Advil internal analgesic tablets
7.	Tylenol internal analgesic tablets
8.	Listerine mouthwash and dental rinse
9.	Dove nondeodorant bar soap
10.	Depend adult incontinence products
11.	Private label adult incontinence products
12.	Private label first-aid ointments and antiseptics
13.	Aleve internal analgesic tablets
14.	Ensure weight control or nutritionals, liquid or powder
15.	Private label multivitamins
16.	Nicorette antismoking gum
17.	Poise adult incontinence products
18.	Private label first-aid tape, bandages, gauze, or cotton
19.	Gillette Mach3 cartridges
20.	Private label laxative tablets
21.	Claritin cold, allergy, and sinus tablets or packets
22.	Claritin D cold, allergy, and sinus tablets or packets
23.	Tampax Pearl tampons
24.	Private label baby wipes
25.	Private label antacid tablets
26.	Benadryl cold, allergy, and sinus tablets or packets
27.	Private label antismoking gum
28.	Mucinex cold, allergy, and sinus tablets or packets
29.	Nature's Bounty mineral supplements
30.	Tampax tampons
31.	Crest toothpaste
32.	Degree deodorant
33.	Nature Made mineral supplements
34.	Private label cotton balls and cotton swabs
35.	Gillette Fusion cartridges
36.	Playtex Gentle Glide tampons
37.	Private label one- and two-letter vitamins
38.	Loreal Superior Preference hair coloring
39.	Olay Regenerist facial antiaging
40.	Airborne cold, allergy, and sinus tablets or packets
41.	Tylenol PM internal analgesic tablets
42.	Nature Made one- and two-letter vitamins
43.	Alli weight control candy or tablets
44.	Crest Whitening Plus Scope toothpaste
45.	Mucinex DM cold, allergy, and sinus tablets or packets
46.	Sudafed PE cold, allergy, and sinus tablets or packets
47.	Stayfree sanitary napkins or liners
48.	Private label cold, allergy, and sinus liquid or powder
49.	Private label nasal spray, drops, or inhaler
50.	Bayer internal analgesic tablets
51.	Loreal Excellence hair coloring
52.	Private label eye or lens care solutions
53.	Kotex sanitary napkins or liners
54.	Centrum Silver multivitamins
55.	PediaSure weight control or nutritionals, liquid or powder
56.	Colgate Total toothpaste
57.	Secret Platinum deodorants
58.	Private label sanitary napkins or liners
59.	Huggies Natural Care baby wipes
60.	Vicks Nyquil cold, allergy, and sinus liquid or powder
61.	Private label mouthwash or dental rinse
62.	Q-tips cotton balls and cotton swabs
63.	Colgate toothpaste
64.	Tylenol cold, allergy, and sinus tablets or packets
65.	Just For Men hair coloring
66.	Clairol Nice 'n Easy hair coloring
67.	Alcon Opti-Free Replenish eye or lens care solutions
68.	Band-Aid first-aid tape, bandages, gauze, or cotton
69.	Slim Fast Optima weight control or nutritionals, liquid or powder
70.	Gillette Mach3 Turbo cartridges
71.	Alcon Opti-Free Express eye or lens care solutions
72.	Osteo Bi-Flex mineral supplements

Rank	Product
73.	Motrin IB internal analgesic tablets
74.	Private Label weight control or nutritionals, liquid or powder
75.	LifeScan OneTouch glucose
76.	Gillette Fusion Power cartridges
77.	Zantac 150 antacid tablets
78.	Clairol Natural Instincts hair coloring
79.	Serenity adult incontinence products
80.	Commit antismoking tablets
81.	Kleenex Cottonelle moist towelettes
82.	Softsoap Liquid Hand Soap
83.	Private label anti-itch treatments (including calamine)
84.	Nicroderm CQ antismoking patch
85.	Revlon Colorsilk hair coloring
86.	Crest Pro Health toothpaste
87.	Abreva lip balm or cold sore medication
88.	Children's Motrin internal analgesic liquids
89.	Neosporin first-aid ointments and antiseptics
90.	Huggies baby wipes
91.	L'Oréal Feria hair coloring
92.	Dove liquid body wash and all other
93.	Old Spice High Endurance deodorants
94.	Private label pregnancy test kits
95.	Breathe Right nasal strips
96.	Centrum multivitamins
97.	Vaseline Intensive Care hand and body lotion
98.	Imodium AD diarrhea tablets
99.	Garnier Nutrisse hair coloring
100.	Crest Pro Health mouthwash or dental rinse
101.	Theraflu cold, allergy, and sinus tablets or packets
102.	Boost weight control or nutritionals, liquid or powder
103.	Pampers baby wipes
104.	Futuro muscle and body support devices
105.	Sensodyne toothpaste
106.	Private label suntan lotion and oil
107.	Crest Whitestrips tooth bleaching or whitening powder or pills
108.	Excedrin internal analgesic tablets
109.	Icy Hot external analgesic rubs
110.	Kotex Security tampons
111.	Pepcid AC antacid tablets
112.	Pepto-Bismol stomach remedy liquid or powder
113.	Metamucil laxative or stimulant liquid, powder, or oil

Rank	Product
114.	Bausch & Lomb ReNu MultiPlus eye or lens care solutions
115.	Vicks humidifiers or vaporizers
116.	Private label vaginal treatments
117.	Ensure Plus weight control or nutritionals, liquid or powder
118.	Alka Seltzer Plus cold, allergy, and sinus liquid or powder
119.	Private label manual toothbrushes
120.	Private label internal analgesic liquids
121.	Coppertone suntan lotion and oil
122.	Dove deodorants
123.	Coppertone Sport suntan lotion and oil
124.	Zicam nasal spray, drops, or inhaler
125.	Right Guard Sport deodorants
126.	Secret deodorants
127.	Dulcolax laxative tablets
128.	Pepcid Complete antacid tablets
129.	ThermaCare heat or ice packs
130.	Tylenol Arthritis internal analgesic tablets
131.	Omron blood pressure kit
132.	Old Spice Red Zone deodorants
133.	Private label hand and body lotion
134.	Monistat 1 vaginal treatments
135.	Private label disposables
136.	Tylenol internal analgesic liquids
137.	Maybelline Great Lash mascara
138.	First Response pregnancy test kits
139.	Children's Tylenol cold, allergy, and sinus liquid or powder
140.	One A Day multivitamins
141.	Private label laxative or stimulant liquid, powder, or oil
142.	Ace muscle and body support devices
143.	Always Fresh sanitary napkins or liners
144.	Fixodent denture adhesives
145.	Crest Whitening Expressions toothpaste
146.	Private label liquid hand soap
147.	Slim-Fast Optima Meal On-the-Go weight control or nutritionals, liquid or powder
148.	Irish Spring deodorant bar soap
149.	Scope mouthwash or dental rinse
150.	Gax-X antacid tablets
151.	Cologate Max Fresh toothpaste
152.	Axe liquid body wash and all other
153.	Private label antismoking patch

(continued)

Rank	Product
154.	Vicks Dayquil cold, allergy, and sinus tablets or packets
155.	Preparation H hemorrhoidal cream, ointment or spray
156.	Pampers Sensitive baby wipes
157.	Mennen Speed Stick deodorants
158.	Kotex Lightdays sanitary napkins or liners
159.	Tylenol Sinus cold, allergy, and sinus tablets or packets
160.	Claritin RediTabs cold, allergy, and sinus tablets or packets
161.	Excedrin Migraine internal analgesic tablets
162.	Private label tampons
163.	Gillette M3 Power cartridges
164.	Wet Ones moist towelettes
165.	Dial deodorant bar soap
166.	Monistat 3 vaginal treatments
167.	L'Oréal Natural Match hair coloring
168.	Bengay external analgesic rubs
169.	Advanced Listerine mouthwash or dental rinse
170.	Secret Clinical Strength deodorants
171.	Gillette Venus cartridges
172.	Alavert cold, allergy, and sinus tablets or packets
173.	Children's Tylenol internal analgesic liquids
174.	Rogaine hair growth products
175.	Tums E-X antacid tablets
176.	Advil PM internal analgesic tablets

Rank	Product
177.	Robitussin cold, allergy, and sinus liquid or powder
178.	Mucinex D cold, allergy, and sinus tablets or packets
179.	Imodium Advanced diarrhea tablets
180.	Vicks VapoRub chest rubs
181.	Ban deodorants
182.	Afrin nasal spray, drops, or inhaler
183.	Private label diarrhea tablets
184.	Olay Definity facial antiaging
185.	Skintimate shaving cream
186.	Private label moist towelettes
187.	e.p.t. pregnancy test kits
188.	Olay Complete facial moisturizers
189.	Nature's Bounty one-and two-letter vitamins
190.	Midol feminine pain relievers
191.	Lever 2000 deodorant bar soap
192.	Private label glucose
193.	Purell hand sanitizers
194.	Chapstick lip balm or cold sore medication
195.	Gillette Custom Plus disposables
196.	Rolaids antacid tablets
197.	Alcon Systane eye or lens care solutions
198.	Suave Naturals regular shampoo
199.	Gillette Sensor Excel cartridges
200.	Banana Boat suntan lotion and oil

Reference

Top 200 OTC/HBC brands in 2007. *Drug Topics*. Available at: http://drugtopics.modernmedicine.com/drugtopics/data/articlestandard//drugtopics/ 082008/492702/article.pdf.

Appendix F

Drugs Excreted in Breast Milk

The following list is not comprehensive; generics and alternate brands of some products may exist. When recommending drugs to pregnant or nursing patients, always check product labeling for specific precautions.

Accolate	Bactrim	CombiPatch	Dilantin	Foradil	Lamictal
Accuretic	Baraclude	Combipres	Dilaudid	Fortamet	Lamisil
Aciphex	Benadryl	Combivir	Diovan	Fortaz	Lamprene
Actiq	Bentyl	Combunox	Diprivan	Fosamax	Lanoxicaps
Activella	Betapace	Compazine	Diuril	Fosamax Plus D	Lanoxin
Actonel	Bextra	Cordarone	Dolobid	Furosemide	Lariam
Actonel with	Bexxar	Corgard	Dolophine	Gabitril	Lescol
Calcium	Bicillin	Cortisporin	Doral	Galzin	Letairis
ActoPlus Met	Blocadren	Corzide	Doryx	Garamycin	Levbid
Actos	Boniva	Cosopt	Droxia	Glucophage	Levitra
Adalat	Brethine	Coumadin	Duraclon	Glucovance	Levlen
Adderall	Brevicon	Covera-HS	Duragesic	Glumetza	Levlite
Advicor	Brontex	Cozaar	Duramorph	Glyset	Levora
Aggrenox	Byetta	Crestor	Duratuss	Guaifed	Levothroid
Aldactazide	Caduet	Crinone	Duricef	Halcion	Levoxyl
Aldactone	Cafergot	Cyclessa	Dyazide	Haldol	Levsin
Aldomet	Calan	Cymbalta	Dyrenium	Helidac	Levsinex
Aldoril	Campral	Cystospaz	EC-Naprosyn	Hycamtin	Lexapro
Alesse	Capoten	Cytomel	Ecotrin	Hydrocet	Lexiva
Alfenta	Capozide	Cytotec	E.E.S.	Hydrocortone	Lialda
Allegra-D	Captopril	Cytoxan	Effexor	HydroDIURIL	Lindane
Aloprim	Carbatrol	Dapsone	Elavil	Iberet-Folic	Lioresal
Altace	Cardizem	Daraprim	Elestat	Ifex	Lipitor
Ambien	Cataflam	Darvon	EMLA	Imitrex	Lithium
Amerge	Catapres	Darvon-N	Enduron	Imuran	Lithobid
Anafranil	Ceclor	Decadron	Epzicom	Inderal	Lo/Ovral
Anaprox	Cefizox	Deconsal II	Equetro	Inderide	Loestrin
Androderm	Cefobid	Demerol	ERYC	Indocin	Lomotil
Aplenzin	Cefotan	Demulen	EryPed	INFeD	Loniten
Apresoline	Ceftin	Depacon	Ery-Tab	Inspra	Lopressor
Aralen	Celebrex	Depakene	Erythrocin	Invanz	Lortab
Arthrotec	Celexa	Depakote	Erythromycin	Invega	Lotensin
Asacol	Cerebyx	DepoDur	Esgic-plus	Inversine	Lotrel
Ativan	Ceredase	Depo-Provera	Eskalith	Ionsys	Luminal
Augmentin	Cipro	Desogen	Estrogel	Isoptin	Luvox
Avalide	Ciprodex	Desoxyn	Estrostep	Janumet	Lyrica
Avandamet	Claforan	Desyrel	Evista	Kadian	Macrobid
Avandia	Clarinex	Dexedrine	Factive	Kaletra	Macrodantin
Avelox	Claritin	DextroStat	FazaClo	Keflex	Marinol
Axid	Claritin-D	D.H.E. 45	Felbatol	Keppra	Maxipime
Axocet	Cleocin	Diabinese	Feldene	Kerlone	Maxzide
Azactam	Climara	Diastat	Femhrt	Ketek	Mefoxin
Azasan	Clozaril	Diflucan	Fiorinal	Klonopin	Menostar
Azathioprine	Codeine	Digitek	Flagyl	Kronofed-A	Metaglip
Azulfidine	Combigan	Dilacor	Floxin	Kutrase	*(continued)*

Methergine	Norinyl	Ponstel	Sanctura	Tiazac	Vaseretic
Methotrexate	Noritate	Prandimet	Sandimmune	Timolide	Vasotec
MetroCream	Normodyne	Pravachol	Santura XR	Timoptic	Ventavis
MetroGel	Norpace	Premphase	Sarafem	Tindamax	Verelan
MetroLotion	Norplant	Prempro	Seconal	Tobi	Vermox
Mexitil	Norpramin	Prevacid	Sectral	Tofranil	Versed
Micronor	Nor-QD	Prevacid	Semprex-D	Tolectin	Vibramycin
Microzide	Novantrone	NapraPAC	Septra	Toprol-XL	Vibra-Tabs
Migranal	Nubain	Prevpac	Seroquel	Toradol	Vicodin
Miltown	Nucofed	Prinzide	Seroquel XR	Trandate	Vigamox
Minizide	Nydrazid	Pristiq	Sinequan	Tranxene	Viramune
Minocin	Oramorph	Prograf	Slo-bid	Trental	Voltaren
Mirapex	Oretic	Proloprim	Soma	Tricor	Vytorin
Mircette	Ortho-Cept	Prometrium	Sonata	Triglide	Vyvanse
M-M-R II	Ortho-Cyclen	Pronestyl	Soriatane	Trilafon	Wellbutrin
Mobic	Ortho-Novum	Propofol	Spiriva	Trileptal	Xanax
Modicon	Ortho Tri-	Prosed/DS	Sprycel	Tri-Levlen	Xolair
Moduretic	Cyclen	Protonix	Stadol	Tri-Norinyl	Zantac
Monodox	Orudis	Provera	Stavzor	Triostat	Zarontin
Monopril	Ovcon	Prozac	Streptomycin	Triphasil	Zaroxolyn
Morphine	Oxistat	Pseudoephedrine	Stromectol	Trisenox	Zegerid
MS Contin	OxyContin	Pulmicort	Symbyax	Trivora	Zemplar
MSIR	OxyFast	Pyrazinamide	Symmetrel	Trizivir	Zestoretic
Myambutol	OxyIR	Quinidex	Synthroid	Trovan	Zetia
Mycamine	Pacerone	Quinine	Tagamet	Truvada	Ziac
Mysoline	Pamelor	Raptiva	Tambocor	Tygacil	Zinacef
Namenda	Pancrease	Reglan	Tapazole	Tylenol	Zithromax
Naprelan	Paxil	Relpax	Tarka	Tylenol with	Zocor
Naprosyn	PCE	Renese	Tasigna	Codeine	Zoloft
Nascobal	Pediapred	Requip	Tavist	Ultane	Zomig
Naturethroid	Pediazole	Reserpine	Tazicef	Ultram	Zonalon
Necon	Pediotic	Restoril	Tazidime	Unasyn	Zonegran
NegGram	Pentasa	Retrovir	Tegretol	Uniphyl	Zosyn
Nembutal	Pepcid	Rifadin	Tenoretic	Uniretic	Zovia
Neoral	Periostat	Rifamate	Tenormin	Unithroid	Zovirax
Neurontin	Persantine	Rifater	Tenuate	Urimax	Zyban
Niaspan	Pfizerpen	Rimactane	Tequin	Valium	Zydone
Nicotrol	Phenergan	Risperdal	Testoderm	Valtrex	Zyloprim
Niravam	Phenobarbital	Rocaltrol	Thalitone	Vanceril	Zyprexa
Nizoral	Phenytek	Rocephin	Theo-24	Vancocin	Zyrtec
Norco	Phrenilin	Roxanol	Theo-Dur	Vantin	
Nordette	Plan B	Rozerem	Thorazine	Vascor	

Reference

LaGow B, ed. *Drug Topics Red Book*. Montvale, N.J.: Thomson Healthcare; 2009.

Appendix G

Drugs That May Cause Photosensitivity

The drugs in this table are known to cause photosensitivity in some individuals. Effects can range from itching, scaling, rash, and swelling to skin cancer, premature skin aging, skin and eye burns, cataracts, reduced immunity, blood vessel damage, and allergic reactions.

The list is not all inclusive; it shows only representative brands of each generic. When in doubt, always check specific product labeling. Individuals should be advised to wear protective clothing and to apply sunscreens while taking the following medications.

Generic name	Trade name
Acamprosate	Campral
Acetazolamide	Diamox
Acitretin	Soriatane
Acyclovir	Zovirax
Alendronate	Fosamax
Aliskiren-hydrochlorothiazide	Tekturna HCT
Alitretinoin	Panretin
Almotriptan	Axert
Amiloride-hydrochlorothiazide	Moduretic
Aminolevulinic acid	Levulan Kerastick
Amiodarone	Cordarone, Pacerone
Amitriptyline	Elavil
Amitriptyline-chlordiazepoxide	Etrafon, Limbitrol
Amitriptyline-perphenazine	
Amlodipine-atorvastatin	Caduet
Amoxapine	Asendin
Amphetamine aspartate–amphetamine sulfate–dextroamphetamine saccharate–dextroamphetamine sulfate	Adderall XR
Anagrelide	Agrylin
Aripiprazole	Abilify
Atazanavir	Reyataz
Atenolol-chlorthalidone	Tenoretic
Atorvastatin	Lipitor
Atovaquone-proguanil	Malarone
Azatadine-pseudoephedrine	Rynatan, Trinalin
Azithromycin	Zithromax, Zmag
Benazepril	Lotensin
Benazepril-hydrochlorothiazide	Lotensin HCT
Bendroflumethiazide-nadolol	Corzide
Bexarotene	Targretin
Bismuth-metronidazole-tetracycline	Helidac
Bismuth subcitrate potassium-metronidazole-tetracycline	Pylera
Bisoprolol-hydrochlorothiazide	Ziac

Generic name	Trade name
Brompheniramine-dextromethorphan-phenylephrine	Alacol DM, Dimetane DX
Brompheniramine-dextromethorphan-pseudoephedrine	Bromfed-DM
Buffered aspirin–pravastatin	Pravigard PAC
Bupropion	Wellbutrin, Zyban
Candesartan-hydrochlorothiazide	Atacand HCT
Capecitabine	Xeloda
Captopril	Capoten
Captopril-hydrochlorothiazide	Capozide
Carbamazepine	Carbatrol, Equetro, Tegretol, Tegretol-XR
Carbinoxamine-pseudoephedrine	Palgic-D, Palgic-DS, Pediatex-D
Carvedilol	Coreg
Carvedilol phosphate	Coreg CR
Celecoxib	Celebrex
Cetirizine	Zyrtec
Cetirizine-pseudoephedrine	Zyrtec-D
Cevimeline	Evoxac
Chlorhexidine gluconate	Hibistat
Chloroquine	Aralen
Chlorothiazide	Diuril
Chlorothiazide sodium	Diuril I.V.
Chlorpheniramine-hydrocodone-pseudoephedrine	Tussend
Chlorpheniramine-phenylephrine	Rynatan
Chlorpromazine	Thorazine
Chlorpropamide	Diabinese
Chlorthalidone	Thalitone
Chlorthalidone-clonidine	Clorpres
Cidofovir	Vistide
Ciprofloxacin	Cipro, Cipro XR
Citalopram	Celexa
Clemastine	Tavist

(continued)

Generic name	Trade name	Generic name	Trade name
Clindamycin phosphate	Clindagel	Fluorouracil	Efudex
Clonidine-chlorthalidone	Clorpres	Fluoxetine	Prozac, Sarafem
Clozapine	Clozaril, Fazzaclo	Fluoxetine-olanzapine	Symbyax
Coagulation Factor IX (recombinant)	BeneFIX	Fluphenazine	Prolixin
		Flutamide	Eulexin
Cromolyn sodium	Gastrocrom	Fluvastatin	Lescol, Lescol XL
Cyclobenzaprine	Flexeril	Fluvoxamine	Luvox, Luvox CR
Cyproheptadine	Periactin	Fosinopril	Monopril
Dacarbazine	DTIC-Dome	Fosphenytoin	Cerebyx
Dantrolene	Dantrium	Furosemide	Lasix
Demeclocycline	Declomycin	Gabapentin	Neurontin
Desipramine	Norpramin	Gatifloxacin	Tequin
Diclofenac potassium	Cataflam	Gemfibrozil	Lopid
Diclofenac sodium	Voltaren	Gemifloxacin mesylate	Factive
Diclofenac sodium-misoprostol	Arthrotec	Gentamicin	Garamycin
Diflunisal	Dolobid	Glatiramer acetate	Copaxone
Dihydroergotamine	D.H.E. 45	Glimepiride	Amaryl
Diltiazem	Cardizem, Tiazac	Glimepiride–pioglitazone hydrochloride	Duetact
Diphenhydramine	Benadryl		
Divalproex	Depakote	Glimepiride–rosiglitazone maleate	Avandaryl
Doxepin	Sinequan		
Doxycycline hyclate	Doryx, Periostat, Vibramycin, Vibra-Tabs	Glipizide	Glucotrol
		Glyburide	DiaBeta, Glynase, Micronase
Doxycycline monohydrate	Monodox	Glyburide–metformin HCl	Glucovance
Duloxetine	Cymbalta	Griseofulvin	Fulvicin P/G, Grifulvin, Gris-PEG
Efalizumab	Raptiva		
Enalapril	Vasotec	Haloperidol	Haldol
Enalapril-felodipine	Lexxel	Hexachlorophene	pHisoHex
Enalapril-hydrochlorothiazide	Vaseretic	Hydralazine-hydrochlorothiazide	Hydra-Zide
Enalaprilat (injection)	Vasotec IV	Hydrochlorothiazide	HydroDIURIL, Microzide, Oretic
Epirubicin	Ellence		
Eprosartan mesylate–hydrochlorothiazide	Teveten HCT	Hydrochlorothiazide-fosinopril	Monopril HCT
		Hydrochlorothiazide-irbesartan	Avalide
Erythromycin-sulfisoxazole	Pediazole	Hydrochlorothiazide-lisinopril	Prinzide, Zestoretic
Escitalopram oxalate	Lexapro	Hydrochlorothiazide—losartan potassium	Hyzaar
Esomeprazole	Nexium		
Estazolam	ProSom	Hydrochlorothiazide-methyldopa	Aldoril
Estradiol	Estrogel, Gynodiol	Hydrochlorothiazide-metoprolol tartrate	Lopressor HCT
Eszopiclone	Lunesta		
Ethionamide	Trecator-SC	Hydrochlorothiazide-moexipril	Uniretic
Etodolac	Lodine	Hydrochlorothiazide-propranolol	Inderide
Felbamate	Felbatol	Hydrochlorothiazide-quinapril	Accuretic
Fenofibrate	Lofibra, Tricor, Triglide	Hydrochlorothiazide-spironolactone	Aldactazide
Floxuridine	Sterile FUDR	Hydrochlorothiazide-telmisartan	Micardis HCT
Flucytosine	Ancobon	Hydrochlorothiazide-timolol	Timolide

Generic name	Trade name	Generic name	Trade name
Hydrochlorothiazide-triamterene	Dyazide, Maxide	Methyclothiazide	Enduron
Hydrochlorothiazide-valsartan	Diovan HCT	Methyldopa-hydrochlorothiazide	Aldoril
Hydroflumethiazide		Metolazone	Mykrox, Zaroxolyn
Hydroxocobalamin	Cyanokit Antidote	Metoprolol succinate	Toprol-XL
Hydroxychloroquine	Plaquenil	Metoprolol tartrate	Lopressor
Hypericum	Kira, St. John's wort	Minocycline	Dynacin, Minocin, Solodyn
Hypericum–vitamin B$_1$–vitamin C–kava-kava	One-A-Day Tension & Mood	Mirtazapine	Remeron
		Moexipril	Univasc
Ibuprofen	Motrin	Moexipril-hydrochlorothiazide	Uniretic
Imatinib Mesylate	Gleevec	Moxifloxacin	Avelox
Imipramine	Tofranil	Nabilone	Cesamet
Imiquimod	Aldara	Nabumetone	Relafen
Indapamide	Lozol	Nadolol-bendroflumethiazide	Corzide
Interferon alfa-2b, recombinant	Intron A	Nalidixic acid	Neggram
Interferon alfa-n3 (human leukocyte derived)	Alferon-N	Naproxen	Naprosyn, EC-Naprosyn
Interferon beta-1a	Avonex	Naproxen sodium	Anaprox, Anaprox DS, Naprelan
Interferon beta-1b	Betaseron	Naratriptan	Amerge
Irbesartan-hydrochlorothiazide	Avalide	Nefazodone	Serzone
Isocarboxazid	Marplan	Nifedipine	Adalat CC, Procardia
Isoniazid-pyrazinamide-rifampin	Rifater	Nisoldipine	Sular
Isotretinoin	Accutane, Amnesteem	Norfloxacin	Noroxin
Itraconazole	Sporanox	Nortriptyline	Pamelor
Ketoprofen	Orudis, Oruvail	Ofloxacin	Floxin
Lamotrigine	Lamictal	Olanzapine	Zyprexa
Leuprolide acetate	Lupron, Lupron Depot	Olanzapine-fluoxetine	Symbyax
Levamisole	Levamisole	Olmesartan medoxomil–hydrochlorothiazide	Benicar HCT
Levofloxacin	Levaquin		
Levofloxacin–5% dextrose	Levaquin Injection	Olsalazine	Dipentum
Lisinopril	Prinivil, Zestril	Omeprazole–sodium bicarbonate	Zegerid
Lisinopril-hydrochlorothiazide	Prinzide, Zestoretic		
Lomefloxacin	Maxaquin	Oxaprozin	Daypro
Loratadine	Claritin	Oxcarbazepine	Trileptal
Loratadine-pseudoephedrine	Claritin-D	Oxycodone	Roxicodone
Losartan	Cozaar	Oxytetracycline	Terramycin
Losartan-hydrochlorothiazide	Hyzaar	Panitumumab	Vectibix
Lovastatin	Altoprev, Mevacor	Pantoprazole	Protonix
Lovastatin-niacin	Advicor	Paroxetine hydrochloride	Paxil
Maprotiline	Ludiomil	Paroxetine mesylate	Pexeva
Mefenamic acid	Ponstel	Pastinaca sativa	Parsnip
Meloxicam	Mobic	Pentosan polysulfate	Elmiron
Mesalamine	Pentasa	Pentostatin	Nipent
Methazolamide	Glauctabs, Neptazane	Perphenazine	Trilafon
Methotrexate	Trexall	Pilocarpine	Salagen
Methoxsalen	8-MOP, Oxsoralen, Uvadex	Piroxicam	Feldene

(continued)

Generic name	Trade name
Polymyxin B sulfate–trimethoprim sulfate	Polytrim
Polythiazide	Renese
Polythiazide-prazosin	Minizide
Porfimer sodium	Photofrin
Pramipexole dihydrochloride	Mirapex
Pravastatin	Pravachol
Pregabalin	Lyrica
Prochlorperazine	Compazine, Compro
Promethazine	Phenergan
Protriptyline	Vivactil
Pyrazinamide	Pyrazinamide
Pyrimethamine-sulfadoxine	Fansidar
Quetiapine	Seroquel
Quinapril	Accupril
Quinapril-hydrochlorothiazide	Accuretic
Quinidine gluconate	Quinidine
Quinidine sulfate	Quinidex
Rabeprazole sodium	Aciphex
Ramipril	Altace
Rasagiline mesylate	Azilect
Riluzole	Rilutek
Risperidone	Risperdal, Risperdal Consta
Ritonavir	Norvir
Rizatriptan	Maxalt, Maxalt-MLT
Ropinirole	Requip
Rosuvastatin	Crestor
Ruta graveolens	Rue
Saquinavir mesylate	Invirase
Selegiline	Eldepryl, Emsam
Sertraline	Zoloft
Sibutramine	Meridia
Sildenafil	Viagra
Simvastatin	Zocor
Simvastatin-ezetimibe	Vytorin
Sirolimus	Rapamune
Somatropin	Serostim
Sotalol	Betapace, Betapace AF
Sulfamethoxazole-trimethoprim	Bactrim, Septra

Generic name	Trade name
Sulfasalazine	Azulfidine
Sulfisoxazole acetyl	Gantrisin Pediatric
Sulindac	Clinoril
Sumatriptan	Imitrex
Tacrolimus	Prograf, Protopic
Tazarotene	Tazorac
Telmisartan-hydrochlorothiazide	Micardis HCT
Tetracycline	Sumycin
Thalidomide	Thalomid
Thioridazine hydrochloride	Thioridazine HCl
Thiothixene	Navane
Tiagabine	Gabitril
Tigecycline	Tygacil
Tolazamide	Tolinase
Tolbutamide	Orinase
Topiramate	Topamax
Tretinoin	Avita, Retin-A
Triamcinolone acetonide	Azmacort Inhalation
Triamterene	Dyrenium
Triamterene-hydrochlorothiazide	Dyazide, Maxzide
Trifluoperazine	Trifluoperazine
Trimipramine	Surmontil
Trovafloxacin	Trovan
Valacyclovir	Valtrex
Valdecoxib	Bextra
Valproate	Depacon
Valproic acid	Depakene
Valsartan-hydrochlorothiazide	Diovan HCT
Vardenafil	Levitra
Varenicline tartrate	Chantix
Venlafaxine	Effexor, Effexor XR
Verteporfin	Visudyne
Vinblastine	Velban
Voriconazole	Vfend
Zalcitabine	Hivid
Zaleplon	Sonata
Ziprasidone	Geodon
Zolmitriptan	Zomig
Zolpidem	Ambien, Ambien CR

Reference

LaGow B, ed. *Drug Topics Red Book*. Montvale, N.J.: Thomson Healthcare; 2009.

Appendix H

Drug Information Resources by Category

General Drug Information

AHFS Drug Information
(www.ahfsdruginformation.com)
Drug Information Handbook
Facts & Comparisons
(www.factsandcomparisons.com)
Lexi-Comp Online (http://online.lexi.com)
Micromedex DRUGDEX
(www.micromedex.com/products/drugdex/)
Physicians' Desk Reference
UpToDate (www.uptodateonline.com/online)

Adverse Drug Reactions and Specific Uses

Clinical Alerts (www.nlm.nih.gov/databases/alerts/
clinical_alerts.html)
Davies's Textbook of Adverse Drug Reactions
Institute for Safe Medication Practices (www.ismp.org)
Meyler's Side Effects of Drugs
Side Effects of Drugs Annual
U.S. Food and Drug Administration (FDA) MedWatch
Program (www.fda.gov/medwatch/safety.htm)
Vaccine Adverse Event Reporting System
(http://vaers.hhs.gov/professionals/index)

Chemical and Physical Properties

CRC Handbook of Chemistry and Physics
Merck Index
Remington: The Science and Practice of Pharmacy
*Textbook of Organic, Medicinal, and Pharmaceutical
Chemistry*
United States Pharmacopeia–National Formulary
USP Dictionary

Compounding

Allen's Compounded Formulations
Handbook on Extemporaneous Formulations
International Academy of Compounding Pharmacists
(www.iacprx.org)
Trissel's Stability of Compounded Formulations

Drug Interactions

Drug Interaction Facts
Evaluation of Drug Interactions

Facts & Comparisons
(www.factsandcomparisons.com)
*Hansten and Horn's Drug Interactions Analysis and
Management*
Lexi-Comp Online (http://online.lexi.com)
Liverpool HIV Pharmacology Group
(www.hiv-druginteractions.org)
Micromedex DRUG-REAX
(www.micromedex. com/products/drugreax/)

Foreign Drugs

British National Formulary (www.bnf.org/bnf/)
The British Pharmacopoeia
(www.pharmacopoeia.co.uk/)
Drug Facts and Comparisons (Canadian Trade Name
Index)
electronics Medicines Compendium (eMC)
(www.medicines.org.uk)
Martindale: The Complete Drug Reference
Micromedex Index Nominum (www.micromedex.
com/products/indexnominum/)
Royal Pharmaceutical Society of Great Britain
(www.rpsgb.org.uk)

Immunology

Center for Biologics Evaluation and Research (http://
www.fda.gov/BiologicsBloodVaccines/default.htm)
Centers for Disease Control and Prevention (CDC)
(www.cdc.gov/vaccines/)
Concepts in Immunology and Immunotherapeutics
Immunization Action Coalition (www.immunize.org)
ImmunoFacts (www.immunofacts.com)
U.S. Department of Health and Human Services
(www.hrsa.gov/vaccinecompensation/)

Infectious Disease

*Mandell, Douglas, and Bennett's Principles and
Practice of Infectious Disease*
Sanford Guide to Antimicrobial Therapy

Intravenous Compatibility and Stability

Guide to Parenteral Admixtures
Handbook on Injectable Drugs (Trissel's)
Micromedex IV Index (www.micromedex.com/
products/ivindex/) (Trissel's)
Trissel's Tables of Physical Compatibility
King Guide to Parenteral Admixtures

Investigational Drugs

CenterWatch (www.centerwatch.com/
patient/trials.html)
Facts & Comparisons
(www.factsandcomparisons.com)
ImmunoFacts (www.immunofacts.com)
Inteleos (www.inteleos.com)
National Institutes of Health Clinical Trials Database
(www.clinicaltrials.gov)
Pharmaceutical Research and Manufacturers of
America (www.phrma.org)

Laboratory Tests

Basic Skills in Interpreting Laboratory Data
Clinical Guide to Laboratory Tests
Laboratory Tests and Diagnostic Procedures
Laboratory Test Handbook

Legal and Regulatory Issues

Code of Federal Regulations (Title 21)
(www.accessdata.fda.gov/SCRIPTs/cdrh/cfdocs/
cfcfr/CFRSearch.cfm)
Guide to Federal Pharmacy Law
Joint Commission on Accreditation of Healthcare
Organizations (www.jcaho.org)
National Association of Boards of Pharmacy
(www.nabp.net)
Pharmacy Law Digest
United States Pharmacopeia–National Formulary
U.S. Drug Enforcement Administration
(www.usdoj. gov/dea/)
U.S. Food and Drug Administration (www.fda.gov)
USP DI Volume III: Approved Drug Products and
Legal Requirements
World Health Organization (www.who.int/en/)

Literature Search Databases

EMBASE (www.embase.com)
CINAHL (www.ebscohost.com/cinahl/)
IDIS (http://itsnt14.its.uiowa.edu/)
IPA (http://library.dialog.com/bluesheets/html/
bl0074.html)
MEDLINE/PubMed
(www.ncbi.nlm.nih.gov/pubmed/)
Ovid (www.ovid.com)
PsycINFO (www.apa.org/psycinfo/)

Manufacturer Information

American Drug Index
Drug Topics Red Book

Facts & Comparisons
(www.factsandcomparisons.com)
Inteleos (www.inteleos.com)
Manufacturer Web sites (various)
Martindale: The Complete Drug Reference
Micromedex (www.micromedex.com/products/hcs/)
Mosby's GenRX
Physicians' Desk Reference

New Drug Approvals

CenterWatch (www.centerwatch.com/
drug-information/)
Drugs@FDA (www.accessdata.fda.gov/
scripts/cder/drugsatfda)
Medical Letter (www.medicalletter.org)
Pharmacist's Letter (www.pharmacistsletter.com)
The Pink Sheet (www.thepinksheet.com)
U.S. Food and Drug Administration (www.fda.
gov)

Nonpharmacologic Use

Handbook of Nonprescription Drugs
Herbs of Choice
National Center for Alternative and Complementary
Medicine (http://nccam.nih.gov)
National Institutes of Health Office of Dietary Supple-
ments (http://dietary-supplements.info.nih.gov)
Natural Medicines Comprehensive Database
(http:// www.naturaldatabase.com)
PDR for Nonprescription Drugs and Dietary
Supplements
The Review of Natural Products
The Complete German Commission E Monographs
U.S. Food and Drug Administration Center for
Food Safety and Applied Nutrition's Dietary
Supplements (www.fda.gov/Food/
DietarySupplements/default.htm)

Patient Counseling

MD Consult (www.mdconsult.com)
Medication Teaching Manual (American Society of
Health-System Pharmacists)
Micromedex CareNotes (www.micromedex.com/
products/carenotes/)
Professional's Guide to Patient Drug Facts
UpToDate (www.uptodateonline.com/online)

Pharmacokinetics

Applied Pharmacokinetics
Clinical Pharmacokinetics

Pharmacology

Basic Concepts and Clinical Applications
Goodman and Gilman's The Pharmacological Basic of Therapeutics
Melmon and Morrelli's Clinical Pharmacology
Principles of Pharmacology
Textbook of Pharmacology

Poisoning and Toxicology

Clinical Management of Poisoning and Drug Overdose
Clinical Toxicology of Drugs
Goldfrank's Toxicologic Emergencies
Handbook of Poisoning
Micromedex POISINDEX (www.micromedex.com/products/poisindex/)
Physical and Theoretical Chemistry Laboratory Oxford University (http://physchem.ox.ac.uk/MSDS/)
Poisoning and Toxicology Compendium
Principles of Clinical Toxicology
ToxNet (http://toxnet.nlm.nih.gov/)
U.S. Environmental Protection Agency Integrated Risk Information System (http://www.epa.gov/iris/)

Pregnancy and Lactation

Breastfeeding: A Guide for the Medical Profession
Drugs in Pregnancy and Lactation
Drugs in Pregnancy and Breastfeeding (www.perinatology.com/exposures/druglist.htm)
Micromedex REPRORISK (www.micromedex.com/products/reprorisk/)

Product Identification

American Drug Index
Drug Information Online (http://www.drugs.com/imprints.php)
Drug Topics Red Book
Facts & Comparisons (www.factsandcomparisons.com)
Ident-A-Drug (http://identadrug.com)
Micromedex IDENTIDEX (www.micromedex.com/products/identidex/)
RxList (www.rxlist.com)

Renal Dose Adjustments

Drug Prescribing in Renal Failure
GlobalRPh.com (www.globalrph.com/renaldosing.htm)
Handbook of Dialysis

Shortage Information

ASHP Drug Shortage Center (www.ashp.org/shortages)
Drug wholesaler Web sites (various)
FDA Drug Shortage Resource Center (www.fda.gov/cder/drug/shortages/)

Specific Patient Population: Geriatric

Drug Therapy in the Elderly
Geriatric Dosage Handbook
Therapeutics in the Elderly

Specific Patient Population: Pediatric

The Harriet Lane Handbook
Lexi-Comp's Pediatric Dosage Handbook
Micromedex NeoFax (www.micromedex.com/products/neofax/)
Nelson Textbook of Pediatrics
Principles and Practice of Pediatrics
Teddy Bear Book: Pediatric Injectable Drugs

Therapeutics and Drug Therapy

Applied Therapeutics: The Clinical Use of Drugs
Cecil Textbook of Medicine
Harrison's Principles of Internal Medicine
Medical Letter (www.medicalletter.org)
Merck Manual of Diagnosis and Therapy (http://www.merck.com/mmpe/)
Pharmacist's Letter (www.pharmacistsletter.com)
Pharmacotherapy: A Pathophysiologic Approach
Textbook of Therapeutics: Drug and Disease Management
The Washington Manual of Medical Therapeutics

Appendix I

Drugs That Should Not Be Crushed

The following list includes both various slow-release and enteric-coated products that should not be crushed or chewed. Slow-release (SR) products are controlled-release, extended-release, long-acting, or timed-release products. Enteric-coated (EC) products are delayed-release products. In general, capsules containing SR or EC particles may be opened and their contents administered on a spoonful of soft food. However, instruct patients not to chew the particles. (Patients should, in fact, be discouraged from chewing any medication unless it is specifically formulated for that purpose.)

The list should not be considered all inclusive. Generic and alternate brands of some products may exist. Tablets intended for sublingual or buccal administration (not included in this list) should also be administered only as intended, in an intact form.

Drug	Manufacturer	Form	Drug	Manufacturer	Form
Abletex LA	Able	SR	Amibid LA	Amide	SR
Aciphex	Eisai	EC	Amrix	ECR	SR
Adalat CC	Schering-Plough	SR	Anextuss	Cypress	SR
Adderall XR	Shire US	SR	Anti-tussive	Qualitest	SR
Advicor	KOS	SR	Aplenzin	Biovail	SR
Aerohist	Aero	SR	Aquabid-DM	Alphagen	SR
Aerohist Plus	Aero	SR	Aquatab C	Adams	SR
Afeditab CR	Watson	SR	Aquatab D	Adams	SR
Aggrenox	Boehringer Ingelheim	SR	Aquatab DM	Adams	SR
Ala-Hist	Poly	SR	Arthrotec	Pharmacia	EC
Ala-Hist D	Poly	SR	Asacol	Procter & Gamble	EC
Aleve Cold & Sinus	Bayer HealthCare	SR	Ascocid-500-D	Key	SR
Aleve Sinus & Headache	Bayer HealthCare	SR	Ascocid-1000	Key	SR
Allegra-D 12 Hour	Sanofi-Aventis	SR	Ascriptin Enteric	Novartis Consumer	EC
Allegra-D 24 Hour	Sanofi-Aventis	SR	Atrohist Pediatric	Celltech	SR
Allerx	Cornerstone	SR	Augmentin XR	GlaxoSmithKline	SR
Allerx-D	Cornerstone	SR	Avinza	Ligand	SR
Allfen	MCR American	SR	Azulfidine Entabs	Pharmacia	EC
Allfen-DM	MCR American	SR	Bayer Aspirin Regimen	Bayer HealthCare	EC
Alophen	Numark	EC	Biaxin XL	Abbott	SR
Altoprev	First Horizon	SR	Bidex-A	SJ	SR
Ambi 45/800	Ambi	SR	Bidhist	Cypress	SR
Ambi 45/800/30	Ambi	SR	Bidhist-D	Cypress	SR
Ambi 60/580	Ambi	SR	Bisac-Evac	G&W	EC
Ambi 60/580/30	Ambi	SR	Biscolax	Global Source	EC
Ambi 80/700	Ambi	SR	Blanex-A	Blansett	SR
Ambi 80/700/40	Ambi	SR	Bontril Slow-Release	Valeant	SR
Ambi 1000/55	Ambi	SR	Bromfed	Victory	SR
Ambien CR	Sanofi-Aventis	SR	Bromfed-PD	Victory	SR
Ambifed-G	Ambi	SR	Bromfenex	Ethex	SR
Ambifed-G DM	Ambi	SR	Bromfenex PD	Ethex	SR
Amdry-C	Prasco	SR	Bromfenex PE	Ethex	SR
Amdry-D	Prasco	SR	Bromfenex PE Pediatric	Ethex	SR

Drug	Manufacturer	Form	Drug	Manufacturer	Form
Budeprion SR	Teva	SR	Deconex	Poly	SR
Budeprion XL	Teva	SR	Deconex DM	Poly	SR
Buproban	Teva	SR	Deconsal II	Cornerstone	SR
Calan SR	Pharmacia	SR	Depakote	Abbott	EC
Campral	Forest	EC	Depakote ER	Abbott	SR
Carbatrol	Shire US	SR	Depakote Sprinkles	Abbott	EC
Cardene SR	Roche	SR	Despec SR	International Ethical	SR
Cardizem CD	Biovail	SR	Detrol LA	Pharmacia	SR
Cardizem LA	Kos	SR	Dexedrine Spansules	GlaxoSmithKline	SR
Cardura XL	Pfizer	SR	D-Feda II	WE Pharmaceuticals	SR
Carox Plus	Seneca	SR	D-Hist D	Midlothian	SR
Cartia XT	Andrx	SR	Diabetes Trio	Mason Vitamins	SR
Cemill 500	Miller	SR	Diamox Sequels	Duramed	SR
Cemill 1000	Miller	SR	Dilacor XR	Watson	SR
Certuss-D	Capellon	SR	Dilantin	Pfizer	SR
Cevi-Bid	Lee	SR	Dilantin Kapseals	Pfizer	SR
Chlorex-A	Cypress	SR	Dilatrate-SR	Schwarz Pharma	SR
Chlor-Phen	Truxton	SR	Diltia XT	Andrx	SR
Chlor-Trimeton Allergy	Schering-Plough	SR	Dilt-CD	Apotex	SR
Chlor-Trimeton Allergy Decongestant	Schering-Plough	SR	Dilt-XR	Apotex	SR
			Dimetane Extentabs	Wyeth	SR
Cipro XR	Schering-Plough	SR	Disophrol Chronotab	Schering-Plough	SR
Claritin-D	Schering-Plough	SR	Ditropan XL	Ortho-McNeil	SR
Claritin-D 12 Hour	Schering-Plough	SR	Donnatal Extentabs	PBM	SR
Claritin-D 24 Hour	Schering-Plough	SR	Doryx	Warner Chilcott	EC
Coldamine	Breckenridge	SR	D-Phen 1000	Midlothian	SR
Coldex-A	United Research	SR	Drexophed SR	Qualitest	SR
Concerta	McNeil Consumer	SR	Drihist SR	Prasco	SR
Contac 12-Hour	GlaxoSmithKline	SR	Drixoral	Schering-Plough	SR
Coreg CR	GlaxoSmithKline	SR	Drixoral Plus	Schering-Plough	SR
Correctol	Schering-Plough	EC	Drixoral Sinus	Schering-Plough	SR
Cotazym-S	Organon	EC	Drize-R	Monarch	SR
Covera-HS	Pfizer	SR	Drysec	AG Marin	SR
CPM 8/PE 20/MSC 1.25	Cypress	SR	D-Tab	Palm	SR
CPM 12	Brighton	SR	Dulcolax	Boehringer Ingelheim	EC
Creon 5	Solvay	EC	Duomax	Capellon	SR
Creon 10	Solvay	EC	Durahist	Proethic	SR
Creon 20	Solvay	EC	Durahist D	Proethic	SR
Cymbalta	Eli Lilly	EC	Durahist PE	Proethic	SR
Dairycare	Plainview	EC	Duratuss	Victory	SR
Dallergy	Laser	SR	Duratuss CS	Victory	SR
Dallergy-JR	Laser	SR	Duratuss DA	Victory	SR
Deconamine SR	Kenwood Therapeutics	SR	Duratuss GP	Victory	SR

(continued)

Drug	Manufacturer	Form	Drug	Manufacturer	Form
Dynacirc CR	Reliant	SR	Flagyl ER	Pharmacia	SR
Dynahist-ER Pediatric	Breckenridge	SR	Fleet Bisacodyl	C.B. Fleet	EC
Dynex LA	Athlon	SR	Focalin XR	Novartis	SR
Dynex VR	Athlon	SR	Folitab 500	Rising	SR
Dytan-CS	Hawthorn	SR	Fortamet	First Horizon	SR
Easprin	Harvest	EC	Fumatinic	Laser	SR
EC Naprosyn	Roche	EC	Genacote	Wax	EC
Ecotrin	GlaxoSmithKline	EC	GFN 500/DM 30	Cypress	SR
Ecotrin Adult Low Strength	GlaxoSmithKline	EC	GFN 550/PSE 60	Cypress	SR
Ecotrin Maximum Strength	GlaxoSmithKline	EC	GFN 550/PSE 60/DM 30	Cypress	SR
Ecpirin	Prime Marketing	EC	GFN 595/PSE 48	Cypress	SR
Ed A-Hist	Edwards	SR	GFN 595/PSE 48/DM 32	Cypress	SR
Effexor-XR	Wyeth	SR	GFN 600/Phenylephrine 20	Cypress	SR
Efidac 24 Chlorpheniramine	Novartis Consumer	SR	GFN 600/PSE 60/DM 30	Cypress	SR
Efidac 24 Pseudoephedrine	Novartis Consumer	SR	GFN 1000/DM 50	Cypress	SR
Enablex	Novartis	SR	GFN 1200/DM 60	Cypress	SR
Endal	Pediamed	SR	GFN 1200/DM 60/PSE 60	Cypress	SR
Entab-DM	Rising	SR	GFN 1200/Phenylephrine 40	Cypress	SR
Entercote	Global Source	EC	GFN 1200/PSE 50	Cypress	SR
Entex LA	Andrx	SR	Gilphex TR	Gil	SR
Entex PSE	Andrx	SR	Giltuss TR	Gil	SR
Entocort EC	Prometheus	EC	Glucophage XR	Bristol-Myers Squibb	SR
Equetro	Shire US	SR	Glucotrol XL	Pfizer	SR
ERCY	Warner Chilcott	SR	Glumetza	Depomed	SR
Ery-Tab	Abbott	EC	G/P 1200/75	Cypress	SR
Eskalith-CR	GlaxoSmithKline	SR	Guaifenex DM	Ethex	SR
Execof	Larken	SR	Guaifenex GP	Ethex	SR
Exefen-DM	Larken	SR	Guaifenex PSE 60	Ethex	SR
Exefen-DMX	Larken	SR	Guaifenex PSE 80	Ethex	SR
Exefen-PD	Larken	SR	Guaifenex PSE 85	Ethex	SR
ExeTuss-DM	Larken	SR	Guaifenex PSE 120	Ethex	SR
Extendryl G	Fleming	SR	H 9600 SR	Hawthorn	SR
Extendryl JR	Fleming	SR	Halfprin	Kramer	EC
Extendryl SR	Fleming	SR	Hemax	Pronova	SR
Extress-30	Key	SR	Histacol LA	Breckenridge	SR
Extress-60	Key	SR	Hista-Vent DA	Ethex	SR
Feen-a-mint	Schering-Plough	EC	Hista-Vent PSE	Ethex	SR
Femilax	G&W	EC	Humavent LA	WE Pharmaceuticals	SR
Fero-Folic-500	Abbott	SR	Humibid	Adams	SR
Fero-Grad-500	Abbott	SR	Humibid DM	Carolina	SR
Ferro-Sequels	Inverness Medical	SR	Humibid LA	Carolina	SR
Ferrous Fumarate DS	Vita-Rx	SR	Iberet-500	Abbott	SR
Fetrin	Lunsco	SR	Iberet-Folic-500	Abbott	SR

Drug	Manufacturer	Form	Drug	Manufacturer	Form
Icar-C Plus SR	Hawthorn	SR	Mag64	Rising	EC
Imdur	Schering-Plough	SR	Mag-SR Plus Calcium	Cypress	SR
Inderal LA	Wyeth	SR	Mag-Tab SR	Niche	SR
Indocin SR	Forte Pharma	SR	Maxifed	MCR American	SR
Innopran XL	Reliant	SR	Maxifed DM	MCR American	SR
Invega	Janssen	SR	Maxifed DMX	MCR American	SR
Isochron	Forest	SR	Maxifed G	MCR American	SR
Isopro	Rugby	SR	Maxiphen DM	Ambi	SR
Isoptin SR	FSC	SR	Medent DM	SJ	SR
Kadian	Alphagen	SR	Medent PE	SJ	SR
Kaon-Cl 10	Savage	SR	Mega-C	Merit	SR
Keppra XR	UCB	SR	Melfiat	Numark	SR
Klor-Con 8	Upsher-Smith	SR	Menopause Trio	Mason Vitamins	SR
Klor-Con 10	Upsher-Smith	SR	Mestinon Timespan	Valeant	SR
Klor-Con M10	Upsher-Smith	SR	Metadate CD	Celltech	SR
Klor-Con M15	Upsher-Smith	SR	Metadate ER	Celltech	SR
Klor-Con M20	Upsher-Smith	SR	Methylin ER	Mallinckrodt	SR
Klotrix	Bristol-Myers Squibb	SR	Micro-K	Ther-Rx	SR
K-Tab	Abbott	SR	Micro-K 10	Ther-Rx	SR
K-Tan	Prasco	SR	Mild-C	Carlson	SR
Lescol XL	Novartis	SR	Mindal DM	Breckenridge	SR
Levall G	Athlon	SR	Montephen	Monte Sano	SR
Levbid	Alaven	SR	MS Contin	Purdue	SR
Levsinex	Schwarz Pharma	SR	Mucinex	Adams	SR
Lexxel	AstraZeneca	SR	Mucinex D	Adams	SR
Lialda	Shire	EC	Mucinex DM	Adams	SR
Lipram 4500	Global	EC	Multi-Ferrous Folic	United Research	SR
Lipram-PN10	Global	EC	Multiret Folic-500	Amide	SR
Lipram-PN16	Global	EC	Mydex	Larken	SR
Lipram-PN20	Global	EC	Mydocs	Centurion	SSR
Liquibid-D	Capellon	SR	Myfortic	Novartis	EC
Liquibid-D 1200	Capellon	SR	Nacon	Cypress	SR
Liquibid-PD	Capellon	SR	Nalex-A	Blansett	SR
Lithobid	Capellon	SR	Naprelan	Blansett	SR
Lodrane 12 hour	ECR	SR	Nasatab LA	ECR	SR
Lodrane 12D	ECR	SR	New Ami-Tex LA	Amide	SR
Lodrane 24	ECR	SR	Nexium	AstraZeneca	EC
Lodrane 24D	ECR	SR	Niaspan	Kos	SR
Lohist-12	Larken	SR	Nicomide	Sirius	SR
Lohist-12D	Larken	SR	Nifediac CC	Teva	SR
Lusonex	Wraser	SR	Nifedical XL	Teva	SR
Luvox CR	Jazz Pharmaceuticals	SR	Nitrocot	Truxton	SR
Mag Delay	Major	EC	Nitro-Time	Time-Cap	SR

(continued)

Drug	Manufacturer	Form	Drug	Manufacturer	Form
Nohist	Larken	SR	Pentasa	Shire US	SR
Nohist-Plus	Larken	SR	Pentopak	Zoetica	SR
Nohist-Plus JR	Larken	SR	Pentoxil	Upsher-Smith	SR
Norel SR	U.S. Pharmaceuticals	SR	Phenabid	Gil	SR
Norpace CR	Pharmacia	SR	Phenabid DM	Gil	SR
Obstetrix EC	Seyer Pharmatec	EC	Phenavent	Ethex	SR
Omnihist LA	WE Pharmaceuticals	SR	Phenavent D	Ethex	SR
Opana ER	Endo	SR	Phenavent LA	Ethex	SR
Oramorph SR	AAI Pharma	SR	Phenavent PED	Ethex	SR
Oracea	Collagenex	SR	Phendiet-105	Truxton	SR
Oruvail	Wyeth	SR	Phenytek	Mylan Bertek	SR
Oxycontin	Purdue	SR	Phlemex-PE	Cypress	SR
Palcaps 10	Breckenridge	EC	Plendil	AstraZeneca	SR
Palcaps 20	Breckenridge	EC	Poly Hist Forte	Poly	SR
Pancrease	McNeil Consumer	EC	Poly-Vent	Poly	SR
Pancrease MT 10	McNeil Consumer	EC	Poly-Vent Jr	Poly	SR
Pancrease MT 16	McNeil Consumer	EC	Prehist D	Marnel	SR
Pancrease MT 20	McNeil Consumer	EC	Prevacid	Tap	EC
Pancrecarb MS-4	Digestive Care	EC	Prilosec	AstraZeneca	EC
Pancrecarb MS-8	Digestive Care	EC	Prilosec OTC	Procter & Gamble	SR
Pancrecarb MS-16	Digestive Care	EC	Pristiq	Wyeth	SR
Pancrelipase 4500	Mutual	EC	Procanbid	Monarch	SR
Pangestyme CN 10	Ethex	EC	Procardia XL	Pfizer	SR
Pangestyme CN 20	Ethex	EC	Prolex PD	Blansett	SR
Pangestyme EC	Ethex	EC	Prolex D	Blansett	SR
Pangestyme MT 16	Ethex	EC	Pronestyl-SR	Bristol-Myers Squibb	SR
Pangestyme UL 12	Ethex	EC	Proquin XR	Esprit	SR
Pangestyme UL 18	Ethex	EC	Prosed EC	Star	EC
Pangestyme UL 20	Ethex	EC	Proset-D	Blansett	SR
PanMist DM	Pamlab	SR	Protid	Lunsco	SR
PanMist JR	Pamlab	SR	Protonix	Wyeth	EC
PanMist LA	Pamlab	SR	Prozac Weekly	Eli Lilly	EC
Panocaps	Breckenridge	EC	Pseubrom	Alphagen	SR
Panocaps MT 16	Breckenridge	EC	Pseubrom-PD	Alphagen	SR
Panocaps MT 20	Breckenridge	EC	Pseudocot-C	Truxton	SR
Papacon	Consolidated Midland	SR	Pseudocot-G	Truxton	SR
Para-Time SR	Time-Cap	SR	Pseudovent	Ethex	SR
Paser	Jacobus	SR	Pseudovent 400	Ethex	SR
Pavacot	Truxton	SR	Pseudovent DM	Ethex	SR
Paxil CR	GlaxoSmithKline	SR	Pseudovent PED	Ethex	SR
PCE Dispertab	Abbott	SR	Quibron-T/SR	Monarch	SR
PCM LA	Cypress	SR	Quindal	Qualitest	SR
Pendex	Cypress	SR	Ralix	Cypress	SR

Drug	Manufacturer	Form	Drug	Manufacturer	Form
Ranexa	CV Therapeutics	SR	Sudal DM	Atley	SR
Razadyne ER	Ortho-McNeil	SR	Sudal SR	Atley	SR
Reliable Gentle Laxative	Ivex	EC	Sudatex-DM	Larken	SR
Requip XL	GlaxoSmithKline	SR	Sudatex-G	Larken	SR
Rescon-Jr	Capellon	SR	Sudatrate	Larken	SR
Rescon-MX	Capellon	SR	Sudex Tab	Atley	SR
Respa-1st	Respa	SR	Sular	First Horizon	SR
Respa-AR	Respa	SR	Sulfazine EC	Qualitest	EC
Respa-BR	Respa	SR	Symax Duotab	Capellon	SR
Respa-DM	Respa	SR	Symax-SR	Capellon	SR
Respa-PE	Respa	SR	Tarka	Abbott	SR
Respahist	Respa	SR	Taztia XT	Andrx	SR
Respahist-II	Respa	SR	Tegretol-XR	Novartis	SR
Respaire-60 SR	Laser	SR	Tenuate Dospan	Sanofi-Aventis	SR
Respaire-120 SR	Laser	SR	Theo-24	UCB	SR
Rhinacon A	Breckenridge	SR	Theochron	Forest	SR
Risperdal Consta	Janssen	SR	Theo-Time	Major	SR
Ritalin LA	Novartis	SR	Tiazac	Forest	SR
Ritalin-SR	Novartis	SR	Time-Hist	MCR American	SR
Rodex Forte	Legere	SR	Toprol XL	AstraZeneca	SR
Rondec-TR	Biovail	SR	Totalday	National Vitamin	SR
Ru-Tuss	Carwin	SR	Touro Allergy	Dartmouth	SR
Ryneze	Stewart-Jackson	SR	Touro CC	Dartmouth	SR
Rythmol SR	Reliant	SR	Touro CC-LD	Dartmouth	SR
SAM-e	Pharmavite	EC	Touro DM	Dartmouth	SR
Sanctura XR	Allergen	SR	Touro HC	Dartmouth	SR
Scopohist-PE	Larken	SR	Touro LA	Dartmouth	SR
Seroquel XR	AstraZeneca	SR	Touro LA-LD	Dartmouth	SR
Simcor	Abbott	SR	Tranxene-SD	Ovation	SR
Simuc-GP	Cypress	SR	Trental	Sanofi-Aventis	SR
Sinemet CR	Bristol-Myers Squibb	SR	Trikof-D	Respa	SR
Sinutuss DM	WE Pharmaceuticals	SR	Trinalin Repetabs	Schering-Plough	SR
Sinuvent PE	WE Pharmaceuticals	SR	Trituss-ER	Everett	SR
Slo-Niacin	Upsher-Smith	SR	Tussafed-LA	Everett	SR
Slow Fe	Novartis Consumer	SR	Tussall-ER	Everett	SR
Slow Fe with Folic Acid	Novartis Consumer	SR	Tussi-Bid	Capellon	SR
Slow-Mag	Purdue	EC	Tussicaps	Mallinckrodt	SR
Solodyn	Medicis	SR	Tusso-DM	Everett	SR
Stahist	Magna	SR	Tusso-HC	Everett	SR
St. Joseph Pain Reliever	McNeil Consumer	EC	Tylenol Arthritis	McNeil Consumer	SR
Sudafed 12 Hour	Pfizer	SR	Ultrabrom	WE Pharmaceuticals	SR
Sudafed 24 Hour	Pfizer	SR	Ultrabrom PD	WE Pharmaceuticals	SR
Sudahist	Larken	SR	Ultracaps MT 20	Breckenridge	EC

(continued)

Drug	Manufacturer	Form	Drug	Manufacturer	Form
Ultram ER	Ortho-McNeil	SR	We Mist LA	WE Pharmaceuticals	SR
Ultrase	Axcan Scandipharm	EC	We Mist II LA	WE Pharmaceuticals	SR
Ultrase MT12	Axcan Scandipharm	EC	Wellbid-D	Prasco	SR
Ultrase MT18	Axcan Scandipharm	EC	Wellbid-D 1200	Prasco	SR
Ultrase MT20	Axcan Scandipharm	EC	Wellbutrin SR	GlaxoSmithKline	SR
Uniphyl	Purdue	SR	Wellbutrin XL	GlaxoSmithKline	SR
Uni-Tex	United Research	SR	Wobenzym N	Marlyn	EC
Urimax	Xanodyne	EC	Woman's Wellbeing Menopause Relief	Consumer Choice	SR
Uritact-EC	Cypress	EC	Xanax XR	Pharmacia	SR
Urocit-K 5	Mission	SR	Xedec II	Cypress	SR
Urocit-K 10	Mission	SR	Xiral	Hawthorn	SR
Uroxatral	Sanofi-Aventis	SR	Xpect-AT	Hawthorn	SR
Utira	Hawthorn	SR	Xpect-HC	Hawthorn	SR
Veracolate	Numark	EC	Xpect-PE	Hawthorn	SR
Verelan	Schwarz Pharma	SR	Zephrex LA	Sanofi-Aventis	SR
Verelan PM	Schwarz Pharma	SR	Zmax	Pfizer	SR
Videx EC	Bristol-Myers Squibb	EC	Zorprin	Par	SR
Vivitrol	Cephalon	SR	Zotex-12D	Vertical	SR
Vivotif Berne	Berne Products	EC	Zyban	GlaxoSmithKline	SR
Voltaren	Novartis	EC	Zyflo CR	Critical Therapeutics	SR
Voltaren-XR	Novartis	SR	Zymase	Organon	EC
Vospire	Dava	SR	Zyrtec-D	Pfizer	SR
Vospire ER	Dava	SR			

Reference

LaGow B, ed. *Drug Topics Red Book*. Montvale, N.J.: Thomson Healthcare; 2009.

Appendix J

Use-in-Pregnancy Ratings

The U.S. Food and Drug Administration's Use-in-Pregnancy rating system weighs the degree to which available information has ruled out risk to the fetus against the drug's potential benefit to the patient. The following is a list of drugs (by generic name) for which ratings are available.

X: Contraindication In Pregnancy

Studies in animals or humans or investigational or postmarketing reports have demonstrated fetal risk, which clearly outweighs any possible benefit to the patient.

Acetohydroxamic acid
Acitretin
Ambrisentan
Amlodipine besylate–atorvastatin calcium
Anisindione
Atorvastatin calcium
Bexarotene
Bicalutamide
Bosentan
Cetrorelix acetate
Clomiphene citrate
Desogestrel–ethinyl estradiol
Diclofenac sodium–misoprostol
Dihydroergotamine mesylate
Dutasteride
Estazolam
Estradiol
Estradiol acetate
Estradiol cypionate–medroxyprogesterone acetate
Estradiol-levonorgestrel
Estradiol–norethindrone acetate
Estradiol valerate
Estrogens (conjugated)
Estrogens (conjugated)–medroxyprogesterone
    acetate
Estrogens (conjugated, synthetic A)
Estrogens (esterified)
Estrogens (esterified)–methyltestosterone
Estropipate
Ethinyl estradiol–drospirenone
Ethinyl estradiol–ethynodiol diacetate
Ethinyl estradiol–etonogestrel
Ethinyl estradiol–ferrous fumarate–norethindrone
    acetate
Ethinyl estradiol-levonorgestrel
Ethinyl estradiol–norelgestromin

Ethinyl estradiol–norethindrone
Ethinyl estradiol–norethindrone acetate
Ethinyl estradiol–norgestimate
Ethinyl estradiol–norgestrel
Ezetimibe-simvastatin
Finasteride
Fluorouracil
Fluoxymesterone
Flurazepam hydrochloride
Fluvastatin sodium
Follitropin alfa
Follitropin beta
Ganirelix acetate
Goserelin acetate
Histrelin acetate
Hydromorphone hydrochloride
Interferon alfa-2B (recombinant)–ribavirin
Iodine I 131 tositumomab–tositumomab
Isotretinoin
Leflunomide
Leuprolide acetate
Levonorgestrel
Lovastatin
Lovastatin-niacin
Medroxyprogesterone acetate
Megestrol acetate
Menotropins
Mequinol-tretinoin
Mestranol-norethindrone
Methotrexate sodium
Methyltestosterone
Miglustat
Misoprostol
Nafarelin acetate
Niacin-simvastatin
Norethindrone
Norethindrone acetate
Norgestrel
Oxandrolone
Oxymetholone
Plicamycin
Pravastatin sodium
Pravastatin sodium–aspirin (buffered)
Raloxifene hydrochloride
Ribavirin
Rosuvastatin calcium
Simvastatin
Tazarotene
Testosterone
Testosterone enanthate
Thalidomide
Tositumomab
Triptorelin pamoate
Warfarin sodium

D: Positive Evidence of Risk

Investigational or postmarketing data show risk to the fetus. Nevertheless, potential benefits may outweigh the potential risk.

Aliskiren*
Aliskiren-hydrochlorothiazide
Alitretinoin
Alprazolam
Altretamine
Amiodarone hydrochloride
Amlodipine besylate–benazepril hydrochloride
Amlodipine besylate–olmesartan medoxomil
Amlodipine besylate–valsartan*
Anastrozole
Arsenic trioxide
Aspirin (buffered)–pravastatin sodium
Aspirin-dipyridamole
Atenolol
Azacitidine
Azathioprine
Azathioprine sodium
Benazepril hydrochloride*
Benazepril hydrochloride–hydrochlorothiazide*
Bendamustine hydrochloride
Bortezomib
Busulfan
Candesartan cilexetil*
Candesartan cilexetil–hydrochlorothiazide*
Capecitabine
Captopril*
Carbamazepine
Carboplatin
Carmustine (BiCNU)
Chlorambucil
Cladribine
Clofarabine
Clonazepam
Cytarabine liposome
Dactinomycin
Dasatinib
Daunorubicin citrate liposome
Daunorubicin hydrochloride
Demeclocycline hydrochloride
Dexrazoxane
Dexrazoxane hydrochloride
Diazepam
Divalproex sodium
Docetaxel
Doxorubicin hydrochloride
Doxorubicin hydrochloride liposome

Doxycycline
Doxycycline calcium
Doxycycline hyclate
Doxycycline monohydrate
Efavirenz
Enalapril maleate*
Enalapril maleate–hydrochlorothiazide*
Epirubicin hydrochloride
Eprosartan mesylate
Erlotinib
Exemestane
Floxuridine
Fludarabine phosphate
Flutamide
Fosinopril sodium*
Fosinopril sodium–hydrochlorothiazide*
Fosphenytoin sodium
Fulvestrant
Gefitinib
Gemcitabine hydrochloride
Gemtuzumab ozogamicin
Genistein–zinc chelazome–cholecalciferol
Goserelin acetate
Ibritumomab tiuxetan
Idarubicin hydrochloride
Ifosfamide
Imatinib mesylate
Irbesartan*
Irbesartan-hydrochlorothiazide*
Irinotecan hydrochloride
Ixabepilone
Letrozole
Lisinopril*
Lisinopril-hydrochlorothiazide*
Lithium carbonate
Losartan potassium*
Losartan potassium–hydrochlorothiazide*
Mechlorethamine hydrochloride
Melphalan
Melphalan hydrochloride
Mephobarbital
Mercaptopurine
Methimazole
Midazolam hydrochloride
Minocycline hydrochloride
Mitoxantrone hydrochloride
Moexipril hydrochloride*
Moexipril hydrochloride–hydrochlorothiazide*
Mycophenolate mofetil
Mycophenolic acid
Nelarabine

*Category C or D depending on the trimester the drug is given.

Neomycin sulfate–polymyxin B sulfate
Nicotine
Nilotinib
Nilotinib hydrochloride monohydrate
Olmesartan medoxomil
Oxaliplatin
Pamidronate disodium
Paroxetine hydrochloride
Paroxetine mesylate
Pemetrexed
Penicillamine
Pentobarbital sodium
Pentostatin
Perindopril erbumine*
Phenytoin
Procarbazine hydrochloride
Quinapril hydrochloride*
Quinapril hydrochloride–hydrochlorothiazide*
Ramipril*
Sorafenib
Streptomycin sulfate
Sunitinib
Tamoxifen citrate
Telmisartan
Telmisartan-hydrochlorothiazide
Temozolomide
Temsirolimus
Thioguanine
Tigecycline
Tobramycin
Topotecan hydrochloride
Toremifene citrate
Trandolapril*
Trandolapril–verapamil hydrochloride*
Tretinoin
Valproate sodium
Valproic acid
Valsartan*
Valsartan-hydrochlorothiazide*
Vinorelbine tartrate
Voriconazole
Zoledronic acid

C: Risk Cannot Be Ruled Out

Human studies are lacking, and animal studies are either positive for risk or lacking as well. However, potential benefits may outweigh the potential risk.

Abacavir sulfate
Abacavir sulfate–lamivudine
Abacavir sulfate–lamivudine–zidovudine

Abciximab
Acamprosate calcium
Acetaminophen
Acetaminophen-butalbital-caffeine
Acetaminophen–caffeine–chlorpheniramine maleate–hydrocodone bitartrate–phenylephrine hydrochloride
Acetazolamide
Acetazolamide sodium
Acyclovir
Adapalene
Adefovir dipivoxil
Adenosine
Alatrofloxacin mesylate
Albendazole
Albumin (human)
Albuterol
Albuterol sulfate
Albuterol sulfate–ipratropium bromide
Alclometasone dipropionate
Aldesleukin
Alemtuzumab
Alendronate sodium
Alendronate sodium–cholecalciferol
Aliskiren*
Allopurinol sodium
Almotriptan malate
Alpha1-proteinase inhibitor (human)
Alprostadil
Alteplase
Amantadine hydrochloride
Amifostine
Aminocaproic acid
Aminohippurate sodium
Aminolevulinic acid hydrochloride
Aminosalicylic acid
Amlodipine besylate
Amlodipine besylate–benazepril hydrochloride
Amlodipine besylate–olmesartan medoxomil*
Amlodipine besylate–valsartan*
Amoxicillin-clarithromycin-lansoprazole
Amphetamine aspartate–amphetamine sulfate–dextroamphetamine saccharate–dextroamphetamine sulfate
Amprenavir
Anagrelide hydrochloride
Anthralin
Antihemophilic factor (human)
Antihemophilic factor (recombinant)
Anti-inhibitor coagulant complex
Antithymocyte globulin
Apomorphine hydrochloride

*Category C or D depending on the trimester the drug is given.

Aripiprazole

Armodafinil

Arnica montana–herbals (multiple)–sulfur

Asparaginase

Atomoxetine hydrochloride

Atovaquone

Atovaquone–proguanil hydrochloride

Atropine sulfate–benzoic acid–hyoscyamine sulfate–methenamine–methylene blue–phenyl salicylate

Atropine sulfate–hyoscyamine sulfate–scopolamine hydrobromide

Azelastine hydrochloride

Bacitracin zinc–neomycin sulfate–polymyxin B sulfate

Baclofen

BCG (live, intravesical)

Becaplermin

Beclomethasone dipropionate

Beclomethasone dipropionate monohydrate

Benazepril hydrochloride*

Benazepril hydrochloride–hydrochlorothiazide*

Bendroflumethiazide

Benzocaine

Benzonatate

Benzoyl peroxide

Benzoyl peroxide–clindamycin

Benzoyl peroxide–erythromycin

Betamethasone dipropionate

Betamethasone dipropionate–clotrimazole

Betamethasone valerate

Betaxolol hydrochloride

Bethanechol chloride

Bevacizumab

Bimatoprost

Bisacodyl–polyethylene glycol–potassium chloride–sodium bicarbonate–sodium chloride

Bisoprolol fumarate

Bisoprolol fumarate–hydrochlorothiazide

Bitolterol mesylate

Black widow spider antivenin (equine)

Botulinum toxin type A

Botulinum toxin type B

Brimonidine tartrate–timolol maleate

Brinzolamide

Brompheniramine maleate–dextromethorphan hydrobromide–phenylephrine hydrochloride

Budesonide

Bupivacaine hydrochloride

Bupivacaine hydrochloride–epinephrine bitartrate

Buprenorphine hydrochloride

Buprenorphine hydrochloride–naloxone hydrochloride

Bupropion hydrobromide

Bupropion hydrochloride

Butabarbital–hyoscyamine hydrobromide–phenazopyridine hydrochloride

Butalbital-acetaminophen

Butenafine hydrochloride

Butoconazole nitrate

Butorphanol tartrate

Caffeine citrate

Calcipotriene

Calcitonin-salmon

Calcitriol

Calcium acetate

Candesartan cilexetil*

Candesartan cilexetil–hydrochlorothiazide*

Capreomycin sulfate

Captopril*

Carbetapentane tannate–chlorpheniramine tannate

Carbetapentane tannate–chlorpheniramine tannate–ephedrine tannate–phenylephrine tannate

Carbidopa-entacapone-levodopa

Carbidopa-levodopa

Carbinoxamine maleate–dextromethorphan hydrobromide–pseudoephedrine hydrochloride

Carteolol hydrochloride

Carvedilol

Caspofungin acetate

Celecoxib

Cetirizine hydrochloride

Cetuximab

Cevimeline hydrochloride

Chloramphenicol

Chloroprocaine hydrochloride

Chlorothiazide

Chlorothiazide sodium

Chlorpheniramine maleate–methscopolamine nitrate–phenylephrine hydrochloride

Chlorpheniramine maleate–pseudoephedrine hydrochloride

Chlorpheniramine polistirex–hydrocodone polistirex

Chlorpheniramine tannate–phenylephrine tannate

Chlorpropamide

Chlorthalidone–clonidine hydrochloride

Choline magnesium trisalicylate

Ciclesonide

Cidofovir

Cilostazol

Cinacalcet hydrochloride

Ciprofloxacin-dexamethasone

*Category C or D depending on the trimester the drug is given.

Ciprofloxacin hydrochloride
Ciprofloxacin hydrochloride–hydrocortisone
Citalopram hydrobromide
Clarithromycin
Clobetasol propionate
Clonidine
Clonidine hydrochloride
Codeine phosphate–acetaminophen
Colistimethate sodium
Colistin sulfate–hydrocortisone acetate–neomycin sulfate–thonzonium bromide
Corticorelin ovine triflutate
Cyanocobalamin
Cycloserine
Cyclosporine
Cytomegalovirus immune globulin
Dacarbazine
Daclizumab
Dantrolene sodium
Dapsone
Darbepoetin alfa
Darifenacin
Deferoxamine mesylate
Delavirdine mesylate
Denileukin diftitox
Desloratadine
Desloratadine–pseudoephedrine sulfate
Desoximetasone
Desvenlafaxine
Dexamethasone
Dexamethasone sodium phosphate
Dexmethylphenidate hydrochloride
Dexrazoxane
Dextroamphetamine sulfate
Diazoxide
Dichlorphenamide
Diclofenac epolamine
Diclofenac potassium
Diclofenac sodium
Diflorasone diacetate
Diflunisal
Digoxin
Digoxin immune Fab (ovine)
Diltiazem hydrochloride
Dimethyl sulfoxide
Dinoprostone
Diphtheria and tetanus toxoids and acellular pertussis vaccine (adsorbed)
Diphtheria and tetanus toxoids and acellular pertussis vaccine (adsorbed)–hepatitis B Vaccine, (recombinant)–poliovirus vaccine (inactivated)

Dirithromycin
Dofetilide
Donepezil hydrochloride
Dorzolamide hydrochloride
Dorzolamide hydrochloride–timolol maleate
Doxazosin mesylate
Dronabinol
Drotrecogin alfa (activated)
Duloxetine hydrochloride
Echothiophate iodide
Econazole nitrate
Efalizumab
Eflornithine hydrochloride
Eletriptan hydrobromide
Enalapril maleate*
Enalapril maleate–felodipine*
Enalapril maleate–hydrochlorothiazide*
Entacapone
Entecavir
Epinastine hydrochloride
Epinephrine
Epoetin alfa
Eprosartan mesylate
Erythromycin ethylsuccinate–sulfisoxazole acetyl
Escitalopram oxalate
Eszopiclone
Ethionamide
Ethotoin
Etidronate disodium
Exenatide
Ezetimibe
Factor IX complex
Felodipine
Fenofibrate
Fentanyl
Fentanyl citrate
Fentanyl hydrochloride
Ferrous fumarate–folic acid–intrinsic factor concentrate–liver preparations–vitamin B_{12}–vitamin C–vitamins with iron
Fexofenadine hydrochloride
Fexofenadine hydrochloride–pseudoephedrine hydrochloride
Filgrastim
Flecainide acetate
Fluconazole
Flucytosine
Fludrocortisone acetate
Flumazenil
Flunisolide
Fluocinolone acetonide

*Category C or D depending on the trimester the drug is given.

Fluocinolone acetonide–hydroquinone–tretinoin
Fluocinonide
Fluorometholone
Fluorometholone–sulfacetamide sodium
Fluoxetine hydrochloride
Fluoxetine hydrochloride–olanzapine
Flurandrenolide
Flurbiprofen sodium
Fluticasone furoate
Fluticasone propionate
Fluticasone propionate HFA
Fluticasone propionate–salmeterol xinafoate
Fluvoxamine maleate
Fomivirsen sodium
Formoterol fumarate
Fosamprenavir calcium
Foscarnet sodium*
Fosinopril sodium*
Fosinopril sodium–hydrochlorothiazide*
Frovatriptan succinate
Furosemide
Gabapentin
Gallium nitrate
Ganciclovir
Ganciclovir sodium
Gatifloxacin
Gemfibrozil
Gemifloxacin mesylate
Gentamicin sulfate
Gentamicin sulfate–prednisolone acetate
Glimepiride
Glimepiride–rosiglitazone maleate
Glipizide
Glipizide–metformin hydrochloride
Globulin, immune (human)
Globulin, immune (human)–Rho (D) immune
    globulin (human)
Glyburide
Gramicidin–neomycin sulfate–polymyxin B sulfate
Guaifenesin–hydrocodone bitartrate
Haemophilus B conjugate vaccine
Haemophilus B conjugate vaccine–hepatitis B
    vaccine (recombinant)
Halobetasol propionate
Haloperidol decanoate
Hemin
Heparin sodium
Hepatitis A vaccine (inactivated)
Hepatitis A vaccine (inactivated)–hepatitis B
    vaccine (recombinant)
Hepatitis B immune globulin (human)

Hepatitis B vaccine (recombinant)
Homatropine methylbromide–hydrocodone
    bitartrate
Homeopathic formulations
Hydralazine hydrochloride–isosorbide dinitrate
Hydrochlorothiazide
Hydrocodone bitartrate
Hydrocodone bitartrate–acetaminophen
Hydrocodone bitartrate–ibuprofen
Hydrocortisone
Hydrocortisone acetate
Hydrocortisone acetate–neomycin sulfate–
    polymyxin B sulfate
Hydrocortisone acetate–pramoxine hydrochloride
Hydrocortisone butyrate
Hydrocortisone–neomycin sulfate–polymyxin B
    sulfate
Hydrocortisone probutate
Hydromorphone hydrochloride
Hydroquinone
Hyoscyamine sulfate
Ibandronate sodium
Ibutilide fumarate
Iloprost
Imiglucerase
Imipenem-cilastatin
Imiquimod
Immune globulin intravenous (human)
Indinavir sulfate
Indocyanine green
Influenza virus vaccine
Insulin aspart
Insulin aspart protamine (human)–insulin aspart
    (human)
Insulin glargine
Insulin glulisine
Interferon alfa-2B (recombinant)
Interferon alfacon-1
Interferon alfa-N3 (human leukocyte derived)
Interferon beta-1A
Interferon beta-1B
Interferon gamma-1B
Iodoquinol-hydrocortisone
Irbesartan*
Irbesartan-hydrochlorothiazide*
Iron dextran
Isoniazid-pyrazinamide-rifampin
Isosorbide mononitrate
Isradipine
Itraconazole
Ivermectin

*Category C or D depending on the trimester the drug is given.

Ketoconazole
Ketorolac tromethamine
Ketotifen fumarate
Labetalol hydrochloride
Lamivudine
Lamivudine-zidovudine
Lamotrigine
Lanreotide acetate
Lanthanum carbonate
Latanoprost
Levalbuterol hydrochloride
Levalbuterol tartrate
Levamisole hydrochloride
Levetiracetam
Levobunolol hydrochloride
Levofloxacin
Linezolid
Lisdexamfetamine
Lisinopril*
Lisinopril-hydrochlorothiazide*
Lomefloxacin
Lopinavir-ritonavir
Losartan potassium*
Losartan potassium–hydrochlorothiazide*
Loteprednol etabonate
Lubiprostone
Mafenide acetate
Magnesium salicylate tetrahydrate
Measles, mumps, and rubella virus vaccine (live)
Measles virus vaccine (live)
Mebendazole
Mecamylamine hydrochloride
Mecasermin [rDNA origin]
Medrysone
Mefenamic acid
Mefloquine hydrochloride
Meloxicam
Meningococcal polysaccharide diphtheria toxoid
  conjugate vaccine
Meningococcal polysaccharide vaccine
Meperidine hydrochloride
Mepivacaine hydrochloride
Metaproterenol sulfate
Metaraminol bitartrate
Metformin hydrochloride–pioglitazone
  hydrochloride
Metformin hydrochloride–repaglinide
Metformin hydrochloride–rosiglitazone maleate
Methamphetamine hydrochloride
Methazolamide
Methenamine mandelate–sodium acid phosphate

Methocarbamol
Methoxsalen
Methoxy polyethylene glycol–epoetin beta
Methscopolamine nitrate–pseudoephedrine
  hydrochloride
Methyldopa-chlorothiazide
Methyldopa-hydrochlorothiazide
Methylphenidate hydrochloride
Metipranolol
Metoprolol succinate
Metoprolol tartrate
Metoprolol tartrate–hydrochlorothiazide
Metyrosine
Mexiletine hydrochloride
Micafungin sodium
Midodrine hydrochloride
Mivacurium chloride
Modafinil
Moexipril hydrochloride*
Moexipril hydrochloride–hydrochlorothiazide*
Mometasone furoate
Mometasone furoate monohydrate
Morphine sulfate
Morphine sulfate, liposomal
Moxifloxacin hydrochloride
Mumps virus vaccine (live)
Muromonab-CD3
Mycophenolate mofetil
Mycophenolate mofetil hydrochloride
Mycophenolic acid
Nabumetone
Nadolol
Nadolol-bendroflumethiazide
Naloxone hydrochloride–pentazocine
  hydrochloride
Naltrexone hydrochloride
Naphazoline hydrochloride
Naproxen
Naproxen sodium
Naratriptan hydrochloride
Natamycin
Nateglinide
Nebivolol
Nefazodone hydrochloride
Neomycin sulfate–dexamethasone sodium
  phosphate
Neomycin sulfate–polymyxin B sulfate–
  prednisolone acetate
Nesiritide
Nevirapine
Niacin
Nicardipine hydrochloride

*Category C or D depending on the trimester the drug is given.

Nifedipine
Nilutamide
Nimodipine
Nisoldipine
Nitroglycerin
Norfloxacin
Ofloxacin
Olanzapine
Olmesartan medoxomil–hydrochlorothiazide
Olopatadine hydrochloride
Olsalazine sodium
Omega-3-acid ethyl esters
Omeprazole
Oprelvekin
Orphenadrine citrate
Oseltamivir phosphate
Oxcarbazepine
Oxycodone hydrochloride–acetaminophen
Oxycodone hydrochloride–ibuprofen
Oxymorphone hydrochloride
Palifermin
Paliperidone
Palivizumab
Pancrelipase
Paricalcitol
Paroxetine hydrochloride
Paroxetine mesylate
PEG-3350–potassium chloride–sodium bicarbonate–
  sodium chloride
Pegademase bovine
Pegaspargase
Pegfilgrastim
Peginterferon alfa-2A
Peginterferon alfa-2B
Pemirolast potassium
Pentazocine hydrochloride–acetaminophen
Pentoxifylline
Perindopril erbumine*
Phenoxybenzamine hydrochloride
Phentermine hydrochloride
Pilocarpine hydrochloride
Pimecrolimus
Pimozide
Pioglitazone hydrochloride
Pirbuterol acetate
Piroxicam
Plasma fractions (human)–rabies immune globulin
  (human)
Plasma protein fraction (human)
Pneumococcal vaccine (diphtheria conjugate)
Pneumococcal vaccine (polyvalent)
Podofilox

Polyethylene glycol
Polyethylene glycol–potassium chloride–sodium
  bicarbonate–sodium chloride
Polyethylene glycol–potassium chloride–sodium
  bicarbonate–sodium chloride–sodium sulfate
Polymyxin B sulfate–trimethoprim sulfate
Polythiazide–prazosin hydrochloride
Porfimer sodium
Potassium acid phosphate
Potassium chloride
Potassium citrate
Potassium phosphate–sodium phosphate
Pralidoxime chloride
Pramipexole dihydrochloride
Pramlintide acetate
Pramoxine hydrochloride–hydrocortisone acetate
Prazosin hydrochloride
Prednisolone acetate
Prednisolone acetate–sulfacetamide sodium
Prednisolone sodium phosphate
Pregabalin
Promethazine hydrochloride
Propafenone hydrochloride
Proparacaine hydrochloride
Propranolol hydrochloride
Pseudoephedrine hydrochloride
Pyrimethamine
Quetiapine fumarate
Quinapril hydrochloride*
Quinidine sulfate
Rabies vaccine
Raltegravir potassium
Ramelteon
Ramipril*
Ranolazine
Rasburicase
Remifentanil hydrochloride
Repaglinide
Reteplase
Rho (D) immune globulin (human)
Rifampin
Rifapentine
Rifaximin
Riluzole
Rimantadine hydrochloride
Risedronate sodium
Risedronate sodium–calcium carbonate
Risperidone
Rituximab
Rizatriptan benzoate
Rocuronium bromide
Rofecoxib

*Category C or D depending on the trimester the drug is given.

Romiplostim
Ropinirole hydrochloride
Rosiglitazone maleate
Rotigotine
Rubella virus vaccine (live)
Salmeterol xinafoate
Sapropterin dihydrochloride
Sargramostim
Scopolamine
Selegiline hydrochloride
Selenium sulfide
Sertaconazole nitrate
Sertraline hydrochloride
Sevelamer carbonate
Sevelamer hydrochloride
Sibutramine hydrochloride monohydrate
Sirolimus
Sodium benzoate–sodium phenylacetate
Sodium phenylbutyrate
Sodium polystyrene sulfonate
Sodium sulfacetamide–sulfur
Solifenacin succinate
Somatropin
Somatropin (rDNA origin)
Stavudine
Streptokinase
Succimer
Sulfacetamide sodium
Sulfamethoxazole-trimethoprim
Sulfanilamide
Sumatriptan
Sumatriptan succinate
Tacrine hydrochloride
Tacrolimus
Telithromycin
Telmisartan*
Telmisartan-hydrochlorothiazide*
Tenecteplase
Terazosin hydrochloride
Teriparatide
Tetanus and diphtheria toxoids (adsorbed)
Tetanus immune globulin (human)
Theophylline
Theophylline anhydrous
Thiabendazole
Thrombin
Thyrotropin alfa
Tiagabine hydrochloride
Tiludronate disodium
Timolol hemihydrate
Timolol maleate

Timolol maleate–hydrochlorothiazide
Tinidazole
Tiotropium bromide
Tipranavir
Tizanidine hydrochloride
Tobramycin-dexamethasone
Tobramycin–loteprednol etabonate
Tolcapone
Tolterodine tartrate
Topiramate
Tramadol hydrochloride
Tramadol hydrochloride–acetaminophen
Trandolapril*
Trandolapril–verapamil hydrochloride*
Travoprost
Tretinoin
Triamcinolone acetonide
Triamterene
Triamterene-hydrochlorothiazide
Trientine hydrochloride
Triethanolamine polypeptide oleate-condensate
Trifluridine
Trimethoprim hydrochloride
Trimipramine maleate
Tropicamide–hydroxyamphetamine hydrobromide
Trospium chloride
Trovafloxacin mesylate
Tuberculin purified protein derivative (diluted)
Typhoid vaccine (live) oral Ty21a
Unoprostone isopropyl
Urea
Valdecoxib
Valganciclovir hydrochloride
Valsartan*
Valsartan-hydrochlorothiazide*
Varenicline tartrate
Varicella virus vaccine (live)
Venlafaxine hydrochloride
Verapamil hydrochloride
Verteporfin
Vitamin K_1
Yellow fever vaccine
Zalcitabine
Zaleplon
Zanamivir
Zidovudine
Ziprasidone mesylate
Zolmitriptan
Zolpidem tartrate
Zonisamide

*Category C or D depending on the trimester the drug is given.

B: No Evidence of Risk in Humans

Animal findings show risk whereas human findings do not, or, if no adequate human studies have been done, animal findings are negative.

Acarbose
Acrivastine
Acyclovir
Acyclovir sodium
Adalimumab
Agalsidase beta
Alefacept
Alfuzosin hydrochloride
Alosetron hydrochloride
Alvimopan
Amiloride hydrochloride
Amiloride hydrochloride–hydrochlorothiazide
Amoxicillin
Amoxicillin–clavulanate potassium
Amphotericin B
Amphotericin B–cholesteryl sulfate complex
Amphotericin B lipid complex
Amphotericin B (liposomal)
Ampicillin sodium–sulbactam sodium
Anakinra
Antithrombin III
Aprepitant
Aprotinin
Argatroban
Arginine hydrochloride
Atazanavir sulfate
Azelaic acid
Azithromycin
Azithromycin dihydrate
Aztreonam
Balsalazide disodium
Basiliximab
Bivalirudin
Brimonidine tartrate
Budesonide
Bupropion hydrochloride
Cabergoline
Carbenicillin indanyl sodium
Cefaclor
Cefazolin sodium
Cefdinir
Cefditoren pivoxil
Cefepime hydrochloride
Cefixime
Cefoperazone sodium
Cefotaxime sodium
Cefotetan disodium
Cefoxitin sodium

Cefpodoxime proxetil
Cefprozil
Ceftazidime sodium
Ceftibuten dihydrate
Ceftizoxime sodium
Ceftriaxone sodium
Cefuroxime
Cefuroxime axetil
Cephalexin
Certolizumab pegol
Cetirizine hydrochloride
Ciclopirox
Ciclopirox olamine
Cimetidine
Cimetidine hydrochloride
Cisatracurium besylate
Clindamycin hydrochloride–clindamycin phosphate
Clindamycin palmitate hydrochloride
Clindamycin phosphate
Clopidogrel bisulfate
Clotrimazole
Clozapine
Colesevelam hydrochloride
Cromolyn sodium
Cyclobenzaprine hydrochloride
Cyproheptadine hydrochloride
Dalfopristin-quinupristin
Dalteparin sodium
Dapiprazole hydrochloride
Daptomycin
Desflurane
Desmopressin acetate
Dicyclomine hydrochloride
Didanosine
Diphenhydramine hydrochloride
Dipivefrin hydrochloride
Dipyridamole
Dolasetron mesylate
Doripenem
Dornase alfa
Doxapram hydrochloride
Doxepin hydrochloride
Doxercalciferol
Edetate calcium disodium
Emtricitabine
Emtricitabine–tenofovir disoproxil fumarate
Enfuvirtide
Enoxaparin sodium
Eplerenone
Epoprostenol sodium
Ertapenem
Erythromycin
Erythromycin ethylsuccinate

Erythromycin stearate
Esomeprazole magnesium
Esomeprazole sodium
Etanercept
Ethacrynate sodium
Ethacrynic acid
Etravirine
Famciclovir
Famotidine
Fenoldopam mesylate
Fondaparinux sodium
Galantamine hydrobromide
Glatiramer acetate
Glucagon
Glyburide–metformin hydrochloride
Granisetron hydrochloride
Hydrochlorothiazide
Ibuprofen
Indapamide
Infliximab
Insulin aspart
Insulin lispro (human)
Insulin lispro protamine (human)–insulin lispro
    (human)
Ipratropium bromide
Iron sucrose
Isosorbide mononitrate
Lactulose
Lansoprazole
Lansoprazole-naproxen
Laronidase
Lepirudin
Levocarnitine
Levocetirizine dihydrochloride
Lidocaine
Lidocaine hydrochloride
Lidocaine-prilocaine
Lindane
Loperamide hydrochloride
Loracarbef
Loratadine
Malathion
Maraviroc
Meclizine hydrochloride
Memantine hydrochloride
Meropenem
Mesalamine
Metformin hydrochloride
Metformin hydrochloride–sitagliptin phosphate
Methohexital sodium
Methyldopa
Methylnaltrexone bromide
Metolazone

Metronidazole
Miglitol
Montelukast sodium
Mupirocin
Mupirocin calcium
Naftifine hydrochloride
Nalbuphine hydrochloride
Nalmefene hydrochloride
Naloxone hydrochloride
Naproxen sodium
Nedocromil sodium
Nelfinavir mesylate
Nitazoxanide
Nitrofurantoin macrocrystals
Nitrofurantoin macrocrystals–nitrofurantoin
    monohydrate
Nizatidine
Octreotide acetate
Omalizumab
Ondansetron
Ondansetron hydrochloride
Orlistat
Oxiconazole nitrate
Oxybutynin
Oxybutynin chloride
Oxycodone hydrochloride
Palonosetron hydrochloride
Pancrelipase
Pantoprazole sodium
Pegvisomant
Pemoline
Penciclovir
Penicillin G benzathine
Penicillin G benzathine–penicillin G procaine
Penicillin G potassium
Pentosan polysulfate sodium
Permethrin
Piperacillin sodium
Piperacillin sodium–tazobactam sodium
Praziquantel
Progesterone
Propofol
Pseudoephedrine hydrochloride
Pseudoephedrine sulfate
Psyllium preparations
Rabeprazole sodium
Ranitidine hydrochloride
Retapamulin
Rifabutin
Ritonavir
Rivastigmine tartrate
Ropivacaine hydrochloride
Saquinavir mesylate

Sevoflurane
Sildenafil citrate
Silver sulfadiazine
Sitagliptin phosphate
Sodium ferric gluconate
Somatropin
Sotalol hydrochloride
Sucralfate
Sulfasalazine
Tadalafil
Tamsulosin hydrochloride
Tenofovir disoproxil fumarate
Terbinafine hydrochloride
Ticarcillin disodium–clavulanate potassium
Ticlopidine hydrochloride
Tirofiban hydrochloride
Torsemide
Trastuzumab
Treprostinil sodium
Urokinase

Ursodiol
Valacyclovir hydrochloride
Vancomycin hydrochloride
Vardenafil hydrochloride
Zafirlukast

A: No Risk Shown in Controlled Studies

Adequate, well-controlled studies in pregnant women have failed to demonstrate risk to the fetus.

Liothyronine sodium
Liotrix
Nystatin

Reference

LaGow B, ed. *Drug Topics Red Book*. Montvale, N.J.: Thomson Healthcare; 2009.

Appendix K

Sugar-Free Products

The following table, by therapeutic category, is a selection of drug products that contain no sugar. When recommending these products to diabetic patients, keep in mind that many may contain sorbitol, alcohol, or other sources of carbohydrates. This list should not be considered all inclusive. Generics and alternate brands of some products may be available. Check product labeling for a current listing of inactive ingredients.

Product	Manufacturer	Product	Manufacturer
Analgesics		***Cough, cold, and allergy preparations***	
Addaprin tablets	Dover	Accuhist drops	Pediamed
Aminofen tablets	Dover	Accuhist PDX drops solution	Pediamed
Aminofen Max tablets	Dover	Alacol solution	Ballay
Aspirtab tablets	Dover	Alacol DM syrup	Ballay
Back Pain-Off tablets	Medique	Amerifed liquid	Ambi
Backprin tablets	Hart Health and Safety	Amerifed DM liquid	Ambi
Buffasal tablets	Dover	Amerituss AD solution	Ambi
Dyspel tablets	Dover	Anaplex DM syrup	ECR
I-Prin tablets	Medique	Anaplex DMX syrup	ECR
Medi-Seltzer Effervescent tablets	Medique	Anaplex HD syrup	ECR
Methadose solution	Mallinckrodt	Andehist DM NR syrup	Cypress
Methadose Sugar-Free Oral Concentrate	Mallinckrodt	Andehist NR syrup	Cypress
Ms.-Aid tablets	Medique	Aquatab C tablets	Deston
Silapap Children's elixir	Silarx	Aridex solution	Gentex
Antacids and antiflatulents		Baltussin solution	Ballay
Alcalak chewable tablets	Medique	Benadryl-D Allergy & Sinus Children's Solution	Johnson & Johnson
Dimacid chewable tablets	Otis Clapp & Son	Bromhist-DM solution	Cypress
Diotame chewable tablets	Medique	Bromhist Pediatric solution	Cypress
Diotame suspension	Medique	Bromphenex DM solution	Breckenridge
Mylanta gelcaplets	Johnson & Johnson/Merck	Bromphenex HD solution	Breckenridge
Mylanta tablets	Johnson & Johnson/Merck	Bromplex DM solution	Prasco
Neutralin tablets	Dover	Bromplex HD solution	Prasco
Pepto-Bismol tablets	Procter & Gamble	Bromtuss DM solution	Breckenridge
Turns E-X chewable tablets	GlaxoSmithKline Consumer	Broncotron liquid	Seyer Pharmatec
Turns E-X sugar-free tablets	GlaxoSmithKline Consumer	Broncotron-D suspension	Seyer Pharmatec
Antiasthmatic and respiratory agents		B-Tuss liquid	Blansett
Jay-Phyl syrup	Pharmakon	Carbaphen 12 suspension	Gil
Antidiarrheals		Carbaphen 12 Ped suspension	Gil
Diarrest tablets	Dover	Carbatuss-12 suspension	GM
Imogen liquid	Pharm Generic	Carbatuss-CL solution	GM
Blood modifiers and iron preparations		Carbetaplex liquid	Breckenridge
I.L.X. B-12 elixir	Kenwood	Carbetaplex solution	Breckenridge
Nephro-Fer tablets	R & D	Carbofed DM drops	Hi-Tech
Corticosteroids		Carbofed DM liquid	Hi-Tech
Pediapred solution	Celltech	Carbofed DM syrup	Hi-Tech
		Cardec solution	Qualitest

(continued)

Product	Manufacturer	Product	Manufacturer
Cardec DM syrup	Qualitest	Double-Tussin DM liquid	Reese
Cetafen Cold tablets	Hart Health and Safety	Drocon-CS solution	Cypress
Cetafen Cough & Cold tablets	Hart Health and Safety	Duratuss DM elixir	Victory
Cheratussin DAC liquid	Qualitest	Duratuss DM solution	Victory
Chlordex GP syrup	Cypress	Dynatuss HC solution	Breckenridge
Codal-DM syrup	Cypress	Dytan-CS tablets	Hawthorn
Codiclear DH solution	Victory	Dytan-HC suspension	Hawthorn
ColdCough syrup	Breckenridge	Emagrin tablets	Otis Clapp & Son
ColdCough HC syrup	Breckenridge	Emagrin Forte tablets	Otis Clapp & Son
ColdCough PD syrup	Breckenridge	Endacof-DM solution	Larken
ColdCough solution	Breckenridge	Endacof-HC solution	Larken
ColdCough HCM solution	Breckenridge	Endacof-PD solution	Larken
ColdCough PD solution	Breckenridge	Endacof-XP solution	Larken
ColdCough XP solution	Breckenridge	Endal HD Plus liquid	Pediamed
Coldonyl tablets	Dover	Ganidin NR liquid	Cypress
Colidrops Pediatric liquid	A. G. Marin	Gani-Tuss NR liquid	Cypress
Cordron-DM NR solution	Cypress	Gani-Tuss-DM NR liquid	Cypress
Cordron-HC solution	Cypress	Genebronco-D liquid	Pharm Generic
Cordron-HC NR solution	Cypress	Genecof-HC liquid	Pharm Generic
Cordron NR solution	Cypress	Genecof-XP liquid	Pharm Generic
Corfen DM solution	Cypress	Genedel syrup	Pharm Generic
Coughtuss solution	Breckenridge	Genedotuss-DM liquid	Pharm Generic
Crantex syrup	Breckenridge	Genelan liquid	Pharm Generic
Crantex HC syrup	Breckenridge	Genetuss-2 liquid	Pharm Generic
Dacex-DM solution	Cypress	Genexpect DM liquid	Pharm Generic
Dallergy drops	Laser	Genexpect-PE liquid	Pharm Generic
Dallergy solution	Laser	Genexpect-SF liquid	Pharm Generic
De-Chlor DM solution	Cypress	Gilphex TR tablets	Gil
De-Chlor DR solution	Cypress	Giltuss liquid	Gil
De-Chlor HD solution	Cypress	Giltuss Ped-C solution	Gil
Despec liquid	International Ethical	Giltuss Pediatric liquid	Gil
Despec-SF liquid	International Ethical	Giltuss TR tablets	Gil
Diabetic Tussin Allergy Relief liquid	Health Care Products	Guiadex DM liquid	Breckenridge
Diabetic Tussin Allergy Relief tablets	Health Care Products	Guiadex DM solution	Breckenridge
		Guiaplex HC solution	Breckenridge
Diabetic Tussin Cold & Flu gelcaplets	Health Care Products	Halotussin AC liquid	Axiom
		Halotussin DAC solution	Axiom
Diabetic Tussin DM liquid	Health Care Products	Histinex HC syrup	Ethex
Diabetic Tussin EX liquid	Health Care Products	Histinex PV syrup	Ethex
Diabetic Tussin solution	Health Care Products	Hydro-Tussin CBX solution	Ethex
Diphen capsules	Medique	Hydro-Tussin DHC solution	Ethex
Donatussin drops	Laser	Hydro-Tussin DM elixir	Ethex
Donatussin solution	Laser	Hydro-Tussin EXP solution	Ethex

Product	Manufacturer
Hydro-Tussin HC syrup	Ethex
Hydro-Tussin HD liquid	Ethex
Hydro-Tussin XP syrup	Ethex
Jaycof Expectorant syrup	Pharmakon
Jaycof-HC liquid	Pharmakon
Jaycof-XP liquid	Pharmakon
Liquicough DM solution	Breckenridge
Liquicough HC solution	Breckenridge
Lodrane liquid	ECR
Lodrane D suspension	ECR
Lodrane XR suspension	ECR
Lohist-LQ solution	Larken
Lohist-PD solution	Larken
Lortuss DM solution	Proethic
Marcof Expectorant syrup	Marnel
Maxi-Tuss HCG solution	MCR American
Maxi-Tuss HCX solution	MCR American
M-Clear solution	R. A. McNeil
M-Clear JR solution	R. A. McNeil
Metanx tablets	Pamlab
Mintuss NX solution	Breckenridge
Nalex-A liquid	Blansett
Nalex-DH liquid	Blansett
Nasop suspension	Hawthorn
Neo DM drops	Laser
Neo DM suspension	Laser
Neo DM syrup	Laser
Neotuss-D liquid	A. G. Marin
Neotuss S/F liquid	A. G. Marin
Niferex elixir	Ther-Rx
Norel DM liquid	US Pharmaceutical
Nycoff tablets	Dover
Organidin NR liquid	MedPointe
Organidin NR tablets	MedPointe
Pancof EXP syrup	Pamlab
Pancof HC solution	Pamlab
Pancof XP solution	Pamlab
Panmist DM syrup	Pamlab
Pediatex HC solution	Zyber
Phanasin syrup	Pharmakon
Phanasin Diabetic Choice syrup	Pharmakon
Phanatuss syrup	Pharmakon
Phanatuss DM Diabetic Choice syrup	Pharmakon

Product	Manufacturer
Phanatuss-HC Diabetic Choice solution	Pharmakon
Phena-HC solution	GM
Phenabid tablets	Gil
Phenabid DM tablets	Gil
Phena-S liquid	GM
Phena-S 12 suspension	GM
Phendacof HC syrup	Larken
Phendacof Plus solution	Larken
Poly Hist DM solution	Poly
Poly Hist HC solution	Poly
Poly Hist PD solution	Poly
Poly-Tussin solution	Poly
Poly-Tussin DM syrup	Poly
Poly-Tussin HD syrup	Poly
Poly-Tussin XP solution	Poly
Pro-Clear solution	Pro-Pharma
Pro-Red solution	Pro-Pharma
Prolex DM liquid	Blansett
Quintex syrup	Qualitest
Relacon-HC solution	Cypress
Rescon-DM liquid	Capellon
Rindal HD liquid	Breckenridge
Rindal HD Plus solution	Breckenridge
Rondec solution	Alliant
Rondec DM solution	Alliant
Ru-Tuss DM solution	Carwin
Ru-Tuss DM syrup	Carwin
Safetussin liquid	Kramer
Scot-Tussin Diabetes CF liquid	Scot-Tussin
Scot-Tussin DM Cough Chasers lozenges	Scot-Tussin
Scot-Tussin DM solution	Scot-Tussin
Scot-Tussin DM Maximum Strength	Scot-Tussin
Scot-Tussin Expectorant solution	Scot-Tussin
Scot-Tussin Senior solution	Scot-Tussin
Siladryl Allergy solution	Silarx
Sildec syrup	Silarx
Sildec-DM syrup	Silarx
Sildec-PE solution	Silarx
Sildec-PE syrup	Silarx
Sildec PE-DM solution	Silarx
Sildec PE-DM syrup	Silarx
Silexin syrup	Otis Clapp & Son

(continued)

Product	Manufacturer	Product	Manufacturer
Silexin tablets	Otis Clapp & Son	***Fluoride preparations***	
Sil-Tex liquid	Silarx	Fluor-A-Day liquid	Pharmascience
Siltussin DAS liquid	Silarx	Fluor-A-Day tablets	Pharmascience
Siltussin DM DAS Cough Formula syrup	Silarx	Flura-Loz tablets	Kirkman
		Lozi-Flur lozenges	Dreir
Siltussin SA liquid	Silarx	Sensodyne with Fluoride Gel	GlaxoSmithKline Consumer
Siltussin SA syrup	Silarx	Sensodyne with Fluoride Cool Gel	GlaxoSmithKline Consumer
Statuss Green liquid	Magna	Sensodyne with Fluoride Tartar Control Toothpaste	GlaxoSmithKline Consumer
Sudafed Children's solution	Pfizer		
Sudafed Children's Cold & Cough solution	Pfizer	Sensodyne with Fluoride Toothpaste	GlaxoSmithKline Consumer
Sudafed Children's Nasal Decongestant liquid	Pfizer	Sensodyne with Fluoride Toothpaste Original Flavor	GlaxoSmithKline Consumer
Sudafed Children's PE Cough & Cold liquid	Pfizer	Sensodyne Tartar Control with Whitening Toothpaste	GlaxoSmithKline Consumer
Sudanyl tablets	Dover	***Laxatives***	
Sudatuss-SF liquid	Pharm Generic	Benefiber powder	Novartis
Supress DX Pediatric drops	Kramer-Novis	Citrucel powder	GlaxoSmithKline Consumer
Suttar-SF syrup	Gil	Colace solution	Purdue Products
Tanacof XR suspension	Larken	Colace Liquid 1% solution	Purdue Products
Triant-HC solution	Hawthorn	Fiber Choice tablets	CNS
Tricodene syrup	Pfeiffer	Fiber Ease liquid	Plainview
Trituss solution	Everett	Fibro-XL capsules	Key
Tri-Vent DM solution	Ethex	Genfiber powder	Teva
Tri-Vent DPC syrup	Ethex	Konsyl powder	Konsyl
Tusdec-DM solution	Cypress	Konsyl Easy Mix Formula powder	Konsyl
Tusnel solution	Llorens	Konsyl-Orange powder	Konsyl
Tussafed syrup	Everett	Metamucil Smooth Texture powder	Procter & Gamble
Tussafed-EX Pediatric drops	Everett	Reguloid Powder	Rugby
Tussafed-HC syrup	Everett	Reguloid Powder Orange Flavor	Rugby
Tussafed-HCG solution	Everett	Reguloid Powder Regular Flavor	Rugby
Tussall solution	Everett	Senokot Wheat Bran	Purdue Products
Tussi-Organidin DM NR solution	Victory	***Miscellaneous***	
Tussi-Organidin DM-S NR solution	Victory	Acidoll capsules	Key
Tussi-Organidin NR solution	Victory	Alka-Gest tablets	Key
Tussi-Organidin-S NR solution	Victory	Bicitra solution	Ortho-McNeil
Tussi-Pres liquid	Kramer-Novis	Cafergot tablets	Sandoz
Tussplex DM solution	Breckenridge	Colidrops Pediatric drops	A. G. Marin
Vazol solution	Wraser	Cytra-2 solution	Cypress
Vi-Q-Tuss syrup	Qualitest	Cytra-K crystals	Cypress
Welltuss EXP solution	Prasco	Cytra-K solution	Cypress
Z-Cof HC solution	Zyber	Mason Natural Drinkin' Buddy tablets	Mason Vitamins
Z-Cof HCX solution	Zyber		
Z-Tuss DM syrup	Magna	Melatin tablets	Mason Vitamins
Z-Tuss Expectorant solution	Magna	Namenda solution	Forest

Product	Manufacturer
Neutra-Phos powder	Ortho-McNeil
Neutra-Phos-K powder	Ortho-McNeil
Polycitra-K crystals	Ortho-McNeil
Polycitra-K solution	Ortho-McNeil
Polycitra-LC solution	Ortho-McNeil
Prosed-DS tablets	Esprit
Questran Light powder	Par
Soltamox solution	Cytogen
Mouth and throat preparations	
Cepacol Dual Relief Sore Throat spray	Combe
Cepacol Maximum Strength spray	Combe
Cepacol Sore Throat + Coating Relief lozenges	Combe
Cepacol Sore Throat lozenges	Combe
Cheracol Sore Throat spray	Lee
Chloraseptic spray	Prestige
Cylex lozenges	Pharmakon
Diabetic Tussin cough drops	Health Care Products
Diabetic Tussin cough lozenges	Health Care Products
Fisherman's Friend lozenges	Mentholatum
Fisherman's Friend Sugar-Free Mint lozenges	Mentholatum
Fresh N'Free liquid	Geritrex
Larynex lozenges	Dover
Listerine Pocketpaks film	Pfizer
Luden's lozenges	Johnson & Johnson
Luden's Sugar-Free Wild Cherry throat drops	Johnson & Johnson
Medikoff drops	Medique
Medikoff Sugar-Free drops	Medique
N'ice lozenges	Heritage/Insight
Oragesic solution	Parnell
Orajel Dry Mouth Moisturizing gel	Del
Orajel Dry Mouth Moisturizing spray	Del
Orasept Mouthwash and Gargle liquid	Pharmakon
Sepasoothe lozenges	Medique
Thorets Maximum Strength lozenges	Otis Clapp & Son
Throto-Ceptic spray	S.S.S.
Triaminic Sore Throat spray	Novartis
Vitamins, minerals, and supplements	
Action-Tabs Made for Men	Action Labs
Adaptosode for Stress liquid	HVS

Product	Manufacturer
Adaptosode R+R for Stress liquid	HVS
Adaptosode R+R for Acute Stress liquid	HVS
Alamag tablets	Medique
Alcalak tablets	Medique
Apetigen elixir	Kramer-Novis
Apptrim capsules	Physician Therapeutics
Apptrim-D capsules	Physician Therapeutics
Bevitamel tablets	Westlake
Biosode liquid	HVS
Biotect Plus caplets	Gil
Bugs Bunny Complete tablets	Bayer
C & M Caps-375 capsules	Key
Cal-Cee tablets	Key
Calcet Plus tablets	Mission Pharmacal
Calcimin-300 tablets	Key
Cal-Mint chewable tablets	Freeda Vitamins
Cerefolin tablets	Pamlab
Cerefolin NAC tablets	Pamlab
Choice DM liquid	Bristol-Myers Squibb
Chromacaps tablets	Key
Delta D3 tablets	Freeda Vitamins
Detoxosode liquid	HVS
Dexfol tablets	Rising
DHEA capsules	ADH Health Products
Diatx ZN tablets	Pamlab
Diet System 6 gum	Applied Nutrition
Dimacid tablets	Otis Clapp & Son
Diucaps capsules	Legere
DI-Phen-500 capsules	Key
DL-Phen-500 capsules	Key
Electrotab tablets	Hart Health and Safety
Ensure Nutra Shake Pudding	Ross Products
Enterex Diabetic liquid	Victus
Essential Nutrients Plus Silica tablets	Action Labs
Evening Primrose Oil capsules	National Vitamin
Evolve Softgel	Bionutrics Health Products
Ex-L tablets	Key
Extress tablets	Key
Eyetamins tablets	Rexall Consumer
Fem-Cal tablets	Freeda Vitamins
Fem-Cal Citrate tablets	Freeda Vitamins
Fem-Cal Plus tablets	Freeda Vitamins
Ferrocite F tablets	Breckenridge

(continued)

Product	Manufacturer
Ferrocite Plus tablets	Breckenridge
Folacin-800 tablets	Key
Folbee tablets	Breckenridge
Folbee Plus tablets	Breckenridge
Foleve tablets	Cura
Foleve Plus tablets	Cura
Folplex 2.2 tablets	Breckenridge
Foltx tablets	Pamlab
Gabadone capsules	Physician Therapeutics
Gram-O-Leci tablets	Freeda Vitamins
Herbal Slim Complex capsules	ADH Health Products
Hypertensa capsules	Physician Therapeutics
Lynae Calcium with Vitamin C chewable tablets	Boscogen
Lynae Chondroitin/Glucosamine capsules	Boscogen
Lynae Ginse-Cool chewable tablets	Boscogen
Mag-Caps capsules	Rising
Mag-Ox 400 tablets	Blaine
Mag-SR tablets	Cypress
Magimin tablets	Key
Maginex tablets	Logan
Magnacaps capsules	Key
Mag-SR Plus Calcium tablets	Cypress
Mangimin tablets	Key
Medi-Lyte tablets	Medique
Metanx tablets	Pamlab
Multi-Delyn with Iron Liquid	Silarx
Natelle tablets	Pharmelle
Natelle C tablets	Azur
Nephro-Fer tablets	Watson
Neutra-Phos powder	Ortho-McNeil
Neutra-Phos-K powder	Ortho-McNeil
New Life Hair tablets	Rexall Consumer
Niferex elixir	Ther-Rx
Nutrisure OTC tablets	Westlake
Nutrivit solution	Llorens
Ob Complete tablets	Vertical
O-Cal F.A. tablets	Pharmics
Os-Cal 500+D tablets	GlaxoSmithKline
Plenamins Plus tablets	Rexall Consumer

Product	Manufacturer
Powervites tablets	Green Turtle Bay Vitamin
Prostaplex Herbal Complex capsules	ADH Health Products
Prostatonin capsules	Pharmaton Natural Health
Protect Plus liquid	Gil
Protect Plus NR Softgel	Gil
Pulmona capsules	Physician Therapeutics
Quintabs-M Tablets	Freeda Vitamins
Replace capsules	Key
Resource Arginaid powder	Novartis Nutrition
Replace without Iron capsules	Key
Ribo-100 T.D. capsules	Key
Samolinic Softgel	Key
Sea Omega 30 Softgel	Rugby
Sea Omega 50 Softgel	Rugby
Sentra AM capsules	Physician Therapeutics
Sentra PM capsules	Physician Therapeutics
Soy Care for Menopause capsules	Inverness Medical
Span C tablets	Freeda Vitamins
Strovite Forte syrup	Everett
Sunnie tablets	Green Turtle Bay Vitamin
Sunvite tablets	Rexall Naturalist
Super Dec B100 tablets	Freeda Vitamins
Super Quints B-50 tablets	Freeda Vitamins
Supervite liquid	Seyer Pharmatec
Suplevit liquid	Gil
Theramine capsules	Physician Therapeutics
Triamin tablets	Key
Triamino tablets	Freeda Vitamins
Ultramino powder	Freeda Vitamins
Uro-Mag capsules	Blaine
Vitafol tablets	Everett
Vitamin C and Rose Hips tablets	ADH Health Products
Vitrum Jr chewable Tablets	Mason Vitamins
Xtramins tablets	Key
Yohimbe Power Max 100 for Women tablets	Action Labs
Yohimbe Power Max 1500 for Women tablets	Action Labs
Yohimbized 1000 capsules	Action Labs
Ze-Plus Softgel	Everett

Reference

LaGow B, ed. *Drug Topics Red Book*. Montvale. N.J.: Thomson Healthcare; 2009.

Appendix L

Alcohol-Free Products

The following is a selection of alcohol-free products grouped by therapeutic category. The list is not comprehensive. Generic and alternate brands may exist. Always check product labeling for definitive information on specific ingredients.

Product	Manufacturer
Analgesics	
Acetaminophen Infants drops	Ivax
Advil Children's suspension	Wyeth Consumer
APAP elixir	Bio-Pharm
Genapap Children's elixir	Ivax
Genapap Infant's drops	Ivax
Motrin Children's suspension	McNeil Consumer
Motrin Infants' suspension	McNeil Consumer
Silapap Infant's drops	Silarx
Tylenol Children's suspension	McNeil Consumer
Tylenol Extra Strength solution	McNeil Consumer
Tylenol Infants' suspension	McNeil Consumer
Antiasthmatic agents	
Dy-G liquid	Cypress
Jay-Phyl syrup	Pharmakon
Anticonvulsants	
Zarontin syrup	Pfizer
Antiviral agents	
Epivir Oral solution	GlaxoSmithKline
Cough, cold, and allergy preparations	
Accuhist PDX Drops solution	Pediamed
Accuhist PDX syrup	Pediamed
Alacol solution	Ballay
Alacol DM syrup	Ballay
Allanhist PDX syrup	Allan
Altarussin syrup	Altaire
Amerifed liquid	Ambi
Amerifed DM liquid	Ambi
Anaplex DM syrup	ECR
Anaplex DMX suspension	ECR
Anaplex HD syrup	ECR
Andehist DM NR syrup	Cypress
Andehist NR syrup	Cypress
Aquatab DM syrup	Adams
Aridex solution	Gentex
Aridex-D solution	Gentex
Atuss G syrup	Atley

Product	Manufacturer
Baltussin solution	Bailey
Banophen elixir	Major
Benadryl Allergy solution	Pfizer Consumer
Benadryl-D Allergy & Sinus Children's solution	Johnson & Johnson Consumer
Bromaline syrup	Rugby
Bromaline DM elixir	Rugby
Bromatan-DM suspension	Cypress
Bromhist PDX solution	Cypress
Bromhist Pediatric solution	Cypress
Bromhist-DM solution	Cypress
Bromhist-DM Pediatric syrup	Cypress
Bromhist-NR solution	Cypress
Bromhist-PDX syrup	Cypress
Bromphenex DM solution	Breckenridge
Bromphenex HD solution	Breckenridge
Bromplex DM solution	Prasco
Bromplex HD solution	Prasco
Bromtuss DM solution	Breckenridge
Broncotron liquid	Seyer Pharmatec
Broncotron-D suspension	Seyer Pharmatec
B-Tuss liquid	Blansett
Carbaphen 12 suspension	Gil
Carbaphen 12 Ped suspension	Gil
Carbatuss liquid	GM
Carbatuss-12 suspension	GM
Carbatuss-CL solution	GM
Carbetaplex solution	Breckenridge
Carbetaplex TS suspension	Breckenridge
Carbofed DM syrup	Hi-Tech Pharmacal
Cardec solution	Qualitest
Cardec DM solution	Qualitest
Children's Dimetapp Cold & Allergy solution	Wyeth Consumer
Children's Dimetapp DM Cold & Cough solution	Wyeth Consumer
Children's Dimetapp Long Acting Cough Plus Cold solution	Wyeth Consumer
Children's Dimetapp Nighttime Flu syrup	Wyeth Consumer
Children's Mucinex syrup	Adams

(continued)

Product	Manufacturer	Product	Manufacturer
Children's Mucinex Cold solution	Adams	Donatussin DM syrup	Laser
Children's Mucinex Cough syrup	Adams	Double-Tussin DM liquid	Reese
Chlordex GP syrup	Cypress	Drocon-CS solution	Cypress
Chlor-Mes D solution	Cypress	Duratuss AC12 suspension	Victory
Codal-DM syrup	Cypress	Duratuss DM solution	Victory
Codimal DH syrup	Victory	Duratan DM suspension	Proethic
Codimal DM syrup	Victory	Duratuss DM12 suspension	Victory
Codimal PH syrup	Victory	Dynatuss EX syrup	Breckenridge
Complete Allergy elixir	Cardinal Health	Dynatuss HC solution	Breckenridge
Cordron-DM solution	Cypress	Endacof DM solution	Larken
Cordron-DM NR solution	Cypress	Endacof HE solution	Larken
Cordron-D NR solution	Cypress	Endacof XP solution	Larken
Cordron-HC solution	Cypress	Endal HD Plus liquid	Pediamed
Cordron NR solution	Cypress	Father John's Medicine Plus drops	Oakhurst
Corfen DM solution	Cypress	Ganidin NR liquid	Cypress
Coughtuss solution	Breckenridge	Gani-Tuss NR liquid	Cypress
Crantex syrup	Breckenridge	Gani-Tuss-DM NR liquid	Cypress
Crantex HC syrup	Breckenridge	Genebronco-D liquid	Pharm Generic
Creomulsion Cough syrup	Summit Industries	Genecof-HC liquid	Pharm Generic
Creomulsion for Children syrup	Summit Industries	Genecot-XP liquid	Pharm Generic
Dacex-DM solution	Cypress	Genecof-XP syrup	Pharm Generic
Dallergy solution	Laser	Genedel syrup	Pharm Generic
De-Chlor DM solution	Cypress	Genedotuss-DM liquid	Pharm Generic
De-Chlor DR solution	Cypress	Genepatuss liquid	Pharm Generic
De-Chlor HD syrup	Cypress	Genetuss-2 liquid	Pharm Generic
Dehistine syrup	Cypress	Genexpect-DM liquid	Pharm Generic
Despec liquid	International Ethical	Genexpect-PE liquid	Pharm Generic
Dex PC syrup	Boca Pharmacal	Genexpect-SF liquid	Pharm Generic
Diabetic Tussin solution	Health Care Products	Giltuss liquid	Gil
Diabetic Tussin Allergy Relief liquid	Health Care Products	Giltuss HC syrup	Gil
Diabetic Tussin Cough lozenges	Health Care Products	Giltuss Pediatric liquid	Gil
Diabetic Tussin DM liquid	Health Care Products	Gauss Ped-C solution	Gil
Diabetic Tussin DM solution	Health Care Products	H-C Tussive syrup	Vintage
Diabetic Tussin DM Maximum Strength liquid	Health Care Products	Histacol DM Pediatric syrup	Breckenridge
Diabetic Tussin EX liquid	Health Care Products	Histinex HC syrup	Ethex
Diabetic Tussin Night Time Formula solution	Health Care Products	Histinex PV syrup	Ethex
		Histussin HC syrup	Victory
Dimetapp Decongestant Pediatric drops	Wyeth Consumer	Hydramine elixir	Ivax
		Hydrofed solution	Larken
Donatussin solution	Laser	Hydro-Tussin CBX solution	Ethex
Donatussin DC syrup	Laser	Hydro-Tussin DI-IC solution	Ethex
Donatussin DM solution	Laser	Hydro-Tussin DM elixir	Ethex
Donatussin DM suspension	Laser	Hydro-Tussin EXP solution	Ethex

Product	Manufacturer
Hydro-Tussin HC syrup	Ethex
Hydro-Tussin HD liquid	Ethex
Hydro-Tussin XP syrup	Ethex
Jaycof Expectorant syrup	Pharmakon
Jaycof-HC liquid	Pharmakon
Jaycof-XP syrup	Pharmakon
Levall liquid	Andrx Auriga
Levall solution	Andrx Auriga
Levall 5.0 liquid	Andrx Auriga
Lodrane liquid	ECR
Lodrane D suspension	ECR
Lodrane XR suspension	ECR
Lohist D syrup	Larken
Lohist DM syrup	Larken
Lohist-LO solution	Larken
Lortuss DM solution	Proethic
Marcof Expectorant syrup	Marnel
Maxi-Tuss HCG solution	MCR American
Maxi-Tuss HCX solution	MCR American
M-Clear solution	R. A. McNeil
M-Clear JR solution	R. A. McNeil
Medi-Brom elixir	Medicine Shoppe
Mintuss G syrup	Breckenridge
Mintuss MR syrup	Breckenridge
Mintuss MS syrup	Breckenridge
Mintuss NX solution	Breckenridge
Motrin Cold Children's suspension	McNeil Consumer
Myhist-DM solution	Larken
Myhist-PD solution	Larken
Nalex-A liquid	Blansett Pharmacal
Nalex-DH liquid	Blansett Pharmacal
Nasop suspension	Hawthorn
Neotuss-D liquid	A. G. Marin
Neotuss S/F liquid	A. G. Marin
Norel DM liquid	US Pharmaceutical
Novahistine DH solution	Deston
Organidin NR liquid	Medpointe
Pancof syrup	Pamlab
Pancof EXP syrup	Pamlab
Pancof HC solution	Pamlab
Pancof XP solution	Pamlab
PediaCare Children's syrup	Johnson & Johnson Consumer

Product	Manufacturer
PediaCare Cough + Cold Children's liquid	Johnson & Johnson Consumer
PediaCare Decongestant & Cough liquid	Johnson & Johnson Consumer
PediaCare Long-Acting Cough solution	Johnson & Johnson Consumer
PediaCare Multi-Symptom Cold liquid	Johnson & Johnson Consumer
PediaCare Nightrest liquid	Johnson & Johnson Consumer
Pediahist DM syrup	Boca Pharmacal
Pedia-Relief liquid	Major
Phanasin syrup	Pharmakon
Phanasin Diabetic Choice syrup	Pharmakon
Phanatuss syrup	Pharmakon
Phanatuss DM Diabetic Choice syrup	Pharmakon
Phena-HC solution	GM
Phena-HC Diabetic Choice solution	Pharmakon
Phena-S liquid	GM
Phena-S 12 suspension	GM
Pneumotussin 2.5 syrup	ECR
Poly Hist DM solution	Poly
Poly Hist HC solution	Poly
Poly Hist PD solution	Poly
Poly-Tussin solution	Poly
Poly-Tussin DM syrup	Poly
Poly-Tussin HD syrup	Poly
Poly-Tussin XP solution	Poly
Pro-Clear solution	Pro-Pharma
Prolex DM liquid	Blansett Pharmacal
Pro-Red solution	Pro-Pharma
Qual-Tussin DC syrup	Pharmaceutical Associates
Quintex syrup	Qualitest
Q-Tussin liquid	Qualitest
Q-Tussin PE liquid	Qualitest
Relacon-DM NR solution	Cypress
Relacon-HC solution	Cypress
Relasin DM solution	Cypress
Rescon-DM liquid	Capellon
Rescon-GG liquid	Capellon
Rindal HD liquid	Breckenridge
Rindal HD Plus solution	Breckenridge
Robitussin Chest Congestion syrup	Wyeth Consumer

(continued)

Product	Manufacturer	Product	Manufacturer
Robitussin Cough & Allergy solution	Wyeth Consumer	Sudatuss-SF liquid	Pharm Generic
Robitussin Cough & Cold CF syrup	Wyeth Consumer	Triant-HC solution	Hawthorn
		TriTuss solution	Everett
Robitussin Cough & Congestion liquid	Wyeth Consumer	Tri-Vent DM solution	Ethex
		Tri-Vent DPC syrup	Ethex
Robitussin Cough, Cold & Flu Nighttime solution	Wyeth Consumer	Tusdec-DM solution	Cypress
Robitussin Cough DM syrup	Wyeth Consumer	Tusnel solution	Llorens
Robitussin DM syrup	Wyeth Consumer	Tusnel Pediatric solution	Llorens
Robitussin Head & Chest Congestion PE syrup	Wyeth Consumer	Tussafed-EX syrup	Everett
		Tussafed-EX Pediatric drops	Everett
Robitussin PE syrup	Wyeth Consumer	Tussafed-EX Pediatric liquid	Everett
Robitussin Pediatric Cough syrup	Wyeth Consumer	Tussafed-HC syrup	Everett
Robitussin Pediatric Cough & Cold CF solution	Wyeth Consumer	Tussafed-HCG solution	Everett
		Tussall solution	Everett
Robitussin Pediatric Cough & Cold Long-Acting solution	Wyeth Consumer	Tussinate syrup	Pediamed
		Tussi-Organidin DM NR solution	Wallace
Robitussin Pediatric Night Relief liquid	Wyeth Consumer	Tussi-Organidin DM-S NR solution	Victory
		Tussi-Organidin NR solution	Wallace
Rondec solution	Biovail	Tussi-Organidin-S NR solution	Victory
Rondec DM drops	Biovail	Tussi-Pres liquid	Kramer-Novis
Rondec DM solution	Biovail	Tussi-Pres Pediatric solution	Kramer-Novis
Ru-Tuss DM solution	Sage	Tylenol Cold Children's suspension	McNeil Consumer
Scot-Tussin Diabetes CF liquid	Scot-Tussin	Tylenol Cold Infants' drops	McNeil Consumer
Scot-Tussin DM solution	Scot-Tussin	Tylenol Cold Plus Cough Children's suspension	McNeil Consumer
Scot-Tussin Expectorant solution	Scot-Tussin		
Scot-Tussin Original solution	Scot-Tussin	Tylenol Cold Plus Cough Infants' suspension	McNeil Consumer
Scot-Tussin Senior solution	Scot-Tussin	Tylenol Flu Children's suspension	McNeil Consumer
Siladryl Allergy solution	Silarx	Tylenol Flu Night Time Max Strength liquid	McNeil Consumer
Sildec syrup	Silarx		
Sildec-DM syrup	Silarx	Tylenol Sinus Children's suspension	McNeil Consumer
Sildec-PE solution	Silarx	Vazol solution	Wraser Pharm
Sildec PE-DM solution	Silarx	Vicks 44E Pediatric liquid	Procter & Gamble
Sil-Tex liquid	Silarx	Vicks 44M Pediatric liquid	Procter & Gamble
Siltussin DAS liquid	Silarx	Vicks Dayquil Multi-Symptom liquid	Procter & Gamble
Siltussin DM DAS Cough Formula syrup	Silarx	Vicks Nyquil Children's liquid	Procter & Gamble
		Vicks Sinex spray	Procter & Gamble
Siltussin SA syrup	Silarx	Vi-Q Tuss syrup	Vintage
Simply Cough liquid	McNeil Consumer	V-Tann suspension	Breckenridge
Sudafed Children's solution	Pfizer	Welltuss EXP solution	Prasco
Sudafed Children's Cold & Cough solution	Pfizer	Z-Cof 8 DM suspension	Zyber
		Z-Cof 12 DM suspension	Zyber
Sudatuss DM syrup	Pharm Generic	Z-Cof DM solution	Zyber
Sudatuss-2 liquid	Pharm Generic		

Product	Manufacturer
Z-Cof DMX solution	Zyber
Z-Cof HC solution	Zyber
Z-Cof HCX solution	Zyber
Z-Tuss Expectorant solution	Magna
Z-Tuss DM syrup	Magna

Ear, nose, and throat products

Product	Manufacturer
4-Way Saline Moisturizing Mist spray	Bristol-Myers
Ayr Baby Saline spray	B. F. Ascher
Bucalcide spray	Seyer Pharmatec
Bucalsep solution	Gil
Bucalsep spray	Gil
Cheracol Sore Throat spray	Lee
Fresh N'Free solution	Geritrex
Gly-Oxide solution	GlaxoSmithKline
Isodettes Sore Throat spray	GlaxoSmithKline
Larynex lozenges	Dover
Listermint solution	Johnson & Johnson Consumer
Nasal Moist gel	Blairex
Orajel Baby liquid	Del
Orajel Baby Day & Night gel	Del
Orajel Baby Nighttime gel	Del
Orajel Baby Nighttime Teething Pain Medicine gel	Del
Orajel Baby Teething Pain Medicine liquid	Del
OraMagic Plus powder	MPM Medical
OraMagicRx powder	MPM Medical
Orasept Mouthwash/Gargle liquid	Pharmakon
Tanac liquid	Del
Throto-Ceptic spray	S.S.S.
Triaminic Sore Throat spray	Novartis Consumer
Vicks Sinex spray	Procter & Gamble
Vicks Sinex 12 Hour spray	Procter & Gamble
Zilactin Baby Extra Strength gel	Zila Consumer

Gastrointestinal agents

Product	Manufacturer
Axid solution	Braintree
Baby Gasz drops	Lee
Colace solution	Purdue
Colidrops Pediatric drops	Dover
Gas Relief solution	Perrigo
Imogen liquid	Pharm Generic
Kaodene NN suspension	Pfeiffer

Product	Manufacturer
Kaopectate Advanced Formula suspension	Pharmacia Consumer
Liqui-Doss liquid	Ferndale
Mylicon Infants' suspension	Johnson& Johnson/Merck

Miscellaneous

Product	Manufacturer
Cytra-2 solution	Cypress
Cytra-K solution	Cypress
Faslodex solution	AstraZeneca
Fluorinse solution	Oral B
Namenda solution	Forest
Primsol solution	FSC

Topical products

Product	Manufacturer
Aloe Vesta 2-N-1 Antifungal ointment	Convatec
Dermatone Lips 'n Face Protector ointment	Dermatone
Dermatone Moisturizing Sunblock cream	Dermatone
Dermatone Skin Protector cream	Dermatone
Evoclin foam	Connetics
Fleet Pain Relief pads	Fleet
Fresh & Pure Douche solution	Unico
Hendclens solution	Woodward
Joint-Ritis Maximum Strength ointment	Naturopathic
Neutrogena Acne Wash liquid	Neutrogena
Neutrogena Antiseptic liquid	Neutrogena
Neutrogena Antiseptic solution	Neutrogena
Neutrogena Clear Pore gel	Neutrogena
Neutrogena T/Derm liquid	Neutrogena
Neutrogena Toner liquid	Neutrogena
Neutrogena Toner solution	Neutrogena
Podiclens spray	Woodware
Sea Breeze Foaming Face Wash gel	Clairol
Shade Uvaguard lotion	Schering-Plough
Sportz Bloc cream	Med-Derm
Therasoft Anti-Acne cream	SFC/Solvent Free
Therasoft Skin Protectant cream	SFC/Solvent Free
Tiger Balm Arthritis Rub lotion	Prince of Peace Enterprises

Vitamins, minerals, and supplements

Product	Manufacturer
Adaptosode for Stress liquid	HVS
Adaptosode R+R for Acute Stress liquid	HVS
Apetigen elixir	Kramer-Novis
Biosode liquid	HVS

(continued)

Product	Manufacturer	Product	Manufacturer
Detoxosode Products liquid	HVS	Poly-Vi-Sol with Iron drops	Mead Johnson
Genesupp-500 liquid	Pharm Generic	Protect Plus liquid	Gil
Genetect Plus liquid	Pharm Generic	Strovite Forte syrup	Everett
Multi-Delyn liquid	Silarx	Supervite liquid	Seyer Pharmatec
Multi-Delyn with Iron liquid	Silarx	Suplevit liquid	Gil
Nutrivit solution	Llorens	Tri-Vi-Sol with Iron drops	Mead Johnson
Poly-Vi-Sol drops	Mead Johnson	Vitafol syrup	Everett

Reference

LaGow B, ed. *Drug Topics Red Book*. Montvale, N.J.: Thomson Healthcare; 2009.

Appendix M

Common Drug Interactions: Cytochrome P450 Interactions

Substrates (trade name)	Inhibitors (trade name)	Inducers (trade name)	Substrates (trade name)	Inhibitors (trade name)	Inducers (trade name)
CYP1A2			**CYP1A2 (cont)**		
Alosetron (Lotronex)	Artemisinin	Cigarette smoke	Ropivacaine (Naropin)		
Amitriptyline (Elavil)	Atazanavir (Reyataz)	Phenobarbital (Luminal)	R-warfarin (Coumadin)		
Anagrelide (Agrylin)	Cimetidine (Tagamet)	Rifampin (Rifadin, Rimactane)	Selegiline (Eldepryl)		
Aprepitant (Emend)		Ritonavir (Norvir)	Tacrine (Cognex)		
Caffeine	Ciprofloxacin (Cipro)		Tamoxifen (Nolvadex)		
Cinacalcet (Sensipar)	Clarithromycin (Biaxin)		Theophylline, amino-phylline (Aerolate, Aquaphyllin, Asmalix, Bronkodyl, Choledyl, Constant-T, Duraphyl, Elixophyllin, Phyllocontin, Quibron, Respbid, Slo-bid, Slo-Phyllin, Sustaire, Theo-24, Theobid, Theochron, Theoclear, Theo-Dur, Theolair, Theon, Theospan, Theovent, Truphylline)		
Clomipramine (Anafranil)	Enoxacin (Penetrex)				
Clozapine (Clozaril)	Erythromycin (E-Mycin)				
Cyclobenzaprine (Flexeril)	Ethinyl estradiol				
Desipramine (Norpramin)	Fluvoxamine (Luvox)				
Diazepam (Valium)	Grapefruit juice				
Diphenhydramine (Benadryl)	Isoniazid (INH, Nydrazid)				
Duloxetine (Cymbalta)	Ketoconazole (Nizoral)				
Erlotinib (Tarceva)	Mexiletine (Mexitil)		Thiabendazole (Mintezol)		
Flutamide (Eulexin)	Norfloxacin (Chibroxin, Noroxin, Norflox)		Tizanidine (Zanaflex)		
Fluvoxamine (Luvox)			Triamterene		
Frovatriptan (Frova)			Zafirlukast (Accolate)		
Gingko	Tacrine (Cognex)		Zileuton (Zyflo)		
Haloperidol (Haldol)	Thiabendazole (Mintezol)		Zolmitriptan (Zomig)		
Imipramine (Tofranil)	Zafirlukast (Accolate)		**CYP2C9**		
Indiplon	Zileuton (Zyflo)		Alosetron (Lotronex)	Alcohol (intoxicating dose)	Aminoglutethimide (Cytadren)
Lidocaine			Amprenavir (Agenerase)	Amiodarone (Cordarone, Pacerone)	Aprepitant (Emend)
Melatonin			Azapropazone		Barbiturates
Mexiletine (Mexitil)			Bosentan (Tracleer)	Benzbromarone	Bosentan (Tracleer)
Mirtazapine (Remeron)			Candesartan (Atacand)	Cimetidine (Tagamet)	Carbamazepine (Tegretol)
Olanzapine (Zyprexa)			Celecoxib (Celebrex)	Clopidogrel (Plavix)	Phenobarbital (Luminal)
Ondansetron (Zofran)			Chlorpropamide (Diabinese)	Delavirdine (Rescriptor)	Rifampin (Rifadin, Rimactane)
Palonosetron (Aloxi)			Diclofenac (Cataflam, Voltaren)		
Pimozide (Orap)					
Propranolol (Inderal)					
Ramelteon (Rozerem)					
Rasagiline (Azilect)					
Ropinirole (Requip)					

(continued)

Substrates (trade name)	Inhibitors (trade name)	Inducers (trade name)
CYP2C9 (cont)		
Doxepin (Sinequan)	Disulfiram (Antabuse)	
Dronabinol (Marinol)	Doxifluridine	
Fluoxetine (Prozac)	Efavirenz (Sustiva)	
Flurbiprofen (Ansaid)	Fluconazole (Diflucan)	
Fluvastatin (Lescol)	Fluorouracil (5-FU)	
Glimepiride (Amaryl)	Fluoxetine (Prozac)	
Glipizide (Glucotrol)	Fluvastatin (Lescol)	
Glyburide (DiaBeta)	Fluvoxamine (Luvox)	
Ibuprofen (Advil, Motrin)	Gemfibrozil (Lopid)	
Indomethacin (Indocin)	Imatinib (Gleevec)	
Irbesartan (Avapro)	Isoniazid (INH, Nydrazid)	
Losartan (Cozaar)	Leflunomide (Arava)	
Melatonin	Metronidazole (Flagyl)	
Meloxicam (Mobic)	Miconazole (Monistat)	
Montelukast (Singulair)	Modafinil (Provigil)	
Naproxen (Aleve, Naprosyn)	Phenytoin (Dilantin)	
Nateglinide (Starlix)	Sertraline (Zoloft)	
Phenytoin (Dilantin)	Sitaxsentan	
Piroxicam (Feldene)	Sulfamethoxazole (Bactrim, Gantanol, Septra, Sulfatrim)	
Ramelteon (Rozerem)	Sulfaphenazole	
Rosiglitazone (Avandia)	Sulfinpyrazone (Anturane)	
Rosuvastatin (Crestor)	Trimethoprim (Bactrim, Primsol, Proloprim, Septra, Sulfatrim, Trimpex)	
Sildenafil (Viagra)		
Sitaxsentan	Valproic Acid (Depakene)	
Sulfamethoxazole (Bactrim, Gantanol, Septra, Sulfatrim)	Voriconazole (Vfend)	
S-warfarin (Coumadin)	Zafirlukast (Accolate)	
Tolbutamide (Orinase)		
Torsemide (Demadex)		
Valdecoxib (Bextra)		
Valsartan (Diovan)		
Voriconazole (Vfend)		

Substrates (trade name)	Inhibitors (trade name)	Inducers (trade name)
CYP2C19		
Aprepitant (Emend)	Chloramphenicol	Artemisinin
Aripiprazole (Abilify)	Cimetidine (Tagamet)	Barbiturates
Carisoprodol (Soma)	Clopidogrel (Plavix)	Carbamazepine (Tegretol)
Citalopram (Celexa)	Delavirdine (Rescriptor)	Phenytoin (Dilantin)
Clomipramine (Anafranil)	Efavirenz (Sustiva)	Norethindrone
Clopidogrel (Plavix)	Felbamate (Felbatol)	Rifampin (Ramactane)
Clozapine (Clozaril)	Fluconazole (Diflucan)	St. John's wort
Desipramine (Norpramin)	Fluoxetine (Prozac)	
Diazepam (Valium)	Fluvastatin (Lescol)	
Diphenhydramine (Benadryl)	Fluvoxamine (Luvox)	
Doxepin (Sinequan)	Isoniazid (INH, Nydrazid)	
Escitalopram (Lexapro)	Ketoconazole (Nizoral)	
Flunitrazepam	Lansoprazole (Prevacid)	
Fluoxetine (Prozac)	Moclobemide (Manerix)	
Imipramine (Tofranil)	Modafinil (Provigil)	
Lansoprazole (Prevacid)	Omeprazole (Prilosec)	
Mephenytoin (Mesantoin)	Oxcarbazepine (Trileptal)	
Methadone	Ticlopidine (Ticlid)	
Moclobemide (Manerix)	Topiramate (Topamax)	
Nelfinavir (Viracept)	Voriconazole (Vfend)	
Olanzapine (Zyprexa)		
Omeprazole (Prilosec)		
Pantoprazole (Protonix)		
Pentamidine (Pentam)		
Phenobarbital		
Phenytoin (Dilantin)		
Proguanil (active metabolite)		
Propranolol (Inderal)		
Rabeprazole (Aciphex)		
R-warfarin (Coumadin)		
Sertraline (Zoloft)		
Thalidomide (Thalomid)		
Voriconazole (Vfend)		

Substrates (trade name)	Inhibitors (trade name)	Inducers (trade name)	Substrates (trade name)	Inhibitors (trade name)	Inducers (trade name)
CYP2D6			*CYP2D6 (cont)*		
Almotriptan (Axert)	Amiodarone (Cordarone, Pacerone)	Rifampin (Rifadin, Rimactane)	Hydrocodone	Quinidine (Cardioquin, Dura-Tabs, Quinaglute, Quinidex)	
Alprenolol			Imipramine (Tofranil)		
Amitriptyline (Elavil)	Bupropion (Wellbutrin)		Loratadine (Claritin)		
Amprenavir (Agenerase)			Maprotiline (Ludiomil)		
Atomoxetine (Strattera)	Chloroquine (Aralen)		Methadone	Quinine	
Bisoprolol (Zebeta)	Chlorpheniramine		Methamphetamine	Ranolazine (Ranexa)	
Carvedilol (Coreg)	Chlorpromazine (Thorazine)		Metoclopramide (Reglan)	Risperidone (Risperdal)	
Cevimeline (Evoxac)	Celecoxib (Celebrex)		Metoprolol (Lopressor)	Ritonavir (Norvir)	
Chlorpheniramine	Cimetidine (Tagamet)		Mexiletine (Mexitil)	Sertraline (Zoloft)	
Chlorpromazine (Thorazine)			Mianserin		
Cinacalcet (Sensipar)	Cinacalcet (Sensipar)		Mirtazapine (Remeron)	Terbinafine (Lamisil)	
Citalopram (Celexa)	Citalopram (Celexa)		Nortriptyline (Aventyl, Pamelor)	Thioridazine (Mellaril)	
Clomipramine (Anafranil)	Clomipramine (Anafranil)		Olanzapine (Zyprexa)		
Codeine			Ondansetron (Zofran)		
Cyclobenzaprine (Flexeril)	Diphenhydramine (Benadryl)		Oxycodone (Endocodone, OxyContin, OxyIR, Percodan, Percolone, Roxicodone)		
Darifenacin (Enablex)	Duloxetine (Cymbalta)				
Debrisoquin					
Desipramine (Norpramin)	Escitalopram (Lexapro)		Palonosetron (Aloxi)		
Dextromethorphan	Fluoxetine (Prozac)		Paroxetine (Paxil)		
Dihydrocodeine			Perhexiline (Pexid)		
Diphenhydramine (Benadryl)	Halofantrine (Halfan)		Perphenazine (Trilafon)		
Dolasetron (Anzemet)	Haloperidol (Haldol)		Promethazine (Phenergan)		
Donepezil (Aricept)	Hydroxychloroquine		Propafenone (Rhythmol)		
Doxepin (Sinequan)			Propoxyphene (Darvon)		
Duloxetine (Cymbalta)	Imatinib (Gleevec)		Propranolol (Inderal)		
Encainide	Paroxetine (Paxil)		Protriptyline (Vivactil)		
Escitalopram (Lexapro)	Perphenazine (Trilafon)		Ranolazine (Ranexa)		
Flecainide (Tambocor)	Promethazine (Phenergan)		Risperidone (Risperdal)		
Fluoxetine (Prozac)	Propafenone (Rhythmol)		Sertindole (Serlect)		
Fluvoxamine (Luvox)			Sertraline (Zoloft)		
Galantamine (Reminyl)	Propoxyphene (Darvon)		Simvastatin (Zocor)		
Haloperidol (Haldol)	Quinacrine		Tamoxifen (Nolvadex)		
			Thioridazine (Mellaril)		

(continued)

Substrates (trade name)	Inhibitors (trade name)	Inducers (trade name)
CYP2D6 (cont)		
Timolol (Betimol, Blocadren, Timoptic)		
Tolterodine (Detrol)		
Tramadol (Ultram)		
Trazodone (Desyrel)		
Venlafaxine (Effexor)		
Yohimbine		
CYP2E1		
Acetaminophen (Tylenol)	Disulfiram (Antabuse)	Chronic ethanol
Chlorzoxazone (Parafon Forte)		Isoniazid (INH, Nydrazid)
Ethanol, enflurane, halothane, isoflurane, methoxyflurane, sevoflurane		
Theophylline, aminophylline (Aerolate, Aquaphyllin, Asmalix, Bronkodyl, Choledyl, Constant-T, Duraphyl, Elixophyllin, Phyllocontin, Quibron, Respbid, Slo-bid, Slo-Phyllin, Sustaire, Theo-24, Theobid, Theochron, Theoclear, Theo-Dur, Theolair, Theon, Theospan, Theovent, Truphylline)		
CYP3A		
Alfentanil (Alfenta)	Amiodarone (Cordarone, Pacerone)	Aminoglutethimide (Cytadren)
Alfuzosin (Uroxatral)		
Almotriptan (Axert)		Barbiturates
Alosetron (Lotronex)	Amprenavir (Agenerase)	Bexarotene (Targretin)
Alprazolam (Xanax)	Aprepitant (Emend)	Bosentan (Tracleer)
Amiodarone (Cordarone)	Aripiprazole (Abilify)	Carbamazepine (Tegretol)
Amitriptyline (Elavil)		Dexamethasone (Decadron)
Amlodipine (Norvasc)	Atazanavir (Reyataz)	Efavirenz (Sustiva)
Amprenavir (Agenerase)	Chloramphenicol	Glucocorticoids
Aprepitant (Emend)	Cimetidine (Tagamet)	Griseofulvin (Grisactin)
Aripiprazole (Abilify)	Clarithromycin (Biaxin)	Modafinil (Provigil)
Astemizole (Hismanal)	Conivaptan (Vaprisol)	Nafcillin (Unipen)
Atazanavir (Reyataz)		
Atorvastatin (Lipitor)		

Substrates (trade name)	Inhibitors (trade name)	Inducers (trade name)
CYP3A (cont)		
Bepridil (Vascor)	Cyclosporine (Neoral)	Nevirapine (Viramune)
Bexarotene (Targretin)		Oxcarbazepine (Trileptal)
Bosentan (Tracleer)	Danazol (Danocrine)	
Bromocriptine (Parlodel)	Darunavir (Prezista)	Phenobarbital (Luminal)
Budesonide (Entocort)	Dasatinib (Sprycel)	Phenytoin (Dilantin)
Bupivacaine (Sensorcaine)	Delavirdine (Rescriptor)	Primidone (Mysoline)
Buprenorphine (Subutex)		
Buspirone (Buspar)	Diltiazem (Cardizem)	Rifabutin (Mycobutin)
Calcium channel blockers	Erythromycin (E-Mycin)	Rifampin (Rifadin, Rimactane)
Carbamazepine (Tegretol)	Estrogens	St. John's wort
Cevimeline (Evoxac)	Fluconazole (Diflucan)	Topiramate (Topamax)
Chlorpheniramine	Fluoxetine (Prozac)	
Cilostazol (Pletal)		
Cinacalcet (Sensipar)	Fluvoxamine (Luvox)	
Cisapride (Propulsid)	Fosamprenavir (Lexiva)	
Citalopram (Celexa)		
Clarithromycin (Biaxin)	Grapefruit juice	
Clomipramine (Anafranil)	Imatinib (Gleevec)	
Clonazepam (Klonopin)		
Clopidogrel (Plavix)	Indinavir (Crixivan)	
Clozapine (Clozaril)		
Colchicine	Interleukin-10	
Conivaptan (Vaprisol)	Isoniazid (INH, Nydrazid)	
Cyclobenzaprine (Flexeril)		
Cyclophosphamide (Cytoxan)	Itraconazole (Sporanox)	
Cyclosporine (Gengraf, Neoral, Sandimmune)	Ketoconazole (Nizoral)	
Dapsone (Avlosulfon)	Lapatinib (Tykerb)	
Darifenacin (Enablex)	Miconazole (Monistat)	
Darunavir (Prezista)		
Dasatinib (Sprycel)	Mifepristone (Mifeprex)	
Delavirdine (Rescriptor)		
Dexamethasone (Decadron)	Nefazodone (Serzone)	
Dextromethorphan	Nelfinavir (Viracept)	
Diazepam (Valium)	Nicardipine (Cardene)	

Substrates (trade name)	Inhibitors (trade name)	Inducers (trade name)
CYP3A (cont)		
Diclofenac (Voltaren)	Norfloxacin (Chibroxin, Noroxin)	
Dihydroergotamine (D.H.E. 45)		
Diltiazem (Cardizem)	Posaconazole (Noxafil)	
Disopyramide (Norpace)	Propoxyphene (Darvon)	
Docetaxel (Taxotere)	Quinupristin (Synercid)	
Dolasetron (Anzemet)		
Donepezil (Aricept)	Ranolazine (Ranexa)	
Doxorubicin (Adriamycin)	Ritonavir (Norvir)	
Droperidol		
Dutasteride (Avodart)	Saquinavir (Fortovase, Invirase)	
Ebastine (Kestine)		
Efavirenz (Sustiva)	Tamoxifen (Nolvadex)	
Eletriptan (Relpax)		
Eplerenone (Inspra)	Telithromycin (Ketek)	
Ergotamine (Ergomar)	Troleandomycin (TAO)	
Erlotinib (Tarceva)		
Erythromycin (E-Mycin)	Verapamil (Calan)	
Escitalopram (Lexapro)	Voriconazole (Vfend)	
Estazolam (Prosom)		
Estrogens	Zafirlukast (Accolate)	
Eszopiclone (Lunesta)		
Ethosuximide (Zarontin)		
Etoposide (Vepesid)		
Exemestane (Aromasin)		
Felodipine (Plendil)		
Fentanyl (Sublimaze)		
Finasteride (Proscar)		
Flunitrazepam		
Flurazepam (Dalmane)		
Fosamprenavir (Lexiva)		
Galantamine (Reminyl)		
Garlic		
Gefitinib (Iressa)		
Gingko		
Granisetron (Kytril)		
Halofantrine (Halfan)		
Haloperidol (Haldol)		

Substrates (trade name)	Inhibitors (trade name)	Inducers (trade name)
CYP3A (cont)		
Ifosfamide (Ifex)		
Imatinib (Gleevec)		
Imipramine (Tofranil)		
Indiplon		
Irinotecan (Camptosar)		
Isradipine (DynaCirc)		
Itraconazole (Sporanox)		
Ivabradine		
Ixabepilone (Ixempra)		
Ketoconazole (Nizoral)		
Lansoprazole (Prevacid)		
Lapatinib (Tykerb)		
Levomethadyl (Orlaam)		
Lidocaine		
Loperamide (Imodium)		
Loratadine (Claritin)		
Losartan (Cozaar)		
Lovastatin (Mevacor)		
Maraviroc (Selzentry)		
Mefloquine (Lariam)		
Meloxicam (Mobic)		
Methadone		
Methylprednisolone		
Midazolam (Versed)		
Mifepristone (Mifeprex)		
Mirtazapine (Remeron)		
Modafinil (Provigil)		
Montelukast (Singulair)		
Nateglinide (Starlix)		
Nefazodone (Serzone)		
Nicardipine (Cardene)		
Nifedipine (Adalat)		
Nimodipine (Nimotop)		
Nisoldipine (Sular)		
Nitrendipine (Baypress)		
Omeprazole (Prilosec)		
Ondansetron (Zofran)		
Oxybutynin (Ditropan)		
Oxycodone (Percodan)		

(continued)

Substrates (trade name)	Inhibitors (trade name)	Inducers (trade name)	Substrates (trade name)	Inhibitors (trade name)	Inducers (trade name)
CYP3A (cont)			*CYP3A (cont)*		
Paclitaxel (Taxol)			Solifenacin (Vesicare)		
Palonosetron (Aloxi)			Sufentanil (Sufenta)		
Pantoprazole (Protonix)			Sulfamethoxazole (Bactrim)		
Paricalcitol (Zemplar)			Sunitinib (Sutent)		
Pimozide (Orap)			Tacrolimus (Prograf)		
Pioglitazone (Actos)			Tadalafil (Cialis)		
Praziquantel (Biltricide)			Tamoxifen (Nolvadex)		
Prednisolone			Tamsulosin (Flomax)		
Prednisone			Teniposide (Vumon)		
Propoxyphene (Darvon)			Terfenadine		
Protease inhibitors			Testosterone		
Quazepam (Doral)			Theophylline		
Quetiapine (Seroquel)			Tiagabine (Gabitril)		
Quinacrine			Tinidazole (Tindamax)		
Quinidine (Cardioquin, Quinaglute, Quinidex)			Tipranavir (Aptivus)		
Quinine			Tolterodine (Detrol)		
Ramelteon (Rozerem)			Topiramate (Topamax)		
Ranolazine (Ranexa)			Tramadol (Ultram)		
Repaglinide (Prandin)			Trazodone (Desyrel)		
Rifabutin (Mycobutin)			Triamterene		
Risperidone (Risperdal)			Triazolam (Halcion)		
Ritonavir (Norvir)			Valdecoxib (Bextra)		
Ropivacaine (Naropin)			Vardenafil (Levitra)		
R-warfarin (Coumadin)			Venlafaxine (Effexor)		
Selegiline (Eldepryl)			Verapamil (Calan)		
Sertindole (Serlect)			Vesnarinone		
Sertraline (Zoloft)			Vinblastine (Velbane)		
Sibutramine (Meridia)			Vincristine (Oncovin)		
Sildenafil (Viagra)			Voriconazole (Vfend)		
Simvastatin (Zocor)			Yohimbine		
Sirolimus (Rapammune)			Ziprasidone (Geodon)		
Sitaxsentan			Zolpidem (Ambien)		
			Zonisamide (Zonegran)		
			Zopiclone (Imovane)		

References

Hansten PD, Horn JR. *The Top 100 Drug Interactions*. Freeland, Wash.: H&H Publications; 2008.
Micromedex Healthcare Series. Greenwood Village, Colo.: Thomson Healthcare. Available at: www.thomsonhc.com. Updated periodically.